Pharmacological Treatment of Epileptic Seizures

Xuefeng Wang • Liemin Zhou
Editors

Pharmacological Treatment of Epileptic Seizures

Springer

Editors

Xuefeng Wang
Neurology
The First Affiliated Hospital of Chongqing Medical University
Chongqing, China

Liemin Zhou
Neurology
The Seventh Affiliated Hospital of Sun Yat-Sen University
Shenzhen, China

ISBN 978-981-96-8519-6 ISBN 978-981-96-8520-2 (eBook)
https://doi.org/10.1007/978-981-96-8520-2

This Springer imprint is published by the registered company Springer Nature Singapore Pte Ltd.
The registered company address is: 152 Beach Road, #21-01/04 Gateway East, Singapore 189721, Singapore

Preface

Epilepsy is a neurological disorder that has impacted humanity for thousands of years, transcending borders, cultures, and social strata. While advances in medicine have dramatically improved the understanding and management of epilepsy, the social consequences of this condition remain profound. People with epilepsy often face significant stigma, discrimination, and psychological challenges that can be as debilitating as the seizures themselves. In this context, effective treatment is not only a medical imperative but also a social one, crucial for improving the quality of life for millions worldwide.

This book, *Pharmacological Treatment of Epileptic Seizures*, is a comprehensive resource compiled by the leading epileptologists in China, whose work has significantly advanced the field of epilepsy treatment, with the contribution of world-famous experts in epilepsy. It aims to equip healthcare professionals with the knowledge and tools necessary to address both the clinical and social dimensions of epilepsy.

This book begins by defining epilepsy and providing a thorough exploration of the Definition and the Classification and diagnosis of epileptic seizures. Understanding the various forms of epilepsy is essential for developing targeted treatment plans that address the specific needs of each patient. Accurate diagnosis is the first step toward effective management, which can significantly reduce the social burden of the disease.

Section 1.3 offers a broader context for understanding how epilepsy treatment has evolved over time. This historical perspective is crucial for appreciating the advances that have brought us to the present day and for anticipating future developments that may further alleviate the social impact of epilepsy.

Section 1.4, addressing “Research on Animal Models of Epilepsy,” provides insight into the scientific foundations of epilepsy treatment. This research is vital for developing new therapies that are more effective and have fewer side effects, thus improving the overall well-being of patients and their ability to participate fully in society.

The book also delves into the Antiseizure medication mechanisms of action and reviews currently available medications and those in pipeline. This part of the book is focused on the pharmacological interventions that are the cornerstone of epilepsy management. By controlling seizures, these medications play a key role in reducing the social stigma and limitations associated with epilepsy, enabling patients to lead more stable and fulfilling lives.

In Chap. 3 the authors review the fundamentals of selection of antiseizure medications and emphasize the importance of individualized treatment plans in individuals across the life span; the treatment options should be based on not only the medical aspects of epilepsy but also the social and psychological needs of patients. Effective treatment can greatly enhance a patient's ability to engage in everyday activities, pursue education, maintain employment, and build relationships—all of which are crucial for social inclusion.

Chapter 4 offers practical guidance for clinicians, helping them to optimize treatment strategies that improve patient outcomes in different clinical conditions, including epilepsy after stroke, brain trauma, tumor-associated epilepsy, and others.

Special attention is given to Chaps. 5 and 6, both of which are critical for managing more severe forms of epilepsy. These chapters highlight the importance of timely and effective treatment in preventing the long-term clinical, social, and psychological consequences of uncontrolled seizures.

An important part of the book, Chap. 7, addresses the "Diagnosis and Treatment of Epilepsy Comorbidities," recognizing that epilepsy often coexists with other conditions such as depression, anxiety, and cognitive impairments. These comorbidities can exacerbate the challenges faced by individuals with epilepsy, making their management an essential component of comprehensive care. Following the same line, Chap. 8 provides highly relevant information for the successful management on the complex issues surrounding epilepsy treatment in individuals with epilepsy.

Throughout this book, the editors, who are the most distinguished epileptologists in China, and eminent authors bring their extensive clinical experience and research expertise to the readers. Their work reflects a deep commitment to improving both the medical and social outcomes for people with epilepsy.

This book will serve as a vital resource for those dedicated to improving the lives of people with epilepsy, helping to create a future where effective treatment leads not only to better health outcomes but also to greater social acceptance and integration.

Alla Guekht

Director, Moscow Research
and Clinical Center for Neuropsychiatry,
Professor of Neurology
Pirogov Russian Medical Research
University, Treasurer and President-Elect,
International League Against Epilepsy (ILAE)
Moscow, Russia

Acknowledgments

We would like to thank the following authors for their participation in the preparation of this book:

Guanzhong Ni, Hui Zhang, Junhong Wu, Shenglin Wang, Shuda Chen, Xiaowei Xu, Xianyue Liu, Yingfang She, Yuping Zhao, Juan Li.

Contents

Contributors

Richard Shek-kwan Chang Department of Neuroscience, Central Clinical School, Monash University, Melbourne, VIC, Australia

Wen-Hung Chung Department of Dermatology, Xiamen Chang Gung Hospital, Xiamen, China

Zhibin Chen Department of Neuroscience, Central Clinical School, Monash University, Melbourne, VIC, Australia

Ziyi Chen Department of Neurology, The Seven Affiliated Hospital of Sun Yat-sen University, Shenzhen, China

Emma Foster Department of Neuroscience, Central Clinical School, Monash University, Melbourne, VIC, Australia

Yixue Gu Department of Neurology, The First Affiliated Hospital of Chongqing Medical University, Chongqing, China

Yanbing Han Department of Neurology, First Affiliated Hospital of Kunming Medical University, Kunming, China

Zhen Hong Department of Neurology, West China Hospital, Sichuan University, Chengdu, China

Yue Hu Department of Neurology, Children's Hospital of Chongqing Medical University, Chongqing, China

Huapin Huang Department of Neurology, Fujian Medical University Union Hospital, Fuzhou, China

Zhuo Huang State Key Laboratory of Natural and Biomimetic Drugs, Department of Molecular and Cellular Pharmacology, School of Pharmaceutical Sciences, Peking University, Beijing, China

Guohui Jiang Department of Neurology, Affiliated Hospital of North Sichuan Medical College, Nanchong, Sichuan, China

Li Jiang Department of Neurology, Children's Hospital of Chongqing Medical University, National Clinical Research Center for Child Health and Disorders, Chongqing, China

Wei Jing Shanxi Bethune Hospital, Shanxi Academy of Medical Sciences, Third Hospital of Shanxi Medical University, Tongji Shanxi Hospital, Taiyuan, Shanxi, China

Patrick Kwan Department of Neuroscience, Central Clinical School, Monash University, Melbourne, VIC, Australia

Feng Li Department of Neurology, The First Affiliated Hospital of Chongqing Medical University, Chongqing, China

Ling Li Department of Neurology, Qilu Hospital (Qingdao), Cheeloo College of Medicine, Shandong University, Qingdao, China

Tingsong Li Department of Rehabilitation, Children's Hospital of Chongqing Medical University, National Clinical Research Center for Child Health and Disorders, Chongqing, China

Songyan Liu Department of Neurology, China-Japan Union Hospital, Jilin University, Changchun, Jilin, China

Xuewu Liu Department of Neurology, Shandong Provincial Hospital Affiliated to Shandong First Medical University, Jinan, Shandong, China

Rong Luo Department of Pediatrics, West China Second University Hospital, Sichuan University, Chengdu, China

Terence J. O'Brien Department of Neuroscience, Central Clinical School, Monash University, Melbourne, VIC, Australia

Emilio Perucca Department of Medicine (Austin Health), The University of Melbourne, Melbourne, VIC, Australia

Department of Neuroscience, Central Clinical School, Monash University, Melbourne, VIC, Australia

Meizhen Sun Department of Neurology, The First Hospital of Shanxi Medical University, Taiyuan, Shanxi, China

Xin Tian Department of Neurology, The First Affiliated Hospital of Chongqing Medical University, Chongqing, China

Qun Wang Department of Neurology, Beijing Tiantan Hospital, Capital Medical University, Beijing, China

Wei Wang Department of Neurology, The First Affiliated Hospital of Chongqing Medical University, Chongqing, China

Xiangqing Wang Department of Neurology, The First Medical Center of Chinese PLA General Hospital, Beijing, China

Xuefeng Wang Department of Neurology, The First Affiliated Hospital of Chongqing Medical University, Chongqing, China

Yi Wang Department of Neurology, Children's Hospital of Fudan University, National Children's Medical Center, Shanghai, China

Ying Wang Department of Neurology, The First Affiliated Hospital of DaLian Medical University, DaLian, China

Zan Wang Department of Neurology, The first hospital of JIlin University, Changchun, China

Ye Wu Department of Pediatrics, Peking University First Hospital, Beijing, China

Fei Xiao Department of Neurology, The First Affiliated Hospital of Chongqing Medical University, Chongqing, China

Xin Xu Department of Neurology, The First Affiliated Hospital of Chongqing Medical University, Chongqing, China

Zucai Xu Department of Neurology, Affiliated Hospital of Zunyi Medical University, Zunyi, Guizhou, China

Chao Yan Nanjing University, School of Life Sciences, Department of Physiology, Nanjing, Jiangsu, China

Yin Yan Epilepsy Rehabilitation center, The Affiliated Beibei Hospital of Chongqing Medical University, Chongqing, China

Xiaofeng Yang Guangzhou National Laboratory, Guangzhou, China

Haiqing Zhang Department of Neurology, Affiliated Hospital of Zunyi Medical University, Zunyi, Guizhou, China

Hong Zhang Department of Neurology, Shengjing Hospital of China Medical University, Shenyang, China

Liming Zhang Department of Neurology, The First Affiliated Hospital of Harbin Medical University, Harbin, Heilongjiang, China

Liemin Zhou Department of Neurology, The Seven Affiliated Hospital of Sun Yat-sen University, Shenzhen, China

Chapter 1
Overview

Qun Wang, Xuefeng Wang, Emilio Perucca, Zhuo Huang, and Xiaofeng Yang

1.1 Definition of Epilepsy

The definition of a specific disease is one in which professionals use the simplest language to summarize the characteristics of the disease to facilitate communication among peers and more reasonable treatment of the disease. Because of the different cultures in different countries, it is very difficult to formulate a widely accepted definition. Understanding of diseases varies across time and across countries. Therefore, developing a widely accepted definition of disease has become the most important task of international organizations [1].

Epilepsy is an ancient disease, and there have been descriptions of epilepsy since the beginning of the written human record, but many people still do not know what

Q. Wang (✉)
Department of Neurology, Beijing Tiantan Hospital, Capital Medical University, Beijing, China

X. Wang
Department of Neurology, The First Affiliated Hospital of Chongqing Medical University, Chongqing, China

E. Perucca
Department of Medicine (Austin Health), The University of Melbourne, Melbourne, VIC, Australia

Department of Neuroscience, Central Clinical School, Monash University, Melbourne, VIC, Australia

Z. Huang
State Key Laboratory of Natural and Biomimetic Drugs, Department of Molecular and Cellular Pharmacology, School of Pharmaceutical Sciences, Peking University, Beijing, China

X. Yang
Guangzhou National Laboratory, Guangzhou, China

X. Wang, L. Zhou (eds.), *Pharmacological Treatment of Epileptic Seizures*, https://doi.org/10.1007/978-981-96-8520-2_1

epilepsy is. People can only see epileptic seizures. Therefore, the understanding of epilepsy in humans has progressed from the beginning of epileptic seizures, and epileptic seizures are the basis for people to understand epilepsy [1].

The first human description of epileptic seizures appeared in 1046 BC in the Babylonian treatise on the diagnosis of disease. Since then, people have gradually paid more attention to this episodic disease. Although clinical manifestations vary from individual to individual, they all have a clear beginning and end. The duration is also very short. The clinical manifestation is based on the physiological function of the human body, which supports the strengthening of the physiological function of the human body and does not produce activities outside of those caused by brain function. Each seizure is a temporary disorder of brain function. The symptoms are almost identical in each episode in the same individual, indicating that the dysfunction is spread along specific pathologic pathways [1–4].

Some scholars have summarized the common manifestations of seizures: sudden, transient, stereotypical, and repetitive. The term "paroxysmal" indicates that the patient's seizures occur suddenly and end quickly, and the start and end times are very clear. During the non-seizure period, the patient's brain function is normal. Transient refers to the time of each seizure being very short, from a few seconds to a few minutes, and almost never more than 5 minutes according to the guidelines of the International League against Epilepsy. Stereotypical refers to the fact that although the clinical manifestations of epilepsy are very rich and diverse, every seizure in every patient is similar. However, the scope of the spread of epileptic discharge is different, and its main characteristics must be the same. Repetitive means that the seizures of epilepsy patients not include only one attack but will be repeated. Epilepsy is a prominent manifestation of temporary disorders of normal brain function. Due to the different locations of affected neurons, the range of influence varies, and patients can experience sensory, motor, autonomic nerve, consciousness, and emotional disorders [2–5].

However, an isolated seizure is not epilepsy, and there are many seizures similar to those caused by epilepsy, including those caused by convulsive syncope, hyperventilation syndrome, hypertensive encephalopathy, gestational poisoning in women, hysteria, etc. There are dozens of forms of myoclonus similar to seizures; paroxysmal sleep disorders, such as sleepwalking, night terrors, and periodic tendon movements during sleep, also lead to seizures similar to those of epilepsy, but they are not epilepsy. Nor does it develop in the same way as epilepsy [1, 4].

The greatest difference between epilepsy and epileptic seizures is that people with epilepsy have repeated seizures. Some scholars have shown that 50–60% of patients with similar seizures will not have repeated seizures; therefore, they are not epileptic, and real epilepsy patients have repeated epileptic seizures. Early epidemiological surveys have also shown that epilepsy patients often relapse within 3 years, even if it is an epileptic seizure; before there is a recurrence, the seizure can only be called a pre-seizure, and the presence of epilepsy can only be considered after recurrence [1, 4].

Epileptic seizures are used to understand epilepsy for humans, and epileptic seizures are the basis of the existence of epilepsy. Epilepsy patients also have characteristics of epileptic seizures, that is, sudden, transient, stereotypic and repetitive seizures, and their clinical manifestations should also be classified in the category of brain disorders [1, 4, 5].

In 1870, John Hughlings Jackson proposed a possible mechanism for epileptic seizures by comparing them with nonepileptic seizures. He suggested that epileptic seizures were transient brain disorders caused by sudden seizures and transient, over-synchronous discharge of gray matter neurons. The cause is a sudden release of energy from neurons. Epilepsy is synonymous with this bursting overexcitation of gray matter neurons, in what is known as the Jackson hypothesis [1]. In the following century, many studies investigated the mechanisms of seizures. It has been proposed that epilepsy is a transient disorder of one or several functions of the brain, originates from the highly synchronized discharge of neurons in the cortex, thalamus, and upper brainstem, and is characterized by highly excited lower neurons caused by the reduced inhibitory output of the related upper neuron groups to the lower neuron groups [2–5]. These hypotheses emphasize that electrical and chemical abnormalities in neurons, outside neurons or in the environment are the mechanism of epileptic seizures, greatly enriching the content of the study of epileptic pathogenesis [2–5].

Based on extensive research, the International League against Epilepsy has proposed a definition of epilepsy, epileptic seizures and epileptic syndromes. "Epilepsy is a chronic brain disease characterized by epileptic seizures. The highly synchronized abnormal firing of neurons is the root cause of epileptic seizures. Transient brain dysfunction is the main manifestation of epileptic seizures. Due to the different locations of the affected neurons, the range varies, and due to the differences in the functions of different brain areas, patients can present with sensory, motor, conscious, emotional, language, behavioral, or autonomic dysfunction." Epilepsy is characterized by specific clinical and EEG manifestations, is supported by a specific etiology, is usually diagnosed as having prognostic and therapeutic significance, is accompanied by age-dependent and specific comorbidities, and is called epileptic syndrome [2–6].

1.2 Classification and Diagnosis of Epileptic Seizures

The classification and diagnosis of epileptic seizures are extremely important for clinicians and care teams, patients, and families, and researchers. For patients, the classification is helpful for clarifying the disease diagnosis and exploring the cause; for clinicians and care teams, the classification helps to facilitate communication and discussion. From a research perspective, accurate classification of epileptic seizures facilitates a comprehensive and orderly investigation of the different types of antiseizure medications and/or surgical treatment modalities, treatment responses, and the typical clinical course of epileptic seizures.

1.2.1 History of Epileptic Seizure Classification

The classification of epileptic seizures can be traced back to 1815, when Esquirol classified epileptic seizures into Grand Mal and Petit Mal according to clinical severity [7]. In 1937, Gibbs and Lennox et al. classified epileptic seizures into Grand Mal, Petit Mal, and psychomotor epileptic seizures based on clinical manifestations and EEG features [8]. In 1954, for the first time, Gastaut, combined with the study of Penfield et al., established a more systematic classification of epileptic seizures.

At present, there are two main types of epileptic seizure classification. One is the electroclinical classification proposed by the International League Against Epilepsy (ILAE). The other is the seizure symptomatology classification, which is mainly based on patient clinical symptoms.

In 1964, Gastaut et al. proposed the first draft of the ILAE classification and diagnosis of epileptic seizures [9], which was first revised in 1970 [10]. After analyzing and summarizing hundreds of video EEG recordings of epileptic seizures [11], the ILAE revised the manuscript in 1981, and BLUME et al. further standardized the terminology of their descriptions of symptoms during epileptic seizures in 2001 [12]. It should be noted that the 1981 ILAE classification of epileptic seizures is the most far-reaching classification in the world, and it is still widely used in clinical practice and scientific research. With the in-depth analysis of the electroclinical features of an increasing number of epilepsy cases, scholars have found that some epileptic seizure types cannot be distinguished by the traditional classification of 1981, and the Classification and Nomology Committee of the ILAE introduced an updated version of the classification in 2010 [13], which enriched the classification framework. In recent years, rapid advances in related disciplines such as neuroimaging, genomic technology, and molecular biology have led to a further increase in the reported types of epileptic seizures, making it difficult for a broad classification to cover new types of epileptic seizures and hindering the understanding of the underlying development of the disease and the complexity of pathological and physiological processes. To adapt to the rapid development and new understanding in the field of epilepsy, the ILAE proposed a new operational classification of epileptic seizures [14] in 2017, which improved the intuitiveness, transparency, and universality of the classification and proposed descriptive reporting of seizure types, allowing for the inclusion of previously unclassifiable epileptic seizures.

The symptomatologic classification of epileptic seizures, also known as the Lüders classification of epileptic seizures, was first established by Lüders et al. in 1993 from the sole perspective of symptomatology [15] and was revised in 1998 [16] and 2019 [17].

1.2.2 Classification of Epileptic Seizures

1.2.2.1 Classification of Seizures by the ILAE, 1981

The 1981 ILAE classification of epileptic seizures [11] was based on clinical manifestations and electroencephalogram (EEG) features (interictal stage and attack period), and epileptic seizures are divided into the following:

1. *Partial seizure*: Initial clinical seizure and EEG features suggest that "a group of neurons in one cerebral hemisphere are first involved." Based on the level of consciousness, partial seizures can be further divided into simple partial seizures (SPSs), complex partial seizures (CPSs) and secondarily generalized tonic–clonic seizures (SGTCs).
2. *Generalized seizure*: Initial clinical manifestations and EEG features suggest "simultaneous involvement of both cerebral hemispheres;"
3. Unclassified seizures.

1.2.2.2 Classification of Seizures by the ILAE(2017)

Seizure Classification

The 2017 ILAE classification of seizure type [18] is an operational classification of seizure types, emphasizing that the specific refinement of the classification (basic version/extended version) can be selected according to clinical needs, and the basic version (Table 1.1) is a reduced form of the extended version (Table 1.2). This classification applies to seizures in adults and children but not to seizures in newborns (neonatal seizures are a separate classification).

It is important to emphasize that the 2017 ILAE classification of seizure types chart is columnar rather than hierarchical, meaning that levels can be skipped, and seizure classification may also be terminated at either level. Classification begins with determining whether the initial manifestations of the seizures are of focal or generalized onset; if the origin is not observed or obscured, then the seizure should be of unknown origin. The next level of classification is based on the initial sign or symptom of a seizure, even if it is not ultimately the most significant sign or symptom (except behavioral arrest of focal nonmotor onset seizure, because transient behavioral termination is difficult to determine, so a diagnosis of behavioral arrest requires behavioral termination to be the primary symptom throughout the seizure).

Focal onset seizures can be classified as "Aware" or "Impaired Awareness," with "retained awareness" meaning "aware of self and environment during the seizure, even if immobile." Awareness impairment at any time during focal onset seizures

Table 1.1 2017 Classification of seizure type, basic version [18]

Focal onset		Generalized onset	Unknown onset
Aware	Impaired awareness	Motor	Motor
Motor onset		Nonmotor (absence)	Nonmotor
Nonmotor onset			Unclassified[a]
Focal to bilateral tonic–clonic			

[a]Due to inadequate information or inability to be placed in other categories

Table 1.2 2017 Classification of seizure type, expanded version [18]

Focal onset		Generalized onset	Unknown onset
Aware	Impaired awareness	Motor	Motor
Motor onset		Tonic–clonic	Tonic–clonic
Automatisms		Clonic	Epileptic spasms
Atonic		Tonic	Nonmotor
Clonic		Myoclonic	Behavioral arrest
Epileptic spasms		Myoclonic–tonic–clonic	Unclassified[a]
Hyperkinetic		Myoclonic -atonic	
Myoclonic		Atonic	
Tonic		Epileptic spasms	
Nonmotor onset		Nonmotor (absence)	
Autonomic		Typical	
Behavior arrest		Atypical	
Cognitive		Myoclonic	
Emotional		Eyelid myoclonia	
Sensory			
Focal to bilateral tonic–clonic			

[a]Due to inadequate information or inability to be placed in other categories

should be classified as focal impaired awareness seizures; if awareness is unknown during a seizure, the classification of this level ("Aware" or "Impaired Awareness") should be ignored when classifying the seizure and go directly to the next level, that is, the classification of "Motor Onset" or "Nonmotor onset." In the classification of motor or nonmotor, motor signals usually dominate unless nonmotor (such as sensory) symptoms and signs are significant. Therefore, some words can be omitted without causing ambiguity, such as "focal onset tonic," rather than "focal motor onset tonic."

When classifying generalized onset seizures, "awareness" can be omitted because awareness impairment is present in most generalized onset seizures.

An episode of "Unknown Onset" is not a truly separate type of seizure but merely a placeholder for those whose origin is unknown. For example, if a wife is awakened in her sleep and observes her husband's first tonic–clonic seizure, the husband's seizure may be classified as "unknown onset tonic–clonic seizure" in the initial diagnosis; however, if a seizure with a clear focal onset is subsequently observed, the husband's seizure type will be reclassified as "focal to bilateral tonic–clonic." It is recommended that a seizure be classified as having focal or generalized onset only when there is a high degree of confidence (e.g., ≥80%, arbitrarily chosen to parallel the usual allowable beta error) in the accuracy of the determination; otherwise, the seizure should remain unclassified until more information is available. The term "unclassified seizure" means that the nature of the origin of the seizure is not specific, there are no motor or nonmotor characteristics, and the level of awareness is unclear. If any of the above characteristics are known, a certain classification of the seizure can be made.

The major changes and features of the 2017 classification of seizure type compared to those of the 1981 classification include the following:

1. Focusing on the initial symptoms of the seizure and using them as the main basis for detailed classification. With either focal onset or generalized onset, seizures can be roughly divided into motor and nonmotor.
2. The "unknown onset" option was added. Patients with insufficient information about onset can be temporarily classified into this category, and focal or generalized onset can be determined after the information is complete.
3. In terms of the words used to describe the conscious state of focal-onset seizures, the more complex word "consciousness" is replaced by the simple and understandable word "awareness" ["aware of self and environment during the seizure"]. As previously described, "complex partial" can be changed to "focal impaired awareness."
4. New types of focal seizures were identified—myoclonic–atonic, clonic, epileptic spasms, tonic, and myoclonic seizures—which were considered to be either generalized or focal onset seizures. In addition, it also increased the number of types of seizures that are clinically common or may have locational significance, such as automatisms, hyperkinetics, and behavioral arrest.
5. For focal-onset seizures, it is recommended to discard some previously used terms, such as dyscognitive, simple partial, and psychic.
6. New types of generalized seizures—myoclonus-tonic-clonus, myoclonus-atonic, epileptic spasm, and myoclonic and eyelid myoclonia seizures.
7. The previous term "secondarily generalized" was replaced by "focal to bilateral tonic–clonic."

In summary, the 2017 ILAE classification of seizure types does not represent a fundamental change but allows for more flexibility and transparency in the types of names.

Common Seizure Types and Diagnostic Points of the 2017 ILAE Classification of Seizure Types

1. Focal onset seizures.

   (a) Specification of level of awareness (retained awareness means the person is aware of the self and the environment during the seizure, even if immobile, and impaired awareness during any part of the seizure renders it a focal impaired awareness seizure.) is optional for focal seizures. If awareness is not applicable or is unknown, it can be simply described as a "focal onset seizure."

(b) Automatism refers to the repetitive, aimless, or seemingly purposeful, basically coordinated involuntary movements or behaviors usually made by patients with impaired awareness. The common types of automatism include oropharyngeal automatism, hand automatism, oral automatism and hypermotor automatism.

(c) A hypermotor seizure is a type of focal-onset seizure that mainly involves the trunk and the proximal extremities of the limb, and the range of movement is usually large, fast, and intense. For example, fast flapping movements of the upper limbs or repeated pedaling movements of the lower limbs;

(d) Autonomic seizures refer to focal nonmotor seizures characterized by significant changes in autonomic nervous system function. Changes in the autonomic nervous system may involve cardiopulmonary, papillary, gastrointestinal, perspiratory, vasomotor, and thermoregulatory processes and are often characterized as tachycardia, hyperventilation, elevated gastric gas, flushing, pallor, nausea and vomiting, and erect hair.

(e) Focal behavioral arrest seizures are characterized by the cessation of activity being the dominant feature throughout the seizure and the cessation of activity throughout the entire process;

(f) Cognitive seizures imply impaired language or other cognitive domains or positive features such as déja vu, hallucinations, illusions, or perceptual distortions;

(g) Emotional seizures include anxiety, fear, joy, other emotions, or the appearance of affect without subjective emotions;

(h) Sensory seizures refer to self-perceived and experiential seizures induced by nonexogenous stimuli. Common clinical types include somatosensory, visual, auditory, olfactory, gustatory, temperature, or vestibular seizures.

(i) Focal to bilateral tonic–clonic seizure is a special seizure type, corresponding to the 1981 phrase "partial onset with secondary generalization." Focal to bilateral tonic–clonic seizure reflects a propagation pattern of a seizure rather than a unified seizure type, but it is such a common and important presentation that the separate categorization was continued.

In general, the EEGs of these focal seizures are characterized by epileptic activity with focal initiation and evolution, which may vary according to the initial site of discharge, diffusion rate, and extent.

2. Generalized Onset Seizures

(a) Generalized tonic–clonic seizures (GTCSs) are characterized by loss of consciousness and bilateral symmetrical ankylosis followed by clonic movement and are usually accompanied by autonomic nerve involvement. It is the most obvious form of seizure and used to be called Grand Mal seizure.

(b) Tonic seizures are characterized by continuous contraction and stiffness of the muscles in the central axis of the body, the proximal ends of both limbs, or the whole body. It usually lasts 2–10 seconds and occasionally lasts for a few minutes. The EEG features during seizures mainly include bilateral spike rhythm [(20 ± 5 Hz)] or low amplitude (10 Hz) rhythmic discharge activity. Tonic seizures are the most important seizure type of Lennox–Gastaut syndrome (LGS).

(c) Clonic seizures are characterized by bilateral limb rhythmic (1–3 Hz) jerks, with awareness or impaired awareness. During the seizure, the EEG is mostly generalized spikes/polyspike complexes or spike and slow wave complexes/polyspikes and slow wave complex synthesis.

(d) Myoclonic seizures are characterized by involuntary, rapid, transient, electric-like muscle seizures that last from 10–50 milliseconds and rarely exceed 100 milliseconds. These can involve the whole body or be limited to certain local muscle or muscle groups. May recur nonrhythmically. The typical EEG manifestations during seizures include burst generalization polyspikes and slow wave complexes. Myoclonic seizures, such as those related to juvenile myoclonic epilepsy (JEM), can be observed in some idiopathic epilepsy patients with a good prognosis. Myoclonic seizures can also be seen in some cases of epileptic encephalopathy with a poor prognosis and diffuse brain damage, such as Dravet syndrome and LGS.

(e) Atonic seizures are characterized by a sudden loss or reduction in muscle tone in the head, trunk, or limbs, with no significant myoclonus or tonic components. The seizure lasts approximately 1–2 seconds or longer. The clinical manifestations vary in severity, with mild cases consisting only of nodding, while severe cases can lead to sudden falls while standing. During seizures, the EEG shows transient generalization of 2–3 Hz spikes and slow wave complexes/polyspikes and slow wave complexes or sudden voltage reductions. Atonic seizures are more common in LGS and Doose syndrome patients.

(f) Myoclonic–tonic–clonic seizures are characterized by single or multiple clonus or myoclonic jerks of both limbs, which then evolve into tonic–clonic seizures. This type of seizure is more common in juvenile myoclonic epilepsy (JME) patients.

(g) Myoclonic–atonic seizures are a type of seizure characterized by a myoclonic twitch of the limb or trunk followed by hypotonia. These seizures during orthosis may cause the patient to fall. These seizures were formerly known as "myoclonic astatic seizures." This type of seizure is commonly observed in Doose syndrome patients.

(h) Absence seizures include typical absence, atypical absence, myoclonic absence, and eyelid myoclonic absence.

Typical Absence Sudden onset and sudden stop of the seizure, manifested by sudden cessation of movement or significant slowing down, with impaired awareness, with or without mild motor symptoms (such as clonus/myoclonus/rigidity/automatism). The seizure usually lasts 5–20 seconds (<30 seconds). EEG reveals a 3 Hz (2.5–4 Hz) spike and slow wave complex burst with bilateral synchronous symmetry. Hyperventilation can induce a typical absence in approximately 90% of patients. It is mainly observed in children and adolescents, such as children with childhood absence epilepsy (CAE) and juvenile absence epilepsy (JAE), and is rare in adults.

Atypical Absence The onset and end of the seizure are slower than those of a typical absence seizure, with a less severe level of impaired awareness and more complex accompanying motor symptoms (such as automatisms). Muscle tension is usually reduced, and a seizure may last more than 20 seconds. The EEG shows a slow (<2.5 Hz) spike and slow wave complex rhythm during seizures. It is mainly observed in patients with severe neuropsychiatric disorders, such as LGS.

Myoclonic Absence Manifests as absence accompanied by rhythmic 2.5–4.5 Hz myoclonic movements of the limbs, accompanied by tonic components. EEG during the seizure period is similar to that of a typical absence seizure. Mainly seen in myoclonic absence epilepsy.

Eyelid Myoclonic Absence Manifested as a 5–6 Hz myoclonic movement in the muscles of the eyelids and/or forehead simultaneously with the onset of absence. During the seizure period, EEG shows a comprehensive 3–6 Hz polyspike and slow wave complex. This syndrome is commonly observed in Jeavons syndrome patients.

3. Epileptic Spasm

Epileptic spasms were initially clearly classified as a type of seizure in the 2010 ILAE classification report, which can be of focal onset, generalized onset, or unknown onset.

Epileptic spasms are sudden and mainly involve the central axis of the trunk and the proximal muscles of both limbs, with a duration of 0.2–2 seconds and sudden onset cessation. Clinically, spasms can be divided into flexion or extension types, with the former being more common and manifesting as episodic nodding movements, often occurring in clusters after awakening. Interictal EEG signals show hypsarrhythmia, and interictal EEG signals are diverse (such as voltage reduction, high-amplitude biphasic slow waves, or spike and slow wave complexes), often occurring in clusters after awakening. Epileptic spasms, such as those seen in West syndrome, are more common in infants and young children and can also be seen at other ages.

4. Reflex Seizure

Reflex epilepsy is not an independent type of seizure. It can manifest as focal or generalized onset seizures. Its uniqueness lies in the fact that seizures have specific exogenous or endogenous triggering factors; that is, each episode is triggered by a specific sensory stimulus, and there is a close lock-in relationship between seizures and triggering factors. The triggering factors can include nonpathological factors such as vision, thinking, music, reading, eating, and manipulation. These factors can include simple sensory stimuli (such as flashing) or complex intelligence activities (such as reading and playing chess). Seizures induced by pathological conditions such as fever, alcohol or drug withdrawal are not considered reflexive seizures. It should also be noted that both reflexive seizures and spontaneous seizures can occur simultaneously in patients with epilepsy.

Diagnosis and Classification of Seizures in Neonates

The content of the 2017 ILAE classification mainly targets adults and older children and is not suitable for newborns. Given the differences in clinical and electrophysiological manifestations, etiology, diagnostic methods, and other aspects of neonatal epilepsy, the ILAE released a classification of neonatal seizures in 2021 [19]. The overall framework of this classification is generally consistent with the 2017 ILAE classification and can be considered the revised version of the latter for newborns.

The classification and diagnostic processes for neonatal epilepsy are shown in Fig. 1.1 EEG is the "gold standard" for diagnosing neonatal seizures and can be diagnosed solely based on EEG findings. If there are only clinical events without corresponding EEG seizure patterns, the patient cannot be diagnosed with an epileptic seizure. Neonatal seizures can be divided into electroclinical seizures and electrographic seizures. For the former, the seizure type can be further determined based on specific manifestations: motor seizures, such as automatisms; clonic, epileptic spasms; myoclonic, and tonic; and nonmotor seizures, such as autonomic and behavioral arrest. Moreover, it should be emphasized that newborns have only focal seizures and that there are no generalized seizures.

1.2.2.3 Symptomatologic Classification of Seizures

Although new technologies such as EEG, high-resolution magnetic resonance imaging, and magnetoencephalography have played a significant role in the diagnosis and treatment of epilepsy in recent years, detailed medical history records and detailed observations still have important value. The symptomatologic classification of seizures helps to accurately describe the origin of seizures, especially in preoperative evaluation for epilepsy surgery, which is widely used.

According to the 2019 updated classification of paroxysmal events and the four-dimensional epilepsy classification system [11], paroxysmal events need to be classified across four dimensions: ictal semiology, the epileptogenic zone, etiology, and comorbidities. This classification emphasizes that the descriptions of these four imaging features are independent of one another and can be derived based on different diagnostic methods. For example, a patient may have bilateral tonic–clonic seizures (based on ictal semiology), the epileptogenic area is located in the left temporal lobe (based on EEG), the etiology is a tumor in the left frontotemporal lobe (based on MRI and pathological examination), and the case is also complicated by depression. The independence of different dimensions also allows for a certain correlation

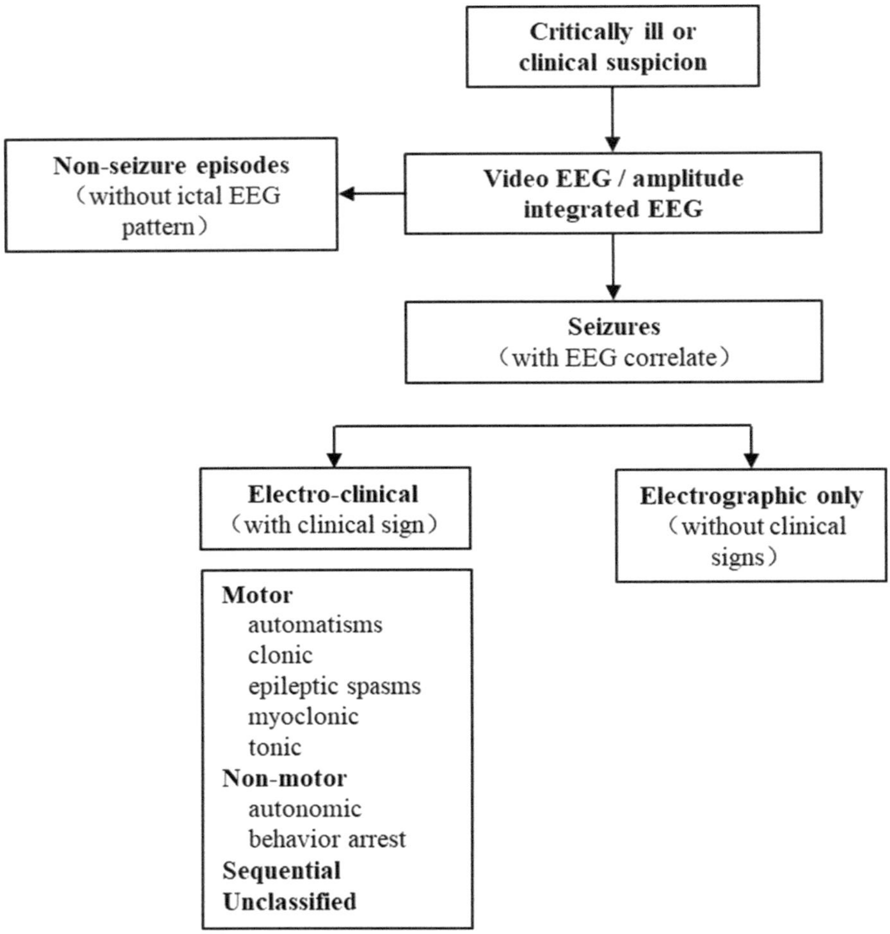

Fig. 1.1 Diagnostic framework of seizures in the neonatal period, including the classification of seizures [13]

between different dimensions (such as the epileptogenic area located in the left temporal lobe or the etiology of a tumor in the left frontal and temporal lobe).

There are six main types of seizures:

1. Auras
   (a) Auditory aura.
   (b) Autonomic aura.
      (i) Abdominal aura/Choking aura.
      (ii) Diaphoretic aura.
      (iii) Disodic aura.
      (iv) Pilomotor aura.

(v) Sialorrheic aura.
(vi) Tachycardic aura.
(vii) Urinary aura.
(viii) Vasomotor aura.

(c) Gustatory aura.
(d) Olfactory aura.
(e) Psychic aura.

(i) Affective aura.

- Pleasure aura (Ecstasy aura/Religious aura/Sexual aura).
- Unpleasant aura (Anger aura/Depression/Sadness aura/Embarrassment aura/Fear/Panic aura/Guilt aura).

(ii) Cognitive aura.
(iii) Experiential aura.
(iv) Familiarity aura.

- Déjà-vu aura.
- Jamais-vu aura.

(v) Illusionary aura.

- Auditory aura.
- Bodily aura.
- Time aura.
- Visual aura.

(f) Somatosensory aura.
(g) Vestibular aura.
(h) Visual aura/Ictal blindness.

2. Autonomic Seizure

(a) Abdominal seizure.
(b) Anisocoric seizure.
(c) Bradycardic seizure.
(d) Emetic seizure.
(e) Fecal incontinence seizure.
(f) Hippus seizure.
(g) Hyperhydrostatic seizure.
(h) Hypertensive seizure.
(i) Lacrimatory seizure.
(j) Pilomotor seizure.
(k) Sexual seizure.
(l) Sialorrheic seizure.
(m) Tachycardic seizure.
(n) Urinary seizure.
(o) Vasomotor seizure.

3. Dyscognitive Seizure
   (a) Amnestic seizure.
   (b) Aphasic seizure.
   (c) Kinetic seizure.
   (d) Dialectic seizure.
4. Motor Seizure
   (a) Simple motor seizure.
      (i) Clonic seizure.
      (ii) Epileptic spasm.
      (iii) Myoclonic seizure.
      (iv) Nystagmoid seizure.
      (v) Tonic seizure.
      (vi) Tonic–clonic seizure.
      (vii) Versive seizure.
      (viii) Vocalization seizure.
   (b) Complex motor seizure.
      (i) Alien limb seizure.
      (ii) Automotor seizure.
      (iii) Dacrystic seizure.
      (iv) Gelastic seizure.
      (v) Hypermotor seizure/Emotional hypermotor seizure.
      (vi) Kissing seizure.
      (vii) Singing seizure.
      (viii) Spitting seizure.
      (ix) Verbalization seizure.
5. Special Seizure
   (a) Astatic seizure.
   (b) Atonic seizure.
   (c) Central apneic seizure.
   (d) Fearful facies seizure.
   (e) Hypnopompic seizure.
   (f) Hypomotor seizure.
   (g) Negative myoclonic seizure.
   (h) Water drinking seizure.
6. Asymptomatic EEG seizure.

2.4 Classification and diagnosis of epileptic syndrome (see Chap. 4).

1.3 History, Present Situation, and Future Perspectives

The first known description of an epileptic seizure is recorded in a 4000-year-old Akkadian tablet from Mesopotamia [19]. At those times, epilepsy was considered to be caused by spirits and gods, and therefore, it was treated with magical rites, including herbal remedies which were not usually ingested, but simply hung around the neck [20]. Herbal remedies as a treatment for epilepsy and seizures have also been used in China for thousands of years, but in traditional Chinese medicine treatments were consumed as part of the diet according to the theory that medicine and food come from the same sources [21]. Plant-derived medicines have been the mainstay of medical therapy for seizures and epilepsy in many other civilizations, and some continue to be used in traditional medicine. Although the evidence base for their efficacy is tenuous [20, 21], and some may even be toxic or interact adversely with modern medicines [22], a number of these treatments deserve to be evaluated through modern methodology [21]. An example of an herbal remedy that withstood the test of scientific scrutiny and was eventually incorporated into the modern pharmacological armamentarium is cannabidiol, which was used as a component of Cannabis to treat epilepsy by Islamic physicians in the twelfth century [23] and is now approved in the United States and Europe for the treatment of seizures associated with Dravet syndrome, Lennox-Gastaut syndrome and tuberous sclerosis complex [24].

Although a myriad of treatments have been applied since the dawn of history as an attempt to control seizures and epilepsy, the modern era of antiseizure medications (ASMs) starts with the introduction of bromide [25, 26]. Accordingly, our description of the history of pharmacological treatments for epilepsy will start from that time.

1.3.1 The Early Period of ASM History: 1857 to 1937

The birth of effective antiseizure treatments has a precise date, May 11, 1857. It was on that date that, at a meeting of the Royal Medical and Chirurgical Society in London, Sir Charles Locock, Queen's Victoria's obstetrician, commented on the excellent efficacy results that he had obtained with potassium bromide in the treatment of young women with 'hysterical epilepsy connected with the menstrual period' [20]. He was probably referring to catamenial epilepsy. Apparently, the rationale for trying bromide in those patients was to exploit its anaphrodysiac properties due to his belief, widely held at that time that epilepsy was caused by masturbation "both in boys and in girls." As we will see later in this chapter, this was not the last time that a wrong hypothesis led to discovery of an effective medications. Within a few years of Charles Locock's presentation, bromides became widely used in the treatment of epileptic seizures. Bromides dominated the therapeutic armamentarium against epilepsy for the last part of the nineteenth century, and continued to do so until the 1920s. When started as initial treatment in newly diagnosed epilepsy, bromides reportedly resulted in long-term remission in about one quarter of patients, and a significant reduction in seizures in about another quarter [27]. Results, however, were less favorable when bromides were used in patients with chronic epilepsy. After the introduction of phenobarbital and phenytoin, bromides were largely replaced by safer and more effective ASMs, although they are still being used today in exceptional cases, especially in children with drug-refractory seizures [28, 29]. Of note, the introduction of bromides did not immediately result in complete disappearance of older, bizarre and often deleterious "treatments" for epilepsy such as tooth removal, ligatures of the extremities, dry cupping, the abstraction of blood, purgatives, mineral tonics, nitromuriatic acid, decoctions of bark and sulphuric acid, and other similar amenities [20]. In fact, more ineffective and toxic treatments were introduced between 1860 and 1910 [20].

The next milestone in ASM history was the introduction of phenobarbital in 1912. Barbiturates had been used for their sedative and sleep-promoting properties for a number of years. Phenobarbital was synthesized in 1904 and joined other barbiturates in the German market in 1911. The discovery of its antiseizure properties can be ascribed again to serendipity. The prevailing story is that Alfred Hauptmann, then a young physician working at a clinic in Freiburg, Germany, lived in an apartment above a ward that housed patients with epilepsy, and his sleep was disrupted by noisy seizures that the patients were having at night [25]. Guided by the erroneous hypothesis that sedation would reduce susceptibility to seizures, he prescribed phenobarbital to his patients and found that their seizure frequency was greatly improved or even suppressed, both at night and during daytime. His meticulous documentation of phenobarbital's efficacy in controlling seizures was published in a local German language scientific journal which was not readily accessible [20]. Because of this, and because of the communication disruption produced by World Word I (1914–1918), phenobarbital started to be known and used outside Germany only in the 1920s [30]. It became increasingly popular in subsequent years, and it continues to be used even in modern times, particularly in low-income countries, because of its low cost. An intravenous formulation of phenobarbital, which provided a valuable tool for the management of status epilepticus, was introduced in 1926. The establishment of phenobarbital as an effective ASM led to subsequent introduction of other barbiturates for the treatment of seizures, namely phenylmethylbarbituric acid (Rutonal®) in 1925 and methylethylphenylbarbituric acid (mephobarbital, Prominal®, Mebaral®) in 1932, but none of these compounds proved to be as successful as phenobarbital [20].It should be emphasized that none of the treatments discussed thus far had undergone rigorous evaluation through controlled trials. Regulatory oversight of the marketing of medicines was minimal at that time. Prior to the approval of the Food and Drug and Cosmetics Act by the American Congress in 1938, medicines could be marketed in America and other parts of the world without any demonstration of safety being required [31]. Moreover, adequate demonstration of efficacy was not a requirement until 1962 in the US, and until several years later in Europe. This explains why during the same period many toxic and ineffective treatments for epilepsy continued to be introduced and used, typically with misleading claims concerning their true effectiveness. For example, a 1940 British textbook cited belladonna, borax and nitroglycerine among medications of definite usefulness for the treatment of epilepsy (Kinnear-Wilson, 1940). In an article by William Lennox (1940), epilepsy treatments used in America in the mid-30 s included not only phenobarbital (and phenytoin, for the last two years of that decade), but also borotartrate, brilliant vital red, and antirabies vaccine! The number of people harmed by these treatments is likely to have been substantial, an observation which highlights the danger of relying on uncontrolled clinical reports without proper evaluation of efficacy and safety [31].

1.3.2 From the Discovery of Phenytoin to the Introduction of Valproic Acid: 1938–1967

The introduction of phenytoin in 1938 represents a true landmark because the discovery of this drug was based on a screening program in an animal model (seizures induced by electrical stimulation of brain) and a paradigm that, with a number of additions and modifications, continues to be used today in ASM discovery. Another landmark advance made with the introduction of phenytoin was the demonstration that antiseizure effects can be achieved without inducing sedation [31]. Interestingly, it took only two years from the first experiments in animal models to the introduction of phenytoin in the market [20]. Overall, the clinical development program of phenytoin lasted about one year, and did not include any controlled trial.

The discovery of phenytoin by Merritt and Putnam is a truly fascinating story that has been described masterfully by [20]. Although based on a rational hypothesis (i.e., the hypothesis that electrically induced seizures could provide a model to identify molecules possessing antiseizure activity), Merritt and Putnam's discovery benefited from a great deal of luck. In fact, phenytoin was one of the very first compounds that underwent screening, and clearly showed very promising activity. Thereafter, Merritt and Putnam screened over 700 molecules, but only four of those reached the stage of being tested clinically and none became commercially available. Should phenytoin not have been among the first 50 or 100 compounds tested, one wonders whether Merritt and Putnam would have continued with their testing program!

Merritt and Putnam's experiments were truly a turning point in the history of ASM discovery, because it led to the introduction of animal models of seizures and, at a later time, models of epilepsy as a standard approach to discover and evaluate novel drug candidates prior to their assessment in the clinic [32, 33]. Intense research efforts in the subsequent 30 years led to the marketing many novel drugs for the treatment of seizure disorders, including (in order of year of introduction for use in epilepsy) trimetadione, paramethadione, mephenytoin, phetenylate, phenacemide, metharbital, beclamide, phensuximide, primidone, methsuximide, allomethadione, acetazolamide, pheneturide, ethotoin, aminoglutethimide, sulthiame, diazepam, carbamazepine, and valproate [31]. This list includes highly valuable ASMs which are still in widely used today as well as compounds that rapidly became obsolete due to poor efficacy or unfavorable tolerability profile. Once more, this reflects the lack of rigorous clinical assessment of these compounds prior to their introduction in the market. Some randomized controlled trials of ASMs were actually conducted during this period, but their application was sparse and trial designs were often suboptimal [31]. This is best summarized by an influential US report on the evidence supporting the efficacy of ASMs introduced prior to the 1970s [20]. Only three of the 110 clinical trials which were closely assessed included an adequate control for bias, and only two had a double-blind design. With respect to modalities of drug discovery, many compounds originated from structural modifications of ASMs, especially phenobarbital and phenytoin, already known to be clinically effective. However, serendipity played again a major role in some instances, the most notable example being valproic acid which was used as a solvent for other drug candidates and discovered by chance when all screening tests done on compounds dissolved in valproic acid turned out to be positive for anticonvulsant activity [34]. In any case, the period between 1938 and 1967 was quite fruitful, because virtually all first-generation ASMs had been introduced by that time. Admittedly, not all of these ASMs became widely available during that period. For example, valproic acid was marketed in France in 1967, but it was approved by the US Food and Drug administration (FDA) in 1978, that is, more than 10 years later.

1.3.3 Establishing the Modern Principles of Epilepsy Treatment and Preparing the Ground for a New Wave of ASMs: 1968–1988

The two decades that followed the introduction of valproic acid were characterized by an improved understanding of the clinical profile of the ASMs existing at the time, as well as the many factors involved in variability in drug response. A number of important developments took place during this period.

First of all, the methodology to evaluate the clinical efficacy and safety of ASMs was greatly improved, with increasing emphasis being placed on high-quality randomized controlled trials. Evaluation of the efficacy of available ASMs was facilitated by the development in the late 1960s of a broadly accepted classification of seizures and epilepsies [35, 36], and reached a high point in the early 1980s with the conduction of a landmark randomized double-blind parallel-group multicenter trial by the US Department of Veterans Affairs (VA) collaborative group [37]. This trial compared the effects of phenytoin, carbamazepine, phenobarbital, and primidone in 622 patients with newly diagnosed (or previously undertreated) focal and/or focal to bilateral tonic–clonic seizures, and demonstrated important differences in the efficacy and tolerability of these drugs. At the same time, smaller-scale studies helped in characterizing the spectrum of efficacy of many ASMs against different seizure types, highlighting the fact that some narrow-spectrum ASMs can paradoxically precipitate or aggravate seizures in patients with certain epilepsy syndromes [38]. Finally, studies conducted in this period led to recognition of the value of monotherapy in the treatment of epilepsy [39], and the appreciation that unnecessary polytherapy can be associated with a major burden of toxicity [40].

A second important advance in this period was the broad recognition that variability in serum drug levels of ASMs contributes to an important extent to differences in clinical response across individuals. Pioneering work on the pharmacokinetics of phenobarbital and phenytoin had been done many years earlier in the USA, and the evaluation of the correlation between serum ASM concentrations and clinical response can be traced back largely to research carried out by Fritz Buchthal and Ole Svensmark in the late 1950s and early 1960s in Copenhagen, Denmark [41]. However, it was only in the 1970s and 1980s that the use of serum ASM concentrations (therapeutic drug monitoring, or TDM) as an aid to dose adjustment became fully established [42–45]. Together with studies on the comparative efficacy and tolerability of existing ASMs, these studies contributed to highlight the importance of tailoring ASM therapy to the characteristics of the individual patient.

Interestingly, not many ASMs were introduced during this period. ASMs marketed between 1968 and 1988 include three benzodiazepine compounds (clonazepam, clobazam and lorazepam), and the GABA-prodrug progabide, which was marketed in France in 1985 but was never widely used because of poor efficacy results and the potential to cause liver toxicity [46–48]. Another investigational drug, cinromide, showed very promising results in Lennox Gastaut syndrome and other seizure disorders, but its development was stopped in 1981 when controlled studies found its efficacy to be similar to that of placebo [20].

In the late 1960s and early 1970s, there was a clear perception that efforts to discover new drugs for epilepsy were relenting, despite an obvious need for safer and more effective treatments. These considerations, coupled with the wisdom and vision of Dr. J. Kiffin Penry at the US National Institute of Neurological Disorders and Stroke, led to the establishment in 1975 of the US Anticonvulsant Screening Program (ASP), with finding from the National Institute of Health (NIH) [20, 49]. The aim of the ASP was to stimulate discovery and development of newer therapies for epilepsy. This program, currently known as the Epilepsy Therapy Screening Program (ETSP), has grown over time into a highly structured testing algorithm that uses a broad range of preclinical models, including models of drug-resistant epilepsy, models of severe genetic epilepsies, and models of epilepsies involving infectious and inflammatory mechanisms [50–52]. Over the years, the ETSP has screened preclinically more than 30,000 drug candidates supplied by the pharmaceutical industry or academia, and has played a role (and often a key role) in the development of many subsequently marketed ASMs, including vigabatrin, lamotrigine, oxcarbazepine, felbamate, gabapentin, topiramate, lacosamide, retigabine, and cannabidiol [20, 49, 53]. In fact, the development of some of these compounds started in the late 1970s or the early 1980s, even though their introduction in the marked occurred at a later time.

1.3.4 The Advent of the New ASMs: 1989–2023

The wave of the so-called "new" ASMs started in 1989 with the introduction in the market of vigabatrin and zonisamide. Since then 21 additional ASMs have been introduced in the European or American market (Table 1.3). These medications differ in mechanism of action, pharmacokinetic profile, drug interaction potential,

Table 1.3 Year of first approval of the most recently developed antiseizure medications (ASMs). For drugs that received earlier approval for other indications, year of first approval refers to initial approval for a seizure-related indication

ASM	Year of first approval	Country (or region) of initial approval
Vigabatrin	1989	UK
Zonisamide	1989	Japan and South Korea
Lamotrigine	1990	Ireland
Oxcarbazepine	1990	Denmark
Felbamate	1993	USA
Gabapentin	1993	UK and USA
Topiramate	1995	UK
Fosphenytoin	1996	USA
Tiagabine	1996	France
Levetiracetam	2000	USA
Pregabalin	2004	European Union and USA
Rufinamide	2007	European Union
Stiripentol	2007	European Union
Lacosamide	2008	European Union and USA
Eslicarbazepine acetate	2009	European Union
Retigabine (ezogabine)[a]	2011	European Union and USA
Perampanel	2012	European Union and USA
Brivaracetam	2016	European Union and USA
Everolimus	2017	European Union
Cannabidiol	2018	USA
Fenfluramine	2020	European Union and USA
Cenobamate	2019	USA
Ganaxolone	2022	USA

[a]Retigabine (ezogabine) was withdrawn from the market in in 2017

spectrum of efficacy against different seizure types, approved indications, and adverse effect profile. Details of their different properties are discussed in Chap. 3 of this volume, and only a few general considerations will be made here.

The first consideration concerns the approach that led to their discovery [54]. Only few of these ASMs were designed rationally to produce the molecular actions underlying their efficacy against seizures. Examples of drugs designed to engage a specific target include vigabatrin (an inhibitor of GABA transaminase), tiagabine (an inhibitor GABA reuptake), perampanel (an AMPA receptor blocker), and ganaxolone (a positive allosteric modulator of the $GABA_A$ receptor mimicking the action of the endogenous neurosteroid allopregnanolone). Some of the other newer ASMs, such as oxcarbazepine, eslicarbazepine acetate, fosphenytoin, pregabalin, and brivaracetam, were developed by structural modification of pre-existing ASMs. The mTOR inhibitor everolimus was approved initially for other indications, and its investigation as an ASM in patients with tuberous sclerosis complex (TSC) was based on the known pathogenic role of mTOR overexpression in TSC patients. The remaining drugs were mainly developed by phenotypic screening in animal models of seizures and epilepsy, in some cases based on erroneous hypotheses. Gabapentin, for example, was synthesized as a GABA derivative, but its primary mechanism of action is not GABA-mediated and consists in inhibition of voltage-sensitive Ca^{2+} channels through an action at the α2δ modulatory subunit of the Ca^{2+} channel [55]. Likewise, lamotrigine, which is not a folate antagonist, originated from structural modification of folate antagonists based on the hypothesis that an action against folate might produce antiseizure effects [56].

The second consideration about progress made during this period stems from the clinical trial designs that led to regulatory approval of the "new" ASMs. Clinical trial designs used in the ASM development evolved markedly during the last 30 years, from small cross-over single-center studies to large parallel-group multicenter trials (Perucca, 1919). Trial endpoints also evolved over time, mainly in order to adapt to changes in regulatory scenario and to address ethical concerns related to the need to minimize prolonged exposure to placebo or ineffective treatments [57].

The third, and most important, consideration is a reflection on the extent to which the ASMs introduced since 1989 improved clinical outcomes for people with epilepsy. As discussed in detail in recent articles, these medications have not increased substantially the proportion of patients with epilepsy who can achieve freedom from seizures [58, 59]. The main contribution of ASMs introduced since 1989 is in permitting better tailoring of drug therapy in order to improve tolerability and safety, although there can also be benefit from reduced seizure frequency or severity. Some of these medications, in particular, are devoid of enzyme-inducing potential, and are therefore, at lower risk of causing adverse drug interactions [60, 61] or some manifestations of chronic drug toxicity [62]. Additionally, some of the newer ASMs, namely lamotrigine, levetiracetam, and oxcarbazepine, also have a well-documented favorable safety record when used in women of childbearing potential [63, 64]. An increase in their utilization, together with a drastic reduction in the use of valproic acid in women with epilepsy of fertile age, has translated over the years into a decrease in the number of births associated with major congenital malformations [65]. However, not all the newer ASMs are safe with respect to risks related to use during pregnancy. Exposure to topiramate, in particular, has been associated with a comparatively high risk of congenital malformations [66] and of postnatal neurodevelopmental disorders in the offspring [67], and there have also been worrisome teratogenicity signals also for zonisamide [68].

1.3.5 The Present Scenario: Managing Epilepsy with an Armamentarium of More than 30 ASMs

No doubt, opportunities to improve outcomes for people with epilepsy are much greater today than they have ever been in the past [20]. There at least three reasons for this: (i) a large armamentarium of effective ASMs [20, 69]; NICE, 2022; Perucca et al., 2023a); (ii) an improved understanding on how to use these ASMs optimally

[20, 70–72]; and (iii) a greater awareness of the important role of epilepsy surgery [73], dietary treatments [74], and neuromodulation [75] in the management of patients with difficult-to-treat epilepsies.

With respect specifically to the role played by ASMs, the availability of so many medications allow to tailor drug choice to the individual's characteristics and preferences. Improved tailoring of treatment is not limited to monotherapy but extends to rational selection of ASM combinations, whenever use of polytherapy is justified [76, 77]. Of note, selecting the best ASM for a given individual is only one component of optimal management. Other key components include tailoring of drug dosage based on individual needs (which may change over time due to a variety of factors, such as intercurrent illness, pregnancy, or drug interactions), and regular monitoring of clinical response. Measurement of serum ASM concentrations can be valuable in clinical management, especially in selected situations, but it is important that these measurements are done and interpreted appropriately, in line with existing guidelines [78].

The availability of many ASMs is an advantage, but it can also complicate clinical management, particularly for non-specialists who find it challenging to become familiar with the indications, contraindications, adverse effects and optimal mode of use of so many drugs. Therefore, the risk of suboptimal use of the available ASMs is substantial, especially in non-specialist settings. This has stimulated the development of tools to assist physicians in choosing the most appropriate ASM for their patient. One example of such tools is a freely accessible Internet-based algorithm that provides suggestions for personalized ASM selection based on individual characteristics such as seizure type, age, gender, comorbidities, and comedications [79]. The algorithm, which is based on input from a group of experts, can be used only for individuals whose epilepsy started at age 10 years or older, and is more easily applicable to patients with newly diagnosed epilepsy. In an external single-center validation study, use of ASMs preferred by the algorithm was associated with higher seizure freedom rates and lower rates of discontinuation due to adverse effects compared with ASMs rated as less desirable by the algorithm [78]. Treatments preferred by this algorithm have also been found to be generally associated with high retention in a national register database [80]. While this tool may be valuable in some settings, it cannot substitute the physician's competent clinical judgement, because individual patients may have features that are not taken into account by the algorithm. Another approach that is likely to be perfected in the future is the use of computerized models to predict response to individual ASMs based on machine learning-assisted big data analysis [81, 82].The machine learning-based prediction models described to date do not appear to have the desirable level of performance, but artificial intelligence-based approaches, discussed in a separate chapter of this volume, are likely to play an important role as an aid to clinical management in the future.

Although progress is being made, epilepsy in many situations the existing level of evidence to guide ASM selection remains very limited. Most randomized controlled trials have been designed to address regulatory requirements [31] or to support drug promotion in the market place [83], not to address important questions faced by clinicians in everyday clinical management. In particular, physicians need to have evidence from controlled studies on the comparative value of different ASMs in a given population. Clearly, this information cannot be derived solely from studies that simply compare one ASM with placebo, often using rigid dosing protocols [84]. In particular, there is a paucity of comparative studies in populations such as infants and children [85], the elderly [86], patients with generalized epilepsies, and patients with combined focal and generalized epilepsy syndromes [84, 87]. Admittedly, in recent years the pharmaceutical interest has shown an increasing interest in developing ASMs for rare epilepsies. As shown in Table 1.3, four of five ASMs introduced in the market since 2017 are drugs that target seizures associated with orphan indications, namely tuberous sclerosis complex (everolimus, cannabidiol), Lennox-Gastaut syndrome (cannabidiol, fenfluramine), Dravet syndrome (cannabidiol, fenfluramine) and CDKL5 deficiency disorder (ganaxolone). For many ultra-rare epilepsies, precision treatments are currently being identified and investigated. These may include not only ASMs, but also dietary treatments and medications approved for other diseases and repurposed for the management of specific epilepsy syndromes [59, 88].

Despite many advances, the pharmacological treatment of epilepsy still faces many unmet needs. In particular, we need (i) better tools to predict drug response; (ii) more effective and better tolerated drugs to achieve freedom from seizures in patients resistant to currently available ASMs; and (iii) drugs that not only suppress the seizures, but also modify favorably the course of the disease (disease modifying epilepsy drugs), and possibly prevent the development of epilepsy (antiepileptogenic drugs). The next section will briefly discuss approached by which these unmet needs could be fulfilled in the future. Although the discussion below only focuses on pharmacological treatments, major advances are also expected to take place in other therapeutic areas, including surgical therapies and neuromodulation-based therapies.

1.3.6 Where Are We Going? A Glimpse into the Future of Drug Treatments for Seizures and Epilepsy

As discussed in the previous section, at the present time ASMs are generally prescribed by a trial-and-error approach which takes into consideration a variety of individual factors, such as seizure types, epilepsy syndrome, age, gender, comorbidities, comedications, and history of response to other drugs. These factors do provide an estimate of the probability of achieving seizure control with the least possible risk of adverse effects with a given ASM [20, 70–72]. However, it would be desirable to have tools that predict with a higher level of confidence the response to specific ASMs, or combinations of ASMs. If such a tool were available, we would be able to prescribe immediately the safest and most efficacious treatment for that individual. As mentioned above, efforts are ongoing to use artificial intelligence to identify individualized predictors of response, based on a large number of clinical variables through a machine learning approach [81, 82]. It is reasonable to expect that future tools based on big data analysis will be strengthened by inclusion of genomic, neuroimaging, electrophysiological, and neurochemical data, and other biomarkers. As an extension of these research efforts, reliable artificial intelligence-based tools could also be developed to predict the risk of seizure recurrence after a first seizure (in order to aid in the decision on whether to start or to defer treatment) or the risk of seizure recurrence after ASM discontinuation in individuals who experienced prolonged seizure freedom and are being considered for possible ASM withdrawal. It might also be possible in the future to develop predictive tools, possibly linked to innovative devices for continuous monitoring of EEG activity, to identify periods of increased seizure susceptibility, which could be managed by appropriate adjustment of antiseizure therapies before seizures occur, or become exacerbated. Similar devices might also be developed to predict the occurrence of individual seizures with sufficient anticipation to permit 'on demand' administration of a rapidly acting ASM in order to prevent or abort the seizure [89, 90].

Accurate predicting tools have the potential to improve the utilization of existing ASMs, but they will not solve the problem of drug-resistant epilepsy. The need for safer and more effective treatments is obvious, and intensive research efforts are ongoing to discover/develop such treatments, which could consist of novel molecules, repurposed drugs currently used for other indications, and non-pharmacological therapies [86]. Research is also ongoing on novel delivery systems for existing ASMs, including direct intracerebroventricular (i.c.v.) infusions of ASMs to maximize their efficacy and limit peripheral adverse effects [91]. Such i.c.v. delivery systems could also permit the utilization of molecules that do not penetrate readily the blood-brain barrier [91]. Rational development of novel and better ASMs will require deeper understanding of mechanisms of epileptogenesis and ictogenesis. For some epilepsies, considerable progress has been made in characterizing not only the underlying cause, but also the functional defects and pathogenic mechanisms involved. This is paving the way to novel paradigms in epilepsy drug discovery that are directed at targeting not the symptoms (seizures), but the underlying cause of the disease. Examples of conditions for which precision treatments are being developed include genetic epilepsies [88, 92], autoimmune seizure disorders [93], and epilepsies in which brain inflammation plays a major role [94–96]. The potential advantage of etiology-targeted therapies is the feasibility of treating/preventing with a single medication (or an appropriate combination of medications) not only the seizures, but also associated comorbidities, particularly if such treatments are started early in the course of the disease. Some highly innovative therapies already in clinical development include gene therapies, antisense oligonucleotides, and direct transplantation of inhibitory interneurons into the epileptogenic brain tissue [20, 86]. Other lines of research that could lead to improved treatments focus on the characterization of the microbiota–gut–brain axis in epilepsy [97, 98]. Many of these investigations and, ultimately, their clinical applications are likely to be guided by biomarkers that could assist in identifying the mechanisms responsible for epilepsy, and their responsiveness to specific treatments, in a given individual. One example of such a biomarker that is receiving attention is High Mobility Group Box 1 (HMGB1), a non-histone DNA-binding protein that is being investigated as a mechanistic biomarker for epilepsy and as a predictor of drug resistance [99, 100].

Treatments that are effective in preventing epilepsy in high-risk individuals, or modify the course of epilepsy (and possibly even cure epilepsy) have been the Holy Grail of epileptology for many years. However, thanks to improved understanding of the mechanisms of epileptogenesis, such treatments are likely to become available in the future, and to vary according to the etiology of epilepsy and underlying mechanisms [20, 26]. Again, development of these treatments will be conditional on the availability of biomarkers to identify as early as possible those individuals who are going to develop epilepsy due to the expression of pathogenic gene variants [92] or after epileptogenic insults such a traumatic brain injury or stroke [101–104]. Biomarkers could also be used to monitor response to treatment. An example of a treatment that in a recent study was suggested to be disease-modifying is provided by the use of vigabatrin before the onset of clinical or electrographic seizures in infants with tuberous sclerosis complex [105]. In that study, appearance of epileptogenic EEG abnormalities was the biomarker that permitted identification of infants at risks, and the initiation of treatment before epilepsy could develop. As it is evident from the considerations above, the identification and use of appropriate biomarkers (or combination of biomarkers) is likely to represent a common denominator to many strategies under investigation aimed at improving clinical outcomes and at discovering novel, safe and effective treatments for seizures and epilepsy,

Although much remains to be done, we have gone a long way since the discovery of bromide's effectiveness in treating epileptic seizures. Thanks to improved knowledge of the causes and mechanisms of epilepsy, there are reasons to expect that major therapeutic breakthroughs will occur in the near future. These breakthroughs will probably generate new challenges. Because of the heterogeneity of the epilepsies, different precision treatments will need to be developed for many rare forms of epilepsy, which requires continuous investment of resources and application of economic models to ensure return on investment. To date, novel medicines for rare diseases have typically been made available at very high, often outrageous prices [106] that only people, or a fraction of people, living in high-income countries are able to afford [107–109]. In the long run, current models for the development and marketing of treatments for rare diseases are not going to be economically and ethically sustainable. New models and new paradigms will need to be implemented to ensure that life-changing medicines for people with epilepsy are not only made available, but also made accessible and affordable everywhere in the world.

1.4 Research on Animal Models of Epilepsy

Epilepsy, characterized by recurrent seizures resulting from highly synchronized abnormal neuronal discharges, is a spontaneous brain dysfunction [2]. The exploration of the underlying mechanisms and abnormal discharge patterns linked to seizures has emerged as a central focus in epilepsy research, with the use of animal models playing a pivotal role. Behavioral assessments and the evaluation of pathophysiological phenotypes in these models contribute to the testing of new antiepileptic drugs, gauging the effectiveness of novel compounds, and discerning molecular and network mechanisms for the treatment of epilepsy and its complications.

1.4.1 An Animal Model of Epilepsy

For an animal model of epilepsy to be considered valid, it must mimic symptoms and phenotypes of human seizures, such as convulsive seizures and abnormal discharges, which is referred to as face validity [110, 111]. Moreover, the model should extend beyond face validity by eliciting molecular, cellular, and connectivity changes specific to distinct types of epilepsy, thereby mirroring the pathogenic mechanisms observed in human diseases—termed construct validity [110, 111]. As the efficacy of targeted treatments for epilepsy faces growing limitations, it is imperative for epilepsy animal models employed in the screening of potential antiepileptic drugs to faithfully reproduce treatment responses observed in clinical settings, known as predictive validity [111]. Currently, no epilepsy animal model perfectly fulfills all three validity criteria.

Epilepsy animal models are developed through the induction or genetic predisposition of specific species to epilepsy [111]. Almost all species with a central nervous system have the potential to develop epilepsy, thereby expanding the pool of species available for epilepsy models [111, 112]. Spontaneous epileptic seizures in many species occur sporadically, making them often unsuitable for experimentation [113]. Ideally, the species chosen for an epilepsy model should readily exhibit spontaneous seizures or be easily induced under controlled experimental conditions. Furthermore, the nervous system of the selected species should closely approximate that of humans in terms of anatomy, physiology, or biochemistry. In the early stages of epilepsy research, emphasis was placed on species such as cats, dogs, and nonhuman primates, which were prioritized for studying experimentally induced seizures [111–113]. Nonhuman primates, including monkeys and baboons, possess brain structures and genomes more akin to those of humans, rendering them invaluable for elucidating neuroanatomical features and genetic foundations [111].

Considering the practical aspects of experimentation, the selection of species for creating epilepsy models should prioritize the ease of breeding, raising, observation, and specimen collection. Rodents, particularly Norway rats (*Rattus norvegicus*) and mice (*Mus musculus*), have progressively become more prominent in epilepsy models, likely owing to their small size, docility, and convenience due to controlled breeding environments [111]. Currently, rodents are the primary species used for constructing epilepsy models [112]. Other species, including fruit flies, zebrafish, birds, sea lions, baboons, chickens, rabbits, hamsters, and pigs, also play roles in epilepsy research [32, 111, 113].

The development of epilepsy animal models has evolved from simple acute seizure models to complex chronic seizure models, progressing from stimulus-induced seizures to spontaneous seizures, closely resembling human epilepsy phenotypes. Epilepsy animal models can be classified based on the causes of seizures into genetic models and acquired epilepsy models (Table 1.4). Genetic models stem from specific genetic changes leading to seizures, while acquired models are induced in healthy animals through the application of specific chemicals, electrical stimulation, or conditions such as trauma, stroke, and infection.

1.4.2 Acute Epilepsy Models

Seizures can be observed following acute injury or genetic manipulation in almost all animals with a nervous system, rendering acute epilepsy models widely applicable. David Ferrier [114], an epilepsy research pioneer in the 1870s, conducted groundbreaking work by directly stimulating the cortices of rabbits, guinea pigs, cats, and dogs, revealing the occurrence of acute tonic–clonic seizure events similar to those seen in human epilepsy. Commonly employed models for screening antiseizure drugs in acute settings include the maximal electroshock seizure (MES) model, the 6 Hz psychomotor seizure model, the acute pentylenetetrazol-induced seizure model, and the local penicillin model.

1.4.2.1 Maximal Electroshock Seizure Model

In 1937, Merritt and Putnam [115] induced seizures in cats using electrical stimulation, revealing the anticonvulsant effects of phenytoin. Swinyard [116] subsequently developed the standardized MES model for rodents, which mimics tonic–clonic seizures in

Table 1.4 Animal models of epilepsy and seizures

Genetic animal models	Acquired animal models
Rodent animal models	Acute seizures
Absence seizure models.	Electrically induced seizures.
Reflex seizure models.	Chemically induced seizures.
Non-rodent animal models	Chronic seizures
Papio papio models.	Electrical kindling models.
Zebrafish models.	Chemical kindling models.
	Optogenetic kindling models.
	Post-status epilepticus models
	Trauma, stroke, infection-induced models

humans, and used this model for drug screening. The MES procedure involves placing electrodes near the eyes or ears of the animal and applying a strong current to induce brief electrical stimulation through the cornea or ears to the brainstem structures, resulting in generalized tonic–clonic seizures in the hind limbs (the endpoint of the test) [117, 118]. The stimulation parameters are generally 50 mA for mice and 150 mA for rats, with corneal electrodes at 60 Hz and a stimulation time of 0.2 seconds [117].

1.4.2.2 6 Hz Psychomotor Seizure Model

The 6 Hz psychomotor seizure model, developed in 1951 by Toman [119], involves prolonged (3 or 4 s) low-frequency (6 Hz) electrical stimulation of the corneas of mice, which induces psychomotor seizures with minimal clonic periods, followed by stereotypical spontaneous behavior, mimicking that of focal epileptic seizures [111]. This model exhibits resistance to drugs such as phenytoin [118]. However, recent experiments suggest that the drug resistance of the 6 Hz psychomotor seizure model should be considered in terms of animal strains and experimental conditions, with CF-1 and B6 mice showing phenytoin resistance, while NMRI mice exhibit a therapeutic response [111].

1.4.2.3 Acute Pentylenetetrazol-Induced Seizure Model

The acute pentylenetetrazol (PTZ)-induced seizure model is utilized to mimic clonic seizures. PTZ, a GABA-A receptor antagonist, reduces the function of inhibitory synapses, increasing neuronal excitability, and triggering generalized seizures [120, 121]. In various animal species, including mice, rats, cats, and primates, PTZ is administered through injection (subcutaneous, intravenous, or intraperitoneal) [122]. Common doses for inducing seizures in mice include 85 mg/kg subcutaneously, 50 mg/kg intravenously, and 50–75 mg/kg intraperitoneally. In the acute PTZ model for rats, observable effects include involuntary movements of the head, forelimbs, or hindlimbs, progressing to falling, clonic–tonic seizures, and complete limb extension, with hindlimb extension as an observation endpoint [112]. Various antiseizure drugs targeting ion channels or receptors, such as trimethadione and ethosuximide [111, 117], have been identified using the acute PTZ model. Notably, the MES model is considered pharmacologically independent, while the acute PTZ model may interact with the tested antiseizure drugs [32, 112].

1.4.2.4 Local Penicillin Model

In 1945, penicillin, initially employed in neurosurgical procedures to prevent postoperative infection, was serendipitously discovered to possess a local proconvulsant effect [123]. Placing cotton balls soaked in 1.7–3.4 mM penicillin on the exposed cortices of rats or cats, followed by the local placement of electrodes, enabled the recording of recurrent interictal spike waves within minutes, resembling those observed in human cortical electroencephalogram recordings [113, 124]. During spike activity, neurons in the focal area tend to synchronize discharges [113]. In the macaque hippocampus, the injection of penicillin established a temporal lobe epilepsy model characterized by behaviors such as motionless staring, head tilting, oral chewing, and lip-smacking [125]. Pathological features, including neuronal loss, glial cell proliferation, and hippocampal sclerosis, were detected [125] Although the local penicillin model is instrumental for studying the neural basis and spread of focal seizure activities, its initiation from known epileptic foci limits its ability to fully replicate the complex mechanisms of human epilepsy [113].

Other compounds used for chemically induced acute seizure models include bicuculline, which induces clonic seizures in mice at a subcutaneous injection dose of 2.7 mg/kg [126, 127]; picrotoxin, which induces seizures at an intraperitoneal injection dose of 7.5 mg/kg [128]; strychnine, which induces seizures at an intraperitoneal injection dose of 2.5 mg/kg; and isoniazid, which induces seizures at an intraperitoneal injection dose of 250 mg/kg [126, 129].

1.4.3 Chronic Epilepsy Models

Acute seizure models are designed to characterize acute seizure events but are lacking in representation of the chronic phenotype of spontaneous recurrent seizures. These models also lack the pathophysiological changes associated with chronic epileptic seizures, such as neuroinflammation and protein expression changes [130]. Consequently, as a chronic epilepsy model, the kindling model has emerged to simulate the complexity of human focal seizures and secondary generalized seizures [131]. Kindling refers to the plasticity phenomenon induced by epileptic seizures [131]. When continuous low-dose electrical or chemical stimulation is applied to specific regions, such as the amygdala or hippocampus, the threshold for epileptic seizures decreases, and seizure susceptibility gradually increases, leading to a kindling response [131]. The kindling model can be categorized into one of three types based on the nature of stimulation: the electrical kindling model, the chemical kindling model, and the optogenetic kindling model.

1.4.3.1 Electrical Stimulation Kindling Model

Electrical stimulation kindling typically involves the implantation of electrodes in specific brain regions of the animal, administering subthreshold stimuli repetitively and intermittently to achieve kindling effects [111, 131–133]. Commonly targeted brain areas for kindling include the amygdala, hippocampus, and perirhinal cortex [111, 131–133]. Even local electrical stimulation of the cornea has been shown to induce kindling [130]. In rats, commonly used stimulation methods include 60 Hz sine-wave or biphasic pulses [132]. The kindling rate and seizure patterns exhibit variation based on strain and age [134]. Racine [135] classified kindling-induced seizures into five stages: (1) mouth and facial movements, (2) head nodding, (3) forelimb clonus, (4) standing, and (5) standing and falling, representing the transition from focal seizures to secondary generalized seizures [3].

The electrical stimulation kindling model allows specific exploration of brain regions to understand their roles in the onset and occurrence of epilepsy. Additionally, it serves as a valuable tool for screening anti-seizure drugs. This kindling process induces progressive changes in the hippocampal neural circuitry [111]. Notably, Goddard et al. [131, 136] reported that kindling-induced epileptic plasticity is similar to learning, implying that healthy brains learn pathological activity patterns during the kindling process.

1.4.3.2 Kindling Model

Both chemical and electrical stimulation can induce a decrease in the seizure threshold in mice, known as the kindling phenomenon [132, 137]. Compared to electrical stimulation, chemical kindling is more straightforward, requires no brain surgery or electrode implantation and is less time-consuming [137]. As mentioned earlier, a single high-dose (suprathreshold dose) injection of PTZ in rodents can induce acute seizures, while multiple low-dose (subthreshold dose) injections can decrease the seizure threshold [138]. Karler et al. [137] reported the kindling response induced by chronic PTZ injections in CF-1 mice. In the PTZ-induced kindling model, a single low-dose injection of PTZ initiated mild epileptic seizures without convulsions [139, 140]. With an increasing number of PTZ injections, the latency period for epileptic seizures decreases, the severity increases, and ultimately, a single low-dose injection can trigger severe tonic–clonic seizures [139, 140]. The commonly used intraperitoneal injection dose for PTZ kindling in mice is 35 mg/kg, and PTZ is administered daily or every other day, with consecutive injections until the manifestation of tonic–clonic seizures [139, 140].

1.4.3.3 Optogenetic Kindling Model

Classic epilepsy models may cause tissue damage and lack the ability to discriminate between neuronal loss and epileptogenesis mechanisms [141, 142]. Moreover, they can only be localized to specific brain areas and cannot activate or parse specific cell populations [141, 142]. The optogenetic kindling model seamlessly integrates the technical advantages of optogenetics with classic kindling practices. By manipulating specific neuronal groups using light-sensitive proteins, such as Channelrhodopsin-2 (ChR2), Halorhodopsin (NpHR), and Archaerhodopsin-3 (Arch) [142], a causal relationship between neuronal groups and epilepsy can be established. ChR2 induces depolarization through cation influx upon exposure to blue light, leading to neuronal activation. NpHR and Arch inhibit neuronal activity by pumping chloride ions into and protons out of the neurons, respectively [143, 144]. Cela et al. [141] expressed ChR2 in the mouse neocortex to develop an optogenetic kindling model. This model reproduces hallmark features of the classic electrical stimulation kindling model, such as gradual increases in epileptic electroencephalogram (EEG) and seizure severity over time and long-term susceptibility to seizures. Unlike the classic model, the optogenetic kindling model circumvents significant brain damage and glial reactions [141].

1.4.4 Poststatus Epilepticus Models

Kindling models typically fail to induce chronic spontaneous seizures in animals. Currently, epilepsy is generally speculated to encompass three stages: (1) initial triggering events, (2) a latent period, and (3) chronic spontaneous seizures (Table 1.5) [145–149].

In the poststatus epilepticus model, status epilepticus (SE) is typically induced by the injection of kainic acid (KA) or pilocarpine, resulting in the development of chronic spontaneous recurrent seizures (SRSs) after an approximately one-month latent period [151–153]. Kainic acid, which was isolated and extracted in 1953 from the red alga Digenea simplex [154], stimulates ionotropic KA receptors, leading to intense neuronal depolarization and eventual neuronal death. The hippocampal damage caused by KA replicates the typical histopathological changes observed in temporal lobe epilepsy (TLE) patients [152]. Administration methods for kainic acid include systemic, intrahippocampal, or intra-amygdalar delivery, with intra-amygdalar administration resulting in a lower survival rate. In rats, stereotaxic injection of kainic acid into the hippocampus induces SE at doses of 0.4–2.0 μg, while systemic administration requires a high single injection dose of 6–15 mg/kg or multiple injections with a low dose of 5 mg/kg [152, 155].

The pilocarpine model also induces hippocampal damage and is used for studying TLE [156]. Pilocarpine acts as an agonist for muscarinic acetylcholine receptors, with the M1 muscarinic acetylcholine receptor speculated to play a role in initiating epileptic seizures [156, 157]. The pilocarpine model induces

Table 1.5 Three hypothesized stages of epileptogenesis

Stage of epileptogenesis	Definitions	Characterizations
Initial precipitating injury or epileptogenic event	An acute insult to the brain that triggers the epileptogenic process [146, 149]	The initial precipitating injury or epileptogenic event includes head trauma, infection, stroke, and prolonged febrile seizures [146]
Latent period	A latent period between the initial injury and the emergence of the first spontaneous seizure [146, 147]	The latent period involves wide cellular and molecular changes, from gene transcription to patterns of neuronal connectivity, which influence the excitability of the neuronal network [146–148, 150]. This period usually lasts for weeks, months or even years [145, 147]
Chronic epilepsy	A period characterized by the emergence of spontaneous recurrent seizures [147, 149]	The cellular and molecular changes have produced reorganized synaptic circuitry, mossy fiber sprouting, and a hyperexcitable state [145]

injuries in the dentate gyrus, thalamus, and amygdala and degeneration of CA1 and CA3 hippocampal neurons, with seizures originating in the hippocampus and spreading to the amygdala and neocortex [112]. The intraperitoneal injection dose for inducing seizures with pilocarpine is 300–400 mg/kg [156], and coadministration of lithium (3 mEq/kg) 24 hours before pilocarpine injection significantly reduces the required pilocarpine dose for inducing seizures to 30 mg/kg [156].

In addition to chemical stimulation, continuous electrical stimulation of the hippocampus or amygdala can also induce SE, leading to spontaneous recurrent seizures after a seizure-free latent period [32, 158]. Compared to chemically induced poststatus epilepticus models, electrical stimulation models offer advantages in testing antiepileptic drugs because they circumvent potential interactions between proconvulsant chemicals and test compounds [158].

1.4.5 Genetic Models

Genetics plays a crucial role in human epilepsy, with the identification of numerous epilepsy-related genes through comprehensive whole-genome association studies and sequencing [159, 160]. Genetic models involving the introduction of gene mutations leading to seizures in animals offer valuable insights into the mechanisms of genetic epilepsy. This, in turn, facilitates the development of antiepileptic therapies and contributes to the progress of precision medicine. Rodents, particularly mice and rats, are species prevalently employed in genetic epilepsy research [110].

1.4.5.1 Rodent Animal Models

Absence Seizure Models

Absence seizures are a representative subtype of inherited generalized epilepsy [159]. Given their hereditary and spontaneous characteristics, genetic models more closely parallel absence epilepsy than experimentally induced seizure models [111]. The tottering (tg) mutant mouse, which was initially utilized for studying hereditary ataxia, has spontaneous epileptic seizures characterized by synchronous burst spike-wave discharges (SWDs) in cortical electroencephalogram recordings concomitant with absence seizures and focal motor seizures [161]. The tottering mouse serves as a valuable animal model due to its analogous electrographic patterns, behavioral manifestations, and pharmacological response to human absence epilepsy [162]. These strains harbor a mutation in the Cacna1a gene, which encodes the CaV2.1 channel α subunit, resulting in reduced CaV2.1 calcium current density [163]. The commonly used Tottering-6j mouse model frequently exhibits absence-like epileptic seizures, with slow-wave discharges in the bilateral cortex and abrupt cessation of behavior and gaze fixation, accompanied by severe ataxia, rendering this model suitable for investigating the pathogenic mechanisms of CaV2.1 channel-related epilepsy and drug screening [164].

In 1982, Vergnes and collaborators [165] introduced the Genetic Absence Epileptic Rats of Strasbourg (GAERs). These rats exhibited spontaneous absence seizures characterized by cortical EEG spike-wave discharges at 6–7 Hz coupled with immobility. Sodium valproate, diazepam, and trimethadione have proven effective in suppressing the spontaneous seizures of this model [166]. Additionally, the GAERs model also exhibits anxiety-like behavior, social impairment, diminished learning capabilities, and heightened contextual and conditioned fear responses, along with deficits in cross-modal recognition memory and visual attention functions [167].

Similarly, Wistar Albino Glaxo strain inbred Rijswijk (WAG/Rij) rats display spontaneous absence seizures, featuring characteristics such as rapid breathing, unexpected eye blinking, whisker twitching, and facial muscle spasms [168]. The spike-wave discharges in WAG/Rij rats can be inhibited by ethosuximide, levetiracetam, and valproic acid. Due to their behavioral, electroencephalographic, and genetic similarities to humans, the WAG/Rij rat model has been widely applied in the study of genetic absence epilepsy, particularly in the context of childhood absence epilepsy [169].

Reflex Seizure Models

Numerous animal models and certain human epilepsies can be experimentally induced by controlled stimuli, referred to as reflex epilepsy [170]. According to Irmen et al. [171], reflex seizures are part of a conceptual continuum with spontaneous seizures. The primary triggers for human reflex epilepsy are visual stimuli, whereas in most rodents, reflex seizures are elicited by auditory stimuli [172]. Consequently, audiogenic seizure (AGS) models have been developed in rodents, notably in Dilute Brown non-Agouti (DBA/2) mice and genetically epilepsy-prone rats (GEPRs).

DBA/2 mice exhibit genetic susceptibility to generalized AGS, increased sensitivity to convulsive seizures, and increased responsiveness to electrically and chemically induced seizures, making them valuable for screening drugs targeting generalized seizures [111]. The sensitivity of DBA/2 mice to audiogenic seizures is greatest in the early life stages (12–17 days of age), peaking between 19 and 24 days of age and gradually decreasing thereafter [172]. By adulthood (>80 days old), they become completely resistant to auditory stimulation [172].

There are two subtypes of GEPRs: GEPR-3 s and GEPR-9 s. In GEPR-3 s, the endpoint of seizures is generalized clonus involving all four limbs, whereas in GEPR-9 s, seizures culminate in tonic hindlimb extension [111]. These heritable reflex models serve as a fundamental foundation for delving into the intricate mechanisms associated with neuronal hyperexcitability in epilepsy.

1.4.5.2 Nonrodent Animal Models

In addition to rodents, earlier research utilized diverse species, such as cats, dogs, and nonhuman primates, as epilepsy animal models [110]. Recent studies have broadened this scope, incorporating species such as fruit flies, zebrafish, birds, sea lions, and baboons [32, 110].

Baboon Photosensitive Epilepsy Model

Killam et al. [173, 174] reported photomyoclonic syndrome in baboons (Papio papio). In the Casamance region of Senegal, a substantial proportion (60% to 80%) of adolescent baboons displayed myoclonic responses to intermittent photic stimulation (25 flashes/second), starting with rapid bilateral eyelid clonus, expanding to facial and neck twitching, followed by limb tonic extension, and potentially evolving into generalized clonus [175]. EEG recordings consistently revealed paroxysmal discharges characterized by multiple spikes or spike-wave patterns, accompanying photosensitive myoclonic seizures [176]. The baboon model of photosensitive epilepsy serves as a valuable tool for replicating human photosensitive myoclonus. Notably, myoclonic responses can be effectively suppressed by primidone, phenobarbital, and benzodiazepine drugs, whereas phenytoin and carbamazepine exhibit limited efficacy [175].

Zebrafish Epilepsy Model

The zebrafish, a straightforward vertebrate model organism, presents notable advantages in replicating genetic forms of epilepsy due to its simplified breeding and maintenance requirements, along with a greater reproductive capacity in comparison to rodent models [110, 177]. The monitoring of zebrafish seizure locomotor activity requires automated behavioral tracking systems, and the characterization of brain activity is accomplished by immobilizing zebrafish in low-melting point agarose and implanting microelectrodes into the optic tectum or forebrain for high-throughput local field potential (LFP) recordings [178–180]. Therefore, the zebrafish epilepsy model is ideal for high-throughput antiseizure drug screening [179, 180]. Baraban and colleagues [181] utilized zebrafish with mutations in the voltage-gated sodium channel Scn1a gene (scn1Lab mutant zebrafish) as a model for Dravet syndrome to screen the effects of stiripentol, an inhibitor of zebrafish seizures [181]. Their findings revealed the action of stiripentol on serotonin receptors, leading to the subsequent screening of topiramate and clonazepam, which target the serotonin signaling pathway and may hold potential for clinical treatment in patients with refractory Dravet syndrome [178]. In addition to scn1Lab mutant zebrafish, diverse mutant zebrafish strains targeting other epilepsy-related genes have been generated. Examples include UBE3A-mutant zebrafish associated with Angelman syndrome, OCRL1-deficient zebrafish linked to Lowe syndrome, UGP2-mutant zebrafish associated with epileptic encephalopathy, and GABRG2-knockout zebrafish associated with light-induced reflex seizures [182–185].

1.4.6 *Trauma, Stroke, and Infection Models*

The most common causes of acquired epilepsy in adults include traumatic brain injury, stroke, and central nervous system infections [32]. These etiologies differ, impacting patient responsiveness to antiepileptic drugs in clinical treatment [32]. Therefore, it is necessary to develop epilepsy animal models that replicate distinct causes [32].

1.4.6.1 Posttraumatic Epilepsy Models

Traumatic brain injury (TBI) is a prevalent cause of refractory epilepsy in temporal lobe epilepsy patients [186]. Common posttraumatic epilepsy (PTE) models include the fluid percussion injury (FPI) model, the controlled cortical impact (CCI) model, and the impact-acceleration model. In comparison to experimentally induced seizure models, posttraumatic epilepsy models exhibit broader brain injuries, accompanied by cognitive and neuropsychiatric symptoms [186, 187].

Fluid Percussion Injury Model

The fluid percussion injury model induces TBI by exposing the intact dura mater to fluid pressure pulses through craniotomy, resulting in neuronal damage and epilepsy [188]. The FPI model primarily induces secondary generalized seizures rather than partial seizures [189]. D'Ambrosio et al. [190] described chronic spontaneous recurrent seizures in rats following fluid percussion-induced traumatic brain injury. The brain damage caused by fluid percussion injury is similar to that caused by temporal lobe epilepsy, including neuronal loss in the hippocampus and mossy fiber sprouting [20, 158, 191]. However, the FPI model has limitations, including a low frequency of spontaneous seizures, a need for prolonged EEG monitoring for spontaneous seizure events, and an apparent lack of predictive validity [189, 192].

Controlled Cortical Impact Model

In 1988, Lighthall and colleagues [193] described controlled cortical impact injury using ferrets as test animals. In the 1990s, the CCI model was adapted for use in various animals, including rats, mice, and primates [189]. The CCI model induces varying degrees of brain injury by compressing the exposed brain using pneumatic or electromagnetic impactors, mimicking various injuries associated with traumatic brain injury, such as cortical tissue loss, acute subdural hematoma, axonal injury, concussion, and blood–brain barrier dysfunction [192]. In addition to seizures, CCI model rats also exhibit cognitive and motor impairments, with motor dysfunction typically resolving within a few months post-CCI induction, while cognitive deficits may persist for an extended period, correlating with brain atrophy and a gradual reduction in cerebral blood flow [112]. Similar to the FPI model, the CCI model has a low frequency of spontaneous seizures [189], but it can exhibit unprovoked seizures and hippocampal pathological changes early after trauma (CCI: 10 weeks postinjury; FPI: several months) [192].

Impact Acceleration Model

The impact acceleration model represents a diffuse traumatic brain injury model [189]. Animals are placed in a stereotactic frame, and a specific weight is dropped from a designated height onto the exposed bare dura mater, also known as the weight-drop model [112, 189]. The severity of brain injury induced by this model can be controlled by adjusting the weight and height of the fall [194]. Despite the simplicity and cost-effectiveness of the impact acceleration model, its shortcomings are conspicuous, including high mortality rates, low reproducibility, and the incapacity to develop spontaneous seizures [189, 192, 194].

1.4.6.2 Poststroke Epilepsy Models

Poststroke epilepsy is a common clinical complication following stroke. Widely used models for poststroke epilepsy include the middle cerebral artery occlusion (MCAO) model and the photothrombotic model [195]. The MCAO model appears to primarily simulate early-stage seizures, with only 1 out of 26 injured rats developing late-stage spontaneous seizures [195]. The photothrombotic model, which is induced by intravenous injection of Rose Bengal dye to induce cortical photothrombosis, results in approximately half of the rats experiencing seizures after 1–2 months [195]. Posttraumatic epilepsy models and poststroke epilepsy models are less commonly used in preclinical pharmacological research, as only 20–50% of the model animals develop seizures, rendering drug screening challenging [32, 195].

1.4.6.3 Postinfection Epilepsy Models

The Theiler's murine encephalomyelitis virus (TMEV) model involves infecting C57BL/6 mice with TMEV, which induces seizures through viral encephalitis [32, 196]. The seizures manifest in two stages: frequent acute seizures during the early infection phase and less frequent late-stage seizures several months after brain inflammation, leading to long-term alterations in seizure susceptibility [32, 196]. The TMEV model alters long-term susceptibility to seizures [196]. This model responds to anti-inflammatory compounds such as minocycline and certain traditional antiseizure medications (e.g., phenytoin and gabapentin), providing a platform to evaluate new compounds for their anti-inflammatory, antiseizure, or combined mechanisms [196]. Another model in which acute seizures are induced through infection utilizes a mature cerebral malaria mouse model in which infected red blood cells are injected intraperitoneally to induce experimental cerebral malaria [186, 197]. Due to the mice succumbing or dying within 1–2 weeks after infection, only early-stage seizures can be analyzed [186, 197]. Additionally, infection with tetanus toxin in a rat motor cortex injection model can lead to long-term seizures characterized by interrupted motor activity, rhythmic facial twitches, and sudden cessation of movement [198]. Limitations of the tetanus toxin model include the absence of typical hippocampal sclerosis and neuronal loss, as well as the limited occurrence of spontaneous seizures [198].

To meet the demands of high-throughput research, epilepsy models have progressively expanded from intact animals to in vitro organotypic preparations, referred to as in vitro models. These models utilize ex vivo brain tissue slices, primary neuronal cultures, human embryonic stem cells (hESCs), or induced pluripotent stem cell (iPSC)-derived neurons or organoids and are increasingly employed for epilepsy modeling and drug screening purposes [199, 200]. iPSC-induced neuronal models are often coupled with multiple electrode array (MEA) technology to assess spontaneous discharge activity, epileptiform burst discharge, and other epilepsy-like phenotypes, enabling high-throughput testing of drug responses [200].

From early acute seizure models to chronic kindling models and further to post-status epilepticus models, genetic models, and trauma-induced models, animal models have replicated distinctive features of epilepsy. However, to date, there is no model that perfectly meets the criteria of face validity, construct validity, and predictive validity. Due to the complexity of epilepsy, the choice of animal model can be tailored based on specific practical needs. With the continuous advancement of new technologies, the future of epilepsy animal models remains promising from face validity to construct validity and potentially expanding to predictive validity. This progression aims to provide valuable insights into the mechanisms underlying epilepsy and the development of new therapies, ultimately enhancing the quality of life for individuals with epilepsy.

1.5 Antiseizure Medication Mechanisms of Action

Epilepsy is one of the most common and disabling chronic neurological disorders. There are 50 to 70 million people with epilepsy worldwide, and the disease traverses the entire lifespan [201]. Antiseizure medications (ASMs) are currently the main treatment modality. They act on various mechanisms and molecular targets involved in neuronal excitability to suppress abnormal hyperexcitability and hypersynchrony in brain circuits, thereby controlling epileptic seizures. In the past century, the discovery of ASMs has progressed from early serendipitous findings to the application of animal model screening and, currently, to rational development [201]. Most of the medications currently used to treat epilepsy control symptoms (seizures), but they have no known effect on the disease processes of patients at risk of developing epilepsy or patients with epilepsy. Therefore, in recent years, we have used the term "antiseizure medications" (ASMs) to replace antiepileptic drugs [202, 203]. To date, there are more than 30 different antiseizure medications available for clinical selection [204]. With the increasing number of antiepileptic drugs, it is essential to understand their mechanisms of action and pharmacokinetics and how they interact with one another for precise individualized drug treatment of epilepsy. This section summarizes the mechanisms of antiseizure medications that have been applied in clinical practice and briefly discusses the interactions between various drugs. Finally, we will briefly outline the future development directions of antiepileptic drugs. Epileptic activity manifests as intermittent and excessive excitation of cortical networks, limbic system networks or more diffuse networks. Existing antiseizure medications have been clearly classified into four major mechanisms: 1) regulation of voltage-gated ion channels, 2) attenuation of glutamate-mediated excitatory neurotransmission, 3) modulation of neurotransmitter release by presynaptic action, and 4) enhancement of γ-aminobutyric acid (GABA)-mediated inhibitory neuronal function. In this chapter, we will discuss the antiseizure medications that have been used clinically, based on the above mechanisms.

1.5.1 Voltage-Gated Ion Channel Modulation Mechanism

1.5.1.1 Blocking Voltage-Gated Sodium Channels

Voltage-gated sodium channels (VGSCs) are transmembrane proteins that can be activated to form ion channels when the nearby membrane potential changes. They are essential for generation and conduction of action potential and expressed throughout the entire neuronal membrane, including that of dendrites and axons [205]. VGSCs exist in one of three basic conformational states: (1) at hyperpolarized potentials, the channel is usually in a resting, closed state; (2) when depolarized, the channel transitions to an open state, allowing sodium ions to permeate; and (3) after depolarization, the channel enters a closed, nonconductive inactivated state [206]. In a single round of depolarization, the channel cycles through these states—from rest to open, from open to inactivated, and from inactivated to rest. When the neuron is at rest or inactivated, sodium ions cannot pass through the channel. Sodium ion channels can be subdivided into fast inactivation channels and slow inactivation channels [207].

Some antiseizure medications are sodium channel inhibitors. They bind to an inactivated voltage-gated channel after neuronal depolarization and change its permeability to sodium ions, thereby reducing the inward flow of sodium ions. This leads to an increase in the inactivation (or refractory) period of frequently firing neurons [208]. The main mechanism of action for drugs such as phenytoin, carbamazepine, oxcarbazepine, lamotrigine, topiramate, zonisamide, phenobarbital, and lacosamide involves controlling the fast inactivation of voltage-gated sodium channels. In contrast, drugs such as lacozamide and eslicarbazepine acetate act by controlling the slow inactivation of sodium channels to reduce neuronal hyperexcitability and, consequently, control seizures [209]. Recent research indicates that cenobamate also has an inhibitory effect on sodium ion channels [210].

Research has shown that a common characteristic of anti-seizure medications that act as sodium channel blockers is their preferential affinity for the channel when it is in an inactivated state [211]. Once bound to the channel, these medications block the process of channel reactivation, thereby limiting the repetitive firing of neurons. This action has little effect on the generation of single action potentials or low-frequency (less than 1 Hz) firing [212]. Rufinamide is a prototypical agent that induces the slow inactivation of sodium ion channels. As epileptic seizure discharges occur on a timescale of seconds, the slow action of rufinamide may confer greater selectivity for epileptogenic action potential discharges than for nonepileptogenic discharges, potentially enhancing efficacy and reducing side effects, thus increasing patient tolerance [213].

1.5.1.2 Blocking Voltage-Gated Calcium Channels

Voltage-gated calcium channels (VGCCs) mediate the influx of calcium ions, leading to membrane depolarization and regulating intracellular processes in many different cell types. The activity of calcium channels is crucial for the coupling of surface electrical signals with intracellular physiological events. Calcium channels are widely expressed in brain tissues, participate in neuronal burst firing, and are responsible for controlling the release of neurotransmitters from presynaptic nerve terminals and neuronal structural plasticity [214, 215]. There are four main types of voltage-gated calcium channels in the human brain. L-type, P/Q-type, and N-type calcium channels are high-voltage-activated calcium channels (high-voltage-activated HVA) that respond to strong depolarization. L-type channels are composed of the α1 subunit of the CaV1 family, while P/Q-type and N-type channels are composed of CaV2.1 and CaV2.2 subunits [216]. Low-voltage-activated T-type calcium channels (low-voltage-activated LVA) include the α1 subunit of the CaV3 family, which opens at the resting membrane potential or undergoes moderate depolarization and then rapidly inactivates, generating transient (hence T-type) currents involved in intrinsic oscillatory activity [217]. Numerous studies have shown that T-type calcium channels play a key role in the generation of thalamocortical hypersynchronous oscillatory activity, which is the basis for epileptic seizures, especially absence seizures [218–220]. Voltage-gated calcium channels are therapeutic targets for several clinical antiepileptic drugs. Zonisamide and ethosuximide block T-type calcium channels in a voltage-dependent manner, have greater affinity for channels in the inactivated state and block voltage-gated sodium channels, thereby increasing the threshold for the generation of action potentials [221]. Zonisamide-mediated blockade of T-type calcium channels is considered one of its mechanisms of action against epileptic seizures. Gabapentin and pregabalin bind with high affinity to the 2–1 subunit of voltage-gated calcium channels, which is considered one of the mechanisms of these drugs against epileptic seizures [221]. Research has shown that inhibiting presynaptic calcium channels reduces the release of excitatory neurotransmitters, which may be one of the mechanisms underlying the antiepileptic activity of gabapentin-like calcium channel blockers, but the underlying mechanism is still unclear [222]. Reports have shown that lamotrigine can block N- and P/Q--type calcium channels at presynaptic nerve terminals, thereby reducing the release of glutamate to exert its anticonvulsant effect [223–225]. In addition, phenobarbital and topiramate can block L-type and N-type calcium currents [215].

1.5.1.3 Voltage-Gated Potassium Channel Enhancement

Potassium ion channels exhibit high heterogeneity and represent a complex class of ion channels. There are multiple subtypes throughout the nervous system, each of which plays different roles in various types of neurons and different brain regions. Therefore, developing drugs targeting specific subtypes is highly challenging. Currently, the only clinically used antiseizure medication that enhances voltage-gated potassium ion channels is retigabine, but many studies are underway to develop novel potassium channel enhancers [226].

Retigabine, acting as a positive allosteric modulator (or opener) of potassium ion channels, is the only clinically approved antiseizure medication that acts on KCNQ channels [227]. It is used to treat focal-onset seizures in adults. Its mechanism of action involves enhancing the voltage-gated potassium channels of the Kv7 subfamily, increasing their repolarization rate, and reducing their subsequent inactivation rate [228].

1.5.2 Blocking Excitatory Neurotransmission

A widespread feature of epilepsy is abnormal neuronal excitability, with glutamate being the primary excitatory neurotransmitter in the adult human brain. Therefore, in the study of antiseizure medications, researchers have shown significant interest in drugs affecting glutamate receptor ion channels, aiming to explore the possibility of controlling seizures by blocking glutamate transmission [229, 230].

Glutamate exerts its excitatory effects through ligand-gated ion channels and metabotropic receptor subtypes. Among the postsynaptic ligand-gated ion channels, α-amino-3-hydroxy-5-methyl-4-isoxazolepropionic acid (AMPA) receptors (AMPARs) are crucial for fast excitatory neurotransmission, while N-methyl-D-aspartate (NMDA) receptors (NMDARs) mediate many globally important slow postsynaptic excitatory potentials [231]. However, the function of kainate receptors, although capable of modulating excitability at both presynaptic and postsynaptic sites, remains unclear [232, 233].

Perampanel is a noncompetitive AMPAR antagonist that reduces neuronal excitability and synchronous features of epileptic-like activity [234, 235]. It was the first drug specifically approved for controlling seizures by blocking glutamate receptors [236–238]. Perampanel binds to the extracellular region of AMPARs, distinct from the glutamate recognition site, in a voltage-independent manner. Its binding induces conformational changes in AMPAR subunits, restricting their ability to convert agonist (i.e., glutamate) binding into channel opening. The ultimate result is a reduction in fast excitatory neurotransmission, limiting the generation of seizures and the spread of epileptic discharges [239]. Experimental evidence has shown that perampanel blocks only a small fraction of AMPAR currents, preserving the majority of normal synaptic transmission while sufficiently slowing epileptic-like discharges [240].

In addition to perampanel, several other antiseizure medications exert their effects by modulating glutamatergic neurotransmission. Although the exact mechanism of action of felbamate is not fully understood, it is speculated to have several potential modes. Its primary antiseizure activity is thought to involve the modulation of NMDA receptors, which reduce glutamate transmission. Other effects include enhancing the action of gamma-aminobutyric acid (GABA) and inhibiting voltage-gated sodium and calcium channels [215, 241, 242].

Topiramate (TPM) demonstrates broad efficacy in refractory partial and secondary generalized seizures. It can reduce the excitatory effects of glutamate through AMPA receptors [243]. Additionally, TPM blocks sodium channels, enhances GABA-A receptor-mediated inhibition, inhibits high-voltage calcium channels, and inhibits carbonic anhydrase [244].

1.5.3 Modulation of Neurotransmitter Release

Because neural functional conduction occurs through electrochemical means, selectively reducing the release of neurotransmitters (such as glutamate) from presynaptic nerve terminals can significantly inhibit the excitability of neural activity. Some antiepileptic drugs act through this pathway to control seizures.

Levetiracetam and brivaracetam primarily achieve their antiepileptic effects by binding to the synaptic vesicle protein SV2A, reducing the release of neurotransmitters [245, 246]. The interaction of levetiracetam with SV2A can decrease the release of synaptic vesicles in rapidly firing neurons during repetitive stimulation. Because levetiracetam restricts the release of glutamate and GABA in an activity-dependent manner, its impact on rapidly firing neurons is most significant, consistent with the selective inhibition of epileptic-like activity [246–249]. However, the exact mechanism by which SV2A inhibits vesicle release remains unclear, mainly due to the uncertain physiological role of SV2A despite extensive research.

Brivaracetam is a selective, high-affinity ligand for SV2A with excellent antiepileptic properties and rapid onset of action. Experiments have shown that brivaracetam has a greater affinity for SV2A than does levetiracetam [250]. Animal studies have demonstrated that, compared to levetiracetam, brivaracetam has a 15- to 100-fold greater affinity for SV2A [250, 251]. Additionally, brivaracetam restricts the release of neurotransmitters in an activity-dependent manner [250].

In addition to the abovementioned antiepileptic drugs that bind to SV2A, lamotrigine can also inhibit the release of neurotransmitters from presynaptic terminals. However, further experimental data are needed to confirm whether this effect is mediated by SV2A [252].

1.5.4 Improving Neuronal GABAergic Inhibitory Function

The inhibitory neurotransmitter gamma-aminobutyric acid (GABA) plays a crucial role in the control of neuronal excitability in the mammalian brain. Disruption of GABAergic neurotransmission has been implicated in the pathogenesis or manifestation of various neurological disorders, including epilepsy.

GABA, an amino acid, serves as the primary inhibitory neurotransmitter in the central nervous system. It induces hyperpolarizing inhibition in nearly all neurons, leading to a reduction in neuronal excitability. GABA exerts its effects on GABA receptors located postsynaptically to GABAergic neurons. These GABA receptors are considered the principal inhibitory receptors in the central nervous system and are classified as GABA-A, GABA-B, and GABA-C receptors [253, 254]. GABA-A receptors are ligand-gated ion channels and are members of the classic "Cys-loop" receptor family. GABA-A receptors mediate transient, fast-desensitizing currents (phasic inhibition) [255]. In contrast to GABA-A receptors, GABA-B receptors couple to potassium channels through G proteins, mediating slow hyperpolarization of the postsynaptic membrane [256]. The most critical component in the regulation of epileptic activity within the GABA system is the GABA-A receptor. Mutations in genes, neurodegeneration causing GABA receptor damage, or the use of GABA receptor antagonists can impair GABAergic transmission and induce seizures, while drugs that enhance GABAergic transmission are used to treat epilepsy [257, 258].

Following GABA release, the extracellular GABA concentration is regulated by GABA transporters. GABA transporters on the cell membrane help regulate the extracellular GABA concentration by reabsorbing GABA. They transiently bind with GABA in the extracellular matrix and transport the neurotransmitter to the cytoplasm, reducing GABA levels in the synaptic cleft. Thus, factors affecting presynaptic GABA release, postsynaptic GABA receptor function, and GABA reuptake and clearance may contribute to neuronal excitation leading to epileptic seizures, and the development of some antiepileptic drugs is targeted at these processes. After GABA is reabsorbed, it can be recycled into the readily releasable neurotransmitter pool or converted to succinic semialdehyde by the mitochondrial enzyme GABA transaminase, rendering it inactive.

In the mature brain, the binding of GABA to GABA-A receptors induces an inward flow of Cl^-, driven by its concentration gradient from a high extracellular level to a low intracellular level. Compared to those in the mature brain, the activation of GABA-A receptors in the immature brain is primarily depolarizing and potentially epileptic due to the flow of chloride ions from a high intracellular level to a low extracellular level [259].

1.5.4.1 Modulation of GABA-A Receptors

Some antiepileptic drugs that act on GABA-A receptors are primarily positive allosteric modulators. In the absence of GABA, they do not activate the receptor [260]. However, when synaptic release of GABA increases, these drugs can enhance inhibitory neurotransmission. Benzodiazepines (such as clonazepam, clorazepate, diazepam, and midazolam) and barbiturates are positive allosteric modulators of GABA-A receptors. Upon binding to the GABA-A receptor, these drugs augment the response to GABA, enhancing chloride ion influx. Barbiturates and benzodiazepines exhibit functional distinctions, with the former prolonging the duration of chloride channel opening and the latter increasing the frequency of channel opening [261]. There are reports suggesting that primidone is also a positive allosteric modulator of GABA-A receptors [262].

1.5.4.2 Increasing GABA Levels and Inhibiting Reuptake and Conversion

Löscher et al. reported that the most convincing mechanism through which primidone exerts its antiepileptic effects is by influencing the content of GABA at synapses, either by increasing GABA neurotransmitter synthesis or release or inhibiting its degradation [263]. Vigabatrin is an irreversible inhibitor of GABA transaminases. It increases brain GABA levels by inhibiting GABA transaminase, the major enzyme responsible for degrading GABA, without significantly affecting other enzymes involved in GABA synthesis and metabolism [264]. Tiagabine is a GABA uptake inhibitor. By selectively inhibiting the GAT-1 GABA transporter, this drug blocks the reuptake of GABA by neurons and glial cells, with little activity against GAT-2, GAT-3, or BGT-1 [265]. By slowing the reuptake of synaptic GABA, it prolongs inhibitory postsynaptic potentials [266]. The temporary prolongation of synaptic endogenous GABA release by blocking GABA uptake is a known mechanism of action for tiagabine in the treatment of seizures [267].

1.5.4.3 Carbonic Anhydrase Inhibitors

Carbonic anhydrase inhibitors (CAIs) are a class of drugs used to treat certain types of seizures. These enzymes act by inhibiting the activity of carbonic anhydrase, an enzyme involved in regulating acid–base balance in the body. CAIs are most commonly used to treat certain types of seizures, such as absence seizures and myoclonic seizures. The exact mechanism by which carbonic anhydrase inhibitors control seizures is not fully understood [268–270].

Acetazolamide (ACZ) is a noncompetitive inhibitor of carbonic anhydrase. Although it has achieved some success as an antiepileptic drug, especially in the treatment of pediatric and chronic epilepsy, its use is limited due to tolerability issues [271]. Acetazolamide induces acidification of intracellular and extracellular environments, thereby activating acid-sensitive ion channels, which may contribute to its antiepileptic effects [268–270]. Topiramate (TPM) and zonisamide (ZNS) are effective antiepileptic drugs. Although their antiepileptic mechanisms are often classified as blockades of voltage-gated sodium ion channels, they are also effective nonspecific CA inhibitors. Therefore, their antiepileptic actions are strongly attributed to their carbonic anhydrase inhibition properties [269, 272, 273].

1.5.5 Other Mechanisms

The mechanisms of action of some clinically used antiepileptic drugs may involve multiple pathways, or their mechanisms are not yet fully understood.

Everolimus is an inhibitor of mammalian target of rapamycin complex 1 (mTORC1) [274, 275]. As a protein kinase, mTOR plays a crucial role in cell growth, differentiation, and metabolism. Everolimus interferes with the abnormal growth and division of cells by inhibiting the activity of mTOR kinase. Therefore, it is used in some cases for the treatment of epilepsy, particularly in patients with tuberous sclerosis complex (TSC), helping to reduce the frequency of seizures in TSC patients [274, 276, 277].

Cannabidiol (CBD, marketed as Epidiolex) is a major component of cannabinoids. It was approved by the US Food and Drug Administration (FDA) as a novel antiepileptic drug in 2018 and is used for the treatment of certain severe pediatric epilepsy syndromes, such as Dravet syndrome, Lennox-Gastaut syndrome, and seizures associated with TSC [278–281]. Despite being the first cannabinoid preparation approved by the FDA for epilepsy treatment, its exact mechanism of action remains unclear.

Studies have indicated that cannabinoids exert their effects by stimulating two receptors in the endocannabinoid system, cannabinoid receptor type 1 (CB1) and type 2 (CB2). CBD reportedly primarily binds to CB1 receptors on presynaptic neurons. This binding leads to the activation of presynaptic T-type calcium channels and subsequent inhibition of neurotransmitter release [282]. Although most recent studies have suggested that cannabinoids act through CB1 receptors for their antiepileptic effects, recent research has reported that CB2 receptors, which are expressed at lower levels in the central nervous system under normal conditions, can be induced to have higher expression under epileptic conditions. Therefore, CB2 receptors might also be a target for antiepileptic drugs [283].

The recently FDA-approved drug cenobamate (CNB) is considered a highly effective treatment for focal-onset seizures, achieving seizure control in more than 20% of drug-resistant epilepsy patients. Because CNB was discovered based on phenotype screening, its mechanism of action is not well-understood. However, it is speculated to have a dual mechanism of action, acting as both a voltage-gated sodium channel inhibitor by blocking sodium ion currents [284] and a positive allosteric modulator of GABA-A receptors, independent of the benzodiazepine binding site [285]. It effectively enhances (tonic) inhibition of hippocampal neurons, which may be a potential molecular mechanism for stabilizing the hippocampal neural circuit in epilepsy. Due to CNB's terminal half-life of 50–60 hours, it can be taken once daily, reducing the frequency of administration and improving patient compliance [286].

Ganaxolone (Ztalmy) is a synthetic neuroactive steroid used to treat seizures in patients with cyclin-dependent kinase-like 5 (CDKL5) deficiency disorder (CDD). Its mechanism of action involves serving as a positive allosteric modulator of

GABA-A receptors [287]. Ganaxolone operates similarly to the endogenous neurosteroid allopregnanolone, binding to a unique recognition site on GABAA receptors distinct from the binding sites of benzodiazepine drugs and barbiturate drugs. Upon binding, ganaxolone produces antiepileptic effects by increasing the inhibitory effect of GABA [287, 288].

1.5.6 Conclusion

In this chapter, we have summarized and determined the mechanisms of action of antiepileptic drugs currently applied in clinical settings. In the early history of human use of antiepileptic drugs, relatively few drug options were available, making the selection process less challenging. However, with the continuous development of novel antiepileptic drugs, there are now more than 30 drugs used in clinical practice. While the emergence of new drugs provides more choices for the treatment of epilepsy patients, it also increases the difficulty for clinicians in selecting appropriate medications. Therefore, understanding the mechanisms of action for each drug, interactions between drugs, how to control side effects, and individualized drug formulation for patients with different etiologies is crucial.

Additionally, despite the continuous development of novel antiepileptic drugs, with reduced drug toxicity and improved patient compliance, neither the rate of seizure control nor the proportion of drug-resistant patients has significantly decreased [289–291].

The reasons for the onset and development of epilepsy are not yet clear, and most antiepileptic drugs are identified through screening in epilepsy animal models. There is currently no treatment that can prevent or terminate epilepsy and its related complications. Therefore, achieving a cure for epilepsy through the application of antiepileptic drugs remains unattainable. Complete control of seizures or addressing the root cause of epilepsy is the ultimate goal of treatment. To achieve this goal, the development of effective and safe antiepileptogenic (AEG), disease-modifying (DM), and/or seizure-preventative treatment drugs has been recognized as a high priority in epilepsy research [292, 293].

References

1. Blume WT. A disease once sacred—a history of the medical understanding of epilepsy. 2001. By Mervyn J. Eadie, Peter F. Bladin. Published by John Libbey & Company Limited. 248 pages. C$61.45 approx. Can J Neurol Sci / J Can Des Sci Neurol. 2002;29:298–9.
2. Fisher RS, Acevedo C, Arzimanoglou A, Bogacz A, Cross JH, Elger CE, et al. ILAE official report: a practical clinical definition of epilepsy. Epilepsia. 2014;55:475–82.
3. Fisher RS, van Emde BW, Blume W, Elger C, Genton P, Lee P, et al. Epileptic seizures and epilepsy: definitions proposed by the International League Against Epilepsy (ILAE) and the International Bureau for Epilepsy (IBE). Epilepsia. 2005;46:470–2.

4. Wang X, Li S. Refractory status epilepticus: diagnosis and treatment. Springer; 2017.
5. Devinsky O, Vezzani A, O'Brien TJ, Jette N, Scheffer IE, de Curtis M, et al. Epilepsy. Nat Rev Dis Prim. 2018;4:18024.
6. Zuberi SM, Wirrell E, Yozawitz E, Wilmshurst JM, Specchio N, Riney K, et al. ILAE classification and definition of epilepsy syndromes with onset in neonates and infants: position statement by the ILAE task force on nosology and definitions. Epilepsia. 2022;63:1349–97.
7. Sidiropoulou K, Diamantis A, Magiorkinis E. Hallmarks in 18th- and 19th-century epilepsy research. Epilepsy Behav. 2010;18:151–61.
8. Gibbs FA, Gibbs EL, Lennox WG. Epilepsy: a paroxysmal cerebral dysrhythmia. Epilepsy Behav. 2002;3:395–401.
9. Arnautova EN, Nesmeianova TN. A proposed international classification of epileptic seizures. Epilepsia. 1964;5:297–306.
10. Gastaut H. Clinical and electroencephalographical classification of epileptic seizures. Epilepsia. 1970;11:102–13.
11. Proposal for revised clinical and electroencephalographic classification of epileptic seizures. From the commission on classification and terminology of the international league against epilepsy. Epilepsia. 1981;22:489–501.
12. Blume WT, Lüders HO, Mizrahi E, Tassinari C, van Emde Boas W, Engel JJ. Glossary of descriptive terminology for ictal semiology: report of the ILAE task force on classification and terminology. Epilepsia. 2001;42:1212–8.
13. Berg AT, Berkovic SF, Brodie MJ, Buchhalter J, Cross JH, van Emde Boas W, et al. Revised terminology and concepts for organization of seizures and epilepsies: report of the ILAE commission on classification and terminology, 2005–2009. Epilepsia. 2010;51:676–85.
14. Fisher RS, Cross JH, French JA, Higurashi N, Hirsch E, Jansen FE, et al. Operational classification of seizure types by the international league against epilepsy: position paper of the ILAE Commission for Classification and Terminology. Epilepsia. 2017;58:522–30.
15. Lüders HO, Burgess R, Noachtar S. Expanding the international classification of seizures to provide localization information. Neurology. 1993;43:1650–5.
16. Lüders H, Acharya J, Baumgartner C, Benbadis S, Bleasel A, Burgess R, et al. Semiological seizure classification. Epilepsia. 1998;39:1006–13.
17. Lüders H, Vaca GF-B, Akamatsu N, Amina S, Arzimanoglou A, Baumgartner C, et al. Classification of paroxysmal events and the four-dimensional epilepsy classification system. Epileptic Disord. 2019;21:1–29.
18. Scheffer IE, Berkovic S, Capovilla G, Connolly MB, French J, Guilhoto L, et al. ILAE classification of the epilepsies: position paper of the ILAE commission for classification and terminology. Epilepsia. 2017;58:512–21.
19. Kaculini CM, Tate-Looney AJ, Seifi A. The history of epilepsy: from ancient mystery to modern misconception. Cureus. 2021;13:e13953.
20. Pitkänen A, Immonen R. Epilepsy related to traumatic brain injury. Neurother J Am Soc Exp Neurother. 2014;11:286–96.
21. Lin C-H, Hsieh C-L. Chinese herbal medicine for treating epilepsy. Front Neurosci. 2021;15:682821.
22. Hassen G, Belete G, Carrera KG, Iriowen RO, Araya H, Alemu T, et al. Clinical implications of herbal supplements in conventional medical practice: a US perspective. Cureus. 2022;14:e26893.
23. Friedman D, Sirven JI. Historical perspective on the medical use of cannabis for epilepsy: ancient times to the 1980s. Epilepsy Behav. 2017;70:298–301.
24. Reddy DS. Therapeutic and clinical foundations of cannabidiol therapy for difficult-to-treat seizures in children and adults with refractory epilepsies. Exp Neurol. 2023;359:114237.
25. Brodie MJ. Antiepileptic drug therapy the story so far. Seizure. 2010;19:650–5.
26. Löscher W, Klein P. The pharmacology and clinical efficacy of Antiseizure medications: from bromide salts to Cenobamate and beyond. CNS Drugs. 2021;35:935–63.
27. Shorvon SD. Drug treatment of epilepsy in the century of the ILAE: the first 50 years, 1909–1958. Epilepsia. 2009;50(Suppl 3):69–92.

28. Ryan M, Baumann RJ. Use and monitoring of bromides in epilepsy treatment. Pediatr Neurol. 1999;21:523–8.
29. Korinthenberg R, Burkart P, Woelfle C, Moenting JS, Ernst JP. Pharmacology, efficacy, and tolerability of potassium bromide in childhood epilepsy. J Child Neurol. 2007;22:414–8.
30. Brodie MJ, Kwan P. Current position of phenobarbital in epilepsy and its future. Epilepsia. 2012;53(Suppl 8):40–6.
31. Perucca E. Antiepileptic drugs: evolution of our knowledge and changes in drug trials. Epileptic Disord. 2019;21:319–29.
32. Löscher W. Animal models of seizures and epilepsy: past, present, and future role for the discovery of Antiseizure drugs. Neurochem Res. 2017;42:1873–88.
33. Rho JM, White HS. Brief history of anti-seizure drug development. Epilepsia Open. 2018;3:114–9.
34. Tomson T, Battino D, Perucca E. Valproic acid after five decades of use in epilepsy: time to reconsider the indications of a time-honoured drug. Lancet Neurol. 2016;15:210–8.
35. Gastaut H. Clinical and electroencephalographical classification of epileptic seizures. Epilepsia. 1969;10(Suppl):2–13.
36. Gastaut H. Classification of the epilepsies. Proposal for an international classification. Epilepsia. 1969;10(Suppl):14–21.
37. Mattson RH, Cramer JA, Collins JF, Smith DB, Delgado-Escueta AV, Browne TR, et al. Comparison of carbamazepine, phenobarbital, phenytoin, and primidone in partial and secondarily generalized tonic-clonic seizures. N Engl J Med. 1985;313:145–51.
38. Shields WD, Saslow E. Myoclonic, atonic, and absence seizures following institution of carbamazepine therapy in children. Neurology. 1983;33:1487–9.
39. Shorvon SD, Chadwick D, Galbraith AW, Reynolds EH. One drug for epilepsy. Br Med J. 1978;1:474–6.
40. Shorvon SD, Reynolds EH. Unnecessary polypharmacy for epilepsy. Br Med J. 1977;1:1635–7.
41. Buchthal F, Svensmark O. Aspects of the pharmacology of phenytoin (dilantin) and phenobarbital relevant to their dosage in the treatment of epilepsy. Epilepsia. 1960;1:373–84.
42. Buchthal F, Svensmark O. Serum concentrations of diphenylhydantoin (phenytoin) and phenobarbital and their relation to therapeutic and toxic effects. Psychiatr Neurol Neurochir. 1971;74:117–36.
43. Lund L. Anticonvulsant effect of diphenylhydantoin relative to plasma levels. A prospective three-year study in ambulant patients with generalized epileptic seizures. Arch Neurol. 1974;31:289–94.
44. Richens A, Dunlop A. Serum-phenytoin levels in management of epilepsy. Lancet (London, England). 1975;2:247–8.
45. Pippenger CE, Penry JK, White BG, Daly DD, Buddington R. Interlaboratory variability in determination of plasma antiepileptic drug concentrations. Arch Neurol. 1976;33:351–5.
46. Crawford P, Chadwick D. A comparative study of progabide, valproate, and placebo as add-on therapy in patients with refractory epilepsy. J Neurol Neurosurg Psychiatry. 1986;49:1251–7.
47. Leppik IE, Dreifuss FE, Porter R, Bowman T, Santilli N, Jacobs M, et al. A controlled study of progabide in partial seizures: methodology and results. Neurology. 1987;37:963–8.
48. Munoz SJ, Fariello R, Maddrey WC. Submassive hepatic necrosis associated with the use of progabide: a GABA receptor agonist. Dig Dis Sci. 1988;33:375–80.
49. Klein BD, Jacobson CA, Metcalf CS, Smith MD, Wilcox KS, Hampson AJ, et al. Evaluation of Cannabidiol in animal seizure models by the Epilepsy Therapy Screening Program (ETSP). Neurochem Res. 2017;42:1939–48.
50. Wilcox KS, West PJ, Metcalf CS. The current approach of the Epilepsy Therapy Screening Program contract site for identifying improved therapies for the treatment of pharmacoresistant seizures in epilepsy. Neuropharmacology. 2020;166:107811.
51. Pernici CD, Mensah JA, Dahle EJ, Johnson KJ, Handy L, Buxton L, et al. Development of an antiseizure drug screening platform for Dravet syndrome at the NINDS contract site for the Epilepsy Therapy Screening Program. Epilepsia. 2021;62:1665–76.

52. Metcalf CS, Vanegas F, Underwood T, Johnson K, West PJ, Smith MD, et al. Screening of prototype antiseizure and anti-inflammatory compounds in the Theiler's murine encephalomyelitis virus model of epilepsy. Epilepsia Open. 2022;7:46–58.
53. Kehne JH, Klein BD, Raeissi S, Sharma S. The National Institute of Neurological Disorders and Stroke (NINDS) Epilepsy Therapy Screening Program (ETSP). Neurochem Res. 2017;42:1894–903.
54. Löscher W. Single-target versus multi-target drugs versus combinations of drugs with multiple targets: preclinical and clinical evidence for the treatment or prevention of epilepsy. Front Pharmacol. 2021;12:730257.
55. Quintero JE, Dooley DJ, Pomerleau F, Huettl P, Gerhardt GA. Amperometric measurement of glutamate release modulation by gabapentin and pregabalin in rat neocortical slices: role of voltage-sensitive Ca2+ α2δ-1 subunit. J Pharmacol Exp Ther. 2011;338:240–5.
56. Wolf P. New antiepileptic drugs already registered. Epilepsia. 1994;35(Suppl 5):S22–4.
57. Perucca E. What clinical trial designs have been used to test antiepileptic drugs and do we need to change them? Epileptic Disord. 2012;14:124–31.
58. Chen Z, Brodie MJ, Liew D, Kwan P. Treatment outcomes in patients with newly diagnosed epilepsy treated with established and new antiepileptic drugs: a 30-year longitudinal cohort study. JAMA Neurol. 2018;75:279–86.
59. Perucca E, Brodie MJ, Kwan P, Tomson T. 30 years of second-generation antiseizure medications: impact and future perspectives. Lancet Neurol. 2020;19:544–56.
60. Perucca E. Clinically relevant drug interactions with antiepileptic drugs. Br J Clin Pharmacol. 2006;61:246–55.
61. Zaccara G, Perucca E. Interactions between antiepileptic drugs, and between antiepileptic drugs and other drugs. Epileptic Disord. 2014;16:409–31.
62. Brodie MJ, Mintzer S, Pack AM, Gidal BE, Vecht CJ, Schmidt D. Enzyme induction with antiepileptic drugs: cause for concern? Epilepsia. 2013;54:11–27.
63. Tomson T, Battino D, Bonizzoni E, Craig J, Lindhout D, Perucca E, et al. Comparative risk of major congenital malformations with eight different antiepileptic drugs: a prospective cohort study of the EURAP registry. Lancet Neurol. 2018;17:530–8.
64. Tomson T, Battino D, Perucca E. Teratogenicity of antiepileptic drugs. Curr Opin Neurol. 2019;32:246–52.
65. Tomson T, Battino D, Bonizzoni E, Craig J, Lindhout D, Perucca E, et al. Declining malformation rates with changed antiepileptic drug prescribing: An observational study. Neurology. 2019;93:e831–40.
66. Cohen JM, Alvestad S, Cesta CE, Bjørk M-H, Leinonen MK, Nørgaard M, et al. Comparative safety of Antiseizure medication monotherapy for major malformations. Ann Neurol. 2023;93:551–62.
67. Bjørk M-H, Zoega H, Leinonen MK, Cohen JM, Dreier JW, Furu K, et al. Association of Prenatal Exposure to Antiseizure medication with risk of autism and intellectual disability. JAMA Neurol. 2022;79:672–81.
68. McCluskey G, Kinney MO, Russell A, Smithson WH, Parsons L, Morrison PJ, et al. Zonisamide safety in pregnancy: data from the UK and Ireland epilepsy and pregnancy register. Seizure. 2021;91:311–5.
69. Elkommos S, Mula M. Current and future pharmacotherapy options for drug-resistant epilepsy. Expert Opin Pharmacother. 2022;23:2023–34.
70. Ackermann S, Wilmshurst JM. Medical management of children with epilepsy. Minerva Pediatr. 2015;67:47–74.
71. Burakgazi E, French JA. Treatment of epilepsy in adults. Epileptic Disord. 2016;18:228–39.
72. Cheng JY, French JA. Intelligent use of antiepileptic drugs is beneficial to patients. Curr Opin Neurol. 2018;31:169–75.
73. Jehi L, Jette N, Kwon C-S, Josephson CB, Burneo JG, Cendes F, et al. Timing of referral to evaluate for epilepsy surgery: expert consensus recommendations from the surgical therapies Commission of the International League Against Epilepsy. Epilepsia. 2022;63:2491–506.

74. Kossoff EH, Zupec-Kania BA, Auvin S, Ballaban-Gil KR, Christina Bergqvist AG, Blackford R, et al. Optimal clinical management of children receiving dietary therapies for epilepsy: updated recommendations of the International Ketogenic Diet Study Group. Epilepsia Open. 2018;3:175–92.
75. Ryvlin P, Rheims S, Hirsch LJ, Sokolov A, Jehi L. Neuromodulation in epilepsy: state-of-the-art approved therapies. Lancet Neurol. 2021;20:1038–47.
76. Gambardella A, Tinuper P, Acone B, Bonanni P, Coppola G, Perucca E. Selection of antiseizure medications for first add-on use: a consensus paper. Epilepsy Behav. 2021;122:108087.
77. Verrotti A, Tambucci R, Di Francesco L, Pavone P, Iapadre G, Altobelli E, et al. The role of polytherapy in the management of epilepsy: suggestions for rational antiepileptic drug selection. Expert Rev Neurother. 2020;20:167–73.
78. Patsalos PN, Berry DJ, Bourgeois BFD, Cloyd JC, Glauser TA, Johannessen SI, et al. Antiepileptic drugs–best practice guidelines for therapeutic drug monitoring: a position paper by the subcommission on therapeutic drug monitoring, ILAE Commission on Therapeutic Strategies. Epilepsia. 2008;49:1239–76.
79. Asadi-Pooya AA, Beniczky S, Rubboli G, Sperling MR, Rampp S, Perucca E. A pragmatic algorithm to select appropriate antiseizure medications in patients with epilepsy. Epilepsia. 2020;61:1668–77.
80. Håkansson S, Zelano J. Big data analysis of ASM retention rates and expert ASM algorithm: a comparative study. Epilepsia. 2022;63:1553–62.
81. de Jong J, Cutcutache I, Page M, Elmoufti S, Dilley C, Fröhlich H, et al. Towards realizing the vision of precision medicine: AI based prediction of clinical drug response. Brain. 2021;144:1738–50.
82. Hakeem H, Feng W, Chen Z, Choong J, Brodie MJ, Fong SL, et al. Development and validation of a deep learning model for predicting treatment response in patients with newly diagnosed epilepsy. JAMA Neurol. 2022;79:986–96.
83. Perucca E, Wiebe S. Not all that glitters is gold: a guide to the critical interpretation of drug trials in epilepsy. Epilepsia Open. 2016;1:9–21.
84. Perucca E. From clinical trials of antiepileptic drugs to treatment. Epilepsia Open. 2018;3:220–30.
85. Sourbron J, Auvin S, Arzimanoglou A, Cross JH, Hartmann H, Pressler R, et al. Medical treatment in infants and young children with epilepsy: off-label use of antiseizure medications. Survey report of ILAE task force medical therapies in children. Epilepsia Open. 2023;8:77–89.
86. Piccenna L, O'Dwyer R, Leppik I, Beghi E, Giussani G, Costa C, et al. Management of epilepsy in older adults: a critical review by the ILAE task force on epilepsy in the elderly. Epilepsia. 2023;64:567–85.
87. Glauser T, Ben-Menachem E, Bourgeois B, Cnaan A, Guerreiro C, Kälviäinen R, et al. Updated ILAE evidence review of antiepileptic drug efficacy and effectiveness as initial monotherapy for epileptic seizures and syndromes. Epilepsia. 2013;54:551–63.
88. Guerrini R, Balestrini S, Wirrell EC, Walker MC. Monogenic epilepsies: disease mechanisms, clinical phenotypes, and targeted therapies. Neurology. 2021;97:817–31.
89. Stirling RE, Maturana MI, Karoly PJ, Nurse ES, McCutcheon K, Grayden DB, et al. Seizure forecasting using a novel sub-scalp ultra-long term EEG monitoring system. Front Neurol. 2021;12:713794.
90. Lehnertz K, Bröhl T, Wrede R von. Epileptic-network-based prediction and control of seizures in humans. Neurobiol Dis. 2023;181:106098.
91. Cook M, Murphy M, Bulluss K, D'Souza W, Plummer C, Priest E, et al. Anti-seizure therapy with a long-term, implanted intra-cerebroventricular delivery system for drug-resistant epilepsy: a first-in-man study. EClinicalMedicine. 2020;22:100326.
92. Knowles JK, Helbig I, Metcalf CS, Lubbers LS, Isom LL, Demarest S, et al. Precision medicine for genetic epilepsy on the horizon: recent advances, present challenges, and suggestions for continued progress. Epilepsia. 2022;63:2461–75.

93. Flammer J, Neziraj T, Rüegg S, Pröbstel A-K. Immune mechanisms in Epileptogenesis: update on diagnosis and treatment of autoimmune epilepsy syndromes. Drugs. 2023;83:135–58.
94. Aronica E, Bauer S, Bozzi Y, Caleo M, Dingledine R, Gorter JA, et al. Neuroinflammatory targets and treatments for epilepsy validated in experimental models. Epilepsia. 2017;58(Suppl 3):27–38.
95. Vezzani A, Ravizza T, Bedner P, Aronica E, Steinhäuser C, Boison D. Astrocytes in the initiation and progression of epilepsy. Nat Rev Neurol. 2022;18:707–22.
96. Villasana-Salazar B, Vezzani A. Neuroinflammation microenvironment sharpens seizure circuit. Neurobiol Dis. 2023;178:106027.
97. Ding M, Lang Y, Shu H, Shao J, Cui L. Microbiota-gut-brain Axis and epilepsy: a review on mechanisms and potential therapeutics. Front Immunol. 2021;12:742449.
98. Kundu S, Nayak S, Rakshit D, Singh T, Shukla R, Khatri DK, et al. The microbiome-gut-brain axis in epilepsy: pharmacotherapeutic target from bench evidence for potential bedside applications. Eur J Neurol. 2023;30:3557–67.
99. Ravizza T, Terrone G, Salamone A, Frigerio F, Balosso S, Antoine DJ, et al. High mobility group box 1 is a novel pathogenic factor and a mechanistic biomarker for epilepsy. Brain Behav Immun. 2018;72:14–21.
100. Walker LE, Sills GJ, Jorgensen A, Alapirtti T, Peltola J, Brodie MJ, et al. High-mobility group box 1 as a predictive biomarker for drug-resistant epilepsy: a proof-of-concept study. Epilepsia. 2022;63:e1–6.
101. Galovic M, Ferreira-Atuesta C, Abraira L, Döhler N, Sinka L, Brigo F, et al. Seizures and epilepsy after stroke: epidemiology, biomarkers and management. Drugs Aging. 2021;38:285–99.
102. Heiskanen M, Das Gupta S, Mills JD, van Vliet EA, Manninen E, Ciszek R, et al. Discovery and validation of circulating microRNAs as biomarkers for Epileptogenesis after experimental traumatic brain injury-the EPITARGET cohort. Int J Mol Sci. 2023;24
103. Yonas AS, Meschia JF, Feyissa AM. Clinical biomarkers and prediction models for Poststroke epilepsy: have we settled the scores yet? Neurol Clin Pract. 2023;13:e200146.
104. Golub VM, Reddy DS. Post-traumatic epilepsy and comorbidities: advanced models, molecular mechanisms, biomarkers, and novel therapeutic interventions. Pharmacol Rev. 2022;74:387–438.
105. Kotulska K, Kwiatkowski DJ, Curatolo P, Weschke B, Riney K, Jansen F, et al. Prevention of epilepsy in infants with tuberous sclerosis complex in the EPISTOP trial. Ann Neurol. 2021;89:304–14.
106. Luzzatto L, Hyry HI, Schieppati A, Costa E, Simoens S, Schaefer F, et al. Outrageous prices of orphan drugs: a call for collaboration. Lancet (London, England). 2018;392:791–4.
107. Crowell JL, Burns TM. Rising drug costs for neurologic diseases. Continuum (Minneap Minn). 2020;26:1392–406.
108. Kamusheva M, Turcu-Stiolica A, Gierczyński J, Subtirelu M-S, Czech M, Petrova G. Do advanced therapies have a future in the low- and middle-income countries – the case of Bulgaria, Romania, and Poland. Front Public Heal. 2021;9:729847.
109. Currie GR, Gerber B, Lorenzetti D, MacDonald K, Benseler SM, Bernier FP, et al. Developing a framework of cost elements of socioeconomic burden of rare disease: a scoping review. PharmacoEconomics. 2023;41:803–18.
110. Grone BP, Baraban SC. Animal models in epilepsy research: legacies and new directions. Nat Neurosci. 2015;18:339–43.
111. Pitkänen L, Montoro Bustos AR, Murphy KE, Winchester MR, Striegel AM. Quantitative characterization of gold nanoparticles by size-exclusion and hydrodynamic chromatography, coupled to inductively coupled plasma mass spectrometry and quasi-elastic light scattering. J Chromatogr A. 2017;1511:59–67.
112. Wang Y, Wei P, Yan F, Luo Y, Zhao G. Animal models of epilepsy: a phenotype-oriented review. Aging Dis. 2022;13:215–31.
113. Fisher RS. Animal models of the epilepsies. Brain Res Brain Res Rev. 1989;14:245–78.

114. Ferrier D. Experimental researches in cerebral physiology and pathology. J Anat Physiol. 1873;8:152–5.
115. Putnam TJ, Merritt HH. Experimental determination of the anticonvulsant properties of some phenyl derivatives. Science. 1937;85:525–6.
116. Swinyard EA. Laboratory assay of clinically effective antiepileptic drugs. J Am Pharm Assoc Am Pharm Assoc. 1949;38:201–4.
117. Löscher W. Critical review of current animal models of seizures and epilepsy used in the discovery and development of new antiepileptic drugs. Seizure. 2011;20:359–68.
118. Löscher W, Klitgaard H, Twyman RE, Schmidt D. New avenues for anti-epileptic drug discovery and development. Nat Rev Drug Discov. 2013;12:757–76.
119. Toman JEP. Neuropharmacologic considerations in psychic seizures. Neurology. 1951;1:444–60.
120. Squires RF, Saederup E, Crawley JN, Skolnick P, Paul SM. Convulsant potencies of tetrazoles are highly correlated with actions on GABA/benzodiazepine/picrotoxin receptor complexes in brain. Life Sci. 1984;35:1439–44.
121. Tourov A, Ferri R, Del Gracco S, Elia M, Musumeci SA, Stefanini MC. Spike morphology in PTZ-induced generalized and cobalt-induced partial experimental epilepsy. Funct Neurol. 1996;11:237–45.
122. Yuskaitis CJ, Rossitto L-A, Groff KJ, Dhamne SC, Zhang B, Lalani LK, et al. Factors influencing the acute pentylenetetrazole-induced seizure paradigm and a literature review. Ann Clin Transl Neurol. 2021;8:1388–97.
123. Arida RM, Passos AA, Graciani AL, Brogin JAF, Ribeiro M de AL, Faber J, et al. The potential role of previous physical exercise program to reduce seizure susceptibility: a systematic review and meta-analysis of animal studies. Front Neurol. 2021;12:771123.
124. Fisher RS, Prince DA. Spike-wave rhythms in cat cortex induced by parenteral penicillin. I Electroencephalographic features. Electroencephalogr Clin Neurophysiol. 1977;42:608–24.
125. Sherdil A, Chabardès S, Guillemain I, Michallat S, Prabhu S, Pernet-Gallay K, et al. An on demand macaque model of mesial temporal lobe seizures induced by unilateral intra hippocampal injection of penicillin. Epilepsy Res. 2018;142:20–8.
126. Bum EN, Schmutz M, Meyer C, Rakotonirina A, Bopelet M, Portet C, et al. Anticonvulsant properties of the methanolic extract of Cyperus articulatus (Cyperaceae). J Ethnopharmacol. 2001;76:145–50.
127. Palmer GC, Murray RJ, Cramer CL, Stagnitto ML, Knowles MK, Freedman LR, et al. [S]-AR-R 15896AR-A novel anticonvulsant: acute safety, pharmacokinetic and pharmacodynamic properties. J Pharmacol Exp Ther. 1999;288:121–32.
128. Lehmann J, Hutchison AJ, McPherson SE, Mondadori C, Schmutz M, Sinton CM, et al. CGS 19755, a selective and competitive N-methyl-D-aspartate-type excitatory amino acid receptor antagonist. J Pharmacol Exp Ther. 1988;246:65–75.
129. Bernasconi R, Klein M, Martin P, Christen P, Hafner T, Portet C, et al. Gamma-vinyl GABA: comparison of neurochemical and anticonvulsant effects in mice. J Neural Transm. 1988;72:213–33.
130. Koneval Z, Knox KM, White HS, Barker-Haliski M. Lamotrigine-resistant corneal-kindled mice: a model of pharmacoresistant partial epilepsy for moderate-throughput drug discovery. Epilepsia. 2018;59:1245–56.
131. Goddard GV. Development of epileptic seizures through brain stimulation at low intensity. Nature. 1967;214:1020–1.
132. Goddard GV, McIntyre DC, Leech CK. A permanent change in brain function resulting from daily electrical stimulation. Exp Neurol. 1969;25:295–330.
133. McNamara JO. Kindling model of epilepsy. Adv Neurol. 1986;44:303–18.
134. Raol YH, Brooks-Kayal AR. Experimental models of seizures and epilepsies. Prog Mol Biol Transl Sci. 2012;105:57–82.
135. Racine RJ. Modification of seizure activity by electrical stimulation. II Motor seizure. Electroencephalogr Clin Neurophysiol. 1972;32:281–94.

136. Goddard GV, Douglas RM. Does the engram of kindling model the engram of normal long term memory? Can J Neurol Sci Le J Can Des Sci Neurol. 1975;2:385–94.
137. Karler R, Murphy V, Calder LD, Turkanis SA. Pentylenetetrazol kindling in mice. Neuropharmacology. 1989;28:775–80.
138. Schmidt J. Changes in seizure susceptibility in rats following chronic administration of pentylenetetrazol. Biomed Biochim Acta. 1987;46:267–70.
139. Dhir A. Pentylenetetrazol (PTZ) kindling model of epilepsy. Curr Protoc Neurosci 2012;Chapter 9:Unit9.37.
140. Shimada T, Yamagata K. Pentylenetetrazole-induced kindling mouse model. J Vis Exp. 2018;136:56573.
141. Cela E, McFarlan AR, Chung AJ, Wang T, Chierzi S, Murai KK, et al. An Optogenetic kindling model of neocortical epilepsy. Sci Rep. 2019;9:5236.
142. Cela E, Sjöström PJ. Novel Optogenetic approaches in epilepsy research. Front Neurosci. 2019;13:947.
143. Zhang F, Wang L-P, Brauner M, Liewald JF, Kay K, Watzke N, et al. Multimodal fast optical interrogation of neural circuitry. Nature. 2007;446:633–9.
144. Chow BY, Han X, Dobry AS, Qian X, Chuong AS, Li M, et al. High-performance genetically targetable optical neural silencing by light-driven proton pumps. Nature. 2010;463:98–102.
145. Reddy DS, Kuruba R. Experimental models of status epilepticus and neuronal injury for evaluation of therapeutic interventions. Int J Mol Sci. 2013;14:18284–318.
146. Sutula TP. Mechanisms of epilepsy progression: current theories and perspectives from neuroplasticity in adulthood and development. Epilepsy Res. 2004;60:161–71.
147. Maguire J. Epileptogenesis: more than just the latent period. Epilepsy Curr. 2016;16:31–3.
148. Pitkänen A, Lukasiuk K, Dudek FE, Staley KJ. Epileptogenesis. Cold Spring Harb Perspect Med. 2015;5
149. Goldberg EM, Coulter DA. Mechanisms of epileptogenesis: a convergence on neural circuit dysfunction. Nat Rev Neurosci. 2013;14:337–49.
150. Lillis KP, Wang Z, Mail M, Zhao GQ, Berdichevsky Y, Bacskai B, et al. Evolution of network synchronization during early Epileptogenesis parallels synaptic circuit alterations. J Neurosci. 2015;35:9920–34.
151. Bragin A, Azizyan A, Almajano J, Wilson CL, Engel JJ. Analysis of chronic seizure onsets after intrahippocampal kainic acid injection in freely moving rats. Epilepsia. 2005;46:1592–8.
152. Lévesque M, Avoli M. The kainic acid model of temporal lobe epilepsy. Neurosci Biobehav Rev. 2013;37:2887–99.
153. Medina-Ceja L, Pardo-Peña K, Ventura-Mejía C. Evaluation of behavioral parameters and mortality in a model of temporal lobe epilepsy induced by intracerebroventricular pilocarpine administration. Neuroreport. 2014;25:875–9.
154. Kondo Y, Hatayama K, Ishiguro T, Takemoto T, Murakami S. Studies on the constituents of Chinese drug "kanzui." 8. KMnO4 oxidation of euphol, tirucallol and beta-euphorbol. Yakugaku Zasshi. 1967;87:21–5.
155. Rogawski MA, Gryder D, Castaneda D, Yonekawa W, Banks MK, Lia H. GluR5 kainate receptors, seizures, and the amygdala. Ann N Y Acad Sci. 2003;985:150–62.
156. Curia G, Longo D, Biagini G, Jones RSG, Avoli M. The pilocarpine model of temporal lobe epilepsy. J Neurosci Methods. 2008;172:143–57.
157. Hamilton SE, Loose MD, Qi M, Levey AI, Hille B, McKnight GS, et al. Disruption of the m1 receptor gene ablates muscarinic receptor-dependent M current regulation and seizure activity in mice. Proc Natl Acad Sci USA. 1997;94:13311–6.
158. Rusina E, Bernard C, Williamson A. The Kainic acid models of temporal lobe epilepsy. ENeuro. 2021:8.
159. Thakran S, Guin D, Singh P, Singh P, Kukal S, Rawat C, et al. Genetic landscape of common epilepsies: advancing towards precision in treatment. Int J Mol Sci. 2020;21
160. Wang J, Lin Z-J, Liu L, Xu H-Q, Shi Y-W, Yi Y-H, et al. Epilepsy-associated genes. Seizure. 2017;44:11–20.

161. Noebels JL, Sidman RL. Inherited epilepsy: spike-wave and focal motor seizures in the mutant mouse tottering. Science. 1979;204:1334–6.
162. Kostopoulos GK. The tottering mouse: a critical review of its usefulness in the study of the neuronal mechanisms underlying epilepsy. J Neural Transm Suppl. 1992;35:21–36.
163. Fletcher CF, Lutz CM, O'Sullivan TN, Shaughnessy JDJ, Hawkes R, Frankel WN, et al. Absence epilepsy in tottering mutant mice is associated with calcium channel defects. Cell. 1996;87:607–17.
164. Kim TY, Maki T, Zhou Y, Sakai K, Mizuno Y, Ishikawa A, et al. Absence-like seizures and their pharmacological profile in tottering-6j mice. Biochem Biophys Res Commun. 2015;463:148–53.
165. Vergnes M, Marescaux C, Micheletti G, Reis J, Depaulis A, Rumbach L, et al. Spontaneous paroxysmal electroclinical patterns in rat: a model of generalized non-convulsive epilepsy. Neurosci Lett. 1982;33:97–101.
166. Marescaux C, Micheletti G, Vergnes M, Depaulis A, Rumbach L, Warter JM. A model of chronic spontaneous petit mal-like seizures in the rat: comparison with pentylenetetrazol-induced seizures. Epilepsia. 1984;25:326–31.
167. Roebuck AJ, An L, Marks WN, Sun N, Snutch TP, Howland JG. Cognitive impairments in touchscreen-based visual discrimination and reversal learning in genetic absence epilepsy rats from Strasbourg. Neuroscience. 2020;430:105–12.
168. Coenen AML, Van Luijtelaar ELJM. Genetic animal models for absence epilepsy: a review of the WAG/Rij strain of rats. Behav Genet. 2003;33:635–55.
169. van Luijtelaar G, van Oijen G. Establishing drug effects on Electrocorticographic activity in a genetic absence epilepsy model: advances and pitfalls. Front Pharmacol. 2020;11:395.
170. Kasteleijn-Nolst Trenité DGA. Provoked and reflex seizures: surprising or common? Epilepsia. 2012;53(Suppl 4):105–13.
171. Irmen F, Wehner T, Lemieux L. Do reflex seizures and spontaneous seizures form a continuum? – triggering factors and possible common mechanisms. Seizure. 2015;25:72–9. https://doi.org/10.1016/j.seizure.2014.12.006.
172. Faingold CL. Role of GABA abnormalities in the inferior colliculus pathophysiology – audiogenic seizures. Hear Res. 2002;168:223–37.
173. Killam KF, Killam EK, Naquet R. Study of responses evoked by intermittent light stimulation in monkeys presenting paroxysmal responses to this type of stimulation. Rev Neurol (Paris). 1966;115:422–3.
174. Killam KF, Killam EK, Naquet R. An animal model of light sensitive epilepsy. Electroencephalogr Clin Neurophysiol. 1967;22:497–513.
175. Löscher W. Genetic animal models of epilepsy BT – genetically defined animal models of neurobehavioral dysfunctions. In: Driscoll P, editor. . Boston: Birkhäuser Boston; 1992. p. 111–35.
176. Wada JA, Naquet R. Proceedings: examination of neural mechanism involved in photogenic seizure susceptibility in epileptic Senegalese baboon: Papio papio. Epilepsia. 1972;13:344–5.
177. Gawel K, Langlois M, Martins T, van der Ent W, Tiraboschi E, Jacmin M, et al. Seizing the moment: zebrafish epilepsy models. Neurosci Biobehav Rev. 2020;116:1–20.
178. Griffin A, Hamling KR, Knupp K, Hong S, Lee LP, Baraban SC. Clemizole and modulators of serotonin signalling suppress seizures in Dravet syndrome. Brain. 2017;140:669–83.
179. Eimon PM, Ghannad-Rezaie M, De Rienzo G, Allalou A, Wu Y, Gao M, et al. Brain activity patterns in high-throughput electrophysiology screen predict both drug efficacies and side effects. Nat Commun. 2018;9:219.
180. Yaksi E, Jamali A, Diaz Verdugo C, Jurisch-Yaksi N. Past, present and future of zebrafish in epilepsy research. FEBS J. 2021;288:7243–55.
181. Baraban SC, Dinday MT, Hortopan GA. Drug screening in Scn1a zebrafish mutant identifies clemizole as a potential Dravet syndrome treatment. Nat Commun. 2013;4:2410.
182. Hortopan GA, Dinday MT, Baraban SC. Spontaneous seizures and altered gene expression in GABA signaling pathways in a mind bomb mutant zebrafish. J Neurosci. 2010;30:13718–28.

183. Ramirez IB-R, Pietka G, Jones DR, Divecha N, Alia A, Baraban SC, et al. Impaired neural development in a zebrafish model for Lowe syndrome. Hum Mol Genet. 2012;21:1744–59.
184. Perenthaler E, Nikoncuk A, Yousefi S, Berdowski WM, Alsagob M, Capo I, et al. Loss of UGP2 in brain leads to a severe epileptic encephalopathy, emphasizing that bi-allelic isoform-specific start-loss mutations of essential genes can cause genetic diseases. Acta Neuropathol. 2020;139:415–42.
185. Liao M, Kundap U, Rosch RE, Burrows DRW, Meyer MP, Ouled Amar Bencheikh B, et al. Targeted knockout of GABA-A receptor gamma 2 subunit provokes transient light-induced reflex seizures in zebrafish larvae. Dis Model Mech. 2019:12.
186. Becker AJ. Review: animal models of acquired epilepsy: insights into mechanisms of human epileptogenesis. Neuropathol Appl Neurobiol. 2018;44:112–29.
187. Kharatishvili I, Immonen R, Gröhn O, Pitkänen A. Quantitative diffusion MRI of hippocampus as a surrogate marker for post-traumatic epileptogenesis. Brain. 2007;130:3155–68.
188. Pitkänen A, Immonen RJ, Gröhn OHJ, Kharatishvili I. From traumatic brain injury to post-traumatic epilepsy: what animal models tell us about the process and treatment options. Epilepsia. 2009;50(Suppl 2):21–9.
189. Mosini AC, Calió ML, Foresti ML, Valeriano RPS, Garzon E, Mello LE. Modeling of post-traumatic epilepsy and experimental research aimed at its prevention. Brazilian J Med Biol Res = Rev Bras Pesqui Medicas e Biol. 2020;54:e10656.
190. D'Ambrosio R, Fender JS, Fairbanks JP, Simon EA, Born DE, Doyle DL, et al. Progression from frontal-parietal to mesial-temporal epilepsy after fluid percussion injury in the rat. Brain. 2005;128:174–88.
191. Kharatishvili I, Nissinen JP, McIntosh TK, Pitkänen A. A model of posttraumatic epilepsy induced by lateral fluid-percussion brain injury in rats. Neuroscience. 2006;140:685–97.
192. Keith KA, Huang JH. Animal models of post-traumatic epilepsy. Diagnostics (Basel, Switzerland). 2019:10.
193. Lighthall JW. Controlled cortical impact: a new experimental brain injury model. J Neurotrauma. 1988;5:1–15.
194. Xiong Y, Mahmood A, Chopp M. Animal models of traumatic brain injury. Nat Rev Neurosci. 2013;14:128–42.
195. Leo A, De Caro C, Nesci V, Tallarico M, De Sarro G, Russo E, et al. Modeling poststroke epilepsy and preclinical development of drugs for poststroke epilepsy. Epilepsy Behav. 2020;104:106472.
196. Barker-Haliski ML, Heck TD, Dahle EJ, Vanegas F, Pruess TH, Wilcox KS, et al. Acute treatment with minocycline, but not valproic acid, improves long-term behavioral outcomes in the Theiler's virus model of temporal lobe epilepsy. Epilepsia. 2016;57:1958–67.
197. Buckingham SC, Ramos TN, Barnum SR. Complement C5-deficient mice are protected from seizures in experimental cerebral malaria. Epilepsia. 2014;55:e139–42.
198. Nilsen KE, Walker MC, Cock HR. Characterization of the tetanus toxin model of refractory focal neocortical epilepsy in the rat. Epilepsia. 2005;46:179–87.
199. Javaid MS, Tan T, Dvir N, Anderson A, O'Brien JT, Kwan P, et al. Human in vitro models of epilepsy using embryonic and induced pluripotent stem cells. Cells. 2022;11:3957.
200. Grainger AI, King MC, Nagel DA, Parri HR, Coleman MD, Hill EJ. In vitro models for seizure-liability testing using induced pluripotent stem cells. Front Neurosci. 2018;12:590.
201. Loscher W, Klein P. New approaches for developing multi-targeted drug combinations for disease modification of complex brain disorders. Does epilepsy prevention become a realistic goal? Pharmacol Ther. 2021:107934.
202. French JA, Perucca E. Time to start calling things by their own names? The case for Antiseizure medicines. Epilepsy Curr. 2020;20(2):69–72.
203. Chen Z, et al. Treatment outcomes in patients with newly diagnosed epilepsy treated with established and new antiepileptic drugs: a 30-year longitudinal cohort study. JAMA Neurol. 2018;75(3):279–86.
204. Devinsky O, et al. Epilepsy. Nat Rev Dis Primers. 2018;4:18024.

205. Johannessen Landmark C, et al. Pharmacological aspects of antiseizure medications: from basic mechanisms to clinical considerations of drug interactions and use of therapeutic drug monitoring. Epileptic Disord. 2023;25(4):454–71.
206. Catterall WA. Forty years of sodium channels: structure, function, pharmacology, and epilepsy. Neurochem Res. 2017;42(9):2495–504.
207. Silva J. Slow inactivation of Na(+) channels. Handb Exp Pharmacol. 2014;221:33–49.
208. Kwan P, et al. Definition of drug resistant epilepsy: consensus proposal by the ad hoc task force of the ILAE commission on therapeutic strategies. Epilepsia. 2010;51(6):1069–77.
209. Pal R, et al. Voltage gated sodium channel inhibitors as anticonvulsant drugs: a systematic review on recent developments and structure activity relationship studies. Bioorg Chem. 2021;115:105230.
210. Roberti R, et al. Pharmacology of Cenobamate: mechanism of action, pharmacokinetics, Drug-Drug Interactions and Tolerability. CNS Drugs. 2021;35(6):609–18.
211. Schwarz JR, Grigat G. Phenytoin and carbamazepine: potential- and frequency-dependent block of Na currents in mammalian myelinated nerve fibers. Epilepsia. 1989;30(3):286–94.
212. Macdonald RL, Kelly KM. Antiepileptic drug mechanisms of action. Epilepsia. 1995;36(Suppl 2):S2–12.
213. Rogawski MA, et al. Current understanding of the mechanism of action of the antiepileptic drug lacosamide. Epilepsy Res. 2015;110:189–205.
214. Catterall WA. Voltage-gated calcium channels. Cold Spring Harb Perspect Biol. 2011;3(8):a003947.
215. Sills GJ, Rogawski MA. Mechanisms of action of currently used antiseizure drugs. Neuropharmacology. 2020;168:107966.
216. Trimmer JS, Rhodes KJ. Localization of voltage-gated ion channels in mammalian brain. Annu Rev Physiol. 2004;66:477–519.
217. Suzuki S, Rogawski MA. T-type calcium channels mediate the transition between tonic and phasic firing in thalamic neurons. Proc Natl Acad Sci USA. 1989;86(18):7228–32.
218. Myers KA, et al. Contribution of rare genetic variants to drug response in absence epilepsy. Epilepsy Res. 2021;170:106537.
219. Casillas-Espinosa PM, et al. Effects of the T-type calcium channel Ca(V)3.2 R1584P mutation on absence seizure susceptibility in GAERS and NEC congenic rats models. Neurobiol Dis. 2023;184:106217.
220. Kim D, et al. Lack of the burst firing of thalamocortical relay neurons and resistance to absence seizures in mice lacking alpha(1G) T-type Ca(2+) channels. Neuron. 2001;31(1):35–45.
221. Thorpe AJ, Offord J. The alpha2-delta protein: an auxiliary subunit of voltage-dependent calcium channels as a recognized drug target. Curr Opin Investig Drugs. 2010;11(7):761–70.
222. Dooley DJ, et al. Ca2+ channel alpha2delta ligands: novel modulators of neurotransmission. Trends Pharmacol Sci. 2007;28(2):75–82.
223. Wang SJ, et al. Presynaptic inhibition of excitatory neurotransmission by lamotrigine in the rat amygdalar neurons. Synapse. 1996;24(3):248–55.
224. Wang SJ, et al. Inhibition of N-type calcium currents by lamotrigine in rat amygdalar neurones. Neuroreport. 1996;7(18):3037–40.
225. Stefani A, Spadoni F, Bernardi G. Voltage-activated calcium channels: targets of antiepileptic drug therapy? Epilepsia. 1997;38(9):959–65.
226. Musella S, et al. Beyond Retigabine: design, synthesis, and pharmacological characterization of a potent and chemically stable neuronal Kv7 channel activator with anticonvulsant activity. J Med Chem. 2022;65(16):11340–64.
227. Zahra A, et al. Identifying the mechanism of action of the Kv7 channel opener, retigabine in the treatment of epilepsy. Neurol Sci. 2023;44:3819.
228. Gunthorpe MJ, Large CH, Sankar R. The mechanism of action of retigabine (ezogabine), a first-in-class K+ channel opener for the treatment of epilepsy. Epilepsia. 2012;53(3):412–24.
229. Plosker GL. Perampanel: as adjunctive therapy in patients with partial-onset seizures. CNS Drugs. 2012;26(12):1085–96.

230. Rogawski MA. Revisiting AMPA receptors as an antiepileptic drug target. Epilepsy Curr. 2011;11(2):56–63.
231. Sobolevsky AI. Structure and gating of tetrameric glutamate receptors. J Physiol. 2015;593(1):29–38.
232. Lerma J, Marques JM. Kainate receptors in health and disease. Neuron. 2013;80(2):292–311.
233. Rodriguez-Moreno A, Herreras O, Lerma J. Kainate receptors presynaptically downregulate GABAergic inhibition in the rat hippocampus. Neuron. 1997;19(4):893–901.
234. Rheims S, Ryvlin P. Profile of perampanel and its potential in the treatment of partial onset seizures. Neuropsychiatr Dis Treat. 2013;9:629–37.
235. Rohracher A, et al. Perampanel in routine clinical use across Europe: pooled, multicenter, observational data. Epilepsia. 2018;59(9):1727–39.
236. Krauss GL, et al. Final safety, tolerability, and seizure outcomes in patients with focal epilepsy treated with adjunctive perampanel for up to 4 years in an open-label extension of phase III randomized trials: study 307. Epilepsia. 2018;59(4):866–76.
237. Krauss GL, et al. Long-term safety of perampanel and seizure outcomes in refractory partial-onset seizures and secondarily generalized seizures: results from phase III extension study 307. Epilepsia. 2014;55(7):1058–68.
238. Krauss GL, et al. Randomized phase III study 306: adjunctive perampanel for refractory partial-onset seizures. Neurology. 2012;78(18):1408–15.
239. Yelshanskaya MV, et al. Structural bases of noncompetitive inhibition of AMPA-subtype ionotropic glutamate receptors by antiepileptic drugs. Neuron. 2016;91(6):1305–15.
240. Rogawski MA. AMPA receptors as a molecular target in epilepsy therapy. Acta Neurol Scand Suppl. 2013;197:9–18.
241. Kleckner NW, et al. Subtype-selective antagonism of N-methyl-D-aspartate receptors by felbamate: insights into the mechanism of action. J Pharmacol Exp Ther. 1999;289(2):886–94.
242. Hanrahan B, Carson RP. Felbamate. In: StatPearls; 2023. Treasure Island (FL) ineligible companies. Disclosure: Robert Carson declares no relevant financial relationships with ineligible companies.
243. Gibbs JW 3rd, et al. Cellular actions of topiramate: blockade of kainate-evoked inward currents in cultured hippocampal neurons. Epilepsia. 2000;41(S1):10–6.
244. Pearl NZ, et al. Narrative review of Topiramate: clinical uses and pharmacological considerations. Adv Ther. 2023;40(9):3626–38.
245. Meehan AL, et al. A new mechanism for antiepileptic drug action: vesicular entry may mediate the effects of levetiracetam. J Neurophysiol. 2011;106(3):1227–39.
246. Yang XF, Weisenfeld A, Rothman SM. Prolonged exposure to levetiracetam reveals a presynaptic effect on neurotransmission. Epilepsia. 2007;48(10):1861–9.
247. Meehan AL, et al. Levetiracetam has an activity-dependent effect on inhibitory transmission. Epilepsia. 2012;53(3):469–76.
248. Yang XF, Rothman SM. Levetiracetam has a time- and stimulation-dependent effect on synaptic transmission. Seizure. 2009;18(9):615–9.
249. Birnstiel S, Wulfert E, Beck SG. Levetiracetam (ucb LO59) affects in vitro models of epilepsy in CA3 pyramidal neurons without altering normal synaptic transmission. Naunyn Schmiedeberg's Arch Pharmacol. 1997;356(5):611–8.
250. Yang X, et al. Brivaracetam augments short-term depression and slows vesicle recycling. Epilepsia. 2015;56(12):1899–909.
251. Klitgaard H, et al. Brivaracetam: rationale for discovery and preclinical profile of a selective SV2A ligand for epilepsy treatment. Epilepsia. 2016;57(4):538–48.
252. Deng Y, et al. A comparison of extracellular excitatory amino acids release inhibition of acute lamotrigine and topiramate treatment in the hippocampus of PTZ-kindled epileptic rats. J Biomed Nanotechnol. 2013;9(6):1123–8.
253. Sigel E, Steinmann ME. Structure, function, and modulation of GABA(a) receptors. J Biol Chem. 2012;287(48):40224–31.

254. Chebib M, Johnston GA. The 'ABC' of GABA receptors: a brief review. Clin Exp Pharmacol Physiol. 1999;26(11):937–40.
255. Belelli D, et al. Extrasynaptic GABAA receptors: form, pharmacology, and function. J Neurosci. 2009;29(41):12757–63.
256. Mott DD, Lewis DV. The pharmacology and function of central GABAB receptors. Int Rev Neurobiol. 1994;36:97–223.
257. Bhagat K, et al. Rational approaches for the design of various GABA modulators and their clinical progression. Mol Divers. 2021;25(1):551–601.
258. Kowalczyk P, Kulig K. GABA system as a target for new drugs. Curr Med Chem. 2014;21(28):3294–309.
259. Liu R, et al. Role of NKCC1 and KCC2 in epilepsy: from expression to function. Front Neurol. 2019;10:1407.
260. Rho JM, Donevan SD, Rogawski MA. Direct activation of GABAA receptors by barbiturates in cultured rat hippocampal neurons. J Physiol. 1996;497(Pt 2):509–22.
261. Twyman RE, Rogers CJ, Macdonald RL. Differential regulation of gamma-aminobutyric acid receptor channels by diazepam and phenobarbital. Ann Neurol. 1989;25(3):213–20.
262. Ticku MK, Davis WC. Effect of valproic acid on [3H]diazepam and [3H]dihydropicrotoxinin binding sites at the benzodiazepine-GABA receptor-ionophore complex. Brain Res. 1981;223(1):218–22.
263. Loscher W. Effects of the antiepileptic drug valproate on metabolism and function of inhibitory and excitatory amino acids in the brain. Neurochem Res. 1993;18(4):485–502.
264. Grant SM, Heel RC, Vigabatrin. A review of its pharmacodynamic and pharmacokinetic properties, and therapeutic potential in epilepsy and disorders of motor control. Drugs. 1991;41(6):889–926.
265. Borden LA, et al. Tiagabine, SK&F 89976-a, CI-966, and NNC-711 are selective for the cloned GABA transporter GAT-1. Eur J Pharmacol. 1994;269(2):219–24.
266. Meldrum BS, Chapman AG. Basic mechanisms of gabitril (tiagabine) and future potential developments. Epilepsia. 1999;40(Suppl 9):S2–6.
267. Suzdak PD, Jansen JA. A review of the preclinical pharmacology of tiagabine: a potent and selective anticonvulsant GABA uptake inhibitor. Epilepsia. 1995;36(6):612–26.
268. Ozsoy HZ. Anticonvulsant effects of carbonic anhydrase inhibitors: the enigmatic link between carbonic anhydrases and electrical activity of the brain. Neurochem Res. 2021;46(11):2783–99.
269. Ciccone L, et al. Carbonic anhydrase inhibitors and epilepsy: state of the art and future perspectives. Molecules. 2021;26(21)
270. Shukralla AA, Dolan E, Delanty N. Acetazolamide: old drug, new evidence? Epilepsia Open. 2022;7(3):378–92.
271. Reiss WG, Oles KS. Acetazolamide in the treatment of seizures. Ann Pharmacother. 1996;30(5):514–9.
272. Villanueva V, Serrano-Castro PJ. Zonisamide in the epilepsy treatment: a literature review from add-on therapy to monotherapy. Rev Neurol. 2013;56(8):429–38.
273. Supuran CT. An update on drug interaction considerations in the therapeutic use of carbonic anhydrase inhibitors. Expert Opin Drug Metab Toxicol. 2020;16(4):297–307.
274. Lechuga L, Franz DN. Everolimus as adjunctive therapy for tuberous sclerosis complex-associated partial-onset seizures. Expert Rev Neurother. 2019;19(10):913–25.
275. Krueger DA, et al. Everolimus treatment of refractory epilepsy in tuberous sclerosis complex. Ann Neurol. 2013;74(5):679–87.
276. Menezes CEG, et al. Everolimus as a therapeutic option in refractory epilepsy in children with tuberous sclerosis: a systematic review. Arq Neuropsiquiatr. 2023;81(4):392–8.
277. Moloney PB, et al. Everolimus precision therapy for the GATOR1-related epilepsies: a case series. Eur J Neurol. 2023;30(10):3341–6.
278. Lattanzi S, et al. Efficacy and safety of adjunctive Cannabidiol in patients with Lennox-Gastaut syndrome: a systematic review and meta-analysis. CNS Drugs. 2018;32(10):905–16.

279. Kuhne F, et al. Real-world data on cannabidiol treatment of various epilepsy subtypes: a retrospective, multicenter study. Epilepsia Open. 2023;8(2):360–70.
280. Devi N, et al. Short-term and long-term efficacy and safety of antiseizure medications in Lennox Gastaut syndrome: a network meta-analysis. Seizure. 2022;99:164–75.
281. Abu-Sawwa R, et al. Effects of Epidiolex(R) (Cannabidiol) on seizure-related emergency department visits and hospital admissions: a retrospective cohort study. Epilepsy Behav. 2022;127:108538.
282. Mirlohi S, et al. Inhibition of human recombinant T-type calcium channels by phytocannabinoids in vitro. Br J Pharmacol. 2022;179(15):4031–43.
283. Ji X, Zeng Y, Wu J. The CB(2) receptor as a novel therapeutic target for epilepsy treatment. Int J Mol Sci. 2021;22(16)
284. Nakamura M, et al. Effects of cenobamate (YKP3089), a newly developed anti-epileptic drug, on voltage-gated sodium channels in rat hippocampal CA3 neurons. Eur J Pharmacol. 2019;855:175–82.
285. Sharma R, et al. Positive allosteric modulation of GABA(a) receptors by a novel antiepileptic drug cenobamate. Eur J Pharmacol. 2020;879:173117.
286. Barbieri MA, et al. Cenobamate: a review of its pharmacological properties, clinical efficacy and tolerability profile in the treatment of epilepsy. CNS Neurol Disord Drug Targets. 2023;22(3):394–403.
287. Lamb YN. Ganaxolone: first approval. Drugs. 2022;82(8):933–40.
288. Nohria V, Giller E. Ganaxolone. Neurotherapeutics. 2007;4(1):102–5.
289. Perucca E, et al. 30 years of second-generation antiseizure medications: impact and future perspectives. Lancet Neurol. 2020;19(6):544–56.
290. Glauser T, et al. Updated ILAE evidence review of antiepileptic drug efficacy and effectiveness as initial monotherapy for epileptic seizures and syndromes. Epilepsia. 2013;54(3):551–63.
291. Baulac M, et al. Efficacy, safety, and tolerability of lacosamide monotherapy versus controlled-release carbamazepine in patients with newly diagnosed epilepsy: a phase 3, randomised, double-blind, non-inferiority trial. Lancet Neurol. 2017;16(1):43–54.
292. Galanopoulou AS, et al. Antiepileptogenesis and disease modification: Progress, challenges, and the path forward-report of the preclinical working group of the 2018 NINDS-sponsored antiepileptogenesis and disease modification workshop. Epilepsia Open. 2021;6(2):276–96.
293. Galanopoulou AS, et al. Joint AES/ILAE translational workshop to optimize preclinical epilepsy research. Epilepsia. 2013;54(Suppl 4):1–2.

Chapter 2
Antiseizure Medications

Wei Jing, Meizhen Sun, and Chao Yan

2.1 Commonly Used Antiseizure Medications

2.1.1 First-Generation Antiseizure Medications (ASMs)

2.1.1.1 Carbamazepine

Drug Characteristics

[Chemical name] 5H-Dibenzo[b,f]azepine-5-formamide

[Chemical structure formula]

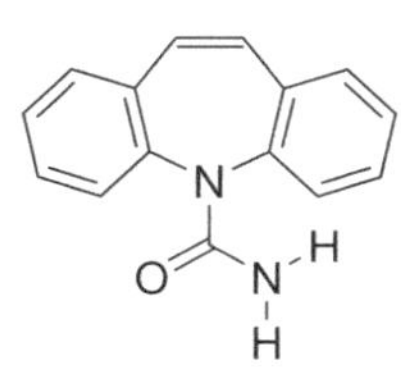

W. Jing (✉)
Shanxi Bethune Hospital, Shanxi Academy of Medical Sciences, Third Hospital of Shanxi Medical University, Tongji Shanxi Hospital, Taiyuan, Shanxi, China

M. Sun
Department of Neurology, The First Hospital of Shanxi Medical University, Taiyuan, Shanxi, China

C. Yan
Nanjing University, School of Life Sciences, Department of Physiology, Nanjing, Jiangsu, China

X. Wang, L. Zhou (eds.), *Pharmacological Treatment of Epileptic Seizures*,
https://doi.org/10.1007/978-981-96-8520-2_2

[Molecular formula] C15H12N2O

[Molecular weight] 236.27

[Indications] This compound is widely utilized for epilepsy and neuralgia treatment, and its application can be extended to diabetes insipidus, muscle tension disorders, schizophrenia, and emotional ailments. It effectively addresses diverse forms of epilepsy, trigeminal and glossopharyngeal neuralgia, diabetes insipidus, muscular tension, schizophrenia, and emotional disorders.

[Specifications]
Tablets: 100 mg and 200 mg doses
Sustained-release tablets: 200 mg dose
Capsules: 200 mg dose

[Usage and dosage] For adults, the initial dosage ranges from 100 to 200 mg once or twice daily. The dose is gradually titrated to achieve optimal efficacy, typically reaching 400 mg/dose, taken two to three times daily, up to a maximum of 1600 mg/day for some patients. For children, 10–20 mg/kg daily is administered based on body weight. For patients less than 12 months of age, the starting dose is 100–200 mg daily; for patients aged 1–5 years, 200–400 mg daily; for patients aged 6–10 years, 400–600 mg daily; and for patients aged 11–15 years, 600–1000 mg daily in divided doses. For children aged 4 or younger, 20–60 mg daily is the initial dose, increasing by 20–60 mg every other day. For those older than 4 years, the initial dose may be 100 mg daily, increasing by 100 mg weekly.

[Adverse reactions] Adverse central nervous system reactions such as dizziness, headache, ataxia, lethargy, fatigue, and double vision may occur. Additionally, gastrointestinal discomfort, such as nausea and vomiting, and skin allergic reactions are possible side effects.

Clinical Application and Basic Research

The History of Carbamazepine

The history of carbamazepine (CBZ) began in 1953 when it was discovered by Swiss chemist Walter Schindler, leading to its commercial release in 1962. Its antiepileptic properties were first described by M. Tchicaloff in 1963 [1]; J. D. Spillane revealed its efficacy in treating trigeminal neuralgia in 1964 [2], while M. Donner reported its benefits in treating epilepsy and psychiatric symptoms in children and adolescents in 1965 [3]. In 1967, V E Fernandez et al. discovered its pharmacological effects [4], and in 1968, T. H. Redpath et al. reported its side effects [5]. In 2022, Roberto Santalucia et al. expanded its electroclinical phenotype for SLC13A5-associated disorders, confirming the safety and efficacy of CBZ in nonstructural early-onset epilepsy [6]. In 2024, Rashid HU et al. identified an association between

ABCB1 gene polymorphisms and the clinical response to CBZ monotherapy in epilepsy patients [7].

Antiepileptic Effect of Carbamazepine

In a study of the antiepileptic effect of CBZ, P. Brittany et al. assessed the antiepileptic effects of CBZ in adults. The authors evaluated its pharmacology, pharmacokinetics, efficacy, safety, dosage, administration methods, potential drug interactions, and therapeutic application. Intravenous CBZ administration serves as a temporary alternative therapy for adult epilepsy patients. Pooling data from a phase 1 trial and two open-label bioavailability studies comparing its effects via oral and intravenous routes of administration, no significant loss of seizure control was observed in patients who switched to intravenous CBZ administration for short-term use. The recommended intravenous dose is 70% of the oral dose and is infused for 30 min every 6 h. Adverse effects were similar to those seen following oral administration, except for increased infusion site reactions. Intravenous CBZ administration is a viable option for adults who are unable to tolerate oral therapy for up to 7 days after oral stabilization, although its use is limited by unknown costs and unavailability in the United States [8]. Additionally, Roberto et al. described a case of a child with a recessive mutation in the SLC13A5 gene causing developmental and epileptic encephalopathy. Early administration of CBZ significantly improved clinical and EEG features in this patient, expanding the understanding of SLC13A5-associated disease and confirming the efficacy and safety of CBZ in treating nonstructural early-onset epilepsy [7].

Studies of Carbamazepine in Special Populations

Ivana Kacirova and colleagues conducted a cohort study to explore the transport of CBZ and its active metabolite, 10,11-epoxide, in mature breast milk and breastfed infants. They observed a highly significant correlation between the levels of CBZ and 10,11-epoxide in both maternal serum and breast milk. When enzyme-induced ASMs were concurrently administered, there was a substantial increase of approximately 130% in the apparent maternal clearance of orally administered CBZ. Combining CBZ treatment with valproic acid resulted in a significant increase in epoxide levels in both breast milk and maternal serum, but this had no impact on breastfed infants. Their findings indicated that the concentration of CBZ in breastfed infants did not reach the lower therapeutic threshold observed in the general epilepsy population, and most epoxide concentrations remained below the lower limit of quantification [9]. Wei Xu et al. conducted a retrospective study to evaluate CBZ misuse, disease duration, and associated health issues among adolescents in China. The median overdose threshold for CBZ was found to be 2000 mg (range from 800 to 5000 mg). The majority of patients resided in urban and suburban areas (76.47% and 52.94%, respectively) exhibited academic performance indicators in the lowest third percentile (52.94%) and lacked parental supervision. Notably, 35.29% of the subjects reported significant euphoria. Neurological symptoms were universal, with six (35.29%) patients experiencing coma (GCS < 8) and five (29.41%) enduring convulsions. Hemodialysis was administered to five patients. Although there was a trend toward a greater incidence of CBZ misuse in younger individuals with repeated usage and lacking parental oversight compared to first-time users (7/4 vs. 10/3428), this disparity was not statistically significant. Repeat users demonstrated a significantly elevated toxic dose of 1035 ± 1470 mg, contrasting with the 646 ± 0 mg dose found in first-time users ($p = 0.001$). The euphoric effects of CBZ may predispose adolescents to its misuse and subsequent overdose. It is imperative to educate vulnerable youth about the dangers of CBZ abuse and overdose to prevent future health complications [10]. Epilepsy, a chronic medical condition, often accompanies adverse physical effects due to either the condition itself or its prolonged treatment. Accurate prediction of oral drug pharmacokinetics in children is crucial for optimizing pediatric drug efficacy and safety. Physiologically based pharmacokinetic (PBPK) models play a key role in this endeavor. However, gaps in our understanding of age-related physiological and anatomical changes hinder the application of these tools. This study aimed to explore age-related disparities in the oral absorption of CBZ, a low-solubility compound, across children, infants, and newborns. Philip et al. developed an oral absorption model using GastroPlus, validated its extrapolation to younger age groups using clinical data, and conducted sensitivity analyses on uncertain model parameters. Their findings underscore the significance of age-specific physiological parameters, particularly clearance, in achieving accurate simulation results. Sensitivity analysis revealed that CBZ absorption was influenced by factors such as solubility, particle size, small intestine transit time, age group, and CBZ dosage. However, in vitro dissolution experiments employing the suggested pediatric biorelevant media exhibited no substantial age-related variations in dissolution kinetics. An improved understanding of oral absorption in pediatric patients is imperative for enhancing exposure prediction accuracy in children and bolstering confidence in oral biopharmaceutical tools [11]. Yuka Miyata-Nozaka et al. enrolled a cohort of 288 epilepsy patients from Malaysia, 63 of whom were prescribed CBZ monotherapy and 85 of whom received valproic acid monotherapy. Notably, none of the patients exhibited drug allergy syndrome. Using the Sequenom MassARRAY genotyping platform, the subject genotypes were determined. This study revealed a significant association between the CYP3A5 rs776746 polymorphism and the response to CBZ treatment ($p = 0.026$), particularly within the Malay subgroup ($p = 0.006$). Furthermore, a modest yet noteworthy correlation was observed between the CYP3A5 rs776746 polymorphism and the response to CBZ treatment among the Malaysian population. Similarly, the CYP3A5 rs776746 polymorphism exhibited an association with the valproic acid response across all patients ($p = 0.037$) and specifically within the Malay population ($p = 0.05$) [12]. In a study, examining challenging-to-treat early-onset epilepsy linked to mutations in the sodium channel 2 subunit alpha (SCN2A), Tatjana Welzel and colleagues described an infant with SCN2A epilepsy who transitioned from phenytoin to CBZ therapy to mitigate potential long-term neurotoxic effects. The transition from high-dose phenytoin (20 mg/kg/day, concentration: ≥20 mg/L) to CBZ (50–75 mg/kg/day, concentration: 9–12 mg/L) treatment during ketogenic diet therapy lasted 85 days, possibly due to significant drug–drug and/or drug–food interactions. Pharmacokinetic modeling analysis indicated that phenytoin-induced CYP3A4 activity, while the CBZ concentration also influenced self-induction, resulting in an apparent clearance time increase of 2.5- to three-fold. Modeling suggested that lower CBZ concentrations were associated with reduced relative bioavailability (44%) during the ketogenic diet, potentially due to decreased absorption (less favorable for this lipophilic drug), heightened intestinal/liver metabolism, and/or reduced binding to ketogenic diet-associated proteins. These findings underscore the importance of monitoring CBZ concentrations during its introduction/removal and highlight the necessity for high CBZ doses to achieve therapeutic levels, particularly in infants undergoing high-dose phenytoin treatment [13].

Side Effects of Carbamazepine

The focus of an observational study led by Bianca Berghuis et al. was on investigating the correlation between adverse reactions in individuals prescribed CBZ or oxcarbazepine and hyponatremia caused by these medications. Data on serum sodium levels and adverse effects were collected from 1370 epilepsy patients treated with CBZ or oxcarbazepine (OXC) between 2017 and 2019. Hyponatremia was defined as sodium levels ≤134 mEq/L, with severe hyponatremia ≤128 mEq/L. Among these patients, 410 had a history of hyponatremia. Symptoms associated with CBZ and OXC use were analyzed in 710 patients (410 with hyponatremia and 300 without), yielding relevant information for 688 patients. This study revealed that 65% of patients with hyponatremia experienced adverse reactions, while 21% of those with normal sodium levels experienced adverse reactions (OR = 7.5, $P \leq 0.001$). Additionally, 83% of patients with severe hyponatremia and 55% with mild hyponatremia experienced adverse reactions ($P \leq 0.001$). Notably, significant predictors of adverse reactions included the number of drugs (OXC vs. CBZ) and concurrent ASMs used. Symptoms such as vertigo (28% vs. 6%), fatigue (22% vs. 7%), instability (19% vs. 3%), and diplopia (16% vs. 4%) were more prevalent in the hyponatremia group than in patients with normal sodium levels. Researchers have concluded that patients with hyponatremia face a sevenfold increased risk of adverse reactions during treatment, emphasizing the importance of clinicians considering sodium levels when prescribing CBZ and OXC [14]. Chan-Wei Pan et al. described a case of CBZ-induced hypersensitivity syndrome in a 35-year-old patient with schizophrenia. Despite lacking previous food or drug allergies and testing negative for the HLA-B1502 genotype, the patient developed high fever (39.4 °C), leukopenia (1670/mm^3), proteinuria, and bilateral pulmonary field infiltration after 19 days of CBZ exposure. These adverse conditions were resolved upon discontinuation of CBZ treatment. This case underscores the relevance of genetic predispositions beyond HLA-B1502 in drug-induced hypersensitivity syndrome [15]. Sherifa et al. conducted a study to assess cochlear function in patients with idiopathic epilepsy following treatment with CBZ. The subjects included 47 patients (mean age 34.56 ± 7.11 years, duration 17.84 ± 7.21 years) and 40 healthy controls. Patients underwent pure tone audiometry and transient evoked otoacoustic emission (TEOAE) analysis. One-third of the patients experienced hearing loss, predominantly mild bilateral loss. Compared to the control group, patients exhibited reduced TEOAE amplitudes, particularly at higher frequencies (3 and 4 kHz). The TEOAE amplitudes showed significant negative correlations with CBZ dosages (3 kHz: $r = -0.554$, $p = 0.008$; 4 kHz: $r = -0.347$, $p = 0.01$), serum concentrations (4 kHz: $r = -0.280$, $p = 0.045$), and treatment durations (3 kHz: $r = -0.392$, $p = 0.008$; 4 kHz: $r = -0.542$, $p = 0.001$). The study concluded that prolonged CBZ usage might result in cochlear dysfunction and hearing impairment [16]. In their study, Caibing Xu et al. identified a total of 1231 reports of Stevens-Johnson syndrome or toxic epidermal necrolysis associated with CBZ or oxcarbazepine. Among these, 1048 cases were linked to CBZ use, comprising 668 cases of Stevens-Johnson syndrome and 380 cases of toxic epidermal necrolysis. Additionally, 183 reports were associated with oxcarbazepine use, including 142 cases of Stevens-Johnson syndrome and 41 cases of toxic epidermal necrolysis. The study revealed a greater risk of Stevens-Johnson syndrome than of toxic epidermal necrolysis, with CBZ use posing a greater risk than that of oxcarbazepine. These findings support clinical observations and underscore the importance of further clinical investigations into Stevens-Johnson syndrome and toxic epidermal necrolysis linked to CBZ or oxcarbazepine use [17]. Wong CSM et al. identified the HLA-B15:11 genotype as a potential risk factor for severe cutaneous adverse drug reactions in Chinese CBZ users negative for the HLA-B15:02 genotype. They recommended additional screening for HLA-B15:11 genotype status in HLA-B15:02-negative patients to mitigate the risk of adverse skin reactions [18]. Ohta K et al. presented a case involving an 11-year-old girl who experienced spontaneous and stimulus-induced focal motor seizures following an overdose of CBZ. The patient had been receiving CBZ (150 mg daily) treatment for focal epilepsy since the age of 6. At 11, she inadvertently consumed 10 CBZ pills (totaling a dose of 1000 mg) in lieu of her normal morning dose, leading to a generalized seizure. Upon arrival at the hospital, she was in a comatose state. She presented with focal to bilateral tonic–clonic seizures triggered by painful stimuli or occurring spontaneously, with focal epileptoid discharge evident on EEG. Her blood CBZ concentration was 40.4 μg/mL, confirming CBZ overdose. Remarkably, the patient's condition improved without specific intervention, and she was discharged without neurological complications. The study concluded that while generalized seizures from CBZ overdose often result in fatal outcomes or necessitate intensive care, the presence of focal seizures induced by stimuli may signify a favorable prognosis for CBZ overdose [19]. Baylis S et al. demonstrated that the combination of continuous venovenous hemofiltration (CVVH) and resin hemoperfusion therapy reduced CBZ levels by 50% within 3 h, from 16 mg/L to 8 mg/L. This approach facilitated a significantly faster CBZ clearance rate than CVVH alone or without in vitro drug elimination during the initial hours. The combined therapy effectively eliminated nearly 35 mg/h CBZ. The study concluded that the combined approach of continuous renal replacement therapy and hemoperfusion is simple to administer, considered safe, and synergistically enhances CBZ clearance by leveraging the efficacy of each modality [20]. Ran D et al. described a case involving a 70-year-old Chinese man who developed pruritic follicular papules and erythema on the trunk and limbs, along with facial, lip, and ear edema and erythema, over a span of 3 days. Initially, the lesions presented as facial edema and erythema, followed by the formation of follicular papules on the body and limbs. The patient experienced no other symptoms. The rash emerged 5 days after initiating CBZ therapy at an oral dose of 100 mg twice daily for trigeminal neuralgia. CBZ treatment was promptly discontinued upon onset of rash. There was no recent history of infection, underlying conditions, or concurrent medication use. Rapid resolution of symptoms ensued following CBZ cessation and administration of systemic corticosteroids. This case underscores the importance of recognizing this rare CBZ-induced rash, known as follicular mucosal disease, and prompting clinicians to remain vigilant for its occurrence [21]. Sarah Perrot et al. described a case of rapidly evolving cerebellar syndrome in a patient with epilepsy after CBZ administration. Serial MRI scans revealed progressive T2/fluid-attenuated inversion recovery signal abnormalities in the posterior fossa, accompanied by enhancement. Routine cerebrospinal fluid analysis was unremarkable. The presence of JC virus DNA in the cerebrospinal fluid confirmed progressive multifocal leukoencephalopathy (PML). The sole immune abnormalities detected were hypogammaglobulinemia and chronic lymphocytopenia. Following discontinuation of CBZ treatment, lymphocyte counts and immunoglobulin levels normalized, and the PML resolved with clinical improvement. The patient did not receive PML-specific treatment. The authors hypothesize that CBZ-induced mild immunosuppression sustained PML and that the discontinuation of CBZ restored immune function, leading to PML resolution. ASMs-associated effects on immune function and infection risk may exacerbate epilepsy-associated morbidity and mortality. Further investigations are warranted to elucidate the prevalence of immune dysfunction and infections in patients receiving treatment with ASMs such as CBZ and explore potential interventions to mitigate infection risk [22]. Bao-Luen Chang et al. observed a decrease in CBZ prescriptions across epilepsy patients from 7% (2000–2003) to 6% (2004–2010) and further to 4% (2011–2017). The screening rates increased from 0% for CBZ nonusers and 0.5% for CBZ users in 2011 to 0.8% and 16%, respectively, in 2017. The mean three-month incidence of severe cutaneous adverse reactions (SCARs) per 10,000 episodes significantly decreased from stage 1 to stage 2 in CBZ users (6.91 vs. 3.09, $p < 0.0001$) and nonusers (1.96 vs. 1.65, $p < 0.0001$). The incidence of Stevens-Johnson syndrome/toxic epidermal necrolysis (SJS/TEN) significantly decreased from stage 1 to stage 2 in CBZ users (2.94 vs. 1.93, $p < 0.001$) but not in nonusers (0.71 vs. 0.74, $p = 0.1492$). In phase 2, the incidence of SCARs was significantly negatively correlated with screening rates in both CBZ users ($r = -0.38$, $p = 0.0342$) and nonusers ($r = -0.180$, $p < 0.001$). However, no significant correlation was found between SJS/TEN incidence and screening rate. The study concluded that identifying HLA-B*1502 alleles in patients with these conditions and avoiding CBZ treatment are crucial for preventing CBZ-induced serious adverse events [23]. I Demir et al. reported that the semi-circular canals (VOR) of gainslateral semi-circular canals (SCCs) were 0.878 ± 0.057 and 0.921 ± 0.045 in patients and healthy controls, respectively ($p = 0.024$). A reduced left-lateral SCCs VOR gain was detected in patients (0.885 ± 0.062 and 0.868 ± 0.063) ($p = 0.011$ and $p = 0.001$). The lateral SSC VOR gain (0.902 ± 0.046) was lower in patients who used CBZ for >10 years than in those who used CBZ for <10 years (0.843 ± 0.055) ($p = 0.008$). Conclusions: Lateral (right/

left) SCCs VOR gain was relatively reduced in epilepsy patients treated with CBZ, especially in those who had used CBZ long term (>10 years) [24].

Basic Research on Carbamazepine

In their study aiming to understand the relationship between genetic variations in drug receptor genes and the response to CBZ in epilepsy patients, Fan-Cheng Kong et al. genotyped adult epilepsy patients ($n = 257$) receiving CBZ monotherapy and combination therapy and divided the patients into drug-sensitive and drug-resistant groups according to the criteria of the International League Against Epilepsy. They examined single nucleotide polymorphisms (SNPs) related to PXR, CAR and AHR treatment, which mainly represent alleles associated with the risk of drug resistance. Moreover, they created a reference sequence set for gene interaction analysis based on SNPS. They did not observe significant effects of PXR- or AHR-related gene polymorphisms. However, the authors observed an interaction between the CAR rs2502815 variant and the CBZ response. In patients receiving CBZ monotherapy or combination therapy, the GG genotype of the CAR rs2502815 variant (homozygous with wild-type) was independently linked to the CBZ response after adjusting for variables [OR = 0.389, 0.203–0.743, 0.389–0.303–0.743, 0.389–0.303–0.743, 0.389–0.2815, 0.389–0.203–0.743; $p = 0.004$]. Case–control analysis of haplotype and gene interactions for CBZ response yielded negative results. These findings offer clinical insights into genetic predispositions influencing drug responses associated with CAR variants in epilepsy patients, highlighting a potential interaction between the CAR rs2502815 polymorphism and CBZ response [25]. In a separate investigation, Timothy A Simeone et al. utilized a multielectrode array to explore the effects of CBZ treatment on hippocampal sharp wave ripples (SPW-Rs) and multiple hippocampal synapses. They discovered that CBZ at treatment-relevant concentrations (IC50 = 37 μM) alters the core characteristics of ripples, which is important for information processing and integration. Furthermore, CBZ inhibited neurotransmission in a synapse-specific manner. CBZ's inhibitory effect was most pronounced at the medial perforant path to CA3 and at mossy fibers to CA3 synapses (IC50 = ~30 and 60 μM, respectively), and it was least effective in the medial perforant path to the dentate granule cell synapse (IC50 = ~120 μM). They suggested that the synapse-specific inhibition of neurotransmission of CBZ diminishes SPW-Rs, potentially contributing to the cognitive impairment observed at therapeutic doses of CBZ [26]. Ming-Liang Zhang et al. investigated the associations between ABCB1, EPHX1 and SCN1A gene polymorphisms and CBZ metabolism and drug resistance. The authors searched the PubMed, EMBASE, Cochrane Library, CNKI, Chinese Science and Technology Journal, Chinese Biomedical CD and Wanfang databases (up to April 2021) to include 18 studies encompassing 3293 epilepsy patients. They found that the ABCB1 c.3435C>T polymorphism correlated significantly with changes in the concentration–dose ratio of CBZ (CDR CBZ) (CC vs. CT, OR = 0.25 (0.08–0.42), $P = 0.004$). The EPHX c.416A>G polymorphism was observed to modify CBZ-10,11-trans-dihydrodiol (CDR CBZD) (AA vs. GG, OR = 0.48 (0.01–0.96), $P = 0.045$; AG vs. GG, OR = 0.68 (0.16–1.20), $P = 0.010$)

and the ratio of CDR CBZD to CBZ-10,11-epoxide (CBZE) (CDR CBZD: CDR CBZE) (AG vs. GG, OR = 0.83 (0.31–1.36), $P = 0.002$). Additionally, the ABCB1 c.3435C>T polymorphism significantly influenced CBZ resistance (CC vs. TT, OR = 1.78 (1.17–2.72), $P = 0.008$; CT vs. TT, OR = 1.60 (1.12–2.30), $P = 0.01$; CC + CT vs. TT, OR = 1.61 (1.15–2.26), $P = 0.006$). These findings suggest that genetic variations in ABCB1 c.3435C>T and EPHX1 c.416A>G may regulate CBZ metabolism and drug resistance in epilepsy patients [27]. Zhang Y et al. examined the adsorption behavior of ubiquitous CBZ (CBZ) and four microplastic (MP) models, including original and aged forms of polyethylene, polyvinyl chloride, polyethylene terephthalate, and polystyrene. They investigated the adsorption isotherms, kinetics, and desorption and analyzed MP changes during aging using various techniques, scanning electron microscopy, contact angle measurements, Fourier transform infrared spectroscopy and X-ray photoelectron spectroscopy. This study revealed that aging increased the MP adsorption capacity for CBZ and extended the desorption lag by altering the surface characteristics. By applying the extended Derjaguin–Landau–Verwey–Overbeek (XDLVO) theory in an innovative manner, they calculated the interfacial free energy, revealing a decrease in hydrophobic interactions and a slight increase in van der Waals forces after aging. Overall, this work elucidated the adsorption mechanism of CBZ on original and aged MPs and provided insights into the adsorption of neutral organic compounds on MPs, providing valuable information for future research [28]. Kanoot Jaruthamsophon et al. employed flow cytometry, proliferation analysis, ELISA, and ELISPOT assays to characterize the phenotype, function, HLA allelic restriction, response pathway, and cross-reactivity of CBZ-specific T-cells. They investigated the association between HLA class II allelic restriction and CBZ hypersensitivity utilizing the allelic frequency network database. Through their study, they generated 44 CD4+ CBZ-specific polyclonal T-cells and observed their restriction to HLA-DR, particularly HLA-DRB107:01. This CD4+-mediated response was attributed to a direct pharmacological interaction between CBZ and HLA-DR molecules. Similar to the CD8+ response, CBZ-stimulated CD4+ clones were found to secrete granulysin, a significant mediator of Stevens-Johnson syndrome (SJS) and toxic epidermal necrolysis (TEN). Database analysis revealed an association between HLA-DRB107:01 and CBZ-induced SJS-TEN. These results imply that HLA class II antigen presentation plays a role in CBZ hypersensitivity. Further investigations into HLA class II molecules and drug-reactive CD4+ T-cells are warranted to enhance our understanding of the pathogenesis of drug hypersensitivity [29].

Carbamazepine in the Treatment of Focal Epilepsy

V A Karlov et al. utilized the epileptiform discharge index (EDI) to assess the efficacy and tolerability of CBZ sustained-release tablets in the treatment of adults with new-onset focal epilepsy (FE). Their study included 62 males (61.3%) and 24 females (38.7%) with new-onset focal epilepsy aged 18–95 years (mean age 42.9 ± 18.4 years). Each patient underwent video EEG monitoring and EDI evaluation at every visit. They observed a significant 4.3-fold reduction in total EDI from baseline to the end of the 12-month follow-up period ($p < 0.001$). The seizure-free rate was 0.3% ($n = 25$), with an effective rate of 21.0% ($n = 13$). They speculate that CBZ demonstrates efficacy and promise as an initial monotherapy for FE [30].

Population Pharmacokinetics of Carbamazepine

Vincent LM Yip et al. investigated the impact of clinical and genetic factors on the pharmacokinetics (PK) of CBZ and its three metabolites, which are known to be chemically reactive or formed through reactive intermediates. They collected a combination of rich and sparse PK samples from healthy volunteers and epilepsy patients and genotyped 20 single nucleotide polymorphisms across 11 genes known to be involved in CBZ and CBZ 10, 11-epoxide metabolism or transport in all subjects. Their study included 248 observations from 80 subjects. The total maternal CBZ clearance was determined to be 1.96 L/h, with a central volume of distribution of 164 L and an absorption rate constant of 0.45 h^{-1}. The coadministration of the total daily dose and of phenytoin was identified as a significant covariate affecting total CBZ clearance. Furthermore, the EPHX1–416 G/G genotype was highlighted as an important covariate for CBZ 10,11-epoxide clearance. The authors concluded that CBZ clearance was influenced by the combined administration of total dose and phenytoin sodium, while CBZ 10,11-epoxide clearance was affected by genetic variants in the microsomal epoxide hydrolase gene [31].

Kacirova I et al. investigated CBZ concentrations in various biological samples, including maternal serum, colostrum, and neonatal serum. They found a range of concentrations in maternal serum (1.0–11.2 mg/L for CBZ and 0.3–4.4 mg/L for epoxide), colostrum (0.5–6.8 mg/L for CBZ and 0.3–2.4 mg/L for epoxide), and neonatal serum (0.5–4.7 mg/L for CBZ and 0.3–1.7 mg/L for epoxide). The median milk/maternal serum concentration ratio of CBZ was 0.45 (epoxide 0.71), the median neonatal/maternal serum concentration ratio of CBZ was 0.20 (epoxide 0.41), and the median neonatal serum/milk concentration ratio of CBZ was 0.38 (epoxide 0.50). They observed a significant correlation between CBZ concentrations in milk and maternal serum, as well as between milk and neonatal serum concentrations. However, they noted that only one CBZ index in the serum of breastfed neonates fell within the reference range for the general epilepsy population, with more than half below the lower limit of quantification. Consequently, the authors concluded that routine monitoring of serum CBZ concentrations in breastfed newborns may not be necessary. Nonetheless, they recommended close observation of newborns for potential adverse effects, with serum concentration measurements warranted if such effects are observed [32]. Yuito Fujita et al. conducted PPK analysis and showed that the couse of CBZ increased the clearance of PER. They found that their PPK models provided a good description of the observed data with low bias, as indicated by the fit quality chart. The mean error, mean absolute error and root-mean-square error values derived from the semimechanical model were smaller than the PER concentrations predicted by the empirical PPK model for CBZ patients. Conclusions: The authors developed two different approaches to PPK models based on electronic medical records data to characterize the pharmacokinetics of PER. They emphasized that their PPK model supports the clinical use of PER, suggesting its efficacy and utility in practice [33].

Additional Studies of Carbamazepine

Amara Gul et al. conducted a case–control study to examine the effects of CBZ on emotional intelligence and mindfulness among patients with epilepsy. They recruited 80 subjects, including 40 epilepsy patients (50%) with an average age of 37.92 ± 9.09 years and 40 control patients (50%) with an average age of 37.80 ± 9.00 years. Emotional intelligence and mindfulness indices were significantly lower in patients with epilepsy than in controls ($p < 0.001$). Patients demonstrated improved emotional intelligence and mindfulness indices following CBZ treatment compared to their baseline scores ($p < 0.05$). Thus, the authors suggest that CBZ may be effective in enhancing emotional intelligence and mindfulness indices among individuals with epilepsy [34].

Jason et al. investigated the potential of the sodium channel blocker CBZ to protect beta cells from inflammatory cytokines in vitro. The authors supplemented LabDiet 5053 female nonobese diabetic (NOD) mice with 0.5% w/w CBZ to assess its effects, resulting in a serum CBZ level of 14.98 ± 3.19 μM. Notably, CBZ-treated animals exhibited an approximately 50% reduction in diabetes incidence at 25 weeks, as indicated by fasting blood glucose levels. Additionally, improved glucose tolerance was observed in CBZ-fed NOD mice at 6 weeks of age, preceding the onset of diabetes in the population. Although fewer islets were detected in CBZ-treated NOD mice at 6 weeks of age, no differences were detected in CD4 and CD8 T-cell composition or circulating inflammatory markers in pancreatic lymph nodes. These findings suggest that CBZ reduces the occurrence of type 1 diabetes in NOD mice by preserving functional beta cell volume. However, due to the growing concern of drug abuse, it has been found that CBZ is discharged into aquatic environments via urban sewage, posing potential harm to aquatic organisms [35]. Bai Zhonghui et al. used zebrafish, an aquatic vertebrate, as a model to comprehensively evaluate the hepatotoxicity of CBZ. Larvae were infected at 72–144 hours postfertilization (hpf) with 0.07, 0.13, or 0.26 mmol/L CBZ and 0.025, 0.05, or 0.1 mmol/L CBZ for 28 days. There were significant changes in liver histopathology and size, indicating that CBZ had severe hepatotoxic effects on larvae and adults. Oil Red O staining revealed substantial lipid deposition in the liver of both larvae and adults exposed to CBZ. Moreover, CBZ exposure promoted hepatocyte apoptosis, as evidenced by TUNEL staining, which was attributed to increased ROS content. The subsequent downregulation of gene expression related to the Wnt pathway in each infected group suggested that CBZ may inhibit liver development through the Wnt/β-catenin signaling pathway. These findings highlight the hepatotoxicity of CBZ in zebrafish and elucidate its mechanism of action, providing valuable insights into environmental issues associated with CBZ exposure [36]. Giulia et al. conducted a retrospective observational study to assess the effectiveness and tolerability of CBZ and oxcarbazepine in a large cohort of patients diagnosed with classic (254 patients), secondary (60 patients), and idiopathic (40 patients) trigeminal neuralgia. Propensity score analysis was employed to address selection bias, and the frequency of side effects linked to CBZ and oxcarbazepine was determined by adjusting the data using the inverse probability of treatment weights. The initial remission rate was 88.3% in the CBZ group and 90.9% in the oxcarbazepine group. Notably, the incidence of refractory cases was significantly greater in patients with idiopathic (15%) and secondary (27%) trigeminal neuralgia than in those with classic trigeminal neuralgia (6%; $p < 0.05$). Among patients treated with CBZ (29.6%) and oxcarbazepine (12.6%), the primary side effects led to treatment interruption or unsatisfactory dose reduction in 53 and 22 patients, respectively. Patients administered CBZ experienced side effects more frequently (43.6%) than those administered oxcarbazepine (30.3%, $p < 0.0001$). Additionally, discontinuation rates were greater in patients with secondary and idiopathic trigeminal neuralgia than in those with classic trigeminal neuralgia ($p < 0.05$). In conclusion, observational evidence indicates that CBZ and oxcarbazepine are effective for the treatment of most patients with trigeminal neuralgia; however, side effects remain a significant concern, particularly in patients with secondary and idiopathic trigeminal neuralgia [37]. *Neisseria gonorrhoeae* has developed resistance to all previously utilized antibiotics, emphasizing an urgent need for novel antimicrobial agents to combat gonococcal infections. Recent investigations have demonstrated that CBZ, a commonly prescribed antiepileptic medication, disrupts the interaction between gonococcal pili and the I-domain of human complement receptor 3 (CR3), which is crucial for cervical infections in women. CBZ effectively eliminates *N. gonorrhoeae* infection in primary human cervical cells. In their study, Lucy et al. quantified CBZ levels in serum, saliva, and vaginal fluid collected from 16 women, comprising both regular and nonregular users of CBZ. Competitive ELISA assays were utilized to detect potential therapeutic levels of CBZ in mucosal secretions of the lower reproductive tract in the experimental group (CBZ users). Moreover, concentrations of CBZ found in the vaginal fluid of CBZ users were sufficient to significantly reduce the number of live *N. gonorrhoeae* bacteria recovered from in vitro and primary cervical cell infections by more than 99% within 24 h. These findings strongly support the potential of CBZ as a novel host-targeted therapy for gonococcal cervicitis [38]. Hamanaka K et al. identified a gain-of-function (GOF) variation in the GRIA3 gene, which encodes the glutamate ionotropic receptor AMPA3 (GluA3), a subunit of a postsynaptic glutamate-gated ion channel crucial for neurotransmission. Unlike the loss-of-function (LOF) variant associated with neurodevelopmental disorders (NDD) in males, this patient exhibited a neonatal hemizygotic missense variant: C.1844C>T (p.LA615VAL). Interestingly, the neurological symptoms observed in this patient, including hypertonia and hyperreflexia, differed from those typically observed in patients with LOF GRIA3 variants. Treatment with CBZ, which is known to inhibit presynaptic glutamate release, improved the patient's seizures and hypertonia. Patch-clamp recordings revealed that the human GluA3 mutant (P.ALAB615VAL) displayed slower desensitization and inactivation kinetics. In a *Drosophila* model expressing the human GluA3 mutant, developmental defects were observed when the flies were mated with a specific mutant, suggesting a gain-of-function effect. This study indicated that the GOF variant of GRIA3 may lead to a distinct NDD phenotype compared to LOF variants, and drugs targeting glutaminergic neurotransmission could ameliorate this phenotype, informing future clinical treatment strategies for GRIA3-associated NDDs [39]. Wang X et al. demonstrated that hydroxide (OH−) ions and chloride (Cl−) ions played significant roles in the degradation of CBZ, with OH− contributing to approximately 50% of the degradation process. Eight transformation products (TPs) were identified during CBZ degradation, showing a decreasing trend in toxicity. The toxic disinfection byproducts (DBPs) generated during CBZ degradation fell within the permissible limits set by the World Health Organization and China's drinking water standards. Although nitrogen-containing DBPs (N-DBPs) exhibited the lowest concentration, they were identified as the main contributors to toxicity, warranting further attention in practical applications. Utilizing advanced oxidation technology involving UV-LED and NH2Cl was shown to be an effective method for degrading active pharmaceutical compounds [40]. Matteo Candeloro et al. conducted a study involving 85 patients (37% female, median age 68 years) receiving treatment with either CBZ (n = 43, 51%) or phenytoin sodium (n = 42, 49%), with 62% initially treated with VKAs and 38% receiving treatment with DOACs. The time in therapeutic range (TTR) for VKA patients was 63%, which improved by year 2. Plasma DOAC levels were lower than expected in a significant portion of the subjects. The thromboembolism rates (95% confidence intervals) in patients treated with VKAs and DOACs were 3.6 (3.1–4.2) and 4.4 (3.5–5.6), respectively. The incidences of major bleeding were 1.8 (1.5–2.1) and 1.5 (1.2–1.9), and the rates of all-cause mortality were 3.6 (3.1–4.2) and 1.5 (1.2–1.9), respectively. The incidences were similar between VKAs and DOACs and between CBZ and phenytoin. Conclusion: The incidence of thromboembolism was greater in patients treated with anticoagulants combined with CBZ or phenytoin sodium. Thrombotic and bleeding events were comparable between VKA and DOAC patients. DOAC levels were lower than expected in 47% of the subjects and did not correlate with clinical outcomes [41]. Wentland L et al. systematically explored methods to enhance the detection of CBZ in undiluted human saliva using polymer lamination devices with screen-printed carbon electrodes. Strategies included adding the anionic surfactant sodium dodecyl sulfate to saliva, filtering saliva to remove larger molecular substances, plasma pretreatment of device electrodes, and sample incubation on electrodes. These techniques enable the quantification of therapeutic CBZ concentrations in saliva without requiring prior dilution [42]. Chan H et al. discovered that vitamin D3 and CBZ mitigate TCDB-induced lysosomal dysfunction, inflammation, and histological damage. They found that during CDI, TcdB inhibits the CTNNB1/MITF axis, leading to lysosomal acidification inhibition and SQSTM1/NF-κB signaling activation downstream of macrophages [43]. Vitamin D3 and CBZ counteract CDI by restoring MITF expression and lysosomal function in mice. Bonaccorso et al. evaluated the design of CBZ nanocrystals (NCSs) for naso-brain delivery. Using ultrasonic precipitation and quality-by-design principles, they optimized CBZ NCS formulation variables to achieve the desired product quality attributes. The CBZ NCS exhibited thermal stability, appropriate crystallinity, morphology, and adhesion. The reactive surface method, which boasts an error rate of only 2.6%, was shown to be a dependable approach for optimizing CBZ nanocrystals (NNMs) with a size not exceeding 300. Additionally, when cultured in artificial cerebrospinal fluid at 37 °C, CBZ nanocrystals do not exhibit aggregation or degradation, further highlighting their stability under physiological conditions. Preliminary biological studies demonstrated the biocompatibility of CBZ NCSs with olfactory nerve cells. The suspension successfully transitioned to a powder form, offering highly concentrated formulations for maximum drug dose delivery in minimal volume [44]. Suwabe S et al. focused on utilizing amorphous solid dispersion (ASD) technology to enhance drug dissolution. They employed CBZ as a model drug and prepared an ASD using the solvent evaporation method (ASD-1). Through the screening of six water-soluble polymer carriers, the ASD-1 formulation based on polyvinyl alcohol (PVA) demonstrated the highest dissolution rate and yield in the nasal cavity (pH 6.0) under experimental conditions. Upon dispersing the CBZ suspension with the PVA-ASD-1 formulation, drug delivery was notably enhanced in rat plasma and brain tissue in vivo. Furthermore, the PVA-ASD spray-dried powder formulation (PVA-ASD-2) exhibited improved drug dissolution and transfer in vivo. Notably, the spray-dried PVA-ASD-2 formulation demonstrated a greater brain/plasma ratio than the PVA-ASD-1 suspension formulation. These findings, supported by physical characterization data, underscore the potential of intranasal agents based on ASD for efficient drug delivery to the brain [45].

2.1.1.2 Clonazepam

Drug Characteristics

[Chemical name] 1,3-Dihydro-7-nitro-5-(2-chlorophenyl)-2H-1,4-benzodiazepine-2-one

[Chemical structure]

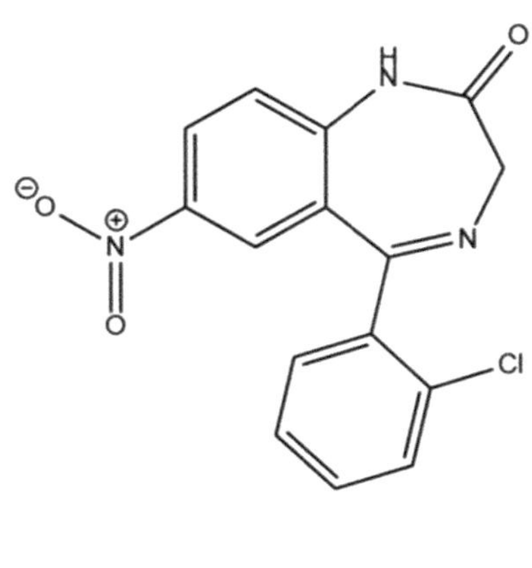

[Molecular formula] C15H10ClN3O3

[Molecular weight] 315.711

[Indications] It is mainly used for the treatment of epilepsy and convulsions and has demonstrated efficacy across all types of epilepsy, especially for petit mal seizures and myoclonic seizures. It is administered via intravenous treatment for status epilepticus. It can also be utilized to address anxiety and insomnia. It is effective in managing chorea and offers therapeutic benefits for conditions such as drug-induced ADHD, chronic multiple convulsions, stiff person syndrome, and various types of neuralgia.

[Specification] 2 mg

[Dosage]
Usual dosage for adults 0.5 mg (1/4 tablet) to begin, three times a day, increased by 0.5–1 mg (1/4–1/2 tablet) every 3 days until the attack is effectively managed or there is an adverse reaction. The dosage should be individualized, with a maximum daily dose of 20 mg (equivalent to ten tablets) for adults.

Usual dosage for children: Children aged 10 years or weighing less than 30 kg start by taking 0.01–0.03 mg/kg of body weight every day, divided two to three times, and then increase by 0.25–0.5 mg (1/8–1/4 tablet) every 3 days until they reach 0.1–0.2 mg/kg/day according to body weight or until any adverse reactions occur. The duration of treatment with clonazepam should not surpass 3–6 months.

[Adverse reactions] Common adverse reactions include drowsiness, dizziness, ataxia, abnormal excitability of behavioral disorders, irritability (which can sometimes paradoxically occur), and muscle weakness. Less commonly, there are behavioral disturbances, difficulty concentrating, irritability (especially in children), confusion, hallucinations, depression, rash or allergies, sore throat, fever or bleeding abnormalities, ecchymosis, or extreme fatigue and fatigue (cytopenia). Symptoms to note include inflexibility, unsteady walking, drowsiness (severe at first and gradually disappears), blurred vision, constipation, diarrhea, dizziness, headache, increased tracheal secretions, nausea, dysuria, and slurred speech.

Clinical Application and Basic Research

Historical Evolution of Clonazepam

In 1969 and 1970, Gastaut et al. conducted a study evaluating the efficacy of a novel nitrate benzodiazepine [7-nitro-5-(2-chlorophenyl)-3H-1′4-benzodiazepine-2(1H)-I (Roche, R05–4023)], clonazepam [46]. Lechat et al. (1970), Fariello and Mutani (1970), and Killam et al. (1970) conducted additional animal experiments on this compound, confirming its anticonvulsant properties in experimental models. In 1983, G. Chouinard et al. discovered that clonazepam had anticonvulsant and anxiolytic effects, leading to its FDA approval for the treatment of epilepsy and panic disorder in the same year [47, 48]. In 2010, the American Academy of Sleep Medicine (AASM) recommended the use of clonazepam for the treatment of rapid eye movement sleep behavior disorder (RBD) [49, 50]. In 2023, clonazepam was found to effectively reduce seizures, promote sleep onset, and stabilize the condition [51].

An Observational Study of Clonazepam for Epilepsy

Monotherapy is the preferred treatment approach for individuals recently diagnosed with epilepsy. To assess the effectiveness and tolerability of oral clonazepam as monotherapy for newly diagnosed epilepsy, various studies have been conducted to compare it with other ASMs. One study evaluated clonazepam and CBZ as singular treatments for newly diagnosed psychomotor epilepsy, which is now recognized as temporal lobe epilepsy. Another study, albeit with only one published abstract, compared clonazepam and ethosuximide as monotherapies for childhood epilepsy. In a small trial comparing clonazepam and CBZ for medial temporal lobe epilepsy, no discernible difference in efficacy or tolerability was observed. However, in a trial examining absence epilepsy in children, clonazepam demonstrated lower tolerability than did ethosuximide, although there was a lack of comparative efficacy data. Presently, there is insufficient evidence to support the use of clonazepam as a standalone therapy for epilepsy [52].

Evidence-Based Medical Research on Clonazepam

A study aimed to compare the safety and effectiveness of trazodone treatment in combination with melatonin and clonazepam for treating sleep problems in Parkinson's disease (PD) patients. This double-blinded, randomized clinical trial conducted at a single center evaluated subjective sleep in PD patients. The results indicated that trazodone 50 mg/day, clonazepam 1 mg/day, and melatonin 3 mg/day were well-tolerated and effective for improving sleep quality among PD patients [46]. Another study evaluated the clinical efficacy of combining N-acetylcysteine (NAC) and clonazepam treatment for treating burning mouth syndrome (BMS). In this study, 160 BMS patients were divided into three groups: Group 1 received NAC (400 mg/day), Group 2 received clonazepam (0.5 mg/day), and Group 3 received both NAC and clonazepam. Symptom relief was assessed after 8 weeks of treatment using a visual analog scale (VAS). The findings suggested that the treatment combination of NAC and clonazepam was more effective at alleviating BMS symptoms than either monotherapy [53].

Side Effects of Clonazepam

Elsevier Inc. et al. reported the first documented case of bilateral parotid gland enlargement associated with clonazepam, suggesting a potential link between benzodiazepine use and salivary gland dysfunction in humans. Peripheral benzodiazepine receptors, previously identified in rodents, have also been found in human salivary glands via receptor ligand 3 photolabeling and positron emission tomography. This study highlighted the importance of further investigations into the mechanisms underlying benzodiazepine-associated salivary gland dysfunction, as different benzodiazepines may impact these glands through different mechanisms. Additionally, the study raised clinical considerations, such as the possibility that switching from clonazepam to diazepam could worsen parotid gland abnormalities [54]. Eric William Lutz et al. described a case of recurrent clonazepam withdrawal delirium in postoperative neurosurgical patients, detailing a middle-aged man who underwent spinal surgery and who experienced benzodiazepine withdrawal delirium. Significant paranoia and hypereuphoria were observed before surgery and on the fourth day postoperatively after the discontinuation of benzodiazepine use. Reintroduction of benzodiazepines alleviated the patient's symptoms, highlighting the importance of considering benzodiazepine withdrawal in the differential diagnosis of acute delirium, even in patients receiving low or moderate doses. Early counseling and preoperative planning for patients with known discontinuation issues, including contacting psychiatric departments for early drug restart, are crucial [55]. Lichenoid drug eruption caused by clonazepam: Clonazepam, commonly administered for anxiety-related disorders and seizures, is generally associated with few adverse skin reactions. However, a single case of lichenoid drug eruption due to clonazepam has been described. An 81-year-old man with Alzheimer's disease developed a lichenoid rash after taking clonazepam, characterized by a purple scaly patch on his lower limbs from hip to foot. The rash subsided 2 months after the discontinuation of clonazepam and the initiation of corticosteroid treatment. This case underscores the importance of recognizing lichenoid drug eruption as a potential adverse reaction to clonazepam administration, emphasizing the need for prompt discontinuation of the medication [56].

Basic Research on Clonazepam

Behrouz et al. utilized an ultrasonic-assisted electric film method to extract clonazepam from plasma and determine its concentration via capillary electrophoresis. They developed an approach combining ultrasound-assisted film extraction (UA-EME) with capillary electrophoresis (CE) and diode array detection (DAD) for clonazepam concentration determination in plasma samples. By comparing conventional EME with UA-EME, they investigated the effect of ultrasound on extraction efficiency. A central composite design was employed to optimize the variables affecting these methods to achieve maximal extraction efficiency. Under optimal conditions, UA-EME exhibited superior extraction recovery in a shorter time (58% over 13 min) than did the EME method (42% over 30 min). Ultrasound decreased the extraction time and enhanced the recovery by reducing the barrier layer thickness. Moreover, UA-EME provided a higher preconcentration factor (203) and a lower limit of detection (3 ng mL^{-1}) with satisfactory repeatability (RSD less than 10.11%) [57]. Polystyrene (PS) electrospun nanofibers were investigated as effective adsorbents for clonazepam. PS nanofibers were prepared by electrospinning for the adsorption of clonazepam from aqueous solutions, with optimization of adsorption conditions such as adsorption time, solution pH, and adsorbent dosage. The kinetic and thermodynamic properties of clonazepam adsorption on PS nanofibers were studied under optimized conditions. The quasi-second-order kinetic model fit well to the adsorption process, suggesting that diffusion within the fibers is the rate-limiting step. Adsorption equilibrium data conformed to the Freundlich isotherm model, indicating a maximum adsorption capacity of 3.2 mg g^{-1}. Thermodynamic analysis revealed that the adsorption process is endothermic and spontaneous. PS electrospun nanofibers therefore demonstrate potential as effective adsorption materials for isolating and purifying clonazepam from water-soluble matrices [58].

Analysis of the regulatory effect of long-term treatment with escitalopram and clonazepam on anxiety-related neuropeptide expression in the rat brain revealed that prolonged administration of clonazepam led to an increase in NMU mRNA expression and the development of NMU-expressing fibers in the amygdala. Conversely, escitalopram treatment resulted in a significant decrease in hypothalamic NPSR mRNA expression levels. The long-term use of escitalopram was found to influence the local expression of the examined neuropeptide mRNA in various ways, depending on the brain structure. The pharmacological effects of escitalopram may be associated with local alterations in NPSR-related expression of the NPS/NMU/NMUR2 gene in selected rat brain regions [59]. In an investigation into the combined antiepileptic effects of cannabidiol (CBD) and clonazepam in a Dravet syndrome-conditioned mouse model, Shu-Hui Chuang et al. studied the treatment combination of the benzodiazepine clonazepam (CLZ) with the nonpsychotropic phytocannabinoid cannabidiol (CBD). They assessed the therapeutic potentials of the two compounds for heat-induced febrile seizures. The results indicated that low doses of CLZ, either alone or in combination with CBD, elevated the threshold temperature for heat-induced seizures. Additionally, compared with treatment by the vehicle or CLZ alone, the combination of CLZ with CBD significantly reduced the duration of seizures but did not impact the severity of seizures. This suggests the potential cumulative effect of CLZ and CBD on seizure duration [60].

Other Studies

Luanna et al. conducted a quasiexperimental study to assess the feasibility of clonazepam treatment in older adults. The results revealed a high prescribing rate and a small correlation with clonazepam withdrawal, indicating the effectiveness of this treatment regimen [61]. In a randomized trial comparing the efficacy and safety of clonazepam and melatonin in REM sleep with RWA and RBD-related symptoms, Jung-Ick Byun et al. demonstrated that clonazepam treatment often resulted in greater improvement in RBD symptoms than did PR melatonin [62]. Clonazepam, known for its muscle relaxant and anxiolytic effects, has been reported to alleviate pain, associated anxiety, and muscle spasms resulting from vertebral compression fractures [63]. Dell'Isola et al. described a case involving PCDH19-associated seizures in a 4-year-old girl with a novel variant of the PCDH19 gene, suggesting that PCDH19-associated seizures can be effectively controlled with clonazepam [64].

2.1.1.3 Ethosuximide

Drug Characteristics

[Chemical name] 3-Methyl-3-ethyl-2,5-pyrrolidinedione

[Chemical structure formula]

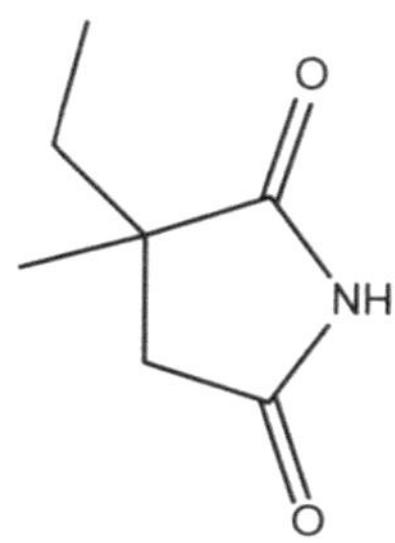

[Molecular formula] C7H11NO2

[Molecular weight] 141.168

[Indications] (1) Ethosuximide is mainly used for absence seizures and myoclonic seizures and is considered the initial option for managing absence minor seizures although it can aggravate major seizures; (2) The use of ethosuximide is combined with that of other ASMs for mixed epileptic seizures; (3) Effective in treating absence epilepsy; (4) It is used to treat acquired epileptic aphasia (Landau–Kleffner syndrome).

[Specifications] Ethosuximide capsules: 250 mg

[Ethosuximide syrup] 5 g/100 mL

[Usage and dosage]
Children under 6 years of age receive an initial dose of 250 mg once daily; depending on the patient's condition and tolerance, the dose can be increased to 1 g/day, usually by 250 mg every 4–7 days.

For children older than 6 years, the initial dose of 250 mg twice a day can be increased to 1.5 g/day depending on the patient's condition and tolerance, usually by 250 mg every 4–7 days.

Adults, 1–2 g/day; children, 15–40 mg/(kg·day). If the daily dose for children over 6 years of age exceeds 0.75–1 g and the daily dose for adults reaches 2 g, it is necessary to take the drug in separate doses. Hemodialysis patients may require additional doses before or after treatment to maintain therapeutic levels. When use of the drug is stopped, the dose should be gradually reduced to avoid triggering absence epileptic status.

[Adverse reactions]

1. Gastrointestinal side effects include nausea, vomiting, anorexia, hematemesis, gastrointestinal discomfort and abdominal pain. Caution is important in patients with liver and kidney diseases because its use may lead to abnormal liver and kidney function. Gastrointestinal side effects are common and usually abate after 1–2 weeks.
2. Common side effects include headache, fatigue, lethargy, insomnia, vertigo, dyskinesia, hiccups, and euphoria. Occasional motor difficulties, personality changes, depression, psychosis.
3. Dermatological reactions: Rash, erythema multiforme and lupus erythema may occur. Sometimes scaly desquamation or blisters, mucositis, conjunctivitis, external genital inflammation, fever, or lymph node enlargement may occur. Stevens-Johnson syndrome, an idiosyncratic reaction, has rarely been reported.
4. Hematological effects, such as the inhibition of hematopoietic function, leading to eosinophilia, leukopenia, granulocyte and platelet reduction, whole cell reduction, and aplastic anemia, have also been reported.
5. Its use may exacerbate tonic–clonic seizures in patients with mixed seizures, so it must be combined with other ASMs.

Clinical Application and Basic Research

Historical Evolution of Ethosuximide

Ethosuximide, a member of the succinimide class, is an antiepileptic medication, although its precise pharmacological mechanism remains somewhat elusive. It is postulated that ethosuximide exerts its effects by diminishing the activation of T-type calcium channels within the thalamus. This action entails the blockade of transient and low-threshold calcium currents in thalamic neurons, consequently elevating the seizure threshold and thwarting the synchronized discharge of corticothalamic neurons implicated in peak wave seizures. Additionally, it is thought to impede neurotransmission in the motor cortex, thereby mitigating seizure activity. Although it has been approved by the FDA for treating absence seizures in individuals over 1 year of age, ethosuximide has been in clinical use since 1958. The pioneering work of L. SOREL in 1960 marked the first documentation of its experimental and clinical efficacy [65]. In 1961, H. M. LOSSIUS first used the new anticonvulsant ethosuximide of the succinimide group [66]. In 1963, J. PROT's findings highlighted its potential for treating refractory minor epilepsy [67]. In 1990, the utilization of ethosuximide in the management of absence epilepsy was further elucidated by J.M. Dooley et al. [68]. Over the years, investigations into its effects have continued. In 2006, Berna Terzioğlu et al. investigated the impact of ethosuximide on amino acids in rats with hereditary epilepsy [69]. A 2010 study by Rezzan Gülhan Aker et al. demonstrated that local cortical administration of ethosuximide suppressed spike-and-wave activity and reduced seizure susceptibility in genetically deficient epileptic rats (GAERS) [70]. In 2022, Anna-Sophia Buschhoff et al. showed the high efficacy of intrathecal ethosuximide administration in suppressing seizures in a genetic model of intractable epilepsy [71].

Ethosuximide in the Treatment of Refractory Epilepsy

Giovanni Mastroianni et al. conducted a comprehensive literature review focusing on the treatment of typical absence seizures, specifically hard-to-treat cases of idiopathic generalized epilepsy. Typical absence seizures are characterized by sudden onset and termination, accompanied by a transient disturbance of consciousness and an electroencephalogram showing a 3 Hz spike slow wave discharge. Ethosuximide, valproic acid, and lamotrigine, whether administered individually or in combination, are regarded as the primary treatment options for these seizures, with studies of moderate to high quality demonstrating their efficacy as monotherapies. However, evidence supporting the use of alternative monotherapies or combination therapies stems largely from poor-quality studies, such as case reports, small case series, or expert opinions. Thus, there is a pressing need for well-designed clinical trials to evaluate the effectiveness of these alternatives in treating hard-to-treat typical absence seizures. In cases where monotherapy is ineffective, alternative monotherapy with ethosuximide, valproic acid, or lamotrigine should be considered. If alternative monotherapy fails, a combination of two of these three ASMs may be necessary, with valproic acid plus lamotrigine or valproic acid plus ethosuximide being the preferred combination. Ethosuximide has emerged as the drug of choice for children with unresponsive epilepsy. In a double-blinded, randomized, controlled clinical trial involving 453 children with childhood absence epilepsy, the incidence-free rate with ethosuximide (53%) and valproic acid (58%) was significantly greater than that with lamotrigine (29%). When these primary ASMs, whether used alone or in combination, fail to achieve adequate seizure control, additional ASMs should be considered [6].

Ethosuximide in the Treatment of Epileptic Syndromes

Michele Ascoli et al. conducted a PubMed literature search on drug-resistant adolescent myoclonic epilepsy (also known as Janz syndrome), in which preliminary studies, systematic reviews, and meta-analyses were reviewed. Adolescent myoclonic epilepsy is a prevalent form of hereditary generalized epilepsy, constituting approximately 10% of all epilepsy cases. Despite receiving appropriate treatment with ASMs, approximately one-third of adolescents with myoclonic epilepsy continue to experience seizures, with approximately 30% exhibiting drug resistance. Sodium valproate is regarded as the drug of choice. For women with reproductive potential, levetiracetam should be the treatment of choice. The use of ethosuximide should be considered for persistent absence episodes [72]. In another review, Debopam Samanta discusses Angelman syndrome (AS), characterized by severe developmental delays, speech disturbances, motor abnormalities (such as ataxia and tremors), and unique behaviors such as frequent laughter. AS is primarily caused by maternal UBE3A gene abnormalities (maternal 15q11–13 deletion, maternal-specific UBE3A mutation, uniparental dimerization, and imprinting defects). Eighty to 90% of patients with AS have intractable seizures in early childhood, accompanied by characteristic EEG abnormalities. Various types of generalized seizures are involved, the most common of which are myoclonic and atypical absence seizures. Seizures are often drug-resistant. Valproic acid, phenobarbital, and clonazepam are commonly used as first-line treatments for AS-associated seizures. However, due to their adverse effects, recent approaches have prioritized the use of ethosuximide in combination with a carbohydrate-restricted diet. Ethosuximide, a T-type calcium ion channel blocker, is preferred for treating typical and atypical absence seizures, and high-dose adjunctive therapy (serum concentration greater than 110 μg/mL) in conjunction with valproate has shown promising results. The serum level of ethosuximide may be elevated by valproic acid, making this combination particularly suitable for refractory epilepsy patients. Furthermore, ethosuximide has demonstrated efficacy in controlling seizures in GABRB3-deficient mice [73].

Application of Ethosuximide in Special Epileptic Populations

Ramzi Shawahna et al. conducted a systematic search across multiple databases, including PubMed, EMBASE, and CINAHL/EBSCO. Their qualitative and comprehensive approach resulted in the inclusion of 15 records focused on evaluating the concentration of ASMs in the breast milk of women with epilepsy during breastfeeding. Qualitative synthetic evidence was used to estimate theoretical doses of ASMs, such as estimated daily intake (EDI) and relative infant dose (RID), and to assess potential risks to infants from exposure to ASMs in breast milk. Recent position papers and guidelines have advocated for exclusive breastfeeding by women with epilepsy, citing the outweighing benefits to the baby compared to potential side effects from drug exposure. The RID for ethosuximide is 31.49%. However, caution is advised, as breastfeeding may need to be restricted or discontinued if signs of excessive sedation, lethargy, or poor weight gain are observed in infants exposed to specific drugs such as phenobarbital or ethosuximide, either alone or in combination with preeclampsia. Healthcare providers and women with epilepsy are encouraged to utilize the findings of this study to make informed decisions about the safety of breastfeeding while taking antiepileptic medications [74].

The Efficacy and Safety of Ethosuximide in the Treatment of Epilepsy

Francesco Brigo and colleagues conducted a comprehensive review of randomized or quasirandomized controlled trials from the Cochrane Research Register and PubMed, aiming to evaluate the efficacy of ethosuximide, valproic acid, and lamotrigine for treating absence seizures in children and adolescents compared to that of placebo or one another. While eight small trials (a total of 691 participants) were included from previous reviews, there were no placebo-controlled trials for ethosuximide or valproic acid; thus, evidence from randomized controlled trials to support their specific effects on absence seizures is lacking. Due to methodological differences among trials comparing ethosuximide, lamotrigine, and sodium valproate, a meta-analysis was deemed inappropriate. In a large randomized, parallel, double-blinded controlled trial involving 453 newly diagnosed children with absence epilepsy, the effectiveness of ethosuximide, lamotrigine, and valproate treatment was compared. At the 12-month mark, patients on ethosuximide exhibited greater seizure freedom than those on lamotrigine, while valproic acid showed comparable effectiveness to ethosuximide. Significant differences in treatment failure rates due to intolerable adverse events were observed among the groups, with the valproic acid group experiencing the greatest proportion of adverse events compared to the ethosuximide and lamotrigine groups. Overall, this extensive study indicates that, in comparison to lamotrigine, ethosuximide and valproic acid demonstrate superior efficacy as initial monotherapies in managing seizures without intolerable adverse effects in children with unresponsive epilepsy. The study's findings provide a high level of confidence in the data's outcomes. Regarding efficacy and tolerability, ethosuximide has emerged as the optimal initial empiric monotherapy for children and adolescents with absence seizures. If absence and generalized tonic–clonic seizures cooccur, valproate is preferred, as ethosuximide may not effectively treat these seizures [75]. A PubMed search was conducted by Victoria Elisa Rinaldi et al. to identify all articles regarding the management and treatment of childhood absence epilepsy (CAE) from 1979 to 2021. The search aimed to summarize recent research and emerging concepts in CAE treatment, with a particular focus on refractory cases. CAE is a common generalized epilepsy syndrome in children. Ethosuximide remains the preferred medication for traditional anticonvulsant therapy for CAE, followed by valproic acid and lamotrigine. If initial treatment has been shown to be ineffective, combination therapy is typically introduced following two single-drug treatments. Ethosuximide is preferred for typical absence seizures due to its lack of inhibition of focal or generalized tonic–clonic seizures. Although its mechanism of action remains unclear, ethosuximide seems to block transient, low-threshold calcium currents in the thalamus, resulting in synchronous activation of spike-and-wave discharges characteristic of absence seizures. The main side effects of ethosuximide include gastrointestinal disturbances, headaches, drowsiness, and less common adverse reactions, such as behavioral and psychiatric disorders, blood dysplasia, and allergic reactions [76]. Barbara Mostacci et al. conducted a review of recent literature on ASMs and assessed their teratogenic potential in idiopathic generalized epilepsy (IGE). In girls and women with reproductive potential, levetiracetam and lamotrigine should be considered the drugs of choice for simple generalized tonic–clonic seizures and adolescent myoclonic epilepsy, and ethosuximide should be considered for children with absence epilepsy. According to the 2013 ILAE evidence review, ethosuximide demonstrated established efficacy for absence episodes (evidence level A). These findings stem from a Class I study involving 446 of the initially enrolled 453 children who were randomly assigned to receive treatment with ethosuximide (n = 156), sodium valproate (n = 148), or lamotrigine (n = 149). The rates of freedom from treatment failure at 16–20 weeks were comparable between ethosuximide and sodium valproate (53% and 58%, respectively), and both rates were greater than that of lamotrigine (29%). Attention deficits were significantly more common in the 2-valproate group than in the ethosuximide group. Although the analysis was based on a limited number of exposures, a systematic review revealed a significantly greater risk of congenital malformations, particularly cleft lip and palate and clubfoot, associated with ethosuximide than in controls. No data regarding cognitive development following intrauterine exposure to ethosuximide are available [77].

Effects of Ethosuximide on EEG and Cognitive Function

Frank M. C. Besag et al. conducted a comprehensive PubMed literature search to evaluate the evidence for cognitive changes linked with antiepileptic medication in children with epilepsy. Epilepsy often accompanies cognitive impairment, which may be induced or exacerbated by ASMs. Conversely, certain antiepileptic medications might exhibit beneficial impacts on cognition. Reliable data concerning cognitive deficits in pediatric patients due to consumption of most ASMs are scarce. Data on ethosuximide are limited; nonetheless, existing evidence indicates that it is not associated with severe cognitive impairment. In a 16-week double-blinded, randomized controlled trial with long-term follow-up, 453 children diagnosed with new-onset absence seizures were compared in terms of treatment efficacy among ethosuximide, 2-valproate, and lamotrigine. None of the children had received ASMs for more than 7 days before randomization. Baseline neuropsychological assessments were conducted in all patients either prior to initiating treatment or within 7 days thereafter. No statistically significant differences were observed in the number of children meeting the Conners Continuous Performance Test criteria for clinical or nonclinical attention deficits (defined as a confidence index score $\geq$0.60) or in the mean full-scale IQ composite score at baseline among the treatment groups. The cognitive abilities of the entire cohort fell within the normal range. Throughout the initial 16–20-week titration phase, children administered 2-valproate exhibited a greater propensity for attention dysfunction than those receiving ethosuximide treatment. Even after adjusting for baseline scores, the difference remained statistically significant ($p < 0.001$). The incidence of attention dysfunction did not significantly differ between the ethosuximide and lamotrigine groups ($p = 0.43$). Even after 12 months, attention dysfunction persisted at a significantly higher level in the 2-valproate group than in the ethosuximide group. This difference persisted even after adjusting for baseline confidentiality index scores ($P = 0.0043$). No significant difference was detected between ethosuximide and lamotrigine ($p = 0.97$). Recently, Ijff et al. delineated the cognitive profile of ethosuximide in 61 children diagnosed with absence epilepsy who underwent ethosuximide monotherapy for an average duration of 1.2 years. Cognitive evaluations comprised the WISC-III and CVST alongside assessments of visual-motor integration, language acquisition, reaction time, and sustained attention. The scores were compared with age-matched reference values. Compared with the control group, the group treated with ethosuximide exhibited notably lower scores for verbal IQ, performance IQ, total IQ, perceptual organization, motor integration, and motor coordination. Markedly slower response times were observed across all reaction time tasks and in certain attentional function evaluations, encompassing search, selective attention, sustained auditory attention, attentional control, switching, and accuracy. Subgroup analyses contrasting children with well-managed seizures for a minimum of 6 months against those with persistent seizures revealed substantially lower IQ, visual perception, and attentional scores in the latter group. The authors posit that this phenomenon could stem from either the direct impact of seizures on cognitive function or underlying pathophysiological effects. Nevertheless, the diminished fuzzy cognitive function (activation, alertness, sustained auditory attention, speed of attentional switching) cannot be solely attributed to persistent seizures, as there was no discernible difference in test outcomes between seizure cohorts, alluding to a plausible direct influence of ethosuximide on cognition. It was concluded that ethosuximide had only a slight effect on cognitive ability [78].

Effects of Ethosuximide Supplementation on Patient Quality of Life

A targeted literature review by Adam Strzelczyk et al. delved into the data on ASMs frequently prescribed for developmental and epileptic encephalopathy, aiming to elucidate the most recent evidence regarding their impacts on behavior, mood, cognition, sedation, and sleep. Current evidence indicates potential adverse effects on specific cognitive aspects associated with topiramate and zonisamide, and ethosuximide seems devoid of detrimental effects. Ethosuximide is associated with sedation to some extent in a randomized controlled trial, and ethosuximide demonstrated superior efficacy compared to lamotrigine in children with refractory epilepsy and exhibited better tolerability (with fewer attention-related adverse effects) than 2-valproate sodium, establishing it as the preferred initial therapy for children with disabled epilepsy. Information concerning the cognitive or behavioral impacts of ethosuximide is scarce. Nevertheless, two studies indicated a potential association between ethosuximide and attention dysfunction, albeit to a lesser degree than or similar to certain other ASMs. In the first study, which compared initial monotherapy in 453 children with absence epilepsy, ethosuximide exhibited significantly fewer attention-related adverse effects at 16–20 weeks and after 1 year than did 2-valproate sodium, while no difference in attention dysfunction was observed between ethosuximide and lamotrigine. Another study on ethosuximide monotherapy involving 61 children with absence episodes revealed markedly lower scores in terms of speech, performance, overall IQ, sensory organs, motor integration, motor coordination, and various attentional function domains than did the control group, although it has been proposed that ethosuximide exerts only minimal effects on certain parameters. Direct literature on sleep parameters is scarce; nevertheless, ethosuximide is associated with sleep-related side effects such as disturbances and night terrors. In summary, although evidence of psychobehavioral adverse events related to ethosuximide is limited, cognitive or sleep alterations, mild attention deficits, and other reactions have also been documented [79]. Ersida Buraniqi et al. conducted a systematic review of Medline studies to evaluate the impacts of ASMs on appetite and weight in children. Eligible studies included randomized controlled trials and open-label studies (open-label extension and intervention) that were conducted on or included pediatric populations (0–18 years of age). The American Academy of Neurology Classification of Therapeutic Research Evidence was employed to classify each study and grade the evidence regarding the effects of each drug on appetite and weight in children. The primary aim was to concentrate on the impacts of epilepsy and ASMs on appetite and weight in children. ASMs have potential adverse effects, several of which may affect appetite and thus normal growth and weight gain. This can increase the incidence of underlying diseases and impede adherence to treatment regimens. Ethosuximide is among the ASMs associated with decreased appetite and/or weight loss. Since the 1960s, ethosuximide has been widely approved for the treatment of children without generalized tonic–clonic seizures.

In the initial randomized controlled trial on absence epilepsy in children, ethosuximide was linked to decreased appetite in 5% of participants; however, this effect was typically transient and did not necessitate treatment discontinuation. There was Grade B evidence of reduced appetite in ethosuximide-treated children, but evidence of weight loss was lacking. In addition to the potential effects of ASMs, other factors related to epilepsy warrant scrutiny, including underlying causes, associated neurological conditions, comorbidities, treatment effects, physical activity levels, and dietary habits [80].

Side Effects of Ethosuximide

Michel Saenz-Farret et al. performed this review by exploring all possible combinations of 15 movement disorders (excluding ataxia) and 24 ASMs. The primary objective was to delineate movement disorders that were treated, worsened, or induced by ASMs. They have summarized the intricate relationship between ASMs and movement disorders, highlighting their mechanism and associated risk factors. Despite the complexity, this relationship remains inadequately reviewed. ASMs can potentially trigger iatrogenic movement disorders, with Parkinson's disease and tremor being the most prevalent. However, identifying movement disorders induced by these drugs is not always straightforward. Ethosuximide is among the medications known to exacerbate or induce dyskinesia. Systemic dancing, including oral facial movements involving the tongue, has been reported following the administration of ethosuximide, which is used to treat loss of consciousness and occasional myoclonic seizures. The resolution of this phenomenology with diphenhydramine suggests a mechanism akin to phenothiazine-associated dyskinesia. Additionally, cases of sedentary disorder concomitant with dyskinesia have been documented. The evidence presented in this review should inform the selection of ASMs for patients with concurrent epilepsy and movement disorders [81]. Hanqing Shang et al. identified acute macroglossia and laryngeal edema as uncommon adverse effects that may lead to life-threatening airway obstruction. They present a case involving a 15-year-old female with severe drug-resistant epilepsy who developed acute macroglossia after initiating ethosuximide. Over the subsequent 2 weeks following the administration of ethosuximide, her condition worsened, hindering extubation. However, upon cessation of the medication, the macroglossia and laryngeal edema improved and completely resolved. The patient was successfully extubated, with prophylactic nasal catheter placement and preextubation dexamethasone administration. In complex patients receiving multiple medications, ASMs should be considered a potential cause of acute macroglossia [82].

Basic Research on Ethosuximide

Priyanka Nagu et al. provided a comprehensive overview of the significance of Wnt signaling in the central nervous system and how its dysregulation disrupts central nervous system function and exacerbates pathological changes during Alzheimer's disease (AD). In the adult brain, Wnt signaling plays a crucial role in neurogenesis, neuronal development, maturation, and proliferation. Impairment of the Wnt signaling pathway, characterized by elevated amyloid-β levels, reduced β-catenin expression levels, and increased GSK-3β enzyme expression, is directly implicated in AD pathogenesis. Studies have indicated that enhancing Wnt signaling through genetic and pharmacological means can enhance cognitive function and restore neurogenesis in the adult brain. Various natural and synthetic compounds, including ethosuximide, have been identified as regulators of Wnt signaling in the adult brain, promoting neurogenesis, and alleviating behavioral dysfunction. Among these compounds is ethosuximide. Ethosuximide and selenomethionine treatment in 3xTg AD mice led to enhanced hippocampal neurogenesis, inhibition of GSK-3β via the PI3K/Akt pathway, elevated β-catenin expression levels, improved cell proliferation, and increased expression of cyclin D1. Ethosuximide also mitigated cognitive decline in the dentate gyri of AD rats, enhanced neuronal diffusion and proliferation, and modulated expression of genes involved in neurogenesis, such as Ngn2 and NeuroD1, as well as other elements of the Wnt signaling pathway. Although this information does not directly imply that ethosuximide regulates neurogenesis by modulating Wnt signaling, some of its connections with β-catenin signaling are evident. Taken together, these findings indicate that targeting Wnt signaling is promising for effective AD management. Further rigorous investigation into Wnt signaling in clinical settings is warranted, as multiple targets are available for comprehending the pathogenesis of AD and devising novel therapeutic interventions to manage the disease [83]. Sean Tatum et al. reported that unilateral or bilateral initiation of spike-wave discharge (SWD) is associated with drug sensitivity akin to absence episodes but differs significantly from complex partial episodes of post-traumatic epilepsy (PTE). Therefore, unilateral SWD seizures following traumatic brain injury (TBI) do not accurately model the complex partial seizures of PTE, in contrast with the relevance of bilateral SWD seizures. Although unilateral SWD seizures in rats have been used to mimic the complex partial seizures of PTE in humans, bilateral SWD seizures are speculated to mirror human absence seizures. Interestingly, both unilateral and bilateral initiation of SWDs after TBI are inhibited by the antiabsence drug ethosuximide but are unaffected by the antiepileptic drug CBZ. Thus, unilateral initiation of SWD is inadequate for investigating the mechanism or treatment of PTE [84].

Other Studies

Sahar M. El-Haggar et al. [85] conducted a prospective, 3-month, randomized, controlled, parallel-group study to assess the additional benefit of ethosuximide, an antiepileptic medication with T-type calcium channel blocking properties, in easing abdominal pain linked to irritable bowel syndrome (IBS). Fifty outpatients who met the inclusion criteria participated in the trial. They were randomly divided into treatment groups, with 25 receiving 135 mg of meperidine three times daily and the other 25 receiving 135 mg of meperidine three times daily alongside 500 mg of ethosuximide three times daily. A gastroenterologist evaluated patients at baseline and 12 weeks after starting treatment. The expression levels of serum tumor necrosis factor, interleukin-6, interleukin-8, fecal myeloperoxidase, and fecal neutrophil gelatin lipocalin (NGAL) were measured before and after treatment. The NRS score for pain was assessed before treatment and 3 months later. This clinical trial is, to the authors' knowledge, the first to compare the efficacy of ethosuximide as an adjunct therapy with that of standard antispasmodic drugs for treating abdominal pain associated with IBS.

The NRS score and the serum tumor necrosis factor, interleukin-6, interleukin-8, fecal NGAL, and fecal myeloperoxidase expression levels were significantly lower in the ethosuximide group than in the meperidine group. It is difficult to determine whether the observed efficacy is solely attributable to meverin alone or in combination with ethosuximide. Further research is required to elucidate the role of ethosuximide in alleviating IBS-related abdominal pain. Nevertheless, the findings suggest that ethosuximide may augment the effects of antispasmodic drugs in patients with IBS, corroborating previous studies indicating that T-type calcium channel blockers could benefit IBS patients. The authors propose that ethosuximide holds promise as an adjunctive treatment for IBS-related abdominal pain, potentially reducing mucosal inflammation and visceral hypersensitivity by lowering the expression levels of serum tumor necrosis factor, interleukin-6, interleukin-8, fecal myeloperoxidase, and fecal lipoprotein-2. Inhibiting T-type calcium channels could be a novel pharmacological approach for alleviating visceral pain associated with low-grade mucosal inflammation in patients with IBS [85]. Léonore Diez et al. conducted a double-phase I study to assess two formulations of ethosuximide granules using lipid multiparticle (LMP) technology. Ethosuximide, the first-line drug for the treatment of childhood absence epilepsy, is currently compounded as a syrup, has a bitter taste and high sugar content, is unsuitable for children and is unsuitable for a ketogenic diet. Two groups of six healthy adult volunteers were subjected to a randomized, placebo-controlled, partially blinded, 3-way crossover trial in which a single 10 mg/kg dose of ethosuximide granules A or B was compared with placebo granules or syrup. This study evaluated the plasma pharmacokinetics, palatability, safety, and tolerability of ethosuximide. Particle A showed suboptimal bitter taste and adherence to the cup wall, while the optimized particle B exhibited good palatability, similar to that of the placebo, with minimal adhesion to glass. The visual analog scale of tolerance indicated a statistically insignificant trend of improvement in transient dizziness (30 min) for all granules, fatigue for granule A, and anxiety for granule B compared to the syrup. The innovative formulation B of ethosuximide granules offers a child-friendly, sugar-free, odorless configuration that is bioequivalent and well tolerated, facilitating precise dosing regulation [86]. Buschhoff AS et al. utilized lateral ventricular injection of the ASMs ethosuximide in a genetic model of absent-seizure epileptic rats from Strasbourg. They observed a significant dose-dependent reduction in spike release without notable abnormal behavior. Moreover, compared with systemic administration, lateral ventricular injection of ethosuximide was more effective at reducing seizures. Compared with standard systemic treatment, local administration minimized systemic drug exposure. Dye distribution tracking throughout the central nervous system supported the notion that lateral ventricular injection delivers drugs to the brain tissue surrounding the ventricle, predominantly remaining at the injection site. These findings suggest that intrathecal administration, which facilitates direct drug penetration from cerebrospinal fluid into brain tissue, is a potential therapeutic avenue for managing generalized epilepsy [71].

2.1.1.4 Phenobarbital

Drug Characterization

[Chemical name] 5-Ethyl-5-phenyl-2,4,6-(1H,3H,5H)-pyrimidinetrione

[Chemical structural formula]

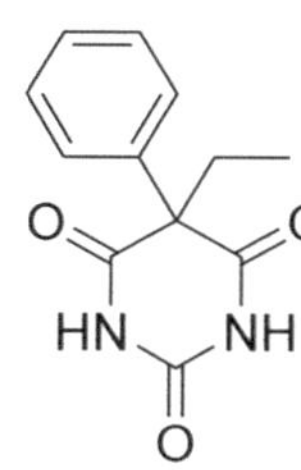

[Molecular formula] C12H12N2O3

[Molecular weight] 232.235

[Indications] Commonly used drugs of choice for treating pediatric epilepsy, including generalized tonic–clonic seizures, focal seizures, acute brain damage combined with epilepsy and status epilepticus.

[Specifications] Phenobarbital tablets: 15 mg; 16.2 mg; 30 mg; 32.4 mg; 60 mg; 64.8 mg; 97.2 mg; 100 mg; phenobarbital oral solution: 20 mg/5 mL; phenobarbital sodium for injection: 50 mg; 100 mg; 200 mg; phenobarbital sodium injection: 100 mg/1 mL; 200 mg/2 mL.

[Usage and dosage]
Adult use:

(1) Oral administration: 90–180 mg once in the evening, or 30–60 mg three times a day; the maximum dose is 250 mg at a time, 500 mg a day. (2) Injection

(intramuscular, subcutaneous, intravenous), 100–200 mg once, one to two times a day; the maximum dose is 250 mg at a time, 500 mg a day; when intravenous administration is used, it is noted that it should be slowly injected. (3) For status epilepticus, 200–300 mg is intravenously injected once (at a rate of no more than 60 mg/min), and this injection is repeated once every 6 h if necessary.

[Children's medication]
(1) Administer orally, 3–5 mg/kg at a time. (2) Intramuscularly, 3–5 mg/kg or 125 mg/m^2 at a time. The doctor's instructions should be followed for details.

[Adverse reactions] Sedation, fatigue, drowsiness, dizziness or spinning sensation, nausea, vomiting, headache, depressed mood, feeling of restlessness or euphoria (especially in children or the elderly), feeling of drunkenness or a "hangover" effect (feeling of fatigue the day after taking phenobarbital).

Clinical Applications and Basic Research

Historical Evolution of Phenobarbital

Phenobarbital (also known as luminal) acts as a positive modulator of the gamma-aminobutyric acid type A (GABAA) receptor. In 1912, the pharmacological effects of phenobarbital (PB) were discovered by French physicians Pierre Émile Dejours and Claude Lavollay, who observed its sedative, hypnotic, and anticonvulsant properties. The biopharmacology of PB was first described in 1980 by R J Porter [87]. In 1987, P D Pigatto discovered PB-induced allergic dermatitis [88]. In 1989, T O Crawford discovered the postphenobarbital state [89]. In 1992, M C Lindberg et al. described acute PB toxicity [90]. In 2012, Martin J Brodie et al. proposed the current role of PB in epilepsy and its future [91]. In 2016, Gian M Pacifici described the clinical effects, metabolism and pharmacokinetics of PB in neonates [92].

Phenobarbital for Epilepsy Syndromes

Benedikt Hofmeister et al. [93] conducted the first global retrospective analysis of anticonvulsant treatment for Nicolaides-Balaise syndrome (NCBRS), marking a significant milestone despite including a limited number of cases. Assessing anticonvulsant therapy for concurrent epilepsy in NCBRS patients holds promise for managing epilepsy associated with this syndrome. Such studies offer valuable insights for clinicians and parents alike, as well as guidance on treatment strategies. NCBRS, stemming from mutations in the SMARCA2 gene, manifests with intellectual disability, facial and limb malformations, and often refractory epilepsy. The study cohort comprised 25 NCBRS patients, 23 of whom experienced epileptic seizures. Among the five most commonly utilized anticonvulsants (valproic acid, levetiracetam, phenobarbital, topiramate, and carbamazepine), PB has emerged as particularly effective, reducing seizure frequency by more than 50% and achieving sustained seizure control (>6 months).

Phenobarbital for Persistent Status Epilepticus

Yingying Su et al. [94] conducted a multicenter, prospective, randomized controlled study to compare the efficacy and safety of PB and valproic acid in the treatment of generalized convulsive status epilepticus (GCSE). They discovered that the GCSE termination rate within 1 h was notably greater in the PB group than in the valproic acid group. However, the rate of nontermination EEG seizure discharge within 1 h was similar between the two groups. The recurrence rates and adverse events were comparable as well. Their conclusion highlighted that the PB regimen demonstrated superior efficacy in terminating GCSE compared to valproic acid. This conclusion is supported by low-quality evidence [95] suggesting that PB effectively halts seizures in benzodiazepine-resistant patients with persistent status epilepticus within 60 min of administration. High-dose levetiracetam, high-dose sodium valproate, and PB may exhibit equivalent efficacy, allowing clinicians to select treatments based on factors such as effectiveness, safety, availability, cost, and systemic comorbidities. Gang Liu et al. [96] observed a better prognosis in the intravenous PB group than in the intravenous valproate group among Chinese adult patients with GCSE during a follow-up period of up to 12 months. This finding may encourage the utilization of intravenous PB, particularly in patients with restricted access to newer anticonvulsants. The rate of GCSE termination within 1 h was notably greater in the PB group than in the valproate group among adult patients, indicating that PB may be a suitable option for countries, regions, and individuals with restricted access to newer anticonvulsant medications or limited economic resources [94].

Phenobarbital in Special Populations with Epilepsy

Ankush Jindal et al. [97] conducted an open-label randomized controlled trial to investigate the effect of early discontinuation of PB on neonatal seizure recurrence. Following a loading dose of PB (20 mg/kg) and achieving seizure freedom for at least 12 h, the children were randomly allocated to groups in which PB administration was either continued or discontinued. They observed comparable rates of seizure recurrence between the groups, along with similar durations for achieving complete enteral feeding, lengths of hospital stay, neurological abnormalities at discharge, and mortality rates. Thus, they concluded that early discontinuation of PB administration does not significantly increase the recurrence rate of neonatal seizures. Julie M. Ziobro et al. [98] discussed the pathophysiology of neonatal seizures and reviewed the currently available evidence for treatment. PB is strongly recommended by the World Health Organization as the primary treatment for neonatal seizures. Analysis of U.S. Pediatric Health Information System hospital data [99] revealed that 97% of neonates with seizures received PB treatment. PB was also the most commonly prescribed medication when neonates were discharged from the hospital on ASMs. These data emphasize the pivotal role of PB in the current approach to managing neonatal seizures. In conclusion, PB remains the first-line standard treatment option for neonatal epilepsy.

Nan Li et al. [100] conducted a study to investigate the characteristics of elderly patients with epilepsy in rural northeast China. They examined patients with convulsive epilepsy (471 patients aged >60 years) from seven counties of Jilin Province, Northeast China, between January 2010 and December 2019. Among these, 329 patients were categorized into the early-onset epilepsy group, and 142 patients were categorized into the late-onset epilepsy group. They found that elderly patients with epilepsy responded well to PB monotherapy, and the difference was similar between the two groups ($p > 0.05$).

Yusuf Cem Kaplan et al. [101] conducted a review to assess the possible risks of four traditional ASMs, phenytoin (PHT), PB, CBZ, and VPA, during pregnancy and lactation in comparison with two newer ASMs commonly used and provided a discussion on the safety of antiepileptic drug use during breastfeeding. A recent analysis from the EURAP registry reported a 6.5% severe malformation rate for PB use during breastfeeding [102]. According to a meta-analysis, PB exposure in utero significantly increased the incidence of major congenital malformations [103]. Severe cases of drowsiness have been reported in infants whose mothers used PB during breastfeeding [104]. Due to the high relative infant dose (RID) and relatively frequent adverse reactions in infants, the American Academy of Pediatrics has categorized PB as a medication to be used cautiously during breastfeeding [105]. Currently, these ASMs should be administered at the lowest effective dose to ensure optimal seizure control in pregnant women.

Efficacy and Safety of the Preferred Addition of Phenobarbital for the Treatment of Epilepsy

Deepak Sharma et al. [106] conducted a literature search through the Cochrane Central Register of Controlled Trials and various other electronic databases to analyze two studies that met the inclusion criteria for systematic evaluation. Both studies showed that levetiracetam is safer than PB for treating neonatal seizures. Although PB has traditionally been used as a first-line ASMs for seizures, concerns have arisen regarding its impact on neuronal cell apoptosis in the developing brain. The literature has shown better seizure control after a single loading dose of levetiracetam than after a single dose of PB, with a greater 24-h seizure cessation rate and fewer side effects. A randomized controlled trial by Gummalla Gyandeep et al. [107] reached the same conclusion. Levetiracetam is as effective as PB in stopping clinical seizures in premature infants, with fewer adverse reactions. A randomized, double-blinded, parallel-group phase III study [108] aimed to evaluate the efficacy of PB sodium injections in participants with clinical seizures. This study was designed to demonstrate the effectiveness of PB in preventing subsequent seizures and to demonstrate better efficacy when it is used at a high dose (40 mg/kg) than at a low dose (20 mg/kg). International surveys of neonatologists worldwide have indicated that PB (used in up to 70% of cases) can serve as a first-line ASMs, irrespective of seizure etiology or gestational age [109].

Evidence-Based Medical Research on Phenobarbital

Jogender Kumar et al. [110] conducted a systematic review and meta-analysis to assess and compare the efficacy and safety of PB with those of other drugs used as first-line medications for the treatment of neonatal seizures. A total of 443 records were screened, and nine eligible studies (719 patients) were identified. Their analysis revealed that PB demonstrated comparable effectiveness and safety to drugs such as phenytoin sodium and levetiracetam. However, the absence of data on long-term neurodevelopmental outcomes suggests that a drug that could replace PB as a first-line medication for antiepileptic seizures in neonates is not yet available.

Claudio Liguori et al. [111] conducted a comprehensive literature review focusing on 25 ASMs to investigate their impact on sleep architecture and daytime sleepiness among individuals with epilepsy. In the initial study, sleep log data from 184 children with febrile convulsions were analyzed and compared with those of children treated with either placebo or PB. No significant difference in total sleep time was observed between the two groups. Subsequently, in a study involving 150 epilepsy patients, a higher prevalence of PB usage was noted among those experiencing excessive daytime sleepiness, suggesting a potential stimulatory effect of PB on daytime somnolence. Another study employing multiple linear regression analysis revealed a weak positive correlation between Pittsburgh Sleep Quality Index scores and PB usage. Taking all factors into account, the authors concluded that PB was associated with poor sleep quality in patients with epilepsy, but the explanation was limited. Overall, PB did not affect or worsen sleep parameters.

Basic Research on Phenobarbital

Marie Johne et al. [112] sought to assess whether higher doses (10 mg/kg) of bumetanide could potentiate the effects of PB in a novel rat model of birth asphyxia. A novel neonatal seizure model was established by inducing intermittent asphyxia with 9% and 5% O2 for 30 min (three 7 + 3 min cycles) in postnatal day 11 (P11) male and female rat pups, respectively, at a constant 20% CO2. Contrary to expectations, bumetanide (10 mg/kg) did not augment the effect of PB (15 mg/kg) on the seizure rate. PB in combination with the ester predrug N,N-dimethylaminoethyl ester (DIMAEB) or bumipramine, a predrug of bumetanide, inhibited neonatal seizures. The bumetanide/phenobarbital combination also prevented asphyxia and postictal hippocampal neurodegenerative changes. Both bumipramine and DIMAEB are promising tools that may help in the development of more effective lead compounds for subsequent clinical trials. In addition, they evaluated the effect of bumetanide/phenobarbital combination treatment on a novel rat model of birth asphyxia (also using P11 rat pups) in another study [113]. They found that when 30 mg/kg PB was applied before asphyxia instead of 15 mg/kg PB, seizures were significantly prevented. In contrast, bumetanide (0.3 mg/kg) alone or in combination with PB (15 or 30 mg/kg) had no significant effect on seizures. They concluded that bumetanide does not enhance the efficacy of PB in this model.

Side Effects of Phenobarbital

The incidence of PB-related adverse reactions was 47%, with sedation and ataxia being the most frequent. These reactions typically manifested within the initial month of treatment and were temporary. Notably, higher initial doses of PB and the introduction of a second ASM were significantly linked to adverse reactions [114].

PB, the oldest ASM currently in widespread use, was developed in 1912 as a short-acting barbiturate. Numerous studies have provided substantial evidence indicating its correlation with various cognitive impairments in children and adolescents. Specifically, memory function tends to be notably affected, often resulting in inferior cognitive performance compared to alternative antiepileptic medications. Jia Liu et al. [115] reported that while there were no significant differences in seizure severity, reductions in number of seizures by 50% or more, or adverse events among levetiracetam (LEV), PB, and lamotrigine (LTG), PB had a detrimental impact on cognitive abilities and mood. Frank M. C. Besag et al. [78] extensively reviewed the literature on PubMed and concluded that PB is particularly linked to cognitive dysfunction, encompassing memory lapses, attention deficits, and comprehension difficulties. Longitudinal studies have consistently shown persistent cognitive impairments even months after the discontinuation of PB. Thus, collective evidence underscores the significant negative cognitive repercussions associated with PB treatment in pediatric patients.

Marta Karaźniewicz-Łada et al. [116] integrated recent literature from PubMed and Google Base to offer insights into ASMs and their interactions with other medications, nutrients, and foods. Notably, as an inducer of ASMs, PB increases the metabolism of oral contraceptives, thereby diminishing their therapeutic efficacy. Additionally, compared to lamotrigine or levetiracetam, PB is associated with increased teratogenicity and neurocognitive deficits. Furthermore, PB treatment may accelerate vitamin D metabolism in the liver, potentially leading to vitamin D deficiency. James Peters et al. [117] studied convulsions induced by ASMs using data from PubMed, Medline, and the Cochrane Library. Examining 43 cases of ASM-induced convulsions from 1984 to 2019, PB use was found to be associated with 7 of 43 (16%) cases. Moreover, not all neuropsychiatric symptoms, either new or exacerbated, were resolved upon discontinuation of PB, with 3 of 43 cases strongly linked to more complex symptoms.

Phenobarbital Use in Other Diseases

PB demonstrates efficacy in depression treatment. Ahmad Shamabadi [118] conducted a literature review revealing that 120 mg/day PB, 20 mg/day diazepam, and 100 mg/day amitriptyline yielded comparable improvements in depression. Notably, PB exhibits enhanced effectiveness in individuals with lower education levels and heightened family stress. In two studies comparing the effects of PB with those of imipramine and amitriptyline, PB was shown to be not only effective in treating depression but also associated with fewer adverse effects.

While benzodiazepines remain the primary treatment for alcohol withdrawal syndrome (AWS), PB serves as an alternative therapy. Treatment with PB for AWS patients demonstrated similar outcomes in terms of intubation rates, ICU lengths of stay, and hospital stays compared to benzodiazepine treatment. However, more robust trials are warranted to validate these findings [119]. In patients with benzodiazepine-resistant AWS, a loading dose of PB significantly reduced the incidence of mechanical ventilation and the need for continuous sedation compared to intermittent low-dose administration [120]. Delayed initiation of PB treatment appears to increase the risk of complications related to AWS [121]. PB is known to induce expression of cytochrome P450 enzymes 3A4 and 2B6, key hepatic metabolic pathways for numerous drugs, and induces glucuronidation, a secondary metabolic pathway. Given that both PB and opioids undergo metabolism via these pathways, their concomitant use may lead to interactions. However, the extent of enzyme induction seems to be dose-dependent and may take days to weeks to reach the maximum effect, potentially decreasing the plasma concentrations of both drugs to subtherapeutic levels, thereby heightening the risk of delayed opioid withdrawal and relapse. Moreover, owing to its long half-life, which averages 80 h in adults, PB's potential for adverse drug interactions may persist for weeks after discontinuation. Consequently, in alcohol withdrawal programs, in which PB is increasingly utilized, caution should be exercised to avoid its use in patients with concurrent opioid use disorders in most instances [122].

2.1.1.5 Primidone

Drug Characteristics

[Drug characteristics] 5-Ethyl-5-phenyl-dihydro-4,6(1H,5H)-pyrimidine dione

[Chemical structure formula]

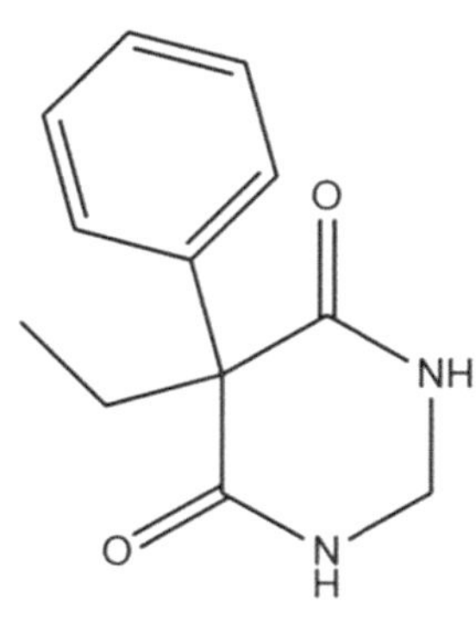

[Molecular formula] C12H14N2O2

[Molecular weight] 325.4242

[Indications] The effect of primidone is similar to that of phenobarbital; approximately 25% of phenobarbital is oxidized in the body, and the other portion of the lytic phenylethylmalamide proeclampone and its metabolites have antiepileptic effects. Clinical agents, mainly other ASMs, are ineffective for treating grand mal seizures and psychomotor seizures and are ineffective for treating minor seizures. Combination treatment with phenytoin sodium can enhance the curative effect.

[Specification] 0.25 g

[Usage and dosage] Primidone is started at a dose of 0.15 g and gradually increased to 0.2 g, three times a day. The maximum 1 day dose is 2 g. Children should take 12.5–25 mg/kg daily, divided two to three times.

[Adverse reactions]
Central nervous system side effects include drowsiness, nausea, vomiting, personality changes, dizziness, ataxia, diplopia, and optic neuritis. The adverse effects on the blood system include folate deficiency, megaloblastic anemia, neonatal hemorrhage, leukopenia, and thrombocytopenia. The skin presents with maculopapulosis and bullous dermatitis. Adverse reactions of the skeletal system include osteoporosis and rickets. There have also been reports of systemic edema due to liver and kidney damage, as well as other syndromes such as lupus erythematosus and malignant lymphoma. The main side effects are sleepiness, personality changes, and folate deficiency. Approximately 10% of patients stopped taking the drug due to severe toxic reactions.

Clinical Application and Basic Research

History of Primidone

In 1953, R HANDLEY first described primidone as a novel antiepileptic agent [123]. In 1954, S GOLDIN described the toxic effects of primidone [124]. In 1954, P W NATHAN et al. discovered primidone for the treatment of nonidiopathic epilepsy [125]. In 1955, V. SCARINCI discovered the pharmacological effects of primidone [126]. In 2005, M Lopez-Gomez et al. reported that primidone was associated with interseizure depression in patients with epilepsy [127]. In 2021, Abhishek Lenka et al. reported that primidone intolerance in essential tremor patients was not just an age-related issue [128]. Primidone is a recognized narrow therapeutic index drug (NTID) and is included in the NTID catalog in China, the United States, and Japan. Its efficacy was described by Desilvey in 1980, with subsequent confirmation of its safety and effectiveness in treating epileptic seizures, supported by four cases reported in China.

Primidone in the Treatment of Epilepsy

An observational study of primidone in the treatment of epilepsy revealed that partial persistent epilepsy, often associated with cerebral cortex lesions, may also stem from subcortical lesions. Trevor et al. described a patient with partial persistent epilepsy who was unresponsive to conventional anticonvulsants but had a significant brief response to alcohol, followed by a response to primidone. This response pattern, akin to that observed in essential tremors, suggests a shared pathology within the same anatomical network. Consequently, a novel pathophysiological model is proposed to explain the development of persistent partial epilepsy in both cortical and subcortical disease processes [129]. To evaluate the concentration of antiseizure medications (ASMs) in the breast milk of women with epilepsy (WWE) during lactation, Ramzi et al. integrated data on estimated daily intake (EDI) and relative infant dose (RID) of ASMs, assessing potential risks to infants. Across the 15 included studies, ASM levels in breast milk were reported, with varying RIDs for different medications. The RIDs of CBZ, lamotrigine, primidone, phenobarbital, gabapentin, valproic acid, ethosuximide, levetiracetam, and topiramate were 3.70%, 36.33%, 4.96%, 3.15%, 4.37%, 1.90%, 31.49%, 12.50%, and 12.18%, respectively. Breastfeeding may be restricted or even stopped when adverse signs of excessive sedation/lethargy and/or weight gain occur in infants exposed to primidone and phenobarbital, ethosuximide/primidone, or ethosuximide/phenobarbital. It was concluded that ASMs can be detected in the breast milk of WWE and in the plasma/serum of infants exposed to breast milk. Healthcare providers and WWE may use the results of this study to make informed decisions about the safety of breastfeeding when taking ASMs. Approximately 70% of individuals with epilepsy can achieve seizure freedom with proper treatment. Discontinuing ASMs when seizures are controlled can mitigate side effects but may increase the risk of recurrence [74]. Jingjing Wang et al. compared the recurrence rates among patients who continued ASMs therapy against those who stopped it. Nevertheless, it remains uncertain whether discontinuing ASMs is correlated with increased seizure recurrence. The primary aim of this meta-analysis was to determine whether there was a discrepancy in epilepsy recurrence rates between seizure-free patients who maintained ASMs usage and those who stopped it. The heterogeneity was assessed via the I2 value, and odds ratios (ORs) and 95% confidence intervals (CIs) were calculated using the Mantel–Haenszel test; seven cohort studies and randomized controlled trials (RCTs) meeting the inclusion criteria were included. The quality of the studies was evaluated with the Newcastle–Ottawa Scale and the Jadad Scale. Their analysis included 1253 patients, revealing a greater recurrence rate among patients who discontinued ASMs than among those who continued therapy. Furthermore, they investigated seizure recurrence rates postdiscontinuation among seizure-free patients treated with various ASMs (CBZ, phenytoin, valproate, and phenobarbital/primidone), incorporating four studies totaling 625 patients. No significant differences in epilepsy recurrence rates were observed among the different ASMs treatment regimens [130]. Inhalation of hyperbaric oxygen can potentially induce seizures akin to epilepsy. Hence, Ivan T et al. conducted experiments to investigate whether pretreatment with an FDA-approved antiepileptic medication could mitigate seizures in a hyperoxic setting with an absolute concentration of 5 atmospheres. Drugs were chosen from two anticipated functional categories: Na+ channel blockers and GABA enhancers. Among the five sodium channel blockers tested, CBZ and lamotrigine exhibited seizure latencies three times greater than those of the solvent control group. However, the effectiveness of primidone, zonisamide, and oxazepane was limited. As these crucial elements of neuronal excitation and inhibition are implicated in the development of various epileptic conditions, including generalized epilepsy, the authors suggest that common pathways might be involved in these pathological processes despite initial divergent damage. Moreover, it remains unclear whether prolonged exposure to high levels of oxygen triggers spontaneous recurrent seizures, a hallmark of clinical epilepsy. Nonetheless, research on hyperbaric oxygen toxicity can shed light on new molecular mechanisms underlying epileptic seizures of diverse origins. Additionally, the neuropathology associated with hyperbaric oxygen exposure lends credence to the hypothesis proposed by some researchers that oxidative stress plays a pivotal role in the onset of clinical epilepsy [131].

Evidence-Based Medical Research on Primidone

Therapeutic drug monitoring (TDM) is crucial for optimizing and tailoring the treatment of ASMs, particularly in vulnerable groups such as pregnant women, elderly individuals, and children. However, the practical application of TDM often faces challenges due to limitations in blood collection methods. Thus, Thierry et al. investigated a novel home sampling technique known as volumetric absorption microsampling (VAMS). Their study aimed to assess VAMS by analyzing and quantifying the concentrations of 16 different ASMs in whole blood samples. Venous blood samples were obtained from 138 patients at the Kempenhaeghe Epilepsy Academic Center. The concentrations of ASMs were measured using both the VAMS method (whole blood) and the conventional method (serum). Additionally, the impact of hematocrit on recovery was evaluated. This study also examined the stability of ASMs in microsampling devices over time and the influence of temperature on their stability using ASMs-infused blood. The results indicated that VAMS could accurately detect 16 different ASMs within a 2-day period. When the recovery deviation was less than 10%, VAMS showed a strong correlation with conventional sampling. Furthermore, hematocrit levels between 0.3 and 0.5 (L/L) did not affect the results. While the storage temperature had an impact on the stability of some ASMs in VAMS, the majority of samples remained unaffected. Conclusion: VAMS can accurately detect multiple ASMs within 2 days [132].

Effect of Primidone Addition on Patient Quality of Life

To characterize the clinical presentation, progression, and management of essential tremor (ET) in children, Debabrata et al. conducted a retrospective analysis of clinical data spanning 27 years from 1984 to 2011. The study included 211 children with ET, comprising 130 males and 81 females. Seven children (14.09 ± 5.0 years) were included, and the age of onset was 9.71 ± 5.62 years. The majority of patients (199) exhibited bilateral hand tremors, with others presenting with asymmetrical or unilateral tremors that later became bilateral. Additional manifestations included leg tremors, head tremors, trunk tremors, and resting tremors. A family history of ET was reported in 35% of patients, predominantly involving parents and siblings. Functional impairments were observed in 55% of patients, affecting activities such as writing, eating, and playing musical instruments. Treatment strategies included propranolol, atenolol, primidone, metoprolol, and nadolol. Follow-up data from 99 patients over an average period of 1.82 ± 2.21 years revealed that untreated tremors remained stable in some patients, while propranolol treatment led to significant short-term improvement in 15 of 20 patients. Overall, this study represents the largest case series of ET in children to date, highlighting the potential for onset at birth, lower familial predisposition compared to adults, and the prevalence of functional disabilities requiring medication in a substantial proportion of cases [133]. Gene expression analysis has been shown to be highly effective in predicting drug responses in cell models, as demonstrated by an endeavor by Charles-Etienne et al. to apply this method in the context of essential tremor (ET), a condition in which many patients respond to two drugs: propranolol and primidone. In this study, cerebellar DAOYs and neural progenitor cells were treated with clinical concentrations of propranolol and primidone for 5 days. Subsequently, RNA sequencing was employed to pinpoint differentially expressed genes that converged during the treatment process. Propranolol was observed to influence the expression of genes previously linked to ET and other movement disorders, including TRAPPC11. Pathway enrichment analysis of these targeted genes revealed multiple terms associated with calcium signaling, endosome sorting, axon guidance, and neuronal morphology. Moreover, the genes affected by ET drugs exhibited enrichment in cell types expressing ET-related genes prominently in cortical and cerebellar tissues. Collectively, these findings shed light on potential cellular and molecular mechanisms linked to tremor alleviation and pinpoint relevant genetic biomarkers for assessing ET drug responsiveness [134].

Side Effects of Primidone

Abhishek et al. proposed that there are limited options available. Among them, primidone stands out as one of only two primary drugs, but it is associated with significant adverse reactions. The reasons why some essential tremor patients using primidone experience adverse reactions while others do not remain unclear, especially considering that these reactions seem to be more common in essential tremor patients than in those with epilepsy who are treated with primidone. Although direct comparative data are lacking, an examination of prior studies involving essential tremor and epilepsy patients suggested that primidone tends to be better tolerated in the former. Moreover, not all essential tremor patients experience adverse reactions of a similar nature or severity. The discussion delves into several potential mechanisms underlying this variability in primidone intolerance, including older age (in both essential tremor and epilepsy patients), potential cross-tolerance in epilepsy patients, and neurobiological abnormalities related to GABA in essential tremor patients [128].

To characterize the clinical manifestations of adverse skin reactions and cross-reactivities induced by antiepileptic medications and to contrast the usage patterns of these drugs among epileptic patients with and without a history of rash, Tallulah et al. conducted an analysis involving patients who developed rashes within 12 weeks of commencing antiepileptic therapy. The occurrence of rash was corroborated through medical records, interviews, and patient identification of lesions via visual aids. The minimum follow-up period was 8 months. The control cohort comprised epileptic individuals who had consistently been taking ASMs for at least 12 weeks without experiencing any rash. A total of 109 patients and 99 controls were enrolled. The findings revealed that cross-reactivity was more prevalent among patients with a history of Stevens-Johnson syndrome (29%) and Stevens-Johnson syndrome/toxic epidermal necrolysis overlap (50%) ($p = 0.01$). While most rashes were mild, the utilization pattern of ASMs differed from that of the control group, with a lower utilization rate of drugs typically associated with severe adverse skin reactions (e.g., CBZ, phenytoin, phenobarbital, primidone, oxcarbazepine, and lamotrigine) ($p < 0.001$). However, cross-sensitization was not prevalent among patients exposed to high-risk drugs. A history of cutaneous adverse reactions could influence the selection of antiepileptic medications. Cross-sensitivity was more frequent in severe cases, yet most patients exhibited mild, self-limiting rashes. Future investigations should explore the significance of mild rashes in managing lifelong epilepsy [135].

Laboratory Studies of Primidone

The transient receptor potential (TRP) channel TRPM3, associated with the melastatin family, functions as a nonselective cation channel present in neurons prone to injury and activated by heat. Given that TRPM3-deficient mice exhibit inflammatory thermal hyperalgesia, inhibiting TRPM3 expression with drugs may confer antinociceptive effects. To identify TRPM3 inhibitors, fluorescence calcium influx assays and screening libraries containing approved or clinically tested drugs were utilized. The biophysical characteristics of channel inhibition were assessed using electrophysiological methods. Diclofenac, a nonsteroidal anti-inflammatory drug; maprotiline, a tetracyclic antidepressant; and primidone, an anticonvulsant, have emerged as highly potent TRPM3 blockers with semimaximum inhibition at concentrations ranging from 0.6 to 6 μM and notable specificity for TRPM3. In particular, primidone exhibited biological activity, effectively inhibiting TRPM3 activation induced by pregnenolone sulfate (PregS) and heat at concentrations significantly lower than the plasma levels typically used in antiepileptic therapy. Primidone inhibited PregS-induced calcium influx through TRPM3 via variable structure regulation and reversed the atypical inward rectifier TRPM3 current caused by the combined action of PregS and clotrimazole. In vivo experiments conducted by Ute et al. revealed the analgesic effects of low-dose primidone using PregS and a heat-induced mouse model of pain, including inflammatory hyperalgesia [136]. The solid-phase FTIR and FT-Raman spectra of primidone were captured within the spectral ranges of 4000–400 cm(−1) and 4000–100 cm(−1), respectively. Following the acquisition, the vibration spectrum underwent thorough analysis, with assignments made and further examination conducted on the underlying principles. The experimental wavenumbers were juxtaposed with their theoretically standardized counterparts determined through DFT. Raman strength was gauged using the B3LYP/6-31G(d,p) method. Furthermore, the B3LYP/6-311++G(d,p) method was employed to determine the total molecular electron density and molecular electrostatic potential surface, revealing the distribution of the electrostatic potential encompassing both electrons and nuclei. The HOMO and LUMO energies were quantified, while the analysis of the natural bond orbitals of primidone indicated the presence of intramolecular charge transfer. Additionally, (1)H and (13)C NMR spectra were recorded, facilitating the computation of chemical shifts for the molecules [137].

Basic Research on Primidone

Theresa et al. investigated RIPK1 inhibitors, culminating in the proposal of an aromatic ASM alongside the FDA-approved primidone as a potent inhibitor of RIPK1 activation both in vitro and in a mouse model of TNF-α-induced shock, replicating the exaggerated inflammatory conditions akin to cytokine release syndrome. These findings advocate for the progression of clinical trials aimed at evaluating the efficacy of RIPK1 inhibition in COVID-19 patients. An application for a clinical trial utilizing primidone to treat a subset of patients with SARS-CoV-2-positive acute respiratory distress syndrome is presently undergoing submission to EudraCT, the European Union Medicines Regulatory Authority Clinical Trials Database. Given the favorable safety profile, tolerability, pharmacokinetics, and pharmacodynamics of primidone, its clinical use in treating diseases caused by pathological RIPK1 activation is straightforward. It is logical to test other drugs that have been approved for other indications and have been marketed on a large scale [138].

Studies of Primidone Use for Other Conditions

Andrew et al. conducted a retrospective review of medical records encompassing all female patients treated with primidone for primary or secondary laryngeal spasm or essential tremor at a tertiary care center. The mean (SD) age of the 30 patients was 71.9 (11.8) years, and the average (SD) treatment duration was 5.25 (7.22) months. Among them, 30% had concurrent dysphonia, with various diagnoses, including spasmodic dysphonia and laryngeal reflux disease. Approximately 40% had received prior treatment. Notably, 54% reported improvement in their vocal symptoms, and 55% continued primidone therapy without discontinuation. However, adverse reactions were experienced by 73% of patients, leading to treatment cessation in a substantial portion of patients. Among those who stopped treatment, there was no significant difference in discontinuation rates between patients who experienced adverse reactions and those who did not. Subsequently, 53% of patients commenced Botox therapy, with variable clinical outcomes. Although 36% reported improvement after primidone treatment, 58% saw no change in symptoms. Overall, this case series suggests that primidone therapy effectively manages idiopathic acoustic tremors in a subset of patients, offering an alternative to Botox neurotoxin therapy [139]. Hitomi et al. investigated the impact of ASMs, including primidone and valproic acid, on the accumulation of free cholesterol (C) in NPC1-empty CHO cells and NPC1* fibroblasts derived from individuals with NPC1 mutations. Like treatment with valproic acid, primidone treatment led to decreased free cholesterol levels in lysosomes/endosomes in NPC1-null/mutant cells. Furthermore, primidone partially restored cholesterol ester levels in NPC1-null cells and upregulated the mRNA expression levels of HMG-CoA reductase and low-density lipoprotein receptor in NPC1* cells. This finding suggested that primidone facilitates the transport of free cholesterol from lysosomes/endosomes to the endoplasmic reticulum in NPC1-null/mutant cells. In NPC1-deficient mice, oral administration of primidone (100 mg/kg/day) extended the lifespan by approximately 5 days, although initial treatment had no effect on ataxia, a classic symptom of neuromotor dysfunction. These findings underscore the therapeutic potential of primidone in the management of nasopharyngeal carcinoma [140].

2.1.1.6 Valproic Acid

Drug Characteristics

[Chemical name] 2-Propylvaleric acid; 2-n-propyl n-valeric acid; 2,2-di-n-propyl acetic acid; A-propylvaleric acid; α-propylvaleric acid

[Chemical structure]

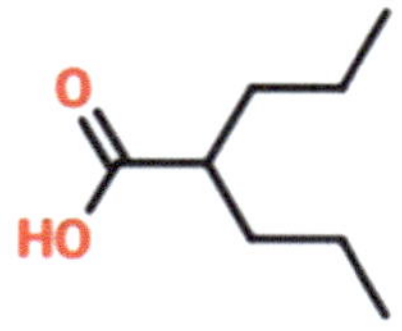

[Molecular formula] C8H16O2

[Molecular weight] 144.21100

[Indications] Valproic acid is suitable for treatment in adults and children over 3 years old. It can be used as a single-drug treatment or as an add-on treatment. It can be used to treat generalized epilepsy: nonmotor seizures (absence), myoclonic seizures, tonic–clonic seizures, atonic seizures, and some types of epilepsy syndromes (West, Lennox–Gastaut syndrome), etc.; it can also be used for the treatment of focal epileptic seizures that progress from focal to generalized seizures.

[Specifications]

Regular tablets:	Sodium valproate tablets	0.1 g 0.2 g
	Magnesium valproate tablets	0.2 g
Sustained-release tablets:	Sodium valproate extended release tablets 0.2 g; 0.5 g (each tablet contains 0.333 g sodium valproate and 0.145 valproic acid, equivalent to 0.5 g sodium valproate)	
	Magnesium valproate extended release tablets 0.25 g	
Oral liquid:	Sodium valproate oral solution	300 mL: 12 g
	Sodium valproate syrup	100 mL: 5 g
Injection:	Sodium valproate for injection	0.4 g

[Dosage]

Syrup and tablets are started at a dose of 5–10 mg/kg, and the dosage is gradually increased. The maintenance dose is 0.6–1.2 g/day for adults, taken orally two to three times, with a maximum dose of 1.8–2.4 g.

Sustained-release tablets: The starting dose for newly diagnosed epilepsy is usually 10–15 mg/kg/day, one to two times a day, and the dose is gradually increased, with an interval of 2–3 days between each dose increase. The maintenance dose is 20–30 mg/kg. This product can be broken in half and taken but cannot be ground or chewed. If the daily dosage exceeds 50 mg/kg, the patient must be closely monitored.

Oral solution: generally starting from 0.6 g/day and taken two times, the usual dosage range is 1–2 g/day, up to 2.5 g/day.

When elderly patients take this product, the dosage should be determined based on seizure control.

For patients whose condition is well-controlled with regular sodium valproate formulations, it is recommended that the current daily dose be maintained when using extended-release tablets as an alternative.

[FDA Black Box Warning]

- Hepatotoxicity: In the general population, frequent serum liver metabolite tests are imperative, especially before and after treatment initiation, particularly within the first 6 months, to monitor for fatal liver failure. Children under 2 years old, especially those taking multiple antiseizure medications, who are afflicted with congenital errors of metabolism, severe epilepsy accompanied by intellectual disability, or organic encephalopathy, face significantly heightened risks of fatal hepatotoxicity. Patients with mitochondrial diseases characterized by mutations in mitochondrial DNA and those with hereditary neurometabolic syndromes such as Alpers-Huttenlocher syndrome caused by POLG gene mutations are particularly prone to valproate-induced acute liver failure and mortality. Therefore, the use of sodium valproate injection is strictly prohibited in children under 2 years old with suspected mitochondrial disease.
- Fetal risk: Valproic acid can cause serious congenital malformations, particularly neural tube defects such as spina bifida. Hence, valproate is contraindicated for

preventing migraines in pregnant women and those of childbearing age who are not practicing effective contraception. It should not be utilized to treat epilepsy during pregnancy or in individuals planning pregnancy, except in cases where other medications fail to control symptoms or are otherwise unsuitable.
- Pancreatitis: Life-threatening cases of pancreatitis have been reported in children and adults. Patients and caregivers should be vigilant for symptoms such as abdominal pain, nausea, vomiting, and anorexia, as these symptoms may indicate pancreatitis and necessitate prompt medical evaluation.

[Adverse reactions]
This product has a range of potential adverse effects, including liver failure, birth defects, intellectual disability, pancreatitis, hyperammonemic encephalopathy, suicidal behavior, bleeding, and various hematopoietic disorders. Additionally, it may lead to hypothermia and has been associated with drug reactions with eosinophilia and systemic symptoms (DRESS), as well as multiple organ hypersensitivity drug reactions.

[Contraindications]
People who are allergic to any ingredient in this product.
Patients with acute or chronic hepatitis.
People with a history or family history of severe hepatitis, especially drug-related hepatitis.
Patients with hepatic porphyria.
Patients with known mitochondrial disease caused by mutations in the mitochondrial DNA polymerase gamma gene (see "FDA Black Box Warning").
Patients with known urea cycle disorders.

[Matters Needing Attention]
- Severe liver injury: Clinical signs are crucial for early diagnosis. This should be considered, especially in the presence of jaundice in at-risk patients; liver function tests should be performed before starting treatment (see "Contraindications") and regularly during the first 6 months, especially in at-risk patients.
- Pancreatitis: When a patient presents with acute abdominal pain, immediate medical evaluation should be performed. If pancreatitis has been diagnosed, valproic acid treatments should be discontinued.
- Girls, female adolescents, women of childbearing age, and pregnant women (see the Special Populations section on the next page).
- Suicidal intent and behavior: Patients should be monitored for signs of suicidal intent and behavior, and appropriate treatment should be considered. Patients (and patient caregivers) should be advised to seek immediate medical help if they notice signs of suicidal intent or behavior.
- Carbapenems: Concurrent use is not recommended.
- Patients with known or suspected mitochondrial diseases: POLG gene testing should be performed according to the clinical diagnostic criteria of the relevant disease.
- Worsening of convulsions: If worsening of convulsions occurs, the patient should be advised to seek immediate medical attention.

- Blood tests (blood count, including platelet count, and bleeding time) are recommended before treatment, before surgery, or when spontaneous bruising or bleeding occurs.
- In patients with systemic lupus erythematosus, the potential benefits should be weighed against the risks.
- Patients with carnitine palmitoyltransferase II deficiency should be warned of an increased risk of rhabdomyolysis when receiving valproic acid treatment.
- Risk of weight gain: Patients should be warned of this risk when initiating treatment, and appropriate measures should be taken to minimize the risk.
- Special groups.

1. For children under 3 years old, monotherapy is advised; however, the potential advantages must be carefully considered in light of the risks of liver injury or pancreatitis before treatment initiation. Due to the risk of hepatotoxicity, simultaneous administration of salicylates should be avoided in this age group.
2. Renal Impairment: dose adjustment may be warranted. Given that plasma concentration monitoring might not accurately reflect the situation, dosage adjustments should be guided by clinical monitoring.

Basic Research and Clinical Applications

History and Prescription Evolution of Valproic Acid

Valproic acid (VPA) stands out as a distinctive drug and ranks among the most commonly prescribed ASMs globally. Originally derived from the low molecular weight carboxylic acid valeric acid, VPA was first synthesized by the American chemist Beverley Burton in 1882 [141]. Initially existing as a clear, colorless to light yellow liquid, it exhibited slight solubility in water but high solubility in organic solvents. However, its anticonvulsant properties remained undiscovered until the early 1960s. VPA debuted in the European market under the brand name Depakine in France in 1967, followed by introduction in the UK in 1973 and in other European countries in the subsequent decade. Its efficacy in treating epilepsy, particularly in children, was established in 1975 by S E Barnes [142]. N Bohlen et al. subsequently identified side effects associated with valproic acid ASMs [143]. After receiving approval from the U.S. Food and Drug Administration (FDA) in 1978, VPA was introduced to the United States. Over the years, VPA has gained widespread acceptance and is now available in more than 100 countries. It is recognized as a primary treatment for both generalized and partial epilepsy in both adults and children. Its utility has extended to include the management of bipolar disorder, preventive care for various disorders, schizophrenia, neuropathic pain, and migraines. Recent research into the effects of VPA on the human body and its novel mechanisms of action with toxic byproducts has led to an expansion of its applications. Consequently, VPA is now considered a crucial component in the treatment of diverse conditions, such as tumors, neurodegenerative diseases (including Huntington's disease, Parkinson's disease, Duchenne progressive muscular dystrophy), and human immunodeficiency syndrome [144].

The European Medicines Agency (EMA) strengthened its recommendations on the use of VPA in women in 2016 and restricted its use in female patients of childbearing potential. A study using the French National Health Insurance Database revealed that among pregnant women with epilepsy (n = 2607), the proportion of those exposed to VPA during pregnancy decreased from 26.4% in 2013 to 9.3% in 2016. Similarly, among pregnant women with bipolar disorder (n = 4278), the proportion of those exposed to VPA decreased from 3.7% in 2013 to 1.9% in 2016 [145]. In Germany, a longitudinal analysis of the individual prescription patterns of 1642 adult patients with epilepsy from 2008 to 2020 revealed that the prescription frequency of VPA decreased significantly (15.4% to 8.7%), and the prescription frequency of VPA also decreased significantly among women of childbearing potential (16.1% to 6.1%) [146]. In China, a survey of the most commonly used ASMs among adult outpatients with epilepsy from 2013 to 2018 revealed that VPA and levetiracetam (LEV) were the most frequently prescribed medications. However, the proportion of VPA usage has declined in recent years, while the proportion of LEV usage has increased in terms of both the number of prescriptions and expenses [147]. In Italy, a study analyzing ASM prescription patterns among pregnant women and women of childbearing age in the Lombardy Region Administrative Health care Database between 2010 and 2019 revealed that the proportion of VPA prescriptions among women of childbearing age decreased from 30.2% in 2010 to 20.0% in 2019 [148]. In Japan, a study investigating the prescription data of pregnant patients with epilepsy aged 16–49 years who visited outpatient clinics between 2016 and 2020 revealed that VPA ranked after LEV and lamotrigine (LTG). The proportion of pregnant patients with epilepsy using VPA prescriptions decreased from 12.4% in 2016 to 10.1% in 2020 [149]. There has been a notable decline in the exposure of women to VPA during and prior to pregnancy. Newer and less-interacting ASMs, such as LEV, LTG, and lacosamide (LCM), have gradually taken the place of VPA, particularly among women of childbearing age, reflecting a shift in prescription patterns aimed at reducing the teratogenic effects of the drug. Nevertheless, some of the aforementioned data highlight that despite the decreasing trend in VPA prescriptions, this medication remains one of the most commonly prescribed ASMs for women of childbearing age. This underscores the importance of educating and raising awareness among health care professionals and the general public, especially women [149]. Supporting this notion is an online survey carried out in Sweden and Norway from May to September 2021. Neurologists from both countries were invited to participate in the survey, which aimed to evaluate their familiarity with VPA restrictions, knowledge of the Marketing Authorization Holder (MAH), and utilization of VPA information resources, as well as their experiences in prescribing VPA to women of childbearing age over the previous 2 years. The results revealed that 51% of the respondents were highly familiar with the EMA restrictions, 49% were acquainted with the educational materials provided by the MAH, and 88 (44%) had prescribed VPA to women of childbearing age in the past 2 years, with only a small fraction consistently using the patient information leaflet and an even smaller number utilizing the VPA risk acknowledgment form. These findings suggest a limited implementation rate of the new EMA restrictions on VPA usage, as well as restricted acceptance and utilization of the information materials and risk acknowledgment forms by doctors. This reminds us that we may need to perform more information campaigns and communicate with those involved in treatment. Doctors must also collaborate more closely [149].

Pharmacokinetics of VPA

VPA is available in various preparations, including oral tablets, sustained-release tablets, film-coated tablets, capsules, and intravenous solutions, with bioavailabilities ranging from 96% to 100%. The drug is primarily distributed in the blood, with rapid exchange with the extracellular fluid. However, VPA can also be distributed in the cerebrospinal fluid (CSF) and brain, with CSF concentrations similar to those of free drugs in plasma. Chronic treatment provides greater bioavailability than does a single dose, with absorption occurring more quickly after a meal. However, taking VPA 2–3 h after a meal can delay absorption, resulting in slower absorption speeds in the afternoon than in the morning. VPA has a high protein binding rate (87–95%), resulting in low clearance rates (6–20 mL/h/kg) [150]. However, protein binding depends on the VPA concentration, and if the serum concentration exceeds the therapeutic range (>600 mol/L, 80 g/mL), protein binding may decrease by 67%. Hypoproteinemia-associated conditions, such as kidney disease, liver disease, old age, pregnancy, and the use of other protein binding drugs, may also reduce VPA protein binding, depending on the affinity of competitors for plasma proteins.

The metabolism of VPA is complex and requires further study. The known metabolic pathways of VPA include glucuronidation, β oxidation, and cytochrome P450 (CYP)-mediated oxidation, with glucuronic acid being the main metabolite in urine (30–50%). However, some products of VPA metabolism produced by mitochondrial and nonmitochondrial pathways are hepatotoxic. A key step in VPA metabolism is the production of 4-ene-VPA, which is toxic to cells and is mediated by CYP2C9, 2A6, and 2B6. The complex metabolism of VPA explains the diversity of active and inactive metabolites that can have therapeutic or toxic effects [144].

The half-life of VPA is 9–18 h and is typically shorter in children. However, when enzyme-induced drugs, such as phenytoin (PHT), CBZ, and barbiturates are used simultaneously, the half-life decreases to 5–12 h [151]. In the treatment of some children with VPA, doses exceeding the therapeutic range (50,100 μg/mL) are sometimes necessary for better epilepsy control. Current guidelines emphasize the importance of therapeutic drug concentration monitoring (TDM) for VPA as a crucial aspect of its treatment. Young et al. [152] conducted a study comparing the occurrence of common adverse reactions (thrombocytopenia, hepatotoxicity, and hyperammonemia) in children across various age groups and various maintenance doses of VPA. This study included 124 children receiving VPA maintenance treatment from January 2013 to January 2021. Among them, 56 patients had concentrations between 50 and 80 μg/mL, 44 patients had concentrations between 80 and 100 μg/mL, and 24 patients had concentrations between 100 and 120 μg/mL. There were 41 prepubertal patients, 57 pubertal patients, and 26 postpubertal patients. The results indicated that the primary endpoint of thrombocytopenia varied across different serum concentration ranges ($P = 0.093$) and age groups ($P = 0.628$). No significant differences were observed in liver dysfunction ($P = 0.099$) or hyperammonemia ($P = 0.548$) among the different concentration groups. Similarly, there were no differences in liver dysfunction ($P = 0.615$) or hyperammonemia ($P = 0.369$) based on age group analysis. The author speculates that according to this study, the serum VPA level of pediatric patients can be considered to be >100 μg/mL. Due to the high protein binding of VPA, in certain clinical scenarios, the unbound (free) portion of VPA might be inaccurately substituted for the total VPA serum level. Therefore, monitoring the serum free VPA concentration may be necessary when assessing the clinical response to VPA treatment. A systematic review was conducted to establish the therapeutic range of free VPA serum levels, investigate the relationship between free VPA serum levels and clinical toxicity and efficacy, and explore factors contributing to discrepancies between free and total VPA levels. This review identified 27 relevant studies from 189 sources, including 14 observational studies, 2 case series, and 11 case reports. Three studies defined the therapeutic range of free VPA levels between 20 and 410 μmol/L. Two studies indicated that hyperammonemia and thrombocytopenia could occur when free VPA levels exceeded 60 μmol/L and 103.3 μmol/L, respectively. Two other studies suggested that the upper limits of neurotoxicity for free VPA were 70 and 207.9 μmol/L, with hypoalbuminemia identified as a predictor of inconsistent results. Consequently, there is a lack of data supporting the clinical efficacy of free VPA at the serum level, necessitating further high-quality studies to confirm the optimal therapeutic range for free VPA [153].

Advances in science and technology have facilitated the translation of personalized drug concepts from theory to clinical practice, leading to the emergence of novel technologies in the TMD field of VPA. Traditional monitoring methods such as chromatography or immunoassays are not suitable for real-time or on-site analysis due to their high cost and extended turnaround time. Some researchers have discovered that ATR-FTMIR combined with nonlinear support vector regression is more effective in real-time TMD monitoring of VPA in clinical settings [154]. Namera et al. [155] also developed a simple and cost-effective method for determining VPA concentrations in human whole blood and urine using gas chromatography–mass spectrometry.

Mechanism of VPA

Various mechanisms have been described to explain the antiepileptic effects of VPA, including increasing GABA synthesis, decreasing GABA turnover, and inhibiting GABA degradation to enhance GABA transmission. Additionally, it reduces the release of excitatory amino acids (such as β-hydroxybutyric acid), inhibits excitatory transmission mediated by the N-methyl-D-aspartic acid (NMDA) receptor, and blocks voltage-gated ion channels (such as sodium, potassium, and calcium channels). VPA also regulates 5-hydroxytryptamine and dopaminergic neurotransmission and inhibits histone deacetylase (HDAC) activity. These mechanisms can explain the broad-spectrum antiepileptic effects of the drug, which are effective for all types of seizures and epilepsy syndromes in children and adults. VPA has been shown to be effective in treating global (tonic–clonic, absence, and myoclonic) and local epileptic seizures, as well as in treating Lennox–Gastaut, West, and Dravet syndromes. It is the first choice for treating coexisting absence seizures and tonic–clonic seizures [75]. Intravenous VPA treatment has also been recognized for its efficacy, safety, and tolerability in treating generalized convulsive status epilepticus (GCSE). Moreover, VPA has strong analgesic and anti-inflammatory effects at low doses, stemming from the inhibition of TNF-α-related pathways, making it useful for preventing migraines and treating bipolar and emotional disorders. In the past few decades, the neuroprotective effects of VPA have been described in various models of acute central nervous system injury, including stroke, hypoxia, traumatic brain injury, and spinal cord injury. Its potential use in new indications, such as cancer treatment and prevention, is also being studied. However, the exact mechanisms underlying the specific clinical effects of VPA are still poorly understood, and many of its functions may also explain its extensive adverse effects [156].

In recent years, increasing evidence has shown the potential influence of microflora on the pathogenesis and course of epilepsy. However, the effects of VPA on the intestinal microflora have not been studied in humans. Gong et al. [157] recruited ten patients who were newly diagnosed with cryptogenic epilepsy and treated with VPA (1000 mg/day) for the first time. Sequencing of 16S rDNA was used to evaluate the microbial community composition after baseline and after 3 months of VPA treatment. The results showed that the intestinal flora characteristics changed in patients treated with VPA and that the intestinal flora were related to weight gain and clinical biochemical indices. These findings suggest that the composition of the intestinal flora may be involved in the mechanism of VPA-induced metabolic disorders.

Basic Research on VPA for the Treatment of Epilepsy

Many experimental studies on comprehensive and local seizures in various epileptic models have confirmed the antiepileptic effect of VPA. In acute seizure models such as the pentylenetetrazol (PTZ) epilepsy model, intraperitoneal VPA administration significantly increases the seizure threshold, and prolonged treatment intensifies its anticonvulsant effects [158]. Another model, the maximal electroshock (MES) model, mimics full-scale tonic–clonic seizures in humans and has shown that VPA reduces seizure frequency in a dose-dependent manner [159].

As a chronic epilepsy model, an amygdala-kindling model simulating local epilepsy was also used. VPA increased the after-discharge (AD) required to induce epileptic seizures in a dose-dependent manner, reduced the duration of AD, effectively prevented epileptic seizures, adjusted membrane permeability, blocked voltage-dependent sodium channels and T-type voltage-activated calcium channels, and enhanced GABA-mediated inhibition. In the kindling model, VPA exhibited neuroprotective effects by safeguarding hippocampal neurons from damage caused by prolonged epileptic seizures, promoting neuroprotection, and preventing behavioral disorders. Data from drug-resistant epilepsy models indicate that VPA can impede both the progression of kindled seizures and their complete manifestation, serving as both a symptomatic control agent and a disease-modifying agent [150, 160].

The critical management of epileptogenesis, particularly in status epilepticus (SE), which can result in neuronal damage and subsequent recurring seizures, relies on the precise adjustment of glutamatergic and GABAergic pathways along with the neuroprotective effects of VPA. By employing neuroprotective mechanisms to curb neuronal harm, VPA represents a promising strategy for preventing epileptogenesis. In the SE kainate model, administering high doses of VPA 40 days post-SE induction not only suppressed spontaneous activity but also safeguarded hippocampal neurons from seizure-induced damage. Furthermore, VPA exposure demonstrated protective effects against seizure-induced cognitive impairments, emphasizing the importance of neuroprotection in both processes. Further experimental evidence supporting the antiepileptic effects of VPA arises from diverse SE models in which VPA displays a preference for AMPA receptor subtypes, preventing neuronal apoptosis in an SE model induced by prolonged electrical stimulation of the basolateral amygdala. Specifically, continuous infusion of VPA 24 h after the end of electrical stimulation conferred significant neuroprotective effects on hippocampal neurons that were comparable to those of antiexcitotoxic and glutamate-depleting agents such as NS1209 [161]. In a genetic epilepsy model derived from a Bsn gene-manipulated mouse epilepsy model characterized by frequent seizures but prolonged survival, VPA significantly decreased both seizure frequency and mortality rates [162]. VPA is a broad-spectrum ASMs with antiabsence effects. Kantarci et al. [163] studied the effect of in utero exposure to VPA on absence epileptic seizures in rats with Strasbourg hereditary absence epilepsy (GAERS). The electroencephalogram of this model displayed bilateral, symmetrical, and synchronized spike-wave discharges (SWDs). However, the study results indicated that VPA did not notably affect the average accumulation time of EEG signals or the average number of SWDs. The authors suggested that the lack of significant differences in SWD parameters might imply that the antiseizure mechanisms of VPA may not be fully operational during the prenatal period. Recently, a study using a rat model investigated the impact of VPA on disrupted sleep patterns in epilepsy patients. In addition to its antiseizure properties, VPA also has hypnotic effects, potentially through leveraging GABAergic mechanisms to mitigate convulsive seizures and promote sleep [164].

Clinical Study of the Effects of VPA on Epileptic Seizures

There are three classic studies on the clinical application of VPA in the Chinese population. The first study included 532 individuals with convulsive epilepsy residing in rural China. VPA monotherapy was administered in primary care facilities, with adults starting at a dose of 600 mg and children starting at a dose of 20 mg/kg. The typical daily maintenance dose ranged from 600 to 1200 mg for adults and 20–30 mg/kg for children, taken thrice daily and monitored for 12 months. The results revealed that 84% of patients experienced at least a 50% reduction in seizure frequency, and 42.6% of patients were seizure-free after 1 year of treatment. The 1-year retention rate for VPA therapy was 96.2%, with 9% of patients reporting mild adverse events. After 1 year of VPA treatment, patients exhibited weight gain, with most adverse events being mild, transient, and not necessitating VPA discontinuation [165]. The second study, conducted in rural Guangxi, China, corroborated the favorable outcomes of VPA. This investigation involved 302 epilepsy patients with various seizure types. All participants received VPA treatment, with retention rates of 100%, 93.56%, 89.05%, and 77.06% at the 6th, 12th, 18th, and 24th months of treatment, respectively. Throughout the 1-year follow-up period, 30 patients displayed mild symptoms, with no severe or serious adverse reactions reported [166]. The third study in China, a multi-center, observational cohort study, enrolled 1008 epilepsy patients, with 519 receiving VPA treatment and 489 receiving topiramate treatment. The primary outcome focused on the time to treatment failure, while the secondary outcomes included the time to first seizure and the time to remission at 12 and 24 months. The findings indicated superior primary and secondary outcomes in the VPA group compared to the topiramate group (28.3% vs. 41.5%, HR = 0.62, $P < 0.0001$; 56.1% vs. 69.3%, HR = 0.73, $P = 0.0002$). Both groups exhibited no significant disparities in remission time between 12 and 24 months or in the incidence of treatment failure or intolerable adverse events [167].

VPA is considered the first-line treatment for patients with newly diagnosed genetic generalized epilepsy (GGE) or difficult-to-classify epilepsy. In most cases of GGE, the lowest daily VPA dose capable of controlling seizures in monotherapy is typically up to 700 mg [168]. Although VPA is recognized as the most effective antiseizure medication (ASM) in studies of GGE, its use in women of childbearing age is significantly restricted due to the heightened risk of teratogenicity and impaired cognitive development following intrauterine exposure. However, there are situations where the use of VPA is unavoidable. Steinbart et al. [169] conducted a retrospective study across tertiary epilepsy centers' outpatient clinics, analyzing GGE patients who visited between January 2015 and April 2020. They compared the proportions of women aged 18–49 years who were taking VPA with men in the same age group and women aged more than 49 years. The study included 125 women of childbearing age, with 28 (22%) receiving VPA, in contrast to 28 (50%) of 56 men aged 49 or younger and 22 (55%) of 40 female patients over 49 years of age. The results indicated that there was no disparity in seizure-free survival between women of childbearing age receiving lower VPA doses and men. Multivariate analysis of women aged 49 or younger revealed age as the sole variable independently linked to VPA use, with no associated variables identified in the other two groups. The authors concluded that despite concerns regarding the teratogenicity and cognitive risks of VPA, the reduction in VPA doses among women of childbearing age with GGE from 2015 to 2020, where nearly a quarter of such women were treated with VPA, seemed adequate to achieve favorable seizure-free rates. Additionally, for GGE, Dibek et al. [170] investigated the rate of reinitiation after discontinuation of VPA treatment in women with GGE and the reasons for such resumption. Among the 199 patients studied, 63 (31.7%) needed reintroduction of VPA. The primary reasons for discontinuing other ASMs were lack of treatment response in 80.0% of patients, adverse drug reactions in 18.3% of patients, and voluntary discontinuation in 1.7% of patients.

Due to the teratogenic nature of VPA and its unsuitability for women of childbearing age, levetiracetam (LEV) is increasingly being utilized for these patient groups. Marson et al. [145] conducted an open-label, randomized controlled trial comparing the efficacy and cost-effectiveness of LEV and VPA as first-line treatments for patients with generalized or unclassifiable epilepsy. The study involved 520 participants aged 5 years or older with at least two noninduced generalized or unclassifiable seizures. The results indicated that, compared with LEV, VPA exhibited superior 12-month remission rates. Adverse events were reported by 37% of participants in the VPA group and 42% in the LEV group. The study concluded that LEV did not demonstrate superior clinical effectiveness or cost-effectiveness compared to VPA. These findings contribute to the ongoing discussion regarding the advantages and disadvantages of avoiding VPA use for girls and women of childbearing potential.

Idiopathic generalized epilepsies (IGEs) are the most common group of syndromes in GGE. Kiiski et al. [171] conducted a retrospective study of patients with IGE treated at Tampere University Hospital between January 1, 2009, and December 31, 2018. The results showed that VPA was more frequently used in males than in females, while LTG and LEV were more commonly used in females than in males. LTG and LEV were used particularly as monotherapies for female epilepsy patients and as a significant part of combination therapy for males. When used as monotherapy in adults, VPA alternatives were as effective as VPA, but VPA remained the most commonly used ASM in the pediatric subgroup. Reducing VPA use in women with epilepsy did not increase the risk of seizure recurrence, suggesting that VPA alternatives could be considered first-line ASMs for women with epilepsy. Patients with juvenile absence epilepsy (JAE) were more likely to return to VPA therapy than those with generalized tonic–clonic seizures (GTCS) subtype alone, with a total of 7.4% of JAE patients switching to VPA therapy experiencing sustained myoclonic seizures, compared with 20.4% of patients treated with alternative medications. The authors concluded that although VPA treatment is not preferred as a first choice for women of childbearing age, there are some patients who can only use VPA for seizure control, especially those with myoclonic seizures and JAE, and that VPA is a commonly used and effective medication for the treatment of juvenile myoclonic epilepsy (JME). Two-thirds of patients with drug-resistant juvenile myoclonic epilepsy are seizure free, and the combination of valproate and lamotrigine is the most effective dual therapy [172]. Overall, patients with IGE who use VPA or other broad-spectrum ASMs as monotherapy have shown favorable clinical outcomes. A study by Kılıç et al. [173] supported the use of VPA as an effective medication for the treatment of JME, although LEV has gradually become the preferred initial ASM in recent years. The study revealed that VPA was the most frequently selected initial ASM (50.9%), followed by LEV (44.4%) and LTG (4.7%), and that VPA was preferred for male children, while LEV was preferred for female children. During the first 5 years of the study period (2010–2015, $n = 66$, 64%), VPA was the most frequently chosen initial ASM, whereas LEV was the most common initial

ASM in the last 5 years ($n = 83$, 53.9%, $p = 0.005$); the most common reasons for discontinuation were the ineffectiveness of LEV and adverse reactions to VPA ($p = 0.001$). During the follow-up period, 237 (92.2%) patients were seizure-free for at least 12 months, and 159 (61.9%) achieved EEG remission, with seizure remission (defined as complete seizure control for at least 12 months) occurring earlier than EEG remission ($p < 0.001$). The authors concluded that LEV has gradually become the preferred initial ASM in the treatment of JME, but VPA seems to be more effective in achieving seizure control than LEV. Moon et al. [174] utilized quantitative EEG (qEEG) to examine alterations in background EEG activity in 17 children with juvenile myoclonic epilepsy (JME) undergoing treatment with VPA. The findings revealed that VPA led to a reduction in background EEG activity in the frontal, parietal, occipital, and limbic lobes, particularly in regions exhibiting low-frequency (δ-θ) background EEG activity. Significant variations were observed in the occipital, parietal, and limbic lobes at δ frequencies, as well as in the frontal, occipital, and limbic lobes at θ frequencies. Notably, the most pronounced differences were noted at δ frequencies in the left occipital and cuneate lobes and at θ frequencies in the left medial frontal gyrus. The authors' conclusion highlighted that this study showcased the anticonvulsant impact of VPA on the neural networks associated with juvenile myoclonic epilepsy (JME). Zöllner et al. [175] conducted a study comparing the impact of VPA and LEV on the EEG alpha peak frequency (APF). Their findings indicated a notable increase in the APF as the VPA dose decreased within the VPA group ($p = 0.005$, $n = 13$), while no significant changes were observed in the LEV group ($p = 0.47$, $n = 18$). In the VPA group, the APF demonstrated a negative correlation with the daily VPA dose ($r = -0.74 \pm 0.12$, $p = 0.0039$), in contrast to the LEV group, where no significant correlation was noted ($r = -0.17 \pm 0.18$, $p = 0.4072$). The researchers concluded that VPA treatment delayed the onset of APF, with this reduction in APF being linked to the daily VPA dose.

In a study by Ozyurek et al. [176], the impact of VPA treatment on cerebral blood flow in children with idiopathic generalized epilepsy (IGE) was investigated. The trial involved 33 children receiving VPA treatment and 34 age-matched controls. Doppler and spectral measurements were conducted on various arteries, including the common carotid artery (CCA), internal carotid artery (ICA), external carotid artery (ECA), anterior cerebral artery (ACA), and middle cerebral artery (MCA), to assess parameters such as the maximal flow velocity (VM), end-diastolic flow velocity (EDV), resistance index (RI), pulsatility index (PI), and flow rate (FR). The mean ages of the VPA and control groups were 9.33 ± 2.11 and 9.74 ± 2 years, respectively, with a follow-up period of 17.7 ± 3.2 months during the VPA treatment phase. No significant differences in VM, EDV, RI, PI, or FR values obtained from the bilateral ICA, ACA, or MCA were observed between the control and VPA groups, suggesting that the dosage of VPA did not impact forebrain blood flow.

It is wellknown that visuospatial ability is the basis for good academic performance and daily functioning; Operto et al. [177] conducted a study to investigate the impact of ASMs, including VPA monotherapy, on visuospatial memory in children. The trial involved 207 children and adolescents with epilepsy (mean age

10.35 ± 2.39 years) and revealed that the mean immediate recall scores in the VPA group significantly worsened. Immediate recall scores were found to be correlated with age, age at seizure, seizure duration, and executive function. This study highlights the importance of monitoring cognitive function in children receiving ASM treatment.

Regarding ASM combinations, VPA has enzyme inhibitory properties and requires caution when used with sodium channel blockers (SCBs), and its combination with topiramate (TPM) or zonisamide (ZNS) may lead to enhanced toxicity [178]. Zhu et al. [179] conducted a review of randomized controlled clinical trials on VPA combined with LEV for children with epilepsy. Their searches included the Cochrane Library (January 1946 to May 2021), PubMed, Web of Science, Chinese Journal Full Text Database (CNKI), WANGFANG DATA, and Sino Med. The review included seven studies with 617 participants who met the data criteria. The results showed that VPA combined with LEV for the treatment of epilepsy in children significantly improved the overall treatment effect (RR = 1.24, 95% CI: 1.16–1.33, $p = 0.927$) and reduced the incidence of adverse events (RR = 0.54, 95% CI: 0.37–0.79, $p = 0.602$). Based on these findings, the authors recommended VPA in combination with LEV for the treatment of pediatric patients with epilepsy.

VPA for the Treatment of SE

Generalized convulsive status epilepticus (GCSE) guidelines recommend stepwise treatment with benzodiazepines followed by second-line ASM therapy, including VPA. Sharshar et al. [180] conducted a multicenter, double-blinded, randomized controlled trial to assess whether VPA, as a stepwise therapeutic strategy for complementary therapy, improves the prognosis of patients with GCSE. The trial involved 244 adults with GCSE treated with ASM in the intensive care units of 16 French hospitals between 2013 and 2018. Patients received standard benzodiazepine therapy and second-line ASM therapy, with patients in the VPA group receiving an intravenous loading dose of 30 mg/kg VPA followed by an infusion of 1 mg/kg/h over 12 h, while those in the placebo group received the same 0.9% saline IV injection and continuous infusion. The primary endpoint was the proportion of patients discharged on Day 15, and the secondary outcomes were seizure control, adverse events, and cognition on Day 90. The results showed no significant differences between groups in patients discharged on Day 15, and there were no differences in secondary outcomes between groups. The authors concluded that VPA was well-tolerated as a recommended regimen for GCSE in adults and did not increase the proportion of patients discharged on Day 15. Liampas et al. [181] conducted a meta-analysis of randomized controlled trials (RCTs) on the use of injectable VPA in patients with status epilepticus (SE). Thirteen RCTs were retrieved, with five comparisons available, four of which involved two or more studies. The results showed no significant differences between VPA and phenytoin sodium in terms of efficacy and tolerability, with phenobarbital being more often associated with multiple adverse effects than VPA. Diazepam was determined to be inferior to VPA in terms of safety issues, including severe respiratory depression and severe hypotension. There were no differences in efficacy between the combination of lorazepam (LZP) and VPA and the combination of LZP and LEV. Based on these conclusions, VPA was determined to be a safe and effective option for the management of SE. Zhang et al. [182] conducted a search for randomized controlled trials aiming to assess the preferred ASMs for pediatric convulsive status epilepticus (SE). They found eight first-line ASM studies involving 1686 pediatric participants and eight second-line ASM studies involving 1711 pediatric participants. VPA was identified as advantageous for preventing SE recurrence within 24 h in these studies. Jain et al. [95] conducted a routine and network meta-analysis of randomized controlled trials in patients (>1 month old) with benzodiazepine-resistant status epilepticus. Their analysis included 17 studies, 16 of which were included in the network meta-analysis. Phenobarbital was identified as having the greatest likelihood of being the best intervention for stopping seizures within 60 min, followed by high-dose LEV and high-dose VPA. This indicates that phenobarbital may be particularly effective in managing benzodiazepine-resistant status epilepticus.

The incidence of valproate-associated encephalopathy in patients with epilepsy receiving long-term treatment ranges from 0.1% to 2.5%. Whereas valproate-associated encephalopathy is frequent and unpredictable in status epilepticus patients, even in the absence of comorbid hyperammonemia, vigilance should be maintained for associated clinical symptoms, and discontinuation of sodium valproate should be considered immediately in suspected patients [183].

VPA and Women with Epilepsy

Issues related to female epilepsy have gained increasing attention in recent years due to increasing scientific research into the multiphasic effects of hormones, seizures, and ASMs, as well as concerns about pregnancy-related fertility, seizure instability, and ASM-related teratogenicity. External hormonal influences, such as gender-affirming medications, hormone replacement therapy, and fertility therapies, can also affect female patients with epilepsy. Although epilepsy itself is not associated with significantly impaired fertility in the absence of preexisting fertility problems, the use of high-dose VPA (≥1500 mg or higher total daily dose) during pregnancy is primarily associated with significant congenital malformations and developmental disorders, several times more so than in the general population. Therefore, careful consideration is needed to choose medication and dosage to mitigate these risks, as well as taking steps such as a pregnancy prevention program (PPP) and the completion of an Annual Risk Acknowledgment Form (ARAF) to reduce the use of VPA in women of potential childbearing age [184, 185]. Eriksson et al. [185] collected data from neurologists registered with the Association of British Neurologists and epilepsy nurse specialists through the Epilepsy Nurses' Association of Great Britain to assess the level of awareness among women of childbearing age taking VPA about the risks of taking VPA during pregnancy, the need for highly effective contraception, and enrolling in the ARAF. The results showed that the majority of women were informed of the risks of taking VPA during pregnancy and the need for highly effective contraception, but there were still individuals whose data were not available. The authors concluded that further work is needed to facilitate the identification of women taking VPA and to implement signing up for the ARAF. For clinicians, careful emphasis needs to be placed on informing women of the teratogenic risks of continuing to take VPA and the risk of worsening seizure control if VPA is discontinued, which is particularly true in women with focal epilepsy. It may be necessary to switch to a safer, equally effective alternative to ASMs. Spoendlin et al. [186] conducted a retrospective descriptive study using the health care claims database of the Swiss health insurance Helsana (2014–2018) to assess VPA use in women of gestational and childbearing age. They found that VPA use decreased from 28/10,000 women in 2014 to 21/10,000 women in 2018, and the rate of VPA exposure during pregnancy in Swiss women of childbearing age was comparable to that in Denmark but lower than that in other European countries. Despite the decrease in exposure rates, VPA use in Swiss women of childbearing age appears to be greater than the actual clinical need. A study by Atalar et al. [187] provided valuable insights into the outcomes and predictors of decision-making regarding the discontinuation/switching or continuation of VPA therapy in women with epilepsy (WWE). They followed 214 WWE for an average of 9.57 ± 7.04 years, 142 of whom had used VPA during their childbearing years, and 72 were still using VPA. The main reasons for remaining on VPA were a high risk of seizure recurrence (63.9%), cognitive impairment (27.8%), and no desire for pregnancy (8.3%). In the group that successfully discontinued VPA, 47.1% of patients maintained seizure remission, with 38.8% experiencing relapse during follow-up. The incidence of side effects associated with the new drugs LEV and LTG was 36.6%.

The rate of discontinuation failure was significantly lower in focal epilepsy patients (13.9%) than in generalized epilepsy patients (86.1%). In patients with generalized epilepsy, all three types of seizures were associated with discontinuation failure, as well as the presence of ASM resistance. Women with focal epilepsy, although more likely to be ASM resistant and have sustained seizures, did not typically experience worsening of their condition after discontinuation of VPA, making it unnecessary to expose them to teratogenic risk. In generalized epilepsy, certain predictive factors, such as known ASM resistance and the presence of three seizure types, should be considered before attempting to discontinue VPA.

SE during pregnancy is a critical medical emergency for both mothers and fetuses. The management of SE during pregnancy is complex due to pregnancy-related pharmacokinetic changes and fetal risks associated with ASM and anesthetic drugs. Although there is no standardized treatment regimen for pregnant patients with SE, benzodiazepines are typically the drug of choice. LEV and phenytoin are considered the most appropriate second-line medications. VPA should only be used when other ASMs have failed and should be avoided during the first trimester of pregnancy to minimize teratogenic risks. This underscores the importance of careful management and consideration of ASM use in pregnant women with epilepsy [188].

VPA and Breastfeeding

Some studies have shown that breastfed infants have higher IQs and better verbal skills at age 6 than nonbreastfed infants. Breast milk has previously been found to contain very low levels of VPA, and infant serum levels of VPA range from undetectable to very low; moreover, breastfeeding during VPA monotherapy does not appear to adversely affect infant growth or development. A safety scoring system study showed that VPA can be used during breastfeeding, and there have been no reports of definite adverse effects of VPA use in breastfed infants. However, it is theoretically possible for breastfed infants to develop VPA-induced hepatotoxicity, so infants should be monitored for jaundice and other signs of liver damage during maternal VPA therapy. Suspected cases of thrombocytopenia have also been reported, so infants should be monitored for unusual bruising or bleeding.

VPA Use in Epilepsy Comorbidities with Somatic Disorders

Epilepsy is a chronic disease, and comorbidity with somatic disorders is common. In recent years, there has been increasing interest in and research on epilepsy comorbidities.

Patients with epilepsy who have preexisting cardiac arrhythmias are at increased risk of sudden death, and appropriate ASM therapy should be administered to manage comorbidities of cardiovascular disorders. However, the concomitant use of antiarrhythmic agents and ASM therapy can cause potential drug–drug interactions due to their similar mechanisms of action. Studies have shown that interactions between antiarrhythmic drugs and ASMs are most likely to occur when the drug components block sodium channels and have membrane-stabilizing properties. Like VPA, mexiletine is an antiarrhythmic drug that blocks sodium channels and has membrane-stabilizing properties. When mexiletine is combined with VPA, mexiletine can attenuate the antiepileptic seizure effect of VPA, as shown in studies conducted using the MES test in mice [189]. It is important to note that VPA also affects coagulation and platelet counts, and antiplatelet agents associated with the treatment of heart disease, in which salicylic acid increases the free dispersion of VPA, can potentially interact with VPA. European guidelines do not recommend the use of VPA in patients taking oral anticoagulants (DOACs). A prospective multicenter cohort study showed that patients with nonvalvular AF treated with both DOACs and ASMs, including VPA, had a relatively high incidence of thromboembolic events [190]. However, intravenous application of VPA is a safe and effective therapeutic option for the treatment of SE patients with epilepsy comorbid with cardiovascular or respiratory diseases.

For SE treatment, VPA is contraindicated in patients with liver disease due to its potential hepatotoxicity. Similarly, in chronic antiepileptic therapy, VPA is not recommended for patients with hepatic insufficiency and should be avoided if possible. VPA is mainly eliminated by the liver and is therefore recommended for renal injury and hemodialysis.

Patients with poststroke comorbid epilepsy are more susceptible to ASM-induced adverse effects, and elevated lipoprotein levels and weight gain, which are associated with an increased risk of cerebrovascular disease, have been found in VPA-treated patients; therefore, VPA is generally less recommended for stroke patients. Despite these drawbacks, intravenous injections of VPA remain a better choice for use in acute situations. Patients with multiple sclerosis appear to be at three times greater risk of seizures than the general population, and seizures may be a symptom of this disease that does not affect motor or cognitive function. Low doses of VPA may be the drug of choice.

When using VPA in patients with brain tumors, drug interactions with chemotherapeutic agents should be considered, as some agents can reduce VPA levels and lead to poor seizure control. For example, methotrexate can reduce VPA levels and lead to seizure recurrence [191]. VPA can reduce the metabolism of cisplatin, etoposide, and teniposide drugs, leading to toxic drug aggregation effects. However, VPA still shows good efficacy and tolerability in the treatment of epilepsy in patients with brain tumors, and IV injections are still a good choice for patients with brain tumors in cases of SE.

In infectious diseases, ASMs and anti-infectives often need to be used in combination, and clinically significant interactions between them may lead to adverse drug reactions or treatment failure. The European Medicines Agency (EMA), in its drug safety report, suggests that concomitant use of carbapenems and VPA should be avoided and that interactions between the two cannot be monitored by determining VPA plasma concentrations or by adjusting the dose, but if they are already used in combination, it is recommended that other ASMs be added and that VPA concentrations be continuously monitored. A recent retrospective study showed that the interaction between VPA and carbapenems results in lower plasma concentrations of VPA and possibly liver injury. The study involved data from 141 patients in the Department of Neurosurgery, Baiqiu'en Hospital, Shanxi, China, from January 2018 to December 2019. The results showed that the serum concentration of VPA in the VPA + meropenem group was significantly lower than that in the VPA monotherapy group. The difference in the incidence of liver injury between the VPA monotherapy group, the VPA + meropenem group, and the VPA + imipenem group was statistically significant, and the liver injury rate in the VPA + meropenem group was greater than that in the VPA + imipenem and VPA monotherapy groups. Although there was no significant difference in the rate of hepatic injury between the VPA + imipenem group and the VPA monotherapy group, the ALT value in the VPA + imipenem group was significantly greater than that before. These findings suggest that the interaction between VPA and carbapenems can result in lower plasma concentrations of VPA and possibly liver injury. Clinicians should be aware of this potential interaction and closely monitor VPA concentrations and liver function when using carbapenems in combination with VPA. Different carbapenems used in combination with VPA may have different effects on blood concentrations and liver function, so careful consideration is needed when using these drugs together [192]. Clinicians should be aware of this potential interaction and closely monitor VPA concentrations and liver function when using carbapenems in combination with VPA. Chen et al. [193] assessed the risk factors for seizures or SE resulting from the combination of VPA and carbapenem antibiotics in adult patients in the ICU. The results showed that 104 out of 162 patients (64.2%) experienced seizures and 45 (27.8%) experienced SE. The risk factors for seizures were age, initial antiepileptic regimen, and serum concentration of VPA after concomitant administration of carbapenems, while the independent risk factor for SE was the combined VPA serum concentration after application of carbapenems. The concomitant administration of imipenem/cilastatin did not significantly reduce VPA blood concentrations compared with meropenem or ertapenem. Patients with concomitant seizures or SE had a significantly increased length of stay and days of ventilation after concomitant carbapenems in the ICU. The authors concluded that carbapenem antibiotics reduced VPA blood levels and increased the risk of seizures and SE, thereby prolonging ICU hospitalization. Furthermore, there have been case reports of the use of meropenem to lower blood levels of VPA to treat acute VPA poisoning [194]. In another study by Yang et al. [195], LC–MS/MS was used to determine the interactions of VPA and its six metabolites in human serum with carbapenems in patients with epilepsy. The method was found to be simple, rapid, accurate, and precise for routine clinical analysis of VPA and its metabolites in human serum. Müller et al. [196] investigated the differences between VPA intravenous therapy for SE in diabetic and nondiabetic patients. The study revealed that the tolerability of VPA therapy was comparable in both groups and that diabetes, as a relevant comorbidity, may portend a post-SE potential increased risk of adverse outcomes in diabetic patients presenting with SE.

Approximately 25% of patients with intellectual disability (PwID) have comorbid epilepsy, and up to two-thirds of these patients are resistant to treatment. Epigenetic pathways are also thought to be associated with altered cognitive function. VPA has been reported to inhibit the expression of aminorhodamine 2,3 dioxygenase (IDO), the tryptophan pathway that regulates tryptophan metabolism. However, the complex epigenetic cascade of VPA-induced responses implies long-term beneficial and deleterious effects on intraneuronal homeostasis and plasticity. BSN-mutant mice are commonly used as a model for long-term synaptic plasticity deficits in the hippocampus, leading to hippocampal learning deficits. VPA treatment reversed the physiological long-term potentiation effect but did not reverse the morphological alterations in dendritic spines or the impairment of nonspatial hippocampal memory. Although VPA inhibited neurogenesis in an animal model of SE, thereby preventing cognitive decline, it failed to improve cognitive performance in rats in the Morris water maze swim test.

Prospective studies in humans have consistently demonstrated that VPA is associated with an increased risk of cognitive impairment and in utero malformations in young children. Dose-dependent negative effects of VPA were found in children of mothers receiving VPA monotherapy. The children performed a number of cognitive tests, including those related to IQ, verbal and nonverbal abilities, memory, and executive function. However, Snoeijen-Schouwenaars et al. [197] conducted an exploratory, retrospective study of patients with intellectual disabilities in England and the Netherlands and found that the most commonly prescribed medication in both centers was still VPA. This is the first observational study to reveal the unique characteristics of epilepsy management in this complex population.

Kessing et al. [198] studied 154 patients with bipolar disorder and comorbid epilepsy and 8381 patients with bipolar disorder without comorbid epilepsy identified in Denmark between 1995 and 2017. The authors concluded that patients with bipolar disorder with comorbid epilepsy should be prioritized for treatment with VPA and LTG. They also emphasized the need for close clinical monitoring and psychological support for patients with bipolar disorder and comorbid epilepsy, as well as further long-term studies on the effects of interventions.

VPA Use in Other Diseases

Mental Illness

The drug insert included in VPA packaging notes that valproic acid (VPA) can effectively manage manic episodes in bipolar disorder patients and exerts a stabilizing influence on mood [199]. Hsieh et al. [200] used data from the National Health Insurance Research Database (NHIRD) in Taiwan to conduct a correlation analysis to study the effect of long-term use of VPA on the mortality of patients with bipolar disorder and found that the long-term use of VPA reduces the mortality of patients with BD risk, especially in the male population and the 65-years-or-older population. Xie et al. [201] conducted a study involving 30 Sprague–Dawley (SD) rats to explore the effects of VPA on hippocampal magnetic resonance imaging (MRI) images, neurocognition, and activity of the JAK1/STAT3 pathway in depressed rats. Their results demonstrated the efficacy of VPA in enhancing hippocampal volumetric features, memory, and neurocognitive function in a model of depression.

In addition, VPA has been increasingly used to treat delirium. Cuartas et al. [202] systematically reviewed 21 abstracts spanning 1946 to January 12, 2021, and included 10 studies (252 patients) evaluating the efficacy of VPA for the treatment of delirium. Notably, patients showed improvement in delirium symptoms within 1–3 days, with a mean starting dose of 733 mg/day and a mean follow-up dose of 1061 mg/day. Common side effects included hyperammonemia (12–19%) and thrombocytopenia (9–13%), with no reported VPA-related deaths.

Although intravenous (IV) VPA is not officially recommended for psychiatric disorders, the literature suggests its potential efficacy. Olivola et al. [203] systematically reviewed studies on intravenous VPA for agitation treatment and concluded that it effectively reduces agitation in psychiatric patients and is generally safer than other antipsychotics or ASMs. However, the evidence is limited due to the reliance on open-label studies or case series reports.

Migraine Prevention

The use of ASMs, including VPA, in the treatment of migraines has been supported by evidence from numerous randomized controlled studies [148]. VPA, an FDA-approved drug, may work in migraine prevention and treatment by blocking neurogenic inflammatory responses and responses to trigeminal vascular system activation. Its mechanism of action involves effects on voltage-gated sodium channels, γ-aminobutyric acid receptors, glutamate-mediated neurotransmission, and calcium channels. By modulating the central nervous system pain mechanism and inhibiting nociceptive modulation loops, VPA can help prevent migraine attacks. When used alone, VPA has shown a migraine headache relief rate of 68–73%, with the ability to reduce accompanying symptoms and cause fewer adverse reactions. It can be effective within 1–4 h of oral intake due to its high bioavailability.

Ischemic Stroke

The findings we have highlighted regarding valproic acid (VPA) in a rodent model of ischemic stroke are significant in demonstrating the potential neuroprotective effects of VPA in this context. Despite the typical caution in using VPA for stroke patients due to its association with lipid metabolism and weight gain, the results from an MCAO model suggest promising therapeutic implications for VPA in ischemic stroke patients. In tan MCAO model, VPA has been shown to inhibit histone deacetylase (HDAC), leading to the suppression of NF-κB and metalloproteinase-9 activation. This inhibition plays a crucial role in reducing postischemic cerebral blood barrier disruption and cerebral edema, which are important factors in the pathophysiology of ischemic stroke. Additionally, VPA has been demonstrated to reduce infarct size and improve clinical deficit symptoms by upregulating the expression of heat shock proteins, particularly of heat shock protein-70, while inhibiting caspase-3 expression and activation. These mechanisms collectively contribute to the neuroprotective effects of VPA in ischemic stroke. Moreover, evidence from in vitro studies on ischemic injury further supports the neuroprotective potential of VPA. Specifically, in an in vitro model of oxygen and glucose deprivation, VPA treatment has shown protective effects against ischemic injury. These findings suggest that VPA may have a significant impact on mitigating neuronal damage and promoting cell survival under ischemic conditions [150]. VPA has been found to exhibit neuroprotective effects against ischemic stroke, as demonstrated by Gao et al. [204] in a rat model of cerebral ischemia–reperfusion injury. After 4 weeks of VPA treatment, the volume of brain atrophy was significantly reduced, and behavioral deficits improved. In vitro studies also showed that VPA treatment protected against OGD/Re-induced astrocyte death and reduced the expression of GFAP, neurocalcitonin, and phosphatidylinositol. These findings suggest that VPA exerts neuroprotective effects and inhibits glial scarring during recovery from ischemic stroke by inhibiting HDAC activity and inducing expression of heat shock protein-70.1B.

Atherosclerosis is a recognized risk factor for ischemic stroke, and abnormal vascular smooth muscle cell (VSMC) proliferation is a key factor in the development of vascular diseases, including atherosclerosis. Research has shown that VPA stimulates the phosphorylation of the Thr389 locus in VSMCs by inhibiting specific protein phosphatase 2A (PP2A) and modulating platelet-derived growth factor (PDGF) levels (p-p70S6K-Thr(389)). This mechanism reduces VSMC proliferation, suggesting that VPA may be useful for the treatment and prevention of atherosclerosis and in-stent restenosis [205]. These findings provide additional support for the potential positive effect of VPA in the context of ischemic stroke.

Trauma and Hemorrhage

Treatment with valproic acid (VPA) has exhibited promising results in enhancing survival rates in animal models of severe trauma, particularly traumatic brain injury (TBI), and cerebral hemorrhage, which pose significant health and socioeconomic challenges and are leading causes of mortality. Clinical trials have revealed that administering 150 mg/kg VPA can mitigate brain damage and expedite neurological recovery. In recent studies, the efficacy of currently FDA-approved VPA doses of up to 60 mg/kg has been assessed in pigs with TBI and hemorrhagic shock [206]. These findings suggest that treatment with VPA within the approved dosage range reduces both the extent of brain injury and neurological impairment. Moreover, investigations indicate that doses exceeding FDA-approved limits may further enhance survival rates in trauma models. Proteomic analyses comparing a single high dose of VPA (140 mg/kg) to the FDA-approved dose (30 mg/kg) in healthy subjects revealed significant cytoprotective alterations induced by the higher dosage. These changes, which are absent at lower doses, likely contribute to the protective effects of VPA against injury [207]. In addition, VPA is metabolically detected in tissues surrounding the injury site, eliciting metabolic alterations in the brain to foster a neuroprotective milieu during the initial hours following TBI [208]. Animal studies using rats have demonstrated the ability of VPA to expedite axonal healing in TBI patients [209]. Additionally, in a porcine model of polytrauma and hemorrhagic shock, a single administration of VPA (150 mg/kg) exhibited notable protective effects against acute kidney injury. These collective findings underscore the potential of VPA as a therapeutic agent for managing severe trauma-related conditions [210].

Tumors

VPA has garnered significant interest as a potential adjuvant therapy in oncology over the past several decades. Numerous lines of evidence suggest that VPA may act as a "booster" in the treatment of various cancers. Preclinical data have described the anticancer effects of VPA in more than 20 solid tumors, ranging from melanoma to colon cancer cells, and these data continue to accumulate annually [211]. In particular, in animal models, VPA modulates the transcription of genes such as ABCA1, ABCA3, and ABCA7, increasing the sensitivity of non-small cell lung cancer cells to cisplatin [212]. The epigenetic effects of VPA have also been suggested for use in the treatment of breast cancer, squamous cell tumors, and human hepatocellular carcinomas (HepG2 cells). In the near future, VPA could be useful as an HDAC inhibitor in conjunction with standard anticancer drugs that target oncogenes through different pathways. Moreover, VPA has been shown to improve the efficacy of radiotherapy in glioblastoma patients and protect hippocampal neurons from radiotherapy-induced apoptosis in the subgranular zone, thus preventing cognitive deficits associated with brain radiotherapy [213]. However, further clinical studies are needed to determine the efficacy of VPA as an adjuvant therapy for solid tumors.

Others

VPA-mediated neuroprotection has garnered significant attention across various animal models of neurodegenerative diseases. For instance, VPA has demonstrated neuroprotective effects in a rat model of Parkinson's disease, where damage to the ventral tegmental area and substantia nigra (SN) occurs. Similar effects have been observed in other neurodegenerative conditions, such as Huntington's disease and amyotrophic lateral sclerosis. Moreover, VPA has shown promise in treating Charcot-Marie-Tooth 2W (CMT2W) disease associated with HARS1 mutation by alleviating the inhibition of neuronal cellular morphological differentiation [214]. CMT2W, characterized by autosomal dominant inheritance, presents as peripheral neuropathy. At the cellular level, VPA has potential as a therapeutic agent for this condition, although further research is warranted to assess its clinical efficacy in humans. Kurishima et al. [215] described the case of a 68-year-old man who was hospitalized with symptomatic epilepsy after cerebral infarction. The patient had a history of superior mesenteric artery occlusion, and only 30 cm of the jejunum was intact. Gastrointestinal absorption remained high after the administration of VPA and LEV. The mechanism of action of VPA involves inhibiting CMT2W through histone deacetylase (HDAC) inhibition, facilitating histone acetylation, modifying DNA and histone methylation status, regulating gene expression, and inducing chromatin remodeling. As an epigenetic drug approved for clinical use, VPA exhibits potent antiviral and anti-inflammatory effects [216]. Saiz et al. [217] showed that VPA intervenes in crucial processes underlying the severity of COVID-19, including downregulating ACE2 and NRP1 expression, reducing SARS-CoV-2 infectivity, and potentially impacting viral replication or stability, thereby curbing viral production and dampening the resultant inflammatory response. These findings suggest that VPA has potential as a candidate drug for combating COVID-19. However, contrasting views exist. Farazdaghi et al. [218] studied 241 patients and found no evidence supporting the protective effect of VPA against COVID-19 infection or its disease-modifying role in patients with active infection. These findings underscore the need for further research to clarify the role of VPA in COVID-19 management.

Mechanisms of Drug Resistance

Drug-resistant epilepsy (DRE) affects approximately one-third of epilepsy patients, with VPA resistance being a significant predictor of DRE and a major challenge for epilepsy treatment. However, the pathogenesis of VPA-resistant epilepsy remains unclear. Many patients with VPA-resistant epilepsy exhibit significant inflammatory responses and localized hypoxia. Hypoxia-inducible factor (HIF)-1α is a key effector molecule of hypoxia and inflammation and may play a crucial role in the development of VPA-resistant epilepsy. Fu et al. [219] systematically investigated the role of HIF-1α in children and mice with VPA-resistant epilepsy and examined the microRNAs that regulate the expression of HIF-1α. They established VPA-sensitive and VPA-resistant epilepsy models in mice and confirmed significant differences in epileptic behavior and EEG data through proteomic analysis. The results showed that HIF-1α was overexpressed in VPA-resistant epileptic mice and regulated the expression of interleukin-1β and tumor necrosis factor-α. Increased expression of HIF-1α led to an increase in the number of microglia and induced their polarization from the M2 phenotype to the M1 phenotype, which triggered the release of proinflammatory mediators. Bioinformatics analysis of public databases revealed that miR-221-3p expression was reduced in VPA-resistant epilepsy and negatively regulated HIF-1α expression. Treatment with miR-221-3p mimics significantly reduced HIF-1α expression and inhibited microglial activation and inflammatory mediator release, resulting in the relief of seizures in VPA-resistant epilepsy patients. These findings suggest that the miR-221-3p/HIF-1α pathway is a critical component in the pathogenesis of VPA-resistant epilepsy and represents a potential therapeutic target for antiepileptic treatment. Wang et al. [220] explored the potential mechanism of VPA resistance by administering VPA (250 mg/kg) to rats with chronic epilepsy induced by pentylenetetrahydroxybenzene (Penta) for 14 days. The seizure stage (seizure score [before Day 14] $\leq$ 0) and latency time (latency time [before Day 14] $\geq$ 0) were evaluated, and rats with controlled seizures were considered responsive to VPA treatment, while the others were considered unresponsive. Differentially expressed genes (DEGs) were identified in the hippocampal transcriptomes of rats that responded to VPA and those that did not respond to VPA treatment, and their functions were evaluated. The roles of the postsynaptic dense region (PSD) and the Homer1 protein were determined. Homer1 was more highly expressed in the hippocampi of rats unresponsive to VPA treatment than in that of rats responsive to VPA treatment. Homer1b/c overexpression blocked the therapeutic effects of VPA by increasing reactive oxygen species production, lactate dehydrogenase release, and calcium levels. In addition, Homer1b/c overexpression induced mGluR1 and mGluR5 overexpression. These findings suggest that Homer1b/c overexpression affects the therapeutic effect of VPA and that Homer1b/c overexpression is a potential marker for improving the efficacy of this treatment.

Adverse Reactions to Valproic Acid

Although patients generally tolerate valproic acid (VPA) well, its efficacy and safety may be constrained by adverse drug reactions (ADRs). Numerous systematic reviews, clinical trials, and postmarketing literature assessments have evaluated the prevalence and clinical relevance of VPA-associated ADRs, encompassing hepatic, gastrointestinal, neurological, hematologic, dermatological, teratogenic, and metabolic disorders. Among patients receiving VPA treatment, gastrointestinal disturbances are relatively common, with prevalent symptoms including nausea, vomiting, dysphagia, and diarrhea. Additionally, dizziness, memory impairment, insomnia, and nystagmus are frequently reported side effects that are often mitigated by adjusting the drug dosage or discontinuing treatment. Notably, VPA is generally not linked to somnolence or cognitive impairment, with rare instances of adverse effects on cognition. Moreover, compared to other ASMs, such as lamotrigine (LTG) or topiramate (TPM), VPA is associated with a notably lower incidence of ADRs in epilepsy patients [221]. VPA toxicity can arise accidentally or therapeutically. In individuals with metabolic disorders, drug interactions, or intentional overdose, toxic reactions may manifest when doses are manipulated to achieve therapeutic levels. Acute VPA overdose typically presents with symptoms such as central nervous system dysfunction, electrolyte imbalances (e.g., hypernatremia), elevated liver enzymes, hyperammonemia, and hepatotoxicity. Severe overdoses may lead to hypotension, tachycardia, respiratory depression, metabolic acidosis, cerebral edema, and VPA-induced hyperammonemic encephalopathy, potentially progressing to coma and fatal outcomes without prompt intervention. Conventional management strategies for VPA toxicity typically involve administering levothyroxine, activated charcoal, and hemodialysis.

Hepatic Impairment

Hepatotoxicity is a known complication in patients undergoing VPA treatment, and drug-induced liver injury (DILI) poses a significant threat. The incidence of hepatotoxicity is less than 1% in approximately 20,000 patients treated with VPA. Studies have shown that the risk of hepatotoxicity is much lower in the general population (1/20,000–1/40,000 patients) than in those with specific risk factors (1/500) who are taking VPA [222]. Monitoring for hepatotoxicity risk factors is crucial because these can lead to severe idiosyncratic side effects. Hepatotoxicity is age-dependent, with a significantly greater risk observed in children under 2 years of age, particularly those with severe seizures or other neurological disorders. The onset of hepatotoxicity typically occurs within the first 6 months of VPA therapy. Although liver function tests can be conducted before initiating treatment, they may not always predict hepatotoxic episodes. Therapeutic drug monitoring, regular serum aminotransferase level assessments, blood ammonia concentration checks, and lipid parameter monitoring during VPA therapy can help improve drug safety profiles and prevent DILI progression [223]. VPA is contraindicated in individuals with a greater risk of hepatotoxicity, especially those with metabolic disorders or mitochondrial disorders. Clinical manifestations of hepatotoxicity include apathy, altered mental status, anorexia, vomiting, jaundice, and potential exacerbation of seizures, particularly during febrile episodes.

The mechanisms through which VPA induces hepatic injury include the release of Δ4VPA metabolites, depletion of glutathione stores leading to oxidative stress, inhibition of fatty acid β-oxidation causing mitochondrial DNA depletion, and interference with various metabolic pathways. Studies have shown that VPA can induce fatty liver through multiple mechanisms involving different enzymes and receptors. Meseguer et al. [224] conducted a retrospective case–control study on patients treated with VPA, revealing factors associated with an increased risk of VPA-induced DILI. Mei et al. [225] described a fatal case of VPA-induced liver failure combined with thrombotic microangiopathy, emphasizing the importance of recognizing and managing such severe adverse reactions promptly.

Succinic acid (SA), a natural polyphenolic compound, has shown potential for mitigating VPA-induced hepatotoxicity by inhibiting hepatic aminotransferase activity, reducing oxidative stress, and suppressing proinflammatory markers in hepatic tissues, as demonstrated in a rat model study by Gheena et al. [226]. This finding suggested that SA could serve as a promising agent for preventing VPA-related liver injury.

Weight and Metabolic Disorders

Weight gain is a common adverse effect associated with valproic acid (VPA) treatment and is frequently highlighted in research studies. Notably, there is considerable variability among patients receiving VPA, with a greater likelihood of weight gain observed in female patients, particularly during adolescence. This weight gain can have significant implications for treatment adherence and overall quality of life, especially in adolescent girls, where excessive weight gain may lead to profound psychological disturbances and the development of significant endocrine abnormalities. The mechanisms underlying VPA-induced weight gain remain unclear, and several hypotheses have been proposed. Among these, dysregulation of the hypothalamic system, alterations in adipokine levels, hyperinsulinemia, and increased insulin resistance (IR) are among the most widely supported. Studies have also indicated alterations in gut flora characteristics in patients treated with VPA, with correlations observed between gut flora composition, weight gain, and clinical biochemical markers. This suggests the potential involvement of microbiome composition in the metabolic disturbances induced by VPA [157].

To investigate the IR-related adverse effects of VPA, George et al. [227] compared the incidence of IR in children receiving VPA monotherapy versus those receiving phenytoin sodium monotherapy for more than a year. Their findings revealed a significantly greater incidence of IR and nonalcoholic fatty liver disease in the VPA group, irrespective of age, sex, puberty, or nutritional status. Furthermore, metabolic complications are common in children undergoing VPA treatment, emphasizing the importance of close monitoring for early detection and intervention. Recent cohort studies have linked VPA treatment in adults to an increased risk of developing type 2 diabetes (T2D), underscoring the metabolic implications of VPA therapy [228].

Yaryari et al. [229] investigated the serum levels of leukoilipin, a newly identified adipokine derived from white adipose tissue involved in gluconeogenesis, in epileptic patients treated with VPA through a cross-sectional study. They discovered significantly elevated mean values of various metabolic markers, including body mass index (BMI), fasting serum glucose, glycohemoglobin (HbA1c), insulin, total cholesterol, low-density lipoprotein (LDL-C), triglycerides, and fasting serum leukocidin, in the VPA-treated group compared to both the lamotrigine-treated and untreated groups. Moreover, a greater proportion of subjects in the VPA group met the criteria for insulin resistance (defined as HOMA-IR > 2.5), and the mean fasting leukocidin serum concentration was notably greater in the VPA group than in the other groups, indicating a potential role for elevated leukocidin levels in the development of obesity, insulin resistance, and metabolic disorders associated with VPA treatment. Yan et al. [230] demonstrated that VPA increased the expression of the nuclear receptor pregnane X receptor (PXR) and fatty acid-binding protein 4 (FABP4) in a dose-dependent manner. This upregulation of PXR-mediated FABP4 expression was identified as the mechanism underlying VPA-induced lipid accumulation. Additionally, a meta-analysis evaluating the long-term effects of valproic acid treatment on the lipid profiles of children with epilepsy revealed that VPA treatment led to reductions in both total cholesterol and LDL cholesterol levels [231].

Adverse effects, such as hepatic steatosis, have been observed in patients undergoing VPA treatment, with most being mild and reversible. Recent research has revealed that VPA increased lipid peroxidation parameters and induced significant microvesicular steatosis throughout hepatic lobules in all alveolar regions. However, coadministration of the natural flavonoid antioxidant naringenin mitigated perifollicular steatosis. Naringenin also acts as a modulator of crucial lipid metabolism pathways [232].

Various factors related to ASMs may impact the growth and development of children with epilepsy. Medications affecting appetite can disrupt normal growth and weight gain. Buraniqi et al. [80] systematically reviewed randomized controlled trials and open-label studies involving children aged 0–18 years from the Medline database. Their findings indicated that VPA was the ASM most strongly associated with increased appetite and/or weight gain. Furthermore, metabolic syndrome, characterized by weight gain, insulin resistance, hyperinsulinemia, atherosclerotic dyslipidemia, and elevated blood pressure, was identified as a serious clinical condition linked to VPA use. Although precise data on the frequency of these adverse events are limited, chronic VPA use has been associated with hyperandrogenemia, irregular menstruation, and polycystic ovary syndrome in women. Additionally, the antiprogesterone effect of VPA may also contribute to the frequency of anovulatory cycles.

Endocrine disorders affecting reproductive and sexual function can also manifest in men receiving VPA treatment. Reproductive disorders in male patients have seldom been studied, with potential effects including altered sperm mobility, reduced testicular weights, and infertility. Prenatal exposure to VPA has been linked to decreased androgen and gonadotropin levels, along with dose-dependent testicular defects, as demonstrated by reduced testicular weight, sperm viability, and seminiferous tubule degeneration in animal studies [233]. VPA induces oxidative stress and testicular damage, triggering the autophagic responses typically observed after testicular injury. This is associated with changes in steroidogenic gene expression, serum testosterone levels, and histopathological deterioration [234]. Guo et al. [235] conducted a study involving 44 young men with epilepsy (23 treated with VPA and 21 treated with OXC) and 30 age-matched healthy individuals. The authors evaluated sexual function using the International Index of Erectile Function (IIEF-5), sperm quality, and sex hormone levels before and 6 months after treatment. The results revealed a significant reduction in sperm quality after 6 months of VPA treatment in young male patients, confirming the negative impact of VPA on sperm quality in human trials.

Thyroid hormones play a crucial role in both the development of the central nervous system and normal brain function. Alterations in thyroid hormone levels impact cortical excitability; conversely, ASMs are linked to changes in thyroid hormone metabolism. This interaction has been increasingly recognized. Rochtus et al. [236] conducted a systematic review following PRISMA guidelines, focusing on epilepsy, ASMs, and thyroid hormone metabolism. They examined altered thyroid function in elderly patients using ASMs, 25% of whom were taking VPA. Consequently, monitoring thyroid function is advisable for patients on VPA therapy. Comert et al. [237] retrospectively analyzed the serum levels of thyroid-stimulating hormone (TSH), free T3 (fT3), and free T4 (fT4) in patients taking VPA. They observed normal pretreatment and early TSH values but significant differences in late TSH and fT4 serum levels. These findings underscore the importance of monitoring patient thyroid hormone levels, particularly late in treatment, due to potential unique or cumulative effects of VPA. Ilia et al. [238] investigated thyroid hormone levels in children under 16 years of age receiving VPA monotherapy. They performed a systematic evaluation and meta-analysis, revealing a greater prevalence of biochemical thyroid abnormalities with elevated TSH levels in the VPA group. This suggests that caution should be taken when using VPA therapy, especially in children predisposed to thyroid disorders. Carnitine deficiency is associated with VPA treatment because carnitine functions as a cofactor in fatty acid metabolism. An observational study by Masanori Saito et al. [239] found significant correlations between serum free carnitine levels and epilepsy duration, duration of VPA treatment, daily VPA dose, and blood VPA concentration. Carnitine supplementation helps maintain serum-free carnitine levels in VPA-treated patients, potentially mitigating pancreatic injury (lower serum amylase levels in supplemented patients) [240].

Teratogenic and Neurodevelopmental Disorders

VPA, which crosses the placenta, can induce a spectrum of congenital abnormalities. The predominant cause of malformations in infants born to mothers with epilepsy receiving VPA during pregnancy seems to be the direct teratogenic effects of VPA itself rather than the underlying epileptic conditions in the mother. The teratogenicity of VPA is notably heightened when VPA is coadministered with other ASMs. Reported malformations include neural tube or cardiovascular defects, orofacial clefts, subfibular clefts, gastrointestinal atresia, diaphragmatic hernia, and premature closure of cranial sutures. Notably, the usage instructions of VPA have been updated to include teratogenic warnings. Christensen et al. [241] investigated the association between VPA exposure and congenital malformations in children born in Denmark between January 1, 1997, and December 31, 2014. Among 895,507 children (51.3% males), 31,790 (3.6%) were diagnosed with severe congenital malformations within the first year of life. Analysis revealed a 3.95-fold increased risk of severe congenital malformations in children prenatally exposed to VPA compared to unexposed children. Consistent correlations were found between VPA monotherapy during the first trimester of pregnancy and increased risks of specific malformations. Over subsequent years, the teratogenic effects of VPA were further corroborated, with improved precision in estimates (1997–2014: aOR = 2.44, 95% CI = 1.80–3.30).

Exposure to VPA during pregnancy can lead to fetal valproic acid syndrome (FVS), characterized by neural tube defects (NTDs), musculoskeletal abnormalities, and neurodevelopmental deficits. The mechanism underlying VPA-induced developmental toxicity involves oxidative stress, which disrupts redox-sensitive cell signaling and leads to improper cell differentiation. In undifferentiated P19 mouse embryonal carcinoma cells, VPA treatment resulted in increased concentrations of glutathione disulfide (GSSG) and increased oxidative glutathione (GSH)/GSSG redox potential compared to those in control cells, indicating increased intracellular oxidative stress. Remarkably, VPA did not affect GSH or GSSG levels in differentiated P19 neurons. Pretreatment with 3h-1,2-dithiophenol-3-thione (D3T) prevented VPA-induced alterations in the GSH/GSSG pathway in undifferentiated cells. Additionally, pretreatment with D3T before VPA exposure improved neurogenesis in P19 cells at different stages of neuronal differentiation. Furthermore, VPA-treated differentiated P19 cells exhibited increased protein oxidation, while D3T treatment reduced protein oxidation. These findings suggest that VPA impedes neural differentiation, while NRF2-mediated redox homeostasis promotes normal neuronal differentiation, potentially reducing the incidence of FVS [242]. Regarding VPA-induced NTDs, a recent animal study suggested that genetic variants related to low embryonic taurine status or environmental exposure may be determinants of the risk of adverse pregnancy outcomes in VPA-exposed pregnant women at the time of health care needs [243]. The results of an animal study suggested that genetic variants and environmental factors, such as low embryonic taurine status, may influence the risk of adverse pregnancy outcomes in pregnant women exposed to VPA. Zebrafish embryos serve as an in vivo model, confirming the associations between VPA exposure and jitteriness/tremor, sensory organ (eye) malformations, and craniofacial malformations, which may be linked to VPA-induced NTDs in mammals [244]. Similarly, Muhsen et al. [245] investigated the neurotoxic effects of VPA exposure using zebrafish as a model and explored the potential for folic acid (FA) supplementation to mitigate VPA-induced neuronal and behavioral disturbances. Their findings revealed that VPA exposure in zebrafish embryos led to a reduced midbrain volume, increased midline gap in the hindbrain, and disrupted synapse sprouting in secondary motor neurons in a concentration-dependent manner. Additionally, VPA exposure decreased the fluorescence intensity of neuronal progenitor cells during early developmental stages, indicating reduced cell numbers. Moreover, VPA exposure altered embryo twitching activity, resulting in hyperactivity in darkness and hypoactivity in light conditions. The authors concluded that VPA exposure induces specific neurotoxicity in developing zebrafish embryos and that FA supplementation reverses most of the identified defects.

Prenatal exposure to VPA poses an elevated risk of postnatal neurodevelopmental impairments, such as autism spectrum disorder (ASD) and attention-deficit/hyperactivity disorder (ADHD). VPA exposure is recognized as an environmental factor contributing to ASD risk, although its precise mechanism of action in the human brain remains unclear, as most relevant studies are conducted in two-dimensional cell cultures and animal models. Meng et al. [246] utilized human forebrain-like organoids (hFOs) and reported that VPA exposure in three-dimensional cell cultures derived from hFOs altered the expression of genes enriched in neurodevelopmental processes, synaptic transmission, oxytocin signaling, and calcium and potassium signaling pathways (e.g., CAMK4, CLCN4, DPP10, GABRB3, KCNB1, PRKCB, SCN1A, SLC24A2)—all of which are implicated in ASD. The genes whose expression was affected by VPA exposure overlapped significantly with those dysregulated in the brains or organoids of ASD patients, known ASD risk genes, and genes within ASD risk-associated coexpression modules. Single-cell RNA sequencing analysis revealed that VPA exposure influenced gene expression in hFOs, particularly in the choroid plexus, excitatory neurons, immature neurons, and medial ganglionic rongeur cells. Furthermore, microelectrode arrays confirmed that VPA exposure disrupted synaptic transmission in hFOs. This study established a link between VPA exposure and ASD pathogenesis using hFOs, providing valuable insights into the etiology of ASD and potential therapeutic targets. Moreover, fetal exposure to VPA during the first trimester of pregnancy is associated with a greater incidence of autism in offspring. Epigenetic mechanisms are speculated to contribute to VPA-induced ASD, as VPA can affect DNA transcription through epigenetic mechanisms, increasing susceptibility to the transmission of new traits to subsequent generations. The use of VPA has been restricted based on retrospective and prospective studies demonstrating its role as a risk factor for ASD [150]. Conversely, an animal study conducted using pregnant rats [247] revealed that supplementation with vitamin A significantly mitigated VPA-induced autism-related behaviors. Additionally, NONRATT021475.2 and Dhh expression were upregulated in the hippocampi of rats exhibiting autism-like behaviors, suggesting a potential therapeutic role for vitamin A in treating this disorder. Integrating these findings with further clinical evidence will be crucial for fully understanding the impact of VPA on different stages of neurodevelopment and exploring additional therapeutic options. Honybun et al. [248] investigated the influence of sex and drug dosage on the relationship between prenatal VPA exposure and postnatal behavioral outcomes. They examined 121 children aged 4–11 years, including 54 children prenatally exposed to VPA (28 males, 26 females; mean dose +/− SD: 644 +/− 310 mg/day) and 67 children exposed to other ASMs. The results indicated that males exhibited more ASD symptoms ($p = 0.01$), but this sex difference was not observed in VPA-exposed children. Furthermore, there was no evidence of a dose–response relationship between VPA exposure and ASD symptoms. Although males had higher ADHD scores than females did, no association between ADHD symptoms and VPA exposure was found. These initial findings suggest that prenatal VPA exposure may counteract the usual male predominance in ASD incidence, indicating that VPA is a "behavioral teratogen" whose effects may be sex-dependent, with females being particularly sensitive. Additionally, no association was observed between VPA dosage and adverse postnatal behavioral outcomes, possibly due to the relatively low VPA dosage used in the study. In a study by Bjørk et al. [249], Nordic health registry and social registry data from 1996 to 2017 were analyzed to investigate whether prenatal exposure to ASMs, including VPA, increased the risk of neurodevelopmental disorders in children. Among 4,494,926 subjects, children born to epileptic mothers receiving VPA monotherapy had a greater incidence of autism spectrum disorder (ASD) than those born to mothers unexposed to ASMs (2.7% vs. 1.5%).

Feleke et al. [250] employed integrative genomics to elucidate the molecular mechanisms underlying the neurodevelopmental effects of gestational exposure to VPA. Through long-term oral administration to pregnant mothers, gestational VPA exposure was linked to differential gene expression, including splicing dysregulation, in the fetal brain, without evident neuronal gain or loss. The functional implications of VPA-induced gene expression alterations were explored via pathway analyses and integration with genetic risk data for psychiatric disorders and behavioral traits. Notably, a subset of genes downregulated by VPA in the fetal brain was significantly enriched in pathways associated with neurodevelopment and synaptic function. Furthermore, these genes showed significant enrichment in the heritability of human intelligence, schizophrenia, and bipolar disorder. These findings establish a mechanistic connection between chronic fetal exposure to VPA and neurodevelopmental disorders mediated by transcriptional dysregulation induced by VPA. Kowalski et al. [251] conducted a transcriptomic meta-analysis of VPA-exposed human embryonic stem cells (hESCs) and identified 61 genes with downregulated expression and 54 genes with upregulated expression. Ontology and pathway enrichment analyses suggested neurodevelopmental and neuroinflammatory effects, with overexpression of epilepsy-associated genes such as SCN1A and GABRB2. Upregulation of expression of NDNF genes, which are involved in neuronal migration and survival during development, was also observed. Subnetwork analyses indicated activation of the TGFβ and BMP pathways. These results indicate the involvement of VPA in epilepsy-related genes and its potential interference with multiple developmental pathways, even in embryonic cells in which neurodevelopmental genes are upregulated. These mechanisms may help elucidate the spectrum of congenital abnormalities induced by VPA and its molecular effects on neurodevelopment.

Hyperammonemia (HA)

VPA-induced hyperammonemia (HA) is a rare adverse reaction that can occur with both short-term and long-term use of valproic acid. While long-term mild hyperammonemia is often asymptomatic, encephalopathy may develop, and severe hyperammonemia can also present acutely, leading to encephalopathy. Symptoms of hyperammonemic encephalopathy include acute impairment of consciousness, confusion, somnolence, neurological signs, worsening seizures, and severe ataxia up to coma, although fatal outcomes are rare. Psychoneurobehavioral changes may be misinterpreted as postictal effects or psychosis, leading to inappropriate increases in VPA dosage. Intravenous VPA administration can also induce hyperammonemia. Hosseini et al. [252] studied 316 patients treated with VPA for neuropsychiatric disorders and reported that 17% of patients developed HA, 15 of whom were symptomatic. Interestingly, there were no significant demographic differences between the symptomatic and asymptomatic HA groups, except for the number of coadministered medications. VPA treatment duration, dosage, and serum levels did not significantly differ between the two groups. However, patients using risperidone alongside VPA had significantly higher VPA levels, which correlated with blood ammonia levels and symptomatic HA. A recent paper by Dong Won Kwack et al. [253] highlighted that the total dosage of ASMs and the use of topiramate were independent predictors of hyperammonemia in epilepsy patients treated with VPA. Levocarnitine is the preferred therapeutic agent for hyperammonemia associated with VPA toxicity. Pagali et al. [254] presented a case of a 20-year-old woman who intentionally overdosed on VPA, demonstrating a recurrence of hyperammonemia and symptoms after discontinuing levocarnitine supplementation. The authors recommended at least 72 h of levocarnitine treatment and an additional 24 h of monitoring to prevent hyperammonemia recurrence post-discontinuation. Another case presented in the literature involved a 56-year-old man who developed hyperammonemia after intentionally overdosing on VPA and was treated with leucovorin. In severe refractory cases, intermittent hemodialysis may be utilized, and recent studies advocate the use of carbapenem antibiotics, particularly meropenem, for treatment [255].

Dyskinesia

Dyskinesia, including tremor and Parkinson's disease symptoms, are recognized adverse effects of VPA. Tremor typically presents as postural tremor, and there is no definitive correlation between VPA dosage and tremor occurrence. Lan et al. [256] conducted a study on the risk factors associated with VPA-induced tremor and reported that female sex, a family history of tremor, a daily dose of VPA exceeding 1000 mg, and a therapy duration exceeding 24 months were associated with VPA-induced tremor. However, the relationship between the development of resting tremors and other symptoms of Parkinson's disease in patients taking VPA remains unexplored. In a study evaluating 125 patients treated with VPA for epilepsy or migraine headaches using the Fahn-Tolosa-Marin Tremor Rating Scale (FTM-TRS), 11.2% of the patients exhibited resting tremors, with significantly greater FTM-TRS scores than did the controls ($p < 0.001$). However, only one patient was diagnosed with Parkinson's disease, suggesting possible VPA-induced Parkinson's disease or exacerbation of motor features of Parkinson's disease by VPA. The incidence of Parkinson's syndrome in this cohort study was 1.6%, which contrasts with a previously reported pooled incidence of 3%. The occurrence of resting tremors in 11.2% of VPA-treated patients was linked to VPA-induced tremor rather than to the presence of Parkinson's disease [257].

VPA is associated with various other movement disorders. Rissardo et al. [258] evaluated the clinico-epidemiological features, pathophysiological mechanisms, and treatment of VPA-related movement disorders (MDs). Among the 362 subjects with MD secondary to VPA across 138 publications, the identified MDs included Parkinson's syndrome (252 cases), myoclonus (54 cases), dystonia (17 cases), dyskinesia (16 cases), stuttering (4 cases), tics (3 cases), and inability to sit still (1 case). Discontinuation of VPA treatment was the most common management approach, with an 80.61% full recovery rate. Additionally, there has been a case report of VPA-induced reversible lateralized manual dexterity in a 24-year-old woman who was diagnosed with Rasmussen's encephalitis at the age of 6. She developed persistent left-sided hemiparesis at the age of 11 years after the addition of VPA to CBZ and phenobarbital treatment, and motor cessation was observed the day after VPA cessation [259].

Others

Yıldız et al. [260] investigated the potential cardiac effects of both low-dose (LD) and high-dose (HD) VPA treatment in seizure-free rats. These findings revealed a dose-dependent increase in caspase-3 staining intensity, accompanied by a notable reduction in connexin 43 and troponin T staining intensity in the VPA-treated group. Biochemically, high-dose VPA administration led to a significant increase in malondialdehyde (MDA) levels within myocardial tissues. These observations underscore the potential risk of cardiovascular complications associated with VPA treatment. In addition, Liang et al. [261] examined the risk of all-cause mortality and mortality specifically from heart failure (HF) in individuals receiving a combination of VPA and LEV/LTG. Their analysis confirmed that VPA treatment was linked to higher rates of both all-cause mortality and mortality attributable to heart failure.

Moreover, VPA has been implicated in renal injury. Anguissola et al. [262] reviewed the literature and identified 28 case reports documenting the cases of 48 epileptic patients who had used VPA for 7 months or longer and exhibited features consistent with significant renal tubular injury. These manifestations included hypophosphatemia, urinary glucose, proteinuria, metabolic acidosis, hyperuricemia, renal tubular proteinuria, hypokalemia, and hypocalcemia. Biopsies from six patients revealed altered proximal renal tubular cells accompanied by large, malformed mitochondria. Notably, mild or asymptomatic renal injury was described in eight patients. Isolated renal tubular proteinuria, primarily of N-acetyl-β-aminoglucosidase, was frequently observed in 285 subjects who had taken VPA for 7 months or more. Thus, valproic acid may induce significant tubular injury, often associated with proximal tubular mitochondrial toxicity; prolonged treatment, typically exceeding 7 months, is commonly linked to asymptomatic or less symptomatic tubular injury. Additionally, VPA has been implicated in lung injury through oxidative stress mechanisms [263].

The long-term administration of VPA has been linked to acute pancreatitis, a potentially life-threatening condition. Monica C M Bischof et al. [264] conducted an extensive literature review on VPA-induced acute pancreatitis, highlighting its unpredictable onset and high fatality rate.

Although the effects of sodium phenytoin on oral health have been extensively studied, information regarding the impact of VPA remains scarce. A study noted a 44% correlation between VPA and gingival hyperplasia, emphasizing the need for dentists treating epilepsy patients to consider the potential for VPA-induced gingival overgrowth [265]. In addition, VPA has been specifically associated with an elevated risk of urinary tract infections [266]. Coagulation disorders are among the most commonly reported adverse effects of VPA, with platelet dysfunction being predominant [267]. Pediatric patients are particularly susceptible to VPA-induced hematotoxicity due to their increased risk of leukemia. Riahi-Zanjani et al. [268] conducted a systematic literature review, identifying 36 relevant articles involving 1381 pediatric patients, which revealed that VPA therapy can lead to severe hematologic toxicity, including neutropenia, thrombocytopenia, and myelosuppression, even at therapeutic doses. Discontinuation of VPA or dose reduction typically results in complete resolution of hematologic impairment within 2 weeks. The authors stressed the importance of monitoring hematological parameters during VPA treatment and suggested that combining VPA with antioxidants may mitigate hematologic side effects by targeting potential mechanistic pathways.

Drug-induced lupus erythematosus (DILE) constitutes 10–15% of systemic lupus erythematosus (SLE) cases and can be caused by more than 100 drugs. The clinical and serologic manifestations of DILE vary widely depending on the drug, often leading to its oversight in clinical practice. In June 2021, Papadopoulou et al. [269] searched for VPA-induced DILE cases in the PubMed and Embase databases and identified 15 articles meeting the inclusion criteria. While SLE predominantly affects women, VPA-induced lupus appears to be more prevalent in men. Half of the patients developed DILE within the initial 3 months of VPA treatment, while four patients experienced DILE onset between 1 and 5 years after commencing VPA therapy. The presentation of lupus was generally mild, with polyarthritis, pleural effusion, or pericarditis being the most common manifestations. Notably, one patient exhibited Rowell syndrome, a rare variant of lupus erythematosus characterized by erythema multiforme and sporadic antinuclear antibodies (ANAs). Involvement of the central nervous system, kidneys, or skin was minimal or absent, although seven patients displayed cytopenia. Immunological assessments revealed positive ANAs in the majority of patients (86.7%), with five patients testing positive for antihistone antibodies, three for anti-dsDNA antibodies, and two showing hypocomplementemia. Despite the rapid resolution of clinical symptoms upon discontinuation of VPA, serologic abnormalities persisted for up to 18 months. Corticosteroids were administered to eight patients during VPA cessation. The authors underscored the association between VPA and DILE, urging clinicians to be vigilant to ensure optimal patient outcomes. Although some potential pathophysiologic mechanisms have been proposed, further research is needed for a comprehensive understanding of the syndrome.

Additionally, a few cases of drug reaction eosinophilia and systemic syndrome (DRESS), characterized by cutaneous symptoms, fever, eosinophilia, thrombocytopenia, and multiorgan involvement, have been linked to VPA [270]. Furthermore, VPA-associated Fanconi syndrome (FS), though rare, should be considered in epilepsy patients, particularly if the patient has severe psychomotor disorders, uses feeding devices, and receives ASM treatment other than VPA [271].

Summary

Since its introduction as an antiseizure medication (ASM), VPA has been subjected to more than 50 years of experimental research and clinical use, establishing it as one of the most potent ASMs available. Its remarkable efficacy extends beyond neurological disorders, demonstrating promising therapeutic benefits in various other fields. This broad potential warrants continued investigation and exploration, not only within the realm of neurology but also across diverse medical domains.

2.1.1.7 Phenytoin Sodium

Drug Characteristics

[Chemical name] 5,5-Diphenylhydantoin sodium salt

[Chemical structure]

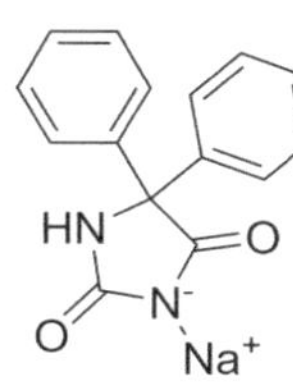

[Molecular formula] C15H11N2NaO2

[Molecular weight] 274.25

[Indications] This drug can be used for the treatment of generalized tonic–clonic seizures, focal seizures, and status epilepticus and for the prevention and treatment of epileptic seizures during and after neurosurgery.

[Specification] Phenytoin sodium tablets (mostly tablets): 50 mg; 100 mg. Phenytoin sodium for injection: 0.1 g; 0.25 g.

[Dosage]
Typical dosages for adults usually start at 100 mg (1 tablet) twice daily, increasing gradually to 250–300 mg/day over 1–3 weeks. The total daily dose is usually divided into three equal doses, with a maximum of 300 mg/dose or 500 mg/day. However, personalized dosing should consider individual patient characteristics and pharmacokinetic profiles. Once seizure control is achieved and steady blood drug levels are reached, long-acting (controlled release) formulations may be used once daily. In cases of frequent seizures, an initial dose of 12–15 mg/kg body weight, divided into

two to three doses every 6 h, may be administered. Starting from the following day, 100 mg (or 1.5–2 mg/kg body weight) may be given three times daily until the appropriate dosage is established.

Regarding children, VPA should generally be avoided in infants and young children due to challenges in monitoring side effects. If necessary, the initial dose is typically 5 mg/kg/day, divided into two to three doses, with adjustments made as necessary. The maximum daily dose is 250 mg. Maintenance dosages typically range from 4 to 8 mg/kg or, according to body surface area, do not exceed 250 mg/m^2, with consideration given to monitoring blood concentrations.

[Adverse reactions]

Gingival hyperplasia is common, with a high incidence in children. If hyperplasia is severe, surgical removal may be needed.

Adverse intestinal effects include nausea, vomiting, constipation, epigastric pain, dysphagia, loss of taste, anorexia, and weight loss.

Adverse central nervous system reactions include confusion, ataxia, blurred vision, diplopia, toxic amblyopia, vertigo, headache, insomnia, transient nervousness, tremor, ataxia, chorea, dystonia, slurred speech and confusion, transient neurosis, chorea, dystonia, tremor, and asterixis.

Hematopoietic system adverse reactions include granulocytopenia or thrombocytopenia, aplastic anemia, and megaloblastic anemia.

Adverse skin reactions include allergic reactions, common rashes with high fever, and rare severe skin reactions, such as exfoliative dermatitis and erosive erythema multiforme.

Adverse reactions of the rheumatic immune system include systemic lupus erythematosus and fatal hepatic necrosis.

Adverse reactions to the lymphatic system include Hodgkin's disease.

Long-term use in children can cause rickets or bone abnormalities, and use by pregnant women can occasionally cause teratogenesis.

In addition, phenytoin has also been reported to increase blood sugar and cause cancer.

Clinical Applications and Basic Research

Historical Evolution of Phenytoin Sodium

Heinrich Biltz first synthesized phenytoin in 1908, initially believing it to possess analgesic and sedative properties, without recognizing its potential as an antiepileptic medication. It was not until 1936 when American doctor H. Houston Merrit and chemist Tracy Putnam first utilized phenytoin sodium for treating epilepsy, observing its inhibitory effects on seizures in patients. This discovery identified phenytoin as a significant drug for epilepsy treatment. In 1946, L.S. Goodman conducted further research on the anticonvulsant properties of phenytoin sodium [272]. B Bashinski proposed the use of phenytoin sodium for treating epilepsy in children [273]. In 1949, J. P. McGovern described phenytoin poisoning [274]. In 1950, R D

Sweet et al. investigated a fixed skin rash caused by phenytoin [275]. In 1981, C.E. Pfeifle and colleagues described the solubility of phenytoin in three different intravenous injection solutions. Their study concluded that 0.9% sodium chloride and lactated Ringer's solution were suitable for intravenous administration of phenytoin [276]. In 2020, Yi Kang discovered that phenytoin improves gingival fibroblast aging and is related to autophagy [277].

Adverse Reactions of Phenytoin Sodium

M Kathiravan et al. [278] conducted a cross-sectional study aiming to address anemia induced by long-term phenytoin treatment in epilepsy patients. They categorized epilepsy patients into groups of cases (duration >2 years) and controls (<1 year) based on the duration of phenytoin treatment. The study revealed that the levels of folic acid and vitamin B12 were significantly lower in the case group than in the control group. This suggests that prolonged use of phenytoin may significantly affect the concentrations of folic acid and vitamin B12 in epilepsy patients.

Y Han et al. [83] performed a systematic review and comprehensive evaluation of thyroid hormone levels in epilepsy patients and controls receiving monotherapy. They assessed the long-term effects of oral ASMs on thyroid hormone levels in epilepsy patients. The findings indicated that patients with treated chronic epilepsy are at a greater risk of developing thyroid dysfunction, such as subclinical or clinical hypothyroidism, than the general population. CBZ and phenytoin treatment were found to decrease T4 levels and have little effect on TSH secretion, making them the drugs most strongly associated with reduced T4 and T3 levels.

Sangeetha et al. [279] conducted a cross-sectional study to assess atherogenic risk factors in young Indian adult epilepsy patients treated with phenytoin. They categorized subjects into three groups: healthy controls, newly diagnosed epilepsy patients, and epilepsy patients treated with phenytoin for more than 6 months. This study revealed that compared to healthy controls, newly diagnosed epilepsy patients exhibited alterations in indicators related to dyslipidemia, oxidative stress, and low-grade inflammation (hsCRP). These changes were further exacerbated in epilepsy patients after 6 months of phenytoin treatment.

C Morán-Mariños et al. [280] conducted a systematic literature review on cases of drug reaction eosinophilia and systemic symptoms (DRESS) syndrome induced by phenytoin and explored the characteristics of patients with this syndrome. DRESS syndrome is a severe adverse skin reaction caused by sensitivity to drugs, including phenytoin. The review identified 40 cases of DRESS syndrome, with all patients presenting with a rash, 50% with lymphadenopathy, and 30% with facial edema. The liver and respiratory tract were the most commonly affected organs, and eosinophilia was a prevalent feature. Given the severity and high mortality rate of DRESS syndrome, the authors emphasized the importance of monitoring for adverse effects of ASMs.

M Sáenz-Farret et al. [81] conducted a comprehensive review aiming to elucidate the intricate relationship between movement disorders and ASMs. They explored various combinations of 15 movement disorders (excluding ataxia) and

24 ASMs, aiming to describe treatable movement disorders, those exacerbated or induced by ASMs, and the complex interaction mechanisms and risk factors involved. The relationship between ASMs and movement disorders is multifaceted. Although ASMs are commonly employed to alleviate tremor, myoclonus, and restless leg syndrome, they can also act as potential triggers for iatrogenic movement disorders, notably Parkinson's disease and tremor. The ASMs that worsen or induce movement disorders include phenytoin. The pathophysiology of phenytoin-induced choreoathetosis is incompletely understood but has been attributed to defects in basal ganglia neurotransmitters. Phenytoin inhibits dopamine uptake in the brain, leading to an increase in homovanillic acid in cerebrospinal fluid, suggesting heightened dopaminergic activity. However, phenytoin treatment may exacerbate Parkinson's disease and tardive dyskinesia, potentially by antagonizing specific dopamine receptor subtypes, thereby potentiating dyskinesia induced by dopamine blockers. Both epileptic and nonepileptic myoclonus have been reported in patients taking phenytoin. Asterixis, a common movement disorder associated with phenytoin use, is frequently observed in patients receiving intravenous phenytoin treatment with transiently elevated drug concentrations. Additionally, generalized athetosis, choreoathetosis, and isolated athetosis may occur, particularly at toxic phenytoin concentrations. In summary, the therapeutic or toxic effects of a drug on motor symptoms can vary depending on factors such as dosage, individual variability, concurrent medication use, and other less understood conditions.

A case report described a 53-year-old woman with recurrent acute ataxia [281]. Although the patient had a history of epilepsy, she had been seizure-free for more than a decade. Complete cranial MRI revealed no evident signs of phenytoin-induced ataxia. Remarkably, her symptoms swiftly ameliorated upon reduction of phenytoin dosage, and no recurrence was noted during the 1-year follow-up period. This finding underscores the importance of considering potential adverse drug effects when patients with epilepsy treated with phenytoin present with ataxia.

A Asadi-Pooya A et al. [282] conducted a systematic review of the literature to comprehensively delineate the cosmetic adverse effects associated with ASMs, focusing particularly on alopecia, hirsutism, acne, and gingival hyperplasia. The most robust evidence for such effects is linked to phenytoin use, which is implicated in causing gingival hyperplasia, hirsutism, and acne, and valproic acid, which is associated with alopecia and hirsutism. Phenytoin-induced gingival hyperplasia is influenced by various factors, including genetic predisposition, activation of collagenase, inflammation and immune changes induced by plaque, and stimulation of growth factors. Maintaining good oral hygiene is crucial for preventing gingival hyperplasia, and patients receiving antiepileptic therapy should prioritize oral health. Some studies suggest that folic acid supplementation may mitigate phenytoin-related gingival hyperplasia, although this remains a topic of debate.

Jana Heidemann [266] investigated the correlation between anticonvulsant drug usage and the risk of urinary tract infections through a case–control study. By matching controls without urinary tract infections with patients with urinary tract infections based on sex, age, and codiagnosis, the study revealed that phenytoin, primidone, carbamazepine, and valproic acid use were associated with an elevated risk of urinary tract infections.

Research by Erika Minowa [283] demonstrated that phenytoin use induces an increase in the intracellular calcium concentration ($[Ca^{2+}]_i$) by impeding calcium efflux in human gingival fibroblasts. Furthermore, phenytoin use was found to augment the small calcium response triggered by low-concentration ATP or histamine stimulation by inhibiting calcium efflux. These findings suggest that phenytoin may contribute to drug-induced gingival overgrowth by interacting with inflammatory bioactive substances in the gingiva.

Matteo Candeloro [41] retrospectively analyzed patient data from 2011 to 2020 to investigate the incidence of thromboembolic events in individuals treated with CBZ or phenytoin in combination with oral anticoagulants. The study revealed a greater occurrence of thromboembolism in patients treated with anticoagulants combined with CBZ or phenytoin than in those not taking ASMs. Thrombotic and bleeding event rates were similar among patients receiving treatment with direct oral anticoagulants (DOACs) or vitamin K antagonists.

Phenytoin Sodium for the Treatment of Refractory and Superrefractory Status Epilepticus

Status epilepticus is a common neurological emergency in children. Rapid treatment is necessary because neuronal death and damage are suspected to be related to the duration of epileptic seizures.

A Klowak J et al. [284] conducted a study to assess the effectiveness and safety of levetiracetam compared to those of phenytoin or fosphenytoin in treating benzodiazepine-refractory status epilepticus in children. Phenytoin is associated with adverse reactions such as hypotension and cardiac arrhythmias, particularly with rapid infusion, and it has a narrow therapeutic window with significant drug interactions. Despite being commonly recommended as a second-line treatment for status epilepticus, this recommendation is based on low-quality evidence, including observational studies and expert opinions. The authors found evidence suggesting that levetiracetam is as effective as phenytoin or fosphenytoin in children with benzodiazepine-refractory status epilepticus. Given their similar efficacy, clinicians and guideline developers should consider the differing safety profiles when choosing between levetiracetam and phenytoin or fosphenytoin.

According to P Jain et al. [95], intravenous phenytoin or phenobarbital administration has traditionally been the preferred treatment for benzodiazepine-resistant status epilepticus. However, the adverse effects of phenytoin, including cardiac arrhythmias, hypotension, extravasation, and purple glove syndrome, as well as limitations on the infusion rate, restrict its use. Based on low-quality evidence, the primary outcome was that phenobarbital was significantly better than phenytoin in children and significantly better than valproate in adults in regard to adverse effects. Levetiracetam is similar to phenytoin or fosphenytoin regarding adverse effects. Mortality rates were comparable between interventions. For intubation in children, phenobarbital is considered safer than phenytoin, levetiracetam is safer than phenytoin, and valproate is superior to both phenobarbital and phenytoin regarding safety, with less cardiovascular instability than phenytoin. Phenobarbital and high-dose levetiracetam were significantly more effective than phenytoin in halting seizures within 60 min. Ultimately, drug selection should take into consideration effectiveness, safety concerns, availability, cost, and systemic comorbidities.

Application of Phenytoin Sodium in Special Populations with Epilepsy

Status epilepticus poses a critical medical emergency with considerable risks to morbidity and mortality. Liver and renal dysfunction can significantly impact the pharmacokinetics of drugs used in its treatment. Phenytoin is often employed as a second-line therapy after benzodiazepines. G Mastroianni et al. [285] reported that severe liver damage can reduce phenytoin clearance, leading to an increased risk of toxic plasma concentrations. However, there are no specific dosage adjustments recommended for patients with mild to severe hepatic disease. Caution should be exercised when using phenytoin in these patients, with frequent monitoring of serum levels advised to mitigate the risk of toxicity. Additionally, phenytoin should be used cautiously in patients with hepatic failure due to its potential for toxicity. In patients with renal disease, it is recommended that lorazepam be administered during the prehospital and early in-hospital stages of status epilepticus and switch to phenytoin when status epilepticus is confirmed. Phenytoin is considered safe for use in individuals with kidney disease.

Status epilepticus during pregnancy poses a life-threatening medical emergency for both the mother and fetus. Managing status epilepticus during pregnancy is challenging due to pregnancy-related pharmacokinetic changes and fetal risks associated with antiepileptic and narcotic drugs. Currently, there is no standardized treatment protocol for status epilepticus during pregnancy, and existing evidence is primarily derived from case reports and small case series. The literature on status epilepticus during pregnancy suggests that benzodiazepines are the preferred first-line treatment, with levetiracetam and phenytoin being the most suitable second-line options [188].

In a single-blinded case–control study conducted by Mahmoud Mohammadi et al. [286], it was observed that phenytoin and levetiracetam had efficacy rates of 83.3% and 86.7%, respectively, in treating neonatal epilepsy, with no statistically significant difference between the two groups. Adverse effects were comparable between the phenytoin and levetiracetam groups, indicating the safety and practicality of both drugs in managing neonatal epilepsy. Veronica Alix [287] conducted a retrospective observational cohort study comparing the acute and long-term efficacy of fosphenytoin and phenobarbital as first-line ASMs for neonatal epilepsy. Although there were no differences in acute outcomes between the two groups, significantly fewer infants in the fosphenytoin group exhibited moderate to severe neurodevelopmental delays at the 18- and 24-month assessments. This suggests that fosphenytoin may have the potential to significantly enhance neurodevelopmental outcomes in neonates aged 18–24 months compared to phenobarbital. In a systematic review by Rui Shi et al. [288], which assessed the effectiveness and safety of levetiracetam and phenytoin as second-line drugs for treating convulsive status epilepticus in children through meta-analysis, levetiracetam was found to be more effective than phenytoin in treating convulsive status epilepticus, with no increase in incidence of adverse reactions. This highlights levetiracetam as a favorable option for managing convulsive status epilepticus in children due to its efficacy and safety profile compared to those of phenytoin.

The Efficacy and Safety of Phenytoin Sodium as the First Choice for the Treatment of Epilepsy

I Guidotti et al. [289] conducted a comprehensive literature review spanning 40 years from 1983 to 2022, focusing on studies describing human regeneration through multichannel video electroencephalography in the treatment of pediatric patients with epileptic seizures. One study compared phenobarbital and phenytoin as first- and second-line treatments and reported that both controlled less than 50% of neonatal seizures. Although phenytoin, or its prodrug fosphenytoin, has been traditionally utilized as a first- or second-line ASM for neonatal seizures due to its effects on voltage-dependent sodium channels, published data do not clearly establish its superiority over phenobarbital. Although phenytoin or its precursor fosphenytoin, which acts on voltage-dependent sodium channels, has traditionally been used as a first- or second-line antiepileptic for neonatal seizures, published data have not definitively confirmed its superiority over phenobarbital. However, phenytoin use poses several risks, including the potential for arrhythmias and hypotension, a narrow therapeutic range due to its nonlinear pharmacokinetics, a short half-life necessitating plasma level monitoring, poor intestinal bioavailability, and interactions with various antibiotics and other epilepsy medications, rendering it potentially unsafe.

J Dell'Aquila et al. [290] reviewed multiple clinical studies comparing the effectiveness of phenytoin and levetiracetam in suppressing seizure activity. Although phenytoin has been a historical mainstay in epilepsy treatment and a second-line option for status epilepticus, its use has declined due to significant side effects, including sedation, hirsutism, gingival hyperplasia, and various other adverse effects. Intravenous phenytoin administration is associated with additional complications, such as hypotension, cardiac arrhythmias, and skin necrosis. Moreover, its narrow therapeutic index and complex pharmacokinetics necessitate careful dose monitoring to prevent toxicity and minimize drug interactions. In contrast, levetiracetam, a second-generation ASM, offers advantages such as fewer adverse reactions, a reduced need for dose monitoring, fewer drug interactions, faster attainment of therapeutic levels, and a wider therapeutic index. Although there was no significant difference in the efficacy of phenytoin or levetiracetam for treating status epilepticus, the incidence of adverse effects of levetiracetam was significantly lower than that of phenytoin.

X Huo et al. [291] explored the efficacy of various antiepileptic medications in preventing early and late posttraumatic epilepsy. Their analysis included 7 randomized controlled trials and 18 nonrandomized controlled trials encompassing six interventions: phenytoin + phenobarbital, levetiracetam, phenytoin, a phenytoin-levetiracetam combination, lacosamide, and valproate. The results indicated that all interventions, except sodium valproate, significantly reduced the incidence of early posttraumatic epilepsy compared to that in the placebo group in patients with traumatic brain injury. Additionally, four treatments (phenytoin + phenobarbital, levetiracetam, phenytoin, and sodium valproate) significantly decreased the occurrence of late seizures in these patients. Phenytoin did not affect mortality rates; however, it was associated with a greater incidence of treatment-related adverse effects than was the placebo.

K Panda P et al. [292] conducted a systematic review of the relevant literature to compare the effectiveness and safety of phenytoin and lacosamide in controlling seizures and improving short-term/long-term function in patients with status epilepticus. Their findings indicated that both drugs demonstrated comparable efficacy, while phenytoin exhibited a greater incidence of serious side effects. Consequently, it can be inferred that lacosamide may serve as a suitable alternative to phenytoin in status epilepticus, offering similar effectiveness with improved tolerability.

Evidence-Based Medical Research on Phenytoin Sodium

Robin Ferner et al. [293] conducted a systematic review to identify the clinical and radiological characteristics and associations of phenytoin's effects on the cerebellum. They analyzed 92 patients, 81 of whom exhibited one or more clinical symptoms, such as ataxia (96%), dysarthria (63%), and nystagmus (70%). Radiological assessment revealed cerebellar atrophy in 41 of 61 patients (67%). Their findings suggested that most patients with cerebellar dysfunction had phenytoin concentrations exceeding the reference range. Moreover, clinical signs of ataxia can persist even in the absence of radiographic evidence of cerebellar atrophy, and cerebellar atrophy can occur without any clinical evidence of cerebellar dysfunction. Clinical evidence indicates that phenytoin can induce the metabolism of voriconazole, potentially leading to reduced efficacy. The coadministration of voriconazole with phenytoin necessitates doubling the voriconazole dose to maintain therapeutic levels. Voriconazole can elevate phenytoin levels, resulting in increased C_{max} and AUC values of approximately 70% and 80%, respectively. These findings underscore the importance of cautious use of voriconazole in patients undergoing phenytoin treatment for epilepsy [294].

Effects of Phenytoin Sodium on Brain Electricity and Cognitive Function

Cognitive changes associated with ASMs treatment in children with epilepsy were thoroughly investigated by Besag FMC et al. [78] through a comprehensive PubMed literature review. Cognitive impairment is a common occurrence in patients with epilepsy, and ASMs may contribute to or exacerbate this condition. Conversely, some ASMs may have positive effects on cognition. However, reliable data on cognitive deficits in pediatric patients are scarce for most ASMs, including phenytoin. Despite its extensive history of use, the cognitive effects of phenytoin in pediatric patients have not been extensively studied. In a randomized comparison involving 64 children undergoing regular cognitive assessments, phenytoin and 2-propylvalerate were not associated with adverse cognitive effects. However, phenytoin was observed to induce greater motor and mental task impairment than CBZ, with these effects persisting even after discontinuation of the drug. Although there is a surprising lack of pediatric studies on the cognitive effects of phenytoin, the available evidence suggests that it may impair neurocognitive function. To address this gap, future studies evaluating ASMs in young adults should incorporate standardized measures of cognition and behavior.

Other Research

A retrospective analysis by A Muñoz-Vendrell et al. [295] examined 121 patients with acute exacerbation of trigeminal neuralgia admitted to a tertiary hospital's emergency department from 2012 to 2020. These patients received intravenous phenytoin or lacosamide for the first time, and the efficacy and safety of intravenous lacosamide and phenytoin for treating acute trigeminal neuralgia were evaluated. Among the 81 patients who received phenytoin injections, 72.8% experienced pain relief, with 12.3% experiencing mild adverse reactions. Specifically, adverse reactions included dizziness, nausea, hypotension, infusion pain, skin rash, abnormal sensation, and pruritus, with some patients experiencing multiple symptoms simultaneously. The study concluded that intravenous lacosamide and phenytoin administration are effective and safe treatments for acute trigeminal neuralgia.

M Karaźniewicz-Łada et al. [116] reviewed recent data on ASMs and their interactions with other medications, nutrients, and food. Phenytoin was found to reduce the levels of various medications, including calcium channel blockers, digoxin, quinidine, hormonal contraceptives, proton pump inhibitors, ibrutinib, nilotinib, sirolimus, and several statins. During the SARS-CoV-2 pandemic, concerns arose regarding the interaction of phenytoin with antiretroviral drugs used to treat COVID-19. Combining phenytoin with lopinavir/ritonavir led to a 30% reduction in antiretroviral drug levels. Consequently, patients with COVID-19 and epilepsy may require a 50% increase in the dose of lopinavir/ritonavir to maintain therapeutic levels.

2.1.1.8 Nitrazepam

Drug Characteristics

[Chemical name] 5-Phenyl-7-nitro-1,3-dihydro-2H-1,4-benzodiazepine-2-one

[Chemical structure]

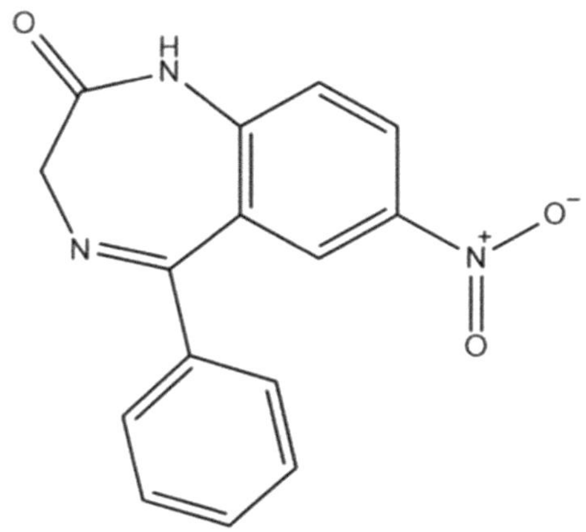

[Molecular formula] C15H11N3O3

[Molecular weight] 281.27

[Indications] (1) Treatment of insomnia and convulsions; (2) Second-line adjuvant drug for various types of epilepsy and adjuvant treatment for different types of refractory epilepsy; mainly used for petit mal seizures, especially myoclonic seizures and infantile spasms.

[Specifications] 5 mg 10 mg

[Dosage] 15–30 mg/day

The dosage varies depending on the ailment being addressed. When treating insomnia, the recommended dosage is 5–10 mg to be taken orally before bedtime. For individuals with severe insomnia, especially among psychiatric patients, an effective therapeutic dosage is 20 mg to be taken orally before sleep. However, adverse reactions and side effects, including severe hangovers, may manifest at this dosage, thereby limiting its application. Regarding convulsions, the recommended dosage for adults ranges from 10 to 20 mg, while for children, it ranges from 5 to 10 mg, depending on the cause, whether it is fever-induced or due to poisoning. For epilepsy, the recommended dosage is 5–10 mg (1–2 tablets) taken three times daily. Children are typically administered a daily dosage of 0.5–3.5 mg/kg, with an average of 1.5 mg/kg, divided into two doses per day. The maintenance dose is usually 5–10 mg/day. For muscle spasms, the recommended dosage is 2–15 mg/day to be taken orally in divided doses. In cases of severe spasticity, such as cerebral palsy, the dosage may be increased to 60 mg/day for adults and 40 mg/day for children. Patients with low tolerance to this medication should begin with a small initial dose to mitigate the risk of addiction from prolonged heavy use. After prolonged administration, it is advisable to gradually taper the dosage to prevent withdrawal symptoms. Abrupt cessation should be avoided, particularly for epilepsy patients, as it may precipitate status epilepticus.

[Adverse reactions] The most common adverse reactions to this product are drowsiness, sedation, muscle weakness, ataxia, disorientation and behavioral disorders. These adverse reactions are caused by the suppression of the central nervous system and can be gradually tolerated and alleviated with continued treatment. Less common adverse reactions include headache, dizziness, confusion, depression, slurred speech or dysarthria, changes in libido, tremor, visual disturbances, acral paresthesia, urinary retention or incontinence, gastrointestinal disorders, decreased appetite, decreased salivary secretion, excessive bronchial secretions, decreased calculation ability, and memory impairment. Rash, liver damage, and bone marrow suppression are occasionally observed. After taking the drug, patients may experience nightmares, hangover reactions, hostility, aggressive behavior and behavioral disinhibition. High-dose parenteral administration may occasionally cause respiratory depression and hypotension. Patients with chronic obstructive bronchitis may experience aggravated respiratory failure symptoms when using this drug. There have been reports of dysphagia, aspiration pneumonia, and death in infants and children after using this product. The side effects of this product are almost always dose-dependent and disappear with a temporary dose reduction or discontinuation of treatment. The main side effects of long-term use are tolerance and dependence. Stopping use of the drug may produce mild but obvious withdrawal symptoms, and a series of disease syndromes may also occur. Therefore, the dosage should be adjusted slowly during use and formulated according to the patient's response. An individualized medication regimen is needed.

Clinical Application and Basic Research

Historical Evolution of Nitrazepam

Nitrazepam is a benzodiazepine drug that was first described as a hypnotic drug in 1969. In 1975, it was reported that nitrazepam could be used as a treatment for children with infantile spasms and myoclonic quiescent seizures [296]. In 1977, L Kangas et al. reported that the half-life of nitrazepam in plasma ranged from 16.5 to 48.3 h (mean 28.8 h) [297]. In 1981, A B Khrana et al. discovered that nitrazepam can treat mood disorders in children [298]. In 1998, Ebata et al. reported that nitrazepam could reduce the frequency of nocturnal scratching in adults with atopic dermatitis [299]. In 2022, nitrazepam was recognized as a safe and viable alternative treatment option for children with drug-resistant West syndrome [300]. Recently, nitrazepam has obtained approval from the Central Drug Standards Organization in India for the treatment of epilepsy. However, it has not received approval from the US Food and Drug Administration (FDA) for marketing in the United States due to the presence of small quantities excreted into breast milk.

An Observational Study of Nitrazepam in the Treatment of Epilepsy

Zhongshu et al. conducted a study focusing on phenylketonuria (PKU) and its association with West syndrome (WS-PKU) to explore the incidence and clinical characteristics of WS-PKU, as well as the significance of early combined therapy involving a hypophenylalanine (PHE) diet alongside use of ASMs. Their findings revealed that the onset of spasms began to diminish upon initiation of the diet, but recurrences were frequent (78%) in the absence of ASMs [301]. However, the recurrence rate of seizures significantly decreased to 18.2% when valproic acid or nitrazepam was administered concurrently with the diet. Another extensive retrospective study conducted by Kaushik et al. examined children with West syndrome. This study utilized a retrospective chart analysis of children who were diagnosed with West syndrome between January 2008 and January 2012 and whose clinical profiles and treatment outcomes were documented at a tertiary care center in northern India. Among the 148 children included (120 boys), the mean (SD) ages at onset and onset of spasms were 5.3 (4.6) months and 13.1 (7.3) months, respectively. Perinatal asphyxia (61.4%), neonatal sepsis/meningitis (10.6%), and postnatal meningitis (11.4%) were identified as the primary causes, while the cause remained undetermined in 16.6% of the patients. The rate of cessation of spasms among 45 children (30.4%) treated with prednisolone was 25.4%. The final outcome was not influenced by factors such as age at onset, sex, treatment delay, the presence of perinatal asphyxia, or comorbid cerebral palsy [302].

Nitrazepam Is Added for the Treatment of Refractory Epilepsy

Beran suggested that stress can act as a catalyst for seizures, and benzodiazepines offer a dual advantage by alleviating anxiety and elevating the seizure threshold in individuals with epilepsy. Many patients attributed their seizures to stress without realizing the connection until after the event. To validate this correlation and enable preemptive measures, meticulous diaries must be maintained and reviewed. Intermittent use of benzodiazepines, such as clobazam, clonazepam, diazepam, or nitrazepam, can effectively prevent subsequent seizures and should be continued for a period even after the risk diminishes [303].

Nitrazepam for the Treatment of Epilepsy Syndrome

Iyer et al. conducted an overview of emerging treatment strategies for infantile spasms, particularly in the context of West syndrome, a prevalent epileptic encephalopathy. Early identification and intervention can enhance neurodevelopmental outcomes in some cases. Currently, corticosteroids, adrenocorticotropic hormone (ACTH), or prednisolone, in combination with vigabatrin, are the preferred initial treatment options. Combining steroids with vigabatrin may offer greater efficacy in suppressing spasms and normalizing EEG patterns. Additional ASMs, such as levetiracetam, nitrazepam, valproate, topiramate, and zonisamide, are commonly used as adjunctive therapies in refractory patients who are resistant to initial treatment or who are experiencing spasm recurrence. Nitrazepam, a benzodiazepine anticonvulsant, is rarely used in epilepsy treatment compared to clobazam and clonazepam. Its primary application is managing infantile spasms, with reported efficacy rates of up to 35% in observational studies. The typical starting dose is 0.2 mg/kg/day and gradually increases to 1–1.5 mg/kg/day. However, adverse effects such as excessive drooling, sedation, and hypotonia may restrict its use to a few weeks or months. Alternative medications for refractory patients include sodium valproate, topiramate, and zonisamide [304]. Hosain et al. described positive outcomes in 14 patients with drug-resistant Lennox–Gastaut syndrome, suggesting that nitrazepam serves as an effective adjunctive ASMs for managing mixed seizures in refractory patients. Unlike other benzodiazepines, its efficacy and tolerability remain consistent over time, making it a preferred option for patients with Lennox–Gastaut syndrome [305]. Tan Wang et al. similarly noted that nitrazepam offers a safe and viable treatment approach for children with tolerable West syndrome, resulting in sustained relief from spasms and electroclinical response improvement in nearly half of the patients.

Nitrazepam in the Treatment of Refractory and Super Refractory Status Epilepticus

Kagitani-Shimono et al. investigated the trajectory of epilepsy, seizure manifestations, and effective pharmacotherapy in patients with Wolf-Hirschhorn syndrome through an examination of 11 patients (ranging from 2 to 25 years old, with a mean age of 7.2 years). This syndrome is commonly associated with intractable seizures and episodes of status epilepticus. Febrile or afebrile seizures were prevalent among all patients, encompassing alternating hemiplegic seizures, generalized tonic–clonic seizures, focal clonic seizures, tonic–clonic seizures, and epileptic spasms. The authors noted a gradual reduction in seizure frequency and seizure burden in most individuals with Wolf-Hirschhorn syndrome after the age of 5. However, during infancy, status epilepticus can lead to irreversible impairment or even mortality. Sodium bromide is recommended as an initial therapeutic option to prevent the onset of status epilepticus linked to Wolf–Hirschhorn syndrome [306].

The Use of Nitrazepam in Special Populations with Epilepsy

Shields et al. documented a case involving a 6-month-old with asthma who developed spasticity and prominent arrhythmias on EEG shortly after commencing oral theophylline therapy. Theophylline levels were slightly elevated at that time. Upon discontinuation of theophylline and initiation of nitrazepam therapy, spasticity ceased, and the EEG returned to baseline. Nitrazepam was tapered by 10 months of age, and EEG during wakefulness and sleep normalized by 14 months of age. Over the subsequent 3 years of follow-up, no seizure recurrence occurred, and the child's neurodevelopment remained unaffected. The authors attributed the infant's spasticity to theophylline toxicity, emphasizing the potential severity of seizures, particularly of the generalized tonic–clonic type, as a consequence of theophylline overdose. Given the prognostic implications of delayed treatment for infantile spasms and heightened arrhythmias, the authors advocate for prompt initiation of nitrazepam therapy [307].

The Efficacy and Safety of Nitrazepam in the Treatment of Epilepsy

Zahan et al. assessed the efficacy, tolerability, and safety of oral nitrazepam in 41 children with drug-resistant West syndrome (WS) who underwent nitrazepam therapy. Nitrazepam has emerged as a safe and viable treatment modality for children with refractory WS, leading to the cessation of spasms and improvements in electroclinical responses in nearly half of the patients [300]. Dreifuss et al. conducted a multicenter randomized controlled trial to compare the effectiveness and safety of nitrazepam and adrenocorticotropic hormone in treating infantile spasms. The study enrolled 52 patients in a 4-week, randomized, multicenter trial, with 48 patients under 2 years of age undergoing assessment for drug efficacy. The research revealed a statistically significant reduction in spasm frequency with both treatments compared to baseline, although there was no significant difference between the two treatments. The incidence of side effects was similar in both groups, but adverse effects were more severe in patients treated with adrenocorticotropic hormone, leading to treatment discontinuation in six patients. The authors noted that the study duration was insufficient to assess the long-term impact of either treatment on the developmental status of patients [308].

Evidence-Based Medical Research on Nitrazepam

Song et al. conducted a systematic review of the literature from the past decade to outline current treatments for infantile spasms. Their findings indicate that topiramate, levetiracetam, zonisamide, and sodium valproate, along with benzodiazepines such as clonazepam or nitrazepam, show promise in treating West syndrome. Other effective treatments include adrenocorticotropic hormone, steroids, vigabatrin, and dietary interventions such as a ketogenic diet and a modified Atkins diet [309].

Effect of Nitrazepam on EEG and Cognitive Function

Saarelainen et al. investigated the incidence of benzodiazepines and related drugs (BZDR) in patients with Alzheimer's disease (AD) compared to non-AD patients over a 5-year follow-up period. They found that BZDR use was greater in AD patients than in control patients, peaking at 6 months after diagnosis and remaining significantly elevated up to 3 years postdiagnosis. BZDRs are associated with impaired cognitive function, which may complicate monitoring of treatment effects in AD patients [310].

Effect of Nitrazepam Addition on Patient Quality of Life

Jan et al. investigated the anticonvulsant properties of nitrazepam in 31 children exhibiting various seizure patterns. Their findings suggest that nitrazepam is a relatively safe and efficacious medication for managing mild motor spasms, particularly infantile spasms, and may even be more beneficial than adrenocorticotropic hormone therapy in this specific epilepsy subtype. In older children, nitrazepam demonstrates utility primarily for myoclonic seizures; however, its effectiveness appears to be constrained in terms of both its scope and duration [311].

Side Effects of Nitrazepam

Kagota et al. assessed the direct vasodilatory effects of benzodiazepines (BZDs) and nonbenzodiazepines (non-BZDs). Zolpidem and tandospirone induced more than 80% relaxation at a concentration of 10 μM, while diazepam, etizolam, etizolam, and toxosone caused 60–70% relaxation. However, 18 other BZDs, including alprazolam, clonazepam, nitrazepam, and triazolam, along with zaleplon, exhibited less than 50% relaxation. Additionally, the decrease in blood pressure observed in patients taking BZDs or non-BZDs may be attributed in part to direct vasodilation [312]. Iqbal et al. conducted a population-based longitudinal case–control study to explore the association between benzodiazepine use and cancer risk in individuals over 20 years old. BZDs are categorized into safe and unsafe groups based on their carcinogenicity. Among the BZDs examined, diazepam, chlordiazepoxide, mezepam, nitrazepam, and oxazepam were deemed safer. However, clonazepam was associated with a greater risk of cancer. In addition, the risk of specific cancers associated with BZD use was significantly increased by 98% in the brain, 25% in colorectal cancer, and 10% in the lungs compared to non-BZD use. Diazepam, chlorodiazole epoxide, medazepam, nitrazepam, and oxazepam are safe for the treatment of cancer [313]. Dennis et al. conducted a case record study involving 90 children with tuberous sclerosis complexes. Among the 86 children with seizures, there was a significant association between walking impairment at 5 years of age and early seizures along with nitrazepam treatment. Significantly more children who were unable to walk were taking nitrazepam, indicating potential adverse effects on motor and cognitive development in disabled children [314]. Lim et al. utilized nitrazepam to manage drug-resistant myoclonic epilepsy in 38 children. The authors speculate that caution must be exercised when using nitrazepam and suggest that esophageal manometry may be beneficial in identifying patients at greater risk of sudden death. Oral motor dysfunction, particularly in the presence of significant neurological deficits, may increase the likelihood of severe nitrazepam side effects. The authors recommended conducting routine baseline esophageal manometry and titrating anticonvulsants before initiating pharmacological intervention to mitigate esophageal spasm and minimize respiratory complications associated with nitrazepam or other benzodiazepines [315].

Basic Research on Nitrazepam

Zhao et al. devised a novel animal model of epilepsy to investigate behavioral alterations, electrocorticogram (ECoG) patterns, and the effects of five classic anticonvulsant drugs. Among these drugs, phenobarbital (30 mg/kg) and nitrazepam (3 mg/kg) completely suppressed seizures, while CBZ showed moderate efficacy. Phenytoin and sodium valproate exhibited limited effectiveness. Despite complete seizure suppression with phenobarbital sodium and nitrazepam, no improvement in mortality within the first 48 h was observed compared to that in untreated rats. CBZ antagonized 60% of seizures, with the treated mice displaying improved mobility and feeding behavior and a seemingly longer lifespan than those in the other groups. Valproate failed to suppress seizures or reduce mortality. Additionally, another study revealed that 30 mg/kg phenytoin could counteract zinc-induced seizures in rabbits [316].

Other Studies

Liao et al. conducted an analysis examining the correlation between various types of hypnotics and the risk of chronic kidney disease (CKD) and end-stage renal disease (ESRD), aiming to elucidate the potential association between hypnotic drug usage and CKD risk, as well as the progression of CKD to ESRD, necessitating dialysis. Their study revealed that the use of sleeping pills was linked to an elevated risk of CKD after adjusting for underlying comorbidities. With the exception of hyperlipidemia, most comorbid conditions were associated with a heightened CKD risk. Furthermore, continuous use of hypnotic drugs following a CKD diagnosis heightened the risk of concurrent ESRD. Subgroup analysis focusing on sleeping pill use revealed significant associations with increased CKD risk for several hypnotic drugs, including brotizolam, chlordiazepoxide, clonazepam, diazepam, diimidazole, etizolam, fludiazepam, flunitrazepam, nitrazepam, trazodone, zolpidem, and zopiclone [317]. Kassie et al. compared the utilization of anxiolytics, sedatives, hypnotics, opioid analgesics, and antidepressants in hip or knee surgery patients without postoperative delirium. Their findings indicated that preoperative benzodiazepine reduction planning may mitigate postoperative psychosis risk. Medications with notable precipitating risks, such as antidepressants and nitrazepam, should be temporarily discontinued or substituted with safer alternatives in older surgical patients to minimize adverse outcomes [318].

2.1.2 *Second-Generation Antiseizure Drugs*

2.1.2.1 Lamotrigine

General Characteristics

[Chemical name] 3,5-Diamino-5,6-(2,3-dichlorophenyl)-1,2,4-triazine

[Structure formula]

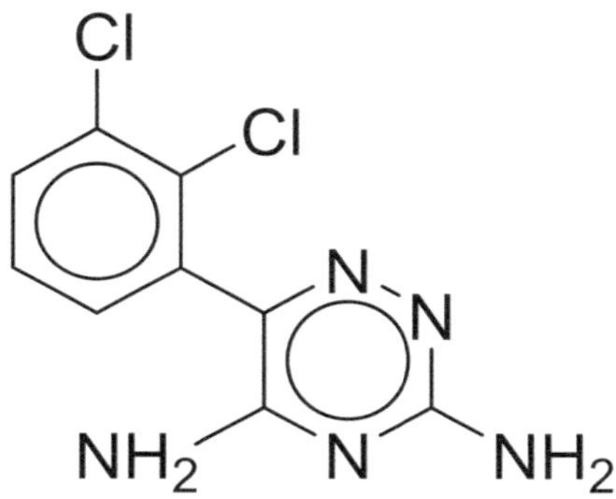

[Molecular formula] $C_9H_7N_5Cl_2$

[Molecular weight] 256.09

[Indications]

- Monotherapy for simple partial seizures, complex partial seizures, and primary and secondary generalized tonic–clonic seizures in children older than 12 years and adults.
- Adjunctive therapy for simple partial seizures, complex partial seizures, and primary and secondary generalized tonic–clonic seizures in children older than 2 years and adults.
- It is also indicated for the treatment of epileptic seizures associated with Lennox–Gastaut syndrome.

[Dosage form]
Film-coated tablets: 50 mg
Dispersible tablets: 5 mg, 50 mg

[Dosage and administration]
For monotherapy in patients over the age of 12, the initial dose is 25 mg once daily for 2 weeks or 12.5 mg twice daily for 2 weeks; then, the dose is increased to 50 mg once daily or 25 mg twice daily for another 2 weeks. After this period, the dose may be increased every 1–2 weeks by a maximum of 50–100 mg until the optimal therapeutic effect is achieved. The usual maintenance dose is 100–200 mg/day, administered either once daily or twice a day.

[Adverse effects]
Rash, Headache, Fatigue, Nausea, Vomiting, Dizziness, Lightheadedness, Drowsiness, Insomnia, Blurred or Double Vision, Irritability and Impulsive Behavior, Ataxia (Loss of Coordination), Anxiety. A minority of patients may experience leukopenia, anemia, thrombocytopenia or tremor.

Fundamental and Clinical Research

Historical Evolution

Lamotrigine (LTG) is a broad-spectrum antiseizure medication that was developed and synthesized in the UK in 1978 and came to market in 1990 for the adjunctive treatment of intractable epilepsy. In 1994, it was approved for the adjunctive treatment of partial seizures in adults, and in 2003, the FDA approved it for monotherapy of partial-onset seizures in patients aged 16 and older, as well as for adjunctive therapy in children aged 2 years and older with focal seizures. That same year, it was also approved for treating acute manic episodes and for the maintenance treatment of bipolar disorder in adults. Its current indications are as monotherapy for simple and complex partial seizures, primary and secondary generalized tonic–clonic seizures in children older than 12 years and adults, and as adjunctive therapy for partial seizures and primary generalized tonic–clonic seizures in children older than 2 years and adults. It is also suitable for treating seizures associated with Lennox–Gastaut syndrome. Lamotrigine acts mainly as a sodium channel blocker and has some effect on calcium channels (N, P-type). Clinically, it is also used to treat generalized absence seizures, infantile spasms, and other seizure types.

Management of Different Seizure Types

The International League Against Epilepsy's Commission on Epilepsy and Gender in their latest techniques and guidelines for clinicians states that after careful consideration of the teratogenic effects and impact of sodium valproate on women of childbearing age during pregnancy, the working group considers lamotrigine and levetiracetam to be the drugs of choice for primary generalized tonic–clonic seizures and juvenile myoclonic epilepsy in women of childbearing age, with lamotrigine being the preferred medication for juvenile absence epilepsy. Another guideline focused on the relationship between patient compliance and antiseizure medication (ASM) intake, seizure control, and potential toxicity. Long half-life immediate-release (IR) medications and extended-release (ER) formulations (such as lamotrigine [IR, ER]) that allow for once-daily dosing have many advantages over short half-life drugs that require multiple daily doses. These advantages include simplified dosing regimens, reduced medication burden, and less fluctuation in serum concentrations, which may decrease the risk of adverse reactions and seizures.

A recent randomized, open-label, controlled trial compared the effectiveness of levetiracetam and zonisamide with that of lamotrigine as a first-line treatment for newly diagnosed focal epilepsy patients. The initial recommended maintenance doses for participants aged 12 and above were 50 mg (morning) and 100 mg (evening) of lamotrigine, 500 mg of levetiracetam twice daily, and 100 mg of zonisamide twice daily. For children aged 5–12 years, the recommended initial daily maintenance dose was 1.5 mg/kg lamotrigine twice daily, 20 mg/kg levetiracetam twice daily, and 2.5 mg/kg zonisamide twice daily. A total of 990 participants were recruited over 4 years and were followed up for another 2 years. Patients were randomly assigned to receive lamotrigine (n = 330), levetiracetam (n = 332), or zonisamide (n = 328). The results suggest that lamotrigine is more cost-effective and has greater net health benefits. It should remain a first-line treatment for patients with focal epilepsy and should be the standard treatment in future trials [319].

Lamotrigine is widely used to treat epilepsy. Chinese scholars [147] assessed the national trend of ASM prescriptions for adult epilepsy outpatients in China over 6 years from 2013 to 2018. Among 225,767 prescriptions available for analysis, the three most common combination therapy schemes observed were lamotrigine/valproate, levetiracetam/oxcarbazepine, and valproate/levetiracetam.

Medication in Special Populations

Clavenna A. and colleagues [148] described the prescription patterns of ASMs among pregnant women and women of childbearing age in the Lombardy region of Italy from 2010 to 2019. The results showed that the proportion of women of childbearing age taking valproic acid (VPA) decreased from 30.2% in 2010 to 20.0% in 2019; over the decade, the proportion of pregnant women using VPA also decreased from 24.9% to 14.1%. Starting in 2017, lamotrigine and levetiracetam became the most frequently used drugs among pregnant women.

Spoendlin J. and others [186] studied the usage of ASMs in Switzerland during pregnancy and among women of childbearing age from 2014 to 2018 and found lamotrigine to be the most commonly used ASM during pregnancy, followed by levetiracetam and pregabalin. Another study aimed at assessing pregnant women receiving polytherapy, particularly prenatal exposure to different combinations of ASMs, suggested that the combination of lamotrigine and levetiracetam could control seizures well without increasing the risk of fetal malformations [320].

Cohen JM et al. [321] also suggested that lamotrigine use does not increase the risk of major congenital malformations (MCMs), and Pekoz MT et al. [322] reached similar conclusions; meanwhile, Bromley R. and colleagues [103] speculated that lamotrigine might slightly increase the aforementioned risk.

Many scholars have focused on the fluctuations in the serum concentrations of lamotrigine during pregnancy and the exposure of newborns to lamotrigine during breastfeeding. Barry JM and others [323] assessed the potential impact of specific dosing regimens of lamotrigine on the increased risk of epilepsy or toxicity. Simulation studies revealed that metabolic changes in pregnant women could lead to blood concentrations that are either too low or too high, potentially increasing the risk of seizures or toxicity; hence, there is a need for individualized monitoring and management of lamotrigine dosing during pregnancy.

Freund B and associates [324] reported that the dose-normalized concentration (DNC) of lamotrigine significantly decreased during the first half of early pregnancy. However, the timing and frequency of drug serum concentration monitoring during pregnancy may not have a significant overall effect on seizure control, with preventive dose adjustments showing similar seizure control outcomes to those based on clinical or laboratory results.

Kacirova I et al. [325] analyzed the exposure of breastfeeding newborns to lamotrigine and reported relatively low drug concentrations in breast milk. However, the concentrations of lamotrigine in maternal serum and breast milk significantly increased after delivery, which could lead to newborn serum concentrations approaching general therapeutic levels for epilepsy, suggesting the need to monitor newborn serum levels for potential adverse events.

Pedersen S and collaborators [326] investigated changes in the serum concentrations of ASMs in children with drug-resistant epilepsy receiving ketogenic diet therapy. The results indicated that after 12 weeks of ketogenic diet therapy, the serum concentration of lamotrigine significantly decreased, potentially increasing the risk of seizures.

Another study focused on the impact of ASM use on bone metabolism in children with self-limited epilepsy with centrotemporal spikes (SeLECTS). Lamotrigine use improved the levels of several bone metabolism indicators in epilepsy patients [327]. In elderly patients, Assis T. and others [328] examined medication usage among hospitalized elderly epilepsy patients between 2009 and 2010 and between 2015 and 2019, during which lamotrigine prescriptions increased from 5.5% to 33.6%.

A randomized double-blinded trial in newly diagnosed epilepsy patients aged ≥65 years showed that lamotrigine was as effective as CBZ (with more than 60% of patients in both groups achieving seizure freedom), but lamotrigine was better tolerated [329].

Lamotrigine for Treating Symptomatic Epilepsy and Epilepsy Syndromes

Lamotrigine plays an important role in treating symptomatic epilepsy and various epilepsy syndromes. However, in comparative studies of juvenile myoclonic epilepsy (JME), sodium valproate and levetiracetam showed comparable effectiveness. Lamotrigine was associated with a greater failure rate in terms of epilepsy control, myoclonic seizures, and adverse drug reactions, suggesting that it is not a suitable sole treatment option for JME patients [330].

Larsson D. et al. [331] noted a lack of evidence guiding antiseizure medication selection for poststroke epilepsy patients. By analyzing Swedish registry data of acute adult stroke patients from July 2005 to December 2010 and individual data on seizures before 2015, they found that compared to CBZ, lamotrigine had the lowest risk for all-cause mortality (risk ratio 0.72, 95% CI 0.60–0.86) and cardiovascular mortality (risk ratio 0.76, 95% CI 0.61–0.95) among drugs such as LEV, VPA, PHT, and OXC. Another study showed that more than 60% of poststroke epilepsy patients were treated with levetiracetam, followed by CBZ, lamotrigine and sodium valproate [332].

Van Opijnen MP et al. [333] studied lamotrigine, a non-enzyme-inducing sodium channel blocker, assessing its effectiveness compared to that of lacosamide as a second-line treatment for epilepsy in patients with diffuse glioma. After a 1-year follow-up of 139 patients, no significant difference in the cumulative incidence of treatment failure or adjusted risk ratios was found between lamotrigine and lacosamide, indicating similar efficacy.

Mahamud Z. et al. [334] analyzed the treatment of 129 patients with multiple sclerosis who developed symptomatic epilepsy. Among drugs such as CBZ, LTG, LEV, VPA, and PHT, lamotrigine had the highest 1-year and 5-year retention rates and was the only antiseizure medication (ASM) showing a lower risk of discontinuation (HR 0.41, 95% CI 0.17, 0.99). Le Roux M. et al. [335] described 18 patients with new or hereditary CACNA1A mutations who presented with seizures, commonly induced by fever or manifesting as absence/motion arrest. ASMs, including lamotrigine, can halt seizures. Nevertheless, lamotrigine is not always the first choice for syndrome treatment. Milano C. et al. [336] examined 28 patients with juvenile myoclonic epilepsy (JME) who switched from VPA to LTG or LEV due to potential teratogenicity or adverse reactions and reported that LEV was significantly more effective than LTG for both myoclonic and generalized tonic–clonic seizures, with similar tolerabilities for both drugs.

Adverse Effects

Adverse reactions to aromatic ASMs have always been a focal point for physicians, especially since the early detection and of life-threatening serious adverse effects and intervention can greatly improve patient outcomes.

Chinese scholar Zhang N and others [337] compared two different titration schedules for lamotrigine (LTG)—once daily versus twice daily—in newly diagnosed epilepsy patients. They found no significant difference between the two groups in terms of the efficacy and safety of LTG. However, the retention rate of patients in the once-daily dosing group was significantly greater than that in the twice-daily dosing group.

Cutaneous Adverse Effects

Korean scholar Chung SJ et al. [338] used a nationwide health claims database to assess the incidence of serious cutaneous adverse reactions (SCARs) caused by seven commonly used antiseizure drugs and found that lamotrigine had an incidence rate of 3860/100,000 person-years. Fukasawa T. et al. [339] reported the first study in Japan to document the different risks of Stevens-Johnson syndrome (SJS)/toxic epidermal necrolysis (TEN) caused by ASMs in an observational setting, with the risk of SJS/TEN significantly increased in patients newly using CBZ (OR 68.00) and lamotrigine (OR 36.00). For the Asian population, several genetic loci associated with cutaneous adverse drug reactions (cADRs) have been thoroughly studied, including significant associations between HLA-A*24:02 and HLA-A*30:01 in the southern Han Chinese population and aromatic antiseizure drug-induced cADRs

[340]. HLAB*15:02, which increases susceptibility to SJS induced by lamotrigine and CBZ, has been found in Chinese and other Southeast Asian populations, and HLAB*31:01 in Japanese patients and HLA-B*44:03 in Koreans increases the risk of SJS when taking the aforementioned drugs [341]. Mortazavi H. et al. [342] reported that HLA-B*38 and HLA-DRB1*13 are significantly associated with lamotrigine-induced SJS/TEN in Iranian intensive care patients.

The occurrence of cADRs also involves cross-reactivity and many variations. A history of adverse skin reactions may affect the use of antiseizure drugs, with cross-reactivity being more common in severe cases, and most patients being affected by mild, self-limiting rashes [135]. Packard E. et al. [343] described a case of drug reaction with eosinophilia and systemic symptoms (DRESS) caused by cross-reactivity between lamotrigine and lacosamide. Considering age differences in patient populations, Shirzadi M. et al. [344] assessed 236 adults and 167 children during their first exposure to LTG, with seven children (4.2%) judged to have "skin reactions less likely caused by LTG hypersensitivity mechanisms" compared to 0.8% (two cases) in adults. Early rashes during LTG treatment are not always drug allergies, and other potential causes, especially in children, should be considered. Alfares I. et al. [345] conducted a systematic review and reported that females are more likely to develop cADRs due to ASM use (odds ratio (OR) 1.76, 95% confidence interval (CI) 1.55–1.99), with the largest difference occurring in those treated with lamotrigine (OR 2.17, 95% CI 1.53–3.08), and the pathophysiological mechanisms underlying this difference remain unclear.

Hematological Adverse Effects

Zhu X. and colleagues [346] described the case of a 15-year-old female epilepsy patient who developed asymptomatic leukopenia after combined treatment with lamotrigine (LTG) and valproic acid (VPA). In this patient, leukopenia was clearly related to increased LTG serum levels and was reversed after the discontinuation of VPA, highlighting the importance of therapeutic drug monitoring (TDM) because of the interaction between these two drugs. Wang C. and others [347] reviewed the occurrence of hemophagocytic lymphohistiocytosis (HLH) in patients using lamotrigine, with the main clinical features including fever, cytopenia, rash, and hyperferritinemia, and bone marrow showing increased numbers of hemophagocytes. Of the 17 patients, two died from severe adverse reactions.

Cardiovascular Adverse Effects

Lamotrigine has a potential risk of causing arrhythmias in patients with heart disease. In 2020, the FDA issued a warning about the risk of this medication prolonging the QRS interval, thereby increasing the risk of arrhythmias and sudden death in high-risk populations. European researchers used the novel PHARMACOM-EPI framework to evaluate the relationship between plasma concentrations of lamotrigine in elderly patients and the risk of death. The results showed that in patients with plasma concentrations within the toxic range, there was a significant increase in the risk of all-cause mortality and cardiovascular-related deaths [348]. However, Christensen J and others [349] conducted a 2-year study of patients newly treated with lamotrigine and reported that the use of lamotrigine did not increase the risk of heart conduction disorders or all-cause mortality in patients with conduction disorders and preexisting heart disease compared to patients with no prior history of heart disease. To date, there is no support from human or animal studies or postmarketing data for this conclusion [350, 351].

A study by Aboukaoud M and others [352] compared the risk of arrhythmias caused by lamotrigine in patients with epilepsy to that caused by other antiseizure drugs. The results indicated that lamotrigine use did not significantly increase the risk of cardiac arrest in patients with epilepsy compared to that of other drugs; however, in patients with psychiatric disorders, the use of lamotrigine might be associated with cardiac arrest, potentially related to the combined use of other medications, overdose, and suicide attempts.

Bunschoten JW and others [353] conducted a systematic review including 26 studies, nearly half of which concluded that there was no obvious increase in the risk of sudden unexpected death in epilepsy (SUDEP), and an additional four reports on sudden death also did not confirm an increased risk of death with lamotrigine use. Researchers speculate that mild prolongation of the PR interval and QT interval is more likely related to cardiac structure rather than to medication. Another study compared patients taking lamotrigine and other sodium channel-modulating antiseizure medications with a control group, showing that the use of lamotrigine or other NaM-ASMs was not significantly associated with an increased risk of SUDEP over a period of up to 16 years after hospital admission [354].

Miscellaneous

Kamitaki BK and others [182] analyzed 2.6 million adverse event reports submitted to the FDA's Adverse Event Reporting System (FAERS) database from July 2018 to March 2020 for drug-induced liver injury (DILI). A total of 2175 DILI cases were attributed to antiseizure medications (ASMs), with the reported odds ratio (ROR) for each individual ASM compared to all non-ASM reports calculated for DILI. Lamotrigine had an ROR of 2.06, higher than that of diazepam, levetiracetam, and clobazam. Scholars have also focused on the data on ocular-related adverse reactions to new antiseizure drugs in the FAERS database [355]. Oxcarbazepine use is mainly associated with several cornea-related side effects, levetiracetam tends to cause adverse reactions related to neuromuscular diseases, and lacosamide rarely causes any serious ocular adverse reactions. In contrast, topiramate and lamotrigine are more likely to cause serious ocular-related adverse reactions.

A study assessing gingival overgrowth in patients with epilepsy revealed that, in addition to that of phenytoin sodium, lamotrigine, oxcarbazepine, and phenobarbital use were also associated with an increased incidence of gingival overgrowth. The incidence rate of this effect following lamotrigine use is between that of oxcarbazepine and that of phenobarbital [265].

Chen Y and others [356] reported that in patients treated with LTG, blood ammonia levels were elevated and positively correlated with plasma LTG concentrations. This abnormal laboratory indicator may be related to factors such as concurrent use of sodium valproate, epileptic seizures, and increased neutrophil counts. Tran DH and others [357] described the case of a 27-year-old woman who developed a range of symptoms, including fever, rash, meningitis, and joint pain, after using lamotrigine. Laboratory tests revealed an immune system abnormality, and the patient was ultimately diagnosed with hemophagocytic lymphohistiocytosis (HLH). A 32-year-old African American male patient developed rapidly progressing drug-induced pneumonia during treatment for depression after taking 25 mg of lamotrigine. Despite the absence of other potential etiological signs, the onset of pneumonia had a clear temporal association with lamotrigine [358]. In addition to common adverse reactions, Ge J and others [359] described a rare side effect in which lamotrigine caused persistent erections in an 11-year-old boy. Previous studies have suggested that lamotrigine may improve sexual function in adult male patients.

Fundamental Research

Huang J. et al. [360] used cryogenic electron microscopy to reveal the structure of lamotrigine (LTG) in complex with a human Nav1.7 channel and showed that LTG blocks Nav channels through a dual-pocket mechanism, thereby providing a significant molecular basis for understanding the pharmacological mechanism of lamotrigine. Chmielewska N and others [361] investigated whether reduced responsiveness to lamotrigine is associated with the expression of sodium channel subunits and miRNAs. The results showed that in drug-resistant rats, miR-9a-5p was the only miRNA with its expression significantly downregulated, and bioinformatics analysis revealed that miR-9a-5p targets expressed in the hippocampus were most significantly associated with epilepsy and were involved in regulating pathways related to neurotrophic factors, inflammatory responses, cell proliferation, and apoptosis.

Faustmann, T. J. and colleagues [362] studied the effects of LTG on the pathophysiological processes of astrocyte and microglial inflammatory responses and showed that LTG reduces the viability of glial cells in a concentration-dependent manner but does not cause significant changes in microglial phenotype. Although LTG may convey neuroglial toxicity, it can reduce inflammatory activity and may have a positive effect on neuroinflammatory changes underlying the pathogenesis of epilepsy.

Regarding the interaction between lamotrigine and other drugs, Filiz AK et al. [363] proposed that a combination of lamotrigine with vitamin B12 could prevent behavioral deficits, hippocampal damage, and oxidative and proinflammatory states during the development of epilepsy. Their study revealed that this combination could reduce the total oxidative status (TOS), oxidative stress index (OSI), and IL-1β and TNF-α levels and increase the total antioxidant status (TAS) in the hippocampus and cerebral cortex of a PTZ-induced epilepsy model.

Another study evaluating the effects of anakinra, lamotrigine, and their combination on the mechanisms of temporal lobe epilepsy showed that the severity of seizures was significantly reduced, which may be related to a reduction in neuronal loss in the hippocampal CA1 area caused by these two drugs [364].

Łuszczki JJ and others [365] attempted to find effective drug combinations in a study of intractable epilepsy; they used a maximal electroshock-induced seizure (MES) model to validate the combination of three antiseizure drugs. The combination of "lamotrigine + phenobarbital + oxcarbazepine" had an additive anticonvulsant effect, which could be beneficial for further translation into clinical trials for patients with intractable epilepsy.

To explore the role of lamotrigine in status epilepticus (SE), Onishi K et al. [366] conducted experiments using a mouse model and found that lamotrigine could extend the latency period of SE, reduce mortality, decrease nitric oxide and malondialdehyde levels, and increase glutathione concentrations. The study also revealed that the antioxidant action of lamotrigine may not entirely depend on the NMDA-related pathway.

With increasing attention being given to prehospital emergency care and nonintravenous routes of administration, Abdelmonem R. et al. [367] aimed to use Spanlastics nanovesicular carriers as a drug carrier to deliver lamotrigine through the intranasal route for brain targeting to improve its solubility and therapeutic effect. This method revealed a high efficacy of brain targeting in a rat model and is promising as a prospective brain-targeted treatment for epilepsy. Mohsen AM and others [368] prepared a cubosomal dispersion of LTG and loaded it into a thermosensitive intranasal gel to enhance intranasal absorption and efficacy. This novel formulation increased the antiseizure effects of LTG through pathways such as those related to increasing GABA release and inhibiting calcium ions and GFAP activity.

Lamotrigine in Psychiatric Disorders

Lamotrigine is also a standard medication for the treatment of bipolar disorder and is often used as a mood stabilizer in psychiatric diseases [369]. Research by Vieta E. et al. [370] revealed that in women of childbearing age with type I bipolar disorder, lamotrigine delayed the onset of mood episodes and particularly delayed the intervention time for depressive episodes. Although it had no significant effect on manic episodes, lamotrigine showed good tolerance in this population. The long-term response to lithium is reduced in patients with bipolar disorder combined with epilepsy, emphasizing a preference for valproate salts and lamotrigine as first-line treatments [198]. Thompson SI et al. [371] described two veterans with war-related posttraumatic stress disorder (PTSD) who exhibited significant anger, aggression, and excitement; these symptoms were not controlled by selective serotonin reuptake inhibitors (SSRIs) but were eventually successfully managed with lamotrigine.

Cuomo A and others [372] summarized the literature and concluded that lamotrigine shows significant efficacy in preventing or delaying depressive episodes of bipolar disorder, with a standard dose of 200 mg/day and slow titration to ensure good tolerance and a lower risk of side effects. After the risk-benefit ratio is assessed, LTG can be used in patients who are pregnant or lactating or who have liver or kidney disease.

2.1.2.2 Levetiracetam

Drug Characteristics

[Chemical name] (S)-α-ethyl-2-oxo-1-pyrrolidine acetamide

[Chemical structure formula]

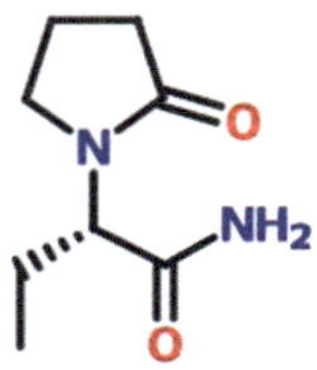

[Molecular formula] C8H14N2O2

[Molecular weight] 170.21

[Indications] For the treatment of partial seizures in adults and children over 4 years old.

[Packing specifications] Tablets: 250 mg, 500 mg, 1000 mg; oral liquid: 150 mL (15 g) per bottle; Injection: 5 mL (500 mg)

[Usage and dosage]
For adults (>18 years) and adolescents (12–17 years) weighing ≥50 kg: 500 mg/dose, twice daily. 500 mg/dose can be added every 2–4 weeks, twice daily; the maximum daily dose is 1500 mg, twice daily.

Children aged 4–11 years and adolescents weighing less than 50 kg (12–17 years): The initial therapeutic dose is 10 mg/kg twice daily. The dose can be increased by 10 mg/kg twice daily every 2 weeks. The maximum starting dose is 30 mg/kg twice daily. The maximum daily dose is 1500 mg twice daily. Patients with impaired renal function may adjust the dose according to creatinine clearance.

[Adverse reactions]
The common adverse reactions are drowsiness, fatigue and dizziness, irritability, emotional instability, hostility, aggressive behavior, dyspepsia, vertigo, double vision, tremor, etc.

Clinical Application and Preclinical Research

The Historical Evolution of Levetiracetam

Levetiracetam (LEV), a piracetam derivative, was originally approved by the FDA in 1999 for adults with partial seizures, and it was approved in oral tablets and solutions for the adjunctive treatment of partial seizures in children at least 4 years of age in 2005. It was released in China in 2007 (product name: Caplan). As a new antiseizure medication (ASM), LEV has a unique biochemical structure and a novel mechanism of action (blocking synaptic vesicles 2A to prevent the presynaptic release of neurotransmitters), and has a rapid effect, showing good antiseizure efficacy, tolerance and safety. In addition to adjuvant therapy for refractory epilepsy, its indications have gradually expanded to include monotherapy for newly diagnosed epilepsy. This product has the characteristics of high bioavailability, linear pharmacokinetics, low protein binding rate, low liver metabolism, rapid acquisition of stable blood drug concentration and few drug interactions, etc., which makes it a relatively safe drug for clinical application.

Application of Levetiracetam in Different Seizure Subtypes

Levetiracetam (LEV) was first approved for the additive treatment of focal seizures in adults and children over 4 years old. Studies have shown that it can also be used in adults with partial seizures and general seizures. It shows efficacy in children with absence epilepsy, juvenile myoclonic epilepsy (JME), refractory epilepsy, and status epilepticus (SE). In addition, LEV has the best efficacy across ASMs in Alzheimer's disease, Down syndrome, and PCDH19-associated epilepsy, although it may show a negligible effect in cortical developmental malformation [373].

A systematic review of two randomized controlled trials involving 574 newly diagnosed focal epilepsy patients treated with levetiracetam or oxcarbazepine monotherapy showed that the seizure free rate of LEV at week 24 was not lower than OXC, but the rate of adverse event (AE)-induced drug withdrawal in adults was also higher than that of OXC [374].

Lucia Gerstl et al. [375] systematically reviewed 19 clinical studies. The objective was to assess the rate of childhood epilepsy remission in children with benign epilepsy of childhood with centrotemporal spikes (BECTS) receiving ASMs. The results suggest that LEV results in a higher remission rate than CBZ, oxcarbazepine and topiramate in the treatment of BECT, and is recommended as a first-line treatment for BECT.

A review of the efficacy and tolerability of levetiracetam or valproate alone in 60 children with epilepsy (2–12 years old) showed that LEV monotherapy was equally effective and tolerated as VPA monotherapy for new idiopathic generalized tonic–clonic seizures in infants and children. Its efficacy was not related to age, EEG characteristics or epileptic syndrome [376].

A multicenter, randomized, double-blinded, placebo-controlled, phase III trial was designed to evaluate the efficacy and safety of levetiracetam as an additive treatment for focal epilepsy in children and adults (4–65 years old). It was performed in 114 patients receiving up to three ASMs treatments. The primary efficacy analysis was based on the proportion of patients with ≥50% reduction in the mean number of focal attacks per week over the 16-week treatment period. The results showed that levetiracetam was significantly more efficacious than placebo. Levetiracetam has been shown to be effective and safe in children and adults with refractory focal epilepsy [377].

Alejandro Ballve [378] observed 26 women of childbearing age (16–45 years) with idiopathic generalized epilepsy (IGE) including four cases of juvenile myoclonic epilepsy, eight cases of tonic–clonic seizures and four cases of adolescent absence epilepsy. The patients were first treated with levetiracetam as monotherapy and were followed for more than 24 months. Ultimately, the one-year retention rate was 78.1%, and the 5-year retention rate was 51%, suggesting that LEV is effective in treating idiopathic generalized epilepsy and can be used as a first-line treatment for IGE in women of childbearing age.

Regarding the treatment of epilepsy associated with brain tumors, a European study of neurooncologist medication questionnaires found that ASMs were most commonly used to treat glioma patients with epilepsy, followed by patients with brain metastases and meningiomas. 86% of the respondents started antiseizure medications in brain tumor patients at the first seizure, and levetiracetam was the most effective drug to reduce the frequency of seizures (72%) and showed fewer adverse effects than other ASMs. Meanwhile, the effective rates of other ASMs selected for the first time were lacosamide (33%), lamotrigine (22%), and valproic acid (21%) [379]. In a study comparing the effects of levetiracetam with those of enzyme-induced anticonvulsants in the treatment of glioma patients with epilepsy [380] that included 808 patients, LEV was significantly more effective than enzyme-induced anticonvulsants with fewer treatment failures due to any cause or adverse effects.

A meta-analysis [291] evaluated the effectiveness of ASM therapy in preventing seizures in patients with brain injury. A total of seven randomized controlled trials and 18 nonrandomized controlled trials were included. The results showed that both LEV and phenytoin sodium (PHT) prevented early and late posttraumatic seizures (PTS), and PHT also reduced the mortality of patients with traumatic brain injury (TBI). The treatment-related adverse effects of LEV and PHT were higher than those of placebo. However, LEV carries a slightly lower incidence of treatment-related adverse effects than PHT. Compared with PHT, LEV did not reduce the length of hospital stay, but it did shorten the length of ICU stay. Based on the results of the meta-analysis, it is speculated that LEV is the best treatment option for patients with TBI. However, further high-quality randomized controlled trials are required to confirm these findings. Regarding LEV dose, studies suggest that LEV (>1000 mg/day) may reduce the incidence of clinical and electroencephalitic seizures in patients with TBI [381].

Another randomized, double-blinded, placebo-controlled phase 3 clinical trial [382] investigating the safety and efficacy of levetiracetam in preventing seizures during acute cerebral hemorrhage showed that clinical or electrical seizures were observed in 3 of 19 patients (16%) in the levetiracetam group within the first 72 h. This was compared to an incidence of 10 of 23 patients (43%) in the placebo group.

It is suggested that levetiracetam is effective in preventing acute seizure caused by cerebral hemorrhage.

Application of Levetiracetam in Refractory Epilepsy and Epileptic Syndrome

LEV can be used to treat Dravet syndrome, epilepsy, and eyelid myoclonus. Expert consensus supports LEV as a common drug used in the treatment of Angelman syndrome [73]. An observational study randomly divided 102 patients with juvenile myoclonic epilepsy into a valproic acid group, a levetiracetam group and a lamotrigine group. The results indicated that levetiracetam had the same efficacy as valproate sodium, and was significantly more effective than lamotrigine in the control of seizures and myoclonic jerks, and had fewer adverse effects than valproic acid and lamotrigine. It is suggested that levetiracetam is a good substitute for valproate in JME patients, especially in women of childbearing age [330].

Pathogenic variants in the gene encoding the proline-rich transmembrane protein 2 (PRRT2) have been identified as the primary cause of self-limiting sporadic and familial infantile epilepsy. A multicenter, retrospective, cross-sectional cohort study [383] included 52 patients with infantile convulsions with a genetic diagnosis of a probable/pathogenic PRRT2 variant. Observation showed that in PRRT2-related infant epilepsy, sodium channel blockers CBZ and oxcarbazepine are associated with reduced seizure frequency, while levetiracetam has poor efficacy and low retention rate, and LEV is not recommended for this type of patient.

Familial adult myoclonic epilepsy (FAME) is a genetic disorder characterized by cortical tremors, myoclonus, and epilepsy. The current clinical treatment is mainly symptomatic treatment and is based on ASM use. LEV is the drug of choice, and other drugs used include valproate, benzodiazepines and perampanel; sodium channel blockers are prohibited [384].

In addition to treatment for refractory focal seizures in children, a systematic review and network meta-analysis [385] showed that lamotrigine and levetiracetam were more effective than other ASMs (gabapentin, Topamax, lacosamide, perampanel, oxcarbazepine, and eslicarbazepine). Levetiracetam is more likely to allow patients to be seizure-free.

However, during LEV treatment, there may be an increase in the frequency of seizures, an increase in the severity of seizures, or incidence of a new type of seizures, which is called an anomalous effect. Especially in patients with drug-resistant focal epilepsy, rhythmic epileptiform discharges upon electroencephalogram is an independent influencing factor for abnormal effects of LEV [386].

Wolf-Hirschhorn syndrome (WHS) is caused by the deletion of a region at the end of the short arm of chromosome 4 and is often associated with refractory epilepsy. The most effective ASM for WHS treatment is levetiracetam [387].

Syntaxin binding protein 1 (STXBP1) is located on chromosome 9q34.11 and encodes STXBP1. STXBP1-associated encephalopathy is a type of brain dysfunction caused by STXBP1 variants, which play an important role in the release of synaptic vesicles. Qiu-Hong Wang et al. [388] studied 40 patients with multicenter pathogenic STXBP1 mutation, whose clinical manifestations were Otahara syndrome, West syndrome, early-onset epileptic encephalopathies (EOEE), and epilepsy of infancy with migrating focal seizures (EIMF). The group systematically analyzed medical histories, video EEGs, imaging data, and antiseizure medication histories. After 6 months of LEV treatment (39.6 mg/kg/day), seizure frequency was reduced by 50% in 88.5% of patients, and seizure freedom was achieved in 53.8% of patients.

Application of Levetiracetam in the Treatment of Status Epilepticus

Phenytoin (PHT), phenobarbital (PB), and valproic acid are the second-line treatments for status epilepticus (SE) after first-line treatment with benzodiazepines fails. In recent years, more and more evidence has shown that the efficacy of levetiracetam as a second-line treatment for SE is comparable to that of classic drugs.

After LEV (2500 mg) was injected intravenously in 20 patients with early SE, LEV blood concentrations were 81.6 μg/mL at 15 min, and the median valley concentrations after 12, 48, and 96 h were 28.8, 10.5, and 9.1 μg/mL, respectively. About 95% of patients had valley concentrations higher than the lower limit of therapeutic plasma concentration (>12 μg/mL) after 12 h, and seizures were suppressed in 83% of patients and 92% of nonintubated patients at 15 min to 48 h, respectively. The elevated levels of aspartate aminotransferase (AST)/alanine aminotransferase (ALT) returned to normal in two patients without treatment, without affecting vital signs [389].

A meta-analysis of 11 studies (1933 patients) evaluated the efficacy and safety of levetiracetam and phenytoin in the treatment of patients with confirmed SE. LEV was significantly more effective than PHT in overall seizure cessation and conveyed fewer severe side effects than PHT, suggesting that LEV could replace phenytoin sodium as the drug of choice for benzodiazepine-resistant status epilepticus [390]. The efficacy of LEV as a second-line ASM in the treatment of convulsive SE in children is similar to that of PHT. However, the recurrence rate of seizures and the proportion of intubation and mechanical ventilation from 1 to 24 h in the PHT group were significantly higher than those in the LEV group [391].

In a retrospective, observational, cohort study, adult patients received at least one dose of undiluted LEV intravenously. Three thousand six hundred seventy-four patients (42.9%) received more than 1000 mg LEV and the maximum was 4500 mg, often administered through a peripheral vein (79.1%), and adverse effects were limited to local injection site reactions (such as redness, burning and loss of peripheral vein lines) [392].

A systematic review [393] that included five studies comparing intravenous levetiracetam with valproic acid and phenytoin in adult SE patients showed no statistically significant difference in efficacy or safety outcomes. There were more cases of hypotension and respiratory failure in phenytoin users and more cases of psychiatric side effects (such as postictal psychosis) in levetiracetam users.

Mehmet Tolga Kole et al. [394] conducted a retrospective study comparing intravenous LEV and PTH as second-line treatment for children aged 1–18 years with convulsive status epilepticus (CSE) and acute repetitive seizures (ARS). The results suggested that LEV is as effective as intravenous PTH and can be used as second-line treatment for CSE and ARS in children.

Application of Levetiracetam in Special Populations

The teratogenic rate of antiseizure medication therapy in pregnant women has always been concerning. A retrospective study from India involved the observation of 103 patients with active epilepsy taking levetiracetam during pregnancy, and the results showed no significant increase in the teratogenic rate, suggesting that levetiracetam monotherapy is a better drug for women with epilepsy of childbearing age than other options [395]. However, due to the decrease in ASM plasma concentration during pregnancy, scMS et al. [396] conducted a retrospective cohort study of 29 pregnant patients treated with LEV. The results showed that decreased LEV concentration was associated with increased seizure frequency in the nonepileptic remission group. It is recommended that LEV concentration should be controlled at higher than 65% of prepregnancy concentration for patients who are not in remission. For patients without seizures, LEV concentration is recommended to be controlled at 46% of the prepregnancy concentration.

By establishing a physiological pharmacokinetic (PBPK) model, scholar Jiarui Chen [397] predicted that the recommended dose of levetiracetam in the first trimester, second trimester and third trimester was 1.2, 1.6 and 1.5 times of the baseline dose, respectively, and should not exceed 4000 mg/day in the third trimester due to fetal safety considerations. An observational study [320] analyzed the effects of combined treatment with different antiseizure meidications on pregnancy outcomes in 110 pregnant women with epilepsy. The results showed that a combination of lamotrigine and levetiracetam helped control seizures and achieve fetal safety.

Phenobarbital has been the preferred treatment for epilepsy following full-term neonatal asphyxia for decades. A nonblinded, single-center, randomized, controlled and practical clinical study included 103 neonates with acute seizures, 29 (65.9%) of whom were in the levetiracetam group and 13 (34.2%) of whom were in the phenobarbital group with clinical seizures controlled. The difference between groups was statistically significant. Of the infants in the phenobarbital group who did not respond to the original drug, 57.8% showed seizure control after the addition of levetiracetam. It is suggested that levetiracetam may be used as the first and second line drug for asphyxiation epilepsy in full-term infants [398]. For acute symptomatic seizures caused by neonatal stroke, a systematic review found that the use of ASMs acting through the GABAergic mechanism was insufficient to control seizures secondary to stroke in full-term newborns. Lidocaine and levetiracetam appear to be very effective and have a clear safety profile in both the short and long term [399].

For patients with epilepsy complicated by liver and kidney function impairment, a study [400] based on a physiologic pharmacokinetic model (PBPK) predicted that the LEV dose should be reduced to 70%, 60%, and 45% in patients with mild, moderate, and severe kidney impairment, respectively. Drug concentrations of 95%, 80%, and 57% of the adult dose were administered to impaired populations with low, medium, and high cirrhosis mortality scores, respectively. Dose adjustment is not required for healthy elderly people, but corresponding dose reduction is required for elderly people with organ dysfunction, to a similar extent as that in adults.

A multicenter retrospective study compared seizure frequency and seizure-free rate in women with focal and generalized epilepsy treated with CBZ, lamotrigine, and levetiracetam monotherapy during the first 3 months of pregnancy, the entire pregnancy, and the postpartum period. A total of 57 patients with epilepsy (45 with focal epilepsy and 12 with generalized epilepsy) were enrolled on monotherapy (29 with CBZ, 11 with LTG, and 17 with LEV). The frequency of seizures in the first trimester of pregnancy was significantly lower than before pregnancy in all participants, and was more pronounced in patients with generalized epilepsy and in the LEV group. In patients overall and in the LEV group, there was a significant increase in seizure-free rates in the first trimester compared to the prepregnancy period, and this continued into the postpartum period. In addition, 88.57% of women without seizures remained seizure-free during pregnancy and postpartum. There was 1 case of major heart malformation in an infant of the CBZ group, while no major heart malformation was found in the LTG and LEV groups, suggesting that levetiracetam is effective and safe in treating gestational epilepsy [401].

Levetiracetam can also be used as a first-line treatment for neonatal epilepsy. A retrospective cohort study comparing the efficacy of levetiracetam to that of phenobarbital in the initial treatment of epileptic seizures showed that initial treatment of levetiracetam reached a seizure-free status more quickly than phenobarbital in neonatal epilepsy [402].

A randomized, double-blinded trial compared controlled-release CBZ, levetiracetam, and lamotrigine for the initial treatment of new localized epilepsy in elderly patients ≥60 years of age. The efficacy of the three drugs was similar, but the retention rate of LEV was significantly higher than that of controlled-release CBZ, similar to that of LTG [403]. Another randomized trial comparing the efficacy of LEV and that of controlled-release CBZ in elderly patients with new poststroke epilepsy showed no difference in the number of seizure-free patients, but a significant reduction in side effects caused by LEV was observed [404].

Safety and Adverse Effects of Levetiracetam

The common adverse reactions of levetiracetam are neuropsychiatric symptoms, hallucinations, delusions, aggressive behavior, and irritability. Some patients also showed suicidal and self-harming behavior. Other reported side effects include drowsiness, nausea, weight gain, and rashes. A case–control study [405] observed 120 adolescent epileptic patients treated with levetiracetam to analyze irritability and its relationship with psychosocial symptoms and quality of life. The results showed that self-reported and parent-reported levels of irritability were significantly higher in the levetiracetam group than in the control group. Irritability was positively correlated with behavior, emotion and attention/hyperactivity problems, and negatively correlated with psychosocial quality of life. In a large prospective registry study involving 38,661 fetuses of pregnant women with epilepsy, prenatal exposure to levetiracetam was associated with anxiety and attention deficit/hyperactivity disorder [406].

Rashes caused by antiseizure medications are another side effect concerning to clinicians. One study [407] compared the incidence of drug-related rash in 353 patients with glioma and 125 patients with meningioma who received LEV or lacosamide (LCM) treatment from 2017 to 2019. The results showed that the incidence of ASM-associated rash was higher in glioma patients (11%) than in meningioma patients (1.6%). Multifactor regression analysis showed that radiotherapy adjuvant therapy and drug allergy were significant risk factors for ASM-associated rash. Patients with both of these factors should be carefully checked for a rash.

The negative effects of ASMs on bone metabolism are also common side effects. A cross-sectional study [408] evaluated the effects of monotherapy on bone metabolism by measuring bone mineral density and biochemical markers 5 years after LEV administration. The results showed that no harmful effects on bone metabolism were observed in long-term LEV treatment, and no significant difference was observed between outcomes at 1 and 5 years, suggesting that LEV is relatively safe for patients with osteoporosis.

ASMs have long been studied for their side effects of inducing thyroid dysfunction. A systematic review and meta-analysis of 945 pediatric patients [238] evaluated the prevalence of thyroid disease in children under 16 years of age treated with valproate (VPA), CBZ, and levetiracetam (LEV) monotherapy. The overall prevalence of thyroid abnormalities was higher in children treated with ASM. In subgroup analysis, the prevalence of thyroid biochemical abnormalities with elevated TSH levels was higher in patients in the VPA and CBZ groups compared with those of the control group. This study suggests a higher prevalence of thyroid biochemical abnormalities in children treated with VPA and CBZ monotherapy, while there is no such evidence for LEV. It is suggested that LEV should be selected for children with thyroid predisposition if they meet the epileptic seizure type and epilepsy syndrome medication. In another meta-analysis [409] involving 4135 participants in 35 studies, eight antiseizure medications and thyroid hormone levels were analyzed, and LEV was associated with subclinical hypothyroidism. In terms of its impact on children's growth and development, LEV has the smallest impact on children's weight and appetite [80] of ASMs and can reduce children's blood phosphorus concentration [410].

For patients with poststroke epilepsy, a cohort study from Sweden used association registry data for all acute adult stroke patients in Sweden from 2005 to 2010, with 2577 patients receiving continuous ASM monotherapy enrolled in the study. Results showed that compared with CBZ, levetiracetam could reduce the risk of cardiovascular death in patients with epilepsy after stroke, but there was no significant difference in overall mortality between the two drugs [331]. A Danish registry study of 1345 patients aged 65 years and older with epilepsy with heart failure showed that VPA treatment was associated with higher all-cause mortality and heart failure mortality compared with LTG and LEV treatment [261]. Therefore, elderly patients with epilepsy should choose lamotrigine or levetiracetam as ASMs.

Neuropsychiatric side effects of levetiracetam should be monitored. Up to 13% of children taking LEV reported irritability, aggression, personality changes, emotional instability, anxiety, and depression [411]. Adel Mahmoud et al. [412] studied 105 children with epilepsy taking levetiracetam (as monotherapy or adjunctive therapy) who developed behavioral symptoms at the beginning of levetiracetam therapy. Patients were randomly and blindly treated to determine whether pyridoxine therapy could reverse or ameliorate behavioral side effects of levetiracetam in children 1–17 years of age with epilepsy. The results suggested that children who received a therapeutic dose of pyridoxine had a more significant improvement in neuropsychiatric symptoms than the control group.

A population-based matched case–control study in Catalonia, Spain, using data from primary health care electronic records, showed that levetiracetam monotherapy showed a higher risk of ischemic stroke, and further research is warranted due to the lack of data related to epilepsy diagnosis and severity of epilepsy in this study [413]. In a retrospective cohort study, LEV was not found to be associated with insufficient anticoagulation due to drug interactions, and no increased risk of ischemic stroke was found when combined with new oral anticoagulants [414].

In terms of the effects of LEV on the heart, studies [415] have observed the electrocardiogram parameters (PR interval, QTc, QT interval, and QRS duration) of levetiracetam before treatment and at the sixth month of treatment, and the results showed no significant changes, suggesting that levetiracetam had no effect on electrocardiogram parameters.

Preclinical Research

By binding to synaptic vesicles 2A and inhibiting L-type calcium channels, LEV inhibits neurotransmitter release and reduces neuronal overexcitation. There are also other molecular targets, including calcium homeostasis, the GABA energy system, and AMPA receptors. Kouji Niidome et al. [416] showed that LEV reduced the expression of FosL1 and the activity of AP-1 in activated microglia, thereby inhibiting neuroinflammation.

Acute brain inflammation following status epilepticus (SE) is involved in blood–brain barrier (BBB) dysfunction and brain edema, leading to the occurrence of symptomatic epilepsy after SE. Levetiracetam (LEV) inhibited the neutrophil and monocyte infiltration into the hippocampus, which may be involved in the suppression of brain inflammation and the incidence of spontaneous recurrent seizures induced by SE [417].

In lipopol ysaccharide-treated rats, levetiracetam increased TGFβ and IL-10 levels, decreased COX-2, NF-κB, TNF-α and IL-6 expression, and decreased BCL2 expression and malondialdehyde levels. LEV improved neuroinflammation-related memory impairment by enhancing cholinergic activity while reducing neuroinflammation, apoptosis, and oxidative stress [418].

Harun DEMIRC et al. [209] examined whether ASMs can contribute to axonal healing after traumatic brain injury. Levetiracetam (80 mg/kg, intraperitoneal injection) was given to a rat model with biparietal area brain injury, which can increase the expression of neuron-glial cell antigen 2 (NG2), suggesting that LEV can accelerate axonal healing.

Early administration of levetiracetam after injury in in vitro trauma sections and in in vivo controlled cortical impact (CCI) models may prevent or reduce the occurrence of posttraumatic epilepsy and suggest that the therapeutic window for successful preventive intervention may be narrow [419].

Other Effects of Levetiracetam besides the Antiseizure Effect

Levetiracetam improved cognition in Alzheimer's disease (AD) patients with epilepsy. KeithVossel et al. [420] conducted a phase 2a randomized double-blinded placebo-controlled crossover clinical trial on levetiracetam in 34 adults with AD, and the results showed that levetiracetam could improve spatial memory and executive function in patients with AD and epileptiform activities.

Nalini R et al. [421] showed that long-term treatment with levetiracetam resulted in a decrease in Aβ42 levels and amyloid plaque burden by normalizing presynaptic endocytoprotein levels and altering the tendency of amyloid precursor protein (APP) to cleave. It provides new evidence for the treatment of levetiracetam to alleviate the pathology of AD.

In rat models of AD, levetiracetam alleviates STZ-induced hippocampal cell death and memory impairment by reducing oxidative damage, inhibiting the expression of proinflammatory cytokines, and inhibiting abnormal hyperphosphorylation of tau [422].

A review evaluating the role of levetiracetam in the prevention of adult migraine patients showed a significant reduction in the frequency, severity, and duration of migraine, suggesting that levetiracetam appears to be effective in the treatment of migraine with or without aura, with fewer side effects [423].

Stress during adolescence is a major risk factor for schizophrenia. Stress in adolescents produces anxiety-like responses that impair social skills and cognitive function. Levetiracetam reduces stress-induced behavioral and electrophysiological changes in adolescents [424].

2.1.2.3 Topiramate

Characteristics of the Drug

[Name of chemical] 2,3,4,5-Dioxygen-(1-methyl-ethyl)-β-D-fructopyranose sulfonate

[Chemical structure formula]

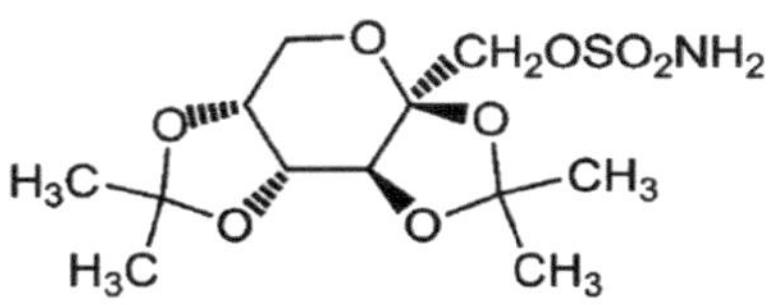

[Molecular formula] $C_{12}H_{21}NO_8S$

[Molecular weight] 339.362

[Indications for use] (1) Monotherapy in patients with newly diagnosed epilepsy or concomitant medication use switched to monotherapy; (2) Add-on therapy for partial seizures in adults and children aged 2–16 years.

[Specification] 25 mg, 100 mg

[Dosage] It is recommended that treatment be started at a low dose and gradually increased to an effective dose. A dose of 25–50 mg can be taken orally every night and increased by 25–50 mg/day at 1- or 2-week intervals. The dose should be adjusted according to clinical efficacy, usually 200–400 mg/day, twice daily.

[Adverse reactions] Ataxia, impaired attention, confusion, dizziness, fatigue, paresthesia, drowsiness, and abnormal thinking.

Clinical Application and Basic Research

Historical Evolution of Topiramate

Approved in the United States in 1996, topiramate (TPM) is a broad-spectrum antiseizure drug authorized for the single and adjuvant treatment of various types of epilepsy, including focal epilepsy, generalized tonic–clonic seizures, juvenile myoclonic epilepsy, epileptic encephalopathy (e.g., West syndrome, Dravet syndrome, and Lennox–Gastaut syndrome), and status epilepticus. In addition, following the in-depth study of the mechanism of epilepsy, the treatment scope of topiramate has also expanded to include other types of epileptic encephalopathy, developmental and epileptic encephalopathy (DEE) and KCNQ2 encephalopathy.

TPM exerts antiseizure effects through several mechanisms of action, including reducing epileptiform discharges through a voltage-dependent Na+ channel block, enhancement of γ-aminobutyrate activity at some subtypes of γ-aminobutyrate receptors, and antagonism of non-N-methyl-D-aspartate (NMDA) glutamate receptors [425].

Application of Topiramate for Different Seizure Types

The antiseizure effects of topiramate in multiple epilepsy subtypes have been widely demonstrated over the past 20 years. There is level 1 evidence that topiramate is effective as an adjunctive treatment for primary generalized tonic–clonic seizures, with a greater reduction in seizure frequency occurring in the topiramate group (56.7%) than in the placebo group (9%) in one study [426]. A systematic review and network meta-analysis of seven randomized controlled trials (1809 patients) comparing the relative efficacy of antiseizure drugs as monotherapy for generalized seizures showed that topiramate had a comparable seizure-free probability (44%) as valproate (38%) in the treatment of generalized tonic–clonic, tonic, and clonic seizures [427]. A Cochrane review of 12 RCTs (1650 participants) revealed that topiramate was almost three times more effective than placebo, reducing seizure frequency by more than 50% when used as an add-on treatment for drug-resistant focal epilepsy [428].

To evaluate the efficacy and tolerability of topiramate in juvenile myoclonic epilepsy (JME), Liu J et al. [429] reviewed three randomized controlled trials that investigated the effects of topiramate versus placebo or sodium valproate in patients with JME, comprising a total of 83 participants. In terms of efficacy, a greater proportion of participants in the topiramate group had a 50% or greater reduction in idiopathic generalized tonic–clonic seizures than did those in the placebo group. There was no significant difference between topiramate and valproate with regard to a 50% or greater reduction in myoclonic seizures versus idiopathic generalized tonic–clonic seizures and no seizures, but topiramate was better tolerated.

In addition, topiramate has good efficacy in treating epileptic encephalopathy. A systematic review of 14 studies conducted by Song JM to evaluate the efficacy of topiramate as a first-line or adjunctive treatment for West syndrome patients revealed that 17–40% of patients were seizure-free and 45–70% had at least a 50% reduction in seizure frequency after taking the drug [309]. In a clinical trial conducted by Knupp KG's team, topiramate treatment reduced seizure frequency by 50% in 35–78% of patients with Dravet syndrome and achieved short-term seizure freedom in 10–17% of patients with Dravet syndrome [430]. A network meta-analysis included a total of eight randomized controlled trials (1171 patients) comparing the efficacy of six antiseizure drugs in patients with LGS, and the results showed that topiramate had a relatively high probability of reducing fall attacks [431]. A retrospective study involving 13 patients showed that topiramate was also effective in the treatment of KCNQ2 encephalopathy [432].

Application of Topiramate in Refractory Epilepsy

Bresnahan R et al. reviewed 12 trials of topiramate as an add-on therapy, including a total of 1650 patients with drug-resistant focal epilepsy. These trials compared the effects of topiramate with those of a placebo drug for up to 18 weeks. The review revealed that topiramate was almost three times more effective than the placebo for reducing the number of drug-resistant focal seizures when used with other drugs. However, adding topiramate to patients' usual treatment increased adverse effects, such as ataxia, concentration difficulties, dizziness, fatigue, "thinking abnormally," paresthesia, and weight loss. Patients taking topiramate were also more than twice as likely to drop out of treatment as those taking placebo, most likely due to adverse effects [428].

A meta-analysis systematically evaluated the clinical effects of valproate alone or in combination with topiramate in the treatment of refractory epilepsy [433]. A total of 10 studies involving 976 patients with epilepsy were included in the analysis, and the results showed that the overall response rate to valproate combined with topiramate was greater than that to valproate alone (OR = 3.52; 95% CI 1.47–8.47). The frequencies of absence seizures, atonic seizures, and tonic–clonic seizures in the combination group were lower than those in the monotherapy group. In addition, there was no clear difference in adverse events between the two groups. Therefore, valproate combined with topiramate is more effective than valproate alone in the treatment of epilepsy.

Application of Topiramate in Refractory Status Epilepticus

To evaluate the efficacy and tolerability of topiramate in patients with refractory status epilepticus (RSE) and superrefractory status epilepticus (SRSE), Fechner A et al. [434] studied a total of 106 patients with a mean age of 67.4 ± 18.1 years. The median latency time from the onset of status epilepticus to the initiation of topiramate treatment was 8.5 days. The median initial topiramate dose was 100 mg/day, which was followed by escalation to a maintenance dose of 400 mg/day. Patients with SE had previously failed to achieve remission with a median of five other antiseizure drugs. Topiramate was the last drug used in 42 of 106 patients (39.6%), with a resultant response attributed to TPM observed in 29 of 106 (27.4%) patients. Topiramate was associated with a response in 21 of 66 RSE patients (31.8%) and 8 of 40 SRSE patients (20%). Topiramate-related adverse events occurred in two patients (pancreatitis and perchloric acid poisoning), and hyperammonemia occurred in 38 patients (35.8%). Based on these results, topiramate could be used to treat RSE and SRSE.

To provide evidence for the use of topiramate in refractory status epilepticus, a systematic review of nine studies of topiramate use in refractory status epilepticus patients using descriptive and qualitative analysis revealed that response rates, defined as the termination of hospitalization within 72 h after topiramate administration, ranged from 27% to 100%. Mortality rates ranged from 5.9% to 68%. Positive long-term functioning was observed in patients in seven of these studies with outcomes including rates of discharge, return to baseline, or recovery between 4% and 55%. Most studies reported no or only mild adverse effects. Thus, topiramate is effective in terminating refractory epilepsy states in patients, has a relatively low mortality rate and is well tolerated [435].

To develop an intravenous topiramate regimen for the treatment of refractory and ultrarefractory status epilepticus, two parenteral formulations of TPM have been developed. One solution is to use sulfobutylether-β-cyclodextrin (SBE-β-CD; Captisol®) as an excipient. A 1% TPM solution in 10% Captisol® was well tolerated in safety studies in healthy volunteers and patients with epilepsy or migraine. Another solution uses the FDA and EMA-approved excipients of the amino sugar meglumine. Meglumine was more effective than Captisol® in dissolving TPM in water. A 1% TPM solution was obtained with 0.5–1% meglumine [436].

Moreover, another team analyzed and compared topiramate dissolved in double-distilled water with or without meglumine for the treatment of SE in rats and found that the amino sugar meglumine significantly enhanced the water solubility of TPM. Comparison with data obtained using sulfobutylether-β-cyclodextrin (Captisol®) for the dissolution of TPM showed that meglumine solubilized TPM to a higher extent. The tolerability of the meglumine-based TPM solution and the combination of meglumine-based TPM in normal rats and rat fluid percussion injury and pilocarpine-induced SE models demonstrated the excellent tolerability of the novel drug solutions. Preclinical studies of antiseizure efficacy in SE models are currently underway [437].

Application of Topiramate in Special Populations

Marissa Vawter-Lee et al. [438] conducted a multicenter retrospective cohort study involving 75 neonates and reported that three (4%) developed necrotizing enterocolitis (NEC) after exposure to topiramate. There was no difference in gestational age, birth weight, etiology of epilepsy, body weight at the initiation of topiramate, or topiramate dose between groups, with the most common side effect being weight loss (5%). Sixty-one percent of patients responded to topiramate, and most infants (72%) continued to take topiramate when they were discharged from the hospital.

Burns et al. [439] evaluated cognitive symptoms in children treated with topiramate, levetiracetam, lamotrigine, oxcarbazepine, or sodium valproate monotherapy for at least 12 months. Children prescribed valproate sodium or topiramate demonstrated weaker working memory and verbal fluency than children prescribed other ASMs. Additionally, parents of children prescribed topiramate reported greater executive functioning and adaptive skills deficits. The pattern of findings suggested that children prescribed valproate sodium or topiramate generally demonstrated a greater risk of cognitive and behavioral impairments than did those prescribed other ASMs.

This systematic review aimed to delineate the impact of in utero exposure to these newer ASMs on child neurodevelopment. Most studies have examined LTG exposure and have reported nonsignificant effects on child neurodevelopment. Fewer high-quality studies on levetiracetam are available, limiting conclusions regarding the findings to date. Data for topiramate, gabapentin, and oxcarbazepine are so limited that firm conclusions could not be drawn. However, no studies have investigated eslicarbazepine, lacosamide, perampanel, or zonisamide. A lack of data cannot be inferred to represent the safety of newer ASMs, which are yet to be investigated [440].

To determine the transplacental transport of topiramate to colostrum, mature breast milk, and breastfed infants, Kacirova I's team examined data from 27 women treated with topiramate between 2004 and 2020 [441]. The results showed that the levels of topiramate in maternal serum and umbilical cord serum were 1.0–7.1 mg/L and 0.8–6.2 mg/L, respectively, for an average umbilical cord/maternal serum ratio of 0.93 ± 0.11. The concentrations of topiramate ranged from 1.4 to 8.4 mg/L in maternal serum, from 1.5 to 8.6 mg/L in breast milk, and from 0.3 to 4.4 mg/L in infant serum at 3–4 days after delivery, with a mean milk/maternal serum ratio of 0.99 ± 0.45 and a mean infant/maternal serum ratio of 0.25 ± 0.15. Maternal serum levels ranged from 1.9 to 9.7 mg/L, breast milk levels ranged from 2.3 to 10.6 mg/L, and infant serum levels ranged from 0.3 to 6.5 mg/L at 7–30 days after delivery. The average milk/maternal serum ratio was 1.07 ± 0.31, and the average infant/maternal serum ratio was 0.51 ± 0.27. The study concluded that the serum concentration of topiramate was lower in breastfed infants than in the mothers.

To determine the adaptive behavioral outcomes of children exposed to topiramate in utero, Knight et al. studied 34 women with epilepsy, 26 of whom completed follow-up, and found significant associations between offspring birth weight, topiramate dose, and VABS-III score in six children exposed to topiramate who were small for gestational age at birth. The topiramate-exposed children were born small for gestational age and showed a significant dose-dependent relationship after correction for parental education level [442].

Topiramate-Related Adverse Reactions

Junyeong Choi's team observationally analyzed adverse events associated with the use of topiramate in South Korea from 2010 to 2017 and reported a total of 1300 adverse events, with the proportion of women of childbearing age in the topiramate group being more than twice that of women in the other antiseizure drug group. Among the cases of topiramate-induced adverse reactions, the most common events involved the central and peripheral nervous systems (29.6%), followed by psychiatric disorders (20.4%), such as cognitive impairment, inattention, memory loss, and sensory loss [443]. Blanka Koristkova did not find an association between plasma levels of topiramate and the occurrence of adverse drug reactions to different concentrations of topiramate in the population [444].

In addition, topiramate has been reported to cause ocular side effects, such as transient myopia or narrowing of the anterior chamber angle [445], bilateral anterior chamber purulent uveitis with choroidal detachment [446], and bilateral angle-closure glaucoma [447].

To understand urinary metabolic disorders in patients taking topiramate and their reversibility after drug withdrawal, Pelzman et al. enrolled 93 patients and analyzed their urine samples. The results showed that 24-h urine samples from 67 patients had a mean citrate excretion of 331 ± 322 mg/day, a mean pH of 6.6 ± 0.5, and a mean calcium phosphate supersaturation of 1.9 ± 1.1. According to the subgroup analysis, urinary citrate excretion increased from 225 to 614 mg/day ($P < 0.01$), and the pH decreased from 6.59 ± 0.54 to 6.33 ± 0.47 ($P = 0.06$) after the discontinuation of topiramate. In addition, 114 stone events occurred in 73 different patients, of which 50% of the stones were composed of pure or high (≥50%) calcium phosphate. This study suggested that hypouricemia and elevated pH occur more often with topiramate use compared with the general population, resulting in a greater rate of calcium phosphate stone formation, and that these metabolic disorders appear to be reversible following discontinuation [448].

Basic Research on Topiramate

One study evaluated the early effects of topiramate and lacosamide treatment on oxidative stress and inflammatory damage in a pilocarpine-induced model of status epilepticus. The experiment revealed that both topiramate and lacosamide were successful at reducing the number of seizures after 30 min of administration. Pilocarpine-induced status epilepticus reduced superoxide dismutase (SOD) activity and glutathione (GSH) levels but increased catalase (CAT) activity and malondialdehyde (MDA) and IL-1β levels compared to those in the control group. Two antiseizure medications restored CAT activity and MDA levels to normal levels. The study suggested that the antioxidant effects of topiramate and lacosamide may contribute to their anticonvulsant effects on pilocarpine-induced status epilepticus [449]. One study evaluated the anticonvulsant effects of systemic use of low-dose gamma rays (LDRs) alone or in combination with topiramate for pantoprazole (PTZ)-induced epilepsy. Male Wistar rats were pretreated with a single dose of low-dose radiation (0.5 Gy), topiramate (50 mg/kg, p.o., 7 days), or topiramate with LDR prior to PTZ injection. The results showed that PTZ treatment induced behavioral changes (high Racine score, short latency and long duration), increased malondialdehyde (MDA) and nitric oxide (NO) levels, and decreased glutathione (GSH) levels. Treatment with topiramate alone or in combination with LDR ameliorated PTZ-induced toxicity and significantly ameliorated behavioral changes, and inhibited the m-TOR signaling pathway, oxidative stress, and histological changes in the hippocampus. LDR may play a role in the treatment of convulsions by modulating the AkT/m-TOR signaling pathway, reducing oxidative stress, and modulating brain amino acids and may ameliorate the oxidative stress side effects of topiramate [450].

The use of topiramate during pregnancy is associated with a significant increase in the risk of cleft lip and palate (OFC) in newborns. To identify the possible underlying mechanism, Syed K Rafi's team [451] first tested the effect of topiramate on human embryonic palatine mesenchymal (HEPM) cells using unbiased antibody array analysis. Among the known OFC-related genes, only expression of TGFβ1 was significantly upregulated. Topiramate can increase the expression of TGFβ1 and phosphorylation of its downstream target gene Smad2 in primary mouse embryonic palatal mesenchymal cells and increase the expression of SOX9 in primary

MEPM cells. Its overexpression in chondrocytes can cause cleft palate in mice. These results suggest that topiramate mediates the upregulation of TGFβ-1 signaling by activating palatal GABA receptors. TGFβ1 and SOX9 expression play important roles in oral and maxillofacial morphogenesis, and their aberrant overexpression provides a possible molecular mechanism for topiramate-related teratogenesis.

Forced exercise acts as a neuroprotective factor and a cognitive enhancer. To evaluate the effects of forced exercise on topiramate-induced cognitive impairment, topiramate antiseizure activity, and the neurodegenerative state after seizures, Zahra Soleimani Meigoni's group measured biomarkers of oxidation, inflammation, and apoptosis after 21 days of forced exercise in adult male rats divided into groups subjected to treatment with saline, topiramate (100 mg/kg), or topiramate combined with forced exercise. The results showed that the combination of forced exercise and topiramate could eliminate the cognitive impairment caused by topiramate and enhance its antiseizure activity. In addition, topiramate treatment decreased malondialdehyde (MDA), tumor necrosis factor α (TNF-α), interleukin-1β (IL-1β), and Bax protein levels while increasing superoxide dismutase (SOD), glutathione peroxidase (GPx), and glutathione reductase (GR) activity. The results of the study propose that forced exercise seems to be useful as an adjunctive therapy to topiramate to manage related cognitive impairment and could also enhance the antiseizure and neuroprotective effects of topiramate [452].

Topiramate was administered daily at a dose of 41 mg/kg to male rats aged 16–28 days. Half of the rats were evaluated at 24 h after birth, and the rest were evaluated in adulthood. There was a reduction in precision ($p = 0.018$), total length ($p = 0.035$), and interstitial tissue volume ($p = 0.018$) but an increase in interstitial cell number/testis number ($p = 0.013$) at postnatal day (PND) 120. The results of this study contribute to the understanding of the effects of topiramate treatment at the juvenile stage on the reproductive system of adult rats, suggesting that rats are more sensitive to topiramate exposure during this period than during puberty [453].

Use of Topiramate in Other Diseases

Koolen-de Vries syndrome (KdVS) is mainly characterized by mild or moderate intellectual disability, especially affecting language development, accompanied by other clinical findings such as seizures, muscle hypotonia, joint hypermobility, or joint dysplasia. Approximately half of patients with KdVS have seizures with a broad phenotype throughout their lives, but most affected children have focal to bilateral tonic–clonic seizures that may not respond to initial medical therapy. Piccinelli Paolo [454] described a case of a female infant with KdVS and epilepsy. At the age of 2 years and 1 month, the patient began to experience epileptic symptoms, which evolved from focal unconsciousness seizures to bilateral tonic–clonic seizures and were not effectively controlled by oral levetiracetam treatment. Seizures were completely controlled with the addition of low-dose topiramate. This case suggests that topiramate may be an antiseizure agent with good efficacy in treating focal epilepsy in patients with KdVS syndrome. However, it is necessary to further extend the follow-up time and perform related studies in children with KdVS in multiple centers to clarify its role.

Impulsivity is an important feature of many psychiatric disorders and a marker of poor prognosis. Topiramate is widely used to reduce impulsivity in individuals with various neuropsychiatric disorders, but no systematic review or meta-analysis has been conducted to explore whether there is evidence to support its clinical use. Sophie Athena Chapron et al. [455] analyzed seven studies involving 578 participants that assessed the efficacy of topiramate in adults with high impulsivity based on psychometric or neuropsychological measures. It was found that topiramate reduced impulsivity levels in two studies using the Barratt Impulsivity Scale (BIS) (401 participants) and one study using neuropsychological measures (63 participants). Four other studies found no effect of topiramate on impulsivity.

Following schizophrenia onset and the use of antipsychotic drugs, cardiovascular disease has a high mortality rate in these patients. Topiramate can be used for weight loss and to improve the psychopathology of schizophrenia patients. In a randomized, double-blinded controlled trial in Sri Lanka, the effects of 100 mg/day topiramate were compared with those of a placebo for weight and mental health improvement in overweight/obese adults with schizophrenia who had been taking antipsychotics for at least 1 year. Compared with placebo, topiramate addition significantly reduced body mass index and improved symptoms, as measured by the Brief Neuropathy Rating Scale (BPRS), but there were more reports of loss of appetite in the topiramate group than in the placebo group [456].

2.1.2.4 Gabapentin

Drug Characteristics

[Chemical name] 11-Aminomethyl-cyclohexaacetic acid

[Chemical structure formula]

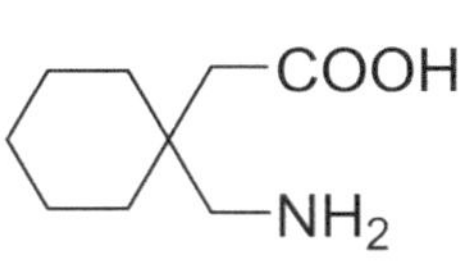

[Molecular formula] C9H17NO2

[Molecular weight] 171.24

[Indications] (1) Postherpetic neuralgia: For the treatment of postherpetic neuralgia in adults. Epilepsy: For the adjuvant treatment of partial seizures in adults and children over 12 years of age with or without secondary generalized tonic–clonic seizures. It can also be used as an adjunct treatment for partial seizures in children aged 3–12 years.

[Packing specifications] 0.1 g, 0.3 g

[Usage and dosage]
Postherpetic neuralgia: 0.3 g once on the first day; on the second day, 0.6 g is taken in two doses. On the third day, 0.9 g is taken in three separate doses. Subsequently, according to need, the dose can be gradually increased to 1.8 g/day, divided into three times; efficacy is comparable in the range of 1.8–3.6 g.

Epilepsy: Patients over 12 years old: 0.3 g on the first day; on the second day, 0.3 g, twice a day; on the third day, 0.3 g, three times a day. The usual dose range is 1.8–2.4 g. Pediatric patients 3–12 years old: Starting dose 10–15 mg/kg/day, three times a day, reaching effective dose in approximately 3 days. The effective dose of gabapentin for patients older than 5 years is 25–35 mg/kg/day, three times a day. The effective dose for pediatric patients aged 3–4 years is 40 mg/kg/day, three times a day. The interval between doses should not exceed 12 h. The first dose in elderly patients is affected by renal function and requires reference to creatinine clearance.

[Adverse reactions] Vertigo, drowsiness, peripheral edema, fatigue, infection, headache, abdominal pain, diarrhea, constipation, dry mouth, nausea, vomiting, flatulence, weight gain, hyperglycemia, ataxia, nystagmus, depression, abnormal thinking, abnormal gait, etc. Aggressive behavior, emotional instability, hyperactivity, and fever have been observed in children under 12 years of old.

Clinical Application and Preclinical Research

The Historical Evolution of Gabapentin

Gabapentin, chemically known as 1-(aminomethyl)-cyclohexane acetic acid, is a synthetic amino acid with a structure similar to 1-aminobutyric acid (GABA). Gabapentin was first developed by the American company Warner-Lanbert and was first marketed in the UK in 1993 as an antiseizure treatment. In 2002, it was approved by the US FDA as a first-line treatment for postherpetic neuralgia. China approved production in 2003. As an analog of the inhibitory neurotransmitter GABA, the original aim of Gabapentin was to increase the lipophilicity of GABA by adding cyclohexyl to the structure of GABA, in order to improve its properties across the central nervous system while retaining its pharmacological properties. The bioavailability of gabapentin is inversely dependent on the dose, and the bioavailability decreases when the dose is increased. The bioavailability of 300 mg oral gabapentin is 60%, and that of 600 mg oral gabapentin is 40%. Gabapentin is mostly unbound to plasma protein in circulation (protein binding rate <3%), the maximum blood concentration is reached by oral administration for 3 h, and the elimination half-life is 5–7 h; patients may require administration three times a day. Gabapentin is not metabolized in the human body, but is cleared by the kidney, and the drug is excreted in the urine.

Gabapentin is mainly used to treat focal seizures and chronic neuropathic pain and postoperative pain; it has a good effect especially for neuropathic pain, diabetic neuralgia, and postherpetic neuralgia.

Application of Gabapentin in Epilepsy

Gabapentin is recommended primarily as a monotherapy or additive treatment for focal seizures and for drug-resistant focal seizures with or without secondary generalized seizures. A review of six studies summarized the evidence from randomized controlled trials of gabapentin as an additional therapy for drug-resistant focal epilepsy. The results suggested that the overall hazard ratio for 50% or greater reduction in seizure frequency in the GBP group compared with the placebo group was 1.89. Dose regression analysis showed that the efficacy of gabapentin as additional therapy for refractory focal epilepsy increased with increasing dose, with 16.0% of patients responding to treatment when the dose was increased to 900 mg and 25.3% of patients responding when the dose was increased to 1800 mg. The adverse reactions with high correlation with GBP use were dizziness, lethargy, ataxia, fatigue, headache, etc. In conclusion, gabapentin is effective and well-tolerated in patients with drug-resistant focal epilepsy, but its efficacy still needs to be confirmed in future long-term clinical studies [457].

A review analyzed five randomized controlled trials (3167 participants) comparing gabapentin with other ASMs for the treatment of focal epilepsy. The results suggested that gabapentin monotherapy may not be as effective in controlling seizures as other ASMs (lamotrigine, CBZ, oxcarbazepine, and topiramate). Compared with CBZ, gabapentin is better-tolerated [458].

Use of Gabapentin for Treating Neuropathic Pain

In 2002, the US FDA approved gabapentin as a first-line treatment for postherpetic neuralgia. Gabapentin and pregabalin are both recommended for the treatment of neuropathic pain. A meta-analysis [459] included 14 RCTs, with a total of 3545 patients, to evaluate the clinical efficacy of pregabalin and gabapentin in the treatment of postherpes zoster neuralgia. The results showed that pregabalin was superior to gabapentin for reducing pain and improving the overall perception of pain and sleep changes, but gabapentin had a lower incidence of adverse reactions and greater safety. Clinicians should consider patient factors comprehensively and prescribe medicine individually.

In a study comparing clinical differences in waist pain, patients were randomized to receive either pregabalin (300 mg/day) or gabapentin (800 mg/day) for 6 weeks. The results showed that pregabalin improved pain relief, and gabapentin improved anxiety, insomnia, and fatigue symptoms [460]. A review summarized the risks and benefits of gabapentin and pregabalin for perioperative pain control. Perioperative gabapentin reduced opioid requirements and pain scores for various procedures. The use of such drugs may reduce postoperative nausea, vomiting and itching, which may be a feature of reduced opioid intake. However, side effects such as dizziness, ataxia and cognitive dysfunction can occur. Gabapentin use also increases the risk of respiratory depression, especially when combined with opioids. Therefore, routine use of these drugs for perioperative pain management is not recommended, and individualized, patient- and surgery-centered treatments are recommended [461]. In women with severe pain after cesarean section, supplemental gabapentin therapy did not reduce opioid withdrawal time, pain, anxiety, depression, or fatigue time or improve physical function [462].

Pain is the main symptom of diabetic foot patients. Network meta-analysis revealed that the most favorable treatments for diabetic foot patients with a benefit/risk ratio were gabapentin, venlafaxine, and pregabalin. Gabapentin not only has the best efficacy but also shows the best balance between efficacy and safety [463]. A systematic review revealed that 1800–3600 mg/day gabapentin provides good analgesic effects in some patients with chronic neuropathic pain (postherpetic neuralgia and diabetic peripheral neuropathy), with side effects including dizziness (19%), drowsiness (14%), peripheral edema (7%), and gait disturbance (14%) [464]. Regarding pain caused by cancer, the National Comprehensive Cancer Network (NCCN) guidelines recommend gabapentin and pregabalin as the most common pain relief drugs [465].

Neuralgia is one of the main factors that affects the quality of life of patients with diabetic peripheral neuropathy. In 2012, a consensus on the diagnosis and treatment of painful peripheral neuropathy formulated by the Neurology Branch of the Chinese Medical Association recommended gabapentin to alleviate neuralgia in patients with diabetic peripheral neuropathy.

Application of Gabapentin in Special Populations

The pregnancy safety rating of gabapentin is Class C. Gabapentin is actively transported through the placenta and may accumulate in the fetus but is not concentrated in breast milk. The plasma concentration of breastfed infants is 12% or less of the mother's plasma concentration, and no adverse effects have been observed [466, 467]. One study examined pregnancy outcomes in 223 gabapentin-exposed pregnancies and 223 unexposed pregnancies. The incidence of major malformations was similar between the two groups. However, the preterm birth rate and low birth weight in the gabapentin group were greater than those in the control group, so gabapentin is not recommended for pregnant women [468].

Adverse Effects of Gabapentin

Common adverse effects of gabapentin are drowsiness, fatigue, double vision, paresthesia, forgetfulness, dizziness, and ataxia. Atopy side effects are rare. Other possible adverse reactions include hyperglycemia and, occasionally, hypoglycemia [469]. Gabapentin is not metabolized in the liver, so the mechanism of liver injury is not clear. However, it has been reported that gabapentin may cause liver toxicity, so it should be considered individually for each patient [470].

Gabapentin and pregabalin are ligands of the $\alpha 2$-δ subunit of voltage-gated calcium channels and have been implicated in the development of peripheral edema and acute heart failure. Pregabalin is more likely to cause peripheral edema and acute heart failure than gabapentin. All cases of peripheral edema or heart failure involving gabapentin or pregabalin reported to the French Pharmacovigilance Centre between 1994 and 2020 were included in a description of their onset patterns. A total of 58 reports were included (gabapentin, $n = 5$; pregabalin, $n = 53$). The male to female ratio was 4:1, and the median age was 77 years (32–95 years). The median onset times of noncardiogenic edema and acute heart failure were 23 days and 17 days, respectively. Cardiogenic and noncardiogenic peripheral edema often occur after the drug dosage is increased, and the disease improved rapidly after gabapentin was discontinued [471].

Gabapentin does not produce euphoria, and there is no evidence of addiction when taken [472]. However, in recent years, there has been a gradual increase in gabapentin abuse. A systematic review of studies in the last 5 years confirmed that gabapentin is being increasingly abused or misused; gabapentin use alone can produce desirable effects but is often used in conjunction with other drugs, and opioid use is the greatest risk factor for gabapentin abuse. There is increasing evidence that abuse of gabapentin and pregabalin is associated with patient harm, including increased rates of hospitalization and increased risk of opioid-related overdose death [473].

Previous case reports and observational studies have suggested that gabapentin use may be associated with an increased risk of atrial fibrillation, especially in patients over 65 years of age with comorbidities. New case reports have suggested that gabapentin can also induce new atrial fibrillation in young people [474].

ASMs such as gabapentin can increase the risk of hypogammaglobulinemia. In case–control studies, hypogammaglobulinemia was associated with the use of antiseizure drugs, with the exception of topiramate. The use of phenytoin sodium, CBZ, and lamotrigine was associated with low IgA levels. If a patient receiving gabapentin or other ASM therapy has an abnormal or recurrent infection, the clinician should check the immunoglobulin levels [475].

In addition, gabapentin is a drug that may induce acute pancreatitis [476]. The type and severity of eye-related adverse reactions vary among different ASMs. Adverse reactions related to macula were associated with gabapentin [355].

Preclinical Research

The exact mechanism of action between gabapentin and GABA receptors is not wellunderstood. Gabapentin is structurally related to the neurotransmitter GABA but does not interact with GABA receptors; it is neither metabolized as GABA nor as a GABA agonist nor is it an inhibitor of GABA uptake or degradation. In vitro studies have shown that the binding sites of gabapentin in the rat brain are distributed in the neocortex and hippocampus, and its high-affinity binding proteins, especially $\alpha 2\delta$-1, have been confirmed to be auxiliary subunits of voltage-gated calcium channels (VGCCs). It appears to inhibit the release of excitatory neurotransmitters in the presynaptic region involved in the development of epilepsy. VGCCs consist of multiple subunits: $\alpha 1$, β, γ, and $\alpha 2\delta$. The $\alpha 1$ subunit allows calcium to enter, and extracellular $\alpha 2\delta$ binds to the γ subunit, where the $\alpha 2\delta$-1 subunit is involved in damage processes. Transgenic mice expressing elevated levels of α2δ-1 developed neuropathic pain even in the absence of nerve damage. Therefore, the analgesic effect of gabapentin is thought to be due to inhibition of the calcium current by its binding to the α2δ-1 subunit, which leads to a reduction in postsynaptic excitability. However, gabapentin has not been shown to consistently inhibit the Ca2+ current [477].

To date, other mechanisms of analgesia are thought to exist [478]: (1) Gabapentin inhibits the accumulation of α2δ-1 expression at the terminus of the presynaptic dorsal horn and reduces the response to pain stimuli; (2) α2δ-1 can enhance the release of neurotransmitters when calcium inflow decreases, and gabapentin can affect pain perception by inhibiting α2δ-1-mediated neurotransmitter release; (3) analgesic effects are mediated by the facilitation of descending noradrenergic inhibition, the inhibition of descending serotonergic facilitation and cortical mechanisms affecting the limbic system; and (4) gabapentin inhibits the formation of new excitatory synapses by blocking the binding of astrocyte-derived thromboreactive proteins to α2δ-1. (5) The uptake of glutamate is stimulated by excitatory amino acid transporters. (6) The inflammatory response is inhibited after injury. (7) Modulation of the affective component of pain.

Other Applications of Gabapentin

In addition to treating focal epilepsy and neuropathic pain, gabapentin can also be used to treat restless leg syndrome, hiccups, drug withdrawal, and other conditions. Persistent hiccups have a significant impact on quality of life and can be a barrier to stroke recovery. Chlorpromazine, the first-line treatment for intractable hiccups, has a sedative effect and may negatively affect participation in rehabilitation. Studies have reported that gabapentin is effective in the treatment of hiccups in both the general population and the poststroke population. The therapeutic dose ranges from 100 mg each time, three times a day, to 400 mg each time, twice a day, and the duration of treatment ranges from 2 days to 5.5 weeks [479].

Gabapentin may assist in benzodiazepine withdrawal treatment. A retrospective study of 172 patients who developed benzodiazepine withdrawal symptoms showed that patients who received gabapentin as a benzodiazepine-assisted treatment took less benzodiazepines and had a shorter hospital stay than did a control group who did not receive gabapentin as a benzodiazepine-assisted treatment. This suggests that gabapentin can be used as an adjunct therapy for patients withdrawing from treatment with benzodiazepines [480].

Gabapentin has protective effects on the myocardium and can reduce ischemia–reperfusion injury, which may be related to the activation of PI3K/Akt in the myocardium and the upregulation of GABAARδ in the spinal cord [481].

Gabapentin can improve sleep quality in patients with sensory nervous system diseases. A meta-analysis showed that compared with the placebo group, the gabapentin group had a significantly lower degree of sleep disturbance, improved sleep quality, and a lower incidence of more than 5 awakenings at night [482].

2.1.2.5 Pregabalin

Drug Characteristics

[Chemical name] (S)-3-(aminomethyl)-5-methylhexanoic acid

[Chemical structure]

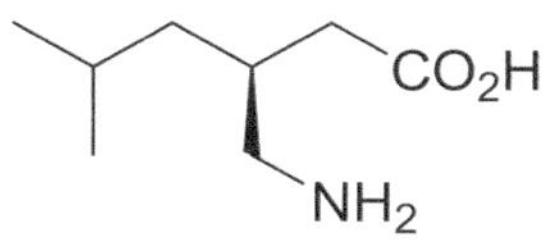

[Molecular formula] $C_8H_{17}NO_2$

[Molecular weight] 159.23

[Indications]
Treatment of adult patients with focal epileptic seizures (with or without secondary generalized seizures).

[Specification] 75 mg, 150 mg

[Dosage]
The therapeutic dose of pregabalin is 150–600 mg/day. The starting dose is 150 mg/day, which is taken two to three times daily. According to the patient's response and tolerance, the dose can be increased to 300 mg/day after 1 week, and then 1 week later, the dose can be increased to the maximum dose of 600 mg/day, which can be taken on an empty stomach or with food.

[Adverse reactions] The most common adverse reactions are dizziness and drowsiness. Other common adverse reactions include dry mouth, edema, blurred vision, weight gain and abnormal thinking.

Clinical Application and Basic Research

Historical Evolution of Pregabalin

Pregabalin (PGB) is a gabapentinoid that is structurally similar to the inhibitory neurotransmitter γ-aminobutyric acid (GABA). It was approved in the United States and the European Union in 2004 as an added medicine for adults with focal epilepsy. Since then, it has been approved for the treatment of focal epilepsy in children older than 4 years in the United States but has not been approved for pediatric use in the European Union. PGB primarily binds to presynaptic voltage-gated calcium channels on the α-2-δ subunit to reduce the release of excitatory neurotransmitters, thereby exerting antiseizure effects.

Pregabalin Monotherapy for Focal Epilepsy

Zhao et al. [483] designed a network meta-analysis (NMA) to compare the effectiveness and safety of different ASMs in the treatment of focal epilepsy, which included 11 pregabalin-related randomized controlled trials (RCTs). The results showed that the efficacy of PGB on focal seizures was relatively high. Compared with patients treated with topiramate and oxcarbazepine, patients treated with PGB had the lowest risk of headache and nausea, although the risk of dizziness, drowsiness and fatigue increased. However, the overall risk of adverse events was low.

French et al. [484] evaluated the efficacy of PGB in the treatment of focal epilepsy by designing with historical controls converted to monotherapy. A total of 161 patients whose disease was poorly controlled by their original antiseizure drugs were included in the study. Finally, 148 patients received 600 mg/day or 150 mg/day pregabalin (4:1) in randomized double-blind monotherapy for 20 weeks (8-week conversion and 12-week monotherapy periods). The results showed that the rate of epilepsy-related withdrawal in the 600 mg/day PGB group was 27.5%, which was significantly lower than that in the historical control group (74% and 68%, respectively) ($p = 0.001$). This finding suggests that PGB is effective for treating focal epilepsy as monotherapy. In addition, eight patients taking 600 mg/day PGB and two patients taking 150 mg/day PGB achieved seizure-free status, and the overall safety was consistent with that of previous trials. The authors concluded that pregabalin monotherapy is safe and effective in patients with poorly controlled focal seizures.

To explore an effective and safe monotherapy regimen for newly diagnosed adult patients with focal epilepsy, Kwan et al. [485] conducted a double-blinded, randomized, noninferiority study comparing pregabalin and lamotrigine. A total of 660 patients with new-onset epilepsy from 105 medical centers were randomly assigned to the treatment groups (330 to pregabalin, 330 to lamotrigine). The initial doses of 150 mg/day PGB and 100 mg/day LTG were administered orally twice a day. As needed, the maximum doses were increased to 600 mg/day PGB and 500 mg/day LTG within 4 weeks and were maintained for 52 weeks. Overall, 622 patients completed the entire therapy (314 with PGB, 308 with LTG). Compared with those in the LTG group, fewer patients in the PGB group achieved 6 months or more without seizures (52% vs. 68%). Dizziness (17% vs. 14%), drowsiness (9% vs. 4%), fatigue (8% vs. 6%), and weight gain (6% vs. 2%) were more common in the PGB group. The overall incidence of adverse events was similar between the two groups. The authors speculated that PGB was similarly tolerable to LTG but might not be as effective as LTG in treating newly diagnosed focal seizures in adults.

Bruin et al. [486] analyzed a total of 66 studies to determine the effectiveness and tolerability of ASMs in the treatment of glioma-related epilepsy. The results showed that phenytoin had the highest seizure-free rate after 6 months of monotherapy. After 12 months, pregabalin and levetiracetam monotherapy showed the greatest efficacy. In addition, levetiracetam was most effective at reducing seizures by ≥50% at 6 and 12 months of treatment. However, phenytoin and pregabalin showed the highest treatment failure rates at 12 months. Based on limited evidence, the authors speculated that levetiracetam, phenytoin and pregabalin monotherapy would be effective in glioma patients with epilepsy, with levetiracetam showing the lowest treatment failure rate compared to the other ASMs studied.

Pregabalin in the Treatment of Generalized Tonic–Clonic Seizures

In a randomized, double-blinded, multicenter study [487] of 219 patients with generalized tonic–clonic seizures, 75, 72, and 72 patients were randomized to receive 5 mg/kg/day pregabalin, 10 mg/kg/day pregabalin, or placebo, respectively. There were 15, 11, and 6 patients who discontinued 5 mg/kg/day, 10 mg/kg/day, and placebo, respectively, due to adverse events (10.7%, 6.9%, and 5.6%, respectively). The results showed that there was no significant change in the average 28-day seizure rate or response rate among the three groups. The most common AEs (≥10%) were dizziness, headache, and somnolence, most of which were mild or moderate. Therefore, pregabalin is not recommended for the treatment of generalized tonic–clonic seizures.

Pregabalin in the Treatment of Refractory Epilepsy

Pregabalin is an effective add-on treatment for focal seizures. The guideline summary recommends that pregabalin can effectively reduce the frequency of seizures in adults with refractory focal epilepsy (Grade A) [488]. To evaluate the efficacy and tolerability of pregabalin as an add-on treatment for drug-resistant focal epilepsy, two groups [489, 490] conducted a systematic review of nine randomized controlled trials. The results showed that pregabalin, as an add-on treatment for refractory focal epilepsy, was significantly more effective than placebo in reducing seizures by 50% or more and attaining seizure freedom. Furthermore, there was a certain dose–response relationship. Doses ranging from 150 to 600 mg/day were effective. As the dose increased from 300 to 600 mg/day, the chance of a response doubled, but tolerability issues occurred at higher doses. Compared with patients taking lamotrigine, patients taking pregabalin were more likely to have a 50% or greater reduction in seizure rates, but there was no significant difference in seizure-free status between patients taking each of the two drugs. Compared with those taking levetiracetam, there was no significant difference in the 50% or greater reduction in seizure rates among patients taking pregabalin, but there was a relatively lower seizure-free rate in patients who received an addition of pregabalin. However, the trials included in this review were short in duration. Longer-term trials are needed to inform clinical decisions.

To compare the efficacy of a new generation of antiseizure drugs in the treatment of refractory epilepsy, Viteva et al. [491] conducted an open, prospective study in which 1259 epilepsy patients participated and 47 patients received pregabalin. The average age of these patients was 34.43 ± 1.65 years. The average duration of epilepsy was 19.96 ± 1.54 years. In addition, the average treatment dose was 333.51 ± 1.47 mg/day. Comparative analysis of the dynamic reduction in seizure severity showed that treatment with PGB reduced seizure severity and frequency to a greater extent than treatment with oxcarbazepine or topiramate, but the retention rate was significantly lower. In addition, at the sixth month of treatment, patients who received PGB had a greater incidence of adverse reactions (25.5%). The authors speculated that pregabalin had a good dynamic improvement effect on the severity and frequency of seizures. It was mainly effective for patients with focal epilepsy, but its tolerability was lower than that of other ASMs.

Mesial temporal lobe epilepsy with hippocampal sclerosis (MTLE-HS) is usually poorly controlled with antiseizure drugs. Androsova et al. [492] conducted a study on the efficacy, tolerability and retention rate of different ASMs in the treatment of MTLE-HS. For comparison, a total of 3249 trials were included, with a total of 767 patients. There were 73 patients who received PGB. The results showed that most (92.1%) of the PGB was added as a third drug, with an average maximum dose of 300 mg/day and an average treatment time of 10 ± 9.8 months. Compared with CBZ and levetiracetam, only 4.7% of patients were seizure free after 12 months of PGB treatment. The therapy failure rate was 41.9%. The incidence of adverse reactions was high (27.4%), and the most common adverse reactions were drowsiness and weight gain. In addition, the retention rate of PGB was the lowest (40%). The authors held that PGB had no obvious advantage in treating seizures in patients with MTLE-HS.

Pregabalin in the Treatment of Refractory Status Epilepticus

There is currently insufficient evidence to support the effectiveness of PGB in the treatment of refractory and superrefractory status epilepticus [493]. It is recommended to combine pregabalin with high-level anesthetics such as propofol, midazolam, thiopental, and ketamine [494].

Novy et al. [495] reported that a clear electroclinical response was observed in 5 of 11 RSE patients treated with PGB. This effect was obvious 24 h after PGB administration. Possible reactions were noted on three occasions when PGB was combined with other antiseizure drugs. The remaining three patients had no obvious response after PGB administration. The response of PGB in the treatment of focal SE appeared to be better than that of generalized convulsive SE.

Swisher et al. [496] administered a combination of intravenous phenytoin (PHT), levetiracetam (median dose of LEV, 3000 mg/day), and oral pregabalin (median dose of PGB, 375 mg/day) for RSE in 23 patients with primary or metastatic brain tumors. The results showed that SE in 16 patients (70%) stopped on average 24 h after the addition of the third antiseizure drug. No related adverse reactions occurred. These findings suggest that the combination of PHT, LEV, and PGB may be safe and efficient for the treatment of RSE in patients with brain tumors.

Another retrospective study [497] included 21 patients with frequent nonconvulsive seizures (NCSs) and nonconvulsive status epilepticus (NCSE). The patients were treated with PGB at an average therapeutic dose of 342 mg/day. Ultimately, 11 patients (52%) achieved an electroclinical response. This result suggests that PGB was more effective for halting NCS (nine patients, 82%) than for preventing NCSE (two patients, 18%). Additionally, seizures were halted in 67% of brain tumor patients. However, none of the patients (four patients) with anoxic injury responded to PGB. In addition, PGB was well-tolerated by most patients after treatment, with only two patients experiencing dizziness and sedation. These findings suggest that pregabalin may be a safe option as an add-on treatment for critically ill patients with nonconvulsive seizures and nonconvulsive status epilepticus when conventional therapy fails.

Pregabalin in Special Populations with Epilepsy

Mann et al. [498] used video electroencephalography (VEEG) monitoring to evaluate the efficacy and safety of pregabalin as an add-on treatment for focal epilepsy in children (1 month to 4 years old). They randomized 175 pediatric patients (mean age 28.2 months, 59% male) at a 2:1:2 ratio to receive 7 mg/kg/day pregabalin, 14 mg/kg/day pregabalin or placebo. The results showed that compared with that in the placebo group ($n = 53$, $P = 0.022$), the 24-h seizure rate was 35% lower in the PGB 14 mg/kg/day ($n = 28$) group. However, the seizure rate in the PGB 7 mg/kg/day ($n = 59$) group did not significantly improve. In addition, the most common AEs in the PGB 7 mg/kg/day, 14 mg/kg/day, and placebo treatment groups were somnolence (11.3%, 17.6%, and 5.7%, respectively) and upper respiratory tract infection (7.0%, 11.8%, and 11.4%, respectively). The severity of all AEs was mild to moderate. The authors considered that 14 mg/kg/day pregabalin could significantly reduce the rate of focal seizures in children. Pregabalin at 7 mg/kg/day and 14 mg/kg/day was generally safe and well tolerated in children aged 1 month to 4 years.

To better understand the efficacy and tolerability of pregabalin as an add-on treatment for focal seizures in children (4–16 years old), Antinew et al. [499] designed a double-blinded, randomized, placebo-controlled study. A total of 295 children (mean age 10.2 years, 55% male) were randomized to receive PGB 2.5 mg/kg/day ($n = 104$), PGB 10 mg/kg/day ($n = 97$), or placebo ($n = 94$). The treatment was double-blinded and lasted for 12 weeks (dose escalation for 2 weeks, fixed dose for 10 weeks). The data showed that the 28-day seizure rate of children in the 10 mg/kg/day PGB group was significantly lower than that in the placebo group (19.9%, $P = 0.0185$). The 2.5 mg/kg/day PGB group showed no significant improvement in seizure frequency ($P = 0.2577$). In addition, the response rate of the PGB 10 mg/kg/day group (40.6%, $P = 0.0068$) was significantly better than that of the PGB 2.5 mg/kg/day group (29.1%, $P = 0.26$) and placebo group (22.6%). Common adverse events (≥10%) in the 10 mg/kg/day PGB, 2.5 mg/kg/day PGB, and placebo groups included somnolence (25.8%, 17.3%, 13.8%), weight gain (13.4%, 3.8%, 4.3%) and increased appetite (10.3%, 6.7%, 4.3%). The authors concluded that 10 mg/kg/day PGB effectively reduced the frequency of focal seizures in children and was well tolerated.

Chan et al. [500] used population pharmacokinetics (PK) and exposure-response (ER) relationships to summarize data related to pregabalin concentration and efficacy. They analyzed and compared the relationship between pregabalin exposure and ER in children and adults with focal epilepsy. Population PK simulations showed that for children aged 4–16 years and weighing ≥30 kg, 2.5–10 mg/kg/day

PGB was required to achieve steady-state exposure concentrations similar to those of adult patients receiving approved doses of 150–600 mg/day. For children aged 4–16 years weighing <30 kg, 3.5–14 mg/kg/day PGB was required to achieve equivalent exposure. The findings support the guidance of PGB dosing provided in the guidelines. Pediatric patients (4–16 years old) weighing <30 kg should receive a 40% higher dose of PGB per kilogram of body weight than patients weighing ≥30 kg to achieve similar exposure.

Regarding the study of pregabalin in the treatment of women, a population-based cohort study was conducted through population registries (2005–2016) in four Nordic countries (Denmark, Finland, Norway, and Sweden). This research examined the association between prenatal exposure to pregabalin and the risk of adverse delivery and postpartum neurodevelopmental outcomes. The results showed that prenatal exposure to pregabalin was not associated with low birth weight, prematurity, small gestational age, low Apgar score, microcephaly, autism spectrum disorder or intellectual disability. The increased risk of any major congenital malformations and ADHD was unlikely to be greater than 1.8 [501].

Effect of Pregabalin on Electroencephalography

Parekh et al. [502] described a rare case of PGB-induced triphasic waves (TWs). The patient was a 74-year-old man with diabetes-related peripheral neuropathy. He had a history of chronic kidney disease and long-term use of PGB (75 mg, twice daily). For pain relief within 8 h, the patient received 450 mg of PGB and subsequently developed altered mental status, somnolence and disorientation. Bedside EEG showed continuous TWs with slow background activity, ruling out nonconvulsive status epilepticus. Forty-eight hours after the discontinuation of PGB, the patient was conscious and alert. Seventy-two hours later, the repeat EEG did not show any TWs. On the fifth day after admission, the patient's mental status fully recovered. The authors determined that this case was acute reversible toxic encephalopathy caused by PGB overdose. Continuous TWs on EEG were successfully treated by drug withdrawal. Therefore, clinicians should use PGB with caution, especially in patients who have impaired renal function and are older.

Anand et al. [503] provided a detailed description of PGB-associated TW cases. The patient was a 41-year-old woman who had received PGB for long-term treatment of neuropathic pain. Three days before admission, the patient developed somnolence, disorientation and abnormal mental status. Renal function tests revealed renal failure. Brain magnetic resonance imaging revealed periventricular and subcortical white matter lesions (diabetic-related). EEG showed generalized periodic discharges with a triphasic morphology and a waveform with three main phases: a positive, sharp transient wave followed by a negative wave of relatively low amplitude. Discharges were bilaterally synchronized, occurred at a frequency of 1–2 s, and were not affected by lorazepam administration. The combined consideration was toxic encephalopathy secondary to renal insufficiency. Three days after the discontinuation of PGB and intravenous fluids, the patient's mental status improved significantly. She was discharged, oriented and able to follow commands. A repeat electroencephalogram showed improvement. The authors suggested that TWs resolved without improvement in renal function, further supporting pregabalin toxicity as the cause of triphasic waves and encephalopathy. Underlying subcortical white matter lesions might be a precipitating factor in the evolution of triphasic waves.

Side Effects of Pregabalin

Most of the adverse reactions caused by pregabalin are mild to moderate in a dose-dependent manner. They mainly occur in the first 2 weeks of initial treatment, with drowsiness and dizziness being the most common. The risk of weight gain increased to 14% for patients receiving 600 mg/day [504]. With rapid or abrupt discontinuation of PGB, symptoms such as insomnia, nausea, headache, anxiety, nervousness, irritability, hyperhidrosis, and diarrhea may occur. The long-term use of PGB can lead to physical dependence. There is a risk of abuse associated with its use, particularly in patients taking opioids or with a history of substance abuse. Baftiu et al. [505] described 593 reports of PGB-related adverse effects. The most common adverse effects included dizziness, weight gain, somnolence, withdrawal syndrome, fatigue, and rash.

Serotonin syndrome (SS) is a potentially fatal clinical syndrome caused by drugs with serotonergic properties. Prakash et al. [506] conducted a systematic review of case reports of SS associated with antiseizure drugs. Of the 76 patients enrolled, seven patients with SS were exposed to pregabalin at a median dosage of 150 mg/day. In four of these studies, there was a temporal association between PGB intake and the occurrence of SS. All patients with pregabalin-induced SS were also treated with another serotonergic agent. The main manifestations of SS induced by PGB include confusion, agitation, hallucinations, tremors, myoclonus, sweating, nausea, diarrhea, fever, hypertension, etc. The authors noted a need to be alert to the possible incidence of SS induced by PGB, especially in patients taking another serotonergic drug at the same time.

Serious cutaneous adverse reactions (SCARs) mainly include Stevens-Johnson syndrome (SJS), toxic epidermal necrolysis (TEN), and drug rash with eosinophilia and systemic symptoms (DRESS). Shukla et al. [507] performed a retrospective analysis of clinical and epidemiological data on SCAR induced by ASMs. Among the patients with drug-related skin and subcutaneous tissue adverse events, 54.1% were female with SJS/TEN/DRESS, 75% of whom were adults (>18 years old). Nearly 64% of drug-related SCARs were severe and resulted in patient death (3.5%), life-threatening conditions (11.5%) or hospitalization/prolonged hospitalization (43.5%). The data from this study showed that pregabalin caused 213 (1.1%) SCAR events in the Asian population and was associated with a significantly increased risk of SCARs in the Asian population (n = 68, $P < 0.0001$). It is one of the most common antiseizure drugs that leads to SCARs in the Asian population.

Hamed et al. [508] explored the frequency and type of sexual dysfunction (SD) caused by PGB and its relationship with duration of use. A total of 75 patients were included, 31 (41.33%) of whom developed PGB-related SD. The patients presented with erectile dysfunction (n = 16, 51.61%), anorgasmia (n = 10, 32.26%), and decreased libido (n = 11, 35.48%). SD mainly occurred within a few weeks at low therapeutic doses of PGB (50–100 mg/day). Its severity was independent of dose. SD improved after several weeks of PGB discontinuation. The authors concluded that although SD is not a common adverse effect of PGB, it is important for clinicians to discuss sexual function with patients and ask about the impact of PGB on sexual function.

Basic Research on Pregabalin

Sobral et al. [509] investigated the effects of PGB and β-caryophyllene (a cannabinoid receptor subtype 2 agonist) on pentylenetetrazol (PTZ)-induced seizures in rats. Adult male Wistar rats received β-caryophyllene (100 mg/kg), PGB (40 mg/kg), or a combination of the two before PTZ (60 mg/kg). Animals were monitored by video-EEG to measure the latency of myoclonic seizures, the latency of tonic–clonic seizures, the duration of tonic–clonic seizures, and the total seizure score. They assessed glial fibrillary acidic protein (GFAP) release and the expression levels of erythroid-associated Factor 2 (Nrf2), c-fos, and 3-nitrotyrosine (3-NT) in the frontal cortex. This study revealed that treatment with β-caryophyllene combined with PGB increased the latency of PTZ-induced myoclonic and tonic–clonic seizures and decreased the durations of tonic–clonic seizures and overall seizure score. Additionally, lower expression levels of GFAP, c-Fos, and 3-NT were observed in animals treated with β-caryophyllene and PGB. The authors suggested that β-caryophyllene and PGB may have synergistic effects on controlling PTZ-induced seizures.

Qureshi et al. [510] evaluated the combined antiseizure effect of pregabalin (PGB) and nimodipine (NMD) in a mouse model of acute seizures. The study showed that the combination of pregabalin and nimodipine treatment had a significant protective effect on death at a dose of 30 ± 2.5 mg/kg. In addition, protection against mortality was highly significant at doses ranging from 35 ± 5 mg/kg to 55 ± 15 mg/kg. This effect was superior to that of PGB, showing a synergistic effect. The authors speculated that NMD and PGB had synergistic anticonvulsant effects. However, clinical studies are needed to determine the effectiveness of this combination in humans.

Imran et al. [511] described the effects of PGB on changes in abundance of acetylcholine-related energy metabolites and oxidative stress during SE. The results showed that acetylcholine (ACh) release increased by a factor of six to eight, glucose levels increased by 30%, lactate levels increased by a factor of four, extracellular glycerol concentrations increased by a factor of 10, and isoprostane levels increased by a factor of more than 20 after SE. Two hours after the administration of pilocarpine, pregabalin (100 mg/kg) was injected intraperitoneally, and the seizures eventually stopped. Within 60–120 min, the release of ACh decreased. The lactate/pyruvate ratio and glycerol and isoprostane levels were also significantly reduced. The authors noted that ACh release in the hippocampus was closely related to seizures in SE. This effect was attenuated upon regression of SE. Pregabalin treatment terminated seizures in a rat model of SE and attenuated cholinergic and metabolic changes within 2 h.

Pregabalin in the Treatment of Pain

Tong et al. [512] evaluated the efficacy and safety of pregabalin for treating spinal cord injury (SCI)-related neuropathic pain. A total of eight RCTs involving four interventions (pregabalin, gabapentin, CBZ, and amitriptyline) were included in this study. Analysis of the results showed that according to the average pain intensity after treatment, the treatments in order of efficacy were pregabalin, gabapentin, amitriptyline, CBZ and placebo. Based on the proportion of patients who discontinued therapy due to adverse reactions, the order of drugs from highest to lowest was pregabalin, amitriptyline, CBZ, gabapentin and placebo. In addition, five studies described the overall incidence of related adverse reactions, with pregabalin, gabapentin, and placebo representing the order of drugs from highest to lowest. The authors concluded that for patients with SCI-related neuropathic pain, pregabalin was most effective for relieving pain, while gabapentin performed better in terms of safety.

Onakpoya et al. [513] conducted a meta-analysis of the benefits and disadvantages of pregabalin for treating neuropathic pain. A total of 28 trials (6087 participants) were reviewed. The types of neuropathic pain explored included diabetic peripheral neuropathy, postherpetic neuralgia, sciatica (radicular pain), poststroke pain and SCI-related pain. The results showed that patients taking pregabalin reported a significant reduction in Numeric Rating Scale (NRS) pain scores compared to those taking the placebo ($p < 0.00001$). The sleep disturbance score of the NRS was significantly reduced ($p < 0.00001$). However, the risk of adverse events significantly increased ($p < 0.00001$). Treatment was more likely to be discontinued due to adverse events ($p < 0.00001$). The authors suggested that pregabalin may be beneficial for certain symptoms of neuropathic pain. However, the increased risk of adverse events and associated discontinuation should be considered.

To understand the analgesic effects of pregabalin on chronic neuropathic pain in adults, Derry et al. [514] reviewed 45 randomized controlled trials (RCTs) with a total of 11,906 participants for 2–16 weeks of treatment. Postherpetic neuralgia, painful diabetic peripheral neuropathy, and mixed neuropathic pain accounted for the majority (85%). Treatment groups for the drug pregabalin were divided into those receiving 150, 300 and 600 mg and compared with the placebo group. Research suggested that pregabalin is effective for treating postherpetic neuralgia, diabetes-related neuralgia and mixed or unclassified posttraumatic neuropathic pain but not for treating HIV-related neuralgia. There is insufficient evidence for the efficacy of PGB in treating central neuropathic pain. It had substantial effects on some patients. A subset of patients achieved moderate improvement. However, many patients do not achieve obvious effects or even stopped treatment.

2.1.2.6 Clobazam

Drug Characteristics

[Chemical name] 7-Chloro-1-methyl-5-phenyl-1,5-diazepine-2,4 (3H)-dione

[Chemical structure]

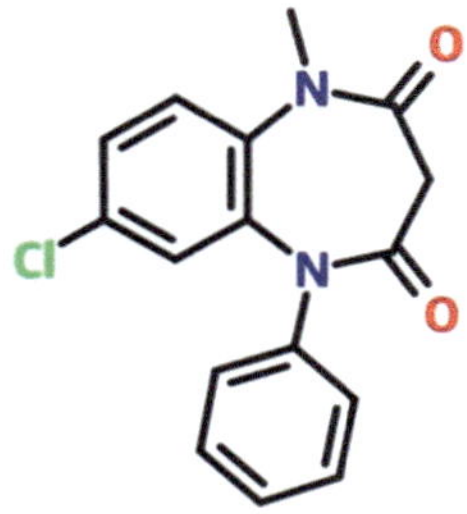

[Molecular formula] C16H13ClN2O2

[Molecular weight] 300.74

[Indications] For the treatment of refractory epilepsy in which other ASMs are ineffective, it can be used alone or as an adjuvant treatment. It is more effective for generalized seizures secondary to complex partial seizures and Lennox-Gaslaut syndrome.

[Specification] 10 mg, 20 mg

[Dosage]
Oral administration is started with a small dose of 20–30 mg (0.5–1 mg/kg) per day, and the dose is gradually increased. When combined with other ASMs, the dose of this product should be reduced, and 5–15 mg (0.1–0.3 mg/kg) should be administered daily.

If it is used continuously, its anticonvulsant effect gradually weakens, and "holiday therapy" can be used; for example, during the onset of menstruation, female patients can start the drug 2–3 days before the onset of menstruation and stop using it after 10 days.

[Adverse reactions]
The adverse effects are similar to those of other benzodiazepines, but they are all mild, with occasional mild sedation, agitation, depression, and muscle weakness.

Clinical Application and Basic Research

Historical Evolution of Clobazam

Clobazam was synthesized in 1966 and began to be used worldwide as an anxiolytic and antiseizure drug in the 1970s. In 2005, clobazam was used in Canada as an additive for epilepsy-related generalized tonic–clonic seizures, myoclonic seizures, and focal-onset perceptual impairment seizures [515]. In 2011, the US Food and Drug Administration (FDA) approved clobazam as an adjunct treatment for seizures in patients ≥2 years of age with Lennox–Gastaut syndrome (LGS) [516]. Indications not approved by the FDA include adjuvant therapy for Dravet syndrome seizures, adjuvant therapy for refractory status epilepticus, and adjuvant therapy for refractory focal epilepsy, menstrual epilepsy, and anxiety disorders [517]. In 2021, Nupur et al. reported that clobazam can be used as an add-on antiseizure medication treatment for tumor-related epilepsy (TRE) [518].

Clobazam Monotherapy Efficacy

A substantial clinical investigation conducted in Canada demonstrated the efficacy of clobazam monotherapy in children afflicted with partial epilepsy or generalized tonic–clonic seizures. Notably, clobazam was found to be as effective as phenytoin and CBZ but exhibited fewer side effects, such as rash, than the other two agents. Consequently, the Canadian Child Epilepsy Study Group has recommended clobazam as the primary treatment option for focal epilepsy and generalized tonic–clonic seizures in children [519]. Despite the scarcity of high-quality randomized controlled trials on clobazam monotherapy, a pooled analysis from a 2018 Cochrane Review of three clinical trials suggested that clobazam monotherapy may be comparably effective to CBZ and phenytoin for new-onset focal or generalized epilepsy [520]. The researchers administered clobazam monotherapy to 25 children with epilepsy for a duration of 26 months, revealing a notable decrease in seizure frequency in 75% of the participants. Although studies on clobazam monotherapy in adults with epilepsy are limited, small-scale investigations have indicated its efficacy in this population as well [521]. Another group conducted a study involving 26 adult patients with epilepsy in which 64% of patients achieved seizure freedom and 84% experienced a reduction of over 50% in seizure frequency following 24 weeks of clobazam monotherapy [522]. Moreover, clobazam has been reported to be effective and well tolerated among pediatric patients, resulting in a significant reduction in seizure rates (57.3%), with a favorable overall treatment response and a low incidence of seizure recurrence [523].

Efficacy and Safety of Clobazam as an Adjuvant Treatment for Epilepsy

Alisha Jami et al. conducted a single-center, retrospective chart review involving patients over 18 years of age with drug-resistant epilepsy who received clobazam therapy between 2010 and 2018. These patients underwent outpatient visits both before and 1 month after commencing clobazam therapy. The findings indicated that clobazam is an effective and safe long-term adjunctive treatment for drug-resistant epilepsy in adults, with off-label use demonstrating efficacy similar to that in Lennox–Gastaut syndrome patients. Level IV evidence from various studies suggests that clobazam is efficacious in treating drug-resistant epilepsy in adults, irrespective of epilepsy classification [524]. Talwar A et al. reported that CBZ is effective as both a stand-alone therapy and in combination with clobazam for controlling seizures in DS, LGS, and TSC patients while limiting side effects [525]. Nagarajan, E. et al. evaluated the tolerability of clobazam in patients aged 50 years and older with drug-resistant epilepsy and concluded that clobazam represents a safe and well-tolerated adjunctive treatment for older individuals with drug-resistant epilepsy [526].

Efficacy of Clobazam in Other Refractory Epilepsy

Clobazam has been utilized in various countries for treating different types of epilepsy, particularly refractory epilepsy. In a retrospective study involving 877 adults and children with refractory epilepsy, the addition of clobazam to a treatment regimen led to a greater than 50% reduction in seizure frequency and demonstrated efficacy across all seizure types [527]. Another single-center retrospective study in the United States spanning 2010–2018 involving 417 adults with refractory epilepsy revealed that approximately half of the patients experienced a 50% reduction in seizure frequency with clobazam treatment, and 17% of patients remained seizure-free after more than 1 year of follow-up. Clobazam was also effective in treating focal epilepsy, generalized epilepsy, and Lennox–Gastaut syndrome [524]. In a study conducted in India involving 88 children with refractory epilepsy, clobazam was found to be effective as an adjunctive therapy for all epilepsy types, with 60.2% of the children achieving complete seizure control [528]. A Cochrane review that pooled data from four clinical studies, predominantly involving individuals with focal refractory epilepsy, concluded that clobazam as an adjunctive therapy may be effective for drug-refractory focal epilepsy. Additionally, numerous small-scale clinical studies have demonstrated the effectiveness of clobazam as an adjunctive therapy for refractory epilepsy in both adults and children. In recent years, clobazam has also been employed for refractory status epilepticus, with control achieved in 76.5% of patients when clobazam is used as an adjunctive therapy.

Observation of the Efficacy of Clobazam as an Adjuvant Treatment for Other Refractory Epilepsy

Brain tumor-associated epilepsy (TRE) often shows resistance to currently available ASMs. While clobazam was initially approved as an adjunct ASMs for patients with Lennox–Gastaut syndrome, it has also shown promise in managing TRE. An observational study investigating the impact of clobazam on seizure frequency in patients with primary CNS tumors revealed that clobazam effectively reduced seizure frequency, yielding a response rate of 93.9% [518]. Moreover, the addition of clobazam not only significantly improved seizure frequency but also aided in reducing the burden of multiple ASMs combinations typically used to manage seizures in this patient population. This simplification of treatment options is particularly beneficial for patients who already have to take numerous medications for cancer treatment or comorbidities. Future research should include prospective studies utilizing clobazam as a first-line agent and comparative studies assessing clobazam against other ASMs as adjunctive therapy in this population. In a separate report, Maille et al. documented successful treatment of drug-resistant seizures through the addition of clobazam in Heidenhain-variant Creutzfeldt–Jakob disease (CJD), suggesting potential clinical benefits of clobazam in patients with suspected CJD [529]. Serrano-Castro PJ et al. showed that the combination of sambicaut (CNB) + clobazam (CLB) may be an individualized regimen for patients with anti-GAD65-associated AAEs [530]. Cannabidiol (CBD) and clobazam (CLB) are important factors for enhancing antiepileptic effects during simultaneous use in patients with refractory epilepsy [531].

Application of Clobazam in Special Populations with Epilepsy

Kamaşak et al. conducted a retrospective cohort study involving 1710 children with epilepsy across eight centers and demonstrated the efficacy and tolerability of clobazam. The study revealed that clobazam significantly reduced seizure rates by 57.3% and exhibited a low rate of seizure recurrence, providing substantial reversible benefits in pediatric patients [523]. Another group reported that clobazam serves as a potent adjunctive antiseizure medication for brain tumor-associated epilepsy (TRE), with 94% of patients experiencing a significant response within 6 months. Sharma et al. identified eosinophilic systemic symptoms syndrome (DRESS syndrome) as a novel symptom associated with clobazam [532].

Side Effects of Clobazam

Regarding the side effects of clobazam, Jeff F. Zhang et al. described a female pediatric patient who developed significant tongue swelling, protruding outside the oral cavity, following treatment for refractory epilepsy with clobazam. Symptoms did not respond to antihistamines or steroids but gradually resolved within a few days after discontinuation of clobazam, with no lasting effects. This suggests that macroglossia may be a potential side effect associated with clobazam in the treatment of drug-resistant epilepsy [533]. Kart PÖ et al. reported that long-term administration of ASMs, including zonisamide, sultiam, lacosamide, clobazam, and rufinamide, from prepuberty to adulthood could lead to follicular apoptosis and disruption of follicular development in nonepileptic rats [534]. Furthermore, a pharmacokinetic trial demonstrated that concurrent administration of sembacot and chlorocazam resulted in a significant increase in the serum concentration of N-desmethylclobazam. While this could have a positive therapeutic effect, it may also lead to unnecessary fatigue [535].

Basic Research on Clobazam

Clobazam, by binding to the γ-aminobutyric acid-A (GABAA) receptor, increases the seizure threshold and enhances GABA action by facilitating chloride-responsive ligand-binding channel conduction. Unlike those of typical benzodiazepines, the nitrogen atoms of clobazam occupy the first and fifth positions of the diazepine ring, resulting in partial agonism of the GABA-A receptor rather than the first and fourth positions found in other benzodiazepines, which act as full agonists. This structural alteration, leading to increased binding affinity for the $\alpha 2\beta 3\gamma 2$ isoform of GABA-A, not only improves side effects but also enhances its anxiolytic and antiepileptic properties [536].

Evidence-Based Medical Studies of Clobazam

Evidence-based medical studies spanning the 1980s have demonstrated the efficacy of clobazam as an ASMs across more than 100 countries. Early clinical trials revealed that more than half of patients experienced a reduction in seizure frequency of more than 50%, with 42% achieving sustained benefits for more than a year. Remarkably, up to 10% of patients with refractory epilepsy achieved remission over a retrospective study period of up to 7 years. Two multicenter controlled studies confirmed the efficacy of clobazam as an adjunctive treatment for seizures in patients with Lennox–Gastaut syndrome (LGS). The participants in these studies exhibited characteristics similar to those of patients treated with other ASMs, including sodium valproate, lamotrigine, levetiracetam, and topiramate. The primary efficacy endpoint was the percentage reduction in weekly fall frequency, encompassing atonic, myotonic, and myoclonic seizures, compared to baseline. Notably, the high-dose clobazam group demonstrated a significant decrease in fall episodes compared to the low-dose group (93% vs. 29%, respectively, $p < 0.05$), with most adverse reactions being mild to moderate and showing no statistically significant differences between the two groups [537]. A meta-analysis examining patients taking clobazam in conjunction with other medications, including CBD, revealed a greater incidence of drowsiness and sedation. Notably, the combination of valproate and clobazam may lead to elevated aminotransferase levels, albeit to a lesser extent. Overall, the addition of CBD and clobazam effectively reduces seizures, albeit with an increased likelihood of drowsiness and sedation in patients taking both medications [538].

2.1.2.7 Felbamate

Drug Characteristics

[Chemical name] 2-Phenyl-1,3-propanediol dicarbamate

[Chemical structural formula]

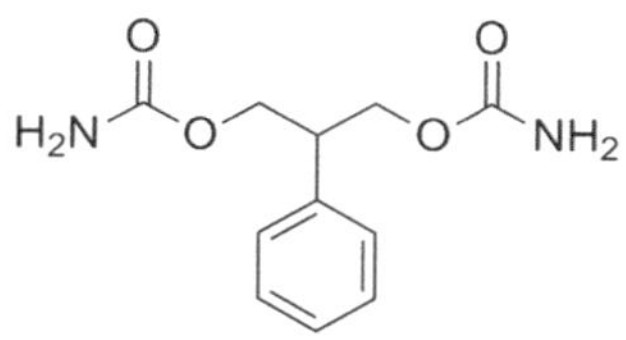

[Molecular formula] C11H14N2O4

[Molecular weight] 238.24

[Adaptation disease] (1) Adjuvant therapy and monotherapy for partial seizures and secondary general seizures in adults and children; (2) Adjuvant treatment of Lennox–Gastaut syndrome and its associated partial and general episodes; (3) Treatment of primary generalized tonic–clonic convulsions or seizures of absence; (4) Adjuvant treatment of refractory incomplete seizures.

[Specification] Tablet: 400 mg, 600 mg
Oral liquid: 600 mg/5 mL

[Usage and dosage]
Felbamate 1200–3600 mg/day.

The initial dose for the treatment of seizures in adults and children over 14 years of age is 1200 mg/day, divided into three to four oral doses, gradually increasing the dose to 600 mg every 2 weeks and up to 3600 mg/day depending on the individual's clinical response and tolerance. The initial dose of adjuvant therapy for the onset of Lennox–Gastaut syndrome in children aged 2–14 years is 15 mg/kg/day in three to four oral doses. It can be increased by 15 mg/kg/day per week, up to 45 mg/kg/day or 3600 mg/day depending on the individual's clinical response and tolerance. In elderly patients or those with renal insufficiency, the amount of felbamate should be reduced as appropriate. When combined with phenytoin, CBZ and valproic acid, the dosage of the latter should be reduced based on clinical observation and steady-state blood concentrations.

[Adverse reactions]

The predominant adverse reactions include mild gastrointestinal and central nervous system symptoms, ranging from loss of appetite, taste alterations, and nausea to vomiting, fatigue, dizziness, and headache. Additionally, insomnia, double vision, ataxia, cognitive impairment, and gait disturbances may occur, as may influenza-like symptoms, palpitations, rashes, and weight loss. These adverse effects typically reverse upon discontinuation or dose adjustment. In postmarketing trials, two rare yet severe adverse events noted were aplastic anemia and hepatotoxicity. Notably, when used in combination therapy, this product tends to elicit more side effects than when it is used as a monotherapy.

Clinical Application and Basic Research

Historical Evolution of Felbamate

The precise mechanism of action of felbamate remains incompletely understood. Felbamate, which was originally developed by the Carter-Wallace Company in the United States, is recognized for its high efficacy and low toxicity as an antiseizure medication. Acting as a 5α-reductase inhibitor, it modulates NMDA and GABA reactions, exhibiting no direct affinity for NMDA receptors but binding to the glycine recognition site of NMDA. In animal models of epilepsy, felbamate has been shown to exhibit broad-spectrum antiepileptic activity. In 1985, A. J. Wilensky et al. evaluated the pharmacokinetics and toxicity of felbamate in 8 adult male patients with epilepsy, laying the groundwork for subsequent research [539]. A pivotal double-blind, randomized, placebo-controlled clinical trial conducted by I. E. Leppik et al. in 1991 demonstrated the safety and efficacy of felbamate as an adjunct treatment for severe refractory epilepsy, with mild adverse reactions primarily comprising nausea and central nervous system effects [540]. This study provides compelling evidence supporting the integration of felbamate into epilepsy treatment protocols. In August 1993, Felbamate received approval from the United States FDA, marking it as the first new antiseizure medication since the approval of valproic acid in 1978 and the first anticonvulsant to exert dual effects on brain excitatory and inhibitory mechanisms. Subsequent research, including a study by M. Gasior et al. in 1998, highlighted Felbamate's distinct profile, including its reduced interaction potential with Ca2+ channel modulators and methylxanthine, thereby broadening the scope of nonammonia ester applications [541]. This, as one of its advantages, broadens the application range of nonammonia esters. In 2004, K K Borowicz et al. conducted a study and reported that the combination of felbamate and CBZ may be useful for patients with drug-resistant partial epilepsy [542]. Further investigations, such as the 2004 study by K. K. Borowicz et al., suggested the potential utility of combining felbamate with CBZ for patients with drug-resistant partial epilepsy [543]. In 2014, Eli Heyman et al. advocated for the early use of felbamate in children with refractory epilepsy based on accumulating efficacy and safety data. More recently, a 2024 study by Laurel Reed et al. highlighted Felbamate's effectiveness in treating epilepsy with myoclonic atonic seizures (EMAtSs), emphasizing its importance in treatment strategies [544]. The continual emergence of research underscores the ongoing exploration of the diverse clinical applications of felbamate in epilepsy management.

Observational Study of Felbamate Treatment for Epilepsy

Between January 1, 2015, and June 30, 2018, samples were collected from three U.S. databases by Wilcox et al. Nine compounds were tested, and five types of liver tests (LTs) were conducted. The aim of this concise investigation was to outline the LT compliance of patients using compounds recommended for monitoring at intervals of 2 weeks or more across three U.S. administrative claims databases. The findings revealed that adherence was less than 33% for patients using each of four drugs (ketoconazole, succinic acid, pentamidine, and felbamate) and exceeded 60% for patients using each of five drugs (oxaliplatin, rifampicin, albendazole, and azathioprine). Among the investigated drugs (excluding succinic acid), patients using oxaliplatin exhibited the highest LT adherence (75.3%), whereas those using pentamidine showed the lowest (20.6%). The researchers concluded that patients using the examined drugs displayed varying levels of adherence to frequent liver tests, with none reaching 80% adherence [545].

Treatment of Refractory Epilepsy with the Addition of Felbamate

The Felbamate Study Group undertook a double-blinded, placebo-controlled, add-on trial to assess the efficacy and safety of felbamate in patients with Lennox–Gastaut syndrome, enrolling 73 patients with the syndrome aged 4–36 years. Patients received conventional antiepileptic therapy over a baseline period of 28 days. Following this phase, patients received an additional 70 days of either felbamate or placebo therapy alongside their existing ASMs. During the initial 14 days of treatment, the nonammonia dose was titrated to 45 mg/kg/day or 3600 mg/day, whichever was lower. Primary efficacy measures included the total number of seizures during a 4-h videotaped period, overall quality of life assessment by the parent or guardian, and total number of atonic seizures reported. The results indicated a 34% reduction in atonic seizure frequency among patients treated with felbamate compared with a 9% reduction in the placebo group ($P = 0.01$). Additionally, the total seizure frequency decreased by 19% in the felbamate group versus a 4% increase in the placebo group ($P = 0.002$). From Day 49 onward, overall assessment scores were significantly greater in the felbamate group than in the placebo group. There was no significant difference in seizure frequency between the control and video monitoring groups ($P > 0.05$), but during the maintenance period, seizures were notably reduced in the nonammonia ester group ($P = 0.017$). The incidence and frequency of adverse reactions were comparable between the two groups. The authors suggest that felbamate is superior to placebo in reducing the frequency of refractory partial seizures and is beneficial for patients with Lennox–Gastaut syndrome. Improved seizure control and quality of life in treatment-resistant patients, along with a favorable safety profile, indicate that felbamate represents a significant advancement in epilepsy treatment [546]. Heyman et al. documented their experience with felbamate in treating drug-resistant epilepsy in children through a retrospective analysis of medical records and EEG recordings of all patients treated with felbamate before May 2012. Despite the introduction of numerous new ASMs over the past two decades, many individuals with epilepsy still experience uncontrolled seizures or significant side effects. Efficacy was assessed by comparing seizure frequency 1 week before starting treatment to that 1 week after reaching the maximum felbamate dose. The study included 50 patients (34 boys) aged between 4 months and 17 years (mean age 5.5 years), nearly one-third of whom were diagnosed with Lennox–Gastaut syndrome. The average duration of epilepsy was 3.4 years (ranging from 1 month to 13 years), with patients having previously tried an average of 7.5 ASMs. The mean follow-up duration was 1.1 years. Of the patients, 29 (58%) experienced at least a 50% reduction in seizure frequency. Side effects were reported in 22 patients (44%), none of whom had aplastic anemia or liver failure. In the group of responders, the maximum felbamate dose was lower, and the patients were older. The authors suggest initiating felbamate after multiple antiseizure medication trials. Early use of felbamate in children with refractory epilepsy is recommended based on its efficacy and safety profile [543]. Shi et al. published a review updating a previous review on "Felbamate as add-on therapy for refractory epilepsy" in the Cochrane Database of Reviews (Issue 7, 2014). This review evaluated the efficacy of felbamate as an adjunct treatment to standard drugs. The efficacy and tolerability of felbamate versus placebo as adjunctive therapy for patients with refractory focal seizures were examined. To gather recent information, the authors searched various databases and contacted manufacturers and experts for data from unpublished or ongoing studies. They included four randomized controlled trials involving 236 participants. The studies varied in design and risk of bias. Due to significant methodological and clinical heterogeneity, as well as differences in outcome measures, a meta-analysis could not be conducted. Only one study reported a 50% or greater reduction in seizure frequency, while others reported reductions in seizure frequency compared to placebo. Adverse reactions were more prevalent in the felbamate phase, especially headache, nausea, and dizziness. Given the methodological limitations and insufficient evidence, the authors call for large-scale randomized controlled trials over longer durations to guide clinical practice [547].

Felbamate Treatment for Epileptic Syndrome

Strzelczyk et al. performed a comprehensive examination of current and forthcoming treatment options for seizures linked with Lennox–Gastaut syndrome (LGS). LGS, a severe developmental and epileptic encephalopathy (DEE) that typically emerges in childhood, encompasses a diverse range of etiologies lacking a singular genetic cause. It manifests with various epilepsy types, abnormal EEG patterns, diffuse slow spike-wave discharges, and cognitive impairment and significantly impacts patient and family quality of life, often manifesting as drug-resistant epilepsy. In the United States, six adjunctive therapies are utilized for LGS-associated epilepsy: lamotrigine, clobazam, rufinamide, topiramate, felbamate, and most recently, cannabidiol. Research findings indicate seizure reduction in 15–68% of trial patients, with response rates (≥50% reduction in seizures) ranging from 37% to 78%. Valproate remains the preferred first-line treatment and is frequently combined with lamotrigine or clobazam. Ongoing clinical development includes the use of felbamate. Nonpharmacological interventions such as a ketogenic diet, vagus nerve stimulation, and surgical procedures also play roles. However, despite these advancements, patients still face significant challenges. Recognizing LGS heterogeneity, treatments must be individualized rather than adopting a one-size-fits-all approach. In conjunction with the approved medication lamotrigine or clobazam, valproate is used as a primary therapy, in combination with other adjunctive options, including rufinamide, topiramate, felbamate, and the recent addition of cannabidiol. Although felbamate is FDA-approved for use in the United States, it lacks approval from the European Medicines Agency (EMA) due to the risks of aplastic anemia and liver failure. However, its anticonvulsant mechanism remains unclear. Early epilepsy models suggest that it increases the seizure threshold and impedes seizure propagation, potentially effectively preventing generalized tonic–clonic or partial seizures. Felbamate primarily reduces glutamate-energy transfer and may inhibit GABA receptor binding to voltage-gated sodium and calcium channels. The authors advocate for further research on the etiology and pathophysiology of LGS and advancements in seizure treatment, encompassing the spectrum of symptoms associated with this intricate syndrome [548].

Felbamate Treats Refractory and Super Refractory Status Epilepsy

Mazarati et al. induced self-sustaining status epilepticus (SSSE) by stimulating the perforant pathway (PPS) through permanent electrode implantation in male adult Wistar rats for 30 min. This was followed by intravenous administration of felbamate (FBM; at doses of 50, 100, and 200 mg/kg), diazepam (DZP; 10 mg/kg), or phenytoin (PHT; 50 mg/kg). They examined the effects of FBM in SSSE animal models and compared them with those of standard ASMs, DZP, and PHT. They analyzed the electrographic manifestations of SSSE and the severity of SSSE-induced neuronal damage. Although both DZP and PHT were highly effective in the initial status epilepticus (SE) model, they failed to halt the SSSE after 10 and 40 min (i.e., seizure duration >30 min). Although FBM did not terminate SSSE under advanced treatment conditions, it was still more effective than PHT. The effects of FBM were enduring, with no subsequent seizure activity observed. The efficacy of FBM was found to be dose dependent, and required high doses of ASMs. The effective dose of FBM in this study surpassed the highest dose used in treatment trials. Administering FBM early in SSSE (10 min after PPS termination) shortened the seizure duration in a dose-dependent manner. The anticonvulsant effect of FBM was validated by the finding of less severe neuronal damage in the FBM group than in the control group. The quantity of FBM needed to halt SSSE exceeded the anticonvulsant dose and resembled the neuroprotective dose. The authors speculate that this is because SE requires more vigorous treatment than standard seizures and because FBM is a relatively weak NMDA receptor antagonist. FBM, a clinically available antiseizure medication with moderate affinity for the glycine site of the NMDA receptor, exhibited robust antiepileptic protective effects in SSSE animal models. These findings suggest that FBM might be beneficial when standard ASMs fail in refractory status epilepticus patients. Drugs that act on the NMDA receptor show promise for treating refractory status epileptic disorder. In addition to its anticonvulsant effect, FBM displays potent neuroprotective effects against excitotoxic injury during hypoxia, global cerebral ischemia, and ischemia, making it a potential candidate for status epilepticus treatment. In conclusion, the high efficacy and low acute toxicity of FBM in the treatment of SSSE make it a promising candidate for SSSE treatment and worthy of further evaluation [549].

Application of Felbamate in Special Epileptic Populations

Yerby et al. described a case involving a 32-year-old man who had been receiving valproate (VPA) monotherapy for epilepsy for 4 years, during which his wife had faced infertility issues. The man's fertility evaluation revealed a severely low sperm count, a lack of sperm motility, 100% structural abnormalities, and normal levels of follicle-stimulating hormone, luteinizing hormone, and testosterone. Due to worsening seizure frequency, he transitioned from VPA monotherapy (at 3500 mg/day) to felbamate monotherapy (at 2400 mg/day) over a 2-month period to enhance seizure control. Four months later, the couple successfully conceived their second child. Upon re-examination, the patient's sperm count significantly improved, with 50% motility [550]. Mishal et al. presented a case study to explore how felbamate monotherapy exerted a potent antiepileptic effect in a unique patient, potentially offering a new treatment avenue for individuals with tuberous sclerosis (TSC) and neurofibromatosis (NF)-associated epilepsy. The patient, a 15-year-old girl, inherited NF1 from her mother and TSC from her father, making her the sole reported case in the literature with both conditions inherited simultaneously rather than due to sporadic mutations. Intractable epilepsy began at the age of 5, with seizures resistant to adequate doses of four ASMs until felbamate therapy was initiated at age 7. Since then, she has remained seizure-free on felbamate monotherapy. Although felbamate acts through multiple mechanisms, its most potent antiepileptic effect is believed to occur via N-methyl-D-aspartate receptor (NMDAR) inhibition. Studies have indicated alterations in NMDARs in various epileptic syndromes, particularly cortical nodules, in patients with TSC. The authors advocate for further research on the potential role of felbamate or other NMDAR antagonists in epileptic syndromes with NMDAR alterations [551]. Rabinowicz S et al. conducted a retrospective analysis of the medical records of patients treated with felbamate at a tertiary pediatric epilepsy clinic from 2009 to 2021. Among the 53 children treated with felbamate, 16 received treatment for epileptic states during sleep, and six received treatment during both wakefulness and sleep. Of these, 37 patients (51%) achieved a ≥50% response to treatment, with nine patients (12%) experiencing a complete response. Adverse reactions occurred in 19 patients (25%), including three patients with elevated liver enzymes and one patient with neutropenia. However, treatment could be continued in all patients. All the children with refractory epilepsy after herpetic encephalitis responded to felbamate. Thus, felbamate has emerged as a safe and effective antiseizure medication for children [552].

Felbamate Is a Preferred Addition for the Treatment of Epilepsy Due to its Efficacy and Safety

Hussain et al. conducted a comprehensive retrospective evaluation of the efficacy, safety, and tolerability of felbamate in a large single-center cohort of children with epileptic spasms. Among 476 infants, 62 children treated with felbamate were identified, all of whom had video-EEG-confirmed epileptic spasms, 58 of had previously failed to respond to hormone therapy. Nonammonia exposure was assessed by calculating the peak and weighted doses per average body weight. Clinical response was defined as remission of epileptic spasms for at least 28 days, starting no more than 3 months after initiating felbamate. An electroclinical response was defined as a clinical response accompanied by a nighttime video EEG showing the absence of epileptic spasms and a high degree of arrhythmia. The median peak dose and weighted average dose of felbamate were 47 and 40 mg/kg/day, respectively. Five children (8%) were classified as clinical responders, and two (3%) were classified as electroclinical responders. Four of 17 patients (24%) were observed to be clinical responders with a latency period of less than 12 months from seizure spasmodic onset to nonammonia initiation. The authors suggest that felbamate may be effective in treating epileptic spasms, but further rigorous studies are warranted. They posited that a higher dose or faster titration may lead to a greater response rate [553]. Dozieres-Puyravel et al. conducted a 10-year retrospective study of infants with epileptic spasms who underwent continuous EEG recordings after first-line treatment to evaluate the efficacy of felbamate in refractory infantile spasms/West syndrome. A total of 29 infants were enrolled, with a mean age of 13.8 months. Starting felbamate therapy after continuous administration or in combination with oral steroids, 23 infants were transitioned to a ketogenic diet. Eight infants continued to experience spasms after a mean dose of 34.6 mg/kg/day of felbamate. Among the 19 infants who discontinued felbamate, the average duration of use was 19 months, and no serious side effects were observed. Reversible neutropenia led to felbamate discontinuation in six patients. One patient experienced spasm relapse upon felbamate discontinuation. The authors highlighted the sustained seizure control achieved by patients with refractory infantile spasms syndrome, underscoring the need to assess the benefit–risk ratio for each patient when considering felbamate use. This study also underscores the potential of targeting NMDA receptors for the treatment of infantile spasm syndrome, potentially paving the way for the development of novel therapeutic agents [554]. de Jong et al. conducted a literature review and identified 30 articles that met the inclusion criteria to investigate potential associations between various newer ASMs and specific congenital abnormalities. This study focused on lamotrigine, topiramate, levetiracetam, gabapentin, oxcarbazepine, CBZ, felbamate, pregabalin, rufinamide, tiagabine, and zonisamide. Congenital abnormalities were classified according to the European Surveillance for Congenital

Abnormalities subgroups. The prevalence of specific congenital abnormalities in fetuses exposed to individual ASMs was compared with the prevalence in the general population reference database. A significantly higher incidence, based on three or more abnormal fetuses, was considered a signal. Compared with other newer ASMs topiramate was associated with a greater rate of congenital abnormalities, with a strong association between topiramate and cleft lip with/without cleft palate and hypospadias. A link between lamotrigine and anencephaly and transposition of large blood vessels was observed in one study but was not supported by others. No congenital abnormalities were found in fetuses exposed to felbamate, pregabalin, tiagabine, or zonisamide. No signal was found for other newer ASMs, or the data were too limited to draw conclusions. The authors recommend further investigation of topiramate and its association with cleft lip with/without cleft palate and hypospadias in pregnancies during the first trimester with the use of newer ASM monotherapy. Due to the low number of observations, no conclusions could be drawn about the risk of congenital abnormalities with other newer ASMs [555]. One study reported an average reduction in number of seizures of 35.8% with the addition of felbamate, while another reported a smaller reduction of 4.2%. Both studies noted an increase in seizure frequency with the addition of a placebo. Significantly, there was a notable difference in seizure reduction between the felbamate and placebo groups, with the discontinuation rate remaining low (below 10%) in the felbamate group, indicating good tolerability of felbamate [556].

Evidence-Based Medical Research Regarding Felbamate

Zhang et al. undertook a systematic review and network meta-analysis, pooling data from eight randomized controlled trials (RCTs) involving 1171 patients with Lennox–Gastaut syndrome (LGS), to assess the effectiveness and safety of ASMs (ASMs) for LGS. The analysis included six RCTs investigating lamotrigine, rufinamide, cannabidiol, topiramate, clobazam, and felbamate. The efficacy and safety of felbamate have been reported to reduce the monthly frequency of seizures by at least 50% in terms of reduced seizures, drop-outs, and serious adverse events. The results were ranked using the surface under the cumulative ranking curve (SUCRA). Felbamate, cannabidiol, and topiramate emerged as having the highest likelihood of efficacy according to the calculated SUCRA values. However, no significant differences were detected among these treatments. Cannabidiol, topiramate, and felbamate were associated with higher rates of withdrawal. Additionally, patients treated with cannabidiol had a significantly greater rate of premature discontinuation than those receiving placebo or lamotrigine. The response rates were significantly greater in all ASM groups than in the placebo group. The SUCRA rankings suggested that felbamate and cannabidiol were more effective than other treatments in reducing epilepsy, although there were no significant differences between them. In the five RCTs with no reported seizures, no significant disparities were found among treatments, nor were they deemed more effective than placebo. SUCRA rankings indicated that topiramate, felbamate, and cannabidiol outperformed the other ASMs. However, lamotrigine, cannabidiol, and felbamate were associated with a higher incidence of serious adverse events [431]. Another group conducted a comprehensive review of the literature, encompassing randomized controlled trials (RCTs) and open-label extension (OLE) studies, to compare ASMs with either placebo or other ASMs in patients with Lennox–Gastaut syndrome (LGS), aiming to assess the short- and long-term comparative efficacy and safety of ASMs in this context. Their analysis involved 15 studies comprising 1263 LGS patients aged 2–54 years who received treatment with six different ASMs (CBD, clobazam (CLB), felbamate (FLB), lamotrigine (LTG), rufinamide (RFM), topiramate (TPM)), or placebo. A reduction of ≥50% in seizure frequency from baseline and the occurrence of therapeutic emergent adverse events (TEAEs) were the primary efficacy and safety outcomes. High doses of CLB (1.0 mg/kg/day; CLB_H) [or: 4.9; 95% confidence interval: 2.3–10.8] reduced seizure frequency by ≥50% compared with placebo and obtained a high probability (0.89) based on SUCRA values (despite overlap between the effect sizes of CLB, RFM, and CBD) compared with high doses of CBD (20 mg/kg/day; CBD_H) [or: 3.8; 95% confidence interval: 1.6–9.0], which had a greater chance of any treatment-related emergent adverse event (TEAEs) and the highest ranking probability (0.85). Long-term use of CLB was associated with a greater proportion of patients experiencing reduced seizures (78%; 95% CI: 70–85%), while long-term use of CBD was linked to a greater frequency of TEAE occurrence (96%; 95% CI: 95–98%). Short-term results, reported as odds ratios (ORs) using a network meta-analysis (NMA), were accompanied by 95% confidence intervals (CIs) and levels of competitive intervention (cumulative ranking under the curve (SUCRA)). Additionally, the ratio of long-term outcomes to 95% CIs was calculated using a random effects model. The authors propose that CLB_H, CBD, and RFM are the most effective and safest options in both the short and long term, with CLB_H likely exhibiting superior efficacy. Future comparative trials directly comparing these ASMs are needed to further elucidate their comparative effectiveness and safety profiles [557].

Effects of Felbamate on EEG and Cognitive Function

To evaluate the evidence concerning cognitive changes linked with ASM therapy in children with epilepsy, Beyag et al. conducted an extensive review of the literature indexed in PubMed. Cognitive impairment frequently accompanies epilepsy and might be induced or exacerbated by ASMs, although certain ASMs may have beneficial effects on cognition. The ASM under scrutiny aligns with the current edition of the UK National Prescription (BNF). Although there is a paucity of reliable data on cognitive deficits in pediatric patients for most ASMs, some studies have indicated that phenobarbital treatment may be associated with cognitive impairment. Similarly, negative impacts on cognition, particularly word recognition differences and other language deficits, have been linked to topiramate and phenytoin, although specific data regarding children are scarce. On the other hand, lamotrigine and levetiracetam have been shown to be associated with improvements in certain cognitive domains, albeit whether these deficits stem directly from drug treatment or improved seizure management remains ambiguous. Available evidence suggests that phenobarbital, phenytoin, and topiramate impair neurocognitive functioning, while levetiracetam, felbamate, and particularly lamotrigine may be linked to cognitive improvements. CBZ, ethosuximide, lacosamide, oxcarbazepine, perampanel, and valproate do not seem to pose significant risks of cognitive deterioration. Data on cannabidiol, clobazam, eslicarbazepine, eslicarbazepine acetate, rufinamide, vigabatrin, and zonisamide are limited, but existing studies suggest that these drugs are not associated with severe cognitive impairments. Insufficient data exist to draw firm conclusions regarding brivaracetam, felbamate, gabapentin, pregabalin, retigabine, stiripentol, and tiagabine. Felbamate, a second-generation ASM, received initial regulatory approval in 1993 as an adjunct treatment for focal and generalized seizures associated with Lennox–Gastaut syndrome (LGS). However, subsequent limitations on felbamate use stemmed from concerns regarding liver toxicity and the risk of aplastic anemia, limiting its usage to patients with severe refractory epilepsy. Felbamate has various modes of action, primarily by modulating N-methyl-D-aspartate (NMDA) receptors to inhibit glutaminergic transmission for its antiepileptic effect. Limited information is available on the cognitive deficits associated with felbamate, and no studies have specifically evaluated cognitive ability in pediatric patients receiving felbamate treatment. An open-label study involving children with LGS treated with felbamate indicated enhancements in cognitive and behavioral function based on responses to a parent/caregiver questionnaire. Notably, improvements in social, intellectual, and motor functions; attention; alertness; initiative; performance; and memory variability were observed. However, upon discontinuation of felbamate, these symptoms tended to diminish, possibly correlating with reduced seizure frequency. The authors emphasize the inadequacy of data on felbamate to draw definitive conclusions and advocate for future studies on ASMs in young individuals to incorporate standardized assessments of cognition and behavior. They recommend routine monitoring of patients undergoing ASM treatment, including evaluation of underlying cognitive deficits, with dosage adjustments or medication changes as needed to mitigate adverse cognitive outcomes [78].

Effect of the Addition of Felbamate on Patient Quality of Life

Buraniqi et al. conducted a systematic study reviewing the impact of antiseizure medication (ASM) use on appetite and weight in children. Randomized controlled trials and open-label studies (open-label extension and intervention studies) involving children aged 0–18 years were included. Each study was classified according to the American Academy of Neurology (AAN) Classification of Evidence for Therapeutic Research and was graded based on its effect on children's appetite and weight. ASMs linked to reduced appetite and/or weight loss include fenfluramine, topiramate, zonisamide, felbamate, rufinamide, stiripentol, cannabidiol, brivaracetam, and ethosuximide. Those with minimal impact on children's weight and appetite include oxcarbazepine, eslicarbazepine, lamotrigine, levetiracetam, lacosamide, CBZ, vigabatrin, and clobazam. Valproic acid is the ASM most closely associated with increased appetite and/or weight gain, with pregabalin and perampanel potentially causing moderate weight gain or increased appetite in children. Felbamate, which inhibits N-methyl-D-aspartic acid receptor currents and enhances GABAA activity, was approved by the FDA in 1993 for the treatment of focal epilepsy and Lennox–Gastaut syndrome in both adults and children. It was proposed as an adjunctive treatment for refractory infantile spasms. Rare but potentially life-threatening reactions such as aplastic anemia and liver failure with felbamate use typically manifest 6–12 months after treatment initiation, with one study indicating that patients with aplastic anemia are often older (17+ years) and have a history of ASM allergy, cytopenia, and/or autoimmune disease. Major pediatric studies have reported that 23–44% of patients experience decreased appetite and weight loss. In a randomized, placebo-controlled trial involving patients with Lennox–Gastaut syndrome, anorexia was significantly greater in nonamino acid-treated patients than in placebo-treated patients, although no significant weight loss was observed. Similar findings have been noted in other open-label studies including both adults and children. The authors assert that epilepsy ranks among the most common neurological disorders in children, with numerous potential factors influencing the growth of children with epilepsy, necessitating evaluation in cases of appetite and weight issues. ASMs carry potential adverse effects, many of which can impact appetite, thereby affecting normal growth and weight gain, potentially increasing the risk of underlying diseases and compromising treatment adherence. In addition to ASM-related effects, other factors to consider include potential causes, associated neurological disorders, comorbidities and their treatment impact, as well as physical activity levels and dietary habits [80].

Side Effects of Felbamate

Vidaurre et al. investigated the acute and chronic management of seizures in patients with advanced liver disease and examined the hepatotoxic potential of specific ASMs. Hepatotoxicity, a rare and unexpected side effect of ASMs treatment, poses challenges in selecting appropriate medications for patients with acute, symptomatic seizures or epilepsy complicating liver disease, given that most drugs are metabolized by the liver. The study recommended the use of novel ASMs with minimal or no liver metabolism, such as levetiracetam, lacosamide, topiramate, gabapentin, and pregabalin, as first-line treatments. Conversely, drugs extensively metabolized by the liver, such as valproic acid, phenytoin, and felbamate, should be reserved as last-option agents. In specific scenarios, such as acute intermittent porphyria, where exposure to most ASMs may trigger seizures; bromides, levetiracetam, gabapentin, and vigabatrin were deemed safer choices. For status epilepticus, levetiracetam and lacosamide are recommended as second-line treatments if benzodiazepines fail to control seizures. Notably, certain drugs, including valproic acid, phenytoin, and felbamate, are associated with well-established hepatotoxicity. Felbamate, primarily prescribed for Lennox–Gastaut syndrome or refractory epilepsy, inhibits enzymes of the P450 system, posing risks of liver toxicity and significant drug interactions. Studies have indicated a risk of liver failure with felbamate use ranging between 1:26,000 and 1:34,000, potentially lower than that of valproic acid-related hepatotoxicity. However, the factors contributing to this risk remain unidentified, although female sex and use of multiple concomitant therapies may elevate it. Liver failure can occur abruptly without warning signs. The authors emphasized the importance of physicians exercising vigilance regarding the pharmacokinetic characteristics and hepatotoxic potential of different ASMs in liver disease patients, recommending heightened awareness of clinical symptoms [558]. In a separate review, Jacob et al. explored the potential of therapeutic drug monitoring (TDM) for new ASMs, including eslicarbazepine acetate, felbamate, gabapentin, lacosamide, lamotrigine, levetiracetam, perampanel, pregabalin, rufinamide, retigabine, stiripentol, tiagabine, topiramate, vigabatrin, and zonisamide. This review detailed the relationships between serum drug concentrations, clinical effects, and adverse drug reactions for each ASMs, as well as various analytical methods for serum drug quantification. Retrospective and prospective data on serum drug concentration efficacy were also discussed. Additionally, the pharmacokinetic parameters, oral bioavailability, reference concentration ranges, and active metabolites of the new ASMs were proposed. TDM is considered crucial in epilepsy management because it aids in the treatment of uncontrolled seizures and clinical toxicity, enables personalized therapy, and accommodates variable or nonlinear pharmacokinetics. Serum concentrations of nonammonia drugs exhibited wide variability, with higher levels in patients with renal impairment and a dependence on age and renal function for an extended half-life. Clearance values were notably greater in children than in adults (20–65%). Propionaldehyde, an intermediate metabolite, poses risks of serious reproductive toxicity, rendering this drug contraindicated for patients with liver damage. Limited pharmacokinetic data during pregnancy and the presence of life-threatening adverse effects, such as hepatotoxicity and aplastic anemia, severely restrict felbamate use. Enzyme-induced ASMs may decrease the serum felbamate concentration, while enzyme inhibitors such as VPA can increase the serum felbamate concentration [559].

Basic Research on Felbamate

Celli et al. utilized PubMed to conduct a cross-search on "glutamate receptor and epilepsy," resulting in an outcome of 3170 reports. They further searched for "ionic glutamate receptor," "AMPA receptor," "NMDA receptor," "kainate receptor," "convulsive seizure," and "nonconvulsive seizure," selecting relevant papers for this review. This comprehensive review explored the involvement of ionotropic glutamate (iGlu) receptors in convulsive and nonconvulsive seizures and their duration and severity, with the aim of informing new strategies for treating drug-resistant epilepsy. Research has identified glutamate neurotransmission dysfunction as pivotal in seizure genesis. Glutamate serves as the primary excitatory neurotransmitter in the cerebral cortex, where seizures manifest. Its action is mediated through iGlu receptors, which are ligand-gated ion channels that facilitate rapid excitatory synaptic transmission. Experimental studies have demonstrated that iGlu receptor antagonists mitigate seizures, while agonists exacerbate seizures in various animal models. Clinical progress in development of iGlu receptor antagonists has been impeded by adverse effects stemming from the inhibition of rapid excitatory synaptic transmission. Currently, perampanel is the sole drug that selectively targets iGlu receptors and is utilized in focal epilepsy treatment. Other drugs, such as topiramate and felbamate, also inhibit iGlu receptors via other mechanisms. The authors propose that this review aids in analyzing steps triggered by iGlu receptor activation, offering insights into potential alterations in antiepileptic efficacy without compromising essential brain physiological functions, thus enhancing the safety and tolerability of iGlu receptor-targeted ASMs. The glycine B site is crucial for ion-mediated glutamate-induced epileptic activity, potentially contributing to the transition of seizures to a state of sustained epilepsy. For instance, in DBA/2 mice, administration of the glycine B site antagonist MNQX exhibited protective effects against kindling-induced status epilepticus. It is widely accepted that felbamate, ramacemide, and riluzole exert at least some of their anticonvulsant effects through glycine B site antagonism. However, glycine B site antagonists with weak intrinsic activity may paradoxically promote convulsive activity [560].

Other Studies Involving Felbamate

Li et al. explored the antidepressant-like effects of felbamate, an anticonvulsant primarily prescribed for epilepsy, in mice. Initially, they employed the forced swimming test (FST) and tail suspension test (TST) to evaluate the impact of felbamate and later extended their investigations to chronic unpredictable mild stress (CUMS) and chronic social defeat stress (CSDS) models. This study assessed alterations in the hippocampal brain-derived neurotrophic factor (BDNF) signaling cascade following chronic stress and felbamate treatment. The results indicated that felbamate exhibited antidepressant-like activity in the FST and TST without affecting motor activity in mice. Moreover, felbamate demonstrated effectiveness in both the CUMS and CSDS models of depression. Furthermore, felbamate fully reversed the decrease in BDNF signaling pathway activity in the hippocampi of mice subjected to CUMS and CSDS. The authors posit that felbamate exerts antidepressant effects in mice through modulation of the hippocampal BDNF system. This study underscores the beneficial effects of felbamate on depression and presents a potential novel antidepressant medication. This study deepens the understanding of the pharmacological effects of felbamate and lays the groundwork for the development of new antidepressants [561]. Bayhan et al. conducted a study utilizing 32 male Sprague–Dawley rats to establish a closed head trauma model and compared the immunological, histological, and oxidative effects of felbamate and levetiracetam on head trauma in rats. The rats were divided into four groups, each including eight rats. Following head trauma, Group 1 received normal saline (control), Group 2 received 50 mg/kg levetiracetam, Group 3 received 100 mg/kg felbamate, and Group 4 received a combination of 50 mg/kg levetiracetam and 100 mg/kg felbamate intraperitoneally once daily for 20 days. On Day 20, the rats were euthanized, and blood and tissue samples were collected for biochemical, immunohistochemical, and histological analyses. The findings revealed that serum cytokine levels were lower in Groups 2, 3, and 4 than in the control group, with the lowest levels observed in Group 4 receiving combination therapy. Pial vascular congestion, monocyte infiltration, bleeding, and neurodegeneration were significantly reduced in Groups 2 and 3 compared to controls. In Group 2, vascular congestion and Purkinje cell degeneration in the cerebellum were diminished compared to controls. Group 4 exhibited the most favorable outcomes, with significantly reduced levels of immune markers (IL-1β, IL-4, IL-6, and TNF-α), lower accumulation of TBARS, and a significant increase in SOD and GSH levels, than controls. The authors suggested that both levetiracetam and felbamate individually exhibit benefits in terms of immune, oxidative, and histological changes, with enhanced efficacy observed when used in combination [562].

2.1.2.8 Vigabatrin

Drug Characteristics

[Chemical name] (±) 4-Amino-5-hexenoic acid

[Structural formula]

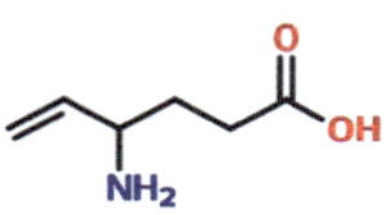

[Molecular formula] C6H11NO2

[Molecular weight] 129.16

[Indications] This product is suitable for many types of seizures. As an adjunct therapy, it is used to treat patients who do not respond to other ASMs, especially those with partial seizures (mainly used to control complex partial seizures). It can also be used in infants with West syndrome (infantile spasm), which usually does not respond to conventional ASMs. As an adjunct therapeutic drug, this product can achieve better curative effects.

[Specifications] Granules/tablets/oral solution powder/oral solution 500 mg

[Usage and dosage] For infants aged 1 month to 2 years with infantile spasms, monotherapy typically involves oral solution powder or oral solution forms. The recommended starting dose is 50 mg/kg/day, which is administered in two divided doses, with subsequent titration upward every 3 days by 25–50 mg/kg/day. The maximum daily dose should not exceed 150 mg/kg/day and should be divided into two doses. Individual dosing should be based on the infant's body weight. Withdrawal from vigabatrin therapy should be gradual, reducing the daily dose by 25–50 mg/kg/day every 3–4 days until it is discontinued. As adjunctive therapy for adult patients with refractory complex partial seizures, common dosage forms include regular tablets, oral solution powder, and oral solutions. Treatment initiation typically involves a daily dose of 1000 mg (500 mg twice daily), with weekly increases of 500 mg based on clinical response. The recommended maintenance dose for adults is 3000 mg/day (1500 mg twice daily). Higher doses of 6000 mg/day have not shown additional benefits compared to 3000 mg/day and are associated with increased incidence of adverse events. When vigabatrin use is discontinued, gradual dose reduction is advised. Vigabatrin can also be used as an adjunctive therapy for children with refractory complex partial epilepsy. The available dosage forms are regular tablets, oral solution powder, and oral solutions. The dosing regimen for pediatric patients aged 2–16 years varies based on body weight. For patients weighing 10–60 kg, the recommended dosage is divided into two doses, with adjustments based on body weight. Pediatric patients aged 17 years and older or weighing more than 60 kg should follow the same dosage regimen as adults.

[Adverse reactions] The most common adverse events associated with vigabatrin in combination with other ASMs were headache, drowsiness, fatigue, dizziness, convulsion, nasopharyngitis, weight gain, upper respiratory tract infection, visual field loss, depression, tremor, nystagmus, nausea, diarrhea, memory impairment, insomnia, irritability, abnormal coordination, blurred vision, double vision, vomiting, influenza, fever, and rash. The most common adverse effects of misusing vigabatrin were convulsions and depression. Among patients with infantile spasm, the most common adverse effects of discontinuing vigabatrin use were infection, epileptic status, developmental coordination disorder, dystonia, hypotonia, hypertonia, weight gain, and insomnia. Clinical attention should be given to permanent visual impairment, magnetic resonance imaging (MRI) abnormalities in infants, neurotoxicity, suicidal behavior and ideation, withdrawal syndrome associated with ASMs, anemia, salivation and fatigue, peripheral nerve disease, weight gain, and edema.

Clinical and Basic Research

Historical Evolution

In 1977, Schechter PJ et al. described for the first time the role of vigabatrin in animals [563]; in 1980, Gale K et al. reported that vigabatrin had an effect on epileptic seizures in animals [564]; in 1981, Gale K et al. identified the antiepileptic action site of vigabatrin. It was found to be related to the action of gamma-aminobutyric acid (GABA) [565]. Subsequently, Kalichman MW et al. reported that vigabatrin had an effect on the occurrence and development of epilepsy in animals with amygdala ignition [566]. In 1983, Gram L et al. reported the results of administration of vigabatrin to patients with epilepsy. They administered it to 15 patients with refractory epilepsy and found that it could significantly reduce the seizure frequency of epilepsy patients, which initially confirmed its antiseizure effect [567]. Since 1989, vigabatrin has been widely utilized in Europe for the management of infantile spasms. Its approval for the treatment of infantile spasms and refractory epilepsy in the United States followed in August 2009. In 2010, vigabatrin was recommended as a first-line therapy for infantile spasms associated with tuberous sclerosis. Acting as an analog of GABA, vigabatrin exhibits specificity in binding to GABA aminotransferase, irreversibly increasing the GABA concentration in the brain and thereby exerting an antiepileptic effect. In 2023, Tierradentric-Garcia and colleagues employed magnetic resonance technology to investigate the effects of vigabatrin on brain damage in epilepsy patients [568]; in 2024, Kuchenbuch M et al. summarized the results of the use of vigabatrin in the treatment of infantile spasm, deepening people's understanding of the use of vigabatrin in the treatment of epilepsy [569].

Observational Research on the Treatment of Epilepsy

From 2012 to 2018, the National Infantile Spasm Association conducted a prospective study at 23 U.S. centers to compare the efficacy of various initial treatments for infantile spasms in children aged 2–24 months. Zachary M. Grinspan et al. utilized propensity score weighting and in-center correlation generalized estimation equations to address treatment selection bias. The study revealed the following failure rates without treatment: adrenocorticotropin (ACTH) 88/190 (46%), oral steroids 42/95 (44%), vigabatrin 32/87 (37%), and nonstandard treatment 4/51 (8%). Transitioning from use of oral steroids to that of ACTH was not predicted to impact remission rates (44% observed, estimated 44% [95% confidence interval 34–54%]). However, switching from nonstandard therapy to ACTH therapy was estimated to increase the response rate from 8% to 39% (17–67%), and transitioning to oral steroid therapy was expected to increase the response rate from 8% to 38% (15–68%). Although statistically insignificant, switching from vigabatrin to ACTH (29–42% [15–75%]), from vigabatrin to oral steroids (29–42% [28–57%]), and from nonstandard treatment to vigabatrin (8–20% [6–50%]) demonstrated substantial estimated effects. Notably, among patients treated with vigabatrin, those with tuberous sclerosis (TSC) exhibited a greater response rate than did the other patients (62% vs. 29%; $p < 0.05$). The researchers concluded that use of ACTH and oral steroids offer advantages over nonstandard treatment for initial infantile spasm therapy. Although the estimated effectiveness of vigabatrin fell between that of ACTH/oral steroids and that of nonstandard treatment, the statistical confidence in the sample was inadequate. Vigabatrin showed optimal efficacy against TSC. This study provides Class III evidence indicating that use of ACTH or oral steroids outperforms nonstandard treatment for children with new-onset infantile spasms [570].

Addition of Treatment for Refractory Epilepsy

In a study conducted by Taylor N. Gatson et al., the terms "vigabatrin" and "sabril" were utilized to search English literature spanning from 1999 to 2023, in an aim to identify relevant studies and review articles. The objective of this study was to examine the pharmacokinetics, efficacy, and adverse reactions associated with sabril and its role in treating refractory focal involuntary seizures in adults. A double-blinded, placebo-controlled multicenter study conducted in 2000 involving

90 adult patients revealed that 48% of those treated with vigabatrin experienced a 50% or greater reduction in the frequency of complex partial seizures, compared to 26% of those receiving placebo. The study also revealed that vigabatrin was well tolerated by 72.4% of patients and had common side effects, including drowsiness, dizziness, headache, and fatigue. Subsequent studies have highlighted the significant risk of visual field loss associated with vigabatrin, suggesting that it may only be an option for refractory patients. Despite these potential risks, studies have indicated that adult patients tend to continue with long-term vigabatrin use. Vigabatrin serves as an adjunctive treatment for patients aged at least 10 years with intractable complex partial seizures who are unresponsive to alternative therapies. Numerous clinical trials have demonstrated its efficacy in reducing seizure frequency when used alongside existing treatments. However, cautious monitoring for adverse reactions, particularly during prolonged use, is imperative, with discontinuation recommended upon the occurrence of serious side effects [571].

Treatment of Epilepsy Syndrome

West syndrome is a prevalent form of epilepsy in infants and young children, often leading to significant neurodevelopmental challenges. A panel of pediatric neurologists and epileptologists led by SUVASINI SHARMA and colleagues collaborated to establish guidelines for the management of West syndrome. Through focused group discussions supplemented by email and phone interactions, the experts reached a consensus based on the reviewed evidence. When uncertainties arose, the Delphi consensus method was employed. The finalized guidelines underwent expert review for approval. The diagnosis of West syndrome relies on clinical identification through history or home video observation of spasms, coupled with EEG findings indicating arrhythmia or variants. Brain magnetic resonance imaging is the preferred neuroimaging modality, with the use of additional tests, such as genetic and metabolic screenings, contingent upon clinical and radiological results. Hormone therapy, involving either corticotropin or oral steroids, is recommended for patients with conditions other than tuberous sclerosis, while vigabatrin is preferred for patients with tuberous sclerosis. Studies have shown comparable efficacy and adverse reaction profiles for adrenocorticotropin and high-dose prednisolone in West syndrome treatment. Second-line options include ASMs (vigabatrin, sodium valproate, topiramate, zonisamide, nitrazepam, and clobazam), ketogenic diet therapy, and epilepsy surgery [572].

In a related study by Ramantani G et al., a literature review spanning from 2014 to July 2020 was conducted to update infantile spasm (ISS) management practices. Their recommendations build upon evidence from previous guidelines and current research findings. Early electroencephalogram (EEG) assessment is advised when ISS is suspected, followed by immediate initiation of treatment upon confirmation. The response to first-line therapy should be evaluated clinically and via EEG after 14 days. First-line therapy consists of hormone-based monotherapy (adrenocorticotropin or prednisolone) or a combination of hormones and vigabatrin. Vigabatrin is recommended for children with tuberous sclerosis or contraindications to hormone therapy. If first-line treatments fail, second-line options, including ketogenic diet therapy, sulthiame, topiramate, valproic acid, zonisamide, or benzodiazepines, should be considered. Early evaluation for epilepsy surgery is recommended for refractory patients, especially those with focal brain injury. Additionally, providing comprehensive information to parents about the disease, medication efficacy, adverse effects, and available support options is crucial, as is regular follow-up care [573]. Xu, Z et al. conducted a systematic review and meta-analysis to assess the efficacy of vigabatrin (VGB) in treating infantile epileptic spasm syndrome (IESS). The authors systematically searched the PubMed, Embase, Web of Science, MEDLINE, and Cochrane Library databases for reports of relevant randomized controlled trials (RCTs) and observational studies (OSs) investigating VGB for IESS. The primary outcome of this meta-analysis was the cessation of epileptic spasms (ES). Their analysis included five RCTs and nine OSs comparing the efficacy of VGB and hormonal monotherapy for IESS. A meta-analysis of the five RCTs revealed that hormonal monotherapy was significantly more effective than VGB monotherapy in patients with newly diagnosed IESS (OR = 0.37, 95% CI = 0.20–0.67). The results from the meta-analyses of the nine OSs were consistent with those of the RCTs (OR = 0.61, 95% CI = 0.43–0.85). VGB demonstrated greater efficacy in patients with tuberous sclerosis complex (TSC) than in those with other etiologies (5 OS, OR = 5.59, 95% CI = 2.17–14.41). However, there was no significant difference in the effectiveness of VGB combined with hormone therapy compared to that of hormone monotherapy for IESS (two RCTs, OR = 0.75, 95% CI = 0.09–6.45). The researchers concluded that hormonal monotherapy was superior to VGB monotherapy for non-TSC-associated IESS, whereas VGB was preferred for patients with IESS due to TSC. Additionally, combining VGB with hormone therapy did not significantly improve the control rate of ES compared to hormone monotherapy [574].

Application of Vigabatrin in Special Epileptic Populations

Katarzyna Kotulska et al. conducted a multicenter study involving 94 infants with tuberous sclerosis complex (TSC) who were monitored with monthly video electroencephalography (EEG) and who received vigabatrin as routine antiepileptic therapy. Treatment commenced either after the first EEG or clinical seizure or as prophylaxis when epileptiform EEG activity was detected before a seizure. In a randomized controlled trial (RCT) conducted at six sites, participants were randomly assigned to treatment or control groups at a 1:1 ratio. At four sites, the treatment distribution was fixed, constituting an open-label trial (OLT). Subjects were followed until 2 years of age, with the primary endpoint being the time to the first clinical episode. The present study revealed that 54 subjects exhibited epileptiform EEG abnormalities before experiencing seizures. Compared with conventional treatment, prophylactic treatment significantly prolonged the time to the first clinical attack. At 24 months, pooled analyses indicated that preventive treatment reduced the risk of clinical seizures, drug-resistant seizures, and infantile spasms. No adverse events were associated with preventive treatment. Researchers have concluded that prophylactic use of the antiseizure medication vigabatrin is safe and has the potential to alter the natural course of TSC-related seizures, thus mitigating the risk and severity of epilepsy [575]. In a study by Sufang Lin et al., the efficacy and safety of vigabatrin in treating focal epilepsy associated with tuberous sclerosis were evaluated. The review included patients with focal epilepsy and tuberous sclerosis treated with vigabatrin over an 8-year period at a children's epilepsy center. Among the 85 patients, 20 (23.5%) achieved seizure freedom at 12 months, 45 (52.9%) achieved a favorable response (≥50% reduction in seizures), and 20 (23.5%) were unresponsive to treatment. Patients who became seizure-free had a greater median age at seizure onset than did those in the responsive and nonresponsive groups. Additionally, fewer patients in the seizure-free group exhibited the largest nodular calcifications, although the presence of nodular calcifications did not differ significantly between the groups. In children with tuberous sclerosis, vigabatrin was more likely to result in seizure freedom in those with focal seizures beginning in infancy and without calcifications within the largest tubercles [576].

Epileptic spasm is a devastating form of early infantile epileptic encephalopathy (EIEE) with multiple etiologies. Early diagnosis and shorter treatment preparation times are critical for terminating seizures and optimizing neurodevelopmental outcomes. Genetic testing has become an integral part of epilepsy treatment, directly guiding management and family planning and playing a role in the discovery of new targeted treatments. Neuronal Differentiation Factor 2 (NEUROD2) variants have recently been found to be the cause of neurodevelopmental disorders (NDDs) and EIEE with unique characteristics. Kullasate Sakpichaisakul et al. described a case of a Southeast Asian female infant who presented with systemic developmental delays and epileptic spasms shortly after birth. Whole exome sequencing identified a novel de novo heterozygotic pathogenic NEUROD2 variant, p.E130Q. Pretreatment EEG showed multifocal independent spikes primarily in two posterior brain regions, which significantly improved with vigabatrin and high-dose prednisolone treatment. However, several relapses occurred after the discontinuation of ASMs.The researchers suggested that the epileptic spasms associated with the novel NEUROD2 pathogenic variant responded well to combination therapy with vigabatrin and high-dose prednisolone, indicating the potential benefits of using such a regimen for treating NEUROD2-associated neurodevelopmental disorder syndrome [577].

Among children with infantile spasm syndrome (ISS), those with trisomy 21 (T21) and those with normal development and no clear cause at the time of onset (previously called "idiopathic") are expected to have relatively favorable outcomes. Anita N. Datta et al. aimed to determine differences in treatment response, recurrence, and subsequent epilepsy between two groups of children with infantile spasms (ISs) treated with vigabatrin as first-line therapy. The study revealed no significant differences in age of onset, sex distribution, or treatment lag between the two groups. However, the T21 group required a greater average number of antiepileptic treatments, experienced more relapses, and had a greater risk of subsequent seizures than did the control group. These findings suggest that vigabatrin may be less advantageous than steroids as a first-line treatment for T21 and ISS patients [578].

Viral encephalitis (VE) or bacterial meningoencephalitis (BME) in early childhood can cause brain damage and neurological sequelae, including seizures. Postencephalitic epilepsy (PEE), characterized by epileptic spasms (ESs), is a rare but serious condition. There is an urgent need to develop new methods to assess the characteristics of these children and select appropriate treatments. Lin Wan et al. conducted an observational study of 20 patients with postencephalitic epilepsy (PEE) characterized by epileptic spasms (ES) following viral encephalitis (VE) or bacterial meningoencephalitis (BME). Patients were followed for more than 12 months and their prognoses were analyzed. The study revealed that children with PEE with ES were more likely to develop drug-resistant epilepsy (DRE), and the prognosis was worse for VE patients than for BME patients. Further research is needed to evaluate the efficacy of treatments such as adrenocorticotropin (ACTH), a ketogenic diet (KD), vigabatrin, and vagus nerve stimulation (VNS) therapy in these patients [579].

The Efficacy and Safety of Vigabatrin as the Preferred Treatment for Epilepsy

The use of vigabatrin in the treatment of patients with infantile spasm (IS) and tuberous sclerosis (TSC) has been extensively studied. Infantile spasm (IS) is an epileptic encephalopathy with a generally poor prognosis, with most patients exhibiting psychomotor delay or intractable epilepsy. However, early and aggressive treatment is associated with better response rates and outcomes, especially in patients with idiopathic IS. Dina Amin Saleh et al. conducted a retrospective chart review to investigate the different treatment modalities and outcomes of patients diagnosed with IS at a pediatric neurology clinic in Abu Dhabi, United Arab Emirates. The authors analyzed the medical history, demographics, etiology, neurodiagnostic tests, treatment modalities, and outcomes of patients diagnosed with IS between September 2014 and September 2019. Three treatment modalities were identified as first-line options: prednisolone (UKISS), ASMs, and vigabatrin. The study revealed that complete response rates to vigabatrin as a first-line therapy showed the greatest statistical significance. Patients with idiopathic IS responded to treatment similarly to patients with symptomatic IS. In patients who showed partial or no response to first-line therapy, an additional response to second-line therapy was noted with the prednisolone UKISS regimen and vigabatrin. None of the patients received adrenocorticotropin therapy. All patients with desirable outcomes had idiopathic IS and did not develop symptoms. The researchers concluded that more than one-third of patients showed poor treatment response when they did not receive treatment according to currently available options. This highlights the need for a unified treatment program that considers the availability of medications, expertise, and diagnostic tests outside major tertiary care centers in the region [580]. Fahad A Bashiri et al. conducted a retrospective medical record review to evaluate neurodevelopmental and epileptic outcomes in children with infantile spasms (ISs) at King Khalid University Hospital (KKUH) in Riyadh, Saudi Arabia. Patients who were diagnosed with IS according to the International League against

Epilepsy (ILAE) criteria between January 2000 and December 2017 were included. Patients who were lost to follow-up or were not treated at KKUH were excluded. A total of 53 patients with IS were included in the study and classified into unknown, cryptogenic, and symptomatic types. The majority had symptoms (71.7%). The etiological type and treatment delay were found to be significant predictors of motor and cognitive outcomes but were not predictors of seizure control. Patients with unknown IS who were diagnosed earlier had better neurodevelopmental outcomes. Treatment with vigabatrin in combination with adrenocorticotropin (ACTH) or prednisolone resulted in better seizure control than monotherapy or other combination therapies [581].

An article by M. Kuchenbuch et al. emphasized significant advancements in the treatment of TSC-related epilepsy in children. A European controlled trial involving 94 infants with TSC demonstrated that early treatment with vigabatrin before the onset of seizures can prevent infantile spasms and reduce the risk and severity of subsequent seizures over a 2-year follow-up period. This underscores the importance of proactive management strategies in improving outcomes for children with TSC-associated epilepsy [582].

In clinical drug application, adverse reactions to drugs are the focus of our attention in addition to drug efficacy. Vigabatrin (VGB) is a second-generation antiseizure medication that is effective in the treatment of infantile spasms and focal epilepsy, mainly in patients with tuberous sclerosis (TSC). However, reports of adverse events related to VGB use, including VGB-related visual field loss and brain abnormalities in neuroimaging, have raised concerns about the wider use of VGB, thus significantly limiting its application. Weronika Golec et al. conducted a review focused on summarizing recent treatment guidelines and the use of VGB in focal seizures, particularly in patients with tuberous sclerosis complex (TSC). They also discussed new applications of VGB to improve treatment for patients with TSC and reviewed current views on potential VGB-related toxicity and safety [583]. Although vigabatrin (VGB) is approved as a monotherapy for pediatric patients with infantile spasm (IS), the duration of use of VGB should be limited due to the risk of retinal and neurotoxicity, but the optimal duration of treatment is unclear. Béatrice Desnous et al. aimed to determine the risk of spasticity recurrence in patients assessed as good responders to VGB therapy. They focused on infants with IS who were treated with VGB as first-line therapy and who did not exhibit clinical spasms or arrhythmias after 4 weeks of treatment. These infants were divided into two groups based on the duration of VGB treatment: a 6-month treatment group and a >6-month treatment group. The study revealed no recurrence of spasticity in either group. Additionally, in the 6-month treatment group, no other seizure types were observed in patients with nonidentified etiology (NIE). Furthermore, between 6 and 9 months after initiating VGB therapy, only 5 of 37 patients developed advanced epilepsy in the form of focal seizures, with 3 of 30 patients in the 6-month treatment group and 2 of 7 patients in the extended treatment group falling into this category. These findings suggest that a brief 6-month course of VGB may suffice for the treatment and prevention of IS; particularly noteworthy is the absence of spasticity recurrence in NIE children [584].

It is crucial to assess any child experiencing appetite and weight issues due to the potential influences of these factors on their growth and development due to various factors associated with epilepsy. Antiseizure medications (ASMs) can have side effects, some of which may impact appetite, thereby affecting normal growth and weight gain in children. Buraniqi E et al. systematically reviewed studies on the effects of ASM use on children's appetite and weight. They found that certain ASMs, such as oxcarbazepine, eslicarbazepine, lamotrigine, levetiracetam, lacosamide, CBZ, vigabatrin, and clobazam, have minimal impacts on weight and appetite. However, some ASMs may influence both appetite and weight, potentially increasing the risk of related ailments and reducing adherence to treatment regimens [80].

The association between ASMs and suicidal tendencies remains contentious, necessitating further analysis of additional datasets to comprehend this intricate relationship. Leppien EE et al. conducted a study utilizing the U.S. Food and Drug Administration Adverse Event Reporting System (FAERS) database to compare the safety profiles of new and traditional ASMs concerning suicidal tendencies. They identified four new ASMs (lacosamide, clobazam, brivaracetam, and vigabatrin) associated with significantly lower rates of suicide attempts than traditional ASMs, while perampanel was associated with notably higher rates. This case–control study, spanning a decade and including 6309 FDA adverse event reports of suicidal tendencies, enhances the understanding of the safety profiles of novel ASMs [585].

Evidence-Based Medical Research

In tuberous sclerosis (TSC), a prevalent genetic contributor to epilepsy, infantile epileptic spasticity syndrome (IESS) typically manifests as the initial neurological hallmark, progressively transitioning into refractory epilepsy. Vigabatrin (VGB) commonly serves as the primary therapeutic option for patients with TSC with IESS in clinical settings. Giovanni Prezioso et al. conducted a systematic review aimed at gathering and analyzing data concerning the efficacy of VGB in treating TSC with IESS, aiming to evaluate the robustness of the evidence available in the literature. The authors' findings indicate that although all examined studies reported a favorable impact of VGB in TSC patients with IESS, exhibiting a superior response rate compared to IESS patients without TSC, the limited evidence base and substantial heterogeneity in findings do not justify firm treatment recommendations [586].

Effects on EEG and Cognitive Function

Vigabatrin (VGB) is a potent and selective inhibitor of gamma-aminobutyric aminotransferase (GABA-T) and is a nonconventional medication approved for treating individuals with intractable epilepsy. However, its impact on epilepsy development and its potential correlation with cognitive function postepilepsy onset remain obscure. Using a Li-pilocarpine-induced seizure model, Ming-Chi Lai et al. investigated the effects of VGB on epileptogenesis and neuronal impairment in Sprague–Dawley rats following status epilepticus. Cognitive assessment was conducted using the inhibitory avoidance test. Research has revealed that VGB can impede epilepsy onset by mitigating spontaneous recurrent seizures, hippocampal neuron deterioration, and chronic mossy fiber sprouting. Nonetheless, VGB failed to preserve cognitive function. These findings underscore the imperative of delving deeper into the role of VGB in both the genesis and management of epilepsy within clinical settings [587].

Side Effects

Side effects such as imaging abnormalities and visual field defects may occur during the use of vigabatrin.

Vigabatrin (VGB) is an effective antiseizure medication for the treatment of West syndrome. It acts by irreversibly inhibiting gamma-aminobutyric acid (GABA) transaminase and increasing central GABA levels. Vigabatrin-associated brain abnormalities on magnetic resonance imaging (VABAMs), a side effect of VGB, have only been described in children, but the pathophysiology of this effect is unknown. Ikeda Azusa et al. evaluated the relationship between VGB and GABA levels in the brain and the association between VABAMs and GABA. Researchers speculate that elevated levels of GABA in the brain are observed in VABAM patients, suggesting that GABA is involved in the pathogenesis of this condition. In particular, it is characterized by a significant increase in free GABA levels in cerebrospinal fluid. Although the increase in the GABA-to-creatine ratio and phosphocreatine (Cr) peak ratio (GABA/Cr) is mild, it may help in the early identification of patients at risk for VABAM [588]. Gabriela Reyes Valenzuela et al. conducted a retrospective analysis of clinical and EEG epilepsy data from 288 WS patients identified between 2014 and 2020. They assessed the efficacy of a ketogenic diet, valproate, levetiracetam, or topiramate in treating these patients. Vigabatrin (VGB) treatment in children with West syndrome (WS) led to characteristic MRI changes, with most cases being asymptomatic. However, some patients experienced dyskinesia and acute encephalopathy. Of the 288 WS patients who underwent VGB, 44 displayed MRI findings consistent with VGB-related brain abnormalities. The median age at diagnosis was 6.29 months (range 2 weeks to 11 months). The etiology of VGB-associated brain abnormalities on MRI was unknown in 22 patients (52.27%), genetic factors in 7 patients (15.9%), genetic structure in three patients (6.8%), structural malformation in 3 patients (6.8%), and acquired structure in eight patients (18.2%). Twenty-five of the 44 patients had asymptomatic brain abnormalities on MRI related to vigabatrin. Among the infants, 10 (22.7%) experienced worsening movement disorders, while nine (21.4%) exhibited progressive psychomotor deterioration linked to encephalopathy signs and symptoms. The researchers observed dose-dependent MRI abnormalities in infants treated with VGB, with potential risk factors including age below 11 months and higher VGB doses (>165 mg/kg/day). Typically, these brain abnormalities resolved after discontinuing VGB, often within 3 months [589]. Chellamani Harini et al. investigated additional hippocampal signal abnormalities in infant patients showing typical vigabatrin-related MRI changes. Among the 55 patients, 26 (47%) exhibited typical vigabatrin-related MRI changes, with six showing additional signal abnormalities in the hippocampus. Follow-up revealed parallel hippocampal signal changes in four patients, while two patients showed good clinical outcomes without MRI follow-up. There were no differences in clinical parameters, including seizure status, between patients with and without additional hippocampal signaling changes. One patient displayed unilateral thalamic/pedalus signal abnormalities alongside typical vigabatrin changes. Researchers have proposed that typical vigabatrin-related hippocampal changes may occur under appropriate exposure circumstances [590].

Yong Xu et al. investigated the potential risk factors and frequency of vigabatrin-associated brain abnormalities on magnetic resonance imaging (VABAMs), building upon prior research showing the association of VGB exposure with such abnormalities. They also scrutinized whether diffusion-weighted imaging (DWI) should be a standard MRI sequence for children undergoing VGB treatment. This study focused on infants with infantile spasms (ISs) receiving VGB therapy. Participants were categorized into VABAM and non-VABAM groups based on VABAM occurrence. Clinical data and drug exposure information were compiled. This study revealed a VABAM incidence of 32.5%, surpassing most previous reports. Furthermore, the peak VGB dosage was confirmed to be a risk factor for VABAM. The findings suggested that VABAMs could manifest even with standard VGB dosages (i.e., 50–150 mg/kg/day). Consequently, researchers advocate for routine MRI assessments, even when administering typical VGB doses [591].

Vigabatrin therapy is frequently prescribed for infants diagnosed with tuberous sclerosis, particularly in cases of epilepsy. However, it can induce bilateral symmetric sequence changes in deep brain matter and the brain stem on MRI. These abnormalities typically manifest in infancy, are reversible, and may or may not present symptoms. Joseph Franklin Craft et al. highlighted a patient with typical neuroimaging findings, emphasizing the importance of recognizing these patterns to prevent unnecessary follow-up tests. The decision to continue or discontinue vigabatrin therapy should take into consideration the potential risk of extrapyramidal symptoms [592].

Jonsson H et al. conducted a study to assess visual fields using Goldmann or Octopus perimetry and peripapillary retinal nerve fiber layer (RNFL) thickness with spectral-domain optical coherence tomography (OCT) during school age or adolescence. They aimed to investigate the prevalence of vigabatrin-attributed visual field defects (VAVFDs) in infantile spasms and the utility of OCT in detecting vigabatrin-related injury. Of the 88 patients who were exposed to vigabatrin in infancy, 28 underwent formal visual field testing. Two patients had structural visual field defects, four had mild VAVFDs, and one had severe VAVFDs. The duration of vigabatrin treatment was significantly longer in the VAVFD group than in the normal visual field group. Three patients with VAVFDs exhibited RNFL thinning on OCT. The study concluded that the incidence of VAVFDs after infancy was low but increased with treatment duration. Further research is needed to identify susceptible infants and determine the role of OCT in diagnosis [593]. Loretta Giuliano et al. conducted a systematic review of 5164 studies, including 67, five of which involved adult patients. They found that ASM side effects, including retinal toxicity, were more common in girls, with a greater risk observed in boys treated with vigabatrin.

Sex differences in ASM side effects are understudied and may be underestimated, highlighting the need for systematic evaluation of sex as a determinant variable in clinical studies to better understand drug responses [594].

Drug-induced liver injury (DILI) is a risk factor associated with ASMs, especially older-generation ASMs. Brad K. Kamitaki et al. sought to quantify recent reports of DILI attributed to old and new generation ASMs and investigate newly marketed ASM hepatotoxicity using the FDA Adverse Event Reporting System (FAERS) database. They analyzed over 2.6 million adverse event reports of DILI from July 1, 2018, to March 31, 2020, uncovering 2175 cases attributed to ASM; these included mostly severe reactions, including death, hospitalization, disability, and other life-threatening outcomes. Older and newer-generation ASMs were implicated in DILI, but no cases were reported for vigabatrin, tiagabine, or rufinamide, suggesting minimal correlation with DILI for most new-generation ASMs [182].

Basic Research

Vigabatrin (VGB) is the primary choice for managing drug-resistant epilepsy and infantile spasms, although its use often triggers ataxia, tremors, and abnormal gait, indicating potential cerebellar involvement. Marwa Abd El-Kader et al. conducted a groundbreaking study aiming to explore, for the first time, the role of necrosis and apoptosis in VGB-induced cerebellar cell loss and the potential protective effect of combined omega-3 and vitamin B12 supplementation. Their research involved 50 adult male Sprague–Dawley rats (160–200 g) divided into five groups receiving various treatments administered intragastrically daily for 4 weeks. The results revealed that VGB-induced damage to the cerebellar cortex and white matter was dose dependent, indicating the occurrence of apoptosis and necrotic death mechanisms. Notably, supplementation with both B12 and omega-3 PUFAs has the potential to ameliorate or mitigate VGB-induced neurotoxicity. These findings underscore the importance of recommending dietary B12 and omega-3 supplements when prescribing VGB [595].

In another study on the use of vigabatrin, an antiepileptic agent that irreversibly inhibits GABA transaminase activity, male C57Bl/6J mice received continuous infusions of various doses (0, 40, or 80 mg/kg/day) for 12 days. The study design involved pooling retinas, eyes (excluding retinas), whole brains, and plasma from $n = 24$ animals per dosage group, yielding eight triplicates per treatment group. Analysis revealed the distribution of active (S)-(+) VGB to the retina, indicating the involvement of a stereospecific transporter whose identification may unveil new therapeutic strategies to mitigate VGB's well-documented retinal toxicity and broaden its clinical utility [596].

Other Research

Vigabatrin (VGB), an unconventional antiseizure medication (ASM), has shown promise in treating brain tumors, yet its impact on ion channels in glioma cells remains unclear. Te-Yu Hung et al. utilized patch-clamp technology to investigate the effect of VGB on ion currents in the glioblastoma multiforme cell line

13–06-MG. Their findings revealed that VGB reduced the activity of intermediate-conductance Ca2+-activated K+ (IKCa) channels in the cell adhesion state in a concentration-dependent manner. DCEBIO could counteract the inhibitory effect of VGB on IKCa channels. However, VGB did not affect the activity of large-conductance Ca2+-activated (BKCa) channels or inwardly rectifying K+ (KIR) channels in human 13–06-MG cells. Nonetheless, the addition of GAL-021 or BaCl2 effectively suppressed BKCa and KIP channels in the presence of VGB. The results of this study suggested that the inhibition of IKCa channels by VGB may be a crucial mechanism underlying its antitumor effects, particularly its antiglioma effects [597].

Commercial immunoassays currently do not include kits for quantifying valproic acid, vigabatrin, pregabalin, and gabapentin levels without interference from structurally similar substances. Chromatography serves as a viable alternative to immunoassays. Jin P et al. developed a simple, robust nonderivatization gas chromatography–mass spectrometry method for simultaneously determining the aforementioned drugs in human plasma. Their method provides reliable drug monitoring during therapy [598].

Vigabatrin, a second-generation ASM, is used for monotherapy in children aged 1 month to 2 years with spasticity and as an adjunct therapy for adults and pediatric patients aged 10 years and older with intractable complex partial seizures. Optimal vigabatrin therapy aims for seizure freedom without significant adverse effects, with therapeutic drug monitoring (TDM) playing a crucial role. Wang J et al. developed and validated a simple, rapid, and sensitive method for measuring plasma vigabatrin levels. Their method, which was successfully applied to pediatric patients undergoing vigabatrin treatment, offers valuable information to clinicians for monitoring hospital plasma vigabatrin levels [599].

2.1.2.9 Zonisamide

Drug Characteristics

[Chemical name] 1,2-Benzisoxazole-3-methanesulfonamide

[Chemical structural formula]

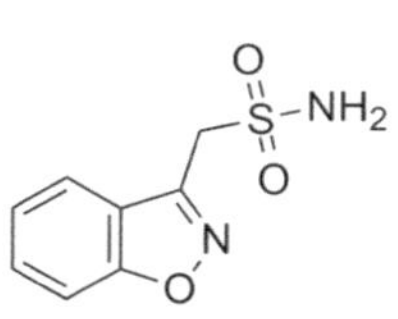

[Molecular formula] C8H8N2O3S

[Molecular weight] 212.23

[Adaptation to disease] For the treatment of major seizures, minor seizures, localized seizures, status epilepticus and psychomotor seizures.

[Specification] 100 mg

[Usage and dosage]
Oral: Adults initially receive 100–200 mg daily, divided into one to three oral doses. Within 1–2 weeks, the dosage is increased to 200–400 mg daily, divided into one to three oral doses. The maximum daily dose is 600 mg. The initial daily dose for children is 2–4 mg/kg orally divided one to three times, which is increased to 4–8 mg/kg orally divided one to three times within 1–2 weeks. The maximum dose for 1 day is 12 mg/kg.

[Adverse reactions]
Common symptoms include drowsiness, anorexia, dizziness, headache, nausea, and anxiety or impatience.

Clinical Application and Basic Research

Historical Evolution of Zonisamide

In 1980, Ito et al. suggested that zonisamide inhibited the activity of epileptogenic foci in the cortex and blocked the transmission of epilepsy from the cortex to subcortical structures [600]. Since its introduction, zonisamide has been the subject of ongoing research. In 1985, J. C. Sackellares et al. conducted a study on zonisamide involving 10 adult patients with intractable partial epilepsy. Their findings indicated that substituting the use of standard ASMs with that of zonisamide led to a decrease in seizure frequency for the majority of patients. Additionally, dose-dependent reversible side effects were observed in both the central nervous system and gastrointestinal system [601]. These early studies laid the groundwork for the clinical application of zonisamide in epilepsy treatment. In 1987, E. J. Hammond et al. further discussed the neuropharmacological aspects of zonisamide. Their findings from preliminary clinical trials demonstrated the efficacy of the drug against various seizure types, including generalized tonic–clonic, simple, and complex partial seizures [602]. Since then, zonisamide has been marketed in Japan since 1989 as an antiseizure medication that acts through multiple mechanisms [603]. In 1996, M K Ito et al. conducted a study examining the impact of zonisamide on the voltage-dependent T-type calcium current (ICa) in cultured human neuroblastoma cells (NB-I). These findings suggested that the blockade of T-type calcium channels by zonisamide could inhibit a critical component of the inward current responsible for triggering epileptoid cell firing, thereby restraining the propagation of epileptic activity [604]. This research provides a solid foundation for further electrophysiological investigations of zonisamide and its role in epilepsy management. Subsequently, the drug received approval for marketing in the United States in 2000 and in Europe in 2005 [603]. In March 2005, zonisamide capsules were authorized for sale in the United Kingdom and Germany as adjunctive therapy for treating partial epileptic seizures, establishing it as a broad-spectrum antiseizure medication [605]. In 2006, Martin J Brodie published an article suggesting that combining zonisamide with commonly used ASMs could offer effective and well-tolerated treatment for patients with intractable partial epilepsy [606]. This is an encouraging result. In 2015, Saori Tsujii et al. studied the neuroprotective effect of zonisamide on endoplasmic reticulum stress [607]. These reports indicate that much of the research on zonisamide is relatively recent. In 2021, Stefano Parravicini et al. described a case of electroclinical improvement in patients with 20-ring chromosome syndrome following zonisamide treatment. Epilepsy associated with this syndrome is often medically challenging to address. When traditional medications such as valproate and lamotrigine fail to yield results, zonisamide may merit further investigation due to its antifocal effect and potential for preventing dopamine depletion [608]. This finding also suggests that combining the pharmacological characteristics of drugs to explore the clinical use of zonisamide to open up new areas is a sound approach.

Efficacy and Safety of Zonisamide in the Adjuvant Treatment of Refractory Epilepsy

A study assessed the efficacy and reliability of zonisamide (ZNS), a novel ASMs, in children with treatment-resistant epilepsy who were already on multiple ASMs. Among the participants, 46 (67.6%) had treatment-resistant generalized epilepsy (RGE), and 22 (32.35%) had treatment-resistant focal epilepsy (RFE). In the RGE group, 26 patients (56.5%) experienced a reduction in seizures of more than 50%, and seven patients (15.2%) achieved complete seizure cessation. In the RFE group, 19 patients (86.4%) experienced a reduction in seizures of more than 50%, and two patients (9.1%) achieved complete seizure cessation. Notably, among patients diagnosed with tuberous sclerosis (TSC) who were followed, four patients experienced significant termination or reduction of seizures by more than 50% [605]. Furthermore, Rubio et al. presented the case of a patient who was diagnosed with Lafora disease and had previously shown a poor response to several ASMs. The patient exhibited a favorable and stable response to zonisamide, suggesting its potential as a treatment option for progressive myoclonic epilepsy (MPE) [609].

Application of Zonisamide in the Treatment of Epilepsy in Special Populations

ZNS has emerged as an effective and dependable adjunctive therapy for children with refractory epilepsy, particularly focal epilepsy, and it may hold promise for patients with tuberous sclerosis (TSC) [605]. However, concerns have been raised regarding the potential teratogenicity of zonisamide during human pregnancy. One study revealed three major congenital malformation (MCM) cases in the ZNS monotherapy group and five in the combined treatment group. The median birth weights for infants in the monotherapy and multidrug groups were 71 and 44 ounces, respectively, and the incidence of small-for-gestational-age babies was notably greater (21% for both groups). These findings warrant attention regarding the potential teratogenic effects of zonisamide during pregnancy [610]. Rebecca et al. described the case of a young female patient with global developmental delay, progressive ataxia, epilepsy, and myoclonus stemming from a truncated mutation in the SEMA6B gene. Recent research has identified DNA truncation variations in the last exon of SEMA6B as the cause of autosomal dominant progressive myoclonic epilepsy. Treatment with zonisamide has shown clinical improvements in patients, particularly in alleviating both positive and negative myoclonus, along with significant enhancements in gait and mobility [611].

Application of Zonisamide in Other Diseases

ZNS exhibits benefits in patients with obesity and metabolic syndrome who are at high risk for vascular diseases. One study evaluated the efficacy of ZNS in reducing obesity and mitigating vascular disease and liver steatosis. The hepatic steatosis index (HSI) was used to assess nonalcoholic fatty liver disease progression. After 12 and 24 weeks of ZNS treatment, 24.6% and 32.8% of patients, respectively, experienced a ≥5% loss of body weight. Generalized estimation equation analysis, adjusting for baseline variables, indicated significant reductions in body weight, BMI, serum HbA1c, triglyceride, and hs-CRP levels and HSI scores [612]. In recent years, zonisamide has been the subject of numerous studies focusing on its potential in Parkinson's disease (PD) management. Naito et al. conducted a comprehensive transcriptome sequencing analysis of PD patients. They selected 23 zonisamide hyperresponders (SRs) and 25 nonresponders (NRs) from among PD patients and analyzed whole-transcriptomic data from peripheral blood samples before and 12 weeks after zonisamide treatment. Differential gene expression analysis of SRs and NRs at each time point revealed that the efficacy of zonisamide in PD patients was correlated with glutamate-related synaptic regulation and p53-mediated dopaminergic nerve loss [613]. Suzuki K. et al. conducted a 3-month open-label study to investigate the effects of zonisamide on motor symptoms, depressive symptoms, and sleep problems in PD patients. Patients receiving zonisamide at doses of 25–50 mg/day underwent corresponding scale assessments and questionnaire surveys. This study demonstrated significant improvements in the Parkinson's Disease Sleep Scale (PDSS-2) score at 3 months in the tremor group and in the Beck Depression Inventory-II (BDI-II) score at 1, 2, and 3 months in the nontremor group following zonisamide treatment. These findings underscore the beneficial effects of zonisamide on motor symptoms and sleep problems in PD patients treated with levodopa experiencing motor fluctuations [614].

Zonisamide has demonstrated efficacy as an adjunct therapy for alleviating motor symptoms in Parkinson's disease (PD) patients. Considering that Lewy body dementia (DLB) and PD are considered subtypes of Lewy body spectrum disorders, zonisamide was investigated for treating Parkinson's symptoms in DLB patients. In Japanese phase II and phase III clinical trials involving DLB patients, participants were randomly assigned to receive zonisamide at doses of

25 or 50 mg/day or placebo for 12 weeks. The results revealed that zonisamide significantly improved the Unified Parkinson's Disease Rating Scale Part III (UPDRS-III) score without affecting cognitive or neuropsychiatric measures at week 12 [615]. Moreover, Manabu et al. conducted a study to compare the efficacy and safety of adding zonisamide (25 mg/day) versus increasing levodopa doses (100 mg/day but ≤300 mg/day) in treating Parkinson's syndrome in DLB patients. At weeks 16 and 24, the adjusted mean change in the Movement Disorder Society Unified Parkinson's Disease Rating Scale Part III (MDS-UPDRS Part III) total score was significantly greater in the zonisamide addition group than in the levodopa dose increase group. These findings suggest that in DLB patients with insufficient levodopa efficacy, the addition of zonisamide (25 mg/day) can moderately improve motor symptoms. However, it remains uncertain whether the addition of zonisamide (25 mg/day) is as effective as increasing the levodopa dose (100 mg/day) [616]. Furthermore, a meta-analysis indicated that zonisamide can enhance motor function in both PD patients and DLB patients, improve activities of daily living and drug efficacy in PD patients, and shorten the duration of motor disorders. These findings collectively support the potential role of zonisamide as a beneficial treatment option for motor symptoms in PD and DLB patients [617].

Zhengguang Wang et al. conducted a study utilizing 40 adult Sprague–Dawley rats to establish a model of degenerative cervical spondylitic myelopathy (DCM). The rats were divided into four groups: the Sham group, the DCM model group, the ZNS group (treated with zonisamide), and the ZNS + CD95 group. Their findings indicated that ZNS treatment facilitated motor recovery and reversed the histopathological injuries and apoptosis observed in DCM rats. Additionally, ZNS was observed to mitigate DCM damage by regulating Fas and FasL signaling, suggesting its beneficial effect on DCM [618].

In a study by Rose JE et al., a novel treatment approach involving the combination of bupropion and zonisamide was explored to aid smokers in transitioning from combustible cigarettes (CCs) to electronic nicotine delivery systems (ENDSs). Twenty-four smokers participated in a 13-week treatment regimen in which they were provided ENDSs, bupropion, and zonisamide. The assessment parameters included CC and ENDS usage, exhaled air carbon monoxide (CO) levels, smoking cessation symptoms, reward scores, and tolerance/side effects. At the conclusion of the study, 33% of participants achieved biochemically confirmed complete abstinence from CCs, indicating the potential efficacy of the bupropion/zonisamide combination in facilitating the transition to ENDSs. This suggests that further randomized controlled trials are warranted to validate this promising approach [619].

Side Effects of Zonisamide

Zonisamide can cause delirium through toxic epidermal necrolysis (TEN) [620]. TEN and Stevens-Johnson syndrome (SJS) are life-threatening reactions marked by extensive skin stripping and mucosal erosion. Samuel et al. described a case of TEN accompanied by delirium and psychosis triggered by zonisamide. Zonisamide has been linked to psychosis and other mental disorders, particularly when it is used concomitantly with other ASMs. For instance, a 61-year-old woman diagnosed with heparin-induced SJS experienced worsening insomnia, persecution delusions, and visual hallucinations.

Pj nar Ozkan Kart et al. examined the histological effects of ZNS and other commonly used ASMs on rat ovarian tissue. ZNS, along with STM, LCM, CLB, and RUF, administered to nonepileptic preadolescent rats had adverse effects on ovarian tissue follicular ability when continued into adulthood. ZNS treatment led to a significant reduction in the number of atretic follicles and corpus luteum in the ovaries, along with an increase in the number of apoptotic follicles. Animal studies suggest potential teratogenic effects and a risk of miscarriage associated with zonisamide use [534]. Furthermore, zonisamide has been linked to decreased appetite and weight loss in children, potentially leading to underlying health issues and poor treatment adherence [80]. Additionally, a case involving a woman in her 20s who developed distal (type 1) renal tubular acidosis due to zonisamide, resulting in severe hypokalemia, corrected QT interval prolongation, and metabolic acidosis, has been reported [621]. Regarding safety concerns, zonisamide use significantly increases the likelihood of contusion in patients with dementia with Lewy bodies (DLB) and may also cause appetite loss in DLB patients and drowsiness in Parkinson's disease (PD) patients [617].

Evidence-Based Medical Research on Zonisamide

A meta-analysis of zonisamide for epileptic spasticity, comprising studies with at least 10 participants, included 401 children with epileptic spasms. They were administered ZNS at doses ranging from 9.9 to 35 mg/kg/day, with few patients experiencing minor adverse effects. The results indicated that 20.8% (95% CI-11.4–29.2%) and 23.4% (95% CI-17.8–29.1%) of patients treated with zonisamide achieved complete cessation of spasticity and at least a 50% reduction in total spasticity frequency compared to baseline, respectively. Additionally, 20.3% (95% CI-10.1–30.5%) of patients exhibited alleviation of EEG rhythms with zonisamide. These findings demonstrate that zonisamide can effectively reduce spasticity in approximately 21% of children with epilepsy, with minimal adverse reactions [622].

Basic Research on Zonisamide

Zonisamide upregulates neuregulin-1 expression and enhances acetylcholine receptor aggregation at neuromuscular junctions in vitro, enhancing the axonal elongation of primary spinal motor neurons (SMNs). Taro et al. investigated the impact of ZNS on AChR clusters at NMJs, given the compensatory role of neuroblastulation in human diseases involving AChR cluster loss. The authors observed that molecules conferring ZNS responsiveness were not secreted into the medium. Moreover, while 10 μM ZNS upregulated Nrg1 expression in cocultured cells, it had no effect on monocultures of C2C12 muscle tubes or NSC34 motor neurons. Inhibition of the Nrg1/ErbB signaling pathway counteracted the enhancement of AChR clustering induced by 10 μM ZNS treatment in NMJs in vitro, and antiagglomerin antibodies mitigated ZNS-mediated AChR clustering enhancement [623]. Zonisamide exhibits a neuroprotective effect on adult rat dorsal root ganglion (DRG) neurons in vitro, countering the toxic effects of the platinum-based drug oxaliplatin (OHP), which is known to induce peripheral neuropathy. Pretreatment with zonisamide (100 μM) significantly reduced OHP-induced death of DRG neurons. Additionally, zonisamide inhibited p38 MAPK phosphorylation in ND7/23 DRG neurons treated with OHP. This neuroprotection against OHP-induced peripheral sensory neuropathy may involve the activation of the MEK/ERK and PI3K/AKT signaling pathways and the concurrent inhibition of the p38 MAPK pathway in DRG neurons [624]. Using an inflammatory astroglia-microglia coculture model, Ismail FS and colleagues investigated the effects of tiagabine (TGB) and zonisamide (ZNS). They investigated glial cell viability, microglial activation, articulin 43 (Cx43) expression, and the coupling of gap junctions. These findings indicate that under inflammatory conditions, TGB exhibits potential anti-inflammatory effects. Conversely, ZNS did not significantly alter the microglial phenotype. Moreover, ZNS might exert supplementary antiseizure effects by interfering with glial gap junction communication during inflammatory states. Notably, there were disparities in the modulation of glial cell characteristics between the TGB and ZNS groups [625]. Tada et al. established a PD mouse model through treatment with 1-methyl-4-phenyl-1,2,3,6-tetrahydropyridine and lipopolysaccharide (LPS). Their aim was to explore the impact of zonisamide on mitochondrial reactive oxygen species generation in microglia. Zonisamide reversed the inhibitory effects of LPS on the mitochondrial oxygen consumption rate (OCR), providing insights into mitigating mitochondrial dysfunction in microglia. This finding supports its potential clinical utility as a treatment for Parkinson's disease [618]. Idiopathic epilepsy (IE) is a prevalent chronic brain disorder in canines. Recent investigations into the efficacy of a medium-chain triglyceride (MCT)-rich diet on seizure frequency in dogs with IE have been conducted. These studies revealed no significant difference in episode frequency between dogs fed a placebo diet (PL) and those fed a Purina ProPlan Veterinary Diet Neurocare (NC) diet. Moreover, concurrent administration of zonisamide alongside the MCT diet did not cause any discernible adverse effects and did not influence the zonisamide concentration. Hence, commercially available MCT-rich diets (NCs) can be safely administered concurrently with zonisamide to IE-afflicted dogs [626].

2.1.3 *Third-Generation Antiseizure Medications*

2.1.3.1 Lacosamide

Medicinal Features

[Chemical name] (R)-2-(acetylamino)-N-benzyl-3-methoxypropionamide

[Structure formula]

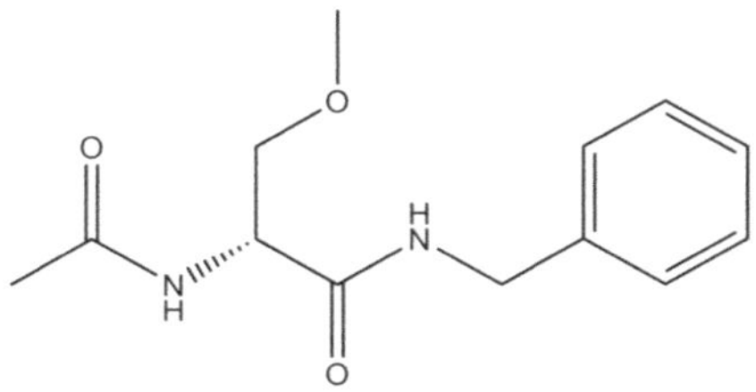

[Molecular formula] $C_{13}H_{18}N_2O_3$

[Molecular weight] 250.30

[Indications] Monotherapy or add-on therapy in the treatment of partial-onset seizures in patients with epilepsy aged 4 years and older.

[Dosage forms]
Film-coated tablets: 50 mg/100 mg/200 mg
Oral solution: 200 mL (2 g)
Injection: 200 mg

[Dosage and administration]
Adults (aged 17 and above) and children weighing ≥50 kg:

Treatment begins with a dosage of 50 mg per administration, which is administered twice daily. The dose is incrementally increased weekly to 50 mg per administration, twice daily, until the maximum permissible dosage of 400 mg/day is reached.

Pediatric and adolescent patients (aged 4 years and above):

Pediatric patients weighing 30–50 kg: Initiate treatment at 1 mg/kg per administration, twice daily. The dosage is adjusted weekly to 1 mg/kg, following a twice-daily regimen, up to a maximum of 8 mg/kg/day.

Pediatric patients weighing ≥11 to <30 kg: Commence with a dosage of 1 mg/kg per administration, twice a day. The dose is increased weekly by 1 mg/kg, adhering to a twice-daily schedule, with a maximum dosage of 12 mg/kg/day.

[Adverse effects]
Dizziness, nausea, diplopia, vomiting, fatigue, blurred vision, ataxia, tremor, etc.

[Historical evolution]
Lacosamide (LCM) is a synthetically manufactured antiseizure medication (ASM). It selectively enhances the slow inactivation of voltage-gated sodium channels without affecting rapid inactivation. Its antiepileptic mechanism is also associated with interactions with collapsin response mediator protein (CRMP-2) [627]. In 2008, the FDA approved it for adjunctive therapy in focal epilepsy in patients aged 17 and older [628]. Initially, approved for adjunctive therapy, it subsequently received approval for monotherapy indications, extending from adult patients to children and adolescents aged 4 years and above.

Inoue Y. et al. [629] conducted a phase III, long-term, open-label extension (OLE) trial to evaluate the long-term safety, tolerability, and efficacy of adjunctive lacosamide (100–400 mg/day) in Chinese and Japanese people with epilepsy (PWE) (16–70 years) who had completed a double-blinded, randomized, placebo-controlled trial of adjunctive lacosamide. The median reduction in focal seizure frequency per 28 days from baseline was 57.1%, and the ≥50% and ≥75% responder rates were 57.1% (269/471) and 29.7% (140/471), respectively. Among people with epilepsy (PWE) who completed 12, 24, and 36 months of treatment, the 12-, 24-, and 36-month seizure-free survival rates were 3.5% (13/375), 3.4% (11/321), and 2.0% (5/247), respectively. The most common treatment-emergent adverse events (≥20% of PWE) were nasopharyngitis, dizziness, and upper respiratory tract infection.

In a phase III, double-blinded, noninferiority trial [630], newly diagnosed adult patients were randomly assigned to receive either controlled-release CBZ or monotherapy with lacosamide, with daily doses of LCM ranging from 200 to 600 mg. By comparing metrics such as the proportion of patients who were seizure-free at 6 months and the incidence of adverse events, researchers considered lacosamide to be a first-line monotherapy for newly diagnosed epilepsy. Another phase III, double-blinded, randomized, placebo-controlled trial [631] included 242 patients (≥4 years old) with idiopathic generalized epilepsy (IGE) with poorly controlled primary generalized tonic–clonic seizures (PGTCS). Compared with placebo, lacosamide significantly differed in terms of the risk of GTCS recurrence within 24 weeks, seizure-free rates at 24 weeks, and reduction in GTCS frequency.

Fundamental and Clinical Research on Lacosamide

Recent Fundamental Research

Studies on the mechanism of lacosamide have focused on its antioxidative and anti-inflammatory protective effects. Lazzarotto, L. et al. [632] investigated the effects of LCM on biochemical and mitochondrial parameters in mice using a PTZ-induced model. These changes included changes in expression levels of superoxide dismutase (SOD), catalase (CAT), mitochondrial complexes, Bcl-2, and cyclooxygenase-2 (COX-2). These results suggest that while LCM does not inhibit seizure generation in vivo, it offers neuroprotection against oxidative stress, bioenergetic dysfunction, and DNA damage. Bilal B et al. [633] studied the neuroprotective effects of lacosamide in a rat model of Parkinson's disease and showed that drug intervention significantly reduced dopaminergic neuron degeneration, decreased malondialdehyde and inflammatory cytokine (TNF-α) levels, and increased dopamine metabolite (HVA) abundance.

Langton RL et al. [634] reported that lacosamide inhibited neocortex epileptiform discharges in neonatal mice without increasing neuronal apoptosis. Other researchers [635] have evaluated the effect of LCM on kynurenine pathway (KP) levels in a mouse model of epilepsy with comorbid depression based on measurements of inflammatory cytokines and oxidative stress markers. They concluded that the antiepileptic effect of LCM is at least partly due to its anti-inflammatory and antioxidative activities. Corvace F. and colleagues [636] concluded that LCM has no significant effect on glial cell activity, and its induced reduction in gap junction protein expression may be related to its antiepileptic activity. LCM also reduced the number of activated microglia, thereby decreasing neuroinflammatory responses and reducing the likelihood of epilepsy.

In regard to status epilepticus (SE), Szewczyk A. et al. [637] used pilocarpine (PILO) to induce SE in mice and assessed the impact of the drug on neurogenic stem cell (NSC) proliferation and cognitive functions. They found that long-term treatment with LCM appeared to have no negative impact on cognitive function or neurogenesis. However, prolonged usage of LCM might reduce the formation of new neurons. Shishmanova-Doseva M. et al. [449] also used a pilocarpine-induced model to determine that the antioxidative mechanisms of LCM and TPM might contribute to their anticonvulsant effects. Sumbul O. et al. [638] used an animal model of penicillin-induced status epilepticus to evaluate the electrophysiological and biochemical effects of lacosamide. Lower doses of lacosamide (10 mg/kg) significantly reduced spike wave frequency, decreased ST-segment elevation to the level of the control group and inhibited the increase in total oxidant status (TOS) and TNF-α levels, while higher doses of LCM (50 mg/kg) not only increased spike wave frequency but also increased ST-segment elevation and the QT and PR intervals.

Wu PM et al. [639] explored the effects of lacosamide on voltage-gated Na^+ currents (INas). They found that lacosamide inhibited both the peak and sustained components of INas and could alter their magnitudes, gating, and voltage dependency, possibly via postbinding interactions with certain amino acid residues in sodium channels.

Application in Critical Care

Among third-generation ASMs, lacosamide is advantageous because of its increasing application in status epilepticus, cluster seizures, and other critical conditions, making it a treatment for convulsive status epilepticus (CSE) with broad application prospects [640].

Schaidle S. et al. [641] studied neurosurgery patients in intensive care units. After first-line antiseizure drug treatments failed, the patients were switched to phenytoin or lacosamide treatment. Lacosamide was associated with similar failure rates but fewer adverse effects when compared with phenytoin for refractory seizures in neurosurgical ICU patients. Another study reported that the outcomes of patients with status epilepticus refractory to treatments such as benzodiazepines and phenytoin were best in terms of response rate, while lacosamide and valproate performed comparably [642]. Chimakurthy AK. et al. [643] reviewed and analyzed data regarding 382 patients with acute epileptic seizures and status epilepticus admitted to the ICU. The dose range of intravenous LCM was approximately 400–1000 mg, and the need to adjust the dose according to body weight was emphasized; 8 mg/kg intravenous LCM can be safely used in ICU patients, and the effective plasma concentration is 15–20 μg/mL.

Both the efficacy and tolerability of intravenous administration have been evaluated. Eilam A. et al. [644] conducted a retrospective study on cluster seizure patients treated with IV LCM from September 2017 to September 2019. The median loading dose was 136.5 mg (range 100–300 mg) among 39 patients, with 9 patients receiving 200–300 mg. The response rate was 89%, with common side effects being mild, and no electrocardiographic changes or other cardiovascular side effects observed. Torian SC et al. [645] observed no additional risk of infusion site reactions, hypotension, or bradycardia with high-dose IV injections of 300 or 400 mg. However, Kim HK. et al. [646] retrospectively analyzed data on 85 patients who received IV LCM over 2 years, and found that 28 (32.9%) experienced at least one adverse cardiac event. The most common events were new-onset first-degree atrioventricular block (19 patients) and hypotension (seven patients), with an average increase in the PR interval (169.3 ms vs. 184.5 ms, $P < 0.01$) and a decrease in the average heart rate (91.7 vs. 86.9, $P = 0.01$) postinjection.

Fong SL et al. [647] reported that only a few children experienced drug-related adverse events, mainly including mild symptoms such as rash and somnolence. Intravenous lacosamide administration showed good tolerance in children and neonates, but there was a doubled risk of rash in the high-dose group compared to the low-dose group. Elderly patients or those with underlying cardiac conditions were more prone to PR interval prolongation after bolus injections. Thus, IV LCM loading doses should be used under strict electrocardiographic monitoring. Another retrospective study [648] comparing the safety of IV administration of LCM and LEV revealed that 6 out of 36 patients (16.6%) in the lacosamide group and 6 out of 50 patients (12.0%) in the levetiracetam group experienced hypotension or bradycardia. There were no reports of PR interval prolongation in patients using lacosamide who underwent 12-lead EKG.

Intranasal administration has always been considered suitable for prehospital emergencies and special situations in emergency departments. A study by Gonçalves J. et al. [649] evaluated intranasal (IN) administration of lacosamide to cross the blood–brain barrier. The results show that IN administration can result in rapid and complete systemic absorption (absolute bioavailability: 120.46%). Compared with intravenous administration, nasal lacosamide administration leads to higher concentrations in the brain and lower concentrations in the kidneys, with lacosamide concentrations in the lungs being significantly greater than those observed after intravenous administration and lasting until 30 min after administration. Intranasal administration has potential applications for intracerebral drug delivery in epilepsy and related emergency situations.

Treatment of Symptomatic Epilepsy/Syndromes and Nonepileptic Diseases

Mo F. et al. [650] analyzed data from 132 patients with primary brain tumors treated with LCM monotherapy. Seizure-free rates at 3 and 6 months were 64.4% and 55%, respectively. Patients with a history of two or more ASMs had poorer outcomes than those who used LCM as the first-line medication. The main side effects included dizziness and somnolence, both of which were mild, with a dropout rate of 1.5%. Van Opijnen MP. et al. [333] analyzed 139 patients with grade 2–4 gliomas with seizures in a multicenter study. After failure of first-line monotherapy with levetiracetam or valproate, patients received lamotrigine or lacosamide. At 12 months, there was no significant difference in the cumulative incidence of treatment failure with lamotrigine or lacosamide, indicating similar efficacy in patients with neuroglioma with epilepsy.

A multicenter observational study [651] collected data from 207 patients with poststroke epilepsy (PSE) who did not change their initial antiseizure monotherapy during a 12-month period. Efficacy was assessed based on standardized three-month seizure frequency and seizure freedom. Safety was estimated based on the reported side effects. ASMs that act via the slow inactivation of sodium channels, such as lacosamide and eslicarbazepine, are well-tolerated and might be associated with better seizure control in PSE patients.

A retrospective study from a tertiary hospital in India [652] revealed that in patients with neurocysticercosis with seizures, LCM and OXC had comparable seizure frequencies at 12 and 24 weeks after beginning treatment, but the OXC group had more severe adverse reactions, with four patients discontinuing treatment due to severe side effects. This indicates a greater relative safety of LCM.

Lacosamide can be considered a first-line drug for benign childhood epilepsy with centrotemporal spikes (BECTs) [653]. One study included 18 BECT patients aged 3–13 years treated with LCM monotherapy for more than 6 months. The results showed that 7, 12, and 13 patients achieved seizure-free status at 0–3, 4–6, and 7–12 months after treatment, respectively, with 15 patients ultimately becoming seizure-free. Only four patients experienced transient tolerable fatigue or somnolence. Numoto S. et al. [654] evaluated the efficacy and tolerability of LCM and LEV in patients with benign infantile epilepsy (BIE). Among 24 children, five who were treated with LCM achieved seizure freedom at the starting dose of 2 mg/kg/day without significant adverse effects, while two patients taking LEV experienced seizure recurrence, one of whom achieved seizure freedom after switching to CBZ. Kobayashi Y et al. [655] described the potential long-term efficacy of lacosamide as an adjunctive therapy in juvenile myoclonic epilepsy patients, but further studies are needed to verify its exact effect on refractory generalized tonic–clonic seizures. Notably, the effective average dose for JME treatment reached 425 mg/day, which is higher than the routine monotherapy dose range. Zawar I. et al. [656] described significant seizure control in a 15-year-old woman with medically refractory Jeavons syndrome after switching to lacosamide treatment. She had failed to respond to treatment with adequate doses of ethosuximide, valproic acid, lamotrigine, topiramate and a ketogenic diet, either as monotherapy or in combination.

The therapeutic effects of lacosamide on cranial nerve diseases have been described. Goldschagg N et al. [657] described a patient with recurrent vertigo, paroxysmal taste disturbances and facial sensory abnormalities whose symptoms significantly decreased after lacosamide treatment, suggesting its potential as an effective option for paroxysmal taste disturbances and vestibulocochlear nerve lesions. Lacosamide monotherapy also performed well in treating facial pain, with significant pain improvement and good tolerability observed in three patients with idiopathic trigeminal neuralgia, tumor-related trigeminal neuralgia and persistent idiopathic facial pain without side effects [658]. Muñoz-Vendrell A et al. [659] administered lacosamide to patients with trigeminal neuralgia for whom first-line treatment failed, and approximately 66% of these patients experienced pain relief and relatively mild adverse effects.

Geng JH. et al. [660] described the first case of LCM effectively treating an epileptic patient with paroxysmal kinesigenic dyskinesia (PKD). The patient had a PRRT2 gene mutation (c.649dupC). Although LEV controlled generalized tonic–clonic seizures, it was ineffective against PKD. Fortunately, the patient's movement symptoms completely disappeared after LCM was added. Fitouchi S et al. [661] described a 60-year-old male patient with repeated syncope accompanied by olfactory or gustatory hallucinations who was diagnosed with limbic encephalitis and treated with lacosamide, resulting in the improvement and disappearance of syncope and hallucinations.

Adverse Effects

Because lacosamide is a new-generation medication in clinical use, its relatively rare adverse reactions are gradually being discovered in case reports, cohort studies, or systematic reviews, all of which are important for long-term practice.

Psychiatric and behavioral disorders are the most prominent types of adverse reactions caused by LCM. Ono-Takiguchi Y. et al. [662] described a 23-year-old female with Lennox–Gastaut syndrome (LGS) who was hospitalized for weight loss and behavioral abnormalities and was diagnosed with forced normalization (FN) induced by LCM. Symptoms improved after reducing the LCM dose, although some mild focal seizures recurred at a dose of 150 mg/day. However, her behavior and diet remained acceptable. Using the Japanese Adverse Drug Event Report database, Japanese researchers found an association between lacosamide treatment and delirium with an adjusted odds ratio of 2.44 (95% CI, 1.24–4.80) [663]. Another 82-year-old male patient with poststroke epilepsy experienced personality changes after the introduction of lacosamide [664]. Within a few days of starting the medication, the usually aggressive patient became gentle and calm. However, there was an insistence and a use of sexualized language toward women. He returned to his previous state after discontinuation of lacosamide. Kawai M. et al. [665] conducted a survey using the Buss-Perry Aggression Questionnaire (BAQ) among 266 patients and suggested that LEV is associated with increased aggression, while LCM showed a reduction effect. This seems to align with the abovementioned case report. Although levetiracetam can cause mental and behavioral abnormalities, it is unclear what effect it may have when it is given in combination with lacosamide. Matsunuma S. et al. [666], in a single-center retrospective cohort study including 44 patients on LEV + LCM and 50 patients on LEV + PER, reported a significantly lower incidence of psychiatric disorders in the former group ($p < 0.001$). These disorders tended to develop within 1 month of therapy and were not dose dependent. Antiseizure drugs should be cautiously prescribed to avoid the induction of psychiatric disorders.

The cardiovascular side effects of lacosamide should receive increased attention because of its sodium channel blocker characteristics. Goodnough R. [667] described one patient with epilepsy who developed a Brugada I-type ECG pattern during sepsis, which normalized after LCM discontinuation. Lu YT et al. [668] retrospectively analyzed data from 38 patients treated with LCM and reported one case of first-degree atrioventricular block and one case of premature atrial contraction, neither of which required clinical intervention. Another patient [669] who developed severe cardiac arrhythmias required life-saving veno-arterial extracorporeal membrane oxygenation (ECMO). Another case of cardiovascular side effects involved severe agranulocytosis [670]. The patient's initial dose of LCM was 100 mg/day, which was increased to 200 mg/day on the ninth day. Severe sinal node dysfunction occurred the next day, and LCM treatment was immediately discontinued. However, he still developed agranulocytosis and died from septic shock on the 15th day after admission.

Zhao X. et al. [671] first described a case of panniculitis induced by LCM. A 9-year-old female epilepsy patient developed red and swollen nodules on the outsides of her arms and the fronts of her legs after receiving LCM treatment for 2 weeks. The biopsy results revealed lobular panniculitis. The lesions spontaneously subsided and disappeared 2 months after lacosamide treatment was discontinued. There was no recurrence during the 1-year follow-up. Tateishi Y et al. [672] reviewed data on 15 children whose neutrophil levels were significantly reduced and whose immunoglobulin A levels were increased after taking lacosamide, which may have an impact on the immune and hematological systems.

Serum Concentrations

Lacosamide, a representative third-generation antiseizure drug, has long been a research focus due to fluctuations seen in its blood concentration levels and its clinical significance in guiding medication use. Li Y et al. [673] investigated the potential factors affecting the blood concentrations of lacosamide in Chinese children with epilepsy. The results indicated that the conventional LCM monitoring reference range is approximately 2.0–7.0 μg/mL and that older children with higher body weights may present with lower blood drug concentrations. Zhao T et al. [674] studied 500 pediatric patients from China and reported that the concurrent use of enzyme-inducing ASMs (EIASMs) significantly reduced the blood concentrations of lacosamide, highlighting the importance of monitoring the blood levels of lacosamide in pediatric clinics. Pozzi, M. et al. [675] conducted a 3-year follow-up of 44 patients and found that the average blood concentration of lacosamide was linearly correlated with the administered dose, and the therapeutic effect was also correlated with the dose of lacosamide. However, the same conclusion cannot be extended to the pediatric population. Ishikawa N. and colleagues [676] divided 51 Japanese children with epilepsy into a responsive group and a nonresponsive group based on therapeutic effects. There was no significant difference in drug dosage between the two groups, but there was a statistically significant difference in blood drug concentration, suggesting a closer relationship between plasma levels and therapeutic effects. Lukka PB. et al. [677] used a pharmacokinetic model to simulate the relationship between dosage and blood concentration in patients under 4 years of age, suggesting that a higher per-kilogram body weight dosage (12–18 mg/kg) is required to match the exposure levels of 4-year-olds as age decreases.

Pregnant women are sensitive to changes in blood concentrations of drugs. Pennell PB. et al. [678] studied pregnancy-related changes in the concentrations of several ASMs: the dose-normalized concentration (DNC) of lacosamide during pregnancy decreased by 39.9% compared to the postpartum value; compared to prepregnancy levels, the DNC significantly decreased with gestational age. Another study [679] involving seven patients reached similar conclusions.

The plasma concentration of lacosamide is associated with certain gene mutations. Zhao T et al. [680] explored the effect of ABCC2 gene mutations on the blood concentration and efficacy of lacosamide in Uyghur children with epilepsy, finding significant correlations between gene variance and the plasma concentration–dose ratio, which may lead to drug resistance, and suggested that ABCC2 gene screening should be conducted before LCM treatment, if possible. A study monitoring the blood concentration of lacosamide in adult patients with epilepsy in Korea [681] showed that the therapeutic concentration reference value was 6–9 μg/mL, with a linear relationship indicated between concentration and dosage and an association between concentration and the presence of genetic polymorphisms of CYP2C19.

Medication in Special Populations

Farkas MK and colleagues [682] evaluated the safety and tolerability of intravenous lacosamide treatment in epileptic patients aged 1 month to 17 years. Only 5 out of 103 patients experienced mild adverse events, mainly hypertriglyceridemia, indicating that intravenous administration is generally well-tolerated in this age group. Another study examined the use of new ASMs in pregnant women and reported an increased use of lacosamide. Moreover, lacosamide exposure during pregnancy did not increase the risk of severe congenital defects or spontaneous miscarriage, but instances of bradycardia in newborns exposed to lacosamide indicate that further in-depth research is needed to assess the safety of lacosamide [683].

Husein N et al. [684] investigated the differing views on treating epilepsy in patients over the age of 65. General neurologists and geriatricians tend to favor the use of levetiracetam and lamotrigine, while epilepsy specialists consider lacosamide more often. This reflects an inconsistency among doctors regarding the view of lacosamide as a first-line treatment option for elderly patients with epilepsy.

2.1.3.2 Perampanel

Characteristics of the Drug

[Name of chemical] Perampanel

[Chemical structure formula]

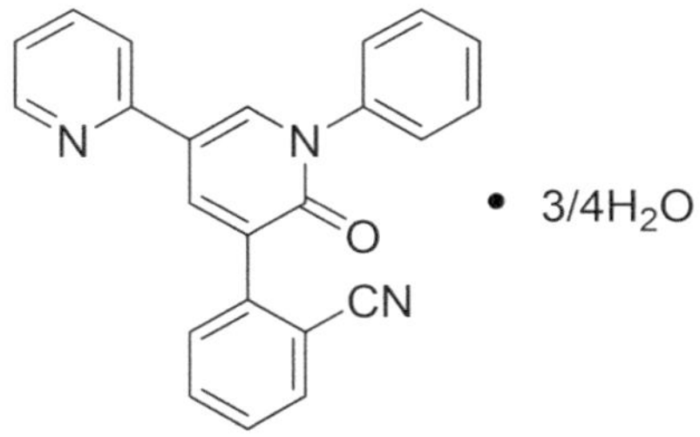

[Molecular formula] $C_{23}H_{13}N_3O \cdot 3/4H_2O$

[Molecular weight] 362.90(3/4 hydrate of water)

[Indications for use] It is indicated as an add-on therapy for adults, adolescents and children 4 years and older with partial seizures with or without secondary generalized seizures.

[Specification] 2 mg, 4 mg

[Dosage] For adults, adolescents and children ≥4 years of age, the recommended starting dose is 2 mg once daily at bedtime, increased by 2 mg/day at 1 or 2 week intervals depending on individual clinical response and tolerance. Recommended maintenance doses range from 6 to 8 mg once daily and the highest dose is 12 mg once daily.

[Adverse reactions] Somnolence, weight gain, dizziness, vertigo, ataxia, headache, fatigue, irritability, falls, nausea, vomiting, contusions, abdominal pain, and anxiety.

Clinical Application and Basic Research

Perampanel is a type of α-amino-3-hydroxy-5-methyl-4-isoxa-zolep-propionate acid (AMPA) receptor antagonist, which was approved by the US FDA in October 2012. It mainly inhibits the activity of postsynaptic AMPA receptors and reduces the excessive excitability of neurons. It is the first antiseizure drug approved by FDA whose mechanism of action is against glutamate receptors.

An Observational Study of Perampanel in Epilepsy

Faught et al. [685] conducted an observational study to understand the hospitalization rate of patients with epilepsy before and after the use of perampanel (PER) and compared it with that of lacosamide. In their analysis of patients in the Symphony Health database who received perampanel treatment, they found that among 1771 patients (mean age, 34 years; 55% women), the hazard ratio for hospitalization for any cause was 0.76 ($P < 0.05$), and the premedication hospitalization rate was 36.2%. The hospitalization rate was 29.5% during the follow-up period. The 1-year hazard ratio for epilepsy-related hospitalization was 0.72 ($P < 0.05$). The previous hospitalization rate of the patients had been 30.8%, and that observed during the follow-up period was 23.9%. The rate of hospitalization due to all causes was reduced by 9.6% in the perampanel cohort and 5.8% in the lacosamide cohort, and the rate of epilepsy-related hospitalization was reduced by 9.9% in the perampanel cohort and 3% in the lacosamide cohort ($P < 0.05$). The authors concluded that perampanel was associated with a significant reduction in the risk of hospitalization for patients with epilepsy during the whole year.

Villanueva et al. [686] conducted a pooled analysis of data from 44 observational studies of PER treatment for epilepsy patients from 17 countries, assessing retention and effectiveness at 3, 6, 12 months and the last follow-up of perampanel treatment. The retention rates of PER treatment at 3, 6, and 12 months were 90.5%, 79.8%, and 64.2%, respectively, with a mean retention time of 10.8 months. At 12 months, 58.3% of the patients had a 50% or greater reduction in seizures, and 50.0% of the patients had a 50% reduction in seizures at the last follow-up, and the corresponding seizure-free rates were 23.2% and 20.5%, respectively. The authors suggest that PER is effective and well-tolerated in daily clinical practice when used to treat patients with focal and/or generalized epilepsy.

A retrospective study regarding retention, dose, efficacy, and safety of perampanel administered to patients during routine clinical care showed that daily oral administration of perampanel during routine clinical care was generally well-tolerated in patients aged 1 to <18 years, with good retention rates for ≤2 years [687]. A large prospective observational study in Japan included 3808 patients. Of these patients, data from 3716 and 3272 patients were analyzed for safety and efficacy, respectively. In the safety analysis dataset, 1247 patients (33.6%) reported adverse reactions, 36.2% of which were younger than 65 years old and 22.2% of which were older than 65 years of age. Drowsiness and dizziness were the most common adverse reactions. The 50% responder rates in patients aged <65 years and those ≥65 years were 60.1% and 89.0%

for those with focal aware seizures (FAS) with motor signs; 48.0% and 60.0% for FAS without motor signs; 47.4% and 80.2% for focal impaired awareness seizures; 70.8% and 93.4% for focal to bilateral tonic–clonic seizures (FBTCS); and 63.6% and 88.9% for generalized tonic–clonic seizures(GTCS), respectively. The results of this study suggest that perampanel was effective for reducing seizure frequency and was safe, especially in older patients. Perampanel may be the clinical treatment of choice for elderly patients with epilepsy [688].

PROVE (NCT03208660) [689] was a multicenter, retrospective, nonintervention study designed to evaluate the retention, efficacy, safety and dosage of PER in patients with epilepsy during routine clinical diagnosis and treatment. Among patients eligible for inclusion in the retention analysis, the median reduction in seizure frequency was 79.3% among adolescents and 70.8% among adults. In the safety analysis data set regarding data on seizure effects, the majority of patients had improvement in the number of seizures at the last follow-up time point (51.4% among adolescents and 52.3% among adults). Adverse effects occurred in 38.4% of the adolescents and 44.3% of the adults. The most common AE was aggression (6.5%) in adolescents and dizziness (9.2%) in adults.

A structured literature search and scope-based assessment of European observational studies of adolescents or adults prescribed perampanel for focal epilepsy or primary generalized tonic–clonic seizures in the setting of idiopathic generalized epilepsy was conducted, and 29 relevant studies were ultimately included. Most patients (76.1%) were receiving two or more other ASMs along with perampanel. The maintenance dose ranges from 2 to 16 mg/day (most commonly 6 mg/day). Retention at 12 months ranged from 46% to 90.5% (median 71.1%). The proportion of patients who were seizure-free while taking PER ranged from 1.8% to 84.6%. Across studies, adverse event (AE) rates ranged from 18.2% to 67.4% (median 37.1%), and discontinuation due to AE ranged from 6.2% to 56% (median 12.5%). The most common individual adverse events were dizziness/vertigo (median incidence 13.7%), somnolence (median 11.9%), aggression (median 9.8%), irritability (median 9.1%), and cognitive impairment (median 7.0%). The overall incidence of adverse events was not related to the perampanel dose, the perampanel plasma level, or the number of concomitant drugs [690].

A retrospective, observational, multicenter study of patients >12 years of age with focal or generalized epilepsy who were consecutively recruited from 52 Italian epilepsy centers showed a very high retention rate across the entire group (89% at 12 months). The rate of treatment-induced adverse events was 25%, which was much lower than that seen in randomized trials of PER, confirming the good efficacy and safety of PER in the treatment of focal or generalized epilepsy in a real-life setting [691]. A 1-year prospective, single-center, observational study of patients with focal epilepsy in Huashan Hospital found a PER retention rate of 70.4%, a mean dosage of 4.3 mg/day, and a significant reduction in seizure frequency at 3, 6, and 12 months compared with baseline [692]. A study designed to define the real-world use of PER monotherapy for epilepsy showed that seizure freedom with PER monotherapy (primary or secondary) was achieved with good retention and safety [693].

Perampanel Use as an Add-on Therapy for Refractory Epilepsy

To understand the role of PER in patients with refractory epilepsy, Sagar et al. [694] conducted a retrospective, multicenter observational study. A total of 387 adult patients were included in the study and followed for a median time of 12.1 months. Focal epilepsy (FE) patients accounted for 79.6% of the cohort, idiopathic generalized epilepsy (IGE) patients accounted for 10.3%, and developmental epileptic encephalopathy (DEE) patients accounted for 10.1%. All patients had drug-resistant epilepsy, and 71.6% had never been seizure-free for 6 months and had taken an average of six antiseizure drugs before PER. The retention rate was 40%, the effective rate was 21.7%, and the seizure-free rate was 9.0% at 12 months of follow-up. The authors suggest that for drug-resistant epilepsy, even a late addition of PER therapy is an effective and well-tolerated approach.

In order to evaluate the clinical efficacy and tolerability, as well as the pharmacokinetic characteristics of PER in patients with drug-resistant epilepsy, Lossius et al. [695] studied the clinical data of 175 patients with drug-resistant epilepsy, mainly adults, who received PER as an adjuvant treatment at the National Epilepsy Center of Oslo University Hospital in Norway, with an average treatment duration of 16.1 months. Forty patients (23%) had a 50% or greater reduction in seizures, four of whom had no seizures, 50 (29%) of whom had no response, and 15 (9%) of whom had an exacerbation of seizures. Logistic regression analysis showed that the efficacy of this drug in treating patients with generalized epilepsy was better than that in the treatment of patients with focal epilepsy. Adverse effects were reported in 135 patients (77%), ranging from mild (34%) to moderate (41%) and severe (2%). These adverse effects led to the discontinuation of PER in 55 patients (41%). The most common adverse effects were psychiatric symptoms (34%), dizziness (31%), and drowsiness (26%). Among the 31 patients for whom serum concentrations were available, the mean daily dose of PER was 6.3 mg, and the mean steady-state serum concentration was 1.03 μmol/L (0.15–3.59 μmol/L). There was a significant difference in concentration/dose (C/D) ratios of 12-fold between patients ranging from 0.06 to 0.69 μmol/L/mg, which was associated with the enzyme inducer. The authors suggest that perampanel has a modest seizure reduction effect in this very resistant patient group and that clinicians may consider increasing the dose of PER above 6 mg/day in patients with no history of psychiatric illness, having taken into consideration combination therapy and blood concentration monitoring.

Identifying factors associated with response may enable clinicians to better help patients benefit from treatment. To this end, L Krauss et al. [696] studied potential predictors of response to PER in patients with drug-resistant focal epilepsy. They found that the best predictors in the multivariate model were the number of seizures during baseline, higher PER plasma concentration, and older age at diagnosis. In the final multivariable model, the best predictors of response were a lower baseline seizure frequency, no focal seizures associated with disturbance of consciousness at baseline, a lower baseline number of antiseizure drugs used, no concomitant use of other antiseizure drugs at baseline, older age at diagnosis, and no structural cause.

The authors suggest that the determination of these factors may help guide clinicians in predicting patient response to treatment and optimizing individual treatment regimens.

In addition, a clinical case report has been described of a patient with AMPA2 receptor-related encephalitis with memory impairment and refractory focal seizures, manifested as paroxysmal convulsions on the right side of the face and dystonic seizures on the right side. A combination of levetiracetam, CBZ, and clonazepam, regular monthly intravenous immunoglobulin, and immunosuppressive therapy for 5 months did not lead to a treatment response of focal seizures. However, adjuvant PER therapy resulted in rapid seizure relief. These results suggest that in the treatment of seizures associated with anti-AMPA receptor encephalitis, PER may be considered to control seizures by directly attenuating the neural excitability caused by the glutamate and Ca2+-permeable GluA4 subunits of AMPA receptors [697].

PER for the Treatment of Epileptic Syndromes

Obara et al. [698] described a long-term surviving patient with Lafora disease. This 34-year-old woman presented with seizures at the age of 11 years. She became bedridden after 20 years of age because of frequent generalized tonic–clonic seizures, myoclonus, and progressive mental decline. The seizures were not terminated despite the administration of multiple high doses of ASMs. At 31 years of age, she began taking PER, which was tapered after the myoclonus and convulsions were controlled, and a homozygous mutation in exon W219R of the NHLRC1 gene was identified. Because PER not only controls seizures but also prevents mental deterioration in patients, the authors suggest that PER should be used from the early stage of the disease.

In order to understand the efficacy and patient tolerance of PER in the treatment of drug-resistant sleep-related hypermotor epilepsy, Siew NaLim et al. [699] selected 36 patients for study, 20 of whom (six women, mean age 34.1 ± 9.0 years) completed adjuvant treatment with PER; it was effective in 10 patients and ineffective in 4. The remaining six patients discontinued use of the drug due to adverse events ($n = 5$) and patient selection ($n = 1$). A seizure-free period lasting 6 months was reported in six of ten responders (60%). The most common adverse events were dizziness (25%) and malaise (10%). The authors suggest that PER may be an effective antiseizure drug for highly resistant patients. Kazuyuki Saito et al. [700] described a 49-year-old man who developed cardiopulmonary arrest induced by a severe bronchial asthma attack; myoclonus then appeared after the onset of Lante-Adams syndrome. The myoclonus was effectively controlled with PER, even 10 years after the onset of the disease. The authors concluded that PER should be considered for refractory myoclonus caused by Lance-Adams syndrome.

Leigh syndrome is a mitochondrial disease characterized by basal ganglia damage and psychomotor delay. There are hardly any effective drugs. Kimura et al. [701] described a 26-year-old male patient who presented with psychomotor delay and short stature at the age of 1 year and was diagnosed with Leigh syndrome based on the results of cerebrospinal fluid examination and high signal intensity on T2 weighted magnetic resonance imaging of bilateral striatum. Psychomotor delay and respiratory disturbance were shown but progressed very slowly. Twenty-four years later, the symptoms of Leigh syndrome suddenly became worse, and seizures occurred. Multiple antiseizure drugs were ineffective, but the seizures were suppressed and the patient's activities of daily living were improved after the use of low dose of PER. The authors speculate that a low dose of PER can be used for the treatment of seizures and the improvement of activities of daily living in patients with Leigh syndrome.

A multicenter, retrospective study of patients with developmental and epileptic encephalopathy (DEEs) [702] found that 51.7% of patients had significant improvement in at least one seizure type. Seizure freedom for each specific type of seizure at 12 months was significantly achieved by 35% of patients with generalized tonic–clonic seizures (GTCS, $p < 0.001$), 17% with tonic seizures (TS) ($p = 0.016$) and 37% with seizure clusters ($p < 0.001$). Patients achieved seizure freedom from other seizure types but with no statistical significance: 7% freedom from focal onset seizures (FOSs), 28% freedom from atypical absences (AAs), 6% freedom from atonic seizures (ATSs), and 18% freedom from myoclonic seizures (MSs). Twenty-nine patients discontinued perampanel: 18 (21%) due to AEs, 8 (9%) due to lack of efficacy, and 3 (3%) due to seizure aggravation. Adverse events, mostly mild or moderate, were reported in 53% of patients, and irritability/mood changes (22%) and somnolence (17%) were the most frequent.

A multicenter retrospective analysis of the long-term efficacy of adding PER treatment for patients with Lennox–Gastaut syndrome (LGS) found that 52 subjects (59.8%) experienced treatment failure at a median time of 12 months. Treatment failure was due to lack of efficacy in 27 patients (52.0%), lack of tolerance in 14 (27.0%), and both reasons in 11 (21.0%). Slower titration times compared to faster titration times are associated with a risk of PER failure, while the occurrence of adverse events increases the risk of treatment failure. At a median follow-up time of 11 months, 36 patients (41.4%) were responders. After a median of 21 months, 13/36 patients (36.1%) had seizure recurrence; the overall rate of seizure responders was 23 of 87 patients (26.4%) at the end of follow-up [703].

Application of PER in Special Populations with Epilepsy

Lattanzi et al. [704] studied the efficacy of adjunctive use of PER in elderly patients with epilepsy under real-world conditions. In a retrospective analysis of the efficacy, adverse events, and patient discontinuation of add-on treatment with PER in elderly patients (≥65 years) with epilepsy at 12 Italian epilepsy centers, they found that among 92 patients enrolled with a median age of 69 (65–88) years, 53 (57.6%) had a response at 12 months. Twenty-two patients (23.9%) were seizure-free. The authors concluded that realistically, the addition of PER was associated with improved seizure control and good tolerance, and could be used as a treatment option for elderly patients with epilepsy.

Macrohon et al. [705] performed a cross-sectional descriptive study in which they reviewed the medical records of children who received PER either as adjunctive therapy or monotherapy for epilepsy by surveying pediatric neurologists. A total of 65 patients aged 1–18 (10.0 ± 5.2) years were included in the study. The follow-up period ranged from 2 weeks to more than 1 year. The results showed that the response rate was 69.2% (45/65), the seizure control rate was 29.2% (19/65), the exacerbation rate was 9.2% (6/65), and the retention rate for PER use was 83.1% (54/65). The authors conclude that the use of PER is effective and relatively safe in Philippine children.

Belousova et al. [706] also conducted an observational study on pediatric patients, in which 47% of the enrolled patients had focal seizures, 65% had focal seizures converted to bilateral tonic–clonic seizures, and 65% had primary generalized tonic–clonic seizures. Seizure cessation occurred in 12%, 19%, and 55% of patients, respectively, after treatment. The most common side effects were fatigue (26%), nasopharyngitis (19%), dizziness (13%), irritability (13%), fever (13%), and vomiting (11%).

To understand the data of PER treatment in adolescents in the real world, Inoue Y et al. [707] conducted a large-scale, prospective observational study with a total of 519 adolescents (12–17 years old) with drug-resistant refractory epilepsy over a period of 104 weeks. The main reasons for discontinuation at 104 weeks were adverse events (48.4%) and inadequate efficacy (46.8%). The retention rate for PER use at 104 weeks was 50.5%. The incidence of adverse reactions and serious adverse reactions was 42.2% and 1.8%, respectively. The most common side effects were somnolence (13.5%), irritability (8.5%), dizziness (5.1%), and agitation (4.8%). The median percentage change in seizure frequency at the last observation was −50.0% for motor focal seizures with conscious retention, −73.3% for nonmotor focal seizures with conscious retention, −28.6% for focal seizures with disturbance of consciousness, and −62.6% for focal to bilateral tonic seizures. Generalized tonic seizures were changed at a rate of −20.0%. These results suggest that PER is well-tolerated and effective in reducing seizure frequency in adolescent patients. No unexpected safety concerns were observed, and slow titration may reduce the incidence of adverse effects.

An international multicenter project based on the NETRE (Rare Epilepsy Treatment Network) framework conducted a retrospective analysis of the data regarding PER in the treatment of hereditary epilepsy. Expression of SCN1A, GNAO1, PIGA, PCDH19, SYNGAP1, POLG1, POLG2, and NEU1 genes were found to respond to therapy. A total of 64.7% of patients with Dravet syndrome caused by pathogenic variants of SCN1A responded to treatment with PER, and 35.3% of these patients had a 90% reduction in seizures. Other epileptic etiologies of patients who experienced a significant 90% reduction in seizure numbers were GNAO1 and PIGA pathogenic variants [708].

PER for Refractory and Superrefractory Status Epilepticus

Siew NaLim et al. [709] retrospectively analyzed the efficacy and safety of PER in the treatment of refractory or superrefractory status epilepticus. A total of 81 patients, including 39 women, with a median age of 64 (17–91) years old, were treated with PER; treatment was effective in 27 and ineffective in 54 patients. The initial dose of PER was positively correlated with the treatment response (OR = 1.27, 95% CI 1.03–1.57, $p = 0.025$), while the maximum dose was negatively correlated with the treatment response (OR = 0.74, 95% CI 0.58–0.96, $p = 0.022$). Hypoxemia caused seizures in six patients, five died in the hospital, and one was severely disabled; no cardiopulmonary adverse events or laboratory abnormalities were noted. The authors concluded that PER is effective and has a satisfactory safety profile in the emergency treatment of confirmed refractory and superrefractory status epilepticus.

An observational study in Chinese patients showed good efficacy, safety, and tolerability of PER in children (aged 4–12 years) with intractable epilepsy. The 50% response rates at 4, 8, 12, 24, 36, and 48 weeks after the addition of PER were 37.50%, 43.75%, 53.13%, 59.38%, 59.38%, and 62.07%, respectively. During the 48-week study period, 44.12% of the patients reported adverse events, and only three patients discontinued treatment because of adverse events. The most common adverse events were aggression (14.7%) and dizziness (8.82%) [710].

The Efficacy and Safety of PER as a Preferred Add-on Treatment for Epilepsy

Nuno Canas et al. [711] analyzed the efficacy and safety of PER in 60 patients after the failures of three antiseizure drugs and compared the efficacy of patients treated with PER as the preferred additional treatment ($n = 21$). At 12 months, there was no significant difference in retention between the preferred add-on therapy group and the last-add-on therapy group (93.8% vs. 66.7%); however, freedom from seizures among patients in the first group who preferred add-on therapy (81.2% vs. 27.8%; $p = 0.002$) and response rate (93.8% vs. 44.4%; $p = 0.002$) were significantly higher. There was no significant difference in tolerability between the two groups. Adverse events were reported in 54.3% of patients; most of these were mild or moderate, and dizziness was the most common.

Fernandes et al. [712] added PER to the treatment regimens of 94 patients (mean age 36.89 years, 51.1% women) for 24 months or more to evaluate the long-term efficacy and tolerability of PER in patients with epilepsy. The results showed that 33 patients (35.1%) were seizure-free at an average dose of 6.02 mg/day. Compared with patients who received two antiseizure drugs, patients who received only one antiseizure drug had a higher rate of seizure freedom. Efficacy was maintained in subgroups of patients who were followed for 36 or 48 months. The authors concluded that PER is effective in combination with one or two antiseizure drugs in pediatric and adult patients without the use of higher doses of drugs, and early addition of PER is more likely to result in seizure freedom.

Labate et al. [713] investigated the efficacy of PER in patients with medial temporal lobe epilepsy in real-world conditions. A total of 37 patients with medial temporal lobe epilepsy older than 12 years of age were enrolled. The patients were divided into two groups: Group 1 (20/37 patients) was treated with PER after failure of the first antiseizure drug, and Group 2 (17/37 patients) was treated with PER after the failure of ≥2 antiseizure drugs. At 3 months, 70% of patients in the first group had a >50% reduction in seizure frequency, including six patients who were seizure-free, compared with 23.5% of patients in the second group who had a >50% reduction in seizure frequency and none who were seizure-free. After the first group of six patients switched to PER monotherapy, five of them remained seizure-free at 12 months. At 1 year of follow-up, the response rate was 70% in the first group and 29.4% in the second. The authors speculate that PER has better efficacy as a preferred add-on therapy in patients with medial temporal lobe epilepsy.

In a 52-week, multicenter, observational cohort study [714], a follow-up analysis of 483 patients found that 227 patients (46.0%) discontinued the study. The most common reason for discontinuation was adverse events (26.4%). Serious treatment-emergent adverse events (TEAEs) occurred in 51 patients (10.6%), including two deaths determined to be unrelated to PER, and clinically significant TEAEs were reported in 153 patients (31.7%); the most common of these were dizziness (13.9%), balance disturbance (5.6%), aggression (5.4%), and weight gain (5.4%). The frequency of clinically significant TEAEs was lower in this study than in previous clinical studies, but rates of suicide (2.1% vs. 1.0%) and aggression (5.4% vs. 5.1%) were not significantly different. Data from this observational study were consistent with the safety profile of PER derived from previous phase II and III clinical studies, with no unexpected TEAEs observed in a real-world clinical practice setting.

A post hoc analysis of the open-label extension (OLEx) study by Trevor Resnick et al. [715] found that 53.8% of patients who received PER treatment during the double-blinded study and did not have FBTCS remained seizure-free for up to 24 months during Study 307. In contrast, 31.6% (6/19) of patients without GTCS in the double-blinded phase of Study 332 remained seizure-free for up to 24 months in the OLEx phase. More than 40% of patients were seizure-free for at least six consecutive months. Multivariate analysis showed that the best predictors of achieving FBTCS seizure freedom for at least 6 months were a lower baseline seizure frequency ($p = 0.0014$) and a lack of enzyme-induced antiseizure drug use at baseline ($p = 0.0056$). In addition, PER was well-tolerated, and no new safety indicator issues were identified. The most common TEAE was dizziness. Based on the Study 332 open-label extension study, a phase study evaluating the long-term efficacy and safety of adjuvant PER treatment (up to 12 mg/day) in patients aged over 12 years with generalized tonic–clonic seizures found a median reduction in GTC episodes per 28 days of 77% (weeks 1–13) and 90% (weeks 40–52), respectively. Retention rates were 88% (6 months) and 75% (12 months), respectively. Freedom from seizures was maintained for at least 2 years regardless of the treatment received during the core study period. The most common pattern daily dose was >4–8 mg/day, indicating that PER is generally well-tolerated and provides a long-term treatment option for patients ≥12 years of age [716].

Evidence-Based Medical Study of PER

Trinka et al. [717] conducted a systematic analysis of the application of PER in clinical practice, and 91 studies met the inclusion criteria, including 15 reports of randomized controlled trials (RCTS), 8 nonrandomized intervention studies, 37 observational studies, 21 case reports, and 10 systematic reviews and meta-analyses. The extracted data included those of 359 patients with secondary generalized tonic–clonic seizures, 251 with myoclonic seizures, 112 with absence seizures, 50 with tonic seizures, and 32 children with epileptic spasms. The most common type of epilepsy was IGE ($n = 378$), and the most common syndromes were juvenile myoclonic epilepsy ($n = 92$), progressive myoclonic epilepsy ($n = 59$), and absence epilepsy ($n = 43$). The RCT provides level I evidence that the addition of PER to treatment is effective for primary generalized tonic–clonic seizures in IGE patients ≥12 years of age. Data from other studies provide observational evidence of its effectiveness in multiple generalized seizure types, including myoclonic, absence, and tonic seizures. There was no indication of worsening or exacerbation of seizures in any seizure or seizure type. The authors speculate that existing studies have shown that PER has great potential as a broad-spectrum antiseizure drug. However, as most of the available data are from nonrandomized, noncontrolled studies and have a high risk of bias, further research is needed to provide more reliable evidence.

To assess the efficacy, tolerability, and safety of PER in focal seizure patients, a systematic review and meta-analysis conducted by Sonia Shinde Mahajan et al. [718] showed that patients treated with PER exhibited a 50% higher response rate compared to patients treated with placebo. The risk of TEAEs was significantly higher with 8 mg and 12 mg doses of PER compared with placebo. Only the number of patients who withdrew from the trial due to the incidence of adverse events was statistically significant in the 12 mg subgroup compared with the placebo group.

A systematic review including 21 studies aimed to assess the role of PER in terminating status epilepticus. It was found that PER was administered in 324 cases and started at a dose of 2–36 mg between 30 min and 59 days after the onset of SE. SE was halted between 1 h and 4 weeks after the initiation of PER. A total of 119 patients (36.6%) were considered PER responders. However, according to the GRADE methodology, the quality of evidence for all outcomes was very low, and further clinical studies are needed to determine the appropriate timing, dosage, and titration methods for safe and effective termination of SE [719].

Effects of PER on EEG and Cognitive Function

Seon-Jae Ahn et al. [706] evaluated the effects of PER on cognitive function and EEG, and studied the effects of PER on neuropsychological tests and quantitative EEG (QEEG) and its relationship with blood concentrations of PER. Seventeen patients with epilepsy were enrolled in the study and underwent electroencephalogram (EEG) and neuropsychological measurements before and after 6 months of treatment. The relative frequency band power, peak α frequency and neuropsychological QEEG test scores were compared before and after treatment. The results showed that there was a positive correlation between blood concentration of PER and QEEG changes. Delayed recall of complex figures was significantly improved with PER treatment, and other cognitive function tests showed no significant differences before and after treatment. The θ band power increased and the α band power decreased in each brain region following treatment, and the θ/α ratio, which represents the slowing of the background EEG, increased in all brain regions following treatment. The peak frequency of the α rhythm decreased significantly after PER ingestion. The difference of relative α power in the central region was positively correlated with the whole blood PER concentration ($r = 0.53$, $P = 0.03$). The authors' findings confirm that PER induced slowing of electrical activity, but no cognitive decline was observed. Because the study had no control group, cognitive test results should be interpreted with caution.

Lanzone et al. [720] studied QEEG changes in patients undergoing adjunctive treatment of epilepsy with PER, analyzed EEG changes in 25 patients with epilepsy before and after medication, and evaluated the correlation of their clinical characteristics. The results showed that θ power increased significantly on QEEG after the use of PER, but there was no significant change in EEG connectivity. Patients who responded to PER treatment had greater α power at T0 and T1, indicating that this parameter can predict the response to treatment. Therefore, the authors suggest that treatment-EEG is a viable tool for studying the neurophysiological changes induced by antiseizure drugs, emphasizing that α power changes can be used as a marker of response to antiseizure drugs.

A systematic review of the effects of PER on seizure control, cognition, behavior, and psychological status in patients with epilepsy was performed by Fong YO et al. [721] Analysis showed the efficacy and tolerability of PER in the treatment of epilepsy, and no negative effects on cognitive function were found, but the side effect of aggressive behavior compared with other antiseizure drugs cannot be ignored.

Effect of Add-on Treatment with PER on Patient Quality of Life

Trigg et al. [722] investigated whether the addition of oral PER treatment had an effect on the quality of life of patients with epilepsy. In this clinical phase III, multicenter, open-label study, the effect of the drug on health-related quality of life was analyzed. A total of 115 patients completed the trial, and it was found that PER as adjunctive therapy did not lead to deterioration in quality of life, thus informing the cost-effectiveness modeling of PER in the treatment of seizures.

Side Effects of PER

Kenaan et al. [723] described a 32-year-old African American man with recurrent generalized tonic–clonic seizures. Cataplexy occurred after the addition of PER to his antiseizure medication, and PER was temporarily discontinued considering his neuropsychiatric symptoms. The authors speculated that it was most likely a side effect of PER affecting projections to the inferolateral putamen nucleus (sublocus coeruleus), which inhibited arousal.

Among 92 patients older than 65 years treated by Lattanzi et al. [704], 20 patients (21.7%) discontinued PER, 12 of which due to adverse events (60%). The most common adverse events were irritability (8.7%), somnolence (4.3%), and dizziness/vertigo (4.3%). Patients with histories of psychiatric comorbidities had higher rates of behavioral and psychiatric adverse events. In an observational study of 387 cases of drug-resistant epilepsy treated with PER, Sagar et al. [694] also found that the most common side effects of PER were neuropsychiatric symptoms (18.86%), followed by dizziness (13.70%), and sleepiness (5.68%). Among 65 patients treated by Macrohon et al. [705], adverse events occurred in 53.8% of children, with somnolence (20.0%), gait problems (12.3%), weight gain (10.8%), and dizziness (9.2%) being the most common adverse events. The incidence of dizziness was significantly higher in children aged 12–18 years.

To evaluate the clinical effects of PER exposure, an analysis of 138 reported exposures by the American Poison Center found that the median age was 20 years (IQR 10–38), and 68 (49.3%) were male. The most common reason for exposure was treatment error (58%), followed by exploratory ingestion (17.4%) and suicidal ingestion (10.1%) [724].

Basic Studies on PER

Pavel Mareš et al. [725] studied the effect of PER in immature animals, examining the response to PER in rats at 12, 18, and 25 days of age, and found that PER selectively suppressed generalized tonic seizures of epilepsy in the two younger groups and suppressed total tonic–clonic seizures in the 25-day group. The authors suggest that PER was an effective anticonvulsant even in the early stages of brain development.

Culjat et al. [726] used 6,7-dimethoxy-4-ethyl-β-carbolin-3-carboxylic acid methyl ester (DMCM) to induce seizures in rats, and studied the antiseizure effects of PER and brivaracetam. The results showed that both PER and brivaracetam failed to inhibit seizures in rats on postnatal day 10 (P10). Both drugs reduced the severity of seizures. This effect was more pronounced with 20–40 mg/kg brivaracetam and 0.9–2.7 mg/kg PER, and the authors suggest that while the efficacy of these drugs against neonatal seizures may be limited, their efficacy increases with postnatal development. Vazquez et al. [727] studied the developmental effects of PER in pregnant rats and rabbits and found that PER may be associated with postimplantation failure and/or some specific delays in physical development, but not with fertility and early embryonic development.

Other Studies

To understand the role of PER in human glioma cell lines, Salmaggi et al. [728] exposed four human glioma cell lines to different concentrations of PER and temozolomide, either alone or in combination. The results showed that PER could significantly inhibit the growth of tumor cells and induce a high level of apoptosis. A stronger synergistic effect of PER in combination with temozolomide was observed in the U87 group but not detected in the U138 group. The authors suggest that PER has a pro-apoptotic effect on human glioblastoma cell lines, which may be related to the increased expression of GluR2/3.

Levetiracetam combined with PER can be used for the treatment of intraoperative seizures in patients with glioma during wakeful surgery. Motomura K et al. [729] conducted a retrospective cohort analysis of 78 consecutive glioma patients who underwent conscious surgery and found 18 cases (36.0%) of intraoperative seizures in the levetiracetam treatment group and two cases (7.1%) in the levetiracetam + PER group. Treatment-related adverse reactions in the two groups were rare and mild. This study demonstrated that treatment with levetiracetam plus PER significantly reduced the risk of intraoperative seizures compared with levetiracetam alone in patients with glioma. These findings will help neurosurgeons to perform safe and reliable wakeful surgeries and reduce the incidence of intraoperative refractory seizures during such procedures.

PER is a selective noncompetitive AMPA antagonist that slows the progression of the amyotrophic lateral sclerosis phenotype and increases anterior horn cell numbers in transgenic mice. Hotait et al. [730] conducted a study in six patients to understand the safety of PER in patients with amyotrophic lateral sclerosis. Subjects were started on 2 mg/day PER with weekly increases of 2 mg/day to a maximum dose of 8 mg/day. It was found that all six volunteers recruited had side effects to varying degrees; these mainly included mental and behavioral abnormalities. Two of the patients completed the trial and the other four withdrew due to the incidence of adverse events. All participants reported resolution of these events after discontinuation of the study regimen. The authors speculate that the use of PER in this amyotrophic lateral sclerosis study was limited by its poor tolerability. Another systematic review and meta-analysis of PER in the treatment of amyotrophic lateral sclerosis found significant improvements in cortical motor hyperexcitability with PER compared to placebo, but not according to the revised ALS Functional Rating Scale score. PER was associated with adverse events, such as irritability, somnolence, anger, and dysarthria [731].

Recent studies have shown that PER can play a neuroprotective role in hemorrhagic and ischemic stroke models by regulating blood–brain barrier function. To understand the neuroprotective effects of PER in neurovascular unit and traumatic brain injury models in vitro, Chen et al. [732] used cultured neurons and found that PER protected the cells from traumatic and excitotoxic damage, and treatment with PER attenuated lipid peroxidation and expression of inflammatory cytokines. In addition, PER increased Sirt3 protein expression, enhanced the activities of mitochondrial enzymes IDH2 and SOD2, and preserved blood–brain barrier (BBB) function in vitro. Sirt3 expression knockdown with a specific siRNA (si-Sirt3) partially preserved the effects of PER on neuronal injury and blood–brain barrier function. The authors suggested that PER could protect neurons and reduce brain damage after TBI by activating the Sirt3 signaling cascade.

In addition, it has been found that AMPAR activation leads to neuronal apoptosis after subarachnoid hemorrhage (SAH), at least in part through periostin expression upregulation. The clinically available AMPAR antagonist PER appears to have neuroprotective effects on early brain injury after SAH through anti-inflammatory and antiapoptotic effects independent of its antiepileptic effects [733].

2.1.3.3 Brivaracetam

Characteristics of the Drug

[Name of chemical] Brivaracetam

[Chemical structure formula]

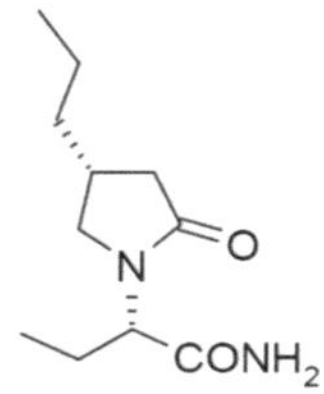

[Molecular formula] C11H20N2O2

[Molecular weight] 212.29

[Indications for use] It is indicated as adjunctive therapy in the treatment of partial-onset seizures in patients 1 month of age and older with epilepsy.

[Specification]

Tablets: 10 mg, 25 mg, 50 mg, 75 mg, and 100 mg
Oral solution: 10 mg/mL
Injection: 50 mg/5 mL single-dose vial

[Dosage] The recommended starting dosage is 50 mg twice daily. Based on individual patient tolerability and therapeutic response, the dosage may be adjusted down to 25 mg twice daily (50 mg/day) or up to 100 mg twice daily (200 mg/day).

Injection may be used when oral administration is temporarily not feasible.

Hepatic Impairment: For all stages of hepatic impairment, the recommended starting dosage is 25 mg twice daily; maximum dosage is 75 mg twice daily.

[Adverse reactions] Most common adverse reactions are somnolence/sedation, dizziness, fatigue, and nausea/vomiting.

Basic Research and Clinical Study of Brivaracetam

Brivaracetam (BRV) is an n-propyl analog of levetiracetam (LEV) developed by UCB Pharma, Belgium. In 2004, it was introduced as a new antiseizure medication (ASM) with high affinity for synaptic vesicle protein 2A (SV2A) [734]. In 2016, BRV was approved in the United States and Europe for the treatment of focal and generalized epilepsy [735]. As a derivative of LEV, BRV also binds to SV2A vesicles with high affinity and linear pharmacokinetic characteristics, but BRV has a 13-fold higher affinity for SV2A than LEV, and has higher selectivity and brain permeability. Many clinical trials with a retrospective and randomized design have demonstrated the efficacy of BRV, even in patients who failed to respond to LEV.

Basic Research on BRV

The antiepileptic/anticonvulsant effect of BRV is thought to be achieved through regulation of SV2A, a prototype protein that specifically recognizes endocrine granules and neuronal synaptic vesicles, and its main role is to regulate synaptic GABA release and inhibit Na+ channels, thereby playing an antiepileptic effect. Although the pharmacological mechanism of BRV is not fully understood, it plays an important role in regulating the release of neurotransmitters, and its metabolism is performed through the hydrolysis of acetamide groups to carboxylic acid metabolites. It is also the first ASM discovered whose mechanism of action is optimizing the pharmacodynamic activity of a molecular target [736].

To explore the antiepileptic/anticonvulsant mechanism of BRV associated with SV2A modulation. Motohiro Okada et al. [737] studied concentration-dependent effects of brivaracetam on astroglial L-glutamate release associated with connexin43 (Cx43), tumor necrosis factor-α (TNFα) and α-amino-3-hydroxy-5--methyl-4-isoxazolepropionic acid (AMPA)/glutamate receptor expression of rat primary cultured astrocytes. Furthermore, the interaction among TNF-α levels, elevated extracellular K+ levels and brivaracetam on the expression of SV2A and Cx43 was determined. TNF-α and elevated extracellular K+ levels predominantly enhanced astroglial L-glutamate release associated with respective AMPA/glutamate receptor and hemichannel expression. These effects were enhanced by a synergistic effect of TNF-α levels and elevated extracellular K+ levels in combination. The activation of astroglial L-glutamate release and expression of SV2A and Cx43 in the plasma membrane were suppressed by subchronic brivaracetam administration but were unaffected by acute administration.

These results suggest that migration of SV2A expression to the astroglial plasma membrane by hyperexcitability activates astroglial glutamatergic transmission, perhaps via hemichannel activation. Subchronic brivaracetam administration suppressed TNF-α-induced activation of AMPA/glutamate receptors and hemichannels via inhibition of ectopic SV2A. These findings suggest that combined inhibition of vesicular and ectopic SV2A functions contribute to the antiepileptic/anticonvulsive mechanism of brivaracetam action.

Clinical Practice of BRV in the Treatment of Seizures

To understand the clinical efficacy and tolerability of BRV in patients with epilepsy, Stefanatou et al. [738] performed a retrospective observational multicenter study. Patients were 16 years of age or older with various types of epilepsy and at least one follow-up after dose titration. The 156 enrolled patients had a mean age of 40 years (16–84 years), a mean duration of seizures of 21 years, 81% diagnosed with focal seizures, 16% with generalized seizures and 3% with unclassified seizures. Nine patients received BRV monotherapy. At the first follow-up, 56 patients (36%) showed seizure cessation, 24 patients (15%) had no significant change in seizure frequency, 6 patients (4%) had an increase in seizure frequency, and 9% had a decrease of less than 50% in seizure frequency. Adverse events occurred in 26 patients (17%) but were not life-threatening. The authors concluded that BRV is an effective, easy to use and safe ASM.

Stephen et al. [739] described the practice of BRV treatment in epilepsy clinics. They initiated BRV after 12 weeks of stable ASM treatment in patients older than 16 years with refractory epilepsy, at a target dose of 200 mg/day, and repeated examinations at 12- to 16-week intervals. A total of 108 patients were enrolled in the study, including 38 men and 70 women. Eighty-eight patients presented with focal epilepsy, 20 with hereditary generalized epilepsy, and 53 patients had previously used LEV and discontinued it due to ineffectiveness or side effects. Seizure reduction of more than 50% was observed in 71 patients (65.7%), 23 of whom (21.3%) remained seizure-free for more than 6 months. Four patients with juvenile myoclonic epilepsy had complete control of generalized tonic–clonic seizures, absence seizures and myoclonic seizures. The authors suggest that BRV is effective in various seizure types with a wide range of doses. BRV is also effective for patients who failed to respond to LEV treatment.

Nearly half of patients with epilepsy (PWE) have seizure clusters (SCs) and are at risk of subsequent hospitalization. Orlandi N et al. [740] evaluated the treatment of SCs ($\geq$2 seizures/24 h) with intravenous BRV. Of 97 patients (mean age 62 years) enrolled, 74 (76%) had a history of epilepsy (with drug-resistant seizures in 49% of cases); BRV was administered as first-line therapy in 16% of patients, whereas it was used as a first-line/second-line agent after benzodiazepine failure in 49% and 35% of patients, respectively. It was found that 58% of patients were seizure-free at 24 h after BRV administration, and 75 of 97 patients (77%) were not using other drugs. In patients without a history of epilepsy and who used BRV as a second or third-line agent, a higher likelihood of seizure recurrence and/or evolution to status epilepticus was observed. No serious treatment-emergent adverse events were observed. The authors concluded that intravenous BRV administration was well-tolerated in the treatment of SCs and could be considered as a treatment option, especially in the case of an in-hospital onset.

Long-Term Efficacy and Safety of BRV

To evaluate the long-term efficacy, retention, and tolerability of BRV add-on therapy, Strzelczyk et al. [741] conducted a multicenter, retrospective cohort study of patients treated with BRV between February and November 2016. They analyzed data from a 5-year observation period of 262 patients (mean age, 40 years; range, 5–81 years; 129 men), 227 of whom (87%) were diagnosed with focal epilepsy, 19 (7%) with hereditary generalized epilepsy, and 16 (6%) with other or unclassified epilepsy syndromes. Only 26 patients (10%) had never received LEV and 133 (50.8%) had switched from LEV to BRV. The total duration of BRV treatment was

6829 person-months (569 years). Seizures were reduced by more than 50% in 33.1% (79/239) patients, and 10.9% of them were seizure-free. Twenty-three patients were lost to follow-up. The retention rate was 61.1% at 12 months and 50.8% over the course of the study. At the last follow-up, 133 patients had received BRV at a mean dose of 222 ± 104 mg. Of these patients, 52 (39.1%) exceeded the upper limit of the recommended dose (200 mg). The authors concluded that although 90% of the patients had previously used LEV, there was still a 33% efficacy at 12 months, with an overall retention rate of >50%. They concluded that BRV had a good long-term efficacy and was well-tolerated for those types of epilepsy.

To evaluate the long-term efficacy and safety of BRV in patients with epilepsy, Manuel Toledo et al. [742] conducted a multicenter clinical trial with the use of variable doses of BRV for the treatment of patients with focal or generalized epilepsy. Of 766 patients treated with BRV (753 with focal seizures and 13 with generalized seizures), 51.7% had a >50% reduction in seizure frequency; 26% of patients were seizure-free at 6 months and 17.9% were seizure-free at 12 months, with a median of 52.0% reduction in seizure frequency. 42.4% of patients had a clinically meaningful improvement in the weighted Quality of Life Epilepsy Questionnaire 31 total score at 12 months and 46.8% at 24 months. The Kaplan–Meier calculated retention rate was 71.9% at 12 months and 53.7% at 36 months; 257 patients (33.6%) had drug-related adverse events, 49 (6.4%) had somnolence, and 41 (5.4%) had dizziness. Ninety-one patients (11.9%) discontinued BRV due to adverse events. The authors concluded that BRV was safe and generally effective. Simona Lattanzi et al. [743] conducted a network meta-analysis (NMA) to evaluate and compare the efficacy and safety of BRV, cenobamate (CNB), eslicarbazepine acetate (ESL), lacosamide (LCM), and perampanel (PER) for adult focal seizures. They systematic searched MEDLINE, the Cochrane Central Register of Controlled Trials (CENTRAL), and the US National Institutes of Health Clinical Trials Registry (http://www.clinicaltrials.gov). These randomized, double-blinded, controlled, parallel-group studies compared oral administration of the above ASMs with other comparators over a maintenance period of at least 12 weeks. The efficacy outcome was the proportion of patients with ≥50% and 100% reduction in baseline seizure frequency during the maintenance period, and the tolerability outcome was the proportion of participants who experienced at least one treatment-emergent adverse event (TEAE) and who experienced at least one TEAE leading to discontinuation of treatment. A total of 16 trials were included, including an overall enrollment of 4507 patients randomized to ASM treatment (BRV = 803, CNB = 221, ESL = 990, LCM = 1104, PER = 1389) and 2246 patients given placebo. Finally, cenobamate scored best for efficacy, and BRV and LCM were better-tolerated than the other drugs.

Efficacy of BRV on Epileptic Seizures in Children

Ferretjans et al. [744] studied the efficacy and safety of BRV in 66 children with epilepsy. The mean age of the patients was 8.8 years (range 1–16 years). 93.4% of the patients had drug-resistant epilepsy, and 27 of them had epileptic encephalopathy. The median dose of BRV used was 4.3 mg/kg/day. The results showed that 30.3% of the patients had a >50% reduction in seizure frequency, and 9% of the patients became seizure-free. When LEV treatment was ineffective, LEV was switched to BRV, and the efficacy was better in patients receiving higher doses. The authors speculated that BRV was effective for children with refractory epilepsy.

Alberto Verrotti et al. [745] noted that most studies on efficacy and tolerability have been conducted in adult cohorts, while few studies have been conducted in children, especially in those with generalized epilepsy and epilepsy syndromes; BRV is an ASM suitable for focal epilepsy in children. To evaluate the efficacy of BRV in children with epilepsy and epilepsy syndromes, the authors conducted a comprehensive review of the relevant literature and concluded that BRV was effective and safe in children with epilepsy. Among the children, there was more evidence of its effectiveness in children aged 4–16 years with focal seizures. Benefits have also been reported in patients with epileptic encephalopathy, such as Jeavons epilepsy, Dravet syndrome, Lennox–Gastaut syndrome, and juvenile myoclonic epilepsy. Song T et al. [746] searched four databases including PubMed, Embase, Web of Science and Cochrane Library. A total of 1884 articles were obtained on the use of BRV monotherapy or adjuvant therapy in the included children (age ≤18 years), and 9 articles were ultimately included, including 503 children with epilepsy. The retention rate of BRV treatment was 78%, the response rate (≥50% reduction in seizure frequency) was 35%, the seizure freedom rate was 18%, and the incidence of all treatment-related adverse events (TEAEs) was 39%. The most common TEAEs were somnolence (9%) and mental or behavioral disorders (12%). These results suggested that BRV seems to be safe and effective in the treatment of epilepsy in children.

BRV Treatment of Refractory Epilepsy

Ersilia Savastano et al. [747] evaluated the clinical and electroencephalographic effects of BRV (50–200 mg) in 76 patients aged ≥16 years with drug-resistant focal epilepsy. Seizure frequency of the 54 patients remaining in the study at 6 months was reduced >50% in 29.6% of cases (responders), <50% in 31.5% (nonresponders 1), and it remained unchanged in 38.8% (nonresponders 2). Twenty-nine percent of patients discontinued BRV early because of a lack of efficacy or minor adverse effects (AEs) like irritability, asthenia or headache. EEG quantitative analysis showed a significant decrease in α absolute power at 6 months. The θ band power of patients with no response was significantly higher than that of patients who responded. The $\delta + \theta/\alpha + \beta$ index of patients with side effects was higher than that of patients who did not have side effects. The authors speculated that BRV has a good efficacy, safety and tolerability, with a good behavioral profile. The reduction of α band power was related to its sedative effect, the increase of θ band power can be considered as a predictor of inadequate response to treatment, and the increase of $\delta + \theta/\alpha + \beta$ index may be a predictor of adverse events.

Svendsen T et al. [748] retrospectively collected data on patients older than 18 years of age with refractory epilepsy and started to receive BRV treatment from 2016 to

2019, and followed the clinical and laboratory data of the patients for more than 1 year or when the patient stopped BRV treatment. The results suggested that BRV treatment had a response rate of 48% in adults with intractable epilepsy after 1 year, and BRV was generally well tolerated, but psychiatric adverse effects such as increased irritability, anxiety, and depressive symptoms occurred in one-third of patients.

Anniko Snoeren et al. [749] explored whether BRV could significantly improve the treatment effect and reduce treatment-induced adverse events (TEAEs) in patients with refractory epilepsy who had failed to respond to previous LEV treatment. The mean time since the first seizure in the enrolled patients was 25.4 years. Among the 379 patients, 82.8% were diagnosed with focal epilepsy and 9.8% with generalized epilepsy. The median duration of treatment was 39 months for LEV and 20 months for BRV. The mean maximum dose was 1749.9 mg/day for LEV and 144.2 mg/day for BRV. Two hundred and eight patients (54.9%) directly switched from LEV to BRV. There was a certain time interval between LEV withdrawal and BRV initiation in 171 (45.1%) patients. The average interval was 77.7 months. Of the patients who discontinued BRV, 30 (24.8%) switched back to LEV. Discontinuation of initial LEV therapy was due to TEAEs in 63.6% of patients, including behavioral TEAEs in 55.1% of patients. 24.0% of the patients discontinued BRV due to inadequate efficacy, 47.1% due to TEAEs, and 22.3% due to both inadequate efficacy and TEAEs. Regarding efficacy, the analysis showed no significant difference between positive response rates to LEV or BRV. 78.0% of the patients who responded positively to LEV treatment also responded positively to BRV treatment. 46.2% of the nonresponders to LEV had a positive response to BRV. Compared with those treated with LEV, patients treated with BRV reported significantly fewer TEAEs. The difference in TEAEs was greatest in the "behavior" category. Newly discovered behavioral TEAEs after switching from LEV to BRV accounted for 7.1%. The authors suggested that BRV was better tolerated than LEV, especially for behavioral TEAE. Efficacy analysis showed that when patients responded positively to LEV, they were likely to respond positively to BRV. The lack of response to LEV did not affect the positive response to BRV. In summary, BRV appeared to be an alternative treatment option for patients previously treated with LEV.

BRV on Epilepsy with Other Diseases

Patients with intellectual disabilities are often excluded from clinical trials, and little is known about the best way to treat epilepsy in patients with intellectual disabilities. BRV is a new type of ASM and is often used as an adjuvant therapy for focal epilepsy patients with or without secondary generalized seizures. To understand the effect and safety of BRV on seizures in epilepsy patients with intellectual impairment, Ruby M E Gillis et al. [750] investigated the efficacy and tolerability of BRV in patients with epilepsy and intellectual impairment who had or had not previously received LEV treatment. The study enrolled 116 patients (mean age 34.9 years; 44% women). All patients completed 3 months of follow-up, 76 patients completed 6 months of follow-up and 39 patients completed 1 year of follow-up. The median initial dose of BRV was 50 mg/day, and an average of 2.6 other ASMs were simultaneously used. It was found that more than 50% of the patients had a reduction in seizure frequency. The retention rates after 3, 6, and 12 months were 84.4%, 75.5%, and 58.1%, respectively. There were no significant differences in seizure reduction and side effects between patients with and without prior LEV treatment. The authors concluded that BRV was effective and well-tolerated in epilepsy patients with intellectual impairment, and in patients who had failed previous treatment with LEV.

Approximately 13% of cancer patients have seizures. Patients who cannot normally use ASMs are treated by subcutaneous injection of midazolam, but this may cause sedation. BRV is an effective ASM for cancer patients with partial and refractory epilepsy with or without generalized seizures. It has fewer behavioral or psychiatric side effects than LEV, has a very low incidence of drug interactions, can be administered by injection, and thus may be used in patients with seizures that occur secondary to cancer. Bond et al. [751] described three cancer patients in whom subcutaneous BRV injection successfully controlled seizures during inpatient palliative care. The dose of BRV was switched from oral to subcutaneous injection at a ratio of 1:1, and no adverse effects were observed.

Poststroke epilepsy (PSE) is one of the most common causes of acquired epilepsy, accounting for approximately 10–15% of all newly diagnosed epilepsy. Simona Lattanzi et al. [752] evaluated the efficacy and tolerability of adjuvant BRV in the treatment of PSE patients for 12 months. At 12 months, 32 patients (42.7%) had at least a 50% reduction in baseline seizure frequency, and 26 of 75 patients (34.7%) were seizure-free. During the 1-year study period, ten patients (13.3%) discontinued BRV due to poor efficacy in six patients (8.0%) and four patients (5.3%) discontinued BRV due to poor tolerability. Adverse events were reported in 13 patients (20.3%), 84.6% of which were mild and 15.4% were moderate. It can be seen that in clinical practice, adjuvant BRV therapy is significantly effective and generally well-tolerated when used in PSE patients, and BRV can be a suitable treatment option for PSE patients.

Evidence-Based Medical Research

Madhuri Khilari et al. [753] speculated that the efficacy of BRV as a new type of ASM in early addition to treatment was not clear. To evaluate the efficacy and safety of BRV as an early addition treatment for refractory focal epilepsy, six randomized, parallel, and controlled trials were selected from Medline and Cochrane Central databases for meta-analysis. Among 1938 patients with focal epilepsy who received BRV as early add-on therapy, the hazard ratio for a 50% reduction in seizure numbers was 1.88, and the overall hazard ratio was 5.82. The authors suggest that their study provides some evidence for the clinical efficacy of BRV as an adjuvant in the early treatment of focal epilepsy, and that its efficacy in several other indications needs further clinical trials and evaluation. Eleonora Tulli et al. [754] retrospectively analyzed randomized controlled trials, retrospective studies and prospective studies of BRV in the treatment of partial epilepsy published before December 2020 from the MEDLINE, EMBASE and Clinical Trial databases. It was considered that analysis of literature data had demonstrated the safety and efficacy of BRV in pediatric epilepsy patients, with more evidence in children who developed focal epilepsy between the ages of 4–16 years. BRV may also be effective in some patients with epileptic encephalopathy, but comparative efficacy studies with other ASMs are needed to better determine the role and potential of this ASM.

Rebecca Bresnahan et al. [755] published a Cochrane review in 2022 to evaluate the efficacy and tolerability of BRV as an additional treatment for drug-resistant epilepsy patients and included six studies. They found that BRV, when used as an add-on therapy in patients with drug-resistant epilepsy, may be effective in reducing the frequency of seizures and may help patients achieve seizure freedom. However, BRV add-on therapy, compared with placebo, may be associated with treatment discontinuation due to adverse events. Only one eligible study included subjects with generalized epilepsy, none of the included studies involved subjects under 16 years of age, and all were short-term studies. Therefore, the results of this evaluation were mainly applicable to adult patients with drug-resistant focal epilepsy.

Efficacy-Based on Real-World Studies

Simona Lattanziet al. [756] used a time-baseline counting method to evaluate the clinical efficacy of BRV addition in practical applications. A total of 387 patients were included in the study. The overall median time-to-baseline seizure count was 150 days. The median time-to-baseline seizure count was 198 days for LEV-naïve patients, 126 days for patients with prior LEV use and withdrawal due to insufficient efficacy, and 170 days for patients who discontinued LEV due to adverse events ($P = 0.002$). The number of prior ASMs used and baseline monthly seizure frequency were independently associated with the primary endpoint. Add-on BRV treatment improved seizure control in LEV-naïve and LEV-prior use patients. The time-to-baseline seizure count represents an informative endpoint alongside traditional study outcomes and designs.

Due to the aging population, the management of epilepsy in the elderly has become a daily issue. Simona Lattanzi et al. [757] evaluated the effectiveness and tolerability of adjuvant BRV treatment for 12 months in middle-aged and elderly epilepsy patients (≥65 years old) in the real world. A total of 1029 patients with focal epilepsy were included in this multicenter retrospective study. Efficacy outcomes included the rate of seizure remission (≥50% reduction in baseline seizure frequency), freedom from seizures, and treatment discontinuation. Safety and tolerability outcomes included the rate of treatment discontinuation due to adverse events and the incidence of adverse events. Date of patients aged ≥65 years (elderly group, 111 patients, 10.8%) was compared with that of patients aged <65 years (younger group). The results showed that at 3 months, the median daily BRV dose was 100 (100–175) mg in the elderly group and 100 (100–200) mg in the young group. 150 (100–200) mg was the median dose in both groups at 6 months or 12 months. At 12 months, 49 elderly patients (44.1%) and 334 younger patients (36.4%) had at least a 50% reduction in baseline seizure frequency, and seizure-free rates were 35/111 (31.5%) and 134/918 (14.6%), respectively. During the one-year study period, 20 patients (18.0%) in the older group and 245 patients (26.7%) in the younger group discontinued BRV. Discontinuation of treatment because of inadequate efficacy was less common in older patients than in younger patients. Adverse events were reported by 24.2% of the older patients and 30.8% of the younger patients. The most common adverse events were somnolence, nervousness and/or agitation, vertigo, and fatigue in both study groups. The authors concluded that BRV was an effective, well-tolerated adjuvant drug, and no new or unexpected safety issues have emerged in clinical use. In the elderly population, brivaracetam is a suitable treatment option.

BRV for Status Epilepticus

Martellino C et al. [758] evaluated the efficacy and tolerability of intravenous BRV as a second-line treatment for status epilepticus (SE). Twenty-one patients (median age 68 ± 17.28 years) were treated with BRV (50–200 mg) as second-line add-on therapy for SE. Nearly a quarter of the patients had generalized seizures, while the vast majority (76.2%) presented with focal seizures. In 52.4% of the patients, the underlying cause was cerebrovascular disease. Fourteen patients (66.7%) showed a good early response to the drug within 6 h after the onset of seizures, and eight patients (38%) and 11 patients (52.4%) were seizure-free at 12 and 24 h, respectively. This study suggested that BRV can be used as an advantageous weapon for early addition treatment of SE.

Orlandi et al. [759] studied the efficacy and adverse events of intravenous BRV for SE in 24 Italian hospitals. Fifty-six patients were enrolled; their mean age was 62 years, 57% were men, and 21 (38%) had previous epilepsy. Regarding SE etiology classification, 46% of the patients were acute symptomatic, 18% were remote, and 16% were progressive symptomatic. About 80% of the patients had motor seizures. After benzodiazepine treatment failure, BRV was used as a first choice in 21% of patients and as a second or third (or more) choice in 38% of each. The median loading dose of BRV therapy was 100 mg (range 50–300 mg). Responses were found in 32 patients (57%). An early response was documented in 22 patients (39% of the whole sample). The use of the BRV within 6 h from SE onset was independently associated with an early SE resolution. No severe treatment-emergent adverse events were observed. The authors concluded that BRV was safe and effective in the treatment of SE, especially in the early stage of SE.

Alfredo De Liso et al. [760] reported a rare case of successful control of nonconvulsive status epilepticus by enteral administration of BRV. The patient was an 82-year-old woman who presented with elevated blood pressure, severe headache, and two focal motor seizures 4 days after right carotid endarterectomy. A CT scan showed right hemisphere edema with a 5 mm midline shift. EEG monitoring revealed persistent epileptiform discharges in the right hemisphere, consistent with the diagnosis of SE. She was treated with intravenous phenytoin (PHT), lacosamide (LCM), and LEV, but these were not effective. After an experimental treatment with 200 mg BRV administered through a nasogastric tube, her seizures improved significantly. The authors suggested that BRV could improve clinical seizures in patients with refractory status epilepticus. Enteral administration through a nasogastric tube should be considered.

Methodological Studies on Clinical Use of BRV

Junichi Yamamoto et al. [761] conducted intravenous injection of 100 mg BRV, 15 min of infusion, and oral administration in 24 healthy subjects, and found that there was no need to adjust the dose when changing from oral dose to intravenous dose because the response of epilepsy patients to BRV was related to the exposure dose (AUC). Beatriz Chavarria et al. [762] observed electrophysiological changes 10 min after intravenous injection of BRV (100 mg) correlated with its effects on brain dynamics after blood–brain barrier diffusion. They suggest that rapid BRV IV infusion has a favorable safety profile and is effective in controlling seizure series in the short term.

Mark Kristof Farkaset al. [763] evaluated the pharmacokinetics, safety, and tolerability of BRV in children with epilepsy between 15 min intravenous infusion and a single injection (≤2 min injection). Children received up to 5 mg/kg/day BRV (no more than 200 mg/day). No new safety concerns were identified in children 1 month to 16 years of age. Plasma concentrations were within the expected range, and no unanticipated pharmacokinetic differences were observed between patients who received either a 15-min infusion or a one-time injection.

Kiwon Lee et al. [764] also evaluated the clinical pharmacology, safety, tolerability, efficacy, and effectiveness of the use of intravenous BRV in the treatment of acute seizures in critically ill patients. PubMed was searched from its inception to April 13, 2021, and a total of 12 studies were included. The results showed that intravenous BRV was generally well-tolerated in patients with acute seizures in the hospital setting, with a low incidence of individual TEAEs classified as behavioral disorders. Intravenous BRV administration demonstrated efficacy and effectiveness, with a rapid onset of action, clinical and electrophysiological improvement of seizures observed within minutes, and general tolerability in patients with status epilepticus. The authors suggested that intravenous BRV showed efficacy and was generally well tolerated in the treatment of acute epilepsy in hospitalized patients requiring rapid dosing, which represents a possible use of BRV in an intensive care setting.

To understand the effects of different doses of BRV on seizures, Ben-Mnachem et al. [765] analyzed the long-term safety and tolerance of individualized doses of BRV in patients with focal epilepsy or generalized epilepsy or Unverricht-Lundborg disease. Overall, 72.6% patients discontinued the trial, mainly due to lack of efficacy (41.5%), adverse events (11.7%), and patient choice (11.5%). Overall, 720/853 (84.4%) patients reported TEAEs, 451 (52.9%) had a drug-related TEAE, and 95 (11.1%) discontinued BRV due to a TEAE. In the ULD subgroup, 87/94 (92.6%) patients reported TEAEs, 60 (63.8%) had a drug-related TEAE, and 16 (17.0%) discontinued due to a TEAE.

The most commonly used BRV dose was 150 mg/day (48.7%). In the Unverricht-Lundborg subgroup, the most common BRV dose was 100 mg/day (46.8%) and

39.4% of patients took BRV for 96 months. Focal seizure frequency compared to baseline was 43.1%, the 50% responder rate was 43.6%, and 6-and 12-month seizure freedom rates were 22.2% and 15.8%, respectively. The authors concluded that, overall, BRV was well-tolerated as a long-term adjuvant therapy in patients with focal epilepsy, generalized epilepsy, or Unverricht-Lundborg syndrome, with continuous improvement in focal seizure frequency maintained over time.

To understand the relationship between different doses of BRV and the number of ASMs taken before medication and clinical efficacy and safety, Sang-Kun Lee et al. [432] randomly assigned focal epilepsy patients taking 1–2 kinds of ASMs to take 50, 100, or 200 mg/day BRV or a placebo, and evaluated the results after summarizing the data. The results showed that in the subgroups of ≥5 ASMs (50, 100, and 200 mg/day BRV), the percentage of decrease in focal seizure frequency after 28 days of adjustment compared to placebo was 13.0% in the 50 mg/day group, 18.1% in the 100 mg/day group, 19.8% in the 200 mg/day group, and 17.0% in all BRV treatment groups. The 50% reduction rates of epileptic seizures in the 50, 100, 200, and 50–200 mg/day BRV groups were 26.9%, 29.9%, 30.0%, and 29.7%, respectively (placebo: 13.2%); For the 100, 200, and 50–200 mg/day BRV groups, there was a statistically significant difference in the ratio compared to the placebo group. In the immediate administration of 0–4 ASMs subgroups (50, 100, 200 mg/day BRV), all BRV dose groups showed statistical differences in the following three aspects: (1) Compared with the placebo group, the frequency of focal epileptic seizures adjusted for 28 days decreased to 21.4–28.7%; (2) Compared with the placebo group, there was a significant difference in the median percentage reduction of focal seizure frequency from baseline after 28 days of adjustment, with the BRV groups accounting for 35.5–45.9% and the placebo group accounting for 21.3%; (3) Compared to the placebo group, the advantage of a 50% reduction in seizures was more favorable for the BRV groups. Among patients receiving BRV treatment, the incidence of adverse events was 73.8%, with 10.5% discontinuing medication due to adverse events. Adverse events were more common in subgroups using ≥5 ASMs than in subgroups using 0–4 ASMs. Serious adverse reactions were rare in both subgroups (3.1% for past ≥5 ASMs; 2.9% for past 0–4 ASMs), indicating that the addition of BRV in the treatment of focal epilepsy in adults was effective and well-tolerated, regardless of the number and type of ASMs previously taken.

Side Effects of BRV

About 24.2% of 66 patients treated by Ferretjans et al. [744] experienced side effects of varying degrees, the most common of which were irritability and lethargy. In a study of 262 patients using BRV long-term, Strzelczyk et al. [741] found that psychological and behavioral abnormalities occurred in 1/10 patients. Ruby M E Gillis et al. [750] studied the safety of BRV in 116 epilepsy patients with or without previous LEV treatment and intellectual disability, and found that the most-reported side effects were drowsiness, dizziness, and aggression. In a study by Linda Stephen [739], among 108 patients taking BRV, 37 (34.3%) discontinued brivaracetam, 23 of which were due to side effects, four due to ineffectiveness, and 10 due to both.

Sedation was the most common side effect leading to the discontinuation of brivaracetam, followed by mental and behavioral abnormalities. Kuan-Ying Li et al. [766] conducted a literature review using Cochrane Library, PubMed/MEDLINE, and Embase, and the analysis showed that BRV had limited effects on cognition and behavior. For patients who could not tolerate LEV and had side effects of LEV-related behavioral disorders, A switch to BRV may be beneficial.

Cost-Utility of BRV Addition in Patients with Epilepsy

To evaluate the cost-utility of BRV compared with the third generation ASMs, Barrachina-Martinez et al. [767] used the Markov model to simulate the cost-utility of BRV in 2 years of treatment, and found that the incremental cost-utility ratio of BRV was better than that of LCM and zonisamide. Treatment with BRV was considered to be highly cost-effective. However, there were different views. Mehta D et al. [768] compared all-cause and epilepsy-specific pharmacy costs and total costs associated with initiation of eslicarbazepine acetate (ESL) or brivaracetam (BRV) among patients with focal seizures in long-term care (LTC) in the United States. The results suggested that ESL initiation, compared with BRV, was associated with 33.3% lower all-cause pharmacy costs, 34.4% lower epilepsy-specific pharmacy costs, 21.3% lower all-cause total costs and 30.9% lower epilepsy-specific total costs.

2.1.3.4 Rufinamide (RFN)

Drug Characteristics

[Chemical name] 1-(2,6-Difluorobenzyl)-1H-1,2,3-triazole-4-formamide

[Structural formula]

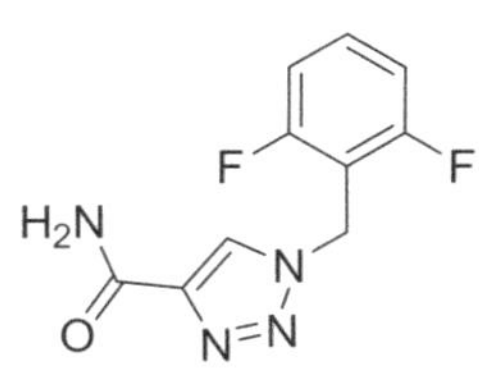

[Molecular formula] C10H8F2N4O

[Molecular weight] 238.193

[Indications] This novel antiepileptic compound can be used as an adjunct therapy for Lennox–Gastaut syndrome.

[Specifications] 100 mg

[Usage and dosage] Orally, twice a day, once in the morning and once in the evening. For patients weighing less than 30 kg, usually 200 mg/day, with a maximum dose of 1000 mg/day. Patients weighing more than 30 kg usually receive 400 mg/day, with a maximum of 3200 mg/day.

[Adverse reactions] Mild neurological symptoms characterized by fatigue, drowsiness, lethargy, and tremors.

Clinical and Basic Research

Historical Development

In 1992, a new potential ASM, rufinamide, was developed, prompting Brunner LA et al. to devise and validate a fully automated method for measuring its concentration in human plasma [769]. By 1996, Perucca E et al. had compiled existing data on the clinical pharmacokinetics of rufinamide [770]. In 1998, Cardot JM et al. investigated how food affects the pharmacokinetics of rufinamide [771]. In 2000, Jain KK assessed rufinamide in phase III trials and discovered that it has a significantly greater protective effect against seizures than other common ASMs in rodent epilepsy models [772]. By 2006, Aldenkamp AP et al. conducted a comprehensive study across multiple centers and countries, employing a double-blind, randomized, placebo-controlled design to explore the impact of rufinamide on cognitive function, ultimately revealing no significant cognitive impairment even with additional treatment and higher doses [773]. In 2009, Brodie MJ et al. organized a multicenter trial employing a double-blinded, placebo-controlled, randomized, parallel group design to evaluate the efficacy and safety of rufinamide as adjuvant therapy for refractory partial epilepsy in individuals aged 16 years and older [774]. With a unique chemical structure among approved ASMs, rufinamide has gained clearance from both the European Union and the FDA for use as adjunctive therapy in patients with seizures associated with Lennox–Gastaut syndrome [775]. In early 2024, research by Chen JL et al. suggested the potential of rufinamide for treating diseases characterized by nerve hyperexcitability [776].

Safety and Efficacy of Rufinamide Adjuvant Therapy in Patients with Epilepsy

In the field of ASMs utilization, considerable attention has been directed toward both efficacy and safety, with drug interactions emerging as a pivotal factor. Monitoring drug concentrations constitutes a crucial aspect of clinical practice. Yoshiaki Yamamoto et al. conducted a study to scrutinize the interplay between rufinamide and concomitant use of ASMs while also delineating the therapeutic threshold for rufinamide. Serum samples (n = 1531) from 178 patients (ranging from 2 to 57 years old) were obtained, and retrospective examination of clinical records was performed to evaluate the safety and efficacy of rufinamide (mean observational duration: 1073 ± 846 days).

Rufinamide demonstrated linear pharmacokinetics at doses up to 60 mg/kg (ranging from 50 to 3200 mg/day). Concurrent administration of ASMs such as phenytoin sodium, CBZ, and phenobarbital led to reductions in the rufinamide concentration of 43.4%, 13.2%, and 30.3%, respectively. Conversely, sodium valproate coadministration significantly increased the rufinamide concentration. Forty-one patients of the cohort (23.0%) exhibited a clinical response, with a median treatment concentration (interquartile range) of 20.6 g/mL (13.3–27.0). Therapeutic concentrations displayed no disparity among seizure types; however, patients experiencing tonic/atonic seizures tended toward higher rufinamide concentrations. Throughout the study duration, 64 patients (35.8%) reported adverse events, including drowsiness, gastrointestinal disturbances, dizziness, and irritability/behavioral alterations. Conditional logistic regression analysis revealed an 8.6-fold greater incidence of adverse events in patients receiving doses greater than 20 g/mL. These findings suggest the utility of therapeutic drug monitoring for rufinamide in predicting interactions between rufinamide and concurrently administered ASMs. In instances of tetanic/atonic seizures, particular attention should be given to whether the titrated concentration exceeds 20 g/mL [777].

Rufinamide, an ASM, is prescribed for treating epilepsy linked with Lennox–Gastaut syndrome and possesses a distinct structural composition compared with traditional ASDs. A presentation by Junaid Humayun et al. offered a succinct and illustrative overview of FDA-approved indications, pharmacodynamics, and pharmacokinetic properties. Additionally, this study shed light on the side effects, contraindications, and dosing regimens of this drug while elucidating the practical aspects of the American Academy of Neurology guidelines regarding its efficacious utilization in clinical settings [778]. Lennox–Gastaut syndrome (LGS) is a type of developmental and epileptic encephalopathy in which the initial symptoms typically manifest in early childhood. Due to its highly variable underlying causes, LGS cannot be categorized as a singular disease; rather, it is considered an electroclinical entity often posing challenges in early diagnosis and tailored treatment. Rufinamide, an antiepileptic medication, is recommended as an adjunctive therapy for LGS patients aged ≥1 year. Alexis Arzimanoglou et al. conducted a post hoc analysis to assess the safety and efficacy of adjuvant rufinamide treatment in the 022 study for total seizures and tetano-atonic seizures in children (<16 years) and adults (≥16 years). The randomized, placebo-controlled phase III 022 studies included LGS diagnosis and various seizure types (including tetano-atonic or standing inability seizures and atypical absence seizures; with ≥90 episodes in the month preceding baseline). The evaluation criteria included monitoring adverse events during treatment (TEAEs), percentage change in tonic-atonic seizure frequency over 28 days of the double-blind phase relative to baseline (primary endpoint), and the proportion of patients experiencing seizure frequency reduction of ≥25%, ≥50%, or ≥75% from baseline. Among the 138 enrolled patients, 74 received rufinamide (<16 years, n = 49 [66%]), and 64 received placebo (<16 years, n = 43 [67%]). The incidence of TEAEs was comparable across age groups. Both younger and older patients exhibited reduced tetanic-atonic episode frequency (per 28 days) with rufinamide treatment compared to placebo. The response rates in patients ≥16 years were 52% and 32% (rufinamide) and 15% and 5% (placebo), respectively. This post hoc analysis demonstrated that LGS patients, irrespective of age, tolerated rufinamide addition well and experienced improved seizure management [779].

Lennox–Gastaut syndrome (LGS) poses a significant challenge as a severe, chronic, and intricate form of early childhood epilepsy characterized by diverse seizure types, generalized slow (≤2.5 Hz) spike-and-wave and other EEG abnormalities, and cognitive impairments. Early seizure control is a pivotal therapeutic objective, and several ASMs are available. Given the limited success of monotherapy in achieving seizure control and the absence of conclusive efficacy data supporting specific ASM combinations for LGS, a judicious selection of combination therapy is imperative to optimize patient outcomes. This approach, termed "rational combination treatment," involves evaluating factors such as safety (including black box warnings), potential drug interactions, and synergistic mechanisms of action. Drawing from the clinical insights of Raman Sankar et al., rufinamide has emerged as the preferred adjuvant therapy for LGS, particularly when combined with clobazam and other newer LGS medications, offering promise in reducing tetano-atonic seizures associated with LGS [780].

A review encompassing 1759 participants in six trials, four of which focused on patients with uncontrolled focal epilepsy (1563 participants) and two of which specifically targeted individuals with identified Lennox–Gastaut syndrome (196 participants). The findings indicated that in patients with refractory focal epilepsy, rufinamide treatment in combination with a conventional ASM (adjunctive to a conventional ASM) significantly outperformed the placebo (adjunctive to a conventional ASM) in reducing seizure frequency by at least 50%. However, the rufinamide treatment group exhibited a greater likelihood of experiencing adverse reactions. Adverse events significantly associated with rufinamide included headache, dizziness, drowsiness, vomiting, nausea, fatigue, and double vision. While rufinamide adjunctive therapy effectively diminishes seizure frequency in patients with drug-resistant focal epilepsy, the reviewed trials were relatively brief in duration and did not provide evidence regarding the long-term utilization of rufinamide [781].

Application of Rufinamide in Epilepsy Patients in Special Populations

Children with epilepsy represent a unique subset within the epilepsy population, necessitating careful consideration of both the efficacy and safety of ASMs and their impact on growth and development.

Numerous factors may influence the growth and development of children with epilepsy, underscoring the importance of assessing any child experiencing appetite and weight issues. ASMs have potential side effects, and many can affect appetite, potentially impeding normal growth and weight gain in children. Buraniqi E et al. conducted a comprehensive review aimed at examining the impact of epilepsy and ASMs on appetite and weight in children. Using the Medline database, researchers systematically analyzed studies investigating the effects of ASMs on appetite and weight in children. The eligible studies included randomized controlled trials and open-label studies (including open-label extensions and interventions) involving children aged 0–18 years. Each study underwent classification based on treatment research evidence from the American Academy of Neurology (AAN) and was graded according to the level of evidence pertaining to children's appetite and weight. ASMs associated with symptoms of decreased appetite and/or weight loss include fenfluramine, topiramate, zonisamide, rufinamide, cannabidiol, ethosuximide, and other medications. Certain ASMs may impact both appetite and weight, potentially resulting in an elevated incidence of related ailments and diminished adherence to treatment regimens [80].

Evidence-Based Medical Research

Research on ASMs plays a crucial role in guiding clinical decision-making. Rufinamide, which acts through sodium channels, has demonstrated efficacy in treating Lennox–Gastaut syndrome (LGS). At the outset of this study, no systematic review had assessed the efficacy and safety of rufinamide in LGS patients. Indar Kumar Sharawat et al. conducted a comprehensive search across various electronic databases for articles detailing rufinamide use in LGS patients. The primary efficacy outcomes were compared to a placebo, encompassing studies with a minimum sample size of 20 to ensure a comprehensive evaluation of efficacy. A total of 557 patients participated in ten studies, five of which were placebo controlled. Among these, 265 patients received rufinamide, while 203 received a placebo. During the double-blinded period, the rufinamide group exhibited a mean percentage reduction of 29.3% in total seizure frequency per 28 days, compared to 8.3% in the placebo group (a significant difference of 20.9%, 95% CI: 14.4–27.3%, $p < 0.00001$). Rufinamide demonstrated superiority over placebo across various seizure types, including tonic–clonic seizures, atypical absence seizures, tetanic seizures, focal seizures, and myoclonic seizures. Notably, a greater proportion of patients receiving rufinamide experienced at least one treatment-related adverse event than did those in the placebo group (60.2% vs. 50.7%, $p = 0.02$, RR 1.24 (95% CI 1.03–1.51)). Nevertheless, the adverse effects were generally mild. In conclusion, as an adjunctive therapy for LGS patients, rufinamide effectively reduces the total seizure frequency with tolerable adverse effects [782].

To assess the efficacy and safety of ASMs in patients with Lennox–Gastaut syndrome (LGS), Zhang et al. conducted a systematic review of randomized controlled trials (RCTs) comparing ASM efficacy against placebo or each other for LGS. Efficacy and safety outcomes included seizure reduction, dropout rates, and serious adverse events with at least a 50% reduction in monthly seizure frequency. The results were ranked by the area under the cumulative ranking curve (SUCRA). The review included 1171 patients from eight RCTs involving six ASM types: lamotrigine, rufinamide, cannabidiol, topiramate, clobazam, and felbamate. SUCRA analysis indicated that rufinamide, cannabidiol, and topiramate were most likely to achieve a favorable response, although no significant differences were found between these treatments. Cannabidiol, topiramate, and rufinamide were associated with higher withdrawal rates, particularly cannabidiol, which exhibited a significantly greater discontinuation rate than placebo, clobazam, and lamotrigine. In conclusion, all ASMs showed significantly greater response rates than did the placebo, with rufinamide and cannabidiol ranking highest in terms of seizure reduction efficacy [431].

Concerning the safety of novel ASMs in children and the risk of movement disorders, Peacock DJSJ et al. conducted a systematic review and meta-analysis. They searched randomized controlled trials on novel antiseizure agents, including lacosamide, perampanel, eslicarbazepine, rufinamide, fenfluramine, cannabidiol, and brivaracetam, in pediatric populations up to October 2020. Among the 1690 nonredundant manuscripts, 23 studies were selected (total studies, $n = 1912$). The analysis revealed a significantly increased risk of movement disorders associated with perampanel use (RD 0.07, 95% CI 0.01–0.13; $N = 133$), albeit based on only one relevant clinical trial. Other ASMs did not increase the risk of movement disorders. This suggests that most new ASMs are generally safe for children with movement disorders, although the quality of evidence is limited by adverse event reporting [783].

Basic Research

Lennox–Gastaut syndrome (LGS) poses a challenge due to its resistance to classic sodium channel inhibitors. Rufinamide, a novel sodium channel inhibitor, has gained the approval of LGS treatment, deviating from conventional ASMs selection criteria. Yun-Chu Lin et al. conducted a quantitative investigation into the effects of rufinamide on Na+ channels, cellular discharge, and seizure behavior in neuronal and mammalian epilepsy models and compared them with those of other sodium channel inhibitors. The study revealed that rufinamide binds Na+ channels at a significantly faster rate than does phenytoin, making it particularly effective against seizures characterized by short pulses and hyperpolarized intervals, such as spikes and spike-wave discharge (SWD) on electroencephalograms. In models such as pentetrazol or AY-9944, rufinamide inhibited SWD-associated seizures, unlike phenytoin. This delineates the electrophysiological and behavioral manifestations of both typical and atypical seizures in LGS. The authors suggest that sodium channel inhibitors with varying binding kinetics and affinities for inactivated channels exhibit different antiepileptic effects, suggesting the rational selection of ASDs based on molecular pharmacology and paroxysmal discharge characteristics [100].

The efficacy of rufinamide in LGS stems from its rapid binding kinetics, as observed by Yun-Chu Lin et al. They found that rufinamide is most effective in altering the Na+ channel inactivation curve when the inactivation pulse duration is 1 s. Rufinamide selectively inhibits burst discharges of 50–300 ms at a platform voltage of −60 mV, which is attributed mechanistically to its selective binding to the intermediate inactivation state. Consequently, as the first molecule with an escape transition gated state, rufinamide may possess unique antiepileptic characteristics, indicating its potential for LGS management [784].

The full extent of the effects of rufinamide, a triazole derivative with a unique structure, on membrane ion currents has not been fully elucidated. Lai MC et al. utilized patch-clamp technology to investigate the impact of rufinamide on the pituitary GH3 lactotroph ion current amplitude, gating, and hysteresis. They observed that rufinamide increased the amplitude of the Ca2+-activated K+ current (IK(Ca)) in GH3 lactating pituitary cells, an effect attenuated by the addition of either bicillin or penicillin. Furthermore, rufinamide enhanced the activity of large conductance Ca2+-activated K+ channels (BKCa channels) when it was added to the cytoplasmic surface of the in vitro membrane, and this effect was reversed by parserine. Rufinamide also intensified the hysteresis exhibited by the BKCa channel under a reverse isosceles triangle ramp pulse. Additionally, rufinamide differentially suppressed the peak and late voltage-gated Na+ current (INa) induced by fast-stepping polarization. Molecular docking analysis revealed that rufinamide binds to the intracellular domain of the KCa1.1 channel through amino acid residues, suggesting functional modulation of BKCa channel activity. This study revealed that rufinamide can alter IK(Ca) and inhibit INa, suggesting that it has an effect on neuronal function and excitability [785].

Moreover, the mechanism by which rufinamide protects against brain injury remains unclear. Huaxu Yu et al. investigated the neuroprotective effects of rufinamide on rhodophyllin (KA)-induced neuronal damage in mice. Rufinamide mitigated KA-induced neuronal damage in a dose-dependent manner, with a significant improvement observed at a dose of 120 mg/kg. Immunohistochemical and Western blot analyses revealed that rufinamide inhibited KA-induced overexpression of IBA-1, preventing microglial overactivation. Additionally, rufinamide treatment attenuated the overexpression of neuroinflammatory cytokines (IL-1β, TNF-α, HMGB1, and NLRP3) in KA mice. Furthermore, rufinamide upregulated the expression of tight junction proteins (occludin and claudin-5) at the mRNA and protein levels, counteracting the KA-induced inhibition of tight junction expression. These findings suggest that rufinamide inhibits microglial overactivation, suppresses neuroinflammatory responses, and reduces blood–brain barrier breakdown, thus alleviating excitatory nerve damage in KA mice [786].

In addition to its pharmacological properties, the study of rufinamide has also extended to the development of novel methods for plasma determination to facilitate therapeutic drug monitoring. This research effort aimed to establish a sensitive and selective reversed-phase high-performance liquid chromatography method for quantitatively determining rufinamide content in human plasma alongside major metabolites. The plasma samples were subjected to protein precipitation with methanol, and the method demonstrated linear concentration ranges from 0.5 to 50 μg/mL. Bioanalytical validation, adhering to European Medicines Agency guidelines, indicated that the precision of the method ranged from 95.97% to 114.13%, with intraday and interday precision coefficients less than 10%. The samples remained stable under the experimental conditions. This method offers utility in therapeutic drug monitoring, pharmacokinetic assessment, and bioequivalence studies [775].

Furthermore, investigations into the effects of rufinamide include morphological and histological evaluations in animal studies. Pınar Ozkan Kart et al. sought to ascertain the morphological and histological impacts of rufinamide alongside other ASMs on follicular genesis in rats. Sixty female Wistar rats were divided into experimental groups and treated with zonisamide, sulthiame, lacosamide, clobazam, rufinamide, or a control regimen via intragastric administration for 90 days. Ovaries were extracted and fixed based on daily vaginal smears indicating the oestrus cycle stage. Immunohistochemistry and apoptosis staining were also performed. The results indicated a significant increase in the healthy follicular count in the control group compared with the ASM group ($p < 0.001$), with a notable decrease in luteinized follicles in the latter group ($p < 0.001$). Additionally, there was a significant difference in the number of TUNEL-positive apoptotic follicles between the control and drug groups ($p < 0.001$). Immunohistochemical analysis revealed stronger immune responses in the control group, suggesting that long-term treatment with ASMs such as rufinamide suppressed ovarian follicle development and increased apoptosis [534].

Other Research

Perampanel, rufinamide, stiripentol, and other newly developed antiepileptic medications have emerged as viable alternatives for managing chronic epileptic conditions. Sara Meirinho et al. conducted a study utilizing HepaRG cells as an in vitro model to investigate the metabolic stability of these drugs. In the experiment, HepaRG cells were exposed to perampanel (1 μM), rufinamide (100 μM), or stiripentol (5 μM) for 12 h. Additionally, HepaRG cells pretreated with known inducers of CYP450 isoenzymes (including rifampicin, phenytoin, phenobarbital, omeprazole, and CBZ) were subjected to the same treatments to evaluate potential drug–drug interactions mediated by CYP450 induction. The findings revealed a significant decrease in the concentrations of perampanel and stiripentol within the 12-h timeframe, whereas the concentration of rufinamide remained unchanged. This study not only provides insights into the metabolic stability and potential drug interactions of novel antiepileptic agents but also underscores the utility of HepaRG cells as dependable in vitro models for predicting in vivo metabolism [787].

2.1.3.5 Tiagabine (TGB)

Drug Characteristics

[Chemical name] (3R)-1-[4,4-bis (3-methylthiophene-2-yl) but-3-enyl] piperidin-3-3-carboxylic acid

[Structural formula]

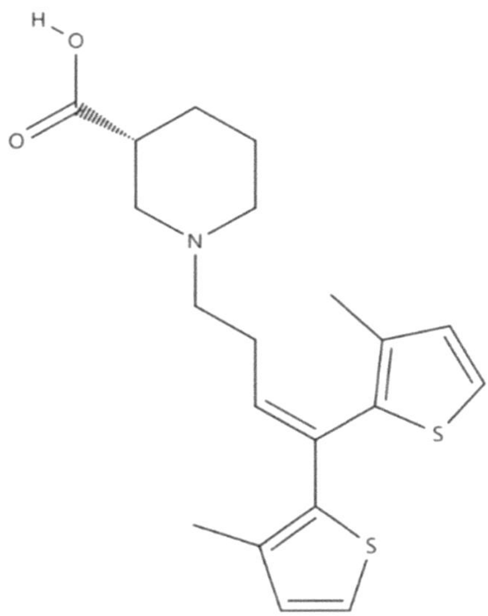

[Molecular formula] C20H25NO2S2

[Molecular weight] 375.55

[Indications] An anticonvulsant. It is a gamma-aminobutyric acid (GABA) absorption inhibitor. For the maintenance treatment of epilepsy in children and adults under 12 years of age.

[Specification] 12 mg

[Usage and dosage] The initial dose is 12 mg/day, divided into two doses, and the dose can be increased by 12–24 mg/week. Usually, the effective dose is 24–60 mg/day, divided into two to four doses. Patients with hepatic insufficiency need a lower dose.

[Adverse reactions] Adverse reactions include drowsiness, dizziness, headache, fatigue, pharyngitis, vomiting, diarrhea, irritability, and lack of concentration. Rare amblyopia, ophthalmia, myasthenia, myalgia, insomnia, mental disorders, depression, pruritus, ataxia, and sensory disorders may occur. It is rare for patients to have forgetfulness, emotional instability, excitement, nystagmus, rash, etc.

Clinical and Basic Research

Historical Development

In 1988, Pertwee RG et al. reported that drugs that stimulate or promote central GABA energy delivery synergistically with δ-9-tetrahydrocannabinol resulted in significant cataplexy in mice, and tiagabine attracted immediate attention [788]. In 1991, Nielsen EB et al. identified tiagabine as a novel centrally acting GABA reuptake inhibitor and conducted a study on its pharmacological properties [789]. In 1992, Coleman MH et al. assessed the protective effects of tiagabine against chronic seizures induced by intraventricular injection of a K+ channel-blocking peptide dendritic toxin (DTX) in mice [790]. In 1994, Sveinbjornsdottir S et al. investigated the neuropsychological effects of tiagabine [791]. In the same year, Walton NY et al. evaluated the potential clinical efficacy of tiagabine in the control of status epilepticus in an experimental model, suggesting the need for further research [792]. By 1995, Schachter SC conducted three trials to evaluate tiagabine hydrochloride (TGB) monotherapy in patients with partial seizures, suggesting its promise as a novel therapeutic approach for refractory partial epilepsy [793]. In October 1997, the FDA approved tiagabine as an adjunctive therapy for partial epilepsy in adults and adolescents aged 12 years and older [794]. In 2021, Kowalska M et al. conducted pharmacological and numerical analyses to assess potential cardiovascular risks associated with tiagabine use [795]. By 2023, experimental findings by Miziak B et al. revealed that subconvulsive doses of caffeine significantly attenuated the efficacy of anticonvulsant drugs in rodents, with tiagabine being an exception [796].

Tiagabine Addition for Refractory Epilepsy Treatment

A study was conducted on the efficacy of tiagabine (TGB) in Bulgarian patients with drug-resistant epilepsy, examining various facets of its effectiveness. TGB served as adjunct therapy for 43 patients, comprising 24 men with a mean age of 39 years. The findings revealed a relatively mild and fleeting dynamic enhancement in seizure severity, coupled with a satisfactory decrease in seizure frequency observed in 32.6% of participants. However, two patients experienced new seizure types. Notably, initial monotherapy yielded superior clinical outcomes. Adverse events, including dizziness/vertigo, sedation, memory impairment, loss of appetite and weight, confusion, psychosis, insomnia, transient diplopia, enlarged lymph nodes, rash, nausea, depression, anxiety, hand tremors, unstable gait, leg edema, thrombocytopenia, and neck muscle tightening, were reported in 26.19% of patients.

In summary, TGB treatment was correlated with diminished and temporary amelioration of epilepsy severity, significant and sustained improvement in seizure frequency, potential exacerbation of seizure control, emergence of new seizure types, and acceptable safety and tolerability profiles [797].

Adjuvant Therapy with Tiagabine for Drug-Resistant Focal Epilepsy

A comprehensive review assessed the efficacy and tolerability of tiagabine as an adjunctive therapy in patients with drug-resistant focal seizures. Enrolled participants, aged 12–77 years, underwent treatment for 12–22 weeks, with tiagabine compared against a placebo. The analysis revealed a significant association between tiagabine administration and adverse effects such as dizziness and tremors. However, the available data on cognitive function and quality of life outcomes suggested no notable impacts on cognition or mood. While tiagabine reduced seizure frequency, it also exhibited certain adverse effects when utilized alongside existing treatments for drug-resistant focal epilepsy. Notably, the review's findings primarily pertained to adults and adolescents, with limited applicability to children, as no trials included participants under 12 years old. Furthermore, no significant disparity was observed between tiagabine and topiramate as adjunctive therapies, although the evidence remains limited [798].

Application of Tiagabine in Special Epileptic Populations

Neonatal hypoxia-induced seizures (HSs) can manifest as spontaneous seizures in adulthood, a phenomenon observed in experimental models such as rats, where early hypoxia predisposes individuals to epilepsy later in life. However, the most effective ASMs for treating adult epilepsy caused by neonatal HS remain unknown. One study aimed to assess the efficacy of three ASMs on spontaneous seizures in adult rats with a neonatal history of HS: (1) phenobarbital (PHB), a longstanding epilepsy medication; (2) levetiracetam (LEV); and (3) tiagabine (TGB). Although LEV and TGB are newer anticonvulsants with limited efficacy in traditional seizure models but significant effectiveness in other models, the study revealed that PHB and LEV-reduced seizures in adult rats with a neonatal HS background, whereas TGB exacerbated seizures [799].

The Efficacy and Safety of Tiagabine as the Preferred Treatment for Epilepsy

A series of experiments involving C57BL/6 mice exposed to 100% oxygen at 5 absolute atmospheres (ATA) aimed to assess the combined efficacy of GABA enhancers (tiagabine and gabapentin) and sodium channel antagonists (CBZ and lamotrigine) in delaying seizures induced by hyperbaric oxygen (HBO2). Initially, the effective dose was determined from a single drug-dose response curve, and subsequently, the combination of tiagabine + CBZ or lamotrigine was examined to ascertain the maximum effective combined dose for subsequent experiments. These experiments were designed to elucidate the type of pharmacodynamic interaction of the three fixed-ratio combinations (1:3, 1:1, and 3:1). This study aimed to investigate whether the benefits of these drug combinations could extend to improving lung function. The results demonstrated that combining tiagabine with carbamazepine or lamotrigine not only conferred greater protection against HBO2-induced seizures but also allowed for the use of lower doses, thereby minimizing side effects and mitigating acute lung damage [800].

Evidence-Based Medical Research

Research on the effects of evidence-based medicine on ASMs provides some evidence for the formulation of clinical drug protocols and the innovation of scientific research ideas.

Gianni Cutillo et al. conducted a systematic review aiming to evaluate the efficacy of ASMs in controlling focal to bilateral tonic–clonic seizures (FBTCS), particularly at night, which are a significant risk factor for sudden death in epilepsy (SUDEP). The researchers searched various online databases for all post-1990 randomized, double-blinded, and placebo-controlled clinical trials of FDA-approved ASMs, specifically describing a reduction in FBTCS. They compared these reductions, where possible, to reductions in the onset of focal impairment of consciousness (FIA). Among the ASMs studied, topiramate (TPM) emerged as the most extensively researched, followed by tiagabine (TGB), brivaracetam (BRV), and lamotrigine (LTG). The TPM trials showed a reduction in FBTCS ranging from 44.8% to 100% (4.5–99% lower than placebo), while TGB exhibited reductions ranging from 21.8% to 46.7% (21.8–61% higher than placebo). BRV and LTG also demonstrated reductions, with BRV ranging from 33.9% to 82.1% (11.6–57.4% higher than placebo) and LTG ranging from 55.2% (20.3–52% higher than placebo). The authors underscored the need for future studies to uniformly report reductions in FBTCS episodes, including nocturnal events, to inform ASM choices effectively and minimize FBTCS occurrences, thereby mitigating the risk of SUDEP [801].

Wei-Chih Yeh et al. conducted a meta-analysis to investigate the effects of ASMs on polysomnography parameters by searching for randomized controlled trials (RCTs) in the PubMed, Embase, and Cochrane Central databases up to February 2021. Among the 18 eligible RCTs identified, the effects of five major categories of ASMs on sleep structure were analyzed: sodium channel blockers, calcium channel blockers, GABA enhancers, synaptic vesicular glycoprotein 2A (SV2A) ligands, and broad-spectrum ASMs. Calcium channel blockers and GABA enhancers were found to significantly increase slow wave sleep (SWS) times compared to placebo. GABA enhancers also decreased the percentage of rapid eye movement (REM) sleep, while calcium channel blockers significantly improved sleep efficiency (SE). Sodium channel blockers, SV2A ligands, and broad-spectrum ASMs did not affect SWS, REM sleep, or SE. Subgroup analysis revealed that gabapentin, pregabalin, and tiagabine increased the percentage of SWS time, while tiagabine also reduced REM sleep time, and pregabalin increased SE. Levetiracetam did not affect SWS, REM sleep, or SE. This meta-analysis highlighted the varying effects of different

ASMs on sleep parameters, indicating the importance of individualized treatment approaches in managing epilepsy [802].

Side Effects

Tiagabine-associated status epilepticus (SE) is a rare but serious complication of tiagabine. A case report described a 30-year-old man who experienced super refractory SE following tiagabine poisoning. After 72 h under general anesthesia, he achieved complete recovery and was discharged from the ICU on the 16th day. Patients with tiagabine-related SE exhibit distinct characteristics. Systemic convulsive SE can arise from voluntary or involuntary tiagabine poisoning, presenting significant treatment challenges. The electroclinical manifestations of tiagabine-associated SE vary depending on the underlying pathophysiological mechanism and may pose life-threatening risks. Typically, recovery occurs following tiagabine discontinuation and SE management, with treatment escalation guided by response to prior anticonvulsant therapy [803].

Use of Tiagabine in Other Diseases

One study revealed that tiagabine protects dopaminergic neurons from neurotoxins by inhibiting microglial activation. Pretreatment with tiagabine decreased microglial activation, partially safeguarded the nigrostriatal axis, and ameliorated motor deficits in a methyl-4-phenyl-1,2,3,6-tetrahydropyridine (MPTP) mouse model of Parkinson's disease (PD). Notably, in MPTP-treated GAT1 knockout mice, the protective effect of tiagabine was abolished. In another PD model, the inhibitory effects of tiagabine and subsequent neuroprotective effects on microglia were confirmed through intranigral infusion of lipopolysaccharide (LPS). Moreover, preconditioning with GABAergic drugs inhibited the LPS-induced inflammatory activation of BV-2 microglia and mitigated the toxicity of conditioned medium to SH-SY5Y cells. A reduction in nuclear translocation of nuclear factor κb (NF-κB) and suppression of inflammatory mediator production are potential mechanisms underlying this effect. These findings suggest that tiagabine can impede the activation of nigrostriatal microglia, potentially representing a novel therapeutic approach for Parkinson's disease [804].

Another study evaluated the role of tiagabine in a kainic acid-induced model of cerebellar injury in rats. Tiagabine was administered intraperitoneally to adult rats with kainic acid-induced cerebellar dystonia. Various assessments, including light beam walking devices, telemetry electromyography (EMG) recording, and histological validation, were performed to confirm postoperative dystonia symptoms in the rats. The study revealed repetitive stiffness indicative of involuntary dystonia spasms, alongside high dystonia scores and amplitudes, confirming twisting movements in rats. The results demonstrated that tiagabine effectively reduced dystonia spasms, as evidenced by EMG recordings and behavioral evaluations of rats walking through the light beam. This finding suggests that tiagabine may serve as an alternative therapeutic agent for dystonia treatment [805].

Basic Research

Tiagabine, a novel antiseizure medication, operates by inhibiting GABA transporter-1, thereby enhancing GABAergic signaling. However, its efficacy in chronic epilepsy models with neurobehavioral and neuroinflammatory conditions has been underexplored. Sana Javaid et al. investigated the real-time effects of tiagabine on electroencephalogram (EEG) activity, behavioral performance, and mRNA expression in mice treated with pentetrazol (PTZ). Male BALB/c mice received tiagabine (0.5, 1, or 2 mg/kg) for 21 days, along with PTZ injections (40 mg/kg) every other day for a total of 11 injections, and seizure progression was monitored via EEG. Behavioral experiments confirmed the anxiolytic and cognition-enhancing effects of tiagabine. In vitro analysis revealed that a 2 mg/kg dose of tiagabine mitigated seizure development and reduced epileptic spike discharge while also exerting a dose-dependent antianxiety effect and protecting against PTZ-induced cognitive impairment. Tiagabine reduced oxidative stress, regulated BDNF/TrkB signaling, and suppressed neuroinflammatory markers by enhancing GABAergic regulation. Overall, tiagabine may reduce epilepsy occurrence and improve associated neuropsychiatric effects by modulating oxidative stress, BDNF/TrkB signaling, and neuroinflammation [806].

During this study, Ismail FS et al. observed limited evidence on the effects of ASMs on glial cells. They investigated the role of tiagabine (TGB) and zonisamide (ZNS) in an inflammatory astroglia-microglia coculture model. Various concentrations of ZNS (10, 20, 40, 100 μg/mL) or TGB (1, 10, 20, 50 μg/mL) were added to cocultures under physiological conditions (M5) or inflammatory conditions (M30). TGB exhibited toxicity under both physiological and pathological conditions, while ZNS had limited effects on glial cell viability, especially at lower concentrations. TGB reduced microglial activation and enhanced resting microglia under inflammatory conditions, suggesting that it has anti-inflammatory effects. ZNS did not significantly alter the microglial phenotype. TGB disrupted gap junction coupling under noninflammatory conditions, possibly contributing to its antiepileptic activity, while ZNS disrupted glial gap junction communication under inflammatory conditions, potentially enhancing its antiseizure effects. TGB and ZNS differentially modulate glial cell characteristics, indicating the potential for new ASMs targeting glial cells as adjunctive therapies to traditional neuron-targeting ASMs [625].

Research has explored whether chronic administration of the GABAergic drug tiagabine and the dopamine mimetic pramipexole following trauma influences behavioral outcomes and plasma levels of corticosterone, testosterone, or 17β-estradiol in both female and male mice. These drugs were investigated for their potential to ameliorate GABAergic and dopaminergic deficits associated with post-traumatic stress disorder (PTSD). The animals underwent a single prolonged stress procedure (mSPS), and after 13 days of treatment with tiagabine (10 mg/kg) or pramipexole (1 mg/kg) once daily, PTSD-like phenotypes were assessed using a fear conditioning paradigm. Plasma hormone levels were measured shortly after the conditioned fear assessment. Exposure to mSPS increased conditioned fear responses in both male and female mice. However, while plasma corticosterone levels decreased in males, elevated levels were observed in females. Trauma led to increased plasma testosterone levels in both sexes but had no significant effect on 17β-estradiol levels. Pramipexole reduced trauma-related behavioral manifestations in both sexes, whereas tiagabine reduced them only in females. Although neither compound affected corticosterone levels in stressed animals, tiagabine further increased testosterone levels in females. The study revealed a sex-dependent effect of tiagabine in a mouse model of PTSD-like symptoms, while pramipexole did not demonstrate such an effect, and steroid hormone levels did not predict the efficacy of PTSD treatment [807].

Other Research

Tiagabine, primarily prescribed as an antiepileptic medication for managing partial seizures in humans, has shown promise in treating various nonepileptic conditions, such as anxiety, chronic pain, and sleep disorders. However, the incidence of tachycardia, a common nonneurological adverse effect, prompted Magdalena Kowalska et al. to conduct pharmacological and numerical studies assessing the potential cardiovascular risks of tiagabine. Molecular docking analysis methods were employed to describe the chemical interaction between tiagabine and human voltage-gated ion channels (VGICs). The in silico results suggested that the reported adverse cardiac effects of tiagabine cannot be directly attributed to its interaction with VGICs, a finding supported by in vitro organ studies and in vivo electrocardiogram measurements. The study concluded that tiagabine-induced tachycardia and other cardiac complications are not directly caused by the drug's effects on ventricular depolarization and repolarization [795].

Moreover, tiagabine hydrochloride overdose, while effective in reducing seizure frequency, can lead to adverse effects such as speech disorders, depression, and suicidal tendencies. Thus, establishing a convenient and sensitive analysis method for tiagabine (TGB) is crucial for guiding its clinical use. Zhen Zou et al. introduced a novel fluorescence initiation detection method for detecting TGB in urine, which also revealed the presence of a fluorescent dye [808]. Additionally, to elucidate the interaction of TGB with plasma proteins, other studies have investigated its binding to human serum albumin (HSA) and bovine serum albumin (BSA). VP capillary differential scanning calorimetry (DSC) measurements indicated that TGB slightly enhanced the thermal stability of these proteins. The isothermal titration calorimetry (ITC) results demonstrated moderate binding between TGB and HSA/BSA, as confirmed by fluorescence analysis. Furthermore, thermodynamic parameters suggested that hydrophobicity plays a significant role in TGB-protein complex formation. Competitive binding experiments with classic fluorescence probes revealed shared binding sites between TGB and dansulfosarcosine on HSA and BSA. Spectral analysis indicated no significant conformational changes in HSA and BSA upon interaction with TGB. Overall, these findings offer valuable insights into the mechanism of the interaction of TGB with serum albumin, aiding its utilization in the biomedical field [809].

2.2 New Antiseizure Medications under Study

2.2.1 Cannabidiol

2.2.1.1 Drug Characteristics

[Chemical name] (−)-trans-2-p-mentha-1,8-dien-3-yl-5-pentylresorcinol

(−)-trans-Cannabidiol,2-(6-Isopropenyl-3-methyl-2-cyclohexen-1-yl)-5-pentyl-1,3-benzenediol

[Chemical formula]

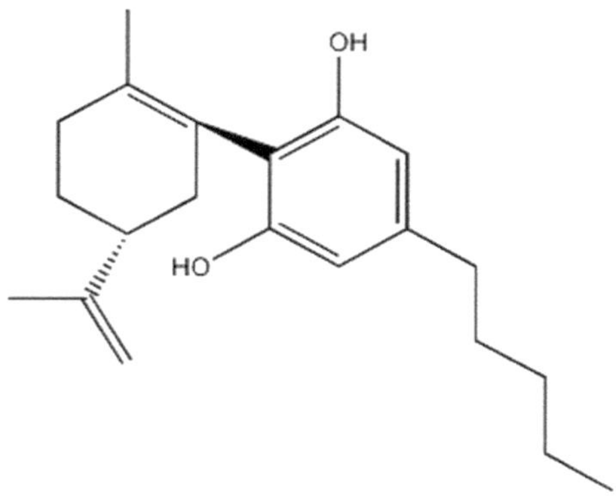

[Molecular formula] $C_{21}H_{30}O_2$

[Molecular weight] 314.462

[Indications] Seizures associated with Lennox–Gastaut syndrome (LGS), Dravet syndrome (DS), or tuberous sclerosis (TSC) in patients 1 year of age and older.

[Packing specifications] 100 mg/mL.

[Usage and dosage] In patients with LGS or DS,the starting dose is 2.5 mg/kg orally twice daily (5 mg/kg/day); after 1 week, the dose can be increased to 5 mg/kg, and finally to a maintenance dose of 10 mg/kg/day twice a day; patients who need to further reduce seizures may benefit from increasing the dose to the recommended maximum maintenance dose of 10 mg/kg twice daily (20 mg/kg/day) if a dose of 5 mg/kg/dose is tolerated, or from increasing the dose 2.5 mg/kg weekly twice daily if tolerated. For those patients who require rapid titration from 10 to 20 mg/kg/day, the dose should be increased at least every other day. The use of a dose of 20 mg/kg/day reduced the rate of seizures to some extent compared with the recommended maintenance dose of 10 mg/kg/day, but there was an increase in adverse reactions.

In patients with TSC, the starting dose is 2.5 mg/kg orally twice daily (5 mg/kg/day); to increase to 2.5 mg/kg twice a day (5 mg/kg/day) per week; if tolerated, it is recommended to increase to the maintenance dose of 12.5 mg/kg twice daily (25 mg/kg/day). For patients requiring a more rapid increase to 25 mg/kg/day, the dose should be increased at least every other day.

[Adverse effects] Common adverse effects include liver injury, drowsiness and sedation, suicidal behavior and thoughts, and hypersensitivity reactions. Elevated serum transaminase levels usually occur in the first 2 months of treatment and are related to drug dosage, especially in patients taking valproate concomitantly. Liver injury can be relieved after discontinuation. Patients with elevated levels of transaminases exceeding three times the ULN and bilirubin exceeding two times the ULN should discontinue medication. Cannabidiol can cause drowsiness and sedation, which are more common in the early stages of treatment and may weaken with continued treatment. The hypersensitivity reactions caused by cannabidiol can manifest as itching, erythema, and vascular edema, which can be treated with corticosteroids and antihistamines.

2.2.1.2 Clinical and Preclinical Research

Cannabidiol (CBD), the main chemical component in cannabis, acts as an antiseizure agent through a complex network of signals. Epidiolex was approved as a CBD-rich drug for the treatment of Dravet syndrome (DS) and Lennox–Gastaut syndrome (LGS) in children by the FDA in 2018. In 2020, the drug was approved by the FDA for the treatment of epilepsy associated with tuberous sclerosis (TSC). In the UK, New Zealand and Israel, standardized medical cannabis has been approved for clinical use, bringing new hope for the treatment of refractory epilepsy.

Cannabidiol for Dravet Syndrome and Lennox–Gastaut Syndrome

An ongoing expanded access program of cannabidiol in treatment-resistant Dravet syndrome and Lennox–Gastaut syndrome was conducted in Italy [810], in which 82 patients in 30 centers with at least 3 months of treatment were included in the effectiveness analysis. They found that at 3 months of follow-up, compared to the baseline, the percentage of patients with at least a 50% reduction in seizure frequency was 40.2% (plus 1.2% seizure-free).

Boudewijn Gunning et al. [538] analyzed four randomized, controlled phase 3 trials, including a total of 396 patients with LGS (49% on clobazam) and 318 patients with DS (64% on clobazam). Patients received plant-derived, highly purified CBD medicine (Epidiolex® in the USA; Epidyolex® in Europe; 100 mg/mL oral solution) at a dose of 10 or 20 mg/kg/day, or placebo for 14 weeks. CBD treatment resulted in a reduction in primary seizure frequency vs. placebo in the overall population and in patients receiving clobazam. The antiseizure efficacy of CBD was also demonstrated across other endpoints vs. placebo (≥50% response rate, total seizure frequency, number of seizure-free days) in the overall populations and in patients receiving clobazam.There were higher incidences of somnolence and sedation in patients taking CBD and clobazam. Most incidences of elevated transaminase levels occurred in patients taking concomitant valproate and, to a lesser extent, clobazam. This study indicates that add-on CBD was effective in reducing seizures in the overall population and in conjunction with clobazam.

To estimate the time to onset of CBD treatment effects in patients with Dravet syndrome (DS), Jennifer Madan Cohen et al. [811] conducted a post hoc analysis of two randomized controlled trials, GWPCARE1 and GWPCARE2. Patients received highly purified CBD (Epidiolex in the United States; 100 mg/mL oral solution) 10 mg/kg/day (CBD10; GWPCARE2) or 20 mg/kg/day (CBD20; GWPCARE 1 & 2), or matching placebo for 14 weeks. Treatment started at 2.5 mg/kg/day, reached 10 mg/kg/day on day 7, and went up to 20 mg/kg/day on day 11 during the 14-day titration period. Overall, 124 patients received placebo and 194 received CBD (CBD10, $n = 64$; CBD20, $n = 130$). Differences in convulsive seizure reduction rates between placebo and CBD emerged during titration and became significant by day 12 for CBD20 and day 13 for CBD10. Additionally, differences in the 50% responder rate between placebo and CBD became apparent during titration.

Onset of the first reported AE occurred during the titration period in 48.4% of placebo patients and 54.1% of CBD patients. The three most common AEs, somnolence, decreased appetite, and diarrhea, resolved within 4 weeks of onset in the majority of CBD-treated patients. The therapeutic effect of CBD for DS may start within 2 weeks of treatment in some patients. Although AEs lasted longer for CBD than placebo, most resolved within the 14-week study period.

Cannabidiol's Effects on Tuberous Sclerosis-Related Epilepsy and Other Epilepsy Syndromes

To evaluate efficacy and safety of 25 mg/kg/day (CBD25) and 50 mg/kg/day (CBD50) cannabidiol dosages vs. placebo against seizures associated with TSC, Elizabeth A Thiele [812] conducted a double-blinded, placebo-controlled randomized clinical trial. Eligible patients were those with a clinical diagnosis of TSC and medication-resistant epilepsy. Of the 224 included patients, 75 were randomized to CBD25, 73 to CBD50, and 76 to placebo, with 201 completing treatment. The percentage reduction from baseline in the type of seizures considered the primary endpoint was 48.6% for the CBD25 group, 47.5% for the CBD50 group, and 26.5% for the placebo group; the percentage reduction from placebo was 30.1% for the CBD25 group and 28.5% for the CBD50 group. The most common adverse events were diarrhea and somnolence, which occurred more frequently with cannabidiol use than that of placebo. Twenty-eight patients taking cannabidiol (18.9%) had elevated liver transaminase levels vs. none taking placebo.

It was revealed that cannabidiol significantly reduced the number of TSC-associated seizures compared with placebo. The 25 mg/kg/day dosage had a better safety profile than the 50 mg/kg/day dosage.

In the subsequent open-label extension experiments [813], median treatment time was 267 days at a 27 mg/kg/day mean modal dose. Most patients had an adverse event (AE). Most common AEs were diarrhea, seizure, and decreased appetite. AEs led to permanent discontinuation in 6% of patients. Median percentage reductions in seizure frequency (12-week windows across 48 weeks) were 54–68%. Seizure responder rates (≥50%, ≥75%, 100% reduction) were 53–61%, 29–45%, and 6–11% across 12-week windows for 48 weeks. Improvement on the S/CGIC scale was reported by 87% of patients/caregivers at 26 weeks. In patients with TSC, long-term add-on CBD treatment was well-tolerated and sustainably reduced seizures through 48 weeks, with most patients/caregivers reporting global improvement.

A retrospective analysis [814] found that CBD takes effect within 6–10 days of treatment. The most common adverse reactions being were diarrhea, decreased appetite, and drowsiness, which disappeared after 16 weeks of treatment.

Simona Lattanzi et al. [815] conducted a systematic review aimed to summarize the effects of pharmaceutical-grade CBD in patients with epileptic conditions, especially developmental and epileptic encephalopathies other than Dravet syndrome and Lennox–Gastaut syndrome. It included 42 studies through database and trial registry searches. CBD was found to be equally effective in treating other epileptic syndromes in children and adults, including CDKL5 deficiency disorder and Aicardi, Dup15q, and Doose syndromes, SYNGAP1 encephalopathy, and epilepsy with myoclonic absences. It is suggested that a highly purified, plant-derived CBD oil-based solution is effective in the treatment of a broad range of epilepsy disorders and etiologies, which provides preliminary support for additional research.

Application of Cannabidiol in Refractory Epilepsy

Tyler E Gaston et al. [816] conducted a 2-year follow-up of 169 participants (89 children and 80 adults) treated with highly purified CBD in order to evaluate the safety, efficacy, and tolerability of CBD for the treatment of seizures in children and adults with medication-resistant epilepsy. The results revealed a significant mean reduction in seizure frequency compared to baseline in children and adults at all time points (1 month, 1 and 2 years). Percentage of children achieving 50% seizure frequency reduction was 44% at month 1, 41% at year 1, and 61% reduction at year 2, while adult responder rates were 34% at month 1, 53% at year 1, and 71% at year 2. Chalfont Seizure Severity Scores (CSSSs) showed a sustained reduction from baseline to all three time points. Children displayed a 52% seizure reduction at month 1, a 51% reduction at year 1, and a 75% reduction at year 2. Seizure reductions in adults were 60%, 81%, and 85% at these time points, respectively (all $P < 0.0001$). While there were no significant differences in seizure frequency reduction between children and adults at all time points, there was a significant difference in seizure severity reduction at year 1, with adults reporting greater improvement in seizure severity ($P < 0.001$). The most commonly reported adverse events in the study were diarrhea, sedation, and decreased appetite.

A study by Sandip Patel et al. [817] also confirmed the long-term efficacy of CBD in the treatment of refractory epilepsy. By following 54 patients with refractory epilepsy for up to 60 months (median 45.5 months), they found that CBD maintained its efficacy for controlling seizures from Year 1 to the most recent study visit. The percentage of seizure responders remained similar at these time points (41.7–42.6%), and the seizure response rate was also maintained. Efficacy was also seen over a broad dose range, and at doses up to 50 mg/kg/day. CBD was particularly effective for controlling seizures in the setting of tuberous sclerosis complex and for reducing epileptic spasms and absence seizures. CBD was generally well-tolerated, with drowsiness and diarrhea as the primary adverse reactions. This study demonstrates that CBD does not lose its efficacy in controlling seizures over a treatment period of up to 60 months and is an effective, safe, and well-tolerated ASM for long-term use.

However, in an observational study of medical marijuana as a treatment for medication-resistant epilepsies, 29 subjects with medication-resistant epilepsies were treated with medical marijuana for ≥24 weeks and no significant differences in convulsive seizure frequency, seizure duration, postictal duration, or use of rescue medications compared to baseline were found. However, the doses of CBD used in this study were lower than those in prior studies. Randomized trials with larger cohorts are needed [818].

Cannabidiol oil (CBD) has been approved as an antiseizure medication for the treatment of uncommon types of epilepsy occurring in children: Dravet syndrome, Lennox–Gastaut syndrome, and Tuberous Sclerosis Complex. There are few publications related to the use of CBD in adult patients with focal drug-resistant epilepsy. The objective of this study was to evaluate the efficacy, tolerability, safety, and changes in quality of life of adjuvant treatment with CBD for at least 6 months in adult patients with drug-resistant focal epilepsy. From a total of 44 patients, 5% of patients were seizure-free, 32% of patients reduced their seizure numbers by more than 80%, and 87% of patients reduced their monthly seizure numbers by 50%. Eleven percent presented a decrease of less than 50% in seizure frequency. The average final dose was 335 mg/day, orally administered. Thirty-four percent of patients reported mild adverse events and no patients reported severe adverse effects. At the end of the study, most patients had a significant improvement in the quality of life in all the items evaluated. Adjuvant treatment with CBD in adult patients with drug-resistant focal epilepsy was effective, safe, well-tolerated, and associated with a significant improvement in their quality of life [819].

Camilo Espinosa-Jovel et al. [820] evaluated the efficacy and safety of CBD for the treatment of drug resistant epilepsy of different etiologies in patients >2 years of age in a multicenter retrospective study. Seventy-eight patients with a median age of 24 years and a wide spectrum of mainly structural and genetic etiologies were included. Patients were using a median of three antiseizure drugs and had a median of 30 monthly seizures before starting CBD. The median treatment time with CBD was 14 months. The efficacy analysis at the last available visit showed that mean percent reduction in seizures, ≥50% reduction in seizure frequency and seizure freedom were achieved in 67.8%, 68.8% and 11.5% of patients, respectively. They found no significant impact of concomitant clobazam use on the efficacy and safety of CBD. In the safety analysis, 28.2% ($n = 22$) of patients presented adverse events related to CBD and the drug-retention rate was 78.2%. Based on these findings, highly purified CBD should be considered as an adjuvant therapy for drug resistant epilepsy, regardless of its underlying cause or specific syndrome. Nevertheless, this assumption should be validated through further controlled trials.

Cannabidiol Effects on EEG and Cognitive Behavior in Patients with Refractory Epilepsy

To assess the longitudinal impact of CBD on the electroencephalogram (EEG) of children and adults, Leslie Grayson et al. [821] evaluated EEG changes before starting CBD, after approximately 12 weeks of CBD (FU1), and after approximately 1 year of CBD therapy (FU2). They found that at FU1, the adult group showed significant decrease in interictal discharge (IED)/minute, while a nonsignificant decrease was observed among children. The difference in changes over time between participant groups was significant after adjusting for last CBD dose. At FU2, both groups showed significant reductions from baseline after controlling for last CBD dose. There was no significant correlation between changes in seizure frequency and EEG IED frequency at each timepoint. This longitudinal EEG study shows that highly purified plant-derived CBD has positive effects on interictal epileptiform discharge frequency but no effects on other EEG measures (background frequency, focal slowing, reactivity, frequency of ictal discharges).

Aline Herlopian et al. [822] analyzed the EEG changes of 52 patients treated with CBD and found that 88.4% of patients had EEG changes. Eighty-nine percent of these patients had changes in their backgrounds, 74% in IEDs, and 46% in ictal findings. At the post-CBD EEG, 83% had a reduction in the frequency of the most predominant seizure type, and 25% reported subjective cognitive improvement. Of these patients, 88% and 92% had corresponding EEG changes, respectively. The study revealed electrographic changes in association with the CBD treatment. Despite these changes, a substantial association between specific electrographic findings and clinical outcomes was not established.

Metternich B, et al. [823] conducted neuropsychological tests on 39 patients with treatment-resistant epilepsy at baseline (T0) and after 3 months of CBD treatment (T1) to determine the cognitive and behavioral effects of CBD on children and adults. No significant cognitive decline was observed in any of the included measures. There was a significant improvement on a measure of selective attention and on a caregiver-rated behavioral measure in patients treated with CBD.

The Role of Cannabidiol in Epilepsy in Children

A retrospective cohort study [824] including 78 patients treated with off-label cannabidiol in Denmark was performed. In 51 patients with seizure frequency registration, 31.4% had ≥50% seizure reduction at 3 months of treatment, 31.1% at 6 months,

28.1% at 12 months and 20.0% at 24 months. At the same periods, the degrees of seizure reduction were 68.6%, 57.8%, 46.9%, and 20.0%, respectively. Seizure reduction was higher with clobazam comedication. In Dravet and Lennox-Gastaut patients, 70.0% had ≥50% seizure reduction at 3 months compared with 22.0% in patients with other epilepsies, in whom the degrees of seizure reduction at 3 months were 80.0% and 65.9%, respectively. The findings suggest that cannabidiol is a treatment option in children and young adults with severe refractory epilepsy outside of Dravet and Lennox–Gastaut syndromes. Clobazam comedication increases seizure reduction.

Roberto Caraballo et al. [825] presented eight patients with West syndrome who were refractory to ASMs, and who were treated with cannabidiol-enriched cannabis oil as add-on therapy. After a follow-up of between 6 and 13 months, a 75–99% decrease in seizure frequency was observed in two patients, a 50–74% decrease was observed in two, a less than 50% decrease was observed in three, and no changes in seizure frequency were seen in the remaining patient. The index of EEG abnormalities improved between 20% and 80% in seven patients concurrently with the reduction in seizures.

A prospective cohort study [826] found that in children with drug-resistant epileptic encephalopathies (DEEs), treatment with CBD-enriched medical cannabis as an adjuvant therapy induced reductions in seizure frequency. At the end of a median follow-up of 20 months, 78% of the children had a ≥50% decrease in seizure frequency and 47.5% had a >75% decrease. Seven patients (11.9%) were seizure-free. Adverse effects were mostly mild or moderate. CBD was discontinued in 17 patients (28.8%) due to lack of response to treatment, increased seizure frequency, intolerance to the drug, or poor compliance. It was indicated that in children with drug-resistant DEEs, long-term treatment with CBD-enriched medical cannabis was found to be safe, well tolerated, and effective as an adjuvant therapy to antiseizure therapy.

Real World Research on Cannabidiol

Katri Silvennoinen [827] described real-world experience with cannabidiol (CBD) in adults with Dravet Syndrome (DS). Adults with genetically confirmed DS had CBD added to existing therapy, titrated up to 20 mg/kg, as tolerated. The primary outcome measure was percentage reduction in convulsive seizures. Secondary outcome measures included changes in myoclonic seizures, and in cognition and quality of life as assessed by the Caregiver Global Impression of Change (CGIC), and incidence of adverse events (AEs). Eighteen adults (median age 27.5 years) were included. Median follow-up was 176 days. 17.6% of patients had a >30% reduction in number of convulsive seizures. AEs occurred in all patients, the most common being transaminitis (52.9%). Behavioral AEs led to discontinuation in 3/18 patients, including a seizure-free responder. In 7/18 patients, CBD was stopped due to lack of effect. 8/18 continued on treatment. Improvements in Caregiver Global Impression of Change (CGIC) were reported in 41.2% and 47.1% of patients by physicians and families, respectively. 17.6% achieved sufficient reduction in convulsive seizure frequency.

Safety of Cannabidiol

The main adverse reactions of cannabidiol included drowsiness, decreased appetite and diarrhea, followed by elevated serum transaminase levels. To determine the effect of cannabidiol on liver biochemical markers, Paul B Watkins et al. [828] evaluated changes in liver-related markers in healthy adults who received therapeutic daily doses of CBD for approximately 3.5 weeks. Seven participants (44%) experienced peak serum alanine aminotransferase (ALT) values greater than the upper limit of normal (ULN). For five participants (31%), the value exceeded 5 × ULN, thereby meeting the international consensus criteria for drug-induced liver injury. There was no correlation between transaminase level elevations and baseline characteristics, CYP2C19 genotype, or CBD plasma concentrations. All ALT level elevations above the ULN began within 2–4 weeks of initial exposure to CBD. The authors concluded that healthy adults consuming CBD may experience elevations in serum ALT levels consistent with drug-induced liver injury. Clinicians should be alert to this potential effect of CBD.

However, a safety study of repeated use of different doses (1, 2, 4, or 12 mg/kg) of plant-derived CBD in healthy adult beagles found that the dogs tolerated repeated administration well, with no clinically meaningful changes in measured safety outcomes. Adverse events were mild in severity. Relative to placebo administration, CBD administration at 12 mg/kg/day resulted in more gastrointestinal adverse events (mainly hypersalivation) and significantly higher serum alkaline phosphatase activity. Total systemic exposure to CBD increased on a dose-dependent basis following both acute (first dose) and chronic (28 days) administration [829].

Giselda Cabral-Pereira et al. [830] examined the behavioral and molecular effects of acute and chronic intraperitoneal administrations of VPA (300 mg/kg) and CBD (100 mg/kg) on the GASH/Sal audiogenic seizures (a reliable experimental model of generalized tonic–clonic seizures in response to intense sound stimulation). They found that acute and chronic CBD treatments have no significant adverse effects on body weight, hematological parameters, and liver function, although locomotor activity was reduced.

In addition to the above common adverse reactions, Ifrah Zawar et al. [831] described two cases of exacerbation of eyelid myoclonia in Jeavons Syndrome (JS) patients, which correlated with CBD use and resolved after CBD discontinuation. These cases highlight that caution should be practiced when using CBD for JS as it can potentially worsen eyelid myoclonia.

Preclinical Research on Cannabidiol

Effects on Seizures in Epileptic Animals

Frías-Soria CL et al. [832] evaluated the effects of cannabidiol use alone or in combination with antiseizure drugs on the expression of recurrent generalized seizures in a rat model. The results revealed that cannabidiol did not modify the expression of the 3-mercaptopropionic acid (MP)-induced seizures but reduced the prevalence of status epilepticus (SE) in both experimental groups. Phenytoin decreased the expression of major seizures but did not modify the prevalence of SE. Cannabidiol combined with phenytoin did not modify these effects. Phenobarbital diminished the expression of major seizures, an effect more evident when combined with cannabidiol. In contrast, CBD use in association with appropriate antiseizure drugs reduces the severity and prevalence of generalized seizures.

Merrick S Fallah et al. [833] assessed the efficacy of cannabidiol (CBD) and 9-tetrahydrocannabinol (THC) for suppressing focal and secondarily generalized seizures in an amygdala-kindling rat. It was found that CBD alone produced a partial suppression of both generalized seizures and focal seizures. THC alone also produced partial suppression of generalized and focal seizures, but doses of 10 mg/kg and above produced hypolocomotion. The addition of a low dose of THC to CBD (15:1) has antiseizure properties in the amygdala-kindling model. The addition of small amounts of THC greatly improves the effectiveness of CBD. A combination of CBD and THC might be useful for the management of focal impaired awareness seizures (FIASs).

Antiepileptic Mechanisms of Cannabidiol

José Carlos Pastrana-Trejo et al. [834] evaluated the effects on the posttranslational modification (PTM) of histones H3K4Me3, H3K9ac, H3K9Me2, H3K27Me3, and H3K36Me2 levels in the cerebral cortex, hypothalamus and pons of CBD-treated rats. It was found that CBD increased the PTM levels on the histones H3K4Me3, H3K9ac, and H3K27Me3 in the cerebral cortex. In addition, in the hypothalamus, CBD decreased the contents of H3K9ac. In the pons, CBD-treated rats showed a significant decline on the PTM levels of H3K4Me3. The study showed that CBD induced differential effects in levels of PTMs on the histones H3K4Me3, H3K9ac, H3K9Me2, H3K27Me3, and H3K36Me2 in several brain regions.

Willian Lazarini-Lopes et al. [835] studied the effects of chronic CBD administration in chronic models of seizures. Chronic CBD administration twice a day attenuated brainstem tonic–clonic seizures, prevented limbic recruitment, and suppressed limbic kindled seizures. Additionally, CBD prevented chronic neuronal hyperactivity, suppressing FosB immunostaining in the brainstem (inferior colliculus and periaqueductal gray matter) and forebrain (basolateral amygdala nucleus and piriform cortex), structures associated with tonic–clonic and limbic seizures, respectively. Chronic seizures increased cannabinoid receptor type 1 (CB1R) immunostaining in the hippocampus and in the BLA, while CBD administration prevented changes in CB1R expression induced by the AuK. The results strongly suggested chronic CBD anticonvulsant and antiepileptogenic effects associated with reduced chronic neuronal activity and modulation of CB1R expression.

Giselda Cabral-Pereira et al. [830] examined acute and chronic CBD administration in a hamster model of hereditary auditory convulsion, and found that chronic treatment with CBD caused abnormal mRNA expression levels for Trpv1, Adora1, Slc29a1, and Cnr1 genes. The study constituted a basis on which to develop further studies on the pharmacological effects of CBD and its interactions with other anticonvulsants.

Claudia Taborda Gómez et al. [836] performed experiments in the laboratory showing that CBD has an inhibitory role on P-glycoprotein excretory function, highly related to RE. CBD is considered a multitarget drug that could act throughout the canonical endocannabinoid receptors (CB1-CB2) or multiple noncanonical pathways. Since CB2 is expressed mainly in immune cells, they hypothesized that CBD treatment could alter the activity of polymorphonuclear neutrophils (PMNs) in a similar way to microglia/macrophages and other circulating leukocytes. In vitro, CBD induced PMN cytoplasmatic vacuolization and proapoptotic nuclear condensation associated with a significantly decreased viability in a concentration-dependent manner, while low CBD concentration decreased PMN viability in a time-dependent manner. At a functional level, CBD reduced the chemotaxis and oxygen consumption of PMNs related with superoxide anion production, while the singlet oxygen level was increased, suggesting oxidative stress damage. These results are in-line with the well-known CBD anti-inflammatory effect and support a potential immunosuppressor role on PMNs that could promote an eventual defenseless state during chronic treatment with CBD in RE.

Zhang HB. et al. [837] used a fluorescence-based thallium flux assay and found enhancement of flux through heterologously expressed human Kv7.2/7.3 channels by CBD. Patch-clamp recordings showed that CBD acts at submicromolar concentrations to shift the voltage dependence of Kv7.2/7.3 channels in the hyperpolarizing direction. The potent enhancement of Kv2/7.3 channels by CBD may contribute to its effectiveness as an antiseizure medication by reducing neuronal hyperexcitability.

2.2.2 *Fenfluramine*

2.2.2.1 Characteristics of the Drug

[Name of chemical] Fenfluramine

[Chemical structure formula]

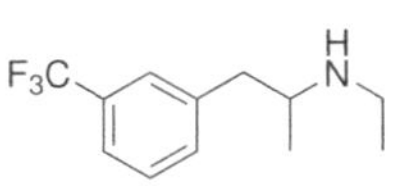

[Molecular formula] C12H16F3N

[Molecular weight] 231.257

[Indications for use] It is indicated for the treatment of seizures associated with Dravet syndrome and Lennox–Gastaut syndrome in patients 2 years of age and older.

[Specificatication] Oral solution: 2.2 mg/mL fenfluramine; 360 mL/bottle.

[Dosage]
The initial starting and maintenance dosage is 0.1 mg/kg twice daily, which can be increased weekly based on efficacy and tolerability. The maximum daily maintenance dosage of fenfluramine is 0.35 mg/kg twice daily (maximum daily dosage of 26 mg).

Dose adjustment is required in patients taking concomitant stiripentol plus clobazam: the maximum daily maintenance dosage of fenfluramine is 0.2 mg/kg twice daily (maximum daily dosage of 17 mg).

Dosage adjustment is recommended in patients taking strong CYP1A2 or CYP2D6 inhibitors, with severe renal impairment, or with mild, moderate, or severe hepatic impairment.

[Adverse reactions]
The most common adverse reactions (incidence at least 10% and greater than placebo) in patients with Dravet Syndrome were decreased appetite, somnolence, sedation, lethargy, diarrhea, constipation, abnormal echocardiogram, fatigue, malaise, asthenia, ataxia, balance disorder, gait disturbance, blood pressure increase, drooling, salivary hypersecretion, pyrexia, upper respiratory tract infection, vomiting, decreased weight, fall, status epilepticus.

The most common adverse reactions (incidence at least 10% and greater than placebo) in patients with Lennox–Gastaut syndrome were diarrhea, decreased appetite, fatigue, somnolence, and vomiting.

2.2.2.2 Clinical Application and Basic Research

Fenfluramine (3-trifurimethyl-n-ethylamphetamine) is a derivative of amphetamine that primarily affects serotonin neurotransmitter levels [838]. Fenfluramine (FFA) was initially used as an antidepressant and later as an appetite suppressant, but was withdrawn from the market in 1997 due to incidence of valvular heart disease and pulmonary hypertension in patients taking doses up to 220 mg/kg/day of fenfluramine [839–842].

However, the oral solution of fenfluramine was approved by the Food and Drug Administration of the United States and the European Union for the treatment of seizures associated with Dravet syndrome on June 25, 2020 and on December 21, 2020, respectively, completing the "new life of an old drug" [843]. On March 28, 2022, the FDA approved the drug for the treatment of seizures associated with Lennox–Gastaut syndrome (LGS). Since 2021, international research on fenfluramine in the treatment of epilepsy has made significant progress.

Fenfluramine for Dravet Syndrome

Sullivan et al. [844] analyzed longitudinal data from two phase 3 studies to calculate the numbers needed to treat (NNT) with fenfluramine to achieve "clinically meaningful" (50%) or "profound" (75%) monthly convulsive seizure frequency (MCSF) reductions in patients with Dravet syndrome (DS). In Study 1, NNTs to achieve

50% and 75% MCSF reduction were 1.8 and 2.1 at 0.7 mg/kg/day fenfluramine. In Study 2, these NNTs were 2.0 and 3.1, respectively. These results were seen as early as weeks 6–7 and were sustained through weeks 14–15.

They concluded that in both trials, one in every two to three DS patients treated with fenfluramine achieved a reduction in the number of episodes of ≥50% or ≥75% compared to placebo. Respondent analysis and NNTs can provide important information for clinical decision-making, supplementing the average number of individuals achieving meaningful levels of improvement in MCSF.

To investigate the association between reduced seizure frequency and daily executive function (EF) dose in children and young adults on fenfluramine adjuvant therapy, Bishop et al. [845] performed a postmortem analysis of data from patients 5–18 years of age with DS who were enrolled in a randomized, placebo-controlled Phase 3 clinical trial. A minimum 1 year fenfluramine Open Label Extension (OLE) study was subsequently completed. They found that a reduction of ≥50% in the daily frequency of attacks in 78% of patients. Overall, there was a significant correlation between change in MCSF and change in the Behavior Rating Inventory of Executive Function (BRIEF) 2 T scores for emotional regulation index (ERI) ($p = 0.008$). The 50% MCSF reduction group was significantly more likely to achieve clinically meaningful improvement in ERI ($p = 0.002$) and in cognitive regulation index (CRI) ($p = 0.001$) than the <50% MCSF reduction group. In summary, in children and young adults with DS, the magnitude of reduction in MCSF after long-term treatment with adjunctive fenfluramine was associated with clinically meaningful levels of improvement in everyday EF. Seventy-eight percent of children and young adults treated with adjunctive fenfluramine for 1 year in the OLE study achieved a 50% reduction in MCSF, for a magnitude of efficacy associated with a significantly greater likelihood of experiencing clinically meaningful improvement in emotion regulation and cognitive regulation.

Strzelczyk et al. [846] conducted a multicenter, retrospective, observational study to describe the efficacy, tolerability, and retention of fenfluramine (FFA). Patients received add-on therapy with oral FFA gradually titrated to a target dose between 0.13 and 0.7 mg/kg/day. Overall, 78 patients with DS (median age = 8.0 years, range = 2.1–46; 53% female) were treated with FFA for a median duration of 255.5 days (range = 31–572). Responder rates (≥50% reduction; $n = 78$) and seizure freedom rates at 3 months were 68% and 14% for total seizures, respectively, and 67% and 23% for generalized tonic–clonic seizures. Responder rates were consistent at 6 and 12 months ($n = 66$ and $n = 43$, respectively). Median seizure days per month significantly decreased from 10 (range = 0.5–30) to 3 (range = 0–30) in the 3-month period before and after FFA treatment ($p < 0.001$). Significantly fewer patients reported at least one episode of status epilepticus (28% vs. 14% patients before and after FFA initiation, $p = 0.005$). During FFA treatment, 35 patients (45%) were able to discontinue a concomitant ASM. At the last follow-up date, 66 (85%) patients remained on treatment with FFA. The most common adverse events were somnolence (36%), decreased appetite (22%), and ataxia (8%). Forty-eight patients (62%) were reported to have a meaningful global clinical improvement. They concluded that fenfluramine significantly reduced the number of seizures and was well tolerated, providing valuable information for real-world practice.

Sullivan et al. [847] analyzed data from two phase 3 placebo-controlled trials of fenfluramine adjuvant therapy for DS. They enrolled patients aged 2–19 years who were randomized to receive placebo or the addition of fenfluramine (Study 1: 0.7 mg/kg/day or 0.2 mg/kg/day; In Study 2: 0.4 mg/kg/day and stepentol). The proportion of patients who never reached baseline seizure frequency was greater with fenfluramine than with placebo (Study 1: fenfluramine 0.7 mg/kg/day, 60%; fenfluramine 0.2 mg/kg/day, 31%; placebo, 13%; Study 2: fenfluramine 0.4 mg/kg/day, 58%; placebo, 2%). Median time-to-nth seizure was longer after fenfluramine than after placebo ($p < 0.001$). The longest duration of convulsive seizure-free days was increased in fenfluramine groups versus the placebo group ($p < 0.05$). The most common adverse events included decreased appetite, pyrexia, upper respiratory tract infection, diarrhea, and fatigue. The results demonstrate that fenfluramine significantly reduces day-to-day seizure burden in patients with DS, providing prolonged periods of convulsive seizure-free days, which may reduce the physical and emotional disease toll while improving health-related QOL for patients and caregivers.

Evidence-Based Medical Research on Fenfluramine in the Treatment of Epilepsy

Zhang et al. [840] searched the Web of Science, MEDLINE (Ovid and PubMed), Cochrane Library, EMBASE, and Google. A meta-analysis of randomized placebo-controlled trials for the treatment of Dravet syndrome in the Scholar database obtained data from 206 patients receiving fenfluramine, which showed that fenfluramine was an effective antiseizure agent for the treatment of Dravet syndrome in children.

Fenfluramine for CDKL5 Deficiency Disorder Epilepsy

CDKL5 Deficiency Disorder (CDD) is an X-linked drug-resistant neurogenetic disorder characterized by global developmental delays and hard-to-control seizures. Devinsky et al. [848] studied six CDD patients (five women); the efficacy of fenfluramine in the treatment of CDD was evaluated in 83% of patients whose seizures had failed with 5–12 ASMs or other treatments. The median age at enrollment was 6.5 years (range 2–26 years). They found that fenfluramine reduced the median seizure frequency of five patients with tonic–clonic seizures by 90% (range 86–100%). Two patients experienced a 50–60% reduction in the frequency of the episodes. One patient had reduced numbers of myoclonic seizures. They believe fenfluramine may be a promising antiseizure drug for the treatment of CDD.

Basic Research of Fenfluramine in the Treatment of Epilepsy

Parthena et al. [849] examined the modulatory activity of fenfluramine on the S1R-mediated antiamnesic response in mice using combination analyses. Fenfluramine and norfenfluramine, racemate and isomers, were combined with either the S1R agonist PRE-084 or the S1R-acting neuroactive steroids pregnenolone sulfate (PREGS), dehydroepiandrosterone sulfate (DHEAS), or progesterone.

They reported that fenfluramine racemate or (+)-fenfluramine, in the 0.1–1 mg/kg dose range, attenuated the dizocilpine-induced learning deficits in spontaneous alternation and passive avoidance, and showed low-dose synergies in combination with PRE-084. These effects were blocked by the S1R antagonist NE-100. Dehydroepiandrosterone sulfate or PREGS attenuated dizocilpine-induced learning deficits in the 5–20 mg/kg dose range. Cotreatments at low doses between steroids and fenfluramine or (+)-fenfluramine were synergistic. Progesterone blocked fenfluramine's effect. Finally, fenfluramine and (+)-fenfluramine effects were prevented by the addition of the 5-HT1A receptor antagonist WAY-100635 or the 5-HT2A antagonist RS-127445, but not by the 5-HT1B/1D antagonist GR 127935 or the 5-HT2C antagonist SB 242084, confirming a 5-HT1A and 5-HT2A receptor involvement in the drug effect on memory.

They therefore confirmed the positive modulation of fenfluramine racemate or dextroisomer on S1R and showed that, under physiological conditions, the drug potentiated the low-dose effects of neuroactive steroids and endogenous S1R modulators. The latter are potent modulators of the excitatory/inhibitory balance in the brain, and their levels must be considered in the antiepileptic action of fenfluramine.

References

1. Tchicaloff M, Pennetti F. [Therapeutic results with a new antiepileptic, tegretol]. Schweiz Med Wochenschr. 1963;93:1664–6.
2. Spillane JD. The treatment of trigeminal neuralgia: preliminary experience with "tegretol". Practitioner. 1964;192:71–7.
3. Donner M, Frisk M. Carbamazepine treatment of epileptic and psychic symptoms in children and adolescents. Ann Paediatr Fenn. 1965;11(2):91–7.
4. Fernandez VE. [Pharmacology of carbamazepine]. Rev Neuropsiquiatr. 1967;30(3):273–89.
5. Redpath TH, Gayford JJ. The side effects of carbamazepine therapy. Oral Surg Oral Med Oral Pathol. 1968;26(3):299–303.
6. Mastroianni G, Ascoli M, Gasparini S, et al. Therapeutic approach to difficult-to-treat typical absences and related epilepsy syndromes. Expert Rev Clin Pharmacol. 2021;14(11):1427–33.
7. Santalucia R, Vilain C, Soblet J, et al. Carbamazepine efficacy in a severe electro-clinical presentation of SLC13A5-epilepsy. Ann Clin Transl Neurol. 2022;9(7):1095–9.
8. Vickery PB, Tillery EE, DeFalco AP. Intravenous carbamazepine for adults with seizures. Ann Pharmacother. 2018;52(3):285–9.
9. Kacirova I, Grundmann M, Brozmanova H. Therapeutic monitoring of carbamazepine and its active metabolite during the 1st postnatal month: influence of drug interactions. Biomed Pharmacother. 2021;137:111412.

10. Xu W, Chen YL, Zhao Y, et al. A clinical study of toxication caused by carbamazepine abuse in adolescents. Biomed Res Int. 2018;2018:3201203.
11. Kohlmann P, Stillhart C, Kuentz M, et al. Investigating oral absorption of carbamazepine in pediatric populations. AAPS J. 2017;19(6):1864–77.
12. Miyata-Nozaka Y, Tan HJ, Wong SW, et al. CYP3A5 genetic variants and their associations with carbamazepine and valproic acid response in Malaysian epileptic patients. Int J Clin Pharmacol Ther. 2021;59(1):8–16.
13. Welzel T, Ziesenitz VC, Weber P, et al. Drug-drug and drug-food interactions in an infant with early-onset SCN2A epilepsy treated with carbamazepine, phenytoin and a ketogenic diet. Br J Clin Pharmacol. 2021;87(3):1568–73.
14. Berghuis B, Hulst J, Sonsma A, et al. Symptomatology of carbamazepine- and oxcarbazepine-induced hyponatremia in people with epilepsy. Epilepsia. 2021;62(3):778–84.
15. Pan CW, Yu CH, Liao DL. Carbamazepine-induced hypersensitivity syndrome in chronic schizophrenia. Gen Hosp Psychiatry. 2013;35(5):575.e9–e10.
16. Hamed SA, Oseilly AM. Cochlear function in adults with epilepsy and treated with carbamazepine. Audiol Neurootol. 2018;23(1):63–72.
17. Xu C, Pan L, Zhang Y, et al. Assessing carbamazepine and oxcarbazepine-associated Stevens-Johnson syndrome/toxic epidermal necrolysis: data mining the public version of the FDA adverse event reporting system. Int J Clin Pract. 2021;75(8):e14273.
18. Wong CSM, Yap DYH, Ip P, et al. HLA-B*15:11 status and carbamazepine-induced severe cutaneous adverse drug reactions in HLA-B*15:02 negative Chinese. Int J Dermatol. 2022;61(2):184–90.
19. Ohta K, Okanishi T, Kanai S, et al. Stimulus-induced focal motor seizure in a pediatric patient with carbamazepine overdose. Brain Dev. 2022;44(10):765–8.
20. Baylis S, Costa-Pinto R, Hodgson S, et al. Combined hemoperfusion and continuous veno-venous hemofiltration for carbamazepine intoxication. Blood Purif. 2022;51(9):721–5.
21. Ran D, Wang N, Bao F, et al. Carbamazepine-induced follicular mucinosis-like drug eruption. Indian J Dermatol Venereol Leprol. 2022;88(6):826–8.
22. Perrott S, Khan QI, Counsell CE, et al. Progressive multifocal leukoencephalopathy associated with carbamazepine-induced immune dysfunction and recovery after carbamazepine cessation. BMJ Case Rep. 2023;16(7):e255119.
23. Chang BL, Liu JR, Chang SH, et al. Impact on carbamazepine usage and cutaneous adverse reactions before and after the reimbursement of HLA-B*1502 genotyping in Taiwan, 2000-2017: a nationwide longitudinal study. Epilepsia. 2023;64(10):2679–89.
24. Demir I, Adiguzel A. Assessment of vestibulo-ocular reflex with video head impulse test in epilepsy patients undergoing carbamazepine monotherapy. Eur Rev Med Pharmacol Sci. 2023;27(17):8013–8.
25. Kong FC, Ma CL, Lang LQ, et al. Association of xenobiotic receptor polymorphisms with carbamazepine response in epilepsy patients. Gene. 2021;771:145359.
26. Simeone TA, Heruye SH, Kostansek J, et al. Carbamazepine reduces sharp wave-ripple complexes and exerts synapse-specific inhibition of neurotransmission in ex vivo hippocampal slices. Brain Sci. 2021;11(6):787.
27. Zhang ML, Chen XL, Bai ZF, et al. ABCB1 c.3435C > T and EPHX1 c.416A > G polymorphisms influence plasma carbamazepine concentration, metabolism, and pharmacoresistance in epileptic patients. Gene. 2021;805:145907.
28. Zhang Y, Chen Z, Shi Y, et al. Revealing the sorption mechanisms of carbamazepine on pristine and aged microplastics with extended DLVO theory. Sci Total Environ. 2023;874:162480.
29. Jaruthamsophon K, Thomson PJ, Hammond S, et al. Characterization of drug-specific CD4(+) T-cells reveals possible roles of HLA class II in the pathogenesis of carbamazepine hypersensitivity reactions. Chem Res Toxicol. 2023;36(5):757–68.
30. Karlov VA, Vlasov PN, Kozhokaru AB, et al. [The efficacy and tolerability of extended release carbamazepine in adult patients with new-onset epilepsy using epileptiform activity index]. Zh Nevrol Psikhiatr Im S S Korsakova. 2021;121(3):31–8.

31. Yip VLM, Pertinez H, Meng X, et al. Evaluation of clinical and genetic factors in the population pharmacokinetics of carbamazepine. Br J Clin Pharmacol. 2021;87(6):2572–88.
32. Kacirova I, Grundmann M, Brozmanova H. Carbamazepine and carbamazepine-epoxide concentrations in mothers, colostrum, and breastfed newborns: comparison with concentrations determined during delivery and in the mature milk period. Biomed Pharmacother. 2022;151:113176.
33. Fujita Y, Murai M, Muraki S, et al. Population pharmacokinetic analysis of drug-drug interactions between perampanel and carbamazepine using enzyme induction model in epileptic patients. Ther Drug Monit. 2023;45(5):653–9.
34. Gul A, Mehreen S. Effect of carbamazepine on emotional intelligence and mindfulness in patients with partial epilepsy. J Pak Med Assoc. 2021;71(4):1103–6.
35. Lee JTC, Shanina I, Chu YN, et al. Carbamazepine, a beta-cell protecting drug, reduces type 1 diabetes incidence in NOD mice. Sci Rep. 2018;8(1):4588.
36. Bai Z, Jia K, Chen G, et al. Carbamazepine induces hepatotoxicity in zebrafish by inhibition of the Wnt/beta-catenin signaling pathway. Environ Pollut. 2021;276:116688.
37. Di Stefano G, De Stefano G, Leone C, et al. Real-world effectiveness and tolerability of carbamazepine and oxcarbazepine in 354 patients with trigeminal neuralgia. Eur J Pain. 2021;25(5):1064–71.
38. Shewell LK, Day CJ, De Bisscop X, et al. Repurposing carbamazepine to treat gonococcal infection in women: oral delivery for control of epilepsy generates therapeutically effective levels in vaginal secretions. Antimicrob Agents Chemother. 2023;67(1):e0096822.
39. Hamanaka K, Miyoshi K, Sun JH, et al. Amelioration of a neurodevelopmental disorder by carbamazepine in a case having a gain-of-function GRIA3 variant. Hum Genet. 2022;141(2):283–93.
40. Wang X, Ao X, Zhang T, et al. Ultraviolet-light-emitting-diode activated monochloramine for the degradation of carbamazepine: kinetics, mechanisms, by-product formation, and toxicity. Sci Total Environ. 2022;806(Pt 4):151372.
41. Candeloro M, Eikelboom JW, Chan N, et al. Carbamazepine, phenytoin, and oral anticoagulants: drug-drug interaction and clinical events in a retrospective cohort. Res Pract Thromb Haemost. 2022;6(2):e12650.
42. Wentland L, Downs C, Fu E. Comparison of signal enhancement strategies for carbamazepine detection in undiluted human saliva using an electrochemical sensor with stencil-printed carbon electrodes. Anal Methods. 2022;14(32):3103–14.
43. Chan H, Li Q, Wang X, et al. Vitamin D(3) and carbamazepine protect against Clostridioides difficile infection in mice by restoring macrophage lysosome acidification. Autophagy. 2022;18(9):2050–67.
44. Bonaccorso A, Gigliobianco MR, Lombardo R, et al. Nanonized carbamazepine for nose-to-brain delivery: pharmaceutical formulation development. Pharm Dev Technol. 2023;28(2):248–63.
45. Suwabe S, Tagami T, Ogawa K, et al. Improved drug transfer into brain tissue via the "nose-to-brain" approach using suspension or powder formulations based on the amorphous solid dispersion technique. Eur J Pharm Biopharm. 2023;185:137–47.
46. Mogavero MP, Ferri R, Marelli S, et al. Polysomnographic features associated with clonazepam and melatonin treatment in isolated REM sleep behavior disorder: time for new therapeutic approaches? CNS Neurosci Ther. 2024;30(2):e14569.
47. Cloos JM. The treatment of panic disorder. Curr Opin Psychiatry. 2005;18(1):45–50.
48. Chouinard G. The search for new off-label indications for antidepressant, antianxiety, antipsychotic and anticonvulsant drugs. J Psychiatry Neurosci. 2006;31(3):168–76.
49. Aurora RN, Zak RS, Maganti RK, et al. Best practice guide for the treatment of REM sleep behavior disorder (RBD). J Clin Sleep Med. 2010;6(1):85–95.
50. Khouzam HR. Identification and management of tardive dyskinesia: a case series and literature review. Postgrad Med. 2015;127(7):726–37.

51. Alghamdi SA. Hypnic jerks, major depressive disorder, and antidepressant use: a possible relationship. Cureus. 2023;15(10):e47436.
52. Brigo F, Igwe SC, Bragazzi NL, et al. Clonazepam monotherapy for treating people with newly diagnosed epilepsy. Cochrane Database Syst Rev. 2022;2(2):CD013028.
53. Han S, Lim JH, Bang J, et al. Use of a combination of N-acetylcysteine and clonazepam to treat burning mouth syndrome. Oral Surg Oral Med Oral Pathol Oral Radiol. 2021;132(5):532–8.
54. Gautam M, Kaur M, Sivananthan M. Parotid gland enlargement associated with clonazepam: a case report. J Acad Consult Liaison Psychiatry. 2021;62(6):657–8.
55. Lutz EW, Hines C. Recurrent clonazepam withdrawal delirium in a postoperative neurosurgical patient: a case report. BMJ Case Rep. 2021;14(6):e240804.
56. Muramatsu K, Ujiie H, Natsuga K, et al. Lichenoid drug eruption caused by clonazepam. J Eur Acad Dermatol Venereol. 2017;31(2):e117–e8.
57. Seyfinejad B, Ozkan SA, Jouyban A. Ultrasound-assisted electromembrane extraction of clonazepam from plasma and determination using capillary electrophoresis. J Chromatogr B Analyt Technol Biomed Life Sci. 2021;1181:122928.
58. An J, Wang X, Li Y, et al. Polystyrene nanofibers as an effective sorbent for the adsorption of clonazepam: kinetic and thermodynamic studies. RSC Adv. 2022;12(6):3394–401.
59. Piwowarczyk-Nowak A, Pałasz A, Bogus K, et al. Modulatory effect of long-term treatment with escitalopram and clonazepam on the expression of anxiety-related neuropeptides: neuromedin U, neuropeptide S and their receptors in the rat brain. Mol Biol Rep. 2022;49(9):9041–9.
60. Chuang SH, Westenbroek RE, Stella N, et al. Combined antiseizure efficacy of cannabidiol and clonazepam in a conditional mouse model of Dravet syndrome. J Exp Neurol. 2021;2(2):81–5.
61. da Silva LGR, da Silva Pinto AW, de Queiroz WE, et al. Deprescribing clonazepam in primary care older patients: a feasibility study. Int J Clin Pharm. 2022;44(2):489–98.
62. Byun JI, Shin YY, Seong YA, et al. Comparative efficacy of prolonged-release melatonin versus clonazepam for isolated rapid eye movement sleep behavior disorder. Sleep Breath. 2023;27(1):309–18.
63. French JF, Rapoport RM, Matlib MA. Possible mechanism of benzodiazepine-induced relaxation of vascular smooth muscle. J Cardiovasc Pharmacol. 1989;14(3):405–11.
64. Dell'Isola GB, Vinti V, Fattorusso A, et al. The broad clinical spectrum of epilepsies associated with protocadherin 19 gene mutation. Front Neurol. 2021;12:780053.
65. Sorel L. [Experimental antipileptic action and clinical action of zarontin]. Acta Neurol Psychiatr Belg. 1960;60:551–9.
66. Lossius HM. Experience with a new anti-convulsant of the succimide group, zarontin. Acta Psychiatr Scand Suppl. 1961;36(150):200–8.
67. Prot J, Saper J, Stroinska B. [Zarontin therapy of petit mal epilepsy resistant to anticonvulsants]. Neurol Neurochir Psychiatr Pol. 1963;13:487–90.
68. Dooley JM, Camfield PR, Camfield CS, et al. Once-daily ethosuximide in the treatment of absence epilepsy. Pediatr Neurol. 1990;6(1):38–9.
69. Terzioğlu B, Aypak C, Onat FY, et al. The effects of ethosuximide on amino acids in genetic absence epilepsy rat model. J Pharmacol Sci. 2006;100(3):227–33.
70. Gülhan Aker R, Tezcan K, Carçak N, et al. Localized cortical injections of ethosuximide suppress spike-and-wave activity and reduce the resistance to kindling in genetic absence epilepsy rats (GAERS). Epilepsy Res. 2010;89(1):7–16.
71. Buschhoff AS, Scherliess R, de Mooij-van Malsen JG, et al. Intrathecal application of ethosuximide is highly efficient in suppressing seizures in a genetic model of absence epilepsy. Epilepsy Res. 2022;184:106967.
72. Ascoli M, Mastroianni G, Gasparini S, et al. Diagnostic and therapeutic approach to drug-resistant juvenile myoclonic epilepsy. Expert Rev Neurother. 2021;21(11):1265–73.
73. Samanta D. Pharmacotherapeutic management of seizures in patients with Angleman syndrome. Expert Opin Pharmacother. 2022;23(13):1511–22.

74. Shawahna R, Zaid L. Concentrations of antiseizure medications in breast milk of lactating women with epilepsy: a systematic review with qualitative synthesis. Seizure. 2022;98:57–70.
75. Brigo F, Igwe SC, Lattanzi S. Ethosuximide, sodium valproate or lamotrigine for absence seizures in children and adolescents. Cochrane Database Syst Rev. 2021;1(1):CD003032.
76. Rinaldi VE, Di Cara G, Mencaroni E, et al. Therapeutic options for childhood absence epilepsy. Pediatr Rep. 2021;13(4):658–67.
77. Mostacci B, Ranzato F, Giuliano L, et al. Alternatives to valproate in girls and women of childbearing potential with idiopathic generalized epilepsies: state of the art and guidance for the clinician proposed by the Epilepsy and Gender Commission of the Italian League Against Epilepsy (LICE). Seizure. 2021;85:26–38.
78. Besag FMC, Vasey MJ. Neurocognitive effects of antiseizure medications in children and adolescents with epilepsy. Paediatr Drugs. 2021;23(3):253–86.
79. Strzelczyk A, Schubert-Bast S. Psychobehavioural and cognitive adverse events of antiseizure medications for the treatment of developmental and epileptic encephalopathies. CNS Drugs. 2022;36(10):1079–111.
80. Buraniqi E, Dabaja H, Wirrell EC. Impact of antiseizure medications on appetite and weight in children. Paediatr Drugs. 2022;24(4):335–63.
81. Sáenz-Farret M, Tijssen MAJ, Eliashiv D, et al. Antiseizure drugs and movement disorders. CNS Drugs. 2022;36(8):859–76.
82. Shang H, Glaun M, Ongkasuwan J. Ethosuximide induced macroglossia and oropharyngeal edema. Int J Pediatr Otorhinolaryngol. 2021;140:110498.
83. Nagu P, Sharma V, Behl T, et al. Molecular insights to the Wnt signaling during Alzheimer's disorder: a potential target for therapeutic interventions. J Mol Neurosci. 2022;72(4):679–90.
84. Tatum S, Smith ZZ, Taylor JA, et al. Sensitivity of unilateral- versus bilateral-onset spike-wave discharges to ethosuximide and carbamazepine in the fluid percussion injury rat model of traumatic brain injury. J Neurophysiol. 2021;125(6):2166–77.
85. El-Haggar SM, Hegazy SK, Abd-Elsalam SM, Bahaa MM, et al. Open-label pilot study of ethosuximide as adjunctive therapy for relieving abdominal pain related to Irritable Bowel Syndrome. J Clin Pharm Ther. 2022;47(3):306–12.
86. Gadotti VM, Zamponi GW. Ethosuximide inhibits acute histamine- and chloroquine-induced scratching behavior in mice. Mol Brain. 2021;14(1):46.
87. Porter RJ, Penry JK. Phenobarbital: biopharmacology. Adv Neurol. 1980;27:493–500.
88. Pigatto PD, Morelli M, Polenghi MM, et al. Phenobarbital-induced allergic dermatitis. Contact Derm. 1987;16(5):279.
89. Crawford TO, Mitchell WG. Phenobarbital for status. Neurology. 1989;39(4):609.
90. Lindberg MC, Cunningham A, Lindberg NH. Acute phenobarbital intoxication. South Med J. 1992;85(8):803–7.
91. Brodie MJ, Kwan P. Current position of phenobarbital in epilepsy and its future. Epilepsia. 2012;53(Suppl 8):40–6.
92. Pacifici GM. Clinical pharmacology of phenobarbital in neonates: effects, metabolism and pharmacokinetics. Curr Pediatr Rev. 2016;12(1):48–54.
93. Hofmeister B, von Stülpnagel C, Betzler C, et al. Epilepsy in Nicolaides-Baraitser syndrome: review of literature and report of 25 patients focusing on treatment aspects. Neuropediatrics. 2021;52(2):109–22.
94. Su Y, Huang H, Jiang M, et al. Phenobarbital versus valproate for generalized convulsive status epilepticus in adults (2): a multicenter prospective randomized controlled trial in China (China 2-P vs. V). Epilepsy Res. 2021;177:106755.
95. Jain P, Aneja S, Cunningham J, et al. Treatment of benzodiazepine-resistant status epilepticus: systematic review and network meta-analyses. Seizure. 2022;102:74–82.
96. Liu G, Wang Y, Tian F, et al. Long-term follow-up of phenobarbital versus valproate for generalized convulsive status epilepticus in adults: a randomized clinical trial. Epilepsy Res. 2023;195:107187.

97. Jindal A, Angurana SK, Suthar R, et al. Effect of early withdrawal of phenobarbitone on the recurrence of neonatal seizures: an open-label randomized controlled trial. Epilepsy Behav. 2021;117:107875.
98. Ziobro JM, Eschbach K, Shellhaas RA. Novel therapeutics for neonatal seizures. Neurotherapeutics. 2021;18(3):1564–81.
99. Dizon MLV, Rao R, Hamrick SE, et al. Practice variation in anti-epileptic drug use for neonatal hypoxic-ischemic encephalopathy among regional NICUs. BMC Pediatr. 2019;19(1):67.
100. Lin YC, Lai YC, Chou P, et al. How can an Na(+) channel inhibitor ameliorate seizures in Lennox-Gastaut syndrome? Ann Neurol. 2021;89(6):1099–113.
101. Kaplan YC, Demir O. Use of phenytoin, phenobarbital carbamazepine, levetiracetam lamotrigine and valproate in pregnancy and breastfeeding: risk of major malformations, dose-dependency, monotherapy vs polytherapy, pharmacokinetics and clinical implications. Curr Neuropharmacol. 2021;19(11):1805–24.
102. Tomson T, Battino D, Bonizzoni E, et al. Comparative risk of major congenital malformations with eight different antiepileptic drugs: a prospective cohort study of the EURAP registry. Lancet Neurol. 2018;17(6):530–8.
103. Bromley R, Adab N, Bluett-Duncan M, et al. Monotherapy treatment of epilepsy in pregnancy: congenital malformation outcomes in the child. Cochrane Database Syst Rev. 2023;8(8):CD010224.
104. Zuppa AA, Carducci C, Scorrano A, et al. Infants born to mothers under phenobarbital treatment: correlation between serum levels and clinical features of neonates. Eur J Obstet Gynecol Reprod Biol. 2011;159(1):53–6.
105. Verstegen RHJ, Anderson PO, Ito S. Infant drug exposure via breast milk. Br J Clin Pharmacol. 2022;88(10):4311–27.
106. Sharma D, Hussain AM, Sharma SS. Efficacy of levetiracetam in neonatal seizures: a systematic review. J Matern Fetal Neonatal Med. 2022;35(20):3923–30.
107. Gyandeep G, Behura SS, Sahu SK, et al. Comparison between phenobarbitone and levetiracetam as the initial anticonvulsant in preterm neonatal seizures – a pilot randomized control trial in developing country setup. Eur J Pediatr. 2023;182(5):2133–8.
108. Soul JS, Bergin AM, Stopp C, et al. A pilot randomized, controlled, double-blind trial of bumetanide to treat neonatal seizures. Ann Neurol. 2021;89(2):327–40.
109. Variane GFT, Dahlen A, Pietrobom RFR, et al. Remote monitoring for seizures during therapeutic hypothermia in neonates with hypoxic-ischemic encephalopathy. JAMA Netw Open. 2023;6(11):e2343429.
110. Kumar J, Meena J, Yadav J, et al. Efficacy and safety of phenobarbitone as first-line treatment for neonatal seizure: a systematic review and meta-analysis. J Trop Pediatr. 2021;67(1):fmab008.
111. Liguori C, Toledo M, Kothare S. Effects of anti-seizure medications on sleep architecture and daytime sleepiness in patients with epilepsy: a literature review. Sleep Med Rev. 2021;60:101559.
112. Johne M, Käufer C, Römermann K, et al. A combination of phenobarbital and the bumetanide derivative bumepamine prevents neonatal seizures and subsequent hippocampal neurodegeneration in a rat model of birth asphyxia. Epilepsia. 2021;62(6):1460–71.
113. Johne M, Römermann K, Hampel P, et al. Phenobarbital and midazolam suppress neonatal seizures in a noninvasive rat model of birth asphyxia, whereas bumetanide is ineffective. Epilepsia. 2021;62(4):920–34.
114. Marsh O, Corsini G, Van Dijk J, et al. Prevalence and clinical characteristics of phenobarbitone-associated adverse effects in epileptic cats. J Feline Med Surg. 2021;23(2):59–66.
115. Liu J, Wang LN. Treatment of epilepsy for people with Alzheimer's disease. Cochrane Database Syst Rev. 2021;5(5):CD011922.
116. Karaźniewicz-Łada M, Główka AK, Mikulska AA, et al. Pharmacokinetic drug-drug interactions among antiepileptic drugs, including CBD, drugs used to treat COVID-19 and nutrients. Int J Mol Sci. 2021;22(17):9582.

117. Peters J, Vijiaratnam N, Angus-Leppan H. Tics induced by antiepileptic drugs: a pragmatic review. J Neurol. 2021;268(1):321–36.
118. Shamabadi A, Karimi H, Arabzadeh Bahri R, et al. Emerging drugs for the treatment of irritability associated with autism spectrum disorder. Expert Opin Emerg Drugs. 2024;29(1):45–56.
119. Pourmand A, AlRemeithi R, Kartiko S, et al. Evaluation of phenobarbital based approach in treating patient with alcohol withdrawal syndrome: a systematic review and meta-analysis. Am J Emerg Med. 2023;69:65–75.
120. Shah P, Stegner-Smith KL, Rachid M, et al. Front-loaded versus low-intermittent phenobarbital dosing for benzodiazepine-resistant severe alcohol withdrawal syndrome. J Med Toxicol. 2022;18(3):198–204.
121. Pham C, Goldenberg-Sandau A, Sensenig R, et al. Phenobarbital for the management of alcohol withdrawal syndrome in critically ill, surgical-trauma patients. J Surg Res. 2023;283:965–72.
122. Terasaki D, Kulick B, Calcaterra S, et al. Phenobarbital for alcohol withdrawal in the context of the opioid epidemic: a neglected caveat. Addiction. 2023;118(7):1198–200.
123. Handley R, Stewart AS. Mysoline; a new drug in the treatment of epilepsy. Lancet. 1952;1(6711):742–4.
124. Goldin S. Toxic effects of primidone. Lancet. 1954;266(6802):102–3.
125. Nathan PW. Primidone in the treatment of non-idiopathic epilepsy. Lancet. 1954;266(6801):21–3.
126. Scarinci V. [Pharmacology of mysoline (primidone)]. Arch Ital Sci Farmacol. 1955;5(1):10–5.
127. Lopez-Gomez M, Ramirez-Bermudez J, Campillo C, et al. Primidone is associated with interictal depression in patients with epilepsy. Epilepsy Behav. 2005;6(3):413–6.
128. Lenka A, Louis ED. Primidone intolerance in essential tremor: is it more than just age? Tremor Other Hyperkinet Mov (N Y). 2021;11:57.
129. Steve TA, Gross DW. Alcohol-responsive epilepsia partialis continua. Epileptic Disord. 2014;16(1):107–11.
130. Wang J, Huang P, Song Z. Comparison of the relapse rates in seizure-free patients in whom antiepileptic therapy was discontinued and those in whom the therapy was continued: a meta-analysis. Epilepsy Behav. 2019;101(Pt A):106577.
131. Demchenko IT, Zhilyaev SY, Moskvin AN, et al. Antiepileptic drugs prevent seizures in hyperbaric oxygen: a novel model of epileptiform activity. Brain Res. 2017;1657:347–54.
132. Canisius T, Soons J, Verschuure P, et al. Therapeutic drug monitoring of anti-epileptic drugs – a clinical verification of volumetric absorptive micro sampling. Clin Chem Lab Med. 2020;58(5):828–35.
133. Ghosh D, Brar H, Lhamu U, et al. A series of 211 children with probable essential tremor. Mov Disord Clin Pract. 2017;4(2):231–6.
134. Castonguay CE, Liao C, Khayachi A, et al. Transcriptomic effects of propranolol and primidone converge on molecular pathways relevant to essential tremor. NPJ Genom Med. 2022;7(1):46.
135. Tensini TS, Von Glehn CQC, Bettinotti MP, et al. Cutaneous adverse reactions associated with antiseizure medication: clinical characteristics and implications in epilepsy treatment. Epileptic Disord. 2021;23(3):466–75.
136. Krügel U, Straub I, Beckmann H, et al. Primidone inhibits TRPM3 and attenuates thermal nociception in vivo. Pain. 2017;158(5):856–67.
137. Arjunan V, Santhanam R, Subramanian S, et al. Primidone--an antiepileptic drug--characterisation by quantum chemical and spectroscopic (FTIR, FT-Raman, 1H, 13C NMR and UV-Visible) investigations. Spectrochim Acta A Mol Biomol Spectrosc. 2013;109:282–97.
138. Riebeling T, Jamal K, Wilson R, et al. Primidone blocks RIPK1-driven cell death and inflammation. Cell Death Differ. 2021;28(5):1610–26.
139. Nida A, Alston J, Schweinfurth J. Primidone therapy for essential vocal tremor. JAMA Otolaryngol Head Neck Surg. 2016;142(2):117–21.

140. Ashikawa H, Mogi H, Honda T, et al. Beneficial effects of primidone in Niemann-Pick disease type C (NPC)-model cells and mice: reduction of unesterified cholesterol levels in cells and extension of lifespan in mice. Eur J Pharmacol. 2021;896:173907.
141. Burton B. On the propyl derivatives and decomposition products of ethyl acetoacetate. Am Chem J. 1881;3:385–95.
142. Barnes SE, Bower BD. Sodium valproate in the treatment of intractable childhood epilepsy. Dev Med Child Neurol. 1975;17(2):175–81.
143. Bohlen N, Hertl M. [Adverse effects of anti-epileptic drugs]. Dtsch Med Wochenschr. 1975;100(38):1904–6.
144. Shnayder NA, Grechkina VV, Khasanova AK, et al. Therapeutic and toxic effects of valproic acid metabolites. Metabolites. 2023;13(1):134.
145. Marson A, Burnside G, Appleton R, et al. The SANAD II study of the effectiveness and cost-effectiveness of valproate versus levetiracetam for newly diagnosed generalised and unclassifiable epilepsy: an open-label, non-inferiority, multicentre, phase 4, randomised controlled trial. Lancet. 2021;397(10282):1375–86.
146. Hochbaum M, Kienitz R, Rosenow F, et al. Trends in antiseizure medication prescription patterns among all adults, women, and older adults with epilepsy: a German longitudinal analysis from 2008 to 2020. Epilepsy Behav. 2022;130:108666.
147. Yu L, Zhu W, Zhu X, et al. Anti-seizure medication prescription in adult outpatients with epilepsy in China, 2013-2018. Front Neurol. 2021;12:649589.
148. Clavenna A, Campi R, Putignano D, et al. Changes in antiepileptic drug prescriptions over a decade in childbearing women in Lombardy region, Italy. Br J Clin Pharmacol. 2022;88(3):1152–8.
149. Kikuchi D, Obara T, Miura R, et al. Trends in the prescription of anti-seizure medicines for pregnant women outpatients with epilepsy during 2016-2020 in Japan. Seizure. 2022;98:101–4.
150. Romoli M, Mazzocchetti P, D'Alonzo R, et al. Valproic acid and epilepsy: from molecular mechanisms to clinical evidences. Curr Neuropharmacol. 2019;17(10):926–46.
151. Perucca E. Pharmacological and therapeutic properties of valproate: a summary after 35 years of clinical experience. CNS Drugs. 2002;16(10):695–714.
152. Young MR, Bisaccia EK, Romantseva L, et al. Valproic acid serum concentration and incidence of toxicity in pediatric patients. J Child Neurol. 2022;37(6):461–70.
153. Lin K, Cao VFS, Au C, et al. Clinical pharmacokinetic monitoring of free valproic acid levels: a systematic review. Clin Pharmacokinet. 2022;61(10):1345–63.
154. El Orche A, Cheikh A, Johnson JB, et al. A novel approach for therapeutic drug monitoring of valproic acid using FT-IR spectroscopy and nonlinear support vector regression. J AOAC Int. 2023;106(4):1070–6.
155. Namera A, Uekusa K, Saito T, et al. A method for determining valproic acid in human whole blood and urine via gas chromatography-mass spectrometry and small-scale inter-laboratory trial. Leg Med (Tokyo). 2022;59:102133.
156. Tomson T, Battino D, Perucca E. Valproic acid after five decades of use in epilepsy: time to reconsider the indications of a time-honoured drug. Lancet Neurol. 2016;15(2):210–8.
157. Gong X, Liu Y, Liu X, et al. Analysis of gut microbiota in patients with epilepsy treated with valproate: results from a three months observational prospective cohort study. Microb Pathog. 2022;162:105340.
158. Kandratavicius L, Balista PA, Lopes-Aguiar C, et al. Animal models of epilepsy: use and limitations. Neuropsychiatr Dis Treat. 2014;10:1693–705.
159. Luszczki JJ, Trojnar MK, Ratnaraj N, et al. Interactions of stiripentol with clobazam and valproate in the mouse maximal electroshock-induced seizure model. Epilepsy Res. 2010;90(3):188–98.
160. Srivastava AK, White HS. Carbamazepine, but not valproate, displays pharmacoresistance in lamotrigine-resistant amygdala kindled rats. Epilepsy Res. 2013;104(1–2):26–34.

161. Langer M, Brandt C, Zellinger C, et al. Therapeutic window of opportunity for the neuroprotective effect of valproate versus the competitive AMPA receptor antagonist NS1209 following status epilepticus in rats. Neuropharmacology. 2011;61(5–6):1033–47.
162. Sgobio C, Ghiglieri V, Costa C, et al. Hippocampal synaptic plasticity, memory, and epilepsy: effects of long-term valproic acid treatment. Biol Psychiatry. 2010;67(6):567–74.
163. Can Kantarci B, Sanli A, Gavas S, et al. Effects of in utero exposure to valproate or levetiracetam on the seizures and newborn histopathology of genetic absence epilepsy rats. Neurosci Lett. 2022;776:136574.
164. Ayala-Guerrero F, Castro-Domínguez D, Mateos-Salgado EL, et al. Effect of valproate on sleep patterns disturbed by epilepsy. Physiol Behav. 2023;259:114054.
165. Wang W, Wu J, Li S, et al. Sodium valproate for epilepsy in rural China: an efficacy and safety assessment in primary care. Epilepsy Res. 2012;102(3):201–5.
166. Huang DH, Zheng JO, Chen J, et al. Treatment gaps of epilepsy and retention rates of sodium valproate in rural Guangxi, China. Genet Mol Res. 2014;13(3):6202–12.
167. Hu Y, Huang X, Shen D, et al. Outcomes of sustained-release formulation of valproate and topiramate monotherapy in patients with epilepsy: a multi-centre, cohort study. PLoS One. 2012;7(12):e47982.
168. Marques VD, Hackbart BA, Guilhoto LM, et al. Minimum effective sodium valproate dose in genetic generalized epilepsies. Seizure. 2023;108:53–9.
169. Steinbart D, Gaus V, Kowski AB, et al. Valproic acid use in fertile women with genetic generalized epilepsies. Acta Neurol Scand. 2021;144(3):288–95.
170. Mermi Dibek D, Öztura İ, Baklan B. Our reasons for converting to valproic acid treatment in female patients with genetic generalized epilepsy: a retrospective, single-centre study. Neurol Sci. 2022;43(1):517–23.
171. Kiiski R, Basnyat P, Raitanen J, et al. Treatment outcomes in women with idiopathic generalized epilepsy. Acta Neurol Scand. 2022;145(4):423–33.
172. Baheti N, Rathore C, Bansal AR, et al. Treatment outcomes in drug resistant juvenile myoclonic epilepsy: valproate resistance may not be the end of the road. Seizure. 2021;92:112–7.
173. Kılıç B, Serdaroğlu E, Polat BG, et al. Trends in the choice of antiseizure medications in juvenile myoclonic epilepsy: a retrospective multi-center study from Turkey between 2010 and 2020. Seizure. 2022;99:48–53.
174. Moon JU, Lee JY, Kim KY, et al. Comparative analysis of background EEG activity in juvenile myoclonic epilepsy during valproic acid treatment: a standardized, low-resolution, brain electromagnetic tomography (sLORETA) study. BMC Neurol. 2022;22(1):48.
175. Zöllner JP, Strzelczyk A, Rosenow F, et al. Valproate but not levetiracetam slows the EEG alpha peak frequency – a pharmaco-EEG study. Clin Neurophysiol. 2021;132(6):1203–8.
176. Ozyurek H, Bayrak I, Yayici Koken O, et al. Effect of chronic valproic acid use on anterior cerebral blood flow of children with idiopathic generalized epilepsy. Acta Neurol Taiwanica. 2022;31(2):72–6.
177. Operto FF, Pastorino GMG, Di Bonaventura C, et al. Effects of antiseizure monotherapy on visuospatial memory in pediatric age. Eur J Paediatr Neurol. 2021;32:106–14.
178. Zaccara G, Lattanzi S, Brigo F. Which treatment strategy in patients with epilepsy with focal seizures uncontrolled by the first anti-seizure medication? Epilepsy Behav. 2021;121(Pt A):108031.
179. Zhu Y, Yang J, Zhu X. Combined effects of levetiracetam and sodium valproate on paediatric patients with epilepsy: a systematic review and meta-analysis. Seizure. 2022;95:17–25.
180. Sharshar T, Porcher R, Asfar P, et al. Valproic acid as adjuvant treatment for convulsive status epilepticus: a randomised clinical trial. Crit Care. 2023;27(1):8.
181. Liampas I, Siokas V, Brotis A, et al. Intravenous sodium valproate in status epilepticus: review and meta-analysis. Int J Neurosci. 2021;131(1):70–84.
182. Kamitaki BK, Minacapelli CD, Zhang P, et al. Drug-induced liver injury associated with antiseizure medications from the FDA Adverse Event Reporting System (FAERS). Epilepsy Behav. 2021;117:107832.

183. Loser V, Novy J, Beuchat I, et al. Acute valproate-induced encephalopathy in status epilepticus: a registry-based assessment. CNS Drugs. 2023;37(8):725–31.
184. Bui E. Women's issues in epilepsy. Continuum (Minneap Minn). 2022;28(2):399–427.
185. Eriksson SH, Tittensor P, Sisodiya SM. National compliance with UK wide guidelines for usage of valproate in women of childbearing potential. Seizure. 2022;98:8–12.
186. Spoendlin J, Blozik E, Graber S, et al. Use of valproate in pregnancy and in women of childbearing age between 2014 and 2018 in Switzerland: a retrospective analysis of Swiss healthcare claims data. Swiss Med Wkly. 2021;151:w20386.
187. Atalar A, Şirin NG, Bebek N, et al. Predictors of successful valproate withdrawal in women with epilepsy. Epilepsy Behav. 2021;119:107980.
188. Roberti R, Rocca M, Iannone LF, et al. Status epilepticus in pregnancy: a literature review and a protocol proposal. Expert Rev Neurother. 2022;22(4):301–12.
189. Borowicz-Reutt KK. Effects of antiarrhythmic drugs on antiepileptic drug action-a critical review of experimental findings. Int J Mol Sci. 2022;23(5):2891.
190. Giustozzi M, Mazzetti M, Paciaroni M, et al. Concomitant use of direct oral anticoagulants and antiepileptic drugs: a prospective cohort study in patients with atrial fibrillation. Clin Drug Investig. 2021;41(1):43–51.
191. Cherian A, Shetty SC, Divya KP, et al. Weekly methotrexate may reduce valproate levels causing relapse of genetic generalized epilepsy. Epilepsy Behav Rep. 2021;16:100457.
192. Li Z, Gao W, Liu G, et al. Interaction between valproic acid and carbapenems: decreased plasma concentration of valproic acid and liver injury. Ann Palliat Med. 2021;10(5):5417–24.
193. Chen IL, Lee CH, Hsiao SC, et al. Interactions between carbapenems and valproic acid among the patients in the intensive care units. J Crit Care. 2021;62:151–6.
194. Cunningham D, Clark K, Lord K. Treatment of valproic acid overdose with meropenem in an epileptic patient. Am J Emerg Med. 2022;53:284.e1–3.
195. Yang X, Jiang Z, Jiang Y, et al. Determination of valproic acid and its six metabolites in human serum using LC-MS/MS and application to interaction with carbapenems in epileptic patients. Biomed Chromatogr. 2023;37(3):e5572.
196. Müller A, von Hofen-Hohloch J, Awissus C, et al. Does diabetes mellitus affect the safety profile of valproic acid for the treatment of status epilepticus? A retrospective cohort study. Neurol Res Pract. 2022;4(1):52.
197. Snoeijen-Schouwenaars FM, Young C, Rowe C, et al. People with epilepsy and intellectual disability: more than a sum of two conditions. Epilepsy Behav. 2021;124:108355.
198. Kessing LV, Ziersen SC, Gerds T, et al. Response to lithium and anticonvulsants among patients with bipolar disorder with and without comorbid epilepsy – a nation-wide population-based longitudinal study. J Affect Disord. 2022;308:369–74.
199. Pisani F, Rosa Pisani L, Barbieri MA, et al. Optimization of therapy in patients with epilepsy and psychiatric comorbidities: key points. Curr Neuropharmacol. 2023;21(8):1755–66.
200. Hsieh TC, Lin CC, Wu LS. Long-term use of valproic acid reduced mortality in bipolar disorder patients in a Taiwanese population: an association analysis using the national health insurance research database (NHIRD). J Psychiatr Res. 2022;149:339–43.
201. Xie T, Li R, Long X, et al. Magnetic resonance imaging features of hippocampus and mechanism of neurocognitive dysfunction for antiepileptic drugs in treatment of depression rats. Bioengineered. 2022;13(3):4646–57.
202. Cuartas CF, Davis M. Valproic acid in the management of delirium. Am J Hosp Palliat Care. 2022;39(5):562–9.
203. Olivola M, Civardi S, Damiani S, et al. Effectiveness and safety of intravenous valproate in agitation: a systematic review. Psychopharmacology. 2022;239(2):339–50.
204. Gao X, Zeb S, He YY, et al. Valproic acid inhibits glial scar formation after ischemic stroke. Pharmacology. 2022;107(5–6):263–80.
205. Lee H, Hwang YJ, Park JH, et al. Valproic acid decreases vascular smooth muscle cell proliferation via protein phosphatase 2A-mediated p70 S6 kinase inhibition. Biochem Biophys Res Commun. 2022;606:94–9.

206. Wakam GK, Biesterveld BE, Pai MP, et al. Administration of valproic acid in clinically approved dose improves neurologic recovery and decreases brain lesion size in swine subjected to hemorrhagic shock and traumatic brain injury. J Trauma Acute Care Surg. 2021;90(2):346–52.
207. Bhatti UF, Remmer H, Williams AM, et al. Assessment of the cytoprotective effects of high-dose valproic acid compared to a clinically used lower dose. J Surg Res. 2021;266:125–41.
208. Bhatti UF, Karnovsky A, Dennahy IS, et al. Pharmacologic modulation of brain metabolism by valproic acid can induce a neuroprotective environment. J Trauma Acute Care Surg. 2021;90(3):507–14.
209. Demirci H, Kuzucu P, Seymen CM, et al. The effect of antiepileptic drugs on re-myelinization of axons: phenytoin, levetiracetam, carbamazepine, and valproic acid, used following traumatic brain injury. Clin Neurol Neurosurg. 2021;209:106911.
210. Biesterveld BE, Siddiqui AZ, O'Connell RL, et al. Valproic acid protects against acute kidney injury in hemorrhage and trauma. J Surg Res. 2021;266:222–9.
211. Duenas-Gonzalez A, Candelaria M, Perez-Plascencia C, et al. Valproic acid as epigenetic cancer drug: preclinical, clinical and transcriptional effects on solid tumors. Cancer Treat Rev. 2008;34(3):206–22.
212. Chen JH, Zheng YL, Xu CQ, et al. Valproic acid (VPA) enhances cisplatin sensitivity of non-small cell lung cancer cells via HDAC2 mediated down regulation of ABCA1. Biol Chem. 2017;398(7):785–92.
213. Happold C, Gorlia T, Chinot O, et al. Does valproic acid or levetiracetam improve survival in glioblastoma? A pooled analysis of prospective clinical trials in newly diagnosed glioblastoma. J Clin Oncol. 2016;34(7):731–9.
214. Memezawa S, Sato T, Ochiai A, et al. The antiepileptic valproic acid ameliorates Charcot-Marie-Tooth 2W (CMT2W) disease-associated HARS1 mutation-induced inhibition of neuronal cell morphological differentiation through c-Jun N-terminal kinase. Neurochem Res. 2022;47(9):2684–702.
215. Kurishima A, Hayashi M, Shimozato R, et al. Successful treatment of symptomatic epilepsy with oral valproic acid and levetiracetam in a patient with short-bowel syndrome. Intern Med. 2022;61(9):1457–61.
216. Santos DS, Rocha MA, Mello MLS. Epigenetic studies in insects and the valproic acid perspective. Braz J Biol. 2022;84:e256045.
217. Saiz ML, DeDiego ML, López-García D, et al. Epigenetic targeting of the ACE2 and NRP1 viral receptors limits SARS-CoV-2 infectivity. Clin Epigenetics. 2021;13(1):187.
218. Farazdaghi M, Razavizadegan SMA, Moghimi M, et al. Efficacy of valproic acid against coronavirus disease 2019 infection or severity: a pilot study. Clin Neuropharmacol. 2022;45(6):175–6.
219. Fu M, Zhu Y, Zhang J, et al. MicroRNA-221-3p suppresses the microglia activation and seizures by inhibiting of HIF-1α in valproic acid-resistant epilepsy. Front Pharmacol. 2021;12:714556.
220. Wang Y, Li Y, Wang G, et al. Overexpression of Homer1b/c induces valproic acid resistance in epilepsy. CNS Neurosci Ther. 2023;29(1):331–43.
221. Romoli M, Costa C, Siliquini S, et al. Antiepileptic drugs in migraine and epilepsy: who is at increased risk of adverse events? Cephalalgia. 2018;38(2):274–82.
222. Wartman C, VandenBerg A. Valproate: not all boxed warnings are created equal. Ann Pharmacother. 2022;56(12):1349–55.
223. Ezhilarasan D, Mani U. Valproic acid induced liver injury: an insight into molecular toxicological mechanism. Environ Toxicol Pharmacol. 2022;95:103967.
224. Meseguer ES, Elizalde MU, Borobia AM, et al. Valproic acid-induced liver injury: a case-control study from a prospective pharmacovigilance program in a tertiary hospital. J Clin Med. 2021;10(6):1153.
225. Mei X, Wu HC, Ruan M, et al. Acute liver failure with thrombotic microangiopathy due to sodium valproate toxicity: a case report. World J Clin Cases. 2021;9(17):4310–7.

226. Gheena S, Ezhilarasan D, Shree Harini K, et al. Syringic acid and silymarin concurrent administration inhibits sodium valproate-induced liver injury in rats. Environ Toxicol. 2022;37(9):2143–52.
227. George LJ, Singh P, Aneja S, et al. Insulin resistance in children on sodium valproate – a hospital based cross-sectional study in Indian children. Trop Doct. 2023;53(1):91–6.
228. Sun JW, Young JG, Sarvet AL, et al. Comparison of rates of type 2 diabetes in adults and children treated with anticonvulsant mood stabilizers. JAMA Netw Open. 2022;5(4):e226484.
229. Yaryari AM, Mazdeh M, Mohammadi M, et al. Evaluation of serum levels of asprosin and other metabolic profiles in patients with idiopathic tonic-clonic generalized epilepsy on treatment with valproic acid. Eur J Clin Pharmacol. 2022;78(3):393–403.
230. Yan L, Yang K, Wang S, et al. PXR-mediated expression of FABP4 promotes valproate-induced lipid accumulation in HepG2 cells. Toxicol Lett. 2021;346:47–56.
231. Guo HL, Dong N, Chen F, et al. Effect of long-term valproic acid therapy on lipid profiles in paediatric patients with epilepsy: a meta-analysis. Epileptic Disord. 2022;24(5):822–30.
232. Jutrić D, Đikić D, Boroš A, et al. Effects of naringin and valproate interaction on liver steatosis and dyslipidaemia parameters in male C57BL6 mice. Arh Hig Rada Toksikol. 2022;73(1):71–82.
233. Conei D, Rojas M, Santamaría L, et al. Valproic acid during pregnancy decrease the number of spermatogenic cells and testicular volume in the offspring of mice: stereological quantification. Histol Histopathol. 2021;36(11):1189–98.
234. Alsemeh AE, Ahmed MM, Fawzy A, et al. Vitamin E rescues valproic acid-induced testicular injury in rats: role of autophagy. Life Sci. 2022;296:120434.
235. Guo Y, Chen L, Wu D, et al. A comparative study of the effects of valproate and oxcarbazepine on sexual function, sperm quality, and sex hormones in males with epilepsy. Biomed Res Int. 2021;2021:6624101.
236. Rochtus AM, Herijgers D, Jansen K, et al. Antiseizure medications and thyroid hormone homeostasis: literature review and practical recommendations. Epilepsia. 2022;63(2):259–70.
237. Comert E, Celebi U, Piri Cinar B, et al. Thyroid functions as a parameter in monitoring of antiepileptic drugs. Neurol Res. 2022;44(7):614–21.
238. Ilia TS, Dragoumi P, Papanikolopoulou S, et al. Is the prevalence of thyroid disease higher in children receiving antiepileptic medication? A systematic review and meta-analysis. Seizure. 2022;94:117–25.
239. Saito M, Takizawa T, Miyaoka H. Factors associated with blood carnitine levels in adult epilepsy patients with chronic valproic acid therapy. Epilepsy Res. 2021;175:106697.
240. Okumura A, Takagi M, Numoto S, et al. Effects of l-carnitine supplementation in patients with childhood-onset epilepsy prescribed valproate. Epilepsy Behav. 2021;122:108220.
241. Christensen J, Trabjerg BB, Sun Y, et al. Prenatal exposure to valproate and risk of congenital malformations-could we have known earlier?-a population-based cohort study. Epilepsia. 2021;62(12):2981–93.
242. Piorczynski TB, Larsen MW, Lee SJ, et al. NRF2 activation protects against valproic acid-induced disruption of neurogenesis in P19 cells. Differentiation. 2022;123:18–29.
243. Steele JW, Lin YL, Chen N, et al. Embryonic hypotaurine levels contribute to strain-dependent susceptibility in mouse models of valproate-induced neural tube defects. Front Cell Dev Biol. 2022;10:832492.
244. Brotzmann K, Wolterbeek A, Kroese D, et al. Neurotoxic effects in zebrafish embryos by valproic acid and nine of its analogues: the fish-mouse connection? Arch Toxicol. 2021;95(2):641–57.
245. Muhsen M, Youngs J, Riu A, et al. Folic acid supplementation rescues valproic acid-induced developmental neurotoxicity and behavioral alterations in zebrafish embryos. Epilepsia. 2021;62(7):1689–700.
246. Meng Q, Zhang W, Wang X, et al. Human forebrain organoids reveal connections between valproic acid exposure and autism risk. Transl Psychiatry. 2022;12(1):130.

247. Liu Z, Wang J, Xu Q, et al. Vitamin A supplementation ameliorates prenatal valproic acid-induced autism-like behaviors in rats. Neurotoxicology. 2022;91:155–65.
248. Honybun E, Thwaites R, Malpas CB, et al. Prenatal valproate exposure and adverse neurodevelopmental outcomes: does sex matter? Epilepsia. 2021;62(3):709–19.
249. Bjørk MH, Zoega H, Leinonen MK, et al. Association of prenatal exposure to antiseizure medication with risk of autism and intellectual disability. JAMA Neurol. 2022;79(7):672–81.
250. Feleke R, Jazayeri D, Abouzeid M, et al. Integrative genomics reveals pathogenic mediator of valproate-induced neurodevelopmental disability. Brain. 2022;145(11):3832–42.
251. Kowalski TW, Lord VO, Sgarioni E, et al. Transcriptome meta-analysis of valproic acid exposure in human embryonic stem cells. Eur Neuropsychopharmacol. 2022;60:76–88.
252. Hosseini H, Shafie M, Shakiba A, et al. Valproic acid-induced hyperammonemia in neuropsychiatric disorders: a 2-year clinical survey. Psychopharmacology. 2023;240(1):149–56.
253. Kwack DW, Kim DW. Risk factors of hyperammonemia in epilepsy patients with valproic acid therapy. Clin Neurol Neurosurg. 2023;233:107962.
254. Pagali S, Edquist C, O'Rourke N. Managing valproic acid toxicity-related hyperammonaemia: an unpredicted course. BMJ Case Rep. 2021;14(4):e241547.
255. Patel J, Berezowski I, Mazer-Amirshahi M, et al. Valproic acid overdose: case report and literature review. J Emerg Med. 2022;63(5):651–5.
256. Lan L, Zhao X, Jian S, et al. Investigation of the risk of valproic acid-induced tremor: clinical, neuroimaging, and genetic factors. Psychopharmacology. 2022;239(1):173–84.
257. Baizabal-Carvallo JF, Alonso-Juarez M. Valproate-induced rest tremor and parkinsonism. Acta Neurol Belg. 2021;121(2):515–9.
258. Rissardo JP, Caprara ALF, Durante Í. Valproate-associated movement disorder: a literature review. Prague Med Rep. 2021;122(3):140–80.
259. de Oliveira-Costa GVC, Machado Torres C, Ávila Duarte J, et al. Valproate-induced reversible hemichoreoathetosis in a patient with Rasmussen encephalitis. Neurology. 2022;98(21):894–5.
260. Yıldız A, Vardı N, Parlakpınar H, et al. Effects of low- and high-dose valproic acid and lamotrigine on the heart in female rats. Cardiovasc Toxicol. 2022;22(4):326–40.
261. Liang D, Gardella E, Kragholm K, et al. The relationship between valproate and lamotrigine/levetiracetam use and prognosis in patients with epilepsy and heart failure: a Danish register-based study. J Card Fail. 2022;28(4):630–8.
262. Anguissola G, Leu D, Simonetti GD, et al. Kidney tubular injury induced by valproic acid: systematic literature review. Pediatr Nephrol. 2023;38(6):1725–31.
263. Bayrak BB, Yilmaz S, Hacihasanoglu Cakmak N, et al. The effects of edaravone, a free-radical scavenger in lung injury induced by valproic acid demonstrated via different biochemical parameters. J Biochem Mol Toxicol. 2021;35(9):e22847.
264. Bischof MCM, Stadelmann MIE, Janett S, et al. Valproic acid-associated acute pancreatitis: systematic literature review. J Clin Med. 2023;12(18):6044.
265. Gallo C, Bonvento G, Zagotto G, et al. Gingival overgrowth induced by anticonvulsant drugs: a cross-sectional study on epileptic patients. J Periodontal Res. 2021;56(2):363–9.
266. Heidemann J, Schmitz B, Kostev K. Association between antiseizure medication use and risk of urinary tract infection: a case-control study. Epilepsy Behav. 2021;115:107502.
267. Post DS, van der Veer A, Schijns O, et al. Assessment of need for hemostatic evaluation in patients taking valproic acid: a retrospective cross-sectional study. PLoS One. 2022;17(2):e0264351.
268. Riahi-Zanjani B, Delirrad M, Fazeli-Bakhtiyari R, et al. Hematological consequences of valproic acid in pediatric patients: a systematic review with a mechanistic approach. CNS Neurol Disord Drug Targets. 2022;21(4):316–25.
269. Papadopoulou E, Saroglou M, Ismailos G, et al. Pearls for the diagnosis and possible pathophysiological mechanisms of valproic acid-induced lupus erythematosus: a literature review. Lupus. 2022;31(6):650–8.

270. Dutta P, Das S, Fershko A. Non-aromatic anticonvulsant (divalproex sodium)-induced drug reaction with eosinophilia and systemic symptoms (DRESS) syndrome. Cureus. 2021;13(9):e17860.
271. Sturla Álvarez DA, Sánchez Marcos E, de Lucas Collantes C, et al. Fanconi syndrome secondary to sodium valproate therapy: experience and literature review. Pediatr Neurol. 2022;130:53–9.
272. Goodman LS, Swinyard EA, Toman JE. Studies on the anticonvulsant properties of diphenylhydantoin. Fed Proc. 1946;5(1 Pt 2):180.
273. Bashinski B. Treatment of epilepsy in children with sodium dilantin. J Med Assoc Ga. 1946;35:228.
274. Mc GJ, Martin RE. Dilantin intoxication. Clin Proc Child Hosp Dist Columbia. 1949;5(11):316–9.
275. Sweet RD. A fixed skin eruption due to phenytoin sodium. Lancet. 1950;1(6594):68.
276. Pfeifle CE, Adler DS, Gannaway WL. Phenytoin sodium solubility in three intravenous solutions. Am J Hosp Pharm. 1981;38(3):358–62.
277. Kang Y, Yang R, Wei Z, et al. Phenytoin sodium-ameliorated gingival fibroblast aging is associated with autophagy. J Periodontal Res. 2020;55(5):642–50.
278. Kathiravan M, Kavitha S, Shanthi R. To determine the effect of long-term antiepileptic drug on the serum folate and vitamin B12 among epileptic patients. Sci Rep. 2021;11(1):4393.
279. Sangeetha A, Bobby Z, Wadwekar V, et al. Atherogenic risk factors among young Indian adults with epilepsy on treatment with phenytoin: need for novel therapeutic strategies. Neurol India. 2021;69(4):957–61.
280. Morán-Mariños C, Alva-Diaz C, De la Cruz Ramirez W, et al. Drug reaction with eosinophilia and systemic symptoms (DRESS) induced by phenytoin re-exposure: case report and systematic review. Acta Clin Belg. 2022;77(1):177–85.
281. Urushidani S. A phenytoin-induced ataxia mimicking a stroke. Am J Emerg Med. 2022;60:226.e5–6.
282. Asadi-Pooya AA, Rostaminejad M, Zeraatpisheh Z, et al. Cosmetic adverse effects of antiseizure medications; A systematic review. Seizure. 2021;91:9–21.
283. Minowa E, Hayashi Y, Goh K, et al. Enhancement of receptor-mediated calcium responses by phenytoin through the suppression of calcium excretion in human gingival fibroblasts. J Periodontal Res. 2023;58(2):274–82.
284. Klowak JA, Hewitt M, Catenacci V, et al. Levetiracetam versus phenytoin or fosphenytoin for second-line treatment of pediatric status epilepticus: a meta-analysis. Pediatr Crit Care Med. 2021;22(9):e480–e91.
285. Mastroianni G, Iannone LF, Roberti R, et al. Management of status epilepticus in patients with liver or kidney disease: a narrative review. Expert Rev Neurother. 2021;21(11):1251–64.
286. Mohammadi M, Kadivar M, Sangsari R, et al. Comparing the efficacy and safety of levetiracetam versus phenytoin for treating the acute phase of neonatal seizures. Iran J Child Neurol. 2023;17(1):65–71.
287. Alix V, James M, Jackson AH, et al. Efficacy of fosphenytoin as first-line antiseizure medication for neonatal seizures compared to phenobarbital. J Child Neurol. 2021;36(1):30–7.
288. Shi R, Yin HQ, Wang ZZ. [Efficacy and safety of levetiracetam versus phenytoin as second-line drugs for the treatment of children with convulsive status epilepticus: a meta analysis]. Zhongguo Dang Dai Er Ke Za Zhi. 2021;23(4):356–62.
289. Guidotti I, Lugli L, Ori L, et al. Neonatal seizures treatment based on conventional multichannel EEG monitoring: an overview of therapeutic options. Expert Rev Neurother. 2022;22(7):623–38.
290. Dell'Aquila J, Soti V. Treating status epilepticus: phenytoin versus levetiracetam. Cureus. 2021;13(10):e18515.
291. Huo X, Xu X, Li M, et al. Effectiveness of antiseizure medications therapy in preventing seizures in brain injury patients: a network meta-analysis. Front Pharmacol. 2022;13:1001363.

292. Panda PK, Panda P, Dawman L, et al. Efficacy of lacosamide and phenytoin in status epilepticus: a systematic review. Acta Neurol Scand. 2021;144(4):366–74.
293. Ferner R, Day R, Bradberry SM. Phenytoin and damage to the cerebellum – a systematic review of published cases. Expert Opin Drug Saf. 2022;21(7):957–77.
294. Purkins L, Wood N, Ghahramani P, et al. Coadministration of voriconazole and phenytoin: pharmacokinetic interaction, safety, and toleration. Br J Clin Pharmacol. 2003;56(Suppl 1):37–44.
295. Muñoz-Vendrell A, Teixidor S, Sala-Padró J, et al. Intravenous lacosamide and phenytoin for the treatment of acute exacerbations of trigeminal neuralgia: a retrospective analysis of 144 cases. Cephalalgia. 2022;42(10):1031–8.
296. Degen R, Lässker G, Edelmann R. [Long term therapy with nitrazepam in children with infantile spasms and myoclonic-astatic fits]. Psychiatr Neurol Med Psychol Beih. 1975;20–21:90–3.
297. Kangas L, Kanto J, Syvälahti E. Plasma nitrazepam concentrations after an acute intake and their correlation to sedation and serum growth hormone levels. Acta Pharmacol Toxicol. 1977;41(1):65–73.
298. Khorana AB. Nitrazepam in emotional disorders of childhood. Indian J Psychiatry. 1981;23(1):79–81.
299. Ebata T, Izumi H, Aizawa H, et al. Effects of nitrazepam on nocturnal scratching in adults with atopic dermatitis: a double-blind placebo-controlled crossover study. Br J Dermatol. 1998;138(4):631–4.
300. Zahan S, Sahu JK, Madaan P, et al. Effectiveness and safety of nitrazepam in children with resistant West syndrome. Indian J Pediatr. 2022;89(1):37–44.
301. Zhongshu Z, Weiming Y, Yukio F, et al. Clinical analysis of West syndrome associated with phenylketonuria. Brain Dev. 2001;23(7):552–7.
302. Kaushik JS, Patra B, Sharma S, et al. Clinical spectrum and treatment outcome of West syndrome in children from northern India. Seizure. 2013;22(8):617–21.
303. Beran RG. Use of interval therapy with benzodiazepines to prevent seizure recurrence in stressful situations. Brain Sci. 2022;12(5):512.
304. Iyer A, Appleton R. Improving outcomes in infantile spasms: role of pharmacotherapy. Paediatr Drugs. 2016;18(5):357–66.
305. Hosain SA, Green NS, Solomon GE, et al. Nitrazepam for the treatment of Lennox-Gastaut syndrome. Pediatr Neurol. 2003;28(1):16–9.
306. Kagitani-Shimono K, Imai K, Otani K, et al. Epilepsy in Wolf-Hirschhorn syndrome (4p-). Epilepsia. 2005;46(1):150–5.
307. Shields MD, Hicks EM, Macgregor DF, et al. Infantile spasms associated with theophylline toxicity. Acta Paediatr. 1995;84(2):215–7.
308. Dreifuss F, Farwell J, Holmes G, et al. Infantile spasms. Comparative trial of nitrazepam and corticotropin. Arch Neurol. 1986;43(11):1107–10.
309. Song JM, Hahn J, Kim SH, et al. Efficacy of treatments for infantile spasms: a systematic review. Clin Neuropharmacol. 2017;40(2):63–84.
310. Saarelainen L, Taipale H, Koponen M, et al. The incidence of benzodiazepine and related drug use in persons with and without Alzheimer's disease. J Alzheimers Dis. 2016;49(3):809–18.
311. Jan JE, Riegl JA, Crichton JU, et al. Nitrazepam in the treatmet of epilepsy in childhood. Can Med Assoc J. 1971;104(7):571–5.
312. Kagota S, Morikawa K, Ishida H, et al. Vasorelaxant effects of benzodiazepines, non-benzodiazepine sedative-hypnotics, and tandospirone on isolated rat arteries. Eur J Pharmacol. 2021;892:173744.
313. Iqbal U, Nguyen PA, Syed-Abdul S, et al. Is long-term use of benzodiazepine a risk for cancer? Medicine. 2015;94(6):e483.
314. Dennis J, Hunt A. Prolonged use of nitrazepam for epilepsy in children with tuberous sclerosis. Br Med J (Clin Res Ed). 1985;291(6497):692–3.

315. Lim HC, Nigro MA, Beierwaltes P, et al. Nitrazepam-induced cricopharyngeal dysphagia, abnormal esophageal peristalsis and associated bronchospasm: probable cause of nitrazepam-related sudden death. Brain Dev. 1992;14(5):309–14.
316. Zhao DY, Feng GJ, Wu XR, et al. Seizures induced by intraventricular microinjection of ionized cobalt in the rat--a new experimental model of epilepsy. Brain Res. 1985;342(2):323–9.
317. Liao CY, Chung CH, Lu KC, et al. Taking sleeping pills and the risk of chronic kidney disease: a nationwide population-based retrospective cohort study. Front Pharmacol. 2020;11:524113.
318. Kassie GM, Roughead EE, Nguyen TA, et al. The risk of preoperative central nervous system-acting medications on delirium following hip or knee surgery: a matched case-control study. Drug Saf. 2022;45(1):75–82.
319. Marson A, Burnside G, Appleton R, et al. The SANAD II study of the effectiveness and cost-effectiveness of levetiracetam, zonisamide, or lamotrigine for newly diagnosed focal epilepsy: an open-label, non-inferiority, multicentre, phase 4, randomised controlled trial. Lancet. 2021;397(10282):1363–74.
320. Shi X, Wang Y, Zhang Y, et al. Effects of antiepileptic drugs polytherapy on pregnancy outcomes in women with epilepsy: an observation study in northwest China. Epilepsy Behav. 2022;135:108904.
321. Cohen JM, Alvestad S, Cesta CE, et al. Comparative safety of antiseizure medication monotherapy for major malformations. Ann Neurol. 2023;93(3):551–62.
322. Pekoz MT, Aslan-Kara K, Tekin B, et al. Birth outcomes in pregnant women with epilepsy: a nationwide multicenter study from Türkiye. Epilepsia. 2023;64(9):2310–21.
323. Barry JM, French JA, Pennell PB, et al. Empiric dosing strategies to predict lamotrigine concentrations during pregnancy. Pharmacotherapy. 2023;43(10):998–1006.
324. Freund B, Chen B, Kaplan PW, et al. Managing antiseizure medications in pregnancy: is earlier and more frequent monitoring better? Neurol Clin Pract. 2023;13(4):e200169.
325. Kacirova I, Grundmann M, Brozmanova H. Monitoring of lamotrigine concentrations in mothers, colostrum, and breastfed newborns during the early postpartum period. Biomed Pharmacother. 2022;151:113167.
326. Pedersen S, Kverneland M, Rudi K, et al. Decreased serum concentrations of antiseizure medications in children with drug resistant epilepsy following treatment with ketogenic diet. Epilepsia Open. 2023;8(3):858–66.
327. Shi XY, Ju J, Lu Q, et al. Both epilepsy and anti-seizure medications affect bone metabolism in children with self-limited epilepsy with centrotemporal spikes. Epilepsia. 2023;64(10):2667–78.
328. Assis T, Bacellar A, Côrtes L, et al. Trends in prescribing patterns of antiepileptic drugs among older adult inpatients in a Brazilian tertiary center. Arq Neuropsiquiatr. 2021;79(1):22–9.
329. Brodie MJ, Overstall PW, Giorgi L. Multicentre, double-blind, randomised comparison between lamotrigine and carbamazepine in elderly patients with newly diagnosed epilepsy. The UK Lamotrigine Elderly Study Group. Epilepsy Res. 1999;37(1):81–7.
330. Daneshyar S, Ghiasian M, Moradi S, et al. Efficacy of levetiracetam, lamotrigine and sodium valproate on seizure attacks and EEG disorders in patients with juvenile myoclonic epilepsy: a double blind randomized clinical trial. Caspian J Intern Med. 2022;13(3):617–22.
331. Larsson D, Baftiu A, Johannessen Landmark C, et al. Association between antiseizure drug monotherapy and mortality for patients with poststroke epilepsy. JAMA Neurol. 2022;79(2):169–75.
332. Loikas D, Linnér L, Sundström A, et al. Post-stroke epilepsy and antiepileptic drug use in men and women. Basic Clin Pharmacol Toxicol. 2021;129(2):148–57.
333. van Opijnen MP, van der Meer PB, Dirven L, et al. The effectiveness of antiepileptic drug treatment in glioma patients: lamotrigine versus lacosamide. J Neurooncol. 2021;154(1):73–81.
334. Mahamud Z, Håkansson S, Burman J, et al. Retention of antiseizure medications for epilepsy in multiple sclerosis: a retrospective observational study. Epilepsy Behav. 2021;121(Pt A):108034.

335. Le Roux M, Barth M, Gueden S, et al. CACNA1A-associated epilepsy: electroclinical findings and treatment response on seizures in 18 patients. Eur J Paediatr Neurol. 2021;33:75–85.
336. Milano C, Turco F, Pizzanelli C, et al. Response to levetiracetam or lamotrigine in subjects with Juvenile Myoclonic Epilepsy previously treated with valproic acid: a single center retrospective study. Epilepsy Behav. 2021;115:107706.
337. Zhang N, Yang D, Niu C, et al. Comparison of the retention rate, safety, and efficacy of two different titration protocols for lamotrigine in newly diagnosed epilepsy patients. Expert Rev Neurother. 2022;22(11–12):1025–9.
338. Chung SJ, Ahn KM, Oh JH, et al. Incidence rates of severe cutaneous adverse reactions due to antiseizure medication: a nationwide study using health claims data in Korea. Epilepsia. 2021;62(1):250–7.
339. Fukasawa T, Takahashi H, Takahashi K, et al. Risk of Stevens-Johnson syndrome and toxic epidermal necrolysis associated with anticonvulsants in a Japanese population: matched case-control and cohort studies. Allergol Int. 2021;70(3):335–42.
340. Shi YW, Wang J, Min FL, et al. HLA risk alleles in aromatic antiepileptic drug-induced maculopapular exanthema. Front Pharmacol. 2021;12:671572.
341. Edinoff AN, Nguyen LH, Fitz-Gerald MJ, et al. Lamotrigine and Stevens-Johnson syndrome prevention. Psychopharmacol Bull. 2021;51(2):96–114.
342. Mortazavi H, Rostami A, Firooz A, et al. Association between human leukocyte antigens and cutaneous adverse drug reactions to antiepileptics and antibiotics in the Iranian population. Dermatol Ther. 2022;35(5):e15393.
343. Packard E, Kalayanamitra R, Shahid Z, et al. DRESS is a mess: a case of cross reactivity between lacosamide and lamotrigine. S D Med. 2021;74(7):324–8.
344. Shirzadi M, Saunes M, Reimers A, et al. Rash during lamotrigine treatment is not always drug hypersensitivity: a retrospective cohort study among children and adults. Seizure. 2021;89:12–8.
345. Alfares I, Javaid MS, Chen Z, et al. Sex differences in the risk of cutaneous adverse drug reactions induced by antiseizure medications: a systematic review and meta-analysis. CNS Drugs. 2021;35(2):161–76.
346. Zhu X, Xiao T, Huang S, et al. Case report: predicting the range of lamotrigine concentration using pharmacokinetic models based on Monte Carlo simulation: a case study of antiepileptic drug-related leukopenia. Front Pharmacol. 2021;12:706329.
347. Wang C, Fan Z, He Y, et al. Analysis of the clinical characteristics of lamotrigine-induced haemophagocytic lymphohistiocytosis. J Clin Pharm Ther. 2022;47(6):745–51.
348. Wang W, Battini V, Carnovale C, et al. A novel approach for pharmacological substantiation of safety signals using plasma concentrations of medication and administrative/healthcare databases: a case study using Danish registries for an FDA warning on lamotrigine. Pharmacol Res. 2023;193:106811.
349. Christensen J, Trabjerg BB, Dreier JW. Cardiac morbidity and mortality associated with the use of lamotrigine. Epilepsia. 2022;63(9):2371–80.
350. Auerbach DS, Muniz CF. Cardiac safety of lamotrigine: still awaiting a verdict. Neurology. 2022;98(17):697–8.
351. Restrepo JA, MacLean R, Celano CM, et al. The assessment of cardiac risk in patients taking lamotrigine; a systematic review. Gen Hosp Psychiatry. 2022;78:14–27.
352. Aboukaoud M, Wilf-Yarkoni A, Maor E. Investigation of cardiac arrhythmia events in patients treated with lamotrigine: FDA adverse event reporing system analysis. Epilepsia. 2023;64(9):2322–9.
353. Bunschoten JW, Husein N, Devinsky O, et al. Sudden death and cardiac arrhythmia with lamotrigine: a rapid systematic review. Neurology. 2022;98(17):e1748–e60.
354. Nightscales R, Barnard S, Laze J, et al. Risk of sudden unexpected death in epilepsy (SUDEP) with lamotrigine and other sodium channel-modulating antiseizure medications. Epilepsia Open. 2023;8(2):334–45.

355. Hu W, Chen L, Li H, et al. Eye disorders associated with newer antiepileptic drugs: a real-world disproportionality analysis of FDA adverse event reporting system. Seizure. 2022;96:66–73.
356. Chen Y, Chen J, Zhuang X, et al. Risk factors of elevated blood ammonia level in epilepsy patients treated with lamotrigine. Medicine (Baltimore). 2022;101(26):e29780.
357. Tran DH, Jaggon KS, Mikdashi J, et al. Lamotrigine-induced lupus with aseptic meningitis and hemophagocytic lymphohistiocytosis. Cureus. 2022;14(9):e29629.
358. Watzal V, Godbersen GM, Weidenauer A, et al. Case report: interstitial pneumonitis after initiation of lamotrigine. Front Psych. 2023;14:1203497.
359. Ge J, Cao SS, Cao XY, et al. Lamotrigine induced priapism in children: case analysis and literature review. J Int Med Res. 2022;50(11):3000605221133988.
360. Huang J, Fan X, Jin X, et al. Dual-pocket inhibition of Na(v) channels by the antiepileptic drug lamotrigine. Proc Natl Acad Sci USA. 2023;120(41):e2309773120.
361. Chmielewska N, Wawer A, Wicik Z, et al. miR-9a-5p expression is decreased in the hippocampus of rats resistant to lamotrigine: a behavioural, molecular and bioinformatics assessment. Neuropharmacology. 2023;227:109425.
362. Faustmann TJ, Corvace F, Faustmann PM, et al. Effects of lamotrigine and topiramate on glial properties in an astrocyte-microglia co-culture model of inflammation. Int J Neuropsychopharmacol. 2022;25(3):185–96.
363. Filiz AK, Gumus E, Karabulut S, et al. Protective effects of lamotrigine and vitamin B12 on pentylenetetrazole-induced epileptogenesis in rats. Epilepsy Behav. 2021;118:107915.
364. Zubareva OE, Sinyak DS, Kalita AD, et al. Antiepileptogenic effects of anakinra, lamotrigine and their combination in a lithium-pilocarpine model of temporal lobe epilepsy in rats. Int J Mol Sci. 2023;24(20):15400.
365. Łuszczki JJ, Podgórska D, Kozińska J, et al. Polygonogram with isobolographic synergy for three-drug combinations of phenobarbital with second-generation antiepileptic drugs in the tonic-clonic seizure model in mice. Pharmacol Rep. 2021;73(1):111–21.
366. Onishi K, Kamida T, Fujiki M, et al. Anticonvulsant and antioxidant effects of lamotrigine on pilocarpine-induced status epilepticus in mice. Neuroreport. 2023;34(1):61–6.
367. Abdelmonem R, El-Enin HAA, Abdelkader G, et al. Formulation and characterization of lamotrigine nasal insert targeted brain for enhanced epilepsy treatment. Drug Deliv. 2023;30(1):2163321.
368. Mohsen AM, Salama AAA, Asfour MH. Cubosome-based thermosensitive in situ gelling system for intranasal administration of lamotrigine with enhanced antiepileptic efficacy. Pharm Dev Technol. 2023;28(6):520–34.
369. Jeong JH, Bahk WM, Woo YS, et al. Korean medication algorithm project for bipolar disorder 2022: comparisons with other treatment guidelines. Clin Psychopharmacol Neurosci. 2023;21(1):32–48.
370. Vieta E, Ghorpade S, Biswas A, et al. Lamotrigine efficacy, safety, and tolerability for women of childbearing age with bipolar I disorder: meta-analysis from four randomized, placebo-controlled maintenance studies. Eur Neuropsychopharmacol. 2024;78:81–92.
371. Thompson SI, El-Saden SM. Lamotrigine for treating anger in veterans with posttraumatic stress disorder. Clin Neuropharmacol. 2021;44(5):184–5.
372. Cuomo A, Amore M, Vampini C, et al. [Lamotrigine in bipolar disorder: preventing depression to treat the disease]. Riv Psichiatr. 2021;56(1):1–11.
373. Celdran de Castro A, Nascimento FA, Beltran-Corbellini Á, et al. Levetiracetam, from broad-spectrum use to precision prescription: a narrative review and expert opinion. Seizure. 2023;107:121–31.
374. Kharel S, Ojha R, Khanal S. Levetiracetam versus oxcarbazepine as monotherapy in newly diagnosed focal epilepsy: a systematic review and meta-analysis. Brain Behav. 2022;12(11):e2779.

375. Gerstl L, Willimsky E, Rémi C, et al. A systematic review of seizure-freedom rates in patients with benign epilepsy of childhood with centrotemporal spikes receiving antiepileptic drugs. Clin Neuropharmacol. 2021;44(2):39–46.
376. Abdelmesih SK, Elkhateeb N, Zakaria M, et al. Initial levetiracetam versus valproate monotherapy in antiseizure medicine (ASM)-naïve pediatric patients with idiopathic generalized epilepsy with tonic-clonic seizures. Seizure. 2021;91:263–70.
377. Manreza MLG, Pan TA, Carbone EQ, et al. Efficacy and safety of levetiracetam as adjunctive therapy for refractory focal epilepsy. Arq Neuropsiquiatr. 2021;79(4):290–8.
378. Ballvé A, Salas-Puig J, Quintana M, et al. Levetiracetam as first-line monotherapy for idiopathic generalized epilepsy in women. Acta Neurol Scand. 2021;143(4):407–12.
379. van der Meer PB, Dirven L, van den Bent MJ, et al. Prescription preferences of antiepileptic drugs in brain tumor patients: an international survey among EANO members. Neurooncol Pract. 2022;9(2):105–13.
380. van der Meer PB, Maschio M, Dirven L, et al. First-line levetiracetam versus enzyme-inducing antiseizure medication in glioma patients with epilepsy. Epilepsia. 2023;64(1):162–9.
381. Hedges A, Findlay MC, Davis GE, et al. Levetiracetam dosing for seizure prophylaxis in neurocritical care patients. Brain Inj. 2023;37(10):1167–72.
382. Peter-Derex L, Philippeau F, Garnier P, et al. Safety and efficacy of prophylactic levetiracetam for prevention of epileptic seizures in the acute phase of intracerebral haemorrhage (PEACH): a randomised, double-blind, placebo-controlled, phase 3 trial. Lancet Neurol. 2022;21(9):781–91.
383. Döring JH, Saffari A, Bast T, et al. Efficacy, tolerability, and retention of antiseizure medications in PRRT2-associated infantile epilepsy. Neurol Genet. 2022;8(5):e200020.
384. Coppola A, Dubbioso R, Cuccurullo C, et al. Current treatment options for familial adult myoclonus epilepsy. Epilepsia. 2023;64(Suppl 1):S58–63.
385. Zhang L, Li Y, Wang W, et al. Comparative antiseizure medications of adjunctive treatment for children with drug-resistant focal-onset seizures: a systematic review and network meta-analysis. Front Pharmacol. 2022;13:978876.
386. Takebayashi Y, Neshige S, Shishido T, et al. Paradoxical effects of levetiracetam in people with epilepsy with rhythmic epileptiform discharges. Epilepsy Behav. 2023;143:109225.
387. Horiguchi A, Koichihara R, Kikuchi K, et al. Efficacy of antiseizure medications in Wolf-Hirschhorn syndrome. Neuropediatrics. 2023;54(5):339–43.
388. Wang QH, Cao JJ, Wang YY, et al. Efficacy of levetiracetam in STXBP1 encephalopathy with different phenotypic and genetic spectra. Seizure. 2022;95:64–74.
389. Nagano M, Tagami T, Kaneko J, et al. Blood concentration of levetiracetam after bolus administration in patients with status epilepticus. Seizure. 2021;89:41–4.
390. Yang L, Dong XZ, Cui XH, et al. Comparison of the efficacy and safety of levetiracetam and phenytoin in the treatment of established status epilepticus: a systematic review and meta-analysis. J Clin Neurosci. 2021;89:422–9.
391. Angurana SK, Suthar R. Efficacy and safety of levetiracetam vs. phenytoin as second line antiseizure medication for pediatric convulsive status epilepticus: a systematic review and meta-analysis of randomized controlled trials. J Trop Pediatr. 2021;67(2):fmab014.
392. Haller JT, Bonnin S, Radosevich J. Rapid administration of undiluted intravenous levetiracetam. Epilepsia. 2021;62(8):1865–70.
393. Webb CA, Wanbon R, Otto ED. Levetiracetam for status epilepticus in adults: a systematic review. Can J Hosp Pharm. 2022;75(1):46–53.
394. Köle MT, Sager SG, Zeynel H, et al. Efficacy of intravenous levetiracetam versus phenytoin in convulsive status epilepticus and acute repetitive seizures in children. Childs Nerv Syst. 2022;38(7):1357–64.
395. Sharma SR, Sharma N, Hussain M, et al. Levetiracetam use during pregnancy in women with active epilepsy: a hospital-based, retrospective study from a tertiary care hospital in North Eastern INDIA. Neurol India. 2021;69(3):692–7.

396. Schelhaas M, Wegner I, Edens M, et al. Association of levetiracetam concentration with seizure frequency in pregnant women with epilepsy. Neurology. 2023;100(2):e172–e81.
397. Chen J, You X, Wu W, et al. Application of PBPK modeling in predicting maternal and fetal pharmacokinetics of levetiracetam during pregnancy. Eur J Pharm Sci. 2023;181:106349.
398. Susnerwala S, Joshi A, Deshmukh L, et al. Levetiracetam or phenobarbitone as a first-line anticonvulsant in asphyxiated term newborns? An open-label, single-center, randomized, controlled, pragmatic trial. Hosp Pediatr. 2022;12(7):647–53.
399. Sortino V, Praticò A, Marino S, et al. Efficacy of the anti-seizure medications in acute symptomatic neonatal seizures caused by stroke. A systematic review. Acta Biomed. 2022;93(6):e2022328.
400. Bromley RL, Bullen P, Campbell E, et al. Neurodevelopment of babies born to mothers with epilepsy: a prospective observational cohort study. Epilepsia. 2023;64(9):2454–71.
401. Mari L, Placidi F, Romigi A, et al. Levetiracetam, lamotrigine and carbamazepine: which monotherapy during pregnancy? Neurol Sci. 2022;43(3):1993–2001.
402. Verwoerd C, Limjoco J, Rajamanickam V, et al. Efficacy of levetiracetam and phenobarbital as first-line treatment for neonatal seizures. J Child Neurol. 2022;37(5):401–9.
403. Werhahn KJ, Trinka E, Dobesberger J, et al. A randomized, double-blind comparison of antiepileptic drug treatment in the elderly with new-onset focal epilepsy. Epilepsia. 2015;56(3):450–9.
404. Consoli D, Bosco D, Postorino P, et al. Levetiracetam versus carbamazepine in patients with late poststroke seizures: a multicenter prospective randomized open-label study (EpIC Project). Cerebrovasc Dis. 2012;34(4):282–9.
405. Tekin U, Tekin E, Uçar HN. Irritability and its relationship with psychosocial symptoms and quality of life in adolescents with epilepsy receiving levetiracetam therapy: a case-control study. Epilepsy Behav. 2022;135:108877.
406. Dreier JW, Bjørk MH, Alvestad S, et al. Prenatal exposure to antiseizure medication and incidence of childhood- and adolescence-onset psychiatric disorders. JAMA Neurol. 2023;80(6):568–77.
407. Onodera M, Saito T, Fukui A, et al. The high incidence and risk factors of levetiracetam and lacosamide-related skin rashes in glioma patients. Clin Neurol Neurosurg. 2022;220:107366.
408. Gözükızıl ST, Aydın Z, Yalçın AD. Relationship between bone density and levetiracetam monotherapy in epilepsy patients. Clin Neurol Neurosurg. 2022;218:107270.
409. Han Y, Yang J, Zhong R, et al. Side effects of long-term oral anti-seizure drugs on thyroid hormones in patients with epilepsy: a systematic review and network meta-analysis. Neurol Sci. 2022;43(9):5217–27.
410. Zhuo L, Zhang Y. Effects of new antiseizure medication on bone metabolism and bone mineral density in children: a meta-analysis. Front Pediatr. 2022;10:1015691.
411. Egunsola O, Choonara I, Sammons HM. Safety of levetiracetam in paediatrics: a systematic review. PLoS One. 2016;11(3):e0149686.
412. Mahmoud A, Tabassum S, Al Enazi S, et al. Amelioration of levetiracetam-induced behavioral side effects by pyridoxine. A randomized double blind controlled study. Pediatr Neurol. 2021;119:15–21.
413. Giner-Soriano M, Marsal JR, Gomez-Lumbreras A, et al. Risk of ischaemic stroke associated with antiepileptic drugs: a population-based case-control study in Catalonia. BMC Neurol. 2021;21(1):208.
414. Ip BY, Ko H, Wong GL, et al. Thromboembolic risks with concurrent direct oral anticoagulants and antiseizure medications: a population-based analysis. CNS Drugs. 2022;36(12):1313–24.
415. Aydin H, Korkut O. Effect of levetiracetam therapy on electrocardiographic parameters. Arch Pediatr. 2023;30(3):149–52.
416. Niidome K, Taniguchi R, Yamazaki T, et al. FosL1 is a novel target of levetiracetam for suppressing the microglial inflammatory reaction. Int J Mol Sci. 2021;22(20):10962.

417. Matsuo T, Komori R, Nakatani M, et al. Levetiracetam suppresses the infiltration of neutrophils and monocytes and downregulates many inflammatory cytokines during epileptogenesis in pilocarpine-induced status epilepticus mice. Int J Mol Sci. 2022;23(14):7671.
418. Mani V, Rashed Almutairi S. Impact of levetiracetam on cognitive impairment, neuroinflammation, oxidative stress, and neuronal apoptosis caused by lipopolysaccharides in rats. Saudi Pharm J. 2023;31(9):101728.
419. Yang L, Afroz S, Valsamis HA, et al. Early intervention with levetiracetam prevents the development of cortical hyperexcitability and spontaneous epileptiform activity in two models of neurotrauma in rats. Exp Neurol. 2021;337:113571.
420. Vossel K, Ranasinghe KG, Beagle AJ, et al. Effect of levetiracetam on cognition in patients with Alzheimer disease with and without epileptiform activity: a randomized clinical trial. JAMA Neurol. 2021;78(11):1345–54.
421. Rao NR, Savas JN. Levetiracetam treatment normalizes levels of presynaptic endocytosis machinery and restores nonamyloidogenic APP processing in app knock-in mice. J Proteome Res. 2021;20(7):3580–9.
422. Alavi MS, Fanoudi S, Hosseini M, et al. Beneficial effects of levetiracetam in streptozotocin-induced rat model of Alzheimer's disease. Metab Brain Dis. 2022;37(3):689–700.
423. Azeem GM, Faheem F, Farooq N, et al. Levetiracetam for the prophylaxis of migraine in adults. Cureus. 2021;13(7):e16779.
424. Cavichioli AM, Santos-Silva T, Grace AA, et al. Levetiracetam attenuates adolescent stress-induced behavioral and electrophysiological changes associated with schizophrenia in adult rats. Schizophr Bull. 2023;49(1):68–77.
425. Latini G, Verrotti A, Manco R, et al. Topiramate: its pharmacological properties and therapeutic efficacy in epilepsy. Mini Rev Med Chem. 2008;8(1):10–23.
426. Rheims S, Ryvlin P. Pharmacotherapy for tonic-clonic seizures. Expert Opin Pharmacother. 2014;15(10):1417–26.
427. Campos MSA, Ayres LR, Morelo MRS, et al. Comparative efficacy of antiepileptic drugs for patients with generalized epileptic seizures: systematic review and network meta-analyses. Int J Clin Pharm. 2018;40(3):589–98.
428. Bresnahan R, Hounsome J, Jette N, et al. Topiramate add-on therapy for drug-resistant focal epilepsy. Cochrane Database Syst Rev. 2019;10(10):CD001417.
429. Liu J, Tai YJ, Wang LN. Topiramate for juvenile myoclonic epilepsy. Cochrane Database Syst Rev. 2021;11(11):CD010008.
430. Knupp KG, Wirrell EC. Treatment strategies for Dravet syndrome. CNS Drugs. 2018;32(4):335–50.
431. Zhang L, Wang J, Wang C. Efficacy and safety of antiseizure medication for Lennox-Gastaut syndrome: a systematic review and network meta-analysis. Dev Med Child Neurol. 2022;64(3):305–13.
432. Lee SK, Heo K, Kim SE, et al. Effect of number of previous antiseizure medications on efficacy and tolerability of adjunctive brivaracetam for uncontrolled focal seizures: post hoc analysis. Adv Ther. 2021;38(7):4082–99.
433. Ji ZY, Huang YQ, He WZ. Sodium valproate combined with topiramate vs. sodium valproate alone for refractory epilepsy: a systematic review and meta-analysis. Front Neurol. 2021;12:794856.
434. Fechner A, Hubert K, Jahnke K, et al. Treatment of refractory and superrefractory status epilepticus with topiramate: a cohort study of 106 patients and a review of the literature. Epilepsia. 2019;60(12):2448–58.
435. Welling LC, Rabelo NN, Yoshikawa MH, et al. Efficacy of topiramate as an add-on therapy in patients with refractory status epilepticus: a short systematic review. Rev Bras Ter Intensiva. 2021;33(3):440–4.
436. Löscher W, Trinka E. The potential of intravenous topiramate for the treatment of status epilepticus. Epilepsy Behav. 2023;138:109032.

437. Rundfeldt C, Klein P, Boison D, et al. Preclinical pharmacokinetics and tolerability of a novel meglumine-based parenteral solution of topiramate and topiramate combinations for treatment of status epilepticus. Epilepsia. 2023;64(4):888–99.
438. Vawter-Lee M, Natarajan N, Rang K, et al. Topiramate is safe for refractory neonatal seizures: a multicenter retrospective cohort study of necrotizing enterocolitis risk. Pediatr Neurol. 2022;129:7–13.
439. Burns TG, Ludwig NN, Tajiri TN, et al. Cognitive and behavioral outcomes among seizure-controlled children with partial epilepsy on antiepileptic drug monotherapy. Appl Neuropsychol Child. 2018;7(1):52–60.
440. Knight R, Wittkowski A, Bromley RL. Neurodevelopmental outcomes in children exposed to newer antiseizure medications: a systematic review. Epilepsia. 2021;62(8):1765–79.
441. Kacirova I, Grundmann M, Brozmanova H, et al. Monitoring topiramate concentrations at delivery and during lactation. Biomed Pharmacother. 2021;138:111446.
442. Knight R, Craig J, Irwin B, et al. Adaptive behaviour in children exposed to topiramate in the womb: an observational cohort study. Seizure. 2023;105:56–64.
443. Choi J, Yoon D, Park M, et al. Topiramate-related adverse events: pattern and signals in the Korea Adverse Event Reporting System, 2010-2017. Medicine (Baltimore). 2020;99(42):e22669.
444. Koristkova B, Grundmann M, Brozmanova H, et al. Was it necessary to change the therapeutic range of topiramate? Br J Clin Pharmacol. 2022;88(2):613–8.
445. Khan S, Ashraf A, Javaid H, et al. Topiramate-induced acute transient myopia and angle narrowing. J Coll Physicians Surg Pak. 2021;30(6):728–31.
446. Tyagi M, Behera S, Senthil S, et al. Topiramate induced bilateral hypopyon uveitis and choroidal detachment: a report of two cases and review of literature. BMC Ophthalmol. 2021;21(1):287.
447. Pinto-Gouveia C, Bernardes L, Renca S. Topiramate-associated acute bilateral angle-closure glaucoma. J Clin Psychopharmacol. 2022;42(3):320–1.
448. Pelzman DL, Kazi E, Jackman SV, et al. Urinary metabolic disturbances during topiramate use and their reversibility following drug cessation. Urology. 2022;165:139–43.
449. Shishmanova-Doseva M, Peychev L, Yoanidu L, et al. Anticonvulsant effects of topiramate and lacosamide on pilocarpine-induced status epilepticus in rats: a role of reactive oxygen species and inflammation. Int J Mol Sci. 2021;22(5):2264.
450. Lotfy DM, Safar MM, Hassan SHM, et al. Modulation of PTZ-induced convulsions in rats using topiramate alone or combined with low dose gamma irradiation: involving AKT/mTOR pathway. Toxicol Mech Methods. 2022;32(1):18–26.
451. Rafi SK, Goering JP, Olm-Shipman AJ, et al. Anti-epileptic drug topiramate upregulates TGFβ1 and SOX9 expression in primary embryonic palatal mesenchyme cells: implications for teratogenicity. PLoS One. 2021;16(2):e0246989.
452. Soleimani Meigoni Z, Jabari F, Motaghinejad M, et al. Protective effects of forced exercise against topiramate-induced cognition impairment and enhancement of its antiepileptic activity: molecular and behavioral evidences. Int J Neurosci. 2022;132(12):1198–209.
453. Borges LI, Forcato S, do Nascimento Olanda LC, et al. Treatment with topiramate in rats during childhood causes testicular structural impairment at adulthood. J Dev Orig Health Dis. 2023;14(2):279–85.
454. Paolo P, Matteo F, Rossella L, et al. Koolen-de Vries syndrome: preliminary observations of topiramate efficacy. Child Neurol Open. 2021;8:2329048x211019183.
455. Chapron SA, Nourredine M, Dondé C, et al. Efficacy and safety of topiramate for reducing impulsivity: a transdiagnostic systematic review and meta-analysis of a common clinical use. Fundam Clin Pharmacol. 2022;36(1):4–15.
456. Chandradasa M, Ruwanpriya S, de Silva S, et al. Randomised, placebo-controlled trial on topiramate add-on therapy for weight reduction and symptomatology in overweight/obese persons with schizophrenia. Asian J Psychiatr. 2022;68:102963.

457. Panebianco M, Al-Bachari S, Hutton JL, et al. Gabapentin add-on treatment for drug-resistant focal epilepsy. Cochrane Database Syst Rev. 2021;1(1):CD001415.
458. Ziganshina LE, Abakumova T, Hoyle CHV. Gabapentin monotherapy for epilepsy: a review. Int J Risk Saf Med. 2023;34(3):243–86.
459. Cao X, Shen Z, Wang X, et al. A meta-analysis of randomized controlled trials comparing the efficacy and safety of pregabalin and gabapentin in the treatment of postherpetic neuralgia. Pain Ther. 2023;12(1):1–18.
460. Gammoh O, Al-Smadi A, Shawagfeh MQ, et al. The clinical difference between gabapentin and pregabalin: data from a pilot comparative trial. Rev Recent Clin Trials. 2021;16(3):279–87.
461. Patel AS, Abrecht CR, Urman RD. Gabapentinoid use in perioperative care and current controversies. Curr Pain Headache Rep. 2022;26(2):139–44.
462. Fowler C, Chu AW, Guo N, et al. Outpatient treatment with gabapentin in women with severe acute pain after cesarean delivery is ineffective: a randomized, double-blind, placebo-controlled trial. Anesth Analg. 2023;136(6):1122–32.
463. Rudroju N, Bansal D, Talakokkula ST, et al. Comparative efficacy and safety of six antidepressants and anticonvulsants in painful diabetic neuropathy: a network meta-analysis. Pain Physician. 2013;16(6):E705–14.
464. Wiffen PJ, Derry S, Bell RF, et al. Gabapentin for chronic neuropathic pain in adults. Cochrane Database Syst Rev. 2017;6(6):CD007938.
465. Swarm RA, Paice JA, Anghelescu DL, et al. Adult cancer pain, version 3.2019, NCCN clinical practice guidelines in oncology. J Natl Compr Canc Netw. 2019;17(8):977–1007.
466. Davanzo R, Dal Bo S, Bua J, et al. Antiepileptic drugs and breastfeeding. Ital J Pediatr. 2013;39:50.
467. Ohman I, Vitols S, Tomson T. Pharmacokinetics of gabapentin during delivery, in the neonatal period, and lactation: does a fetal accumulation occur during pregnancy? Epilepsia. 2005;46(10):1621–4.
468. Fujii H, Goel A, Bernard N, et al. Pregnancy outcomes following gabapentin use: results of a prospective comparative cohort study. Neurology. 2013;80(17):1565–70.
469. Hayes WJ, Ferdinand A, Neabore S, et al. Patient case report: gabapentin-induced hypoglycemia. J Pharm Pract. 2022;35(2):298–301.
470. Contreras-Mota M, Rosales-Cortés V. [Hepatotoxicity probably associated with gabapentin]. Rev Med Inst Mex Seguro Soc. 2021;59(2):157–62.
471. Largeau B, Bordy R, Pasqualin C, et al. Gabapentinoid-induced peripheral edema and acute heart failure: a translational study combining pharmacovigilance data and in vitro animal experiments. Biomed Pharmacother. 2022;149:112807.
472. Meaadi J, Obara I, Eldabe S, et al. The safety and efficacy of gabapentinoids in the management of neuropathic pain: a systematic review with meta-analysis of randomised controlled trials. Int J Clin Pharm. 2023;45(3):556–65.
473. Evoy KE, Sadrameli S, Contreras J, et al. Abuse and misuse of pregabalin and gabapentin: a systematic review update. Drugs. 2021;81(1):125–56.
474. Park SH, Hunter K, Berry H, et al. Atrial fibrillation induced by gabapentin: a case report. J Med Case Rep. 2023;17(1):236.
475. Perrott SL, Macleod AD. Associations between antiepileptic use and hypogammaglobulinaemia: findings from a population-based case-control study using data linkage. Neuroepidemiology. 2023;57(6):355–66.
476. Kaurich T. Drug-induced acute pancreatitis. Proc (Baylor Univ Med Cent). 2008;21(1):77–81.
477. Uchitel OD, Di Guilmi MN, Urbano FJ, et al. Acute modulation of calcium currents and synaptic transmission by gabapentinoids. Channels (Austin). 2010;4(6):490–6.
478. Chincholkar M. Gabapentinoids: pharmacokinetics, pharmacodynamics and considerations for clinical practice. Br J Pain. 2020;14(2):104–14.
479. Got T, Vivas L, Fan C, et al. Treatment of hiccups in stroke rehabilitation with gabapentin: a case series and focused clinical review. Top Stroke Rehabil. 2021;28(6):475–80.

480. Leung E, Ngo DH, Espinoza JA Jr, et al. A retrospective study of the adjunctive use of gabapentin with benzodiazepines for the treatment of benzodiazepine withdrawal. J Psychiatr Pract. 2022;28(4):310–8.
481. Wu B, Cao Y, Meng M, et al. Gabapentin alleviates myocardial ischemia-reperfusion injury by increasing the protein expression of GABA(A)Rδ. Eur J Pharmacol. 2023;944:175585.
482. Shen Y, Li W, Ma M, et al. Efficacy and safety of gabapentin in improving sleep quality of patients with sensory nervous system diseases: a meta-analysis. Altern Ther Health Med. 2023;29(5):380–5.
483. Zhao T, Feng X, Liu J, et al. Evaluate the efficacy and safety of anti-epileptic medications for partial seizures of epilepsy: a network meta-analysis. J Cell Biochem. 2017;118(9):2850–64.
484. French J, Kwan P, Fakhoury T, et al. Pregabalin monotherapy in patients with partial-onset seizures: a historical-controlled trial. Neurology. 2014;82(7):590–7.
485. Kwan P, Brodie MJ, Kälviäinen R, et al. Efficacy and safety of pregabalin versus lamotrigine in patients with newly diagnosed partial seizures: a phase 3, double-blind, randomised, parallel-group trial. Lancet Neurol. 2011;10(10):881–90.
486. de Bruin ME, van der Meer PB, Dirven L, et al. Efficacy of antiepileptic drugs in glioma patients with epilepsy: a systematic review. Neurooncol Pract. 2021;8(5):501–17.
487. Driscoll J, Almas M, Gregorian G, et al. Pregabalin as adjunctive therapy in adult and pediatric patients with generalized tonic-clonic seizures: a randomized, placebo-controlled trial. Epilepsia Open. 2021;6(2):381–93.
488. Kanner AM, Ashman E, Gloss D, et al. Practice guideline update summary: efficacy and tolerability of the new antiepileptic drugs II: treatment-resistant epilepsy: report of the Guideline Development, Dissemination, and Implementation Subcommittee of the American Academy of Neurology and the American Epilepsy Society. Neurology. 2018;91(2):82–90.
489. Panebianco M, Bresnahan R, Hemming K, et al. Pregabalin add-on for drug-resistant focal epilepsy. Cochrane Database Syst Rev. 2019;7(7):CD005612.
490. Panebianco M, Bresnahan R, Marson AG. Pregabalin add-on for drug-resistant focal epilepsy. Cochrane Database Syst Rev. 2022;3(3):CD005612.
491. Viteva E, Zahariev Z. Comparative effectiveness of add-on therapy with newer-generation antiepileptic drugs in Bulgarian patients with refractory epilepsy. Epilepsy Behav. 2018;87:137–45.
492. Androsova G, Krause R, Borghei M, et al. Comparative effectiveness of antiepileptic drugs in patients with mesial temporal lobe epilepsy with hippocampal sclerosis. Epilepsia. 2017;58(10):1734–41.
493. Ochoa JG, Dougherty M, Papanastassiou A, et al. Treatment of super-refractory status epilepticus: a review. Epilepsy Curr. 2021;21(6):1535759721999670.
494. Gomes D, Pimentel J, Bentes C, et al. Consensus protocol for the treatment of super-refractory status epilepticus. Acta Med Port. 2018;31(10):598–605.
495. Novy J, Rossetti AO. Oral pregabalin as an add-on treatment for status epilepticus. Epilepsia. 2010;51(10):2207–10.
496. Swisher CB, Doreswamy M, Gingrich KJ, et al. Phenytoin, levetiracetam, and pregabalin in the acute management of refractory status epilepticus in patients with brain tumors. Neurocrit Care. 2012;16(1):109–13.
497. Swisher CB, Doreswamy M, Husain AM. Use of pregabalin for nonconvulsive seizures and nonconvulsive status epilepticus. Seizure. 2013;22(2):116–8.
498. Mann D, Antinew J, Knapp L, et al. Pregabalin adjunctive therapy for focal onset seizures in children 1 month to <4 years of age: a double-blind, placebo-controlled, video-electroencephalographic trial. Epilepsia. 2020;61(4):617–26.
499. Antinew J, Pitrosky B, Knapp L, et al. Pregabalin as adjunctive treatment for focal onset seizures in pediatric patients: a randomized controlled trial. J Child Neurol. 2019;34(5):248–55.
500. Chan PLS, Marshall SF, McFadyen L, et al. Pregabalin population pharmacokinetic and exposure-response analyses for focal onset seizures in children (4-16 years) and adults, to support dose recommendations in children. Clin Pharmacol Ther. 2021;110(1):132–40.

501. Dudukina E, Szépligeti SK, Karlsson P. Prenatal exposure to pregabalin, birth outcomes and neurodevelopment – a population-based cohort study in four Nordic countries. Drug Saf. 2023;46(7):661–75.
502. Parekh M, Dash GK, Ahamed I. Pregabalin toxicity manifesting as reversible encephalopathy with continuous triphasic waves in electroencephalogram. Clin Neuropharmacol. 2017;40(5):226–8.
503. Anand P, Kaplan PW. Triphasic waves and encephalopathy in the setting of pregabalin toxicity. J Clin Neurophysiol. 2018;35(6):515–7.
504. Cross AL, Viswanath O, Sherman AL. Pregabalin. In: StatPearls. Treasure Island: StatPearls Publishing; 2024.
505. Baftiu A, Lima MH, Svendsen K, et al. Safety aspects of antiepileptic drugs-a population-based study of adverse effects relative to changes in utilisation. Eur J Clin Pharmacol. 2019;75(8):1153–60.
506. Prakash S, Rathore C, Rana K, et al. Antiepileptic drugs and serotonin syndrome – a systematic review of case series and case reports. Seizure. 2021;91:117–31.
507. Shukla S, Rastogi S, Abdi SAH, et al. Severe cutaneous adverse reactions in Asians: trends observed in culprit anti-seizure medicines using VigiBase®. Seizure. 2021;91:332–8.
508. Hamed SA. Sexual dysfunctions induced by pregabalin. Clin Neuropharmacol. 2018;41(4):116–22.
509. da Costa Sobral KG, Neuberger B, Mello FK, et al. Anticonvulsant activity of β-caryophyllene in association with pregabalin in a seizure model in rats. Epilepsy Res. 2022;179:106842.
510. Qureshi I, Riaz A, Khan R, et al. Effects of pregabalin, nimodipine, and their combination in the inhibition of status epilepticus and the prevention of death in mice. Turk J Pharm Sci. 2021;18(4):398–404.
511. Imran I, Koch K, Schöfer H, et al. Effects of three antiseizure medications on cholinergic and metabolic activity in experimental status epilepticus. J Pharm Pharm Sci. 2019;22(1):340–51.
512. Tong C, Zhengyao Z, Mei L, et al. Pregabalin and gabapentin in patients with spinal cord injury-related neuropathic pain: a network meta-analysis. Pain Ther. 2021;10(2):1497–509.
513. Onakpoya IJ, Thomas ET, Lee JJ, et al. Benefits and harms of pregabalin in the management of neuropathic pain: a rapid review and meta-analysis of randomised clinical trials. BMJ Open. 2019;9(1):e023600.
514. Derry S, Bell RF, Straube S, et al. Pregabalin for neuropathic pain in adults. Cochrane Database Syst Rev. 2019;1(1):CD007076.
515. GBD 2016 Neurology Collaborators. Global, regional, and national burden of neurological disorders, 1990-2016: a systematic analysis for the Global Burden of Disease Study 2016. Lancet Neurol. 2019;18(5):459–80.
516. Kalilani L, Sun X, Pelgrims B, et al. The epidemiology of drug-resistant epilepsy: a systematic review and meta-analysis. Epilepsia. 2018;59(12):2179–93.
517. Humayun MJ, Samanta D, Carson RP. Clobazam. In: StatPearls. Treasure Island: StatPearls Publishing LLC; 2024. Disclosure: Debopam Samanta declares no relevant financial relationships with ineligible companies. Disclosure: Robert Carson declares no relevant financial relationships with ineligible companies.
518. Brahmbhatt N, Stupp R, Bushara O, et al. Efficacy of clobazam as add-on therapy in brain tumor-related epilepsy. J Neurooncol. 2021;151(2):287–93.
519. Cochrane Central Register of Controlled Trials. Clobazam has equivalent efficacy to carbamazepine and phenytoin as monotherapy for childhood epilepsy. Canadian Study Group for Childhood Epilepsy. Epilepsia. 1998;39(9):952–9.
520. Arya R, Giridharan N, Anand V, et al. Clobazam monotherapy for focal or generalized seizures. Cochrane Database Syst Rev. 2018;7(7):CD009258.
521. Dulac O, Figueroa D, Rey E, et al. [Monotherapy with clobazam in epilepsies in children]. Presse Med. 1983;12(17):1067–9.
522. Mehndiratta MM, Krishnamurthy M, Rajesh KN, et al. Clobazam monotherapy in drug naïve adult patients with epilepsy. Seizure. 2003;12(4):226–8.

523. Kamaşak T, Serdaroğlu E, Yılmaz Ö, et al. The effectiveness and tolerability of clobazam in the pediatric population: adjunctive therapy and monotherapy in a large-cohort multicenter study. Epilepsy Res. 2022;184:106963.
524. Jamil A, Levinson N, Gelfand M, et al. Efficacy and tolerability of clobazam in adults with drug-refractory epilepsy. Neurol Clin Pract. 2021;11(5):e669–76.
525. Talwar A, Estes E, Aparasu R, et al. Clinical efficacy and safety of cannabidiol for pediatric refractory epilepsy indications: a systematic review and meta-analysis. Exp Neurol. 2023;359:114238.
526. Nagarajan E, Lynch TM, Frawley B, et al. Tolerability of clobazam as add-on therapy in patients aged 50 years and older with drug-resistant epilepsy. Neurol Sci. 2023;44(8):2883–8.
527. Canadian Clobazam Cooperative Group. Clobazam in treatment of refractory epilepsy: the Canadian experience. A retrospective study. Epilepsia. 1991;32(3):407–16.
528. Kalra V, Seth R, Mishra D, et al. Clobazam in refractory childhood epilepsy. Indian J Pediatr. 2010;77(3):263–6.
529. Maille JM, Hanna SS, Shah DN. Addition of clobazam successfully treating drug resistant seizures in Heidenhain variant Creutzfeldt Jakob disease: a case report. Epilepsy Behav Rep. 2023;21:100585.
530. Serrano-Castro PJ, Rodríguez-Uranga JJ, Cabezudo-García P, et al. Cenobamate and clobazam combination as personalized medicine in autoimmune-associated epilepsy with anti-GAD65 antibodies. Neurol Neuroimmunol Neuroinflamm. 2023;10(6):e200151.
531. Rana RR, Rajasekaran K, Knappertz V, et al. Pharmacodynamic synergism contributes to the antiseizure action of cannabidiol and clobazam. Exp Neurol. 2023;360:114286.
532. Sharma A, Kumar A. Identification of novel signal of clobazam-associated drug reaction with eosinophilia and systemic symptoms syndrome: a disproportionality analysis. Acta Neurol Scand. 2022;146(5):623–7.
533. Zhang JF, Nickerson K, Piryani R, et al. Macroglossia associated with clobazam administration: a case report and literature review. Front Neurol. 2022;13:900763.
534. Kart P, Gürgen SG, Esenülkü G, et al. An investigation of the effects of chronic zonisamide, sultiam, lacosamide, clobazam, and rufinamide anti-seizure medications on foliculogenesis in ovarian tissue in prepubertal non-epileptic rats. Int J Dev Neurosci. 2022;82(5):436–46.
535. Elakkary S, Hagemann A, Klimpel D, et al. A retrospective non-interventional study evaluating the pharmacokinetic interactions between cenobamate and clobazam. Epilepsia. 2023;64(4):e36–42.
536. Sankar R. GABA(A) receptor physiology and its relationship to the mechanism of action of the 1,5-benzodiazepine clobazam. CNS Drugs. 2012;26(3):229–44.
537. Ng YT, Conry JA, Drummond R, et al. Randomized, phase III study results of clobazam in Lennox-Gastaut syndrome. Neurology. 2011;77(15):1473–81.
538. Gunning B, Mazurkiewicz-Bełdzińska M, Chin RFM, et al. Cannabidiol in conjunction with clobazam: analysis of four randomized controlled trials. Acta Neurol Scand. 2021;143(2):154–63.
539. Wilensky AJ, Friel PN, Ojemann LM, et al. Pharmacokinetics of W-554 (ADD 03055) in epileptic patients. Epilepsia. 1985;26(6):602–6.
540. Leppik IE, Dreifuss FE, Pledger GW, et al. Felbamate for partial seizures: results of a controlled clinical trial. Neurology. 1991;41(11):1785–9.
541. Gasior M, Swiader M, Przybyłko M, et al. Felbamate demonstrates low propensity for interaction with methylxanthines and Ca2+ channel modulators against experimental seizures in mice. Eur J Pharmacol. 1998;352(2–3):207–14.
542. Borowicz KK, Ratnaraj N, Patsalos PN, et al. Effect of felbamate and its combinations with conventional antiepileptics in amygdala-kindled rats. Pharmacol Biochem Behav. 2004;78(1):103–10.
543. Heyman E, Levin N, Lahat E, et al. Efficacy and safety of felbamate in children with refractory epilepsy. Eur J Paediatr Neurol. 2014;18(6):658–62.

544. Reed L, Ciliberto M, Fong SL, et al. Efficacy of felbamate in a cohort of patients with epilepsy with myoclonic atonic seizures (EMAtS). Epilepsy Res. 2024;201:107314.
545. Wilcox MA, Hardin J, Weaver J, et al. Liver test monitoring: real-world compliance for drugs with monitoring requirements at 2-week intervals or more frequently. Pharmaceut Med. 2019;33(5):389–94.
546. Felbamate Study Group in Lennox-Gastaut Syndrome. Efficacy of felbamate in childhood epileptic encephalopathy (Lennox-Gastaut syndrome). N Engl J Med. 1993;328(1):29–33.
547. Shi LL, Dong J, Ni H, et al. Felbamate as an add-on therapy for refractory partial epilepsy. Cochrane Database Syst Rev. 2017;7(7):CD008295.
548. Strzelczyk A, Schubert-Bast S. Expanding the treatment landscape for Lennox-Gastaut syndrome: current and future strategies. CNS Drugs. 2021;35(1):61–83.
549. Mazarati AM, Baldwin RA, Sofia RD, et al. Felbamate in experimental model of status epilepticus. Epilepsia. 2000;41(2):123–7.
550. Yerby MS, McCoy GB. Male infertility: possible association with valproate exposure. Epilepsia. 1999;40(4):520–1.
551. Mishal NM, Arkilo D, Tang J, et al. A potential role for Felbamate in TSC- and NF1-related epilepsy: a case report and review of the literature. Case Rep Neurol Med. 2015;2015:960746.
552. Rabinowicz S, Schreiber T, Heimer G, et al. Felbamate for pediatric epilepsy-should we keep on using it as the last resort? Front Neurol. 2022;13:979725.
553. Hussain SA, Asilnejad B, Heesch J, et al. Felbamate in the treatment of refractory epileptic spasms. Epilepsy Res. 2020;161:106284.
554. Dozières-Puyravel B, Nasser H, Bellavoine V, et al. Felbamate for infantile spasms syndrome resistant to first-line treatments. Dev Med Child Neurol. 2020;62(5):581–6.
555. de Jong J, Garne E, de Jong-van den Berg LT, et al. The risk of specific congenital anomalies in relation to newer antiepileptic drugs: a literature review. Drugs Real World Outcomes. 2016;3(2):131–43.
556. Shi LL, Bresnahan R, Martin-McGill KJ, et al. Felbamate add-on therapy for drug-resistant focal epilepsy. Cochrane Database Syst Rev. 2022;8(8):CD008295.
557. Devi N, Madaan P, Ameen R, et al. Short-term and long-term efficacy and safety of antiseizure medications in Lennox Gastaut syndrome: a network meta-analysis. Seizure. 2022;99:164–75.
558. Vidaurre J, Gedela S, Yarosz S. Antiepileptic drugs and liver disease. Pediatr Neurol. 2017;77:23–36.
559. Jacob S, Nair AB. An updated overview on therapeutic drug monitoring of recent antiepileptic drugs. Drugs R&D. 2016;16(4):303–16.
560. Celli R, Fornai F. Targeting ionotropic glutamate receptors in the treatment of epilepsy. Curr Neuropharmacol. 2021;19(6):747–65.
561. Li X, Wang H, Chen Q, et al. Felbamate produces antidepressant-like actions in the chronic unpredictable mild stress and chronic social defeat stress models of depression. Fundam Clin Pharmacol. 2019;33(6):621–33.
562. Bayhan I, Turtay MG, Ciftci O, et al. Comparison of immunological, histological and oxidative effects of felbamate and levetiracetam in traumatic brain injury. Eur Rev Med Pharmacol Sci. 2020;24(12):7083–91.
563. Schechter PJ, Tranier Y. Effect of GABA-transminase inhibition on rectal temperature in mice. Pharmacol Biochem Behav. 1977;6(6):667–9.
564. Gale K, Iadarola MJ. Seizure protection and increased nerve-terminal GABA: delayed effects of GABA transaminase inhibition. Science (New York, NY). 1980;208(4441):288–91.
565. Gale K, Iadarola M. Drug-induced elevation of GABA after intracerebral microinjection: site of anticonvulsant action. Eur J Pharmacol. 1980;68(2):233–5.
566. Kalichman MW, Livingston KE, Burnham WM. Pharmacological investigation of gamma aminobutyric acid (GABA) and the development of amygdala-kindled seizures in the rat. Exp Neurol. 1981;74(3):829–36.

567. Gram L, Lyon BB, Dam M. Gamma-vinyl-GABA: a single-blind trial in patients with epilepsy. Acta Neurol Scand. 1983;68(1):34–9.
568. Tierradentro-García LO, Zandifar A, Stern J, et al. Magnetic resonance imaging-based distribution and reversibility of lesions in pediatric vigabatrin-related brain toxicity. Pediatr Neurol. 2023;148:86–93.
569. Kuchenbuch M, Lo Barco T, Chemaly N, et al. Fifteen years of real-world data on the use of vigabatrin in individuals with infantile epileptic spasms syndrome. Epilepsia. 2024;65(2):430–44.
570. Grinspan ZM, Knupp KG, Patel AD, et al. Comparative effectiveness of initial treatment for infantile spasms in a contemporary US cohort. Neurology. 2021;97(12):e1217–e28.
571. Gatson TN, Freemont OA, Coleman RL, et al. Vigabatrin (Sabril) for the treatment of refractory complex focal seizures in adults: pharmacologic and clinical considerations. Cureus. 2023;15(10):e46414.
572. Sharma S, Kaushik JS, Srivastava K, et al. Association of Child Neurology (AOCN) – Indian Epilepsy Society (IES) consensus guidelines for the diagnosis and management of West syndrome. Indian Pediatr. 2021;58(1):54–66.
573. Ramantani G, Bölsterli BK, Alber M, et al. Treatment of infantile spasm syndrome: update from the Interdisciplinary Guideline Committee coordinated by the German-Speaking Society of Neuropediatrics. Neuropediatrics. 2022;53(6):389–401.
574. Xu Z, Gong P, Jiao X, et al. Efficacy of vigabatrin in the treatment of infantile epileptic spasms syndrome: a systematic review and meta-analysis. Epilepsia Open. 2023;8(2):268–77.
575. Kotulska K, Kwiatkowski DJ, Curatolo P, et al. Prevention of epilepsy in infants with tuberous sclerosis complex in the EPISTOP trial. Ann Neurol. 2021;89(2):304–14.
576. Lin S, Liao J, Zhao X, et al. Focal epilepsy in children with tuberous sclerosis complex: does vigabatrin control focal seizures? J Child Neurol. 2022;37(5):329–33.
577. Sakpichaisakul K, Boonkrongsak R, Lertbutsayanukul P, et al. Epileptic spasms related to neuronal differentiation factor 2 (NEUROD2) mutation respond to combined vigabatrin and high dose prednisolone therapy. BMC Neurol. 2022;22(1):461.
578. Datta AN, Crawford J, Wong PKH. Infantile spasms and trisomy 21: unfavorable outcomes with first-line vigabatrin therapy. Can J Neurol Sci. 2021;48(6):839–44.
579. Wan L, Li Z, Sun Y, et al. Clinical characteristics and treatment outcomes of pediatric patients with postencephalitic epilepsy characterized by epileptic spasms. Seizure. 2021;84:116–21.
580. Saleh DA, Hassan A. Clinical profile, treatment modalities, and outcomes in patients with infantile spasms: a retrospective study from the United Arab of Emirates (UAE). Epilepsy Behav. 2022;127:108519.
581. Bashiri FA, Al-Sehemi MA, Hamad MH, et al. Neurodevelopmental and epilepsy outcomes of patients with infantile spasms treated in a tertiary care center. Neurosciences (Riyadh). 2021;26(1):21–5.
582. Kuchenbuch M, Chiron C, Milh M. Overview of therapeutic options for epilepsy. Arch Pediatr. 2022;29(5S):5S14–5S9.
583. Golec W, Sołowiej E, Strzelecka J, et al. Vigabatrin – new data on indications and safety in paediatric epilepsy. Neurol Neurochir Pol. 2021;55(5):429–39.
584. Desnous B, Lenoir M, Bitton JY, et al. What is the optimal duration for vigabatrin monotherapy in patients with infantile spasms: 6 months or longer? Seizure. 2021;91:503–6.
585. Leppien EE, Doughty BJ, Hurd KL, et al. Newer antiseizure medications and suicidality: analysis of the Food and Drug Administration Adverse Event Reporting System (FAERS) database. Clin Drug Investig. 2023;43(6):393–9.
586. Prezioso G, Chiarelli F, Matricardi S. Efficacy and safety of vigabatrin in patients with tuberous sclerosis complex and infantile epileptic spasm syndrome: a systematic review. Expert Rev Neurother. 2023;23(7):661–71.
587. Lai MC, Huang CW. The discordance between network excitability and cognitive performance following vigabatrin treatment during epileptogenesis. Life (Basel). 2021;11(11):1213.

588. Ikeda A, Tomiyasu M, Yamamoto A, et al. Elevation of brain gamma-aminobutyric acid levels is associated with vigabatrin-associated brain abnormalities on magnetic resonance imaging. Epilepsy Res. 2022;181:106881.
589. Reyes Valenzuela G, Crespo A, Princich J, et al. Vigabatrin-associated brain abnormalities on MRI and other neurological symptoms in patients with West syndrome. Epilepsy Behav. 2022;129:108606.
590. Harini C, Yuskaitis CJ, Libenson MH, et al. Hippocampal involvement with vigabatrin-related MRI signal abnormalities in patients with infantile spasms: a novel finding. J Child Neurol. 2021;36(7):575–82.
591. Xu Y, Wan L, He W, et al. Risk of vigabatrin-associated brain abnormalities on MRI: a retrospective and controlled study. Epilepsia. 2022;63(1):120–9.
592. Craft JF, Cardenas AM. Vigabatrin-associated reversible MRI abnormalities in an infant with tuberous sclerosis. J Radiol Case Rep. 2021;15(2):1–6.
593. Jonsson H, Lehto M, Vanhatalo S, et al. Visual field defects after vigabatrin treatment during infancy: retrospective population-based study. Dev Med Child Neurol. 2022;64(5):641–8.
594. Giuliano L, Vecchio C, Mastrangelo V, et al. Sex differences in side effects of antiseizure medications in pediatric patients with epilepsy: a systematic review. Seizure. 2022;102:6–13.
595. Abd El-Kader M, Hamza E, El-Gamal R, et al. Modulation of vigabatrin induced cerebellar injury: the role of caspase-3 and RIPK1/RIPK3-regulated cell death pathways. J Mol Histol. 2021;52(4):781–98.
596. Walters DC, Jansen EEW, Salomons GS, et al. Preferential accumulation of the active S-(+) isomer in murine retina highlights novel mechanisms of vigabatrin-associated retinal toxicity. Epilepsy Res. 2021;170:106536.
597. Hung TY, Huang HI, Wu SN, et al. Depressive effectiveness of vigabatrin (γ-vinyl-GABA), an antiepileptic drug, in intermediate-conductance calcium-activated potassium channels in human glioma cells. BMC Pharmacol Toxicol. 2021;22(1):6.
598. Jin P, You YX, Zhao LL, et al. A simple and easy non-derivatization gas chromatography-mass spectrometry method for simultaneous quantification of valproic acid, gabapentin, pregabalin, and vigabatrin in human plasma. J Sep Sci. 2023;46(2):e2200622.
599. Wang J, Zhang YY, Guo HL, et al. Rapid determination of plasma vigabatrin by LC-ESI-MS/MS supporting therapeutic drug monitoring in children with infantile spasms. Anal Methods. 2023;15(10):1365–77.
600. Ito T, Hori M, Masuda Y, et al. 3-Sulfamoylmethyl-1,2-benzisoxazole, a new type of anticonvulsant drug. Electroencephalographic profile. Arzneimittelforschung. 1980;30(4):603–9.
601. Sackellares JC, Donofrio PD, Wagner JG, et al. Pilot study of zonisamide (1,2-benzis oxazole-3-methanesulfonamide) in patients with refractory partial seizures. Epilepsia. 1985;26(3):206–11.
602. Hammond EJ, Perchalski RJ, Wilder BJ, et al. Neuropharmacology of zonisamide, a new antiepileptic drug. Gen Pharmacol. 1987;18(3):303–7.
603. Tousi B, Leverenz JB. The application of zonisamide to patients suffering from dementia with Lewy bodies: emerging clinical data. Drug Des Devel Ther. 2021;15:1811–7.
604. Kito M, Maehara M, Watanabe K. Mechanisms of T-type calcium channel blockade by zonisamide. Seizure. 1996;5(2):115–9.
605. Aslan M, Gungor S. Effectiveness of zonisamide in childhood refractory epilepsy. Childs Nerv Syst. 2022;38(5):971–6.
606. Brodie MJ. Zonisamide clinical trials: European experience. Seizure. 2004;13(Suppl 1):S66–70; discussion S1–2.
607. Tsujii S, Ishisaka M, Shimazawa M, et al. Zonisamide suppresses endoplasmic reticulum stress-induced neuronal cell damage in vitro and in vivo. Eur J Pharmacol. 2015;746:301–7.
608. Parravicini S, Pasca L, Zanaboni MP, et al. Electroclinical improvement in a patient with ring chromosome 20 syndrome treated with zonisamide: a case report. J Pediatr Genet. 2023;12(3):219–23.

609. Rubio-Nazábal E, Álvarez-Pérez P, Cores-Bartolomé C, et al. [Efficacy of zonisamide in Lafora's disease case and brief review of its use in progressive myoclonic epilepsy]. Rev Neurol. 2022;75(6):159–63.
610. McCluskey G, Kinney MO, Russell A, et al. Zonisamide safety in pregnancy: data from the UK and Ireland epilepsy and pregnancy register. Seizure. 2021;91:311–5.
611. Herzog R, Hellenbroich Y, Brüggemann N, et al. Zonisamide-responsive myoclonus in SEMA6B-associated progressive myoclonic epilepsy. Ann Clin Transl Neurol. 2021;8(7):1524–7.
612. Huang CR, Chuang HY, Chen NC, et al. Zonisamide therapy reduces metabolic consequences and diminishes nonalcoholic fatty liver disease in patients with epilepsy. J Clin Med. 2021;10(15):3380.
613. Naito T, Satake W, Cha PC, et al. Comparative whole transcriptome analysis of Parkinson's disease focusing on the efficacy of zonisamide. J Neurol Neurosurg Psychiatry. 2022;93(5):509–12.
614. Suzuki K, Fujita H, Matsubara T, et al. Zonisamide effects on sleep problems and depressive symptoms in Parkinson's disease. Brain Behav. 2021;11(3):e02026.
615. Hasegawa K, Kochi K, Maruyama H, et al. Efficacy and safety of zonisamide in dementia with Lewy bodies patients with parkinsonism: a post hoc analysis of two randomized, double-blind, placebo-controlled trials. J Alzheimers Dis. 2021;79(2):627–37.
616. Ikeda M, Mori E, Orimo S, et al. Efficacy of adjunctive therapy with zonisamide versus increased dose of levodopa for motor symptoms in patients with dementia with Lewy bodies: the randomized, controlled, non-inferiority DUEL study. J Alzheimers Dis. 2023;95(1):251–64.
617. Kong L, Xi J, Jiang Z, et al. Zonisamide's efficacy and safety on Parkinson's disease and dementia with Lewy bodies: a meta-analysis and systematic review. Biomed Res Int. 2022;2022:4817488.
618. Tada S, Choudhury ME, Kubo M, et al. Zonisamide ameliorates microglial mitochondriopathy in Parkinson's disease models. Brain Sci. 2022;12(2):268.
619. Rose JE, Willette PN, Botts TL, et al. Bupropion/zonisamide combination to assist smokers to switch from combustible cigarettes to electronic nicotine delivery systems (ENDS). Drug Alcohol Depend. 2022;234:109346.
620. Reinfeld S, Tejeda CI, Koola MM. Delirium in the context of zonisamide-induced toxic epidermal necrolysis. Prim Care Companion CNS Disord. 2022;24(1):21cr03108.
621. MacMahon T, Kelly YP. Zonisamide-induced distal renal tubular acidosis and critical hypokalaemia. BMJ Case Rep. 2023;16(4):e254615.
622. Panda PK, Sharawat IK, Panda P, et al. Efficacy, tolerability, and safety of zonisamide in children with epileptic spasms: a systematic review and meta-analysis. Seizure. 2021;91:374–83.
623. Inoue T, Ohkawara B, Bushra S, et al. Zonisamide upregulates neuregulin-1 expression and enhances acetylcholine receptor clustering at the in vitro neuromuscular junction. Neuropharmacology. 2021;195:108637.
624. Takaku S, Sango K. Pretreatment with zonisamide mitigates oxaliplatin-induced toxicity in rat DRG neurons and DRG neuron-Schwann cell co-cultures. Int J Mol Sci. 2022;23(17):9983.
625. Ismail FS, Faustmann PM, Förster E, et al. Tiagabine and zonisamide differentially regulate the glial properties in an astrocyte-microglia co-culture model of inflammation. Naunyn Schmiedeberg's Arch Pharmacol. 2023;396(11):3253–67.
626. Nakatsuka K, Zanghi B, Hasegawa D. Efficacy evaluation of a commercially available MCT enriched therapeutic diet on dogs with idiopathic epilepsy treated with zonisamide: a prospective, randomized, double-blinded, placebo-controlled, crossover dietary preliminary study. BMC Vet Res. 2023;19(1):145.
627. Shorvon S, Perucca E, Jerome E Jr. The treatment of epilepsy. 4th ed. Wiley-Blackwell; 2016.
628. Li J, Sun M, Wang X. The adverse-effect profile of lacosamide. Expert Opin Drug Saf. 2020;19(2):131–8.

629. Inoue Y, Liao W, Wang X, et al. Safety and efficacy of adjunctive lacosamide in Chinese and Japanese adults with epilepsy and focal seizures: a long-term, open-label extension of a randomized, controlled trial. Epilepsy Res. 2021;176:106705.
630. Baulac M, Rosenow F, Toledo M, et al. Efficacy, safety, and tolerability of lacosamide monotherapy versus controlled-release carbamazepine in patients with newly diagnosed epilepsy: a phase 3, randomised, double-blind, non-inferiority trial. Lancet Neurol. 2017;16(1):43–54.
631. Vossler DG, Knake S, O'Brien TJ, et al. Efficacy and safety of adjunctive lacosamide in the treatment of primary generalised tonic-clonic seizures: a double-blind, randomised, placebo-controlled trial. J Neurol Neurosurg Psychiatry. 2020;91(10):1067–75.
632. Lazzarotto L, Pflüger P, Regner GG, et al. Lacosamide improves biochemical, genotoxic, and mitochondrial parameters after PTZ-kindling model in mice. Fundam Clin Pharmacol. 2021;35(2):351–63.
633. Bilal B, Kirazlar M, Erdogan MA, et al. Lacosamide exhibits neuroprotective effects in a rat model of Parkinson's disease. J Chem Neuroanat. 2023;132:102311.
634. Langton RL, Sharma S, Tiarks GC, et al. Lacosamide decreases neonatal seizures without increasing apoptosis. Epilepsia. 2022;63(12):3051–65.
635. Agarwal S, Vyas P, Nirwan N, et al. Effect of lacosamide on neuroinflammation-mediated seizures comorbid with depression in C57BL/6 mice- role of kynurenine pathway. Epilepsy Behav. 2021;123:108262.
636. Corvace F, Faustmann TJ, Faustmann PM, et al. Anti-inflammatory properties of lacosamide in an astrocyte-microglia co-culture model of inflammation. Eur J Pharmacol. 2022;915:174696.
637. Szewczyk A, Zagaja M, Szala-Rycaj J, et al. Effect of lacosamide and ethosuximide chronic treatment on neural precursor cells and cognitive functions after pilocarpine induced status epilepticus in mice. Brain Sci. 2021;11(8):1014.
638. Sumbul O, Aygun H. Electrocorticographic and electrocardiographic evaluation of lacosamide in a penicillin-induced status epilepticus model. Epilepsy Res. 2022;180:106866.
639. Wu PM, Lin YC, Chiang CW, et al. Effective modulation by lacosamide on cumulative inhibition of I(Na) during high-frequency stimulation and recovery of I(Na) block during conditioning pulse train. Int J Mol Sci. 2022;23(19):11966.
640. Messahel S, Bracken L, Appleton R. Optimal management of status epilepticus in children in the emergency setting: a review of recent advances. Open Access Emerg Med. 2022;14:491–506.
641. Schaidle S, Greathouse K, McConnell D. Safety and efficacy of lacosamide versus phenytoin for refractory seizures in neurosurgical patients. BMJ Neurol Open. 2021;3(1):e000144.
642. Rollo E, Romozzi M, Dono F, et al. Treatment of benzodiazepine-refractory status epilepticus: a retrospective, cohort study. Epilepsy Behav. 2023;140:109093.
643. Chimakurthy AK, Ramsay RE, Sabharwal V, et al. Safety, tolerability, and pharmacokinetics of weight-based IV loading dose of lacosamide in the ICU. Epilepsy Behav. 2021;114(Pt A):107449.
644. Eilam A, Khmeliov N, Penker D, et al. Intravenous lacosamide in seizure clusters: dose and efficacy. Clin Neuropharmacol. 2021;44(3):85–8.
645. Torian SC, Jones GM. Safety profile of high-dose intravenous push lacosamide. Neurohospitalist. 2023;13(3):278–82.
646. Kim HK, Lee H, Bae EK, et al. Cardiac effects of rapid intravenous loading of lacosamide in patients with epilepsy. Epilepsy Res. 2021;176:106710.
647. Fong SL, Utidjian L, Kaur M, et al. Safety of intravenous lacosamide in hospitalized children and neonates. Epilepsia. 2023;64(9):2297–309.
648. Ragoonanan D, Tran N, Levesque M. Safety and tolerability of intravenous push lacosamide and levetiracetam. J Pharm Pract. 2023;36(5):1056–60.
649. Gonçalves J, Alves G, Fonseca C, et al. Is intranasal administration an opportunity for direct brain delivery of lacosamide? Eur J Pharm Sci. 2021;157:105632.

650. Mo F, Meletti S, Belcastro V, et al. Lacosamide in monotherapy in BTRE (brain tumor-related epilepsy): results from an Italian multicenter retrospective study. J Neurooncol. 2022;157(3):551–9.
651. Winter Y, Uphaus T, Sandner K, et al. Efficacy and safety of antiseizure medication in post-stroke epilepsy. Seizure. 2022;100:109–14.
652. Sharawat IK, Panda PK, Kumar V, et al. Comparative efficacy and safety of lacosamide and oxcarbazepine for seizure control in children with newly diagnosed solitary neurocysticercosis. J Trop Pediatr. 2022;68(3):fmac032.
653. Okanishi T, Fujii Y, Sakuma S, et al. Lacosamide monotherapy for the treatment of childhood epilepsy with centrotemporal spikes. Brain Dev. 2022;44(6):380–5.
654. Numoto S, Kurahashi H, Takagi M, et al. Sodium channel blockers are effective for benign infantile epilepsy. Seizure. 2021;92:207–10.
655. Kobayashi Y, Honda R, Yamada K, et al. Two-year efficacy of lacosamide as adjunctive therapy for generalized tonic-clonic seizures in patients with juvenile myoclonic epilepsy. Brain Dev. 2023;45(8):451–5.
656. Zawar I, Franic L, Knight EP. Response to lacosamide monotherapy in a patient with medically refractory Jeavons syndrome: a case report and review of the literature. Epileptic Disord. 2020;22(5):643–7.
657. Goldschagg N, Brem C, Strupp M. Case report: bitter vertigo. Front Neurol. 2022;13:1028597.
658. Masrour S. Lacosamide for refractory trigeminal neuralgia and other facial pain-case report. Headache. 2022;62(9):1227–30.
659. Muñoz-Vendrell A, Tena-Cucala R, Campoy S, et al. Oral lacosamide for the treatment of refractory trigeminal neuralgia: a retrospective analysis of 86 cases. Headache. 2023;63(4):559–64.
660. Geng JH, Zheng Y, Li QF, et al. Case report: a case of concomitant paroxysmal kinesigenic dyskinesia and epilepsy: can we treat two birds with one stone? Front Neurol. 2022;13:826897.
661. Fitouchi S, Jesel L, Hirsch E, et al. Epileptic seizure-induced syncopal asystole reversed by lacosamide: a case report. Europace. 2023;25(4):1510.
662. Ono-Takiguchi Y, Muramatsu K, Koshu K, et al. Forced normalization of Lennox-Gastaut syndrome using lacosamide: a case report. Brain Dev. 2021;43(9):963–6.
663. Kubo T, Sogawa R, Tsuruhashi S, et al. Risk of delirium with antiepileptic drug use: a study based on the Japanese Adverse Drug Event Report database. Int J Clin Pharm. 2023;45(5):1260–6.
664. Hamard J, Rigal M, Gony M, et al. Lacosamide-induced personality changes: an unexpected adverse effect. Fundam Clin Pharmacol. 2022;36(1):224–6.
665. Kawai M, Goji H, Kanemoto K. Aggression as psychiatric side effect of newer AEDs in patients with epilepsy: cross-sectional study based on Buss-Perry Aggression Questionnaire. Epilepsy Behav. 2021;115:107546.
666. Matsunuma S, Sunaga S, Hoshiai A, et al. Psychiatric disorders of the combination of levetiracetam either with lacosamide or perampanel: a retrospective cohort study. Int J Clin Pharm. 2021;43(6):1516–22.
667. Goodnough R, Badea A, Geier C, et al. Lacosamide induced Brugada I morphology in the setting of septicemia: a case report. Medicine (Baltimore). 2021;100(18):e25577.
668. Lu YT, Lin CH, Ho CJ, et al. Evaluation of cardiovascular concerns of intravenous lacosamide therapy in epilepsy patients. Front Neurol. 2022;13:891368.
669. Takai C, Misumi K, Kaito D, et al. Lacosamide intoxication-induced wide QRS tachycardia successfully treated with veno-arterial extracorporeal membrane oxygenation. Intern Med. 2023;62(8):1185–9.
670. Shibata M, Hoshino R, Shimizu C, et al. Lacosamide-induced sinus node dysfunction followed by severe agranulocytosis. BMC Neurol. 2021;21(1):217.
671. Zhao X, Liu Y, Xu Z. A paediatric case of lacosamide-induced panniculitis. Australas J Dermatol. 2022;63(1):e107–e9.

672. Tateishi Y, Ishikawa N, Kobayashi Y, et al. Effect of lacosamide therapy on blood cells and IgA levels in children and adolescents with epilepsy in a clinical setting. Epilepsy Res. 2022;187:107030.
673. Li Y, Guo HL, Zhang YY, et al. Plasma lacosamide monitoring in children with epilepsy: focus on reference therapeutic range and influencing factors. Front Pediatr. 2022;10:949783.
674. Zhao T, Li HJ, Zhang HL, et al. Therapeutic drug monitoring of lacosamide in Chinese pediatric patients with epilepsy: efficacy and factors influencing the plasma concentration. Eur J Drug Metab Pharmacokinet. 2023;48(1):41–9.
675. Pozzi M, Zanotta N, Epifanio R, et al. Lacosamide effectiveness and tolerability in patients with drug-resistant epilepsy and severe disability under polytherapy: therapy optimization as emerging from an observational study. Epilepsy Behav. 2022;128:108598.
676. Ishikawa N, Eguchi Y, Izumo H, et al. Clinical impact of the dose and blood concentration of lacosamide in Japanese pediatric patients with epilepsy: a cohort study. Epilepsy Behav. 2022;129:108614.
677. Lukka PB, Woods M, Chhim R, et al. Use of real-world data and pharmacometric modeling in support of lacosamide dosing in pediatric patients under 4 years of age. J Clin Pharmacol. 2021;61(7):881–8.
678. Pennell PB, Karanam A, Meador KJ, et al. Antiseizure medication concentrations during pregnancy: results from the maternal outcomes and neurodevelopmental effects of antiepileptic drugs (MONEAD) study. JAMA Neurol. 2022;79(4):370–9.
679. Zutshi D, Millis SR, Basha MM, et al. Lacosamide serum concentrations during pregnancy. Epilepsy Behav. 2021;123:108253.
680. Zhao T, Li HJ, Zhang HL, et al. Impact of ABCC2 1249G>A and −24C>T polymorphisms on lacosamide efficacy and plasma concentrations in uygur pediatric patients with epilepsy in China. Ther Drug Monit. 2023;45(1):117–25.
681. Ahn SJ, Oh J, Kim DY, et al. Effects of CYP2C19 genetic polymorphisms on the pharmacokinetics of lacosamide in Korean patients with epilepsy. Epilepsia. 2022;63(11):2958–69.
682. Farkas MK, Beller C, Bozorg A, et al. Safety and tolerability of short-term infusions of intravenous lacosamide in pediatric patients with epilepsy: an open-label, phase 2/3 trial. Epilepsia Open. 2023;8(1):146–53.
683. Hoeltzenbein M, Slimi S, Fietz AK, et al. Increasing use of newer antiseizure medication during pregnancy: an observational study with special focus on lacosamide. Seizure. 2023;107:107–13.
684. Husein N, Langlois-Thérien T, Rioux B, et al. Medical and surgical treatment of epilepsy in older adults: a national survey. Epilepsia. 2023;64(4):900–9.
685. Faught E, Li X, Choi J, et al. Real-world analysis of hospitalizations in patients with epilepsy and treated with perampanel. Epilepsia Open. 2021;6(4):645–52.
686. Villanueva V, D'Souza W, Goji H, et al. PERMIT study: a global pooled analysis study of the effectiveness and tolerability of perampanel in routine clinical practice. J Neurol. 2022;269(4):1957–77.
687. Segal E, Moretz K, Wheless J, et al. PROVE-Phase IV study of perampanel in real-world clinical care of patients with epilepsy: interim analysis in pediatric patients. J Child Neurol. 2022;37(4):256–67.
688. Inoue Y, Sumitomo K, Matsutani K, et al. Evaluation of real-world effectiveness of perampanel in Japanese adults and older adults with epilepsy. Epileptic Disord. 2022;24(1):123–32.
689. Segal E, Wheless J, Moretz K, et al. Perampanel in real-world clinical care of adolescent and adult patients with epilepsy: results from the retrospective Phase IV PROVE study. Seizure. 2022;98:87–94.
690. Estévez-María JC, Garamendi-Ruiz I. The real-world effectiveness and safety of perampanel in Europe: a scoping review. Epilepsy Behav. 2022;134:108777.
691. Gasparini S, Ferlazzo E, Neri S, et al. Effectiveness of perampanel as the only add-on: retrospective, multicenter, observational real life study on epilepsy patients. Epilepsia Open. 2022;7(4):687–96.

692. Wang Q, Xu Y, Chen Y, et al. Effectiveness and safety of perampanel as adjunctive therapy among Chinese patients with focal-onset epilepsy: a real-world prospective observational study. Epilepsy Behav. 2022;136:108937.
693. Yamamoto T, Gil-Nagel A, Wheless JW, et al. Perampanel monotherapy for the treatment of epilepsy: clinical trial and real-world evidence. Epilepsy Behav. 2022;136:108885.
694. Sagar P, Wawryk O, Vogrin S, et al. Efficacy and tolerability of adjuvant perampanel: an Australian multicenter real-world observational study in refractory focal and generalized epilepsy syndromes. Epilepsy Behav. 2021;119:107935.
695. Lossius IMB, Svendsen T, Sødal HF, et al. Effect and tolerability of perampanel in patients with drug-resistant epilepsy. Epilepsy Behav. 2021;119:107965.
696. Krauss GL, Ben-Menachem E, Wechsler RT, et al. A multivariable prediction model of a major treatment response for focal-onset seizures: a post-hoc analysis of Phase III trials of perampanel. Epilepsy Res. 2021;174:106649.
697. Wang T, Wen B, Chi Z, et al. The well responsiveness of drug-resistant focal seizures in anti-AMPA2 receptor encephalitis to perampanel treatment. Neurol Sci. 2022;43(1):525–32.
698. Obara K, Abe E, Toyoshima I. Frontal hypoperfusion and the effectiveness of perampanel in long-lived patient with Lafora disease. Case Rep Neurol. 2021;13(1):211–7.
699. Lim SN, Cheng MY, Hsieh HY, et al. Treatment of pharmacoresistant sleep-related hypermotor epilepsy (SHE) with the selective AMPA receptor antagonist perampanel. Sleep Med. 2021;81:382–6.
700. Saito K, Oi K, Inaba A, et al. [A case of the successful treatment of severe myoclonus with Lance-Adams syndrome by add-on perampanel showing long term effects]. Rinsho Shinkeigaku. 2021;61(1):18–23.
701. Kimura S, Shiraishi H, Egawa K, et al. Efficacy of perampanel for epileptic seizures and daily behavior in a patient with Leigh syndrome: a case report. Brain Dev. 2021;43(1):157–9.
702. Alonso-Singer P, Aguilar-Amat Prior MJ, Oliva-Navarro J, et al. Perampanel as adjuvant treatment in epileptic encephalopathies: a multicenter study in routine clinical practice. Epilepsy Behav. 2022;134:108836.
703. Matricardi S, Cesaroni E, Bonanni P, et al. Long-term effectiveness of add-on perampanel in patients with Lennox-Gastaut syndrome: a multicenter retrospective study. Epilepsia. 2023;64(6):e98–e104.
704. Lattanzi S, Cagnetti C, Foschi N, et al. Adjunctive perampanel in older patients with epilepsy: a multicenter study of clinical practice. Drugs Aging. 2021;38(7):603–10.
705. Macrohon B, Janette Resurreccion-De La Calzada J, Sanchez-Gan B. Clinical experience on the use of perampanel in epilepsy among child neurologists in the Philippines. Brain Dev. 2021;43(3):411–8.
706. Ahn SJ, Kim TJ, Cha KS, et al. Effects of perampanel on cognition and quantitative electroencephalography in patients with epilepsy. Epilepsy Behav. 2021;115:107514.
707. Inoue Y, Sumitomo K, Matsutani K, et al. Real-world evaluation of perampanel effectiveness in Japanese adolescents with epilepsy. Epileptic Disord. 2022;24(5):813–21.
708. Nissenkorn A, Kluger G, Schubert-Bast S, et al. Perampanel as precision therapy in rare genetic epilepsies. Epilepsia. 2023;64(4):866–74.
709. Lim SN, Wu T, Tseng WJ, et al. Efficacy and safety of perampanel in refractory and super-refractory status epilepticus: cohort study of 81 patients and literature review. J Neurol. 2021;268(10):3744–57.
710. Chu SJ, Li Y, Tang JH. Effectiveness and tolerability of adjunctive perampanel in pediatric patients (aged 4-12 years) with refractory epilepsy: an observational study. Medicine (Baltimore). 2022;101(45):e31408.
711. Canas N, Félix C, Silva V, et al. Comparative 12-month retention rate, effectiveness and tolerability of perampanel when used as a first add-on or a late add-on treatment in patients with focal epilepsies: the COM-PER study. Seizure. 2021;86:109–15.
712. Fernandes M, Dainese F, Operto F, et al. Perampanel effectiveness and tolerability in patients with epilepsy at long-term follow-up. Epilepsy Behav. 2021;121(Pt A):108069.

713. Labate A, Fortunato F, Giugno A, et al. Perampanel as first add-on choice on the treatment of mesial temporal lobe epilepsy: an observational real-life study. Neurol Sci. 2021;42(4):1389–94.
714. Maguire M, Ben-Menachem E, Patten A, et al. A post-approval observational study to evaluate the safety and tolerability of perampanel as an add-on therapy in adolescent, adult, and elderly patients with epilepsy. Epilepsy Behav. 2022;126:108483.
715. Resnick T, Patten A, Ngo LY, et al. Sustained seizure freedom with adjunctive perampanel in patients with convulsive seizures: post hoc analysis of open-label extension studies 307 and 332. Epilepsy Behav. 2022;128:108528.
716. French JA, Wechsler RT, Trinka E, et al. Long-term open-label perampanel: generalized tonic-clonic seizures in idiopathic generalized epilepsy. Epilepsia Open. 2022;7(3):393–405.
717. Trinka E, Lattanzi S, Carpenter K, et al. Exploring the evidence for broad-Spectrum effectiveness of perampanel: a systematic review of clinical data in generalised seizures. CNS Drugs. 2021;35(8):821–37.
718. Mahajan SS, Prakash A, Sarma P, et al. Efficacy, tolerability and safety of perampanel in population with pharmacoresistant focal seizures: a systematic review and meta-analysis. Epilepsy Res. 2022;182:106895.
719. Perez DQ, Espiritu AI, Jamora RDG. Perampanel in achieving status epilepticus cessation: a systematic review. Epilepsy Behav. 2022;128:108583.
720. Lanzone J, Ricci L, Tombini M, et al. The effect of perampanel on EEG spectral power and connectivity in patients with focal epilepsy. Clin Neurophysiol. 2021;132(9):2176–83.
721. Fong YO, Huang P, Hsu CY, et al. Effects of perampanel on seizure control, cognition, behavior, and psychological status in patients with epilepsy: a systematic review. J Clin Neurol. 2022;18(6):653–62.
722. Trigg A, Brohan E, Cocks K, et al. Health-related quality of life in pediatric patients with partial onset seizures or primary generalized tonic-clonic seizures receiving adjunctive perampanel. Epilepsy Behav. 2021;118:107938.
723. Kenaan K, Zafar M, Bond R, et al. Perampanel-induced cataplexy in a young male with generalized epilepsy. HCA Healthc J Med. 2020;1(5):283–8.
724. Minhaj FS, Leonard JB, Klein-Schwartz W. Clinical effects and outcomes of perampanel overdoses reported to U.S. poison centers. Clin Toxicol (Phila). 2022;60(2):239–42.
725. Mareš P, Kubová H. Perampanel exhibits anticonvulsant action against pentylentetrazol-induced seizures in immature rats. Epilepsy Res. 2021;169:106523.
726. Culjat M, Huizenga MN, Forcelli PA. Age-dependent anticonvulsant actions of perampanel and brivaracetam in the methyl-6,7-dimethoxy-4-ethyl-beta-carboline-3-carboxylate (DMCM) model of seizures in developing rats. Pharmacol Rep. 2021;73(1):296–302.
727. Vazquez B, Tomson T, Dobrinsky C, et al. Perampanel and pregnancy. Epilepsia. 2021;62(3):698–708.
728. Salmaggi A, Corno C, Maschio M, et al. Synergistic effect of perampanel and temozolomide in human glioma cell lines. J Pers Med. 2021;11(5):390.
729. Motomura K, Chalise L, Shimizu H, et al. Intraoperative seizure outcome of levetiracetam combined with perampanel therapy in patients with glioma undergoing awake brain surgery. J Neurosurg. 2021;135(4):998–1007.
730. Hotait M, Ismail HH, Saab GE, et al. An open label pilot study of the safety and tolerability of perampanel in amyotrophic lateral sclerosis. Muscle Nerve. 2021;64(4):504–8.
731. Turalde CWR, Moalong KMC, Espiritu AI, et al. Perampanel for amyotrophic lateral sclerosis: a systematic review and meta-analysis. Neurol Sci. 2022;43(2):889–97.
732. Chen T, Liu WB, Qian X, et al. The AMPAR antagonist perampanel protects the neurovascular unit against traumatic injury via regulating Sirt3. CNS Neurosci Ther. 2021;27(1):134–44.
733. Kawakita F, Nakano F, Kanamaru H, et al. Anti-apoptotic effects of AMPA receptor antagonist perampanel in early brain injury after subarachnoid hemorrhage in mice. Transl Stroke Res. 2024;15:462–75.

734. Kenda BM, Matagne AC, Talaga PE, et al. Discovery of 4-substituted pyrrolidone butanamides as new agents with significant antiepileptic activity. J Med Chem. 2004;47(3):530–49.
735. Grande-Martín A, Sopelana-Garay D, Pardal-Fernández JM, et al. Exceptional response to brivaracetam in a patient with refractory idiopathic generalized epilepsy and absence seizures. Epileptic Disord. 2018;20(1):60–4.
736. Gayke M, Narode H, Eppa G, et al. Synthetic approaches toward the synthesis of brivaracetam: an antiepileptic drug. ACS Omega. 2022;7(3):2486–503.
737. Okada M, Fukuyama K, Shiroyama T, et al. Brivaracetam prevents astroglial l-glutamate release associated with hemichannel through modulation of synaptic vesicle protein. Biomed Pharmacother. 2021;138:111462.
738. Stefanatou M, Vasileiadou Kapetanou E, Kimiskidis VK, et al. A multicenter retrospective study evaluating brivaracetam in the treatment of epilepsies in clinical practice. Pharmaceuticals (Basel). 2021;14(2):165.
739. Stephen L, Brodie MJ. Adjunctive brivaracetam – a prospective audit of outcomes from an epilepsy clinic. Epilepsy Behav. 2021;116:107746.
740. Orlandi N, d'Orsi G, Pauletto G, et al. A retrospective multicentric study on the effectiveness of intravenous brivaracetam in seizure clusters: data from the Italian experience. Seizure. 2023;108:72–80.
741. Strzelczyk A, Zaveta C, von Podewils F, et al. Long-term efficacy, tolerability, and retention of brivaracetam in epilepsy treatment: a longitudinal multicenter study with up to 5 years of follow-up. Epilepsia. 2021;62(12):2994–3004.
742. Toledo M, Brandt C, Quarato PP, et al. Long-term safety, efficacy, and quality of life during adjunctive brivaracetam treatment in patients with uncontrolled epilepsy: an open-label follow-up trial. Epilepsy Behav. 2021;118:107897.
743. Lattanzi S, Trinka E, Zaccara G, et al. Third-generation antiseizure medications for adjunctive treatment of focal-onset seizures in adults: a systematic review and network meta-analysis. Drugs. 2022;82(2):199–218.
744. Ferragut Ferretjans F, Soto Insuga V, Bernardino Cuesta B, et al. Efficacy of brivaracetam in children with epilepsy. Epilepsy Res. 2021;177:106757.
745. Verrotti A, Grasso EA, Cacciatore M, et al. Potential role of brivaracetam in pediatric epilepsy. Acta Neurol Scand. 2021;143(1):19–26.
746. Song T, Feng L, Xia Y, et al. Safety and efficacy of brivaracetam in children epilepsy: a systematic review and meta-analysis. Front Neurol. 2023;14:1170780.
747. Savastano E, Pulitano P, Faedda MT, et al. Clinical and electroencephalography assessment of the effects of brivaracetam in the treatment of drug-resistant focal epilepsy. Cureus. 2021;13(5):e15012.
748. Svendsen T, Brodtkorb E, Linge HL, et al. Efficacy, tolerability and pharmacokinetic variability of brivaracetam in adults with difficult-to-treat epilepsy. Epilepsy Res. 2022;183:106946.
749. Snoeren A, Majoie M, Fasen K, et al. Brivaracetam for the treatment of refractory epilepsy in patients with prior exposure to levetiracetam: a retrospective outcome analysis. Seizure. 2022;96:102–7.
750. Gillis RME, Wammes-van der Heijden EA, Schelhaas HJ, et al. Efficacy and tolerability of brivaracetam in patients with intellectual disability and epilepsy. Acta Neurol Belg. 2021;121(3):677–84.
751. Bond KR, Rea E, Lawthom C. Seizures in palliative medicine: brivaracetam. BMJ Support Palliat Care. 2023;13(e2):e308–e10.
752. Lattanzi S, Canafoglia L, Canevini MP, et al. Brivaracetam as add-on treatment in patients with post-stroke epilepsy: real-world data from the BRIVAracetam add-on First Italian netwoRk Study (BRIVAFIRST). Seizure. 2022;97:37–42.
753. Khilari M, Nair PP, Jha BK. Brivaracetam: how well does it fare as an anti-epileptic? A review. Neurol India. 2021;69(2):284–93.
754. Tulli E, Di Cara G, Iapadre G, et al. An update on brivaracetam for the treatment of pediatric partial epilepsy. Expert Opin Pharmacother. 2021;22(11):1387–95.

755. Bresnahan R, Panebianco M, Marson AG. Brivaracetam add-on therapy for drug-resistant epilepsy. Cochrane Database Syst Rev. 2022;3(3):CD011501.
756. Lattanzi S, De Maria G, Rosati E, et al. Brivaracetam as add-on treatment in focal epilepsy: a real-world time-based analysis. Epilepsia. 2021;62(1):e1–6.
757. Lattanzi S, Canafoglia L, Canevini MP, et al. Adjunctive brivaracetam in older patients with focal seizures: evidence from the BRIVAracetam add-on First Italian netwoRk Study (BRIVAFIRST). Drugs Aging. 2022;39(4):297–304.
758. Martellino C, Laganà A, Atanasio G, et al. The real-world effectiveness of intravenous brivaracetam as a second-line treatment in status epilepticus. Epilepsy Behav. 2023;148:109464.
759. Orlandi N, Bartolini E, Audenino D, et al. Intravenous brivaracetam in status epilepticus: a multicentric retrospective study in Italy. Seizure. 2021;86:70–6.
760. De Liso A, Ricci L, Bravi MC, et al. An uncommon case of nonconvulsive status epilepticus successfully treated with enteral brivaracetam. Acta Biomed. 2021;92(S1):e2021156.
761. Yamamoto J, Ikeda K, Stockis A. Bioavailability, safety and tolerability of intravenous brivaracetam in healthy Japanese participants. Xenobiotica. 2022;52(2):146–51.
762. Chavarría B, Zucca R, Principe A, et al. Rapid intravenous loading of brivaracetam during invasive and non-invasive video-EEG monitoring. Epilepsy Res. 2023;192:107145.
763. Farkas MK, Kang H, Fogarasi A, et al. Pharmacokinetics, safety, and tolerability of intravenous brivaracetam in pediatric patients with epilepsy: an open-label trial. Epilepsia. 2022;63(4):855–64.
764. Lee K, Klein P, Dongre P, et al. Intravenous brivaracetam in the management of acute seizures in the hospital setting: a scoping review. J Intensive Care Med. 2022;37(9):1133–45.
765. Ben-Menachem E, Baulac M, Hong SB, et al. Safety, tolerability, and efficacy of brivaracetam as adjunctive therapy in patients with focal seizures, generalized onset seizures, or Unverricht-Lundborg disease: an open-label, long-term follow-up trial. Epilepsy Res. 2021;170:106526.
766. Li KY, Hsu CY, Yang YH. A review of cognitive and behavioral outcomes of brivaracetam. Kaohsiung J Med Sci. 2023;39(2):104–14.
767. Barrachina-Martinez I, Vivas-Consuelo D, Reyes-Santias F. Cost-utility model of brivaracetam in the adjunctive treatment of patients with epilepsy in Spain. Expert Rev Pharmacoecon Outcomes Res. 2021;21(5):1081–90.
768. Mehta D, Lee I, Liu H, et al. Comparative economic outcomes in patients with focal seizures initiating eslicarbazepine acetate versus brivaracetam in the long-term care setting in the USA. J Comp Eff Res. 2022;11(17):1293–308.
769. Brunner LA, Powell ML. An automated method for the determination of a new potential antiepileptic agent (CGP 33101) in human plasma using high performance liquid chromatography. Biomed Chromatogr. 1992;6(6):278–82.
770. Perucca E, Bialer M. The clinical pharmacokinetics of the newer antiepileptic drugs. Focus on topiramate, zonisamide and tiagabine. Clin Pharmacokinet. 1996;31(1):29–46.
771. Cardot JM, Lecaillon JB, Czendlik C, et al. The influence of food on the disposition of the antiepileptic rufinamide in healthy volunteers. Biopharm Drug Dispos. 1998;19(4):259–62.
772. Jain KK. An assessment of rufinamide as an anti-epileptic in comparison with other drugs in clinical development. Expert Opin Investig Drugs. 2000;9(4):829–40.
773. Aldenkamp AP, Alpherts WC. The effect of the new antiepileptic drug rufinamide on cognitive functions. Epilepsia. 2006;47(7):1153–9.
774. Brodie MJ, Rosenfeld WE, Vazquez B, et al. Rufinamide for the adjunctive treatment of partial seizures in adults and adolescents: a randomized placebo-controlled trial. Epilepsia. 2009;50(8):1899–909.
775. Hassib ST, Hashem HMA, Mahrouse MA, et al. Development and bio-analytical validation of chromatographic determination method of rufinamide in presence of its metabolite in human plasma. J Chromatogr Sci. 2021;59(5):458–64.
776. Chen JL, Kuo CC. Inhibition of resurgent Na(+) currents by rufinamide. Neuropharmacology. 2024;247:109835.

777. Yamamoto Y, Inoue Y, Usui N, et al. Therapeutic drug monitoring for rufinamide in Japanese patients with epilepsy: focus on drug interactions, tolerability, and clinical effectiveness. Ther Drug Monit. 2022;44(4):585–91.
778. Humayun MJ, Wadhwa R. Rufinamide. In: StatPearls. Treasure Island: StatPearls Publishing LLC; 2024. Disclosure: Roopma Wadhwa declares no relevant financial relationships with ineligible companies.
779. Arzimanoglou A, Pringsheim M, Kluger GJ, et al. Safety and efficacy of rufinamide in children and adults with Lennox-Gastaut syndrome: a post hoc analysis from study 022. Epilepsy Behav. 2021;124:108275.
780. Sankar R, Chez M, Pina-Garza JE, et al. Proposed anti-seizure medication combinations with rufinamide in the treatment of Lennox-Gastaut syndrome: narrative review and expert opinion. Seizure. 2023;110:42–57.
781. Panebianco M, Prabhakar H, Marson AG. Rufinamide add-on therapy for drug-resistant epilepsy. Cochrane Database Syst Rev. 2020;11(11):CD011772.
782. Sharawat IK, Panda PK, Panda P, et al. Efficacy and safety of rufinamide as adjunctive therapy in patients with Lennox Gastaut syndrome: a systematic review and meta-analysis. Seizure. 2021;91:296–307.
783. Peacock D, Yoneda JRK, Siever JE, et al. Movement disorders secondary to novel antiseizure medications in pediatric populations: a systematic review and meta-analysis of risk. J Child Neurol. 2022;37(6):524–33.
784. Lin YC, Lai YC, Lin TH, et al. Selective stabilization of the intermediate inactivated Na(+) channel by the new-generation anticonvulsant rufinamide. Biochem Pharmacol. 2022;197:114928.
785. Lai MC, Wu SN, Huang CW. Rufinamide, a triazole-derived antiepileptic drug, stimulates ca(2+)-activated K(+) currents while inhibiting voltage-gated Na(+) currents. Int J Mol Sci. 2022;23(22):13677.
786. Yu H, He B, Han X, et al. Rufinamide (RUF) suppresses inflammation and maintains the integrity of the blood-brain barrier during kainic acid-induced brain damage. Open Life Sci. 2021;16(1):845–55.
787. Meirinho S, Rodrigues M, Fortuna A, et al. Study of the metabolic stability profiles of perampanel, rufinamide and stiripentol and prediction of drug interactions using HepaRG cells as an in vitro human model. Toxicol In Vitro. 2022;82:105389.
788. Pertwee RG, Greentree SG, Swift PA. Drugs which stimulate or facilitate central GABAergic transmission interact synergistically with delta-9-tetrahydrocannabinol to produce marked catalepsy in mice. Neuropharmacology. 1988;27(12):1265–70.
789. Nielsen EB, Suzdak PD, Andersen KE, et al. Characterization of tiagabine (NO-328), a new potent and selective GABA uptake inhibitor. Eur J Pharmacol. 1991;196(3):257–66.
790. Coleman MH, Yamaguchi S, Rogawski MA. Protection against dendrotoxin-induced clonic seizures in mice by anticonvulsant drugs. Brain Res. 1992;575(1):138–42.
791. Sveinbjornsdottir S, Sander JW, Patsalos PN, et al. Neuropsychological effects of tiagabine, a potential new antiepileptic drug. Seizure. 1994;3(1):29–35.
792. Walton NY, Gunawan S, Treiman DM. Treatment of experimental status epilepticus with the GABA uptake inhibitor, tiagabine. Epilepsy Res. 1994;19(3):237–44.
793. Schachter SC. Tiagabine monotherapy in the treatment of partial epilepsy. Epilepsia. 1995;36(Suppl 6):S2–6.
794. Tidwell A, Swims M. Review of the newer antiepileptic drugs. Am J Manag Care. 2003;9(3):253–76; quiz 77–9.
795. Kowalska M, Fijałkowski Ł, Kubacka M, et al. Antiepileptic drug tiagabine does not directly target key cardiac ion channels Kv11.1, Nav1.5 and Cav1.2. Molecules. 2021;26(12):3522.
796. Miziak B, Błaszczyk B, Chrościńska-Krawczyk M, et al. Caffeine and its interactions with antiseizure medications-is there a correlation between preclinical and clinical data? Int J Mol Sci. 2023;24(24):17569.

797. Viteva E, Zahariev Z. Various aspects of tiagabine effectiveness as add-on therapy in patients with refractory epilepsy. Folia Med (Plovdiv). 2020;62(1):59–64.
798. Bresnahan R, Martin-McGill KJ, Hutton JL, et al. Tiagabine add-on therapy for drug-resistant focal epilepsy. Cochrane Database Syst Rev. 2019;10(10):CD001908.
799. Dunn R, Queenan BN, Pak DTS, et al. Divergent effects of levetiracetam and tiagabine against spontaneous seizures in adult rats following neonatal hypoxia. Epilepsy Res. 2018;140:1–7.
800. Demchenko IT, Zhilyaev SY, Alekseeva OS, et al. Increased antiseizure effectiveness with tiagabine combined with sodium channel antagonists in mice exposed to hyperbaric oxygen. Neurotox Res. 2019;36(4):788–95.
801. Cutillo G, Tolba H, Hirsch LJ. Anti-seizure medications and efficacy against focal to bilateral tonic-clonic seizures: a systematic review with relevance for SUDEP prevention. Epilepsy Behav. 2021;117:107815.
802. Yeh WC, Lu SR, Wu MN, et al. The impact of antiseizure medications on polysomnographic parameters: a systematic review and meta-analysis. Sleep Med. 2021;81:319–26.
803. Hariri G, Ferre A, Legriel S. Tiagabine-related status epilepticus: a case report and systematic literature review. Acta Neurol Belg. 2020;120(6):1283–8.
804. Liu J, Huang D, Xu J, et al. Tiagabine protects dopaminergic neurons against neurotoxins by inhibiting microglial activation. Sci Rep. 2015;5:15720.
805. Wang TC, Ngampramuan S, Kotchabhakdi N. Tiagabine treatment in kainic acid induced cerebellar lesion of dystonia rat model. EXCLI J. 2016;15:716–29.
806. Javaid S, Alqahtani F, Ashraf W, et al. Tiagabine suppresses pentylenetetrazole-induced seizures in mice and improves behavioral and cognitive parameters by modulating BDNF/TrkB expression and neuroinflammatory markers. Biomed Pharmacother. 2023;160:114406.
807. Malikowska-Racia N, Salat K, Gdula-Argasinska J, et al. Sex, pramipexole and tiagabine affect behavioral and hormonal response to traumatic stress in a mouse model of PTSD. Front Pharmacol. 2021;12:691598.
808. Zou Z, Liao X, Yang L, et al. Human serum albumin-occupying-based fluorescence turn-on analysis of antiepileptic drug tiagabine hydrochloride. Anal Chem. 2020;92(5):3555–62.
809. Zhuo W, Peng X, Lin X. Insights into the interaction mechanism between tiagabine hydrochloride and two serum albumins. RSC Adv. 2018;8(44):24953–60.
810. Iannone LF, Arena G, Battaglia D, et al. Results from an Italian expanded access program on cannabidiol treatment in highly refractory Dravet syndrome and Lennox-Gastaut syndrome. Front Neurol. 2021;12:673135.
811. Madan Cohen J, Checketts D, Dunayevich E, et al. Time to onset of cannabidiol treatment effects in Dravet syndrome: analysis from two randomized controlled trials. Epilepsia. 2021;62(9):2218–27.
812. Thiele EA, Bebin EM, Bhathal H, et al. Add-on cannabidiol treatment for drug-resistant seizures in tuberous sclerosis complex: a placebo-controlled randomized clinical trial. JAMA Neurol. 2021;78(3):285–92.
813. Thiele EA, Bebin EM, Filloux F, et al. Long-term cannabidiol treatment for seizures in patients with tuberous sclerosis complex: an open-label extension trial. Epilepsia. 2022;63(2):426–39.
814. Wu JY, Cock HR, Devinsky O, et al. Time to onset of cannabidiol treatment effect and resolution of adverse events in tuberous sclerosis complex: post hoc analysis of randomized controlled phase 3 trial GWPCARE6. Epilepsia. 2022;63(5):1189–99.
815. Lattanzi S, Trinka E, Striano P, et al. Highly purified cannabidiol for epilepsy treatment: a systematic review of epileptic conditions beyond Dravet syndrome and Lennox-Gastaut syndrome. CNS Drugs. 2021;35(3):265–81.
816. Gaston TE, Ampah SB, Martina Bebin E, et al. Long-term safety and efficacy of highly purified cannabidiol for treatment refractory epilepsy. Epilepsy Behav. 2021;117:107862.
817. Patel S, Grinspoon R, Fleming B, et al. The long-term efficacy of cannabidiol in the treatment of refractory epilepsy. Epilepsia. 2021;62(7):1594–603.
818. Devinsky O, Marmanillo A, Hamlin T, et al. Observational study of medical marijuana as a treatment for treatment-resistant epilepsies. Ann Clin Transl Neurol. 2022;9(4):497–505.

819. Kochen S, Villanueva M, Bayarres L, et al. Cannabidiol as an adjuvant treatment in adults with drug-resistant focal epilepsy. Epilepsy Behav. 2023;144:109210.
820. Espinosa-Jovel C, Riveros S, Bolaños-Almeida C, et al. Real-world evidence on the use of cannabidiol for the treatment of drug resistant epilepsy not related to Lennox-Gastaut syndrome, Dravet syndrome or tuberous sclerosis complex. Seizure. 2023;112:72–6.
821. Grayson L, Ampah S, Hernando K, et al. Longitudinal impact of cannabidiol on EEG measures in subjects with treatment-resistant epilepsy. Epilepsy Behav. 2021;122:108190.
822. Herlopian A, Barnett JR, Nascimento FA, et al. Electroencephalographic changes in purified pharmaceutical cannabidiol therapy. Epilepsy Behav. 2022;128:108558.
823. Metternich B, Wagner K, Geiger MJ, et al. Cognitive and behavioral effects of cannabidiol in patients with treatment-resistant epilepsy. Epilepsy Behav. 2021;114(Pt A):107558.
824. Zilmer M, Olofsson K. Cannabidiol treatment of severe refractory epilepsy in children and young adults. Dan Med J. 2021;68(5):A07200527.
825. Caraballo R, Valenzuela GR. Cannabidiol-enriched medical cannabis as add-on therapy in children with treatment-resistant West syndrome: a study of eight patients. Seizure. 2021;92:238–43.
826. Caraballo R, Reyes G, Demirdjian G, et al. Long-term use of cannabidiol-enriched medical cannabis in a prospective cohort of children with drug-resistant developmental and epileptic encephalopathy. Seizure. 2022;95:56–63.
827. Silvennoinen K, Ritter LM, Nashef L, et al. Two-center experience of cannabidiol use in adults with Dravet syndrome. Seizure. 2021;91:5–8.
828. Watkins PB, Church RJ, Li J, et al. Cannabidiol and abnormal liver chemistries in healthy adults: results of a phase I clinical trial. Clin Pharmacol Ther. 2021;109(5):1224–31.
829. Vaughn DM, Paulionis LJ, Kulpa JE. Randomized, placebo-controlled, 28-day safety and pharmacokinetics evaluation of repeated oral cannabidiol administration in healthy dogs. Am J Vet Res. 2021;82(5):405–16.
830. Cabral-Pereira G, Sánchez-Benito D, Díaz-Rodríguez SM, et al. Behavioral and molecular effects induced by cannabidiol and valproate administration in the GASH/Sal model of acute audiogenic seizures. Front Behav Neurosci. 2020;14:612624.
831. Zawar I, Franic L, Kotagal P, et al. Exacerbation of eyelid myoclonia in patients with epilepsy and eyelid myoclonia receiving cannabidiol. Epileptic Disord. 2021;23(6):906–10.
832. Frías-Soria CL, Pérez-Pérez D, Orozco-Suárez S, et al. Cannabidiol modifies the seizure expression and effects of antiseizure drugs in a rat model of recurrent severe seizures. Seizure. 2021;90:67–73.
833. Fallah MS, Dlugosz L, Scott BW, et al. Antiseizure effects of the cannabinoids in the amygdala-kindling model. Epilepsia. 2021;62(9):2274–82.
834. Pastrana-Trejo JC, Duarte-Aké F, Us-Camas R, et al. Effects on the post-translational modification of H3K4Me3, H3K9ac, H3K9Me2, H3K27Me3, and H3K36Me2 levels in cerebral cortex, hypothalamus and pons of rats after a systemic administration of cannabidiol: a preliminary study. Cent Nerv Syst Agents Med Chem. 2021;21(2):142–7.
835. Lazarini-Lopes W, Do Val-da Silva RA, da Silva-Júnior RMP, et al. Chronic cannabidiol (CBD) administration induces anticonvulsant and antiepileptogenic effects in a genetic model of epilepsy. Epilepsy Behav. 2021;119:107962.
836. Gómez CT, Lairion F, Repetto M, et al. Cannabidiol (CBD) alters the functionality of neutrophils (PMN). Implications in the refractory epilepsy treatment. Pharmaceuticals (Basel). 2021;14(3):220.
837. Zhang H-XB, Heckman L, Niday Z, et al. Cannabidiol activates neuronal Kv7 channels. elife. 2022;11:e73246.
838. Simon K, Sheckley H, Anderson CL, et al. A review of fenfluramine for the treatment of Dravet syndrome patients. Curr Res Pharmacol Drug Discov. 2022;3:100078.
839. Dini G, Tulli E, Dell'Isola GB, et al. Improving therapy of pharmacoresistant epilepsies: the role of fenfluramine. Front Pharmacol. 2022;13:832929.

840. Zhang L, Li W, Wang C. Efficacy and safety of fenfluramine in patients with Dravet syndrome: a meta-analysis. Acta Neurol Scand. 2021;143(4):339–48.
841. Abenhaim L, Moride Y, Brenot F, et al. Appetite-suppressant drugs and the risk of primary pulmonary hypertension. International Primary Pulmonary Hypertension Study Group. N Engl J Med. 1996;335(9):609–16.
842. Connolly HM, Crary JL, McGoon MD, et al. Valvular heart disease associated with fenfluramine-phentermine. N Engl J Med. 1997;337(9):581–8.
843. Odi R, Invernizzi RW, Gallily T, et al. Fenfluramine repurposing from weight loss to epilepsy: what we do and do not know. Pharmacol Ther. 2021;226:107866.
844. Sullivan J, Perry MS, Wheless JW, et al. Fenfluramine responder analyses and numbers needed to treat: translating epilepsy trial data into clinical practice. Eur J Paediatr Neurol. 2021;31:10–4.
845. Bishop KI, Isquith PK, Gioia GA, et al. Improved everyday executive functioning following profound reduction in seizure frequency with fenfluramine: analysis from a phase 3 long-term extension study in children/young adults with Dravet syndrome. Epilepsy Behav. 2021;121(Pt A):108024.
846. Strzelczyk A, Pringsheim M, Mayer T, et al. Efficacy, tolerability, and retention of fenfluramine for the treatment of seizures in patients with Dravet syndrome: compassionate use program in Germany. Epilepsia. 2021;62(10):2518–27.
847. Sullivan J, Specchio N, Devinsky O, et al. Fenfluramine significantly reduces day-to-day seizure burden by increasing number of seizure-free days and time between seizures in patients with Dravet syndrome: a time-to-event analysis. Epilepsia. 2022;63(1):130–8.
848. Devinsky O, King L, Schwartz D, et al. Effect of fenfluramine on convulsive seizures in CDKL5 deficiency disorder. Epilepsia. 2021;62(7):e98–e102.
849. Martin P, Maurice T, Gammaitoni A, et al. Fenfluramine modulates the anti-amnesic effects induced by sigma-1 receptor agonists and neuro(active)steroids in vivo. Epilepsy Behav. 2022;127:108526.

Chapter 3
The Basic Principles and Precautions of Drug Therapy

Qun Wang, Xuefeng Wang, Li Jiang, and Hong Zhang

3.1 The Basic Principles of Antiepileptic Drug Selection

Epilepsy is a chronic brain disease. Epidemiological surveys have shown that the prevalence of epilepsy is 7%, and there are approximately 50 million patients worldwide. Although there are a variety of treatment modalities available, medications are still the main method for controlling epileptic seizures. To achieve the desired results, it is important to follow some rules that researchers have summarized in practice.

3.1.1 When to Start Medication

Deciding when to start medication is one of the first questions that medical professionals need to answer. Considering that epilepsy is not only a chronic brain disease but also a potentially fatal disease, as epidemiological surveys have shown that the

Q. Wang
Department of Neurology, Beijing Tiantan Hospital, Capital Medical University, Beijing, China

X. Wang
Department of Neurology, The First Affiliated Hospital of Chongqing Medical University, Chongqing, China

L. Jiang (✉)
Department of Neurology, Children's Hospital of Chongqing Medical University, National Clinical Research Center for Child Health and Disorders, Chongqing, China
e-mail: ljiang@hospital.cqmu.edu.cn

H. Zhang
Department of Neurology, Shengjing Hospital of China Medical University, Shenyang, China

X. Wang, L. Zhou (eds.), *Pharmacological Treatment of Epileptic Seizures*,
https://doi.org/10.1007/978-981-96-8520-2_3

mortality rate of patients with epilepsy is 2–3 times that of the general population [1], experts argue that once the diagnosis of epilepsy is established, treatment needs to be started. International organizations have three different views on the diagnosis of epilepsy. In 1981, the International League against Epilepsy and the World Health Organization suggested that the presence of epilepsy should not be determined until a second seizure. However, in 2005, the International League against Epilepsy proposed that the first noninduced seizure is diagnosable as epilepsy; for the diagnosis of epilepsy in this case, several important conditions have been established, such as the need to determine whether the epilepsy patient's brain has a susceptibility to recurrent seizures. The determination of this susceptibility includes a family history of epilepsy, a clear epileptoid discharge on the electroencephalogram (EEG), and the existence of factors that have been proven to cause recurrent seizures, such as delayed epilepsy after a head injury, epilepsy left over from encephalitis, and late-onset epilepsy caused by cerebrovascular disease [2]. The 2014 criteria required that the probability of recurrence within 10 years be greater than 60% [3]. However, a large number of studies have suggested that starting treatment after the first or second episode has no effect on the outcome of the patient's treatment [4]. Based on these studies, we argue that (1) when there are ILAE seizure susceptibility preconditions, treatment can be started after the first seizure, and (2) if the collected data are not sufficient to support the above preconditions, waiting for the patient to have a second seizure may be more beneficial to the patient. Existing antiepileptic drugs are mostly for the control of seizures and have no antiepileptic effects; therefore, for patients who only have one attack for more than six months to several years, the pros and cons of starting treatment or no treatment should be explained clearly to the patients and their relatives, and the patients or their families should decide whether to use drugs. If patients or their families seek the advice of doctors, experts believe that drug treatment is safer [4, 5].

3.1.2 How to Choose Anti-Seizure Medication

When deciding on treatment, choosing the right medication is a matter to consider. At present, there are dozens of antiseizure drugs on the market, so there are conditions and a basis for drug selection. Before the advent of evidence-based medicine, traditional drug therapy advocated drug selection according to the epilepsy seizure type, but this view has been questioned by evidence-based medical research. A large number of evidence-based medical research results did not validate this method of drug selection, so although this method of drug selection is still widely used in clinical practice, drug selection based on the seizure type is declining in popularity. It is no longer the only condition for the selection of antiepileptic drugs [6–9]. The experts believe that (1) in addition to special types of seizures, such as absence seizures, there is little difference in the efficacy of different antiepileptic drugs. (2) The selection of antiepileptic drugs needs to take into consideration the "three elements" of drug therapy, that is, disease factors, drug factors, patients and social factors. In clinical practice, in addition to the type of seizure, it is also necessary to comprehensively consider the gender, age, aesthetic, and reproductive requirements of patients, pharmacological and pharmacokinetic characteristics of drugs, and some social factors, such as drug price and the stability of drug sources. The type of seizure is not the only basis for selection. (3) The main basis for drug selection is efficacy and safety. Overall, the safety of new antiseizure drugs is better [5–8]. (4) Some antiepileptic drugs may aggravate the onset of another type of seizure during the treatment of one type of seizure and should be avoided [10]. There may be different responses to antiseizure drugs in patients of different ages [11].

Although the type of seizure is not the only basis for drug selection, it is still an important basis, and the specific selection can be found in (see Chap. 4).

3.1.3 Drug Selection for Pregnant Patients

Chittaranjan Andrade et al. [12] found from routine and online meta-analyses that the risk of major malformation after exposure to VPA in early pregnancy was the highest, the risk ratio was dose-dependent and approximately 10%. Phenobarbital, phenytoin sodium, carbamazepine, and topiramate convey a higher risk of birth defects than other ASMs. The absolute risk of major malformations at conventional doses of lamotrigine, levetiracetam, and oxcarbazepine, and even zonisamide and gabapentin is no more than 2% to 3% in the general population. Torbjorn et al. [13] also reported that different dosages of different antiepileptic drugs have different teratogenic risks. The risk of congenital malformations associated with lamotrigine, levetiracetam, and oxcarbamazepine is similar to that of the offspring of nontreated patients. Therefore, experts suggest that the medication used for pregnant patients should be administered in the following order: lamotrigine > leviracetam > oxazepine > carbamazepine. Teratogenic risk: valproate > topiramate > phenylate sodium > phenobarbital > other drugs [13–15].

3.1.4 Discontinue Anti-Seizure Medications

A systematic review and meta-analysis conducted by Herm J Lamberink et al. [16] suggested that the discontinuation of antiepileptic drugs may be considered in patients whose seizures have been controlled, but there has been no comprehensive overview of prognostic factors, no consistent set of predictors can be identified, and many studies have reported conflicting results as study populations vary widely. A meta-analysis with individual participant data is needed because it allows for (1) correcting for differences in the duration of follow-up between subjects and studies; (2) studying the interaction effect, calculating more accurate estimates and clarifying within what range these estimates are valid; and (3) evaluating the effect size of each predictor. Subsequently, Lamberink et al. [17] conducted a meta-analysis of individual reference data. A total of 1769 patients (25%) were included in 10 meta-analyses, with a median follow-up time of 5.3 years, and 812 patients (46%) relapsed. Independent predictors of epilepsy recurrence included duration of preremission seizures, duration of absence of seizures before ASM discontinuation, age at onset of seizures, history of febrile seizures, number of preremission seizures, nonself-limiting epileptic syndrome, developmental delays, and prediscontinuation electroencephalogram (EEG) epileptoid abnormalities. Independent predictors of epilepsy recurrence in the last year of follow-up included duration of preremission seizures, seizure-free time before discontinuation, number of anti-seizure drugs used before discontinuation, family history of epilepsy, number of preremission seizures, focal seizures, and epileptiform abnormalities on electroencephalogram before discontinuation. Yao et al. [18] used meta-analysis to determine the correlation between EEG and epilepsy recurrence during ASM discontinuation. A study of 703 patients revealed that the recurrence rate of abnormal EEG signals before withdrawal was greater than that of normal EEG signals, and abnormal EEG signals before withdrawal were a risk factor for relapse. According to these findings, experts believe that (1) controlled seizures can be an indication for reducing or stopping the drug, (2) after reducing or stopping the drug, 46% of patients may relapse, (3) recurrence is related to many factors, and (4) patients with refractory epilepsy are more likely to relapse after reduction or withdrawal of medication [17–19]. Although there is evidence to support that patients with abnormal EEG readings before withdrawal are more likely to relapse than those with normal EEG readings, experts still believe that more research is needed to use EEG as an indicator of drug withdrawal in patients with epilepsy. Moreover, there is evidence that children need at least two years of being seizure-free before stopping ASM use, but there is insufficient evidence to determine the optimal time to stop ASM use in children with generalized seizures, and there is no evidence to guide the timing of stopping ASM use in adults without seizures [20]. However, experts stress that the longer it takes to stop an attack, the less likely it is to recur. The longer the drug reduction duration is, the less likely seizure recurrence in epilepsy is to recur.

3.1.5 Drug Choice for Patients with Drug-Resistant Epilepsy

According to the definition of epilepsy by the International League against Epilepsy, the failure of treatment with two or more antiepileptic drugs is called drug-resistant epilepsy. Park KM et al. [21] suggested that for these patients, "rational combination therapy can obtain a greater seizure free rate." Since most of the new antiepileptic drugs have been tested in rigorous randomized double-blind controlled trials for drug-resistant epilepsy in the past few decades, the use of new antiepileptic drugs in combination with other antiepileptic drugs may be more reasonable.

3.1.6 Whether to Continue Alone or in Combination After Initial Drug Treatment Fails

Franck et al. [22] conducted an open, cluster-randomized, prospective, controlled trial in which 143 patients were randomized to receive alternative monotherapy or combination therapy, and the primary aim was to compare the percentages of patients who were seizure free for two months after six months of treatment. Secondary outcomes were the percentage of patients with a 50% reduction in the number of seizures within six months and quality of life based on the Epilepsy Patients Quality of Life Scale, which revealed no significant differences in efficacy, quality of life or tolerance between the two groups. Another multicenter, randomized trial of 157 patients, 76 of whom were randomized to alternative monotherapy and 81 to combination therapy, reported similar retention, seizure-free survival, and adverse reaction rates at 12 months in both groups [23]. Based on this literature, experts suggest the following: (1) To date, there is little high-quality evidence to support the use of monotherapy or combination drugs, and there is no evidence to support the use of one newer ASM over another [24]. (2) After a second failure of monotherapy, it may be more reasonable to combine drugs according to the method used to treat drug-resistant epilepsy.

3.2 Special Precautions for Choosing Antiepileptic Drugs in Children with Epilepsy

Anti-seizure medications (ASMs) are the most basic and important treatment for epilepsy. Standardized ASM therapy is effective for more than two-thirds of children with newly diagnosed epilepsy [25, 26]. If no remission has been achieved after two ASM treatments, it is considered drug-resistant epilepsy [27].

Due to differences in age, epilepsy in children has unique clinical characteristics [3, 28–30]. (1) The phenotype of epilepsy is age-dependent and has a unique seizure pattern, and treatment regimens differ from those used in adults. (2) The pattern of epileptic seizures in infants is not typical, especially in newborns, who have abnormal EEGs but no clinical manifestations and need video-EEG to aid in diagnosis. After medication, the clinical seizures associated with epilepsy are stopped, but EEG can reveal sustained epileptic discharges, called clinical and electrophysiological uncoupling. (3) There are more genetic causes leading to epilepsy in children than in adults, especially developmental or epileptic encephalopathy, which starts in early infancy, and family history needs to be carefully considered; once there is a family history, testing of related genes is necessary. (4) Some epileptic syndromes, such as medial temporal lobe epilepsy, Doose syndrome, and Dravet syndrome, present with a history of febrile convulsions or have febrile convulsions as the first manifestation, so special attention should be given to the relationship between fever and seizures. (5) Children's brains are immature and prone to epilepsy comorbidities. Children have a greater risk of developing neurodevelopmental disorders and mental disorders, especially some patients with epilepsy syndromes such as LKS, infantile spasm, and Dravet syndrome, which often lead to intellectual delay, learning disabilities, cognitive disorders, language development disorders, attention deficit and hyperactivity disorders, autism spectrum disorders, emotional disorders, depression, etc. Some ASMs may cause or aggravate cognitive impairment, so timely identification and the development of appropriate, comprehensive treatment plans can help improve prognosis. 6) Refractory epilepsy is characterized by diverse seizure types, and complex seizures are liable to lead to sudden death in patients with epilepsy. (7) Some refractory epilepsies, such as LGS, often require multidrug combination treatment, so patients are prone to more cognitive disorders, behavioral abnormalities, excessive sedation and other side effects. In addition to controlling seizures, we should also consider minimizing drug-related side effects and improving overall quality of life. Some types of epilepsy, such as self-limited epilepsy, have a good long-term prognosis and do not require long-term ASM treatment. Therefore, when selecting ASMs for children with epilepsy, in addition to following the ILAE treatment guidelines, special attention should also be given to (1) atypical seizures combined with clinical seizures and EEG changes to correctly determine the type of seizures to guide medication. Valproate and topiramate are preferred for patients with multiple seizure types or those with unclear seizure types [29, 31]. (2) Epilepsy in children mostly manifests as epilepsy syndrome. The clinical diagnosis of epilepsy syndrome in children should be made as clear as possible, and individualized treatment should be implemented according to the outcome of epilepsy syndrome. For example, most cases of self-limited epilepsy with centrotemporal spines have a good prognosis, and the time to start treatment should be determined after a full assessment of benefits and risks and full communication with the patient's parents. Carbamazepine, oxcarbamazepine, and levetiracetam can be selected as first-line treatments [31]. Most patients with epileptic encephalopathy are drug resistant, and treatment should be initiated after the first seizure. In addition to commonly used ASMs, other therapeutic drugs may also be needed. For example, valproic acid and clobazam can be used as first-line therapeutic drugs for Dravet syndrome, and fenfluramine and stipentol can be recommended as second-line drugs if they are ineffective [32, 33]. ACTH is the first-line treatment for infantile spasms, and glucocorticoids and aminohexanoic acid can also be used as first-line drugs. When first-line drugs such as valproate and lamotrigine fail to treat Lennox–Gastaut syndrome, topiramate, and cannabidiol can be considered additional therapies [33–35]. (4) The genetic etiology of epilepsy plays a prominent role in childhood epilepsy, and the implementation of precise treatment has become the preferred direction for the treatment of childhood epilepsy syndrome. Aminohexenoic acid is preferred for the treatment of infantile spasms with tuberous sclerosis; sodium channel dysfunction caused by SCN2A gene variation is related to the age of the children. Epilepsy occurring before 3 months of age is mostly related to variations in sodium channel function. Sodium channel blockers such as phenytoin, oxcarbazepine, and lamotrigine are generally effective. However, after 3 months of age, most of the patients show functional inhibitory variation, and the use of sodium ion channel drugs leads to poor or aggravated outcomes. In patients with epilepsy caused by acquired variations in the SCN8A gene, sodium channel blockers such as phenytoin, carbamazepine, and oxcarbazepine are usually effective. Patients with KCNQ2 gene mutations can be treated with carbamazepine and phenytoin. Some GRIN2A gene mutations can be effectively treated with memantine. (5) the use of certain ASMs or targeted treatments should be avoided in epilepsy with partial genetic or metabolic causes; for example, using sodium ion channel blockers to treat most SCN1A gene mutation-related epilepsies can aggravate the condition; treatment of POLG1 gene mutation-related epilepsies with valproic acid can lead to liver failure; and pyridoxine-dependent developmental epileptic encephalopathy should be treated with pyridoxine and folic acid. Patients with glucose transporter 1 deficiency syndrome should be treated with a ketogenic diet [30, 35]. (6) Children's intelligence and cognitive development are rapidly developing, and there is a need to choose ASM treatments that do not affect cognitive development; for example, phenobarbital is currently considered to cause more serious cognitive damage, and lamotrigine and levetiracetam can improve the attention spans of children.

Although the principles of ASM treatment for childhood are similar to those for adults, in view of the fact that children are in a period of growth and development, their brain and organ functions are not mature; therefore, particular attention should be paid to the use of medicines. (1) Drugs have a long half-life in newborns and small infants and a short half-life in infants and preschool children, and children should be given ASMs in accordance with their weight in kilograms; it is best to adjust the dose when the blood concentration of the drug is monitored. (2) In addition to closely monitoring the effects of drugs on the liver, kidneys, blood, cardiovascular system and other important organs, the cognitive and intelligent development of children should be followed, and unnecessary multidrug combinations and long-term and large-dose ASMs should be avoided. (3) Small babies have a high incidence of genetic metabolic diseases, and attention should be given to the impact of ASM use on body metabolism. For example, in children under 2 years of age or with inherited metabolic diseases, valproic acid significantly increases the risk of liver damage. For children with mitochondrial disease and organic acidemia, valproic acid should not be used to treat epilepsy. (4) The efficacy of ASM use should be evaluated regularly after seizure control. Whether drugs are discontinued mainly depends on the type of epilepsy syndrome, etiology, and EEG [20, 36]. For children for whom it is difficult to predict the risk of recurrence, such as those with epilepsy of unknown etiology or partial epilepsy related to some foci, the ASM treatment course needs to be determined according to the individual situation. It is generally speculated that onset before 2 years of age or after 10 years of age, abnormal EEG waves, intellectual disability (IQ <70), a history of status epilepticus, and frequent seizures before and during medication suggest a high risk of relapse [20], and it is important to be cautious in reducing and discontinuing drugs.

3.3 Special Concerns for Epilepsy Prevention and Treatment in Elderly People

Some scholars refer to people over the age of 75 years as elderly individuals; others believe that a cutoff at 65 years is more appropriate, and most studies still consider it more acceptable to refer to people over the age of 60 as elderly individuals. With increasing age, the bodies and psyches of elderly people are changing, and more problems need to be considered in the prevention and treatment of epilepsy.

Epilepsy in elderly individuals is a multiple-cause disease, and its clinical manifestations and prognosis are different from those of young people. Moreover, with increasing age, physiological, and pathological changes also affect the pharmacokinetics and pharmacodynamics of ASMs. Elderly individuals are very sensitive to adverse events from ASMs, and the classification of epileptic seizures is not suitable for assessing epilepsy in elderly individuals [37]. Therefore, seizure treatment strategies for elderly individuals are highly demanding.

3.3.1 The Prevalence of Epilepsy in Elderly Individuals Is Greater

Miskov [38] reported that the prevalence of epilepsy in elderly individuals is 1.0% to 1.5%. However, the prevalence of epilepsy in elderly individuals is related to age. Bongomin F [39] studied people older than 60 years and found that 81 out of 10,334 participants (0.78%) had epilepsy; Lidia M V R Moura [40] surveyed 20,945 patients over 65 years of age enrolled in Medicare and found that 2.1% of patients were diagnosed with seizures. By the time patients reach 80 years of age, the cumulative risk of epilepsy ranges from 1.3% to 4% [41]. According to the relevant literature, the prevalence of epilepsy in elderly individuals ranges from 0.8% to 4%, which is far higher than the prevalence of epilepsy in the general population (7%). Therefore, Sanya EO [42] suggested that the prevalence of epilepsy in elderly people is the highest among all people. Miskov [38] conducted a retrospective analysis of 246 patients with epilepsy and found that 43 patients (17.4%) were over 65 years old.

3.3.2 Most Epilepsy in Elderly Individuals Have a Clear Cause

Miskov [38] analyzed 32 cases of newly diagnosed epilepsy in elderly individuals and reported that 22 (68.8%) patients had cerebrovascular disease, 4 had trauma (12.5%), 3 had primary tumors (9.4%), and 3 had metastatic tumors (9.4%), suggesting that cerebrovascular diseases are the main cause of epilepsy in elderly individuals. Gloria MAS Tedrus [43] studied 50 patients diagnosed with nonconvulsive epilepsy and reported that 41 patients (82%) had structural damage, 5 patients had structural damage caused by metabolic factors, and 4 patients had an unknown etiology. Namitha Narayanan [44] studied 125 newly diagnosed epilepsy patients older than 65 years and reported that the main causes of epilepsy were cerebrovascular diseases, metabolic abnormalities, and alcoholism. Temporal infarcts are the most common, followed by parietotemporal and frontal infarcts, but genetic causes of epilepsy are rare. Roberto A Suastegui Roman [45] investigated the etiology of new-onset epilepsy in 100 elderly patients and reported that 26% had no clear etiology, 42% had stroke, and 10% had neurocysticercosis. Since most epileptic seizures in the elderly have causes, clinicians need to carefully review the patient's medical history and perform a detailed physical examination combined with laboratory and imaging examinations, and carefully rule out potential causes.

3.3.3 The Clinical Manifestations of Epilepsy in Elderly Individuals Are Not Typical

Elderly people with epilepsy are different from those with epilepsy in other age groups, and confusion and falling are the main symptoms of epilepsy. Green [46] studied 207 patients over the age of 60 years and found 103 incidences of seizures, 65 of which were focal seizures with confusion and conscious impairment. Tedrus [43] studied 105 elderly patients with conscious changes and found that 50 elderly patients (47.6%) had nonconvulsive status epilepticus, 6 patients of whom were comatose, and 44 patients were not. Verma [47] investigated 250 hospitalized elderly people ($\geq$60 years old) and reported that 123 patients (49.2%) had epileptic status, 94 patients (37.6%) had acute symptomatic epilepsy, and 13.2% (33) had symptomatic epilepsy. The lack of witnesses, nonspecific symptoms, challenging determination of start and end times, and short duration make the diagnosis of epilepsy in elderly individuals challenging [37, 44]. Lance Watkins et al. [48] even suggested that the diagnosis of new epilepsy in the elderly population requires expert evaluation. Treatment plans need to be customized based on an individual's comorbidities, concurrent medication use, and general health conditions.

3.3.4 Comorbidity of Elderly Individuals

In addition to seizures, elderly people often have other diseases simultaneously, causing contradictions in treatment. Alzheimer's disease, Parkinson's disease, multisystem atrophy, progressive supranuclear palsy, corticobasal ganglia syndrome, diabetes, and cerebrovascular disease are all common in elderly people, and these diseases may cause seizures and become markers of old age [49]. In the treatment of these diseases, the use of multiple drugs often leads to interactions. In addition, it may cause neurotoxicity or cognitive impairment. In the presence of these diseases, the treatment of senile epilepsy must take into consideration comorbidities and combined drugs. These factors make the treatment of epilepsy in elderly individuals particularly challenging [50].

3.3.5 Cognitive Dysfunction in Elderly Patients with Epilepsy

Pervin et al. [51] used the SF-36 questionnaire to explore the impact of epilepsy on quality of life in elderly individuals. A survey of 611 people revealed obvious abnormalities in 9 items of the SF-36, including anxiety, sadness, and social activities. Therefore, in senile epilepsy, phenobarbital, topiramate, and other drugs that can cause cognitive impairment should be avoided as much as possible.

3.3.6 Pharmacokinetic Changes

With increasing age, the pharmacokinetics of epilepsy in elderly patients are significantly altered; these patients are more sensitive to adverse drug reactions, and their cognition, emotions, and bones may be affected. Therefore, when treating elderly patients with epilepsy, changes in drug metabolism and their impact on the aging body must be considered [50]. The use of barbiturates, primidone, clobazam, and calcium channel blockers such as flunarizine should be avoided in the elderly population.

3.3.7 Selection of Antiepileptic Drugs

Rohracher [52] suggested that the selection of antiepileptic drugs for elderly patients with epilepsy is complicated by comorbidities and the need for a combination of drugs. They suggest that ASMs with few interactions and good tolerance should be selected. Levetiracetam and lamotrigine are the first-line antiepileptic drugs. Lattanzi [53] systematically analyzed the use of antiepileptic drugs in 1425 patients and reported that lacosamine, lamotrigine, and levetiracetam may be the best drugs for achieving seizure-free effects. Bernd Pohlmann-Eden [54] compared the efficacy of levetiracetam, sodium valproate sustained-release tablets, and carbamazepine controlled-release tablets in patients over 60 years of age with newly diagnosed epilepsy and reported that Lev was more effective and better tolerated. These results suggest that Lev may be a suitable choice for initial monotherapy in patients over 60 years of age with newly diagnosed epilepsy. Older epileptic patients often respond more sensitively to antiepileptic drugs than younger patients do if the drug is chosen appropriately [41].

3.3.8 Prognosis of Elderly Patients with Epilepsy

Verma [55] analyzed the prognoses of 250 hospitalized elderly people (≥60 years old) and reported that the in-hospital mortality of elderly patients with epilepsy was 21.6%, which was related to an age of over 70 years, having a new-onset epilepsy status, and having a longer hospital stay. Verma [56] analyzed the prognoses of 122 hospitalized elderly (≥60 years old) patients with status epilepticus and reported that the in-hospital mortality of newly diagnosed patients with epileptic status was 38.9%, and the prognosis was related to comorbidities and low Glasgow coma score.

3.4 Precautions Regarding Drug Treatment of Women with Epilepsy

Epilepsy is one of the most common neurological disorders, affecting nearly 70 million patients worldwide, approximately half of whom are women. The global prevalence of epilepsy in women is 6.85/1000 [57]. A woman's life can be divided into the neonatal period, childhood, adolescence, reproductive age, perimenopause, and old age, according to changes in hormone levels and age. Each period has different physiological characteristics. Because physiological characteristics govern the challenges that women with epilepsy may face during drug therapy, it is necessary to consider the effects of ASMs on endocrine hormones. Therefore, an individualized medication regimen is particularly important for female epilepsy patients. This chapter mainly discusses several issues that require attention for drug therapy in women with epilepsy at different periods in their lives.

3.4.1 Physical Characteristics of Women

3.4.1.1 Physiological Stage

From birth to the end of life, women experience functional and physiological changes in their reproductive systems, which can be divided into six stages according to their age and physiological characteristics: (1) Neonatal period: within 4 weeks of birth. At this stage, the ovaries are in a naïve state, and there is no hormone secretion. (2) Childhood refers to the period from 4 weeks of birth to approximately 12 years of age. At this stage, the body continues to grow and develop, but the ovaries and reproductive system remain in a relatively naïve state. In late childhood (after approximately 10 years of age), the follicles in the ovaries develop and secrete sex hormones, and female characteristics begin to appear. (3) Adolescence: The World Health Organization defines adolescence as the age between 10 and 19 years. The physiological characteristics of this period include the rapid development of the body and reproductive organs, the development of secondary sexual characteristics, and the beginning of menstruation. (4) Reproductive years: After puberty, the reproductive age period lasts approximately 30 years, during which the central nervous system and the hypothalamic-pituitary-ovarian axis are fully mature, accounting for the largest proportion of time in a woman's life; during this time, women face many stressors related to marriage, family, childbirth, work and career. (5) Menopause (perimenopausal period): Women's ovarian function gradually declines, and the reproductive organs begin to atrophy. This period usually starts at the age of 40 and lasts for more than 10 years. (6) Old age: Generally, after 60 years of age. During this period, women gradually begin to age, and their ovarian function further declines. This chapter mainly discusses the necessary precautions for drug therapy in women with epilepsy in adolescence, reproductive age, perimenopause, and old age.

3.4.1.2 Hypothalamic-Pituitary-Ovarian Axis

The release of female reproductive endocrine hormones is mainly controlled through a two-way feedback loop of the hypothalamic–pituitary–ovarian axis [58]. Gonadotropin-releasing hormone (GnRH) is secreted by the hypothalamus to stimulate the pituitary gland to release follicle-stimulating hormone (FSH) and luteinizing hormone (LH). FSH stimulates the formation of follicles that secrete estradiol. A surge in LH induces oocyte maturation, ovulation, and transformation of the follicle into a corpus luteum. This marks the end of the follicular phase and the beginning of the luteal phase. After ovulation, the corpus luteum secretes progesterone. Progesterone feedback inhibits the secretion and release of GnRH, FSH, and LH. If no pregnancy occurs, the corpus luteum degenerates, the levels of progesterone and estradiol decrease, the inhibition of GnRH weakens, and the next cycle commences.

3.4.1.3 Menstrual Cycle

The average menstrual cycle for women is 28 days (24–35 days); the first day of bleeding is the first day of the menstrual cycle, and ovulation occurs on the 14th day of the menstrual cycle. The menstrual cycle is divided into the follicular and luteal phases; the follicular phase lasts from Day 1 to 14, and the luteal phase lasts from Day 15 to 28. Periodic changes in the ovaries and uterus are regulated by the hypothalamic–pituitary–ovarian axis [59]. Many studies have shown that estradiol and progesterone have neuro-excitability and neuroinhibitory effects, respectively. Therefore, throughout the menstrual cycle, cyclical changes in the levels of these two hormones lead to changes in the frequency of seizures in women with epilepsy, and epilepsy can occur during menstruation.

3.4.2 *Several Problems in Drug Therapy for Women with Epilepsy During Different Life Periods*

3.4.2.1 ASMs and Reproductive Endocrine Disorders

Key evidence indicates that women with epilepsy are more prone to reproductive endocrine dysfunction than are ordinary women. Patients can present with menstrual disorders, polycystic ovaries, sexual dysfunction, infertility, premature menopause, etc. Reproductive endocrine disorders can also increase the frequency of seizures and the risk of comorbidities such as female cancers, migraine, and mental illness. Therefore, reducing the occurrence of reproductive endocrine disorders in the treatment management of women with epilepsy is critical [60, 61]. The mechanism of reproductive endocrine disorders may be related to epilepsy itself (such as the type and frequency of seizures) and ASM exposure [62, 63]. Here, we focus on the effects of ASMs on the reproductive endocrine system.

ASMs can be divided into liver enzyme-inducing and non-enzyme-inducing antiepileptic drugs, as shown in Table 3.1, with significant differences in their effects on female reproductive hormone levels. Enzyme-inducing antiepileptic drugs (EIASMs), such as phenobarbital, phenytoin sodium, and carbamazepine, can alter liver metabolism and reduce reproductive hormone concentrations. They also induce the production of sex hormone-binding globulin (SHBG), which further reduces plasma free estradiol concentrations, leading to menstrual disorders [59]. The non-EIASM sodium VPA is thought to have a direct effect on the production of follicular steroids in the ovaries. VPA can increase testosterone secretion and reduce

Table 3.1 EIASMs and non-EIASMs

EIASMs	Non-EIASMs
Carbamazepine	Acetazolamide
Eslicarbazepine acetate	Clobazam
Oxcarbazepine	Clonazepam
Phenobarbital	Ethosuximide
Phenytoin	Gabapentin
Primidone	Lacosamide
Rufinamide	Levetiracetam
Topiramate	Piracetam
Perampanel	Pregabalin
	Sodium valproate
	Stiripentol
	Tiagabine
	Vigabatrin
	Zonisamide

EIASMs enzyme-inducing antiepileptic drugs, *non-EIASMs* non-enzyme-inducing antiepileptic drugs estradiol secretion, and the testosterone/estrogen ratio increases. This effect leads to an androgen-dominated microenvironment in the ovaries, which may lead to polycystic changes in the ovaries and menstrual disorders [64].

The most common reproductive endocrine disorder among women with epilepsy is polycystic ovary syndrome (PCOS). Among all antiseizure drugs, VPA is most closely associated with the development of PCOS. In 1993, Isojarvi et al. [65] reported that the incidence of polycystic ovaries and/or hyperandrogenemia was extremely high in epileptic patients treated with VPA alone or in combination and that the age at initial VPA exposure was also an important factor. The risk of PCOS appears to be particularly high when VPA treatment is initiated in childhood or adolescence.

Other reproductive endocrine disorders include infertility, sexual dysfunction, and premature menopause. Infertility is considered to be related to seizures and the effects of ASMs on reproductive hormones. Although most women with epilepsy have a normal sex life, there have been reports of sexual dysfunction in this population, including decreased libido and inadequate orgasm satisfaction. The types of ASMs used may be related to sexual dysfunction [66], but more studies have shown that the etiology of sexual dysfunction in women with epilepsy is multifactorial, including physiological and psychological factors, and that epilepsy-related depression is also an important factor in sexual dysfunction in women with epilepsy [67]. Premature menopause may occur in women with epilepsy, especially when the frequency of seizures is high and multiple EIASMs are used throughout their lifetime [68].

In summary, to reduce the occurrence of reproductive endocrine disorders in women with epilepsy, a reasonable selection of ASMs is essential. Adolescents and women of reproductive age should avoid the use of VPA. If they cannot avoid it, they should try to use the smallest effective dose. Even in women in late childhood (more than 10 years old), it is necessary to consider the adverse effects of VPA on the endocrine system and carefully choose the drug. In addition, choosing non-EIASMs can reduce the risk of reproductive endocrine disorders.

3.4.2.2 ASMs and Contraception

Contraceptive counseling is an important part of managing the treatment of women of childbearing age with epilepsy. Effective contraceptive measures can ensure a planned pregnancy, reduce the occurrence of malformations, and improve the quality of life of patients. A two-way pharmacokinetic interaction between ASMs and hormonal contraceptives can reduce the efficacy of either drug. Moreover, the combined use of hormonal contraceptives and ASMs may lead to unintended pregnancy, increased seizures, and drug-related adverse reactions [69]. Many steroid hormonal contraceptives and ASMs are metabolized by the liver P450 enzyme pathway. Steroid hormones, especially the 3A4 isoenzyme, are substrates of the cytochrome P450 enzyme system. EIASMs, including phenytoin sodium, phenobarbital, and carbamazepine, increase the metabolism of steroid hormones, reduce the concentration of ethinyl estradiol and various synthetic progesterone contraceptive drugs, reduce their efficacy, and increase the risk of unintended pregnancy [70]. The new types of ASMs, felbamate, topiramate, and oxcarbazepine, are weak EIASMs and may also have some effect on steroid hormonal contraceptives. In addition, some ASMs can increase the production of SHBG, resulting in an increased ability to bind to progesterone, ultimately reducing the free concentrations of hormonal contraceptives [71]. Non-EIASMs such as ethosuximide, VPA, gabapentin, lamotrigine, tiagabine, levetiracetam, zonisamide, pregabalin, and linamarin do not activate the CYP3A4 isoenzyme system and therefore do not increase the risk of contraceptive failure.

Thus, non-EIASMs are preferable for women with epilepsy who are using hormonal contraceptives. If EIASMs are used, it is recommended that the dose of contraceptives be increased appropriately. The use of nonhormonal contraceptive measures, such as intrauterine devices, condoms, contraceptive sponges, diaphragms, and cervical caps, is also recommended. For older women who no longer need to maintain fertility, sterilization surgery can also be used [69]. In addition, some hormonal contraceptives also affect ASM metabolism. Lamotrigine is currently the most commonly used drug for women of reproductive age, and studies have shown that in women with epilepsy, the use of contraceptives containing ethinylestradiol significantly increases lamotrigine metabolism and reduces the serum concentration by approximately 50% [72]. Therefore, it may be necessary to adjust the dose of LTG and monitor its concentration.

3.4.2.3 ASMs and Pregnancy

Pregnancy is the most critical and challenging period for women with epilepsy. There may be some variation in seizure frequency throughout pregnancy, and seizure frequency tends to remain stable during pregnancy in most women with epilepsy, increasing in approximately one-third of patients and decreasing in some women [73]. Owing to concerns about the adverse effects of ASMs on the fetus, some women choose to reduce or stop drug therapy during pregnancy, which can cause an increase in seizures, endangering the health of pregnant women and the fetus. Epileptic seizures can increase pregnancy complications, such as premature delivery, miscarriage, obstructed labor, vaginal bleeding, and placental abruption, resulting in an increased risk of death. Epileptic seizures can also lead to intrauterine hypoxia, stillbirth, low birth weight, and an increase in the rate of neonatal malformation. Epilepsy has the greatest impact on the fetus in the first 3 months of pregnancy [74]. Therefore, it is crucial to establish a multidisciplinary cooperation model led by epilepsy specialists and involving obstetricians, geneticists, and psychologists to provide guidance throughout conception, pregnancy, childbirth, and lactation for female reproductive-aged epilepsy patients [75].

Women of reproductive age should consult an epilepsy specialist and an obstetrician before preparing for pregnancy. It is generally recommended that women with epilepsy of reproductive age plan pregnancy after a seizure-free period of at least

9 months. If the patient has been seizure-free in the last 3–5 years and her EEG is normal, gradually reducing and stopping drug treatment can be considered, but the patient should be fully informed of the possibility of epilepsy recurrence. However, most patients need to continue taking ASMs throughout pregnancy, and the goal during pregnancy is to balance the risk of seizures with the potential teratogenic effects of ASMs [74]. The incidence of major congenital malformations (MCMs) in women of reproductive age due to intrauterine exposure to ASMs is 4–9%, which is 2–3 times greater than that in the general population. MCMs mainly include cardiac developmental malformations, neural tube defects, urogenital tract malformations, skeletal malformations, cleft palate, etc. [76].

The teratogenicity of ASMs is related to the drug type, drug dose, and number of drugs used in combination. In a recent prospective EURAP study comparing the incidence of MCMs with monotherapy using eight ASMs, VPA (10.3%) was the most common, followed by phenobarbital (6.5%), phenytoin (6.4%), carbamazepine (5.5%), and topiramate (3.9%). Oxcarbazepine (3.0%), lamotrigine (2.9%), and levetiracetam (2.8%) showed high safety indices, and the incidence of MCMs was comparable to that in pregnant women who did not take ASMs [13]. Generally, the teratogenicity of first-generation ASMs, especially VPA, was significantly greater than that of second-generation ASMs. Another EURAP cohort study showed a 27% decrease in the incidence of MCMs at birth in the 2010–2013 cohort, with reduced use of VPA and carbamazepine and increased use of lamotrigine and levetiracetam compared with the previous cohort from 2000 to 2005 [77]. The safety data of third-generation novel ASMs, including eslicarbazepine, perampanel, and lacosamide, during pregnancy are limited. In addition, the teratogenic risk of ASMs is dose-dependent. When the total daily dose of VPA is less than 650 mg, the incidence of MCMs decreases to 6.3%, and when the dose exceeds this level, the incidence of teratogenic risk increases significantly. The total safe daily doses of carbamazepine and lamotrigine are 700 mg and 325 mg, respectively. The overall incidence of MCMs was significantly greater in women using combination therapy than in those using monotherapy, especially when VPA was included in the regimen. It is also important to note that ASM exposure is not the only factor that increases the risk of MCMs in women of reproductive age. The Australian Pregnancy Antiepileptic Drugs Register study reported that maternal age >31 years, family history of abnormalities, preexisting maternal mental illness, and smoking were all independently associated with a greater risk of MCMs [78].

In addition to the structural teratogenicity of ASMs, postnatal cognitive abnormalities associated with intrauterine exposure to ASMs should also be of concern. The Neurodevelopmental Effects of Antiepileptic Drugs (NEAD) study revealed that 6-year-olds exposed to VPA in utero had lower full-scale IQ scores than did those exposed to carbamazepine, lamotrigine, or phenytoin. In addition, this relationship with VPA was dose-dependent; the higher the dose was, the lower the cognitive score was [79]. A recent systematic review of 35 articles on neurocognitive developmental outcomes in children exposed to novel ASMs was conducted. The results showed that children exposed to lamotrigine and levetiracetam in utero had better cognitive outcomes, similar to those in the control group. Data on oxcarbazepine, gabapentin, and topiramate are limited and contradictory. No studies have assessed cognitive outcomes in children exposed to eslicarbazepine, lacosamide, perampanel, or zonisamide in utero, and more research is needed on the effects of novel ASMs on the development of structural and cognitive abnormalities [80].

Treatment recommendations for pregnant women with epilepsy include choosing ASMs that are effective for the type of seizure the patient has and have the lowest risk of teratogenicity and cognitive impairment in offspring. Maintaining the lowest effective dose of monotherapy during pregnancy preparation, replacing highly teratogenic drugs, and avoiding multidrug combination therapy where possible can effectively optimize the health of offspring [81]. However, replacement or dose reduction of ASMs should be performed before pregnancy, as changing medications during pregnancy may increase the risk of epilepsy recurrence. New ASMs should be preferred during pregnancy preparation, and VPA use should be avoided as much as possible. If the pregnancy is unplanned and the patient is using VPA and seizures are well-controlled, replacing VPA during pregnancy is not recommended, but a lower dose can be administered. If seizures are not well controlled, more rapid-acting ASMs should be attempted. Low levels of folic acid are associated with neural tube defects, abortion, and intrauterine fetal growth inhibition. Daily supplementation with small doses of folic acid plays an important role in preventing fetal neural tube malformations and promoting the cognitive development of offspring. Women with epilepsy taking ASMs need to supplement more folic acid than the general population, especially when ASMs that antagonize folic acid metabolism, such as VPA, phenobarbital, phenytoin, and carbamazepine, are used together. Supplementation with 5 mg of folic acid daily is recommended from 3 months before pregnancy until delivery [82].

Physiological changes in pregnant women during pregnancy can affect the pharmacokinetics of various drugs. These changes include changes in kidney and liver function and changes in serum ALB levels. The glomerular filtration rate increases by 40–50% during pregnancy, which leads to an increase in antiepileptic drugs cleared by the kidneys and a decrease in serum drug concentration. Liver changes occur involving the cytochrome P450 enzyme system and glucosylation, and some cytochrome P450 enzymes (CYP3A4, CYP2D6, and CYP2C9) can increase the metabolism of antiepileptic drugs, with drug concentrations decreasing to varying degrees [83]. During pregnancy, the blood concentrations of levetiracetam, topiramate, and oxcarbazepine can be reduced by 30–50%, and the blood concentration of lamotrigine can be reduced by up to 70% [84, 85]. Therefore, detecting ASM blood concentrations before pregnancy and establishing a reference baseline value for drug dosage adjustment during pregnancy are recommended. Monthly monitoring of the ASM concentration is required during pregnancy, and an appropriate increase in the ASM dose may be required during pregnancy to maintain efficacy and prevent the recurrence of epilepsy. Drug metabolism gradually normalizes after delivery, and the risk of excessive maternal blood drug concentration increases. The blood drug concentration should be assessed 10–14 days after delivery, and the drug dosage should be appropriately reduced by referring to the prepregnancy drug concentration. When mothers use EIASMs (carbamazepine, oxcarbazepine, phenytoin sodium, and topiramate) during pregnancy, the risk of neonatal bleeding increases, and intramuscular injection of vitamin K is recommended at birth [86].

3.4.2.4 ASMs and Breastfeeding

The safety of breastfeeding is important for female patients taking ASMs. Breastfeeding provides infants with nutrients needed for growth and development, reduces the risk of infectious diseases, and improves the parent–child relationship [87]. Most ASMs can be secreted into milk, and the concentration of ASMs in milk depends on the plasma protein binding rate of the ASMs; the concentration of ASMs in milk is generally lower than that in plasma. Therefore, the concentration of ASMs encountered by infants from breast milk is very low; thus, breastfeeding is generally safe for women exposed to ASMs [88].

Assessing the risks of breastfeeding is complex and requires a comprehensive evaluation of multiple aspects. Several parameters are used to calculate an infant's exposure to ASMs during breastfeeding, such as the ASM milk/plasma ratio (M/P), which is the ratio between the concentration of drugs in breast milk and maternal plasma; an M/P ratio greater than 1 indicates a high concentration of drugs in breast milk. However, the M/P ratio does not reflect the actual exposure level of children; therefore, its clinical value is limited [89]. The relative infant dose (RID) is the most important measure for evaluating the risk of breastfeeding, and any drug with an RID of less than 10% of the maternal dose is considered safe. Assuming that the mother weighs 70 kg, the RID is calculated by dividing the dose received by the baby through the milk (mg/kg/day) by the dose in the mother's body (mg/kg/day). The RID values of phenobarbital, ethosuximide, topiramate, and zonisamide exceed 10%, which may not be safe and need to be reduced during breastfeeding [90]. According to a work by Hale et al. [91], *Drugs and Breast Milk*, drugs are classified into five categories of lactation risk, ranging from "safest" to "contraindication" (L1–L5). According to this classification, most ASMs fall into three main risk categories during breastfeeding: "L2—safe," "L3—moderately safe," and "L4—possibly dangerous" (see Table 3.2). Breastfeeding in epileptic patients taking ASMs is generally encouraged because the benefits of infant breastfeeding outweigh the risks of moderate drug exposure.

To further guarantee the safety of breastfeeding, measures should be taken to reduce the risk of side effects in infants. For example, phenobarbital has a long half-life, a high plasma protein binding rate, accumulation in milk, and sedative side effects; therefore, infants should be carefully monitored during breastfeeding. In particular, monitoring plasma drug concentrations is recommended for premature infants or infants with lethargy, sucking difficulties, or poor weight gain. If significant side effects occur, breastfeeding should be restricted or switched to mixed/artificial feeding [92]. In addition, for drugs with short half-lives, breastfeeding can

Table 3.2 Clinical parameters and main pharmacokinetic characteristics of each ASM and assessment of their lactation risk

ASMs	PB (%)[a]	Oral Bioavailability[b] (%)	RID[c] (%)	T½[d] (hours)	M/P[e]	Hale 2012[f]
Clonazepam	50-86	100	2.8	18–50	0.33	L3
Carbamazepine	74	100	3.8–5.9	18–54	0.69	L2
Diazepam	99	100	7.1	43	0.2–2.7	L3
Ethosuximide	NA	100	31.4–71.5	30–60	0.94	L4
Phenytoin	89	70–100	0.6–7.7	6–24	0.18–0.45	L2
Phenobarbital	51	80–100	24	20–133	0.4–0.6	L3
Valproate	94	100	1.4–1.7	14	0.42	L3
Primidone	25	90	8.4–8.6	5–18	0.72	L3
Topiramate	15	75	24.5	18–24	0.86–1.1	L3
Lamotrigine	55	98	9.2	29	0.057–1.47	L3
Gabapentin	<3	50–60	1.3–6.6	5–7	0.7–1.3	L2
Vigabatrin	NA	50	1.5–2.7	7	<1	L3
Tiagabine	96	90	NA	7–9	NA	L3
Zonisamide	40	NA	28.9–36.8	63	0.93	L4
Levetiracetam	<10	100	3.4–7.8	6–8	0.76–1.55	L3
Pregabalin	NA	90	NA	6	NA	L3
Oxcarbazepine	40	100	1.5–1.7	9	0.5	L3

[a]PB: maternal plasma protein binding expressed as a percentage

[b]Oral bioavailability: intestinal absorption after oral administration expressed as a percentage of the administered dose

[c]RID relative infant dose

[d]T ½: half-life of the drug

[e]M/P: milk-to-plasma ratio of a drug concentration

[f]Hale lactation risk categories: L1: drugs with the highest level of safety, L2: safe, L3: moderately safe; L4: possibly dangerous, L5: contraindicated

be performed before the next dose, when the concentration of drugs in the milk is lower; this can reduce the exposure of the baby [92]. During pregnancy, some ASMs, such as lamotrigine, need to be increased to maintain the effective drug concentration and quickly adjusted after delivery to avoid excessive drug concentrations in the mother's body and breastmilk [92]. Safe breastfeeding techniques are important, and mothers can be advised to breastfeed in a supine position, preferably in the presence of others, to protect the baby from trauma in the event of a seizure [92].

Present study risk categories: The moderately safe category has a less documented safety profile due to limited clinical experience and a lack of studies. Moderately safe ASMs can be used, but the lowest dose of the drug should be chosen, the nursing infant should be clinically monitored, and when possible, his or her plasma level should be checked.

The data were drawn from references [1, 41], except where otherwise specified. NA: indicates that no data are available.

3.4.2.5 ASMs and Women with Epilepsy and Comorbidities

The prevalence of comorbidities is significantly greater in women with epilepsy than in the general population. These comorbidities include nervous system, psychobehavioral, and systemic disease comorbidities. An observational study that analyzed data from eight commercial health plans showed that women with epilepsy had more comorbidities than men did. In terms of prevalence, the top 10 comorbidities in women were mental illness (16%), hypertension (12%), asthma (11%), hyperlipidemia (11%), headache (7%), diabetes (6%), urinary tract infection (5%), hypothyroidism (5%), anemia (5%), and migraine (4%) [93]. Various comorbidities may cause further functional impairment in women with epilepsy, and early screening for common comorbidities is needed. In treatment, it is necessary to fully consider the interaction between epilepsy and comorbidities, the potential side effects of ASMs on comorbidities, and the interaction between ASMs and other therapeutic drugs. For example, EIASMs affect the metabolism of many other shared drugs, and comprehensive consideration of these interactions will greatly help to improve the overall health of female epilepsy patients [94]. Table 3.3 shows the recommended ASMs for women with epilepsy and comorbidities.

Women with epilepsy have a greater risk of anxiety, depression, and other psychiatric disorders. When using ASMs, it is necessary to pay attention to their positive and negative effects on psychiatric symptoms and to consider the interactions between ASMs and antipsychotics. Many ASMs have positive or negative effects on patient emotions. Among the commonly used ASMs, VPA has a mood stabilizing effect and is also used to treat depression and bipolar disorder. Lamotrigine improved depressive symptoms in patients with epilepsy as an additive therapy in a randomized, double-blind study; carbamazepine and oxcarbazepine use did not increase the risk of suicide or depression. The third-generation ASM lacosamide has a positive effect on depression. Some ASMs can aggravate or cause depression, and phenobarbital, cyclohexene acid, zonisamide, topiramate, and levetiracetam have adverse effects on mood [94]. For patients with epilepsy and depression, it is recommended to use mood-stabilizing drugs, such as VPA, lamotrigine, and lacosamide, while avoiding or reducing the use of ASMs that may aggravate depressive mood, depending on the type of seizure. VPA, gabapentin, etc., have anticonvulsant and antianxiety effects because they can effectively control the symptoms of epilepsy. Therefore, such drugs are recommended for treating epilepsy in patients with anxiety. Benzodiazepines such as clonazepam and alprazolam are suitable for short-term use against anxiety symptoms. In addition, attention should be given to the interactions between ASMs and psychiatric drugs. ASMs with enzyme-inducing effects promote the clearance of antidepressants, resulting in reduced efficacy, whereas VPA increases the concentration of these drugs and can lead to poisoning. Tricyclic antidepressants and some selective serotonin reuptake inhibitors, such as fluoxetine, paroxetine, and fluvoxamine, also inhibit the metabolism of ASMs, leading to toxicity symptoms. Other antidepressants, such as citalopram, escitalopram, sertraline,

Table 3.3 Recommendations for the use of ASMs in WWE and other cormobidities

	Most recommended ASMs	Less recommended ASMs	ASMs to be avoided
Heart disease	LEV, LTG, TPM, VPA,	CBZ, OXC, PGB, PHT	–
Lung disease	ZNS. GBP[a]	CBZ, PHT	BZD, PB,
Hepatic impairment	LEV, LTG, OXC, PGB,	BZD, CBZ, ESM, PB, PHT,	PRM
Renal impairment	TPM, VPA, ZNS.GPB[a]	PRM, ZNS	LTG, VPA
Porphyria	LEV, OXC, PGB,	GBP, LEV, LTG, OXC, PB,	–
Liver transplantation	TPM. GBP[a]	PGB, PRM, TPM, ZNS	CBZ, LTG,
Kidney	BZD, CBZ, ESM, PHT,	BZD	PB, PHT,
transplantation	TGB, VPA	CBZ, PB, PHT, PRM	PRM,
Bone marrow	LEV, OXC, PGB. GBP[a]	ASMs with renal excretion	TGB, TPM,
transplantation	LEV, PGB, TPM. GBP[a]	–	VPA, ZNS
Hypothyroidism	BZD, LTG, VPA	OXC, TPM, VPA	VPA
Osteoporosis	LEV, LTG, TPM. GBP[a]	VPA	–
Obesity	BZD, LEV, LTG, PGB,	CBZ, CLB	CBZ, OXC,
HIV	ZNS. GBP[a]	BZD, LTG, OXC, VPA, ZNS	PB, PRM,
Mental disability	BZD, LEV, LTG, PGB,	PGB, ZNS	VPA
Cognitive	ZNS. GBP[a]	CBZ, OXC, VPA, ZNS	CBZ, PB,
impairment	TPM, ZNS	CBZ, OXC, PHT, TPM,	PHT, PRM
Stroke	LEV, PGB, TPM. GBP[a]	VPA	CBZ, PB,
Brain tumor	LEV, LTG, OXC,	CBZ, LTG, OXC, PHT,	PHT, PRM
	VPA. GBP[a]	TPM	GBP, PGB,
	LEV, LTG, PGB. GBP[a]		VPA
	LEV, LTG. GBP[a]		CBZ, PB,
	LEV, VPA. GBP[a]. PGB[a],		PHT, PRM
	ZNS*		BZD, CBZ,
			PB, PHT,
			PRM, TPM
			BZD, PB,
			PHT, PRM,
			TPM
			BZD, PB,
			PRM
			PB, PRM

[a]Useful as an add-on therapy

trazodone, and venlafaxine, have less effect on the pharmacokinetics of ASMs and can be used as a first choice. Most antipsychotics interfere with the liver metabolism of ASMs to varying degrees, and there is a risk of eclampsia. Patients with epilepsy should avoid clozapine and chlorpromazine, whereas olanzapine, quetiapine, and risperidone are relatively safe (Table 3.4).

The risk of pathological fracture is significantly increased in women with epilepsy who have osteoporosis, especially menopausal and postmenopausal women. The adverse effects of ASMs, especially EIASMs, on bone metabolism are the main causes of bone diseases. Phenobarbital, carbamazepine, and phenytoin sodium (EIASMs) can reduce active vitamin D levels, resulting in reduced calcium absorption and secondary hyperparathyroidism. Non-EIASM VPA can also cause

Table 3.4 Optimization of treatment in patients with epilepsy with psychiatric comorbidities

	Antiseizure medications		Psychiatric drugs	
	Recommended	To be avoided	Recommended	To be avoided
Depression	CBZ, GBP, LTG, OXC, PGB, VPA	PB, PHT, PRM, TGB, TPM, PER	Citalopram Escitalopram sertraline trazodone Venlafaxine	Amoxapine Maprotiline bupropion
Anxiety	BZD, GBP, PGB, VPA	LEV, PER	BZD SSRIs	–
Psychosis	LTG, OXC, VPA	ESM, LEV, TPM	Olanzapine quetiapine risperidone	Chlorpromazine clozapine

osteoporosis through other mechanisms. Data on the bone-specific effects of other novel ASMs are limited, but changes in bone metabolism have also been reported in patients treated with oxcarbazepine, gabapentin, and levetiracetam [95]. Therefore, the bone mineral densities of women who take ASMs for a long time should be regularly monitored, and adequate amounts of calcium and vitamin D should be administered prophylactically.

3.4.3 Principles of Individualization in the Long-Term Management of Treatment in Women with Epilepsy

Due to physiological and social factors, women with epilepsy face more difficulties and challenges than men. In formulating drug treatments for these women, the fact that recurrent seizures and long-term ASM treatment may affect female patients should be considered, and their long-term management needs to be strengthened. In long-term management, considering the different physiological characteristics and needs of each life period and providing individualized drug therapy are crucial. For adolescent female patients, the impact of ASM treatment on sex hormones should be considered, the occurrence of menstrual disorders and PCOS should be avoided, and the impact of ASMs on appearance and weight should be considered. For women of childbearing age, reasonable contraception, reducing the teratogenicity of ASMs, and breastfeeding are the main considerations. Menopausal/elderly epilepsy patients face more comorbidity/comedication problems. The effects of ASMs on comorbidities and drug interactions should be considered, and attention should be given to osteoporosis and mental health issues in menopausal women.

3.5 Role of Artificial Intelligence Technology in Drug Therapy of Epilepsy

3.5.1 Introduction

Epilepsy is a prevalent chronic neurological disorder worldwide, affecting people of all ages and ethnic backgrounds. The lifetime risk of epilepsy is approximately 760 per 100,000 individuals. More than 50 million people live with epilepsy, accounting for 13 million disability-adjusted life years (DALYs) globally [96]. The disease burden is significant at both the individual and societal levels. Recurrent seizures can lead to physical and psychosocial disabilities, while comorbidities such as learning disabilities and psychiatric disorders complicate epilepsy management [97]. Premature mortality can be attributed to status epilepticus and Sudden Unexpected Death in Epilepsy (SUDEP). Epilepsy is associated with social stigma, unemployment, and marital problems across different cultural backgrounds [98–100]. Substantial healthcare resources are allocated to epilepsy care, with an average annual cost of over US$ 1000 per person in high-income countries and an estimated global healthcare cost of US$ 119 billion per year [101].

Currently, pharmacological therapies remain the primary treatment modality for epilepsy. ASMs control seizures via various putative mechanisms of action [102], which include sodium channel blockers (e.g., phenytoin and carbamazepine), GABA agonists (e.g., benzodiazepines and barbiturates), calcium channel blockers (e.g., ethosuximide), as well as agents targeting molecular substrates such as synaptic vesicle protein 2A (SV2A) receptors (e.g., levetiracetam and brivaracetam) and AMPA receptors (e.g., perampanel). The number of ASMs available has significantly increased in the past two decades, with more than 20 in the market currently [103]. Newer ASMs generally exhibit improved adverse event profiles and fewer drug interactions. However, the effectiveness of these new ASMs in seizure control does not surpass their older counterparts. Recent studies have shown that the proportion of people with drug-resistant epilepsy (DRE) remains steady at around 30% of all people living with epilepsy, despite the expanded pharmacological options [104]. This implies the ASMs are not effective in reversing the course of the disease.

Currently, the pharmacological management of epilepsy is largely empirical. Once the diagnosis of epilepsy is confirmed, a patient is typically prescribed an ASM. The choice of drug depends on the clinician's discretion, considering factors such as epilepsy classification, patient demographics (e.g., childbearing potential), comorbidities, and potential drug interactions. The decision-making process may vary depending on the individual clinician's experience. If the initial ASM fails to control seizures, a second ASM may be added to, or substitute for the first. According to the criteria of International League Against Epilepsy (ILAE), a diagnosis of DRE can be made if a patient do not achieve sustained (12 months or more) seizure freedom after adequate trials of two appropriately ASMs [105]. Currently, there are no reliable biomarkers available to predict DRE at the time of epilepsy diagnosis. Patients often undergo a trial-and-error process until the right ASM may be selected, which can take months or even years to achieve the goal of seizure freedom or confirm the diagnosis of DRE [106].

On the other hand, the concept of Personalized Medicine or Precision Medicine has gained significant attention in recent years [107]. In the conventional treatment paradigm, various guidelines on selection of ASMs are based on clinical trials conducted with stringently selected patient groups. These studies draw conclusions by using large patient cohorts to ensure sufficient statistical power and minimize confounding factors. However, this evidence-based practice has been criticized as a "one-size-fits-all" approach that neglects the specific characteristics of individuals. In contrast, Personalized Medicine aims to customize therapy on the individual level. By gathering personal profiles, including demographics, genomics, radiographic, and physiological features, the most suitable therapy can be tailored to each patient. In the field of epilepsy, Personalized Medicine promises to be an achievable goal with advances in technology [108, 109]. For example, the development of pharmacogenomic panels may allow the prediction of responsiveness and potential adverse effects of ASMs in an individual patient [110]. Neuroimaging processing can detect subtle structural substrates of epileptogenicity, thereby enhancing the success rate of surgical treatment [111]. Automated analysis of EEG signals can be used to detect seizures and predict the prognosis of epilepsy [112]. All these techniques involve a huge amount of data that overwhelms manual analytical capacity.

3.5.2 Artificial Intelligence and Machine Learning

Artificial intelligence (AI) refers to the capability of a machine to imitate intelligent human thinking and learning. AI has a wide application in medicine. It has the advantage of precision, efficiency, and perpetuity. Hence, investment in AI in health care industry may save cost by reducing medical errors, streamline workflow and reducing manpower [113]. Novel applications emerge continuously; some notable examples are given below.

Robotics powered by AI has revolutionized the surgical field. Robotic-assisted surgery refers to a specialized robotic system to assist or replace the surgeon in certain procedures to enhance precision and minimize complication risk. These robotic systems even allow telesurgery, in which surgeons can operate on patients remotely [114, 115].

In the journey of management, a patient may have multiple consultations with various specialists or receive treatment from different institutes. Reconstruction of a patient's natural history from electronic medical records from different sources is now possible with Natural Language Processing (NLP) [116]. NLP is a subfield of AI that focuses on how computers could understand and generate human language.

An automatic medical image reporting system involves both computer vision and NLP. Computer vision algorithms process and analyze medical images. These algorithms employ various techniques such as image segmentation, object detection, and image classification to identify anatomical structures and abnormalities in the images. The findings of the input image are expressed as a structured and coherent textual report with the help of NLP.

The concept of applying AI in decision-making or problem-solving processes can be traced back to the mid-twentieth century. Clinical Decision Support Systems (CDSS) are software systems designed to facilitate daily clinical decisions [117]. With the incorporation of AI, the capabilities of CDSS can be enhanced. An exemplary example is the MYCIN system developed in the 1970s, which aimed to facilitate the management of bacterial infections [118]. It consisted of three major components: the knowledge base, inference engine, and user interface. The knowledge base contained facts provided by human experts, while the user interface facilitated communication between the computer software and the user. The data input into the inference engine by the user was then interpreted using a preset logic flow. The MYCIN system employed a backward chaining technique, which is a top-to-bottom approach that tracks backward to prove the truth of facts. Other examples of CDSS include an alert warning system in the computerized prescription program, where a warning signal appears if a patient has a potential drug allergy to the prescribed medication. Over the past two decades, there have been spectacular advances in computer technology, including the emergence of high-performance processors, massive storage, the internet, and cloud computing, nurturing the next generation of AI.

Machine Learning (ML) is a branch of AI that may help to solve many practical problems. ML can be broadly divided into supervised learning and unsupervised learning [119]. In supervised learning, a human-labeled training dataset is used to train the ML algorithm [120]. The training dataset consists of labeled input features matched with corresponding categorized outputs. Examples of supervised learning models include regression, random forest (RF), support vector machine (SVM), *k*-nearest neighbor (*k*NN), and Gradient Boosting Tree (GBT) [121–123]. Supervised learning has wide-ranging applications, such as classification, NLP, and image recognition. Classification predicts categorical outputs; NLP is used for analyzing text data (e.g., automated translators); and image recognition is used for recognizing images (e.g., face recognition systems). Unsupervised learning is usually used in hidden pattern recognition and association. Examples of unsupervised learning techniques include K-Means Clustering, Principal Component Analysis (PCA), and Autoencoders. Deep learning is a more advanced type of ML. It does not require manual input in feature selection; rather, the model could extract features from raw data. The algorithm structure is in the form of a multilayered artificial neural network. The inputs go through artificial neuron layers in a non-linear way and map into outputs. The deep learning model can also improve its performance as the size of the training data grows.

To develop an ML model, several key steps are involved, including data preprocessing, algorithm selection, model training, and performance evaluation. In the data preprocessing stage, data is collected from various sources, and any missing or irrelevant data is removed. Sometimes, features or variables in a dataset are transformed, such as conversion from a continuous scale to a categorical value, for the convenience of model fitting.

Next, suitable algorithms are selected based on the specific problem to be solved. In some cases, multiple models are developed and compared to select the one with the best performance.

Once the algorithm is selected, the dataset is divided into a training set and a validation set. The training set is used to teach the supervised learning model to make meaningful predictions. After training is completed, the model will then be validated to assess its performance and generalizability. Various validation techniques can be employed, such as k-fold cross-validation and leave-one-out cross-validation (LOOCV). In k-fold cross-validation, the whole dataset is divided into equal portions or folds of number k. The model is then trained on k-1 folds, and one-fold is left out for validation. The model is trained for k times, so that each of the k folds is used for validation [124]. In LOOCV, each observation is selected as a validation set while the rest of the observations (N-1) are considered as the training set. The choice of validation approach depends on the size of the dataset and the complexity of the computation involved.

Several metrics are commonly used to assess the performance of ML models. For example, in a classification task, performance metrics usually include accuracy, precision, recall, F-score, positive predictive value (PPV), negative predictive value (NPV), and area under the receiver operating characteristic curve (AUC). The AUC varies from zero to one, where one signifies a perfect classifier and 0.5 suggests a random classifier that is not better than chance.

It is valuable to understand the relative contribution of each feature in predicting within an ML model. This provides insights into the relationships between features and outcomes and helps improve the model. Established methods, such as model coefficient and permutation importance, can be used to assess the relative importance of different features in a predictive model. Model coefficient reflects the weight of a feature in a linear model, with the higher coefficient value indicating greater importance. Permutation importance is a model-agnostic approach that measures the impact of shuffling the value of a feature on the model's performance. By evaluating the drop in performance after shuffling each feature, one can determine its relative importance.

ML may be applied to solve problems in the development and clinical use of ASMs. In this chapter, we will focus on two main clinical applications: ASM response and DRE prediction.

3.5.3 Prediction of ASM Response

Devinsky et al. developed an RF model to predict the ASM with the highest likelihood of seizure control for individual patients utilizing claims data [125]. About 6 years of medical claims data were retrieved from a nationwide comprehensive claim database in the US. Adults with epilepsy were identified based on International Classification of Diseases, Ninth Revision (ICD-9) coding and pharmacy claims for ASMs. The researchers recruited cases with any one of the three conditions: (1) initiation of first ever ASM; (2) addition of ASM to an existing regimen; (3) substitution of an ASM by another ASM. The date of these major changes in regimen was defined as the index date. Patient's features and the treatment outcomes were extracted from 12 months before and after the index date, respectively. ASM substitution or addition of ASM to an existing regimen or complete withdrawal of the ASM was presumed to be treatment failure due to either inefficacy or intolerability.

A huge number of features, about 5000, covering demographics, comorbidities, therapeutic mechanism of ASMs, were available in each case. To avoid overfitting, a selection process with statistical criteria was implemented to filter out irrelevant features. The final training dataset included 34,990 patients, and the validation dataset comprised 8292 patients.

The trained RF model selected the ASM with the highest probability of a successful outcome as output. The machine-selected ASM was compared to the ASM chosen by physicians. The RF model achieved an AUC of 0.72. The ASM selected by the model matched with the physician's choice in only 13% of the cases. In this group, the treatment outcomes were found to be better with a lower chance of altering the ASM regimen. Other secondary outcomes, such as health service utilization, also favored ASM selection by the ML model.

This study used a claim database as the data source for developing an ML model. This kind of administrative database has certain advantages. It contains a large number of cases and is readily available. If the database has a broad coverage, the cohort obtained could minimize selection bias.

However, the claim database also has its limitations. Clinical details could not be directly retrieved. Clinical conditions have to be presumed by surrogate markers. In Devinsky's study, any change in ASM was supposed to be treatment failure, but it could not distinguish whether it was due to lack of efficacy or medication intolerance. Moreover, the database could not differentiate whether the ASMs are prescribed for seizure prophylaxis or other purposes, for instance, valproate could be used as a mood stabilizer and prophylaxis of migraine; gabapentin and pregabalin are commonly used to treat neuropathic pain. The diagnosis defined by coding may be subject to the pitfalls of either over-coding or under-coding. Commonly used clinical outcomes, such as seizure freedom or 50% seizure reduction, could not be obtained directly from the claim database.

Ouyang et al. designed an SVM model to identify biomarkers to predict the therapeutic outcomes of ASMs [126]. Quantitative EEG (QEEG) analysis of patients' background EEG was utilized as a biomarker to assess therapeutic efficacy. A total of 20 children living with epilepsy, 11 of whom responded to ASMs and 9 had DRE, were enrolled. EEG recordings were obtained from each patient at different time points before and after initiation or change of the ASM regimen. The EEG recordings were then analyzed by the QEEG technique. Discriminative features of the EEG were selected and fed into the SVM model to classify the treatment outcomes. A ten-fold cross-validation approach was adopted for internal validation. Finally, six EEG feature descriptors were found crucial in differentiating treatment-effective (seizure reduction >50%) and ineffective groups. The performance metric of the model yielded an accuracy of 83%.

This study integrated clinical and electrophysiological features to enhance the predictive capabilities of the ML model. However, there are drawbacks in the study that undermine its generalizability. First, the number of patients was small. Also, the recruited patients had different seizure subtypes, including both focal and generalized seizures. The EEG features of these seizure subtypes are known to have great discrepancies. On the other hand, the ASMs used by the patients could also affect the EEG tracing. In this study, the ineffective group more commonly had patients using ASM combinations, while the effective group more commonly used monotherapy. The effects of multiple ASMs or their drug interactions may cause bias in QEEG analysis when compared to a single ASM. Further study with a larger and more homogeneous patient population is needed to verify the results.

Zhang et al. attempted to estimate the therapeutic outcomes of specific ASMs by using ML [127]. An SVM classifier was developed to predict seizure freedom in epilepsy patients receiving levetiracetam based on both clinical and QEEG features. The study recruited 46 patients receiving levetiracetam from a single center in China. Twenty-two patients achieved seizure freedom while 24 did not. Eleven clinical features were selected as input, including (1) age; (2) duration of epilepsy; (3) family history of epilepsy; (4) seizure subtype (generalized, focal, or unknown onset); (5) seizure frequency in the 12 months before levetiracetam; 6) psychiatric comorbidities; (7) seizure circadian rhythm; (8) temporal lobe epilepsy; (9) time between levetiracetam initiation to the last seizure before levetiracetam; (10) interictal spikes in EEG; (11) positive MRI findings. For the EEG features, Sample Entropy of alpha, beta, theta, and delta frequencies was used to describe the data [128]. Sample entropy is a measurement used in signal processing and time series analysis to quantify the regularity or predictability of a signal. Four frequency bands of alpha, beta, theta, and delta were reconstructed and then used to calculate Sample Entropy for each patient in every channel.

To prevent overfitting, only strictly selective bands were extracted and incorporated into the input dataset. Consequently, four bands from four different channels were selected: beta bands from EEG lead Fp2, alpha bands from F4, theta bands from C3, and beta bands from F8. The 11 clinical and 4 QEEG features (Sample Entropy of alpha, beta, theta, and delta) of all patients formed the dataset and were then used to train and validate the SVM model. The algorithm was validated by five-fold cross-validation, hold-out validation, and jack-knife validation. Mean Impact Value (MIV) then assessed to determine the contribution of each feature to the model [129]. The results showed that the beta band from Fp2 played a crucial role in the classifier model. Clinical features of temporal lobe epilepsy, family history, circadian rhythm of seizure, MRI findings, comorbidity, time between levetiracetam initiation and last seizure, and duration of epilepsy had descending importance. As for QEEG features, beta band from Fp2 has a significant contribution. Interestingly, age, seizure type, interictal spikes, and seizure frequency before levetiracetam did not have a notable impact on the model.

The combined model of both clinical and EEG features yielded an AUC of 0.95 in the training dataset and an AUC of 0.96 in the validation dataset. The researchers tried to compare the performance of the SVM model with input of clinical features only, EEG features only, and combination of clinical and EEG features. The model with combined input demonstrated the best results.

The superior performance of the combined input integrating clinical and EEG inputs made clinical sense, as multiple modalities probably enhanced the accuracy of the classifier's prediction. However, the small number of recruited patients is a main drawback of the study. The specific bands of the four EEG channels showed a significant difference between seizure-free and non-seizure-free groups, but the authors did not postulate the electrophysiological mechanisms behind their findings. The high AUC values in both training and validation may imply the model has high generalizability. It is worthwhile to further evaluate the model in external validation by using an independent cohort.

Yao et al. constructed ML models to predict the outcomes of ASM in new-onset epilepsy [130]. A total of 287 patients with newly diagnosed epilepsy were recruited from a single center. The cohort had at least three years of follow-up. Fourteen demographic and clinical features were selected as input features of the model, including: (1) sex; (2) living area; (3) occupation; (4) education level; (5) age at seizure onset; (6) risk factors of epilepsy (including brain trauma, stroke intracranial infection, perinatal hypoxia, brain tumor); (7) family history of epilepsy; (8) seizure types (focal, generalized, or unknown onset); (9) number of seizures before treatment; (10) history of febrile seizure; (11) duration of previous treatment; (12) presence of multiple seizure types (more than one seizure type including focal aware, focal impaired awareness, focal to bilateral tonic–clonic, generalized onset, and unknown onset seizures); (13) EEG findings; (14) MRI findings.

In their treatment protocol, monotherapy of ASM was selected by the attending epileptologist. One of seven ASMs were selected: carbamazepine, oxcarbazepine, valproate, lamotrigine, levetiracetam, topiramate, and gabapentin. Outcomes from the first ASM were classified into three groups: early remission (less than six months after ASM commencement), late remission (more than six months after ASM commencement), and no remission (ongoing seizures after one year of ASM treatment). In the dataset, there were 207 remission cases, of which 140 were early remission and 67 were late remission, along with 80 cases of no remission.

The researchers compared the performance of five supervised ML models: Decision Tree, RF, SVM, Extreme Gradient Boosting (XGBoost), and Logistic Regression. Two experiments were conducted. In the first experiment, all 287 patients' data were used as a training dataset, aiming to predict remission versus no remission status. In the second experiment, data from 207 patients in the remission group were used as a training dataset, aiming to predict early versus late remission. A five-fold cross-validation was carried out for internal validation.

Among the five models, the XGBoost algorithm achieved the best metrics in predicting remission versus no remission, with an F1 score of 0.95 and an AUC of 0.98. The best predictor for remission versus no remission was the number of seizures before treatment. The XGBoost model also performed the best in predicting early remission versus later remission, with an F1 score of 0.84 and an AUC of 0.92. The presence of multiple seizure types had the most significant impact in predicting early versus late remission.

This study compares different ML models instead of preselection of a single model, therefore enhancing transparency in model selection. Another notable point is that the input features cover investigational results in addition to other clinical features from medical history and demographics. Both the EEG and MRI findings are incorporated as categorical features in the dataset. The XGBoost model achieved impressively high F1 and AUC values in predicting early remission versus late remission and remission versus no remission. One of the contributing factors was the application of grid search to optimize the hyperparameter set in hyperparameter tuning. Hyperparameters are parameters that are not learned during the training process, but are set before training and determine how the model learns and generalizes from the data. Hyperparameter optimization is the process of finding the best set of hyperparameters for an ML model. Of course, grid search also has its drawbacks, such as the requirement of additional computational resources and inability to deal with a large number of hyperparameters or extensive ranges of hyperparameter values.

Two related studies, conducted by Petrovski et al. and Shazadi et al., aimed to predict response to ASM in newly diagnosed epilepsy patients by exploiting pharmacogenomic markers [131, 132].

Petrovski et al. developed a multi-single nucleotide polymorphisms (SNPs) classification model to predict the treatment outcome of the first ASM in patients with newly diagnosed epilepsy [131]. A total of 115 patients with newly diagnosed epilepsy from two hospitals in Australia were enrolled. Treatment response was assessed at the end of the follow-up period of one year. Drug responders were defined as seizure freedom with the first ASM, while non-responders were defined as those with recurrent seizures while on the initial ASM.

Genotyping for 4041 SNPs in 279 candidate genes was performed. These candidate genes were chosen based on their roles in the pathogenesis of epilepsy or drug metabolism, as well as their high expression levels in the brain. The list of SNPs was further narrowed down, and five sophistically selected SNPs were finally included in the ML model development. The algorithm of *k*NN was employed as a classifier.

A five-fold cross-validation approach was employed for internal validation. In addition, the model was further externally validated by two independent validation cohorts. The first validation cohort comprised 63 newly diagnosed epilepsy patients from the same population, and the second cohort comprised 108 community-treated chronic epilepsy patients. The performance of the multi-SNP model was further compared with models based on individual SNAPs alone in each validation cohort.

The performance metrics showed promising results. In the cross-validation, the model achieved an accuracy of 84%. In the validation using the 63 newly diagnosed epilepsy patients, the model yielded a sensitivity of 91% and specificity of 53%. For the chronically treated epilepsy validation cohort, the multi-SNP classifier model achieved a sensitivity of 81% and specificity of 50%. The multi-SNP models consistently outperformed the single-SNP models in both independent validation cohorts.

Shazadi et al. further investigated Petrovski's multi-SNP model by externally validating it with larger independent cohorts [132]. They utilized two cohorts from the UK: the Glasgow cohort, consisting of 281 new-onset epilepsy patients, and a subset of patients from the SANAD study, which included 491 patients with genetic sampling [133]. The genotyping process was the same as in Petrovski's study, focusing on the five specific SNPs. The *k*NN algorithm retained identical input features as the original model. The UK cohorts were used to validate the multi-SNP model in three ways: (1) Petrovski's training dataset served as the training dataset, and each of the two UK cohorts as the test datasets; (2) retraining the *k*NN model using the SANAD cohort as both training and test datasets. A random 70:30 train-test split was adopted. The parameters of *k*NN were identical to those employed in the original Petrovski's model; (3) testing the performance of Petrovski's *k*NN model using an LOOCV approach in the UK cohorts.

The results showed that the multi-SNAPs model could reasonably predict the treatment responses in carbamazepine or valproate in both Glasgow and SANAD cohorts (Glasgow: odds ratio [OR] = 3.1, 95% confidence interval [CI] = 1.4–6.6, $p = 0.018$; SANAD: OR = 2.8, 95% CI: 1.3–6.1, $p = 0.048$). However, the model could not reliably predict lamotrigine and other ASM treatment responses in both UK cohorts.

These two studies tried to predict the response to ASM using genetic approach. The hypothesis that multiple SNPs could have a better prediction than a single SNP is sensible, as response to ASM is probably a trait influenced by multiple genetic variants. The possible reason for the failed external validation of the ML model on the two UK cohorts may be because of different prescription patterns between the Australian and UK cohorts. Carbamazepine and valproate were more commonly used for the new-onset epilepsy in the Australian cohorts, while lamotrigine or other ASMs were used more commonly in the UK cohorts [132]. This highlights the preference for prescription in different institutions or countries could be a source of bias in the dataset. It would be optimal to collect the developmental dataset from a diverse range of institutions and countries.

De Jong et al. combined both clinical and genetic data to develop an ML to predict the response to brivaracetam [134]. The data sources consisted of two patient cohorts from two randomized placebo-controlled clinical trials of adjunctive brivaracetam. The first cohort consisted of 235 patients, while the second cohort consisted of the other 47 patients. The data from the larger cohort was used for the developmental dataset for both training and internal validation, while the smaller group served as the retrospective validation dataset. The treatment response was defined as a > 50% reduction in seizure frequency after 12 weeks. Both the clinical and genetic features were incorporated into the ML models. Whole-genome sequencing (WGS) data of the patient cohorts were available. The huge amount of genetic data from

WGS was robustly narrowed down to a workable list of genetic features that related to mechanisms of epilepsy and drug action. Finally, four data modalities were employed, including: (1) mutational load scores; (2) polygenic risk score; (3) SV2A structural variance (the molecular target of brivaracetam); and (4) clinical data.

As some of the input features may be associated with placebo response, the researchers further validated the models with an extra placebo dataset. A cohort of 235 patients who were assigned to the placebo arm in the same clinical trial was used as the placebo dataset. However, genetic data was not available in this placebo cohort. The researchers assessed the placebo response in the model trained only on clinical data instead.

The researchers compared five different ML models, including sparse multi-block partial least squares discriminant analysis, multimodal neural network, elastic net classifier, GBT, and logistic regression-based stacking. The ML models underwent internal cross-validation and were further validated externally using the validation dataset.

Among the tested models, the GBT achieved the best performance parameters, with an AUC of 0.76 (95% CI: 0.76 ± 0.014) in the training dataset and 0.75 (95% CI: 0.75 ± 0.15) in the validation dataset. Analysis of the placebo cohort ensured that the model trained on the clinical data modality was not associated with a placebo effect.

The researchers demonstrated that the integration of genetic and clinical data modalities improved the model's performance (AUC of 0.76) compared to using clinical data alone (AUC of 0.71). Genetic factors included the presence of structural variants overlapping the SV2A gene and the mutational load in a gene set representing microtubule minus end binding. The only clinical factor that predicted brivaracetam responsiveness was prior levetiracetam use. Failure in levetiracetam use predicted a poor brivaracetam response.

This study has demonstrated that a meaningful model could be developed with a relatively small cohort. Such a drug response prediction model focusing on a single ASM could facilitate enrichment trials. Eligible subjects with a high probability of non-responsiveness could be screened out using an ML model before being recruited into a drug trial. This measure could effectively reduce the sample size by increasing the responder rate, making it easier to achieve statistically significant differences between the treatment and placebo groups in randomized controlled trials. It would also shorten the drug trial process and reduce the cost of drug development. However, the short duration of follow-up (12 weeks) and small absolute difference in seizure frequency in the corresponding clinical trials make the reliability of the developmental dataset questionable. On the other hand, the contribution of genetic data to the final model was surprisingly small, as reflected by the small increase from AUC 0.71 of the model with clinical features alone to AUC 0.76 of the model with a combination of clinical plus genetic features [135]. The cost-effectiveness of incorporating genetic data into the ML model is challenged.

Hakeem et al. have developed and validated a deep learning model to predict the response of the first ASM for new-onset epilepsy [136]. Five cohorts from Scotland,

Malaysia, Australia, and China, comprising 1798 adults with newly diagnosed epilepsy, were included for model development. An attention-based deep learning Transformer model was adopted in this study [137]. The model consists of an encoder and decoder, both of which have a multi-head attention mechanism. In this mechanism, each head is a separate attention layer that learns to attend to different relationships or patterns in the input data. By using multiple heads, the model can extract useful information from complex relationships and make more reliable predictions.

Sixteen clinical features were input into the model: (1) sex; (2) age group at ASM initiation; (3) history of febrile convulsion; (4) history of childhood CNS infection; (5) history of head trauma; (6) History of hypoxic brain injury; (7) history of alcohol abuse; (8) history of alcohol abuse; (9) epilepsy in first-degree relative; (10) history of cerebrovascular disease; (11) intellectual disability; (12) psychiatric disorder; (13) number of pretreatment seizure; (14) type of epilepsy; (15) EEG findings; (16) brain imaging findings. Shapley additive explanations (SHAP) value was used to assess the relative impact of each feature on the model. The output was one of seven ASMs (carbamazepine, lamotrigine, levetiracetam, oxcarbazepine, phenytoin, topiramate, or valproate), being considered as the best choice, giving the highest chance of treatment success as defined as seizure freedom while still using the first ASM within the first year of treatment. The study had two parts. In the first part, data from pooling the five study cohorts was randomly selected for training and validation. Approach of 80:20 train-test split was adopted. In the second part, the ML model was trained by using the Glasgow cohort, which is the largest of the five cohorts. The model was then validated on each of the remaining four cohorts. The researchers compared six different ML models, including transformer, multilayered perceptron (MLP), XGBoost, SVM, RF, and logistic regression, in both parts of the study.

Among the six models, the transformer model attained the best performance with an AUC of 0.65 (95% CI: 0.65 ± 0.02) and a weighted balanced accuracy of 0.62 (95% CI: 0.62 ± 0.02) on the test set.

In the second part of the study, the Transformer model was trained using the largest cohort and achieved AUCs in the range of 0.52–0.60 and a weighted balanced accuracy in the range of 0.51–0.62 in validation cohorts. Several pre-treatment seizures, EEG, and neuroimaging findings had the highest SHAP values in the pooled cohort and hence contributed most to the prediction model.

This study has two remarkable features. First, the dataset in the ML model development was derived from some of the largest, best-characterized adult cohorts of newly diagnosed epilepsy in the world [27, 138]. Second, a deep learning ML model instead of traditional statistical learning models was selected to predict the best ASM in new-onset epilepsy. This transfer learning technique allows their model to expand to diverse patient populations, tasks, and datasets with small sample sizes, with comparable performance to their large developmental dataset [139, 140]. The model could bring clinical implications if it could be further improved and validated.

3.5.4 Prediction of DRE

Silva-Alves et al. attempted to use both clinical and genetic parameters to predict drug responsiveness in patients with mesial temporal epilepsy [141]. They used an RF classifier for prediction. They gathered a cohort of 237 patients with mesial temporal lobe epilepsy, of which 75 were responsive to ASM and 162 were drug-resistant, from a single center in Brazil. ASM responsiveness was defined as seizure freedom for at least 12 months. DRE was regarded as a failure in reaching seizure freedom despite taking two or more ASMs either sequentially or in combination. Clinical features included gender, age of seizure onset, febrile seizures, and presence of hippocampal sclerosis on MRI. They genotyped 119 SNPs in 11 different genes. They ran the algorithm with the clinical features only, the genetic features only, and a combination of both clinical and genetic features. In addition, the researchers tried different combinations of features to train the model to obtain the best results. They validated their model by LOOCV. The mean decreased accuracy (MDA) value is used to show the most relevant features contributing to the best model [142].

The results showed that the clinical plus genetic features contributed model had the best performance. The best model included the presence of hippocampal sclerosis and 56 SNPs. Finally, the model based on a combination of clinical and genetic data achieved an AUC of 0.82, compared with an AUC of 0.46 for the model with clinical data only and an AUC of 0.80 with genetic data only. SNP in the CYP1A2 gene had the greatest MDA value and hence had the greatest contribution in the prediction model, followed by the presence of hippocampal sclerosis on MRI.

In the current study, the genetic component has a dominant contribution. It is reflected in the AUC of 0.80 for the genetic data only model compared with the AUC of 0.46 for the clinical only model. It contrasts with the aforementioned model developed by de Jong et al., in which clinical data bears more weight. This could be explained by the homogeneity of localization of epilepsy focus, that is, the temporal lobe, in this study, while in de Jong's study, the epilepsy foci were variable. It may imply that the epilepsy subtype should be targeted if genetic features are to be incorporated into the ML model.

An et al. aimed to predict DRE by making use of administrative data through an ML model [143]. They made use of a large claim database in the US. The researchers identified epilepsy and DRE cases indirectly. Epilepsy was defined by three criteria: (1) cases with one or more epilepsy diagnosis claim with ICD-9 or ICD-10 for epilepsy and recurrent seizures, or two claims for convulsion with appropriate ICD-9 or ICD-10 codes; (2) cases with more than one claim for an ASM; (3) cases with the first ASM prescribed as monotherapy for at least 60 days of supply. The authors identified 292, 892 epilepsy patients for inclusion in the dataset. Drug-responsive cases were defined as ordering of the same ASM regimen without the need for change for at least a year. Treatment failure was defined as a different ASM and claimed no matter whether it was an add-on, replacement of a current agent, or as rescue therapy. The definition of DRE in this study was different from the widely accepted consensus endorsed by the ILAE, which states failure of two appropriately chosen ASMs [105]. In this study, the failure of three ASMs was considered as DRE instead. Those who just failed one or two ASMs were excluded from the analysis. The proportion of DRE in their cohort was about 13%. For each patient, an index date was defined as the date when the first ASM was claimed. The period preceding the index date, traced back to the commencement of the health care plan, was defined as the observation window. The period following the index date, up until the date of the last claim, was defined as the evaluation window. The data extracted from the observation window was used to predict the drug responsiveness of epilepsy. Three ML algorithms were compared: multivariate logistic regression (MLR), SVM, and RF. A total of 1270 features were extracted from each patient, encompassing the demographics, comorbidities, insurance policy, treatments, and encounters. Half of the extracted features were finally used in the dataset to build the model. The dataset was randomly divided into a training set (60%), a validation set (20%), and a test set (20%). As a reference, the researchers formulated a benchmark model, which only contained two features, namely the age at epilepsy onset and sex. Information Gain value was used to demonstrate the relative contribution of features to the predictive model [144]. They used Brier scores and calibration plots to assess the reliability of the predicted probabilities output by the ML models [145, 146].

The RF was the best model in this study and achieved an AUC of 0.76 (95% CI: 0.76–0.77), outperforming the benchmark model with an AUC of 0.66 (95% CI: 0.65–0.66). Moreover, predicted probabilities for DRE were well-calibrated with the observed frequencies in the data. The research group analyzed the period from the index date to the date of initiation of the third ASM regimen, which was used as a surrogate marker of failure of the second ASM, which fulfilled the ILAE's definition of DRE. The period was 1.97 years on average. In other words, the RF model could predict ILAE-defined DRE approximately two years before a patient failed two ASMs.

The limitation of the study based on the claim database has been discussed before. Another major drawback of this study is that the definition of DRE departs from the definition accepted globally. A proxy of failure of three, rather than two, ASM regimens was considered as DRE. The aim of this may be to enable a greater contrast in data between DRE and non-DRE, and hence enhance the model performance [147]. This may again highlight the limitations of performing a clinical study by employing an administrative database.

Delen et al. aimed to predict DRE by training ML algorithms on data retrieved from a nationwide electronic medical record (EMR) database [148]. The researchers identified epilepsy patients by the ICD code of epilepsy in the diagnosis record. Drug responsiveness was assessed indirectly. DRE was defined by the use of non-ASM treatments, namely epilepsy surgery or VNS, while all cases with solely ASM treatment were assumed to be non-DRE. A total of 37,024 were finally recruited in the cohort. Among them, 806 had DRE and 36,218 had non-refractory disease. The features listed in the dataset included patient's demographic features namely age, gender, race, and marital status; physician's initial diagnosis; total comorbidity count; and presence of eight common comorbidities: hypertension, depression and anxiety, hyperlipidemia, drug abuse, head and neck symptoms, esophageal disease, anemia, and diabetes mellitus. The dataset was randomly split into a 70:30 ratio for training and validation, respectively. The contribution of each feature was evaluated by excluding features one at a time when running the model repeatedly. In each iteration, the performance difference of the model between including and excluding the specific feature could be calculated, reflecting the importance of the feature. Since the cohort was grossly imbalanced with a very small fraction of DRE cases (2.2%), the researchers used additional balancing measures to avoid biases.

Three ML algorithms were compared, including the decision tree, RF, and GBT. The performances of the three classifiers adopting each of the different balancing approaches were compared. The best combination attained an F1-score of 0.59, accuracy of 75%, and AUC of 0.83. The analysis of the relative importance of input features showed that comorbidity count was the most important feature in the prediction of DRE, followed by drug abuse, hypertension, and hyperlipidemia.

This study defines DRE with an unusual criterion; only cases with epilepsy surgery or VNS were considered as DRE. This is a marked discrepancy with the global consensus. It is well known that epilepsy surgery is underused in the DRE population. The reasons are multifactorial, including under-referral, lack of expertise, and low patient acceptance. The pitfall is reflected by the very low proportion (only 2.2%) of DRE in the cohort, compared to the commonly quoted proportion of around 30%. Although complex statistical measures have been employed, trying to balance the biased figure, the limitation could not be overcome. The high AUC but a relatively low F1 may imply a skewed dataset. The findings of comorbidities, including hypertension and hyperlipidemia, play an important role in predicting DRE are not entirely convincing.

The studies discussed above were summarized in Table 3.5.

3.5.5 Conclusions

The application of AI in epilepsy prognosis prediction is still in its infancy, although and growing number of research studies have shown encouraging results. A crucial factor in the successful development of a powerful predictive model lies in the availability of high-quality developmental datasets. An optimal cohort from which the dataset is generated should consist of reliable diagnoses, comprehensive investigations, and a longitudinal follow-up history. It would be ideal if the dataset could be collected from different centers to minimize biases in prescription preferences, patient demographics, and clinical backgrounds. External validation is an essential step to ensure the generalizability of an ML model. It involves testing the model on a new dataset independent of the model development. Unfortunately, this important step is lacking in most of the existing published models. Furthermore, the inclusion of genetics, radiological, and EEG features holds great potential to enhance the performance of the ML model. Similar to therapeutic agents or medical devices, the ultimate assessment of an ML model prior to widespread clinical use is a randomized controlled trial to verify its efficacy and safety in practice.

Table 3.5 Summary of the aim, strengths and limitations of the included studies

Author (year)	Aim of study	Highlights of study design	Number of patients recruited	Strength of study	Limitation of study
Prediction of ASM response					
Devinsky et al. [125] (2016)	To develop an ML model to select the ASM with highest successful outcome for an individual	ML model: RF Retrospective recruitments from claims database for both training and validation Index date of ASM change (initiation of new claim, add-on or substitution) was used to train the ML to predict ASM regimen with lowest likelihood of regimen change	34,990 patients from a claim database	Very large number of recruited cases from a national wide claims database	Important clinical features such as frequency of seizure, indication of ASM, etc. could not be obtained from the claim databases
Ouyang et al. [126] (2018)	To develop a ML model to differentiate ASM effective and ineffective groups	ML model: SVM EEG recorded before and one to three months after ASM initiation or change for QEEG features selection and model training EEG recorded before and six months after ASM initiation or change for model validation	20 patients from single center	Biomarkers of EEG was employed and analyzed by QEEG technique in the ML development	Small number of patients were recruited
Zhang et al. [127] (2018)	To develop a ML model to predict probability of seizure freedom in patients treated with LEV	ML model: SVM Retrospective recruitment of patients on LEV, employing both clinical and EEG sample entropy in various frequency bands as input features	46 patients from single center	Combination of biomarkers of EEG and clinical features were employed in the ML development Comparison of clinical features only model with EEG and clinical combination model proved the better performance of the combined model	Small number of patients were recruited The reasons of why some frequency bands of certain electrodes of EEG had relatively greater contribution to the ML model outcome than the others were not explained

(continued)

Table 3.5 (continued)

Author (year)	Aim of study	Highlights of study design	Number of patients recruited	Strength of study	Limitation of study
Yao et al. [130] (2019)	To develop a ML model to predict the outcomes ASM of patients with newly diagnosed epilepsy	ML models: Decision trees, RF, SVM, logistic Regression, XGBoost Retrospective recruitment of patients, employing 14 clinical features to train and validate the model	287 patients from single center	Different ML models were compared to choose the best performing one	Patients were recruited from single center, prescription preference, disease pattern may affect the model's generalizability
Petrovski et al. [131] (2009) and Shazadi et al. [132] (2014)	To develop and externally validate a ML model to predict the outcomes ASM of patients with newly diagnosed epilepsy	ML model: *k*NN Prospectively recruited patient cohort was employed for genetic data collection. Selected SNPs were input to train the model The model was validated by Australian and then the UK cohorts	115 Australian patients in training dataset; 63 patients from the same hospital population for validation; 108 community-treated patients for external validation; further external validation on two independent UK cohorts (281 from Glasgow and 491 from SANAD trial)	Genetic features were incorporated into the ML model. Multi-SNP model were compared to individual SNPs models and proved to be outperforming	The model failed to predict treatment response other than with CBZ or VPA in other independent cohorts upon external validation

De Jong [134] (2021)	To develop a ML model to predict the response to BRV	ML models: Sparse multi-block PLS-DA, multi-modal neural network, elastic net classifier, GBT, and logistic regression-based stacking Retrospective recruiting patients from two clinical trials on BRV Both clinical and highly selected genetic features were employed to develop the model The placebo dataset was used to train the model to prove the absence of placebo effects in the final results	235 patients from the treatment arm of a multicenter clinical trial as training dataset; 47 patients from the treatment arm of another multicenter clinical trial as validation dataset; 235 patients from the placebo arm of the same study of training dataset as placebo dataset	Both clinical and genetic features including those related specifically to BRV pharmacodynamics were incorporated in the ML model Relative high AUC (0.75) was achieved in external validation in independent cohort Comparison between genetics plus clinical model to the clinical only model proves that the combined model was superior	Small contribution of pharmacogenetics may indicate cost-ineffectiveness of employment of genetic data or a need of improvement of genetic input selection
Hakeem et al. [136] (2022)	To develop a ML model to predict the outcome of first ASM for newly diagnosed epilepsy	ML models: Transformer, MLP, XGBoost, SVM, RF, and logistic regression 16 clinical features as input for model development Two approaches to train and validate in order to select the best model	1798 patients from five cohorts from four countries	Large number of patients from cohorts from different countries were recruited for model development Deep learning model of transformer was employed	Moderate AUC (0.62) suggested room for further improvement
Prediction of DRE					
Silva-Alves et al. [141] (2017)	To develop an ML model to predict drug resistant mesial TLE	ML model: RF Both clinical and genetic (SNP) variables as input to develop the model	237 patients from single center	Employment of both clinical and genetics (multi-SNPs) in ML development Combination of genetics and clinical features greatly improve the model when compare with clinical only model	High sensitivity but low specificity of the model, probably limit its application. It may be more suitable in screening rather than diagnosing.

(continued)

Table 3.5 (continued)

Author (year)	Aim of study	Highlights of study design	Number of patients recruited	Strength of study	Limitation of study
An et al. [143] (2018)	To develop a ML model to predict DRE	ML models: SVM, RF, MLR Retrospective recruitments from claims database for both training and validation Proxy indicators, such as changes in ASM claim, as surrogates for clinical features	292,892 patients from a claim database	A great number of cases from a claim database were employed	Unusual definition of DRE (those who failed three ASMs rather than two) was used
Delen et al. [148] (2020)	To develop a ML model to predict DRE	ML model: Decision trees, RF, GBT Retrospective recruitments from claims database for both training and validation Proxy indicators as surrogates for clinical features	37,024 patients from a EMR database	A great number of cases from a nationwide EMR database were employed	Unusual definition of DRE (those with VNS and epilepsy surgery) was used resulting in very low proportion of DRE

ASM antiseizure medication, *AUC* area under curve, *DRE* drug resistant epilepsy, *EMR* electronic medical record, *GBT* gradient boosting Tree, *kNN* k-Nearest Neighbor, *ML* machine learning, *MLP* multilayer perceptron, *MLR* multivariate logistic regression, *PLS-DA* partial least squares-discriminant analysis, *QEEG* quantitative EEG, *RF* random forest; sparse multi-block partial least squares discriminant analysis, *SNP* single nucleotide polymorphism, *SVM* support vector machine, *TLE* temporal lobe epilepsy, *VNS* vagus nerve stimulation, *XGBoost* extreme gradient boosting

Achieving all these goals requires close collaboration between clinicians, data scientists, and ML specialists. The synergistic efforts of such interdisciplinary teams could lead to a paradigm shift in the management of epilepsy, ultimately achieving the goal of Personalized Medicine for epilepsy.

3.6 Acute Symptomatic Epileptic Seizures

Based on the ancient disease of epilepsy, the International ILAE named the phenomenon of epilepsy epileptic seizure, epileptic syndrome, epileptic status, and epilepsy. Epilepsy can be divided into primary, cryptogenic, and symptomatic epilepsy according to its cause. Recently, the ILAE has defined epilepsy as a chronic brain disease, so the first seizure caused by an acute brain disease is not in the category of epilepsy, but the clinical manifestations of such patients and seizures are almost the same, so it needs to be renamed. Acute symptomatic seizures may be more consistent with the connotation of seizures in such patients [1, 149].

3.6.1 Definition of Acute Symptomatic Epilepsy

No international organization has established an accepted definition of acute symptomatic epilepsy or guidelines for its prevention and treatment. However, this professional term has been described in the literature. A PubMed database search revealed 1110 related studies on acute symptomatic epilepsy as the main topic, indicating that this topic has a basis for publication. According to the literature, acute symptomatic epilepsy refers to the first seizure caused by an acute brain disease (structural or functional). Because it is the first seizure, it is not accepted according to the ILAE definition for the diagnosis of epilepsy. However, epilepsy is clearly defined by the ILAE for such patients if there are repeated seizures in the future, indicating that there is some intrinsic link between them. Therefore, studying the clinical characteristics of acute symptomatic seizures can help us address the presence of such seizures.

3.6.2 Historical Evolution

According to the PubMed database, Feikes et al. [150] first mentioned acute symptomatic seizures in 1964. They mentioned acute symptomatic seizures in patients presenting with hyponatremia after acute surgery. In 1967, Varavithya et al. [151] mentioned the existence of acute symptomatic seizures in their summary of acute hyponatremia in children. In 1984, when studying alcohol abuse, Pilke et al. [152] reported that acute symptomatic seizures occur after alcohol withdrawal. In 1992, Hauser et al. [153] proposed that age is the determining factor for the occurrence of acute symptomatic seizures in a variety of metabolic or central nervous system injuries in their study on epileptic seizures. In 2024, Grau-Lopez et al. [154] summarized the etiology of acute symptomatic epilepsy and proposed prevention and treatment methods, which increased the recognition of acute symptomatic epilepsy.

3.6.3 Etiology of Acute Symptomatic Epilepsy

The occurrence of acute symptomatic epilepsy is mainly related to brain dysfunction, and the causes of brain dysfunction can be divided into two categories: structural and nonstructural damage. Acute symptomatic epilepsy was first reported by Feikes et al. [150], who reported that hyponatremia after surgery could cause acute symptomatic epilepsy. In 2024, Grau-Lopez et al. [154] analyzed the etiology of symptomatic seizures after acute structural brain injury in 194 patients and reported that the identifiable etiologies included hemorrhagic stroke (44.8%), ischemic stroke (19.5%), traumatic brain injury (18.5%), and meningoencephalitis (17%). Subsequently, Pais-Cunha et al. [155] analyzed the etiology of cerebral venous thrombosis and acute symptomatic epilepsy in 54 children and reported that progressive brain injury (8 patients with malignant tumors, 5 with blood disease), head and neck infection, head trauma, intracranial hemorrhage, and cerebral infarction were common causes. Hernandez-Prieto et al. [156] studied 165 newborns and reported that 43 of these patients had acute symptomatic seizures, 19 patients (34%) of whom had hypoxic-ischemic encephalopathy, and 22 patients (40%) had other acute diseases. Of these, 6 (11%) patients were found to have genetic mutations. Cerebral microhemorrhage (CMB) is a marker of small vessel disease and is very common in ischemic stroke patients, but its relationship with acute symptomatic epilepsy has not been well studied. In 2023, Lekoubou et al. [157] conducted a retrospective cohort study on hospitalized patients with precirculation ischemic stroke complicated with microhemorrhage and reported that among 381 patients, 17 (4.5%) had seizures, and the incidence of epilepsy was three times greater in patients with microbleeds than in those without microbleeds. These studies suggest that the incidence of acute symptomatic epilepsy may vary by etiology, but it is not uncommon. Based on animal experiments, Karan et al. [158] confirmed that local brain injury can cause acute symptomatic seizures.

3.6.4 Epidemiological Investigation

Tsur et al. [159] investigated 816,252 newly enlisted soldiers in Israel. In addition to excluding soldiers with a history of epilepsy and no records of seizures, 346 soldiers experienced acute symptomatic epilepsy, and they believed that the incidence of acute symptomatic epilepsy was 16.2 cases/100,000 cases/year. De Stefano et al.

[160] investigated 1010 patients in the emergency department and reported that 501 patients (49.6%) had acute symptomatic seizures. Sinka et al. [161] investigated 4552 adult stroke patients and reported that 226 (5%) had acute symptomatic epileptic seizures, 8 (0.2%) of whom had status epilepticus (SE). Central nervous system infection is also a common cause of acute symptomatic seizures. Hersh et al. [162] studied 23 patients with herpes simplex encephalitis and reported that 58.3% had acute symptomatic seizures. Metabolic and toxic factors can also cause acute symptomatic seizures [150–152].

3.6.5 Clinical Manifestations

Acute symptomatic seizures mainly manifest as epileptic seizures, SE, and electrical abnormalities. Lopez-Espejo et al. [163] studied 207 children and newborns with stroke and found that acute symptomatic epileptic seizures in these children manifested as SE, epileptic seizures, and epileptic discharge on EEG. Meletti et al. [164] studied patients admitted for the first time with focal SE and found 137 independent, self-limited seizures in these patients. Kim et al. [165] studied 2312 stroke patients and reported that 54 (2.3%) had acute symptomatic seizures. The main manifestations were bilateral tonic–clonic seizures (42.6%).

3.6.6 Predictor

Not all acute brain injuries lead to symptomatic seizures, but the occurrence of symptomatic epilepsy is not rare. Therefore, whether to predict the occurrence of acute symptomatic epilepsy has become an important research topic. Cerebral vein thrombosis is a common cause of acute symptomatic epilepsy. Agircan et al. [166] conducted a study on acute symptomatic epilepsy caused by cerebral vein thrombosis and reported that the serum multiple inflammation index (MII) 1–2 was significantly increased in patients with acute symptomatic epilepsy. These findings suggest that MII-1 and MII-2 may serve as novel predictive and prognostic markers for acute symptomatic seizures in patients with cerebral venous thrombosis.

3.6.7 Relationship Between Acute Symptomatic Seizures and Epilepsy

(1) Acute symptomatic seizure: Acute symptomatic seizures are a manifestation of the primary disease and disappear with the improvement of the primary disease in most cases. Therefore, treatment is not necessary, and the impact on the overall

prognosis is not good; however, if noninduced seizures occur after the primary disease improves, chronic epilepsy can develop. Therefore, the recurrence of epilepsy is a key factor affecting the overall prognosis. Among 194 patients with acute symptomatic seizures reported by Grau-Lopez et al. [154], 56 (29%) had a second seizure during a 2-year follow-up, indicating that 29% of patients with acute structural brain injury may develop epilepsy. Among 54 patients with cerebral venous thrombosis described by Pais-Cunhaz et al. [155], 3 experienced seizures. Among 346 patients with acute symptomatic seizures described by Tsur et al. [159], 29.2% experienced recurrent seizures during follow-up. Rodrigo-Gisbert et al. [167] conducted a study on 230 patients with SE and reported that 198 patients (86.1%) had acute symptomatic epileptic status, 55 patients (23.9%) of whom later experienced seizures. Rodrigo-Gisbert et al. [168] followed 360 patients after their first onset of SE for 1.8 years and reported that 109 patients (30.3%) experienced seizures during the follow-up period, suggesting that 5–30% of patients with acute symptomatic seizures with brain injury develop chronic seizures within 1–3 years. (2) Factors related to the development of chronic epilepsy: not all acute symptomatic seizures evolve into chronic epilepsy requiring treatment, so predicting the development of chronic epilepsy has become important for improving patient prognosis. Grau-Lopez et al. [154] conducted a study on 194 patients with acute symptomatic seizures due to acute structural brain injury and found that significant epileptiform discharge on EEG and SE were important markers for epilepsy recurrence within 2 years and progression to chronic epilepsy. Lopez-Espejo et al. [163] studied 207 children and newborns and reported that patients with acute symptomatic SE, abnormal EEG activity, and cortical lesions were more likely to experience epilepsy recurrence. In a prospective cohort study of EEG monitoring of 81 patients with ischemic stroke, Tatillo et al. [169] also reported that patients with highly suggestive rhythmic or periodic patterns on EEG and no delta region attenuation which is an important indicator for predicting the progression of chronic epilepsy, had a greater likelihood of epilepsy recurrence. It is suggested that continuous EEG monitoring can provide useful information for identifying patients at greater risk of epilepsy after stroke, which can aid in individualized treatment and care. Rodrigo-Gisbert et al. [167] studied 198 patients with acute symptomatic SE and reported that etiology, time to start treatment, EEG pattern, and nonresponsiveness were strong predictors of epilepsy formation after new SE. These studies have shown that SE, epileptoid discharge on EEG, and progressive aggravation of etiology (such as tumor, autoimmune encephalitis, and progressive brain injury) are strong predictors of the progression of acute symptomatic epilepsy to chronic epilepsy [170].

3.6.8 Treatment of Acute Symptomatic Seizures

The management of acute symptomatic seizures involves determining whether medication is needed during acute seizures and the primary and secondary prevention of acute symptomatic seizures. (1) Whether ASMs are needed: Whether acute symptomatic epilepsy needs to be treated with medication has always been controversial. Acute symptomatic seizures are a symptom of the primary disease, and as the primary disease improves, most seizures stop on their own. Considering the side effects of drugs and treatment uncertainty, the use of ASMs is not necessary. Kim et al. [165] reported that 54 (2.3%) of 2312 stroke patients had acute symptomatic seizures. They found that seizures could increase NIHSS scores but had no effect on treatment, and the prognosis of patients with epilepsy was the same as that of patients with or without treatment. Tyvaert et al. [171] suggest that epilepsy of immune origin can be divided into two types: acute symptomatic seizures secondary to autoimmune diseases and autoimmune-related seizures; the latter refers to chronic seizures and requires long-term treatment, while the former only refers to acute symptomatic seizures, for which the use of ASMs has little effect [172]. However, Byrnes et al. [173] conducted a study on 465 stroke patients, 101 of whom used ASMs for a long time, mainly due to the abnormal EEG data of the patients. Therefore, they suggested that acute symptomatic epileptic seizures with risk factors still need to be treated with ASMs. Sortino et al. [174] also advocated the selection of ASMs. A comparison of phenobarbital, midazolam, valproic acid, and other drugs revealed that lidocaine and levetiracetam may be more effective for treating acute symptomatic epileptic seizures in children. (2) Primary prevention: Zaccara et al. [175] reviewed the literature on the need for primary prevention of acute symptomatic seizures and found that the evidence supporting primary prevention of acute symptomatic seizures was limited and of low quality, which was not enough for routine recommendation. (3) Secondary prevention: Whether ASMs are needed to prevent acute symptomatic seizures from progressing to chronic seizures has not been determined. A total of 75.7% of the 346 patients described by Tsur et al. [159] took ASMs, and the authors speculate that ASMs are beneficial for reducing seizures during follow-up. Qiang et al. [176] studied 488 patients, 58 (11.9%) of whom had seizures 3 years after intracerebral hemorrhage. They did not find that preventive use of ASMs had an effect on patient seizures, suggesting that secondary prevention of seizures was not necessary, and Zaccara et al. [175] did not recommend secondary prevention of acute symptomatic seizures. (4) Discontinuation of ASMs: Although acute symptomatic epilepsy is unlikely to be followed by chronic epilepsy, secondary prevention has no definite efficacy. Byrnes et al. [170] reported that most patients with acute symptomatic epilepsy were still taking ASMs after discharge, and their survey of clinics specializing in acute symptomatic epilepsy management also revealed that 27% of patients continued to take ASMs even when they did not have seizures or seizure-like abnormalities. Herzig-Nichtweiß et al. [30] reported that acute symptomatic epilepsy is very common in neurological intensive care. To prevent subsequent seizures, long-term treatment with ASMs is often prescribed despite a lack of supporting evidence. It has also been argued that the selective use of ASMs may be appropriate for patients with acute symptomatic seizures with risk factors, so ASMs are chosen [159, 173]. Therefore, patients taking ASMs need to receive personalized management to achieve safe withdrawal of drugs. An online survey showed that the majority of neuro-intensivists suggest that the use of these ASMs should generally not be for more than 3 months [177].

3.7 Amygdala Epilepsy and SUDEP

The amygdala is a group of nuclei located deep inside the temporal lobe. Although its role in seizures has long been recognized, its relationship with sudden, unexplained death in epileptic patients (SUDEP) has been revealed with advances in neuroimaging techniques for detecting brain activity. Further elucidation of its role in SUDEP development will increase our understanding of SUDEP.

3.7.1 Definition of Amygdala Epilepsy

Although it has long been noted that the amygdala plays a role in seizures, research on epilepsy has remained limited to the hippocampus and the surrounding regions. In recent years, owing to the development of functional magnetic resonance and stereotactic electroencephalography (EEG) techniques, the importance of amygdala epilepsy has received renewed attention [178, 179].

Seizures that originate in and around the amygdala are called amygdala epilepsy. A total of 3847 published papers with amygdala epilepsy as the main topic are available in the PubMed database, indicating that amygdala epilepsy is receiving widespread attention.

3.7.1.1 Historical Evolution of Amygdala Epilepsy

In 1954, Kaada [180] discovered for the first time that stimulation of the amygdala complex in unanesthetized cats produced seizure-like manifestations. Subsequently, Sawa et al. [181] successfully induced seizures in dogs through the application of alumina cream to the amygdala, confirming that the amygdala is related to the development of epilepsy and that removal of the amygdala can reduce the occurrence of psychomotor epilepsy [182]. In 1961, De Giacomo [183] described cholinesterase activity in the human amygdala complex, and in 1963, Pagni et al. [184] used deep electrodes to study potentials after human amygdala-hippocampus discharge. With the widespread use of magnetic resonance and stereotactic EEG in clinical practice, a deeper understanding of the anatomical and physiological functions of the amygdala has been gained [178, 179]. In 2024, Dalla Corte [178] described the anatomical structure of the amygdala from a new perspective and emphasized that the amygdala is related to the autonomic nervous system, emotional activity, and network connections. In the same year, Ya-Chin Yang [185] revealed the unique plasticity of amygdala network connections/reconnections and suggested that this telencephalic plasticity leads to the occurrence of epilepsy and many other diseases.

3.7.2 Characteristics of Amygdala Epilepsy

Amygdala epilepsy most often manifests as drug-resistant temporal lobe epilepsy, which is often accompanied by bilateral tonic-clonic seizures and apnea during or after a seizure. Ariane E Rhone [186] studied eight children with intractable epilepsy who underwent intracranial EEG and reported that all eight subjects (ages 3–17) experienced breathing pauses during amygdala nucleus stimulation; the patients were not aware that they had stopped breathing, and no one reported breathing difficulties. This pattern is very similar to the respiratory function in SUDEP. They also reported that in two patients, apnea occurred simultaneously with the spread of epilepsy to the amygdala.

Using machine learning algorithms for 45 stimulation sites and 210 stimulation trials, artificial intelligence technology identified the human amygdala respiratory depression site in the medial region of the basal ganglia, the cortex and medial nuclei, the amygdala transition region, and embedded neurons, which may be valuable for identifying the population at greatest risk of SUDEP and as a therapeutic target. William P Nobis [187] analyzed data from 8 studies with a total of 22 seizures and reported that apnea associated with each seizure was highly correlated with the spread of seizures to the amygdala. Apnea can occur 2.7 ± 0.4 (mean ± SEM) seconds after the seizure spreads to the amygdala, significantly earlier than after the seizure spreads to the hippocampus (10.2 ± 0.7 seconds; $p < 0.01$). These findings suggest that activation of the amygdala network is associated with central apnea during seizures, confirming the role of the amygdala in autonomic respiratory control. Brian J Dlouhy [188] conducted EEG and electrocardiography (ECG) monitoring on a patient with refractory epilepsy and reported that when the seizure affected the amygdala, apnea occurred, and stimulation of the amygdala also caused respiratory arrest in the patient. Moreover, a similar phenomenon was also reported in another study involving two patients. Surprisingly, the patients did not know that they had stopped breathing and did not have difficulty breathing after apnea occurred, unlike patients with non-amygdala seizures, in whom prolonged breathing cessation would result in severe hypoxia.

3.7.3 Relationship Between Amygdaloid Epilepsy and SUDEP

SUDEP is defined as "sudden, unexplained death in a person with epilepsy, and autopsy does not reveal a structural or toxicological cause of death, but there is often evidence of associated seizures" and is an important cause of death in patients with epilepsy. SUDEP is usually not witnessed and is diagnosed after an autopsy. SUDEP has been reported to occur in 1–2 people per 1000 population per year and is the most common cause of seizure-related death [189].

3.7.3.1 Relationships Between Amygdala Seizures and SUDEP

(1) Clinical studies: Most patients with SUDEP exhibit bilateral tonic–clonic seizures; therefore, this type of seizure is generally considered a high-risk factor for SUDEP. To understand the changes in the amygdala in these high-risk SUDEP patients, Antoine Legouhy et al. [190] selected 53 healthy subjects and 143 patients with epilepsy and determined amygdala volumes from structural MR images and tissue microstructure from diffusion MR images to identify differences between the groups. Diffusion tensor imaging (DTI) and neurite direction dispersion and density imaging (NODDI) models were fit to obtain diffusion measures, and the changes in the amygdala were analyzed; compared with healthy subjects, the amygdala was larger in epileptic patients and had a lower neurite density index (NDI), especially on the left side. This finding reflects the impaired microstructure of the amygdala, which decreases the input from the driving sites and regions in the brain that regulate timed breathing and are critical for blood pressure control, indicating that the amygdala is involved in SUDEP. Bilateral tonic–clonic seizures, central apnea during seizures, and post-seizure apnea are the three major risk factors for SUDEP, and the amygdala is a key structure that can trigger apnea in patients with focal epilepsy. To understand the relationship between the amygdala and SUDEP, Claudia Zeicu [191] studied high-resolution T1-weighted anatomic images and diffusion images of 73 patients with single-focal epilepsy and 30 patients with these risk factors and calculated the NODDI index. The results revealed that the volume of the amygdala was increased in patients with risk factors for SUDEP. Patients with bilateral tonic–clonic seizures with central apnea exhibited the greatest increase in bilateral amygdala volume. The amygdaloid NDI values were significantly lower in both the focal seizure group and the focal bilateral tonic–clonic seizures (FBTCS) group than in the healthy control group, with the FBTCS group having the lowest values. Patients with respiratory changes had significantly lower NDI values than patients with tonic–clonic seizures without apnea. The authors suggest that identifying changes in the volume and structure of the amygdala could help identify individuals at risk.
(2) Studies in animals: Cardiovascular alterations are often associated with epilepsy in clinical and experimental models and are hypothesized to be potential risk factors for SUDEP.

To understand the relationship between the amygdala and SUDEP, Poliana Peres Ghazale et al. [192] used a rat model to study the influence of amygdala ignition on the cardiovascular system of animals. In vitro, when vascular reactivity was used as an indicator, amygdala ignition was found to change aortic ring vasodilation. These findings suggest that the analysis of vascular endothelial function in high-risk SUDEP patients may be beneficial. Both human and animal models have shown that respiratory arrest is the leading cause of cases of sudden death; seizures spread to and stimulate the amygdala, leading to apnea, which causes sudden death. To further understand whether the amygdala is involved in epileptic apnea, a study in DBA/1 mice by Anthony Marincovich et al. [193] was conducted and revealed that electrical damage to the amygdala reduced the incidence of respiratory arrest. These results suggest that the amygdala is a key node in the circuit leading to the lower brain stem, and its involvement is necessary for respiratory arrest to occur during seizures. These findings suggest that the amygdala may be a key node in the brainstem respiratory network that leads to apnea during seizures.

3.7.3.2 Relationships Between SUDEP Risk Factors and the Amygdala

Bilateral tonic–clonic seizures, apnea during or after seizures, and arrhythmia are the most obvious risk factors for SUDEP [194, 195].

1. Epileptic seizures: Most people with epilepsy experience significant seizures in the period before death, but not at the time of SUDEP. Alyma Somani et al. [196] conducted a control study on 15 patients with SUDEP, 12 patients with epileptic seizures, and 10 patients with non-epileptic seizures. Quantification of the biomarkers galanin, neuropeptide Y (NPY) and somatostatin (SST) in the basal and parabasal nuclei and amygdala showed that the levels of galanin, NPY and SST in all amygdala regions were significantly lower in SUDEP patients than in seizure patients and that the level of galanin in the lateral nucleus was lower than that in the non-epileptic group. The authors suggest that seizures can induce a significant decrease in or acute depletion of lateral nuclear galanin in patients, thus inducing SUDEP. Therefore, controlling epilepsy, especially seizures in patients with drug-resistant epilepsy, is beneficial for reducing the occurrence of SUDEP [197]. Ryley Collard et al. [198] demonstrated in animal experiments that seizure-induced respiratory arrest was significantly reduced after the administration of galanin simulants in the central brain regions (intraventricular, amygdala) and the whole body (intraperitoneal, subcutaneous). These findings suggest that the central and systemic use of galanin analogs can protect C57BL/6 J mice from cardiac arrest after the first exposure.
2. Apnea during or after seizures: (1) Apnea after seizures in epileptic patients: Nuria Lacuey [199] investigated 19 epileptic patients and reported that 13 patients had central apnea. Ester Tio [200] studied the breathing of 453 patients with epilepsy and reported that apnea occurred during 79.9% of the 164 seizures in 41 patients who underwent multimodal respiratory monitoring. In 33.3% of seizures, central apnea preceded abnormal EEG discharge by 13 ± 11 seconds. A total of 48.7% of the epileptic seizures occurred 18 ± 14 seconds before the EEG abnormality. Walker [201] et al. studied 79 seizures (70 complex partial seizures and 9 systemic seizures) in 37 patients (20 men and 17 women) and reported that apnea occurred during 100% of generalized tonic–clonic seizures (GTCSs) and 39% of complex partial seizures. This central apnea lasted 10–75 seconds (mean duration of 29 seconds) and may be one of the main factors that induce SUDEP. (2) Relationship between apnea and SUDEP after epileptic seizure: Stephan [202] reported a patient with temporal lobe epilepsy whose seizure monitoring device recorded two focal seizures accompanied by

central apnea lasting 57–58 seconds, during which her oxygen saturation dropped to 68% and 62%; the patient subsequently died of SUDEP confirmed postmortem. These findings suggest that apnea after a seizure is the main cause of SUDEP. L So [203] reported that a 20-year-old woman had a convulsive seizure for 56 seconds while undergoing video EEG monitoring, followed by apnea, which lasted for 57 seconds before stopping. The authors suggested that a possible mechanism of SUDEP was central respiratory depression after epileptic seizures. Laura Vilella [204] monitored autonomic and respiratory biomarkers of SUDEP in patients with refractory epilepsy and reported that post-convulsive central apnea (PCCA) occurred in 31 out of 140 seizures (22.1%) in 22 patients, including one patient who died of probable SUDEP during follow-up. Two patients died of suspected SUDEP, and apnea after a seizure was considered a biomarker of SUDEP. (3) Apnea in amygdala epilepsy: Gail Is Harmata [205] used a multimodal approach to study 20 patients with intractable epilepsy to understand the cause of apnea after seizures and reported that amygdala seizures could lead to apnea. Elisa Micalizzi [206] performed a whole-brain voxel-based morphometry (VBM) test on 16 patients with apnea and 30 patients without apnea and reported that the volume of gray matter in the ipsilateral amygdala increased in patients with apnea. The authors suggested that the study results confirmed that the amygdala plays a key role in respiratory changes during seizures.

Using animal experiments, Gail Is Harmata [205] identified a unique region in the amygdala, the electrical stimulation of which can cause long-term respiratory depression lasting after the stimulation is over. They also reported that persistent apnea is resistant to rising carbon dioxide levels, indicating impaired chemical sensitivity to carbon dioxide. Furthermore, using a method combining electrical stimulation with functional MRI, they found that amygdala stimulation altered blood oxygen level-dependent (BOLD) activity in the pontine/medulla oblongata and ventral insula, and these findings suggested that epileptic activity in the amygdala subregion was sufficient to cause prolonged breathing suppression. This activity may be located in the brainstem and insula, which are involved in chemical and visceral sensations. The findings help identify those most at risk and could be a way to prevent SUDEP.

Frida A Teran [207] summarized the relationships among amygdala seizures, post-seizure apnea, and SUDEP and argued that the death of patients during monitoring in hospital epilepsy wards suggested that most SUDEP cases were caused by post-seizure central apnea. Respiratory depression may occur when a seizure invades the amygdala and activates brainstem projections, and there is evidence that the occurrence of this respiratory depression is related to deficits in the serotonin system and central carbon dioxide chemical sensing. These mysterious epilepsy comorbidities cause premature death in 17%–50% of people with epilepsy.

3.7.4 Prediction and Prevention of SUDEP Caused by Amygdala Seizures

Prevention strategies for SUDEP include timely referral of patients with drug-resistant epilepsy for preoperative evaluation and improvement in lifestyle to reduce the occurrence of GTCS; monitoring cardiopulmonary distress by clinical observation and respiratory and heart rate monitoring equipment; preventing airway obstruction with night supervision and safety pillows; reducing central hypoventilation through physical stimulation and enhancing the serotonergic mechanisms of respiratory regulation with selective serotonin reuptake inhibitors (SSRIs); and reducing adenosine- and endogenous opioid-induced brain and brainstem inhibition [197, 208–210].

3.7.4.1 Magnetic Resonance Examination of Amygdala Seizures

SUDEP is closely related to the amygdala. For patients with frequent bilateral tonic–clonic seizures, especially drug-resistant seizures, magnetic resonance examination of the amygdala is needed. If the amygdala of epilepsy patients is enlarged, physicians and patients should be aware of the possibility of SUDEP. In particular, it is necessary to pay more attention to the possibility of SUDEP when the NDI value of the amygdala is significantly reduced. For example, the incidence of SUDEP is very high in patients with post-paroxysmal apnea and bilateral tonic–clonic seizures. Given that most cases of SUDEP occur after a generalized seizure, with patients usually lying in bed in a prone position, sleep monitoring and seizure control may be beneficial in reducing SUDEP [178, 190, 191].

3.7.4.2 Serotonin Transferrin

Serotonin dysfunction is associated with SUDEP. Postmortem examination of SUDEP patients revealed a reduction in the number of medullary serotonergic neurons (respiratory regulators that respond to hypercapnia). Smriti Patodia [36] et al. studied the amygdala of 17 SUDEP patients after death and compared them with those of another 10 non-SUDEP patients and 8 non-epileptic control patients. Through graphical analysis of serotonin transporters in 13 regions of interest, the immunohistochemical labeling index (LI) and axon length (AL) of serotonin transporters were found to be highest in the amygdala and hypothalamic regions; higher LI and AL values were observed in the amygdala and basal and accessory basement of the periamygdala cortex in SUDEP patients than in epileptic controls. Compared with epileptic controls, higher levels of serotonin reuptake inhibitors in the hippocampal subregion in patients with SUDEP risk factors and in the amygdala in postmortem SUDEP patients revealed changes in the function of the serotonergic network supporting the amygdala limbic region in SUDEP patients.

Katelyn G Joyal [179] investigated whether increasing serotonin (5-HT) neurotransmission with drugs prior to seizures could improve post-seizure respiratory depression. They selected 84 amygdala-lit mice that were pretreated with SSRIs or 5-HT2 receptor agonists and reported that, regardless of sleep status, SSRIs inhibited apnea during or after an episode. Citalopram and the 5-HT2 agonist TCB-2, which are SSRIs, reduce respiratory variability at different post-seizure time points, suggesting that 5-HT mechanisms dependent on or independent of the 5-HT2 receptor family can affect normal respiratory recovery processes. Fluoxetine may reduce episodic central apnea, especially in patients with SUDEP risk factors [211].

Central apnea during seizures and after convulsions is related to the pathological mechanism of SUDEP. Previous studies have shown that both serotonin reuptake inhibitors and benzodiazepines may affect breathing. To determine whether these drugs alter the occurrence of central apnea in patients with epilepsy [211, 212], Nuria Lacuey [213] studied 476 seizures in 204 patients from nine epilepsy monitoring units that agreed to participate in the study and reported that patients taking SSRIs had a reduced incidence of apnea during or after seizures. The duration of central apnea during seizures and post-convulsive apnea was shorter in patients treated with long-term benzodiazepines, and the use of SSRIs and/or benzodiazepines to prevent or shorten the duration of central apnea after seizures in patients with epilepsy may reduce the risk of SUDEP.

3.7.4.3 Night Monitoring

Ito Y [214] conducted a study on 132 patients with epilepsy and reported that SUDEP in prone patients was predominant at night and that death was most common in the bedroom (49.2%). Woojun Kim [208] et al. also reported that SUDEP most often occurred at night or during sleep and that frequent nighttime seizures are an obvious risk factor for SUDEP. Therefore, strengthening nighttime monitoring may reduce the occurrence of SUDEP in patients. Zhao H [209] also suggested that the use of remote monitoring devices at night may reduce the risk of SUDEP.

3.7.4.4 Others

The use of epilepsy detection devices to understand the occurrence of systemic tonic–clonic seizures, respiratory and heart rate monitoring devices to detect cardiopulmonary distress, prevention of airway obstruction (safety pillow), and the use of drugs to reduce central ventilation deficiency may also have preventive effects on SUDEP [209]. In addition, studies in animal models of SUDEP have revealed that a variety of neurotransmitters, including 5-HT and adenosine, may be involved in the pathophysiological mechanism of SUDEP, and these neurotransmitters may become targets for future SUDEP drug intervention [209].

References

1. Wang X, Li S. Refractory status epilepticus. Springer Singapore; 2017.
2. Fisher RS, van Emde Boas W, Blume W, et al. Epileptic seizures and epilepsy: definitions proposed by the International League Against Epilepsy (ILAE) and the International Bureau for Epilepsy (IBE). Epilepsia. 2005;46(4):470–2.
3. Fisher RS, Acevedo C, Arzimanoglou A, et al. ILAE official report: a practical clinical definition of epilepsy. Epilepsia. 2014;55(4):475–82.
4. Shih JJ, Ochoa JG. A systematic review of antiepileptic drug initiation and withdrawal. Neurologist. 2009;15(3):122–31.
5. Leone MA, Giussani G, Nevitt SJ, et al. Immediate antiepileptic drug treatment, versus placebo, deferred, or no treatment for first unprovoked seizure. Cochrane Database Syst Rev. 2021;5(5):CD007144.
6. Campos MS, Ayres LR, Morelo MR, et al. Efficacy and tolerability of antiepileptic drugs in patients with focal epilepsy: systematic review and network meta-analyses. Pharmacotherapy. 2016;36(12):1255–71.
7. Campos MSA, Ayres LR, Morelo MRS, et al. Comparative efficacy of antiepileptic drugs for patients with generalized epileptic seizures: systematic review and network meta-analyses. Int J Clin Pharm. 2018;40(3):589–98.
8. Costa J, Fareleira F, Ascencao R, et al. Clinical comparability of the new antiepileptic drugs in refractory partial epilepsy: a systematic review and meta-analysis. Epilepsia. 2011;52(7):1280–91.
9. Nevitt SJ, Marson AG, Tudur Smith C. Carbamazepine versus phenytoin monotherapy for epilepsy: an individual participant data review. Cochrane Database Syst Rev. 2019;7(7):CD001911.
10. Peters J, Vijiaratnam N, Angus-Leppan H. Tics induced by antiepileptic drugs: a pragmatic review. J Neurol. 2021;268(1):321–36.
11. Lezaic N, Gore G, Josephson CB, et al. The medical treatment of epilepsy in the elderly: a systematic review and meta-analysis. Epilepsia. 2019;60(7):1325–40.
12. Andrade C. Major congenital malformations associated with exposure to antiepileptic drugs during pregnancy. J Clin Psychiatry. 2018;79(4)
13. Tomson T, Battino D, Bonizzoni E, et al. Comparative risk of major congenital malformations with eight different antiepileptic drugs: a prospective cohort study of the EURAP registry. Lancet Neurol. 2018;17(6):530–8.
14. Veroniki AA, Rios P, Cogo E, et al. Comparative safety of antiepileptic drugs for neurological development in children exposed during pregnancy and breast feeding: a systematic review and network meta-analysis. BMJ Open. 2017;7(7):e017248.
15. Campbell E, Kennedy F, Russell A, et al. Malformation risks of antiepileptic drug monotherapies in pregnancy: updated results from the UK and Ireland epilepsy and pregnancy registers. J Neurol Neurosurg Psychiatry. 2014;85(9):1029–34.
16. Lamberink HJ, Otte WM, Geleijns K, et al. Antiepileptic drug withdrawal in medically and surgically treated patients: a meta-analysis of seizure recurrence and systematic review of its predictors. Epileptic Disord. 2015;17(3):211–28.
17. Lamberink HJ, Otte WM, Geerts AT, et al. Individualised prediction model of seizure recurrence and long-term outcomes after withdrawal of antiepileptic drugs in seizure-free patients: a systematic review and individual participant data meta-analysis. Lancet Neurol. 2017;16(7):523–31.
18. Yao J, Wang H, Xiao Z. Correlation between EEG during AED withdrawal and epilepsy recurrence: a meta-analysis. Neurol Sci. 2019;40(8):1637–44.
19. Stevelink R, Koeleman BPC, Sander JW, et al. Refractory juvenile myoclonic epilepsy: a meta-analysis of prevalence and risk factors. Eur J Neurol. 2019;26(6):856–64.
20. Strozzi I, Nolan SJ, Sperling MR, et al. Early versus late antiepileptic drug withdrawal for people with epilepsy in remission. Cochrane Database Syst Rev. 2015;2015(2):CD001902.

21. Park KM, Kim SE, Lee BI. Antiepileptic drug therapy in patients with drug-resistant epilepsy. J Epilepsy Res. 2019;9(1):14–26.
22. Semah F, Thomas P, Coulbaut S, et al. Early add-on treatment vs alternative monotherapy in patients with partial epilepsy. Epileptic Disord. 2014;16(2):165–74.
23. Beghi E, Gatti G, Tonini C, et al. Adjunctive therapy versus alternative monotherapy in patients with partial epilepsy failing on a single drug: a multicentre, randomised, pragmatic controlled trial. Epilepsy Res. 2003;57(1):1–13.
24. Wilby J, Kainth A, Hawkins N, et al. Clinical effectiveness, tolerability and cost-effectiveness of newer drugs for epilepsy in adults: a systematic review and economic evaluation. Health Technol Assess. 2005;9(15):1–157. iii–iv
25. Sillanpaa M, Schmidt D. Natural history of treated childhood-onset epilepsy: prospective, long-term population-based study. Brain. 2006;129(Pt 3):617–24.
26. Sillanpaa M, Saarinen M, Schmidt D. Clinical conditions of long-term cure in childhood-onset epilepsy: a 45-year follow-up study. Epilepsy Behav. 2014;37:49–53.
27. Kwan P, Brodie MJ. Early identification of refractory epilepsy. N Engl J Med. 2000;342(5):314–9.
28. Zuberi SM, Wirrell E, Yozawitz E, et al. ILAE classification and definition of epilepsy syndromes with onset in neonates and infants: position statement by the ILAE task force on nosology and definitions. Epilepsia. 2022;63(6):1349–97.
29. Wilmshurst JM, Gaillard WD, Vinayan KP, et al. Summary of recommendations for the management of infantile seizures: task force report for the ILAE Commission of Pediatrics. Epilepsia. 2015;56(8):1185–97.
30. Epi PMC. A roadmap for precision medicine in the epilepsies. Lancet Neurol. 2015;14(12):1219–28.
31. Glauser T, Ben-Menachem E, Bourgeois B, et al. Updated ILAE evidence review of antiepileptic drug efficacy and effectiveness as initial monotherapy for epileptic seizures and syndromes. Epilepsia. 2013;54(3):551–63.
32. Wirrell EC, Hood V, Knupp KG, et al. International consensus on diagnosis and management of Dravet syndrome. Epilepsia. 2022;63(7):1761–77.
33. Besag FMC, Vasey MJ, Chin RFM. Evaluating fenfluramine hydrochloride as an oral solution for the treatment of seizures associated with Lennox-Gastaut syndrome. Expert Rev Neurother. 2024;24(3):235–49.
34. Bergelson I, Walker C, Frank EL, et al. Felbamate urolithiasis. BMJ Case Rep. 2023;16(12):e253883.
35. Reif PS, Tsai MH, Helbig I, et al. Precision medicine in genetic epilepsies: break of dawn? Expert Rev Neurother. 2017;17(4):381–92.
36. Camfield P, Camfield C. The frequency of intractable seizures after stopping AEDs in seizure-free children with epilepsy. Neurology. 2005;64(6):973–5.
37. De Clerck L, Nica A, Biraben A. Clinical aspects of seizures in the elderly. Geriatrie et psychologie neuropsychiatrie du vieillissement. 2019;17(S1):7–12.
38. Miskov S, Roje Bedekovic M, Mikula I, et al. Etiology and treatment of epilepsy in the elderly. Acta medica Croatica : casopis Hravatske akademije medicinskih znanosti. 2005;59(1):63–7.
39. Bongomin F, Katabira E, Sajatovic M, et al. Epilepsy in older people in sub-Saharan Africa: a systematic review. Neuropsychiatr Dis Treat. 2021;17:2309–14.
40. Moura L, Smith JR, Blacker D, et al. Epilepsy among elderly Medicare beneficiaries: a validated approach to identify prevalent and incident epilepsy. Med Care. 2019;57(4):318–24.
41. Beghi M, Savica R, Beghi E, et al. Utilization and costs of antiepileptic drugs in the elderly: still an unsolved issue. Drugs Aging. 2009;26(2):157–68.
42. Sanya EO. Peculiarity of epilepsy in elderly people: a review. West Afr J Med. 2010;29(6):365–72.
43. Tedrus G. Ictal EEG: etiology and mortality in older adults with nonconvulsive status epilepticus. Clin EEG Neurosci. 2024;55(2):278–82.

44. Narayanan N, Selvaraj S, Mohamedkalifa A, et al. Seizure in geriatric population – an unheeded integer. J Family Med Prim Care. 2023;12(4):644–8.
45. Suastegui Roman RA, Lee A, Hernandez Vanegas LE, et al. New-onset geriatric epilepsy in a Latin American country: a multi-centric study from Mexico. Rev Investig Clin. 2023;75(4):203–11.
46. Green SF, Loefflad N, Heaney DC, et al. New-onset seizures in older people: clinical features, course and outcomes. J Neurol Sci. 2021;429:118065.
47. Verma A, Kumar A, Pathak P, et al. Clinical profile and predictors of in-hospital mortality in De novo convulsive status epilepticus in the elderly populace. J Epilepsy Res. 2022;12(2):48–52.
48. Watkins L, O'Dwyer M, Shankar R. New anti-seizure medication for elderly epileptic patients. Expert Opin Pharmacother. 2019;20(13):1601–8.
49. Konickova D, Mensikova K, Klicova K, et al. Cerebrospinal fluid and blood serum biomarkers in neurodegenerative proteinopathies: a prospective, open, cross-correlation study. J Neurochem. 2023;167(2):168–82.
50. Nikl J. Epilepsy in the elderly. Ideggyogyaszati szemle. 2011;64(3–4):78–87.
51. Pervin S, Jicha GA, Bensalem-Owen M, et al. Incident epilepsy in the cognitively normal geriatric population, irrespective of seizure control, impairs quality of life. Epilepsy Behav. 2022;126:108457.
52. Rohracher A, Trinka E. Epilepsy in the aged : challenges in diagnostics and treatment. Zeitschrift fur Gerontologie und Geriatrie. 2021;54(4):395–408.
53. Lattanzi S, Trinka E, Del Giovane C, et al. Antiepileptic drug monotherapy for epilepsy in the elderly: a systematic review and network meta-analysis. Epilepsia. 2019;60(11):2245–54.
54. Pohlmann-Eden B, Marson AG, Noack-Rink M, et al. Comparative effectiveness of levetiracetam, valproate and carbamazepine among elderly patients with newly diagnosed epilepsy: subgroup analysis of the randomized, unblinded KOMET study. BMC Neurol. 2016;16(1):149.
55. Verma A, Prasad Vaishya G, Mathew DJ, et al. Predictors of in-hospital mortality in epilepsy and epileptic seizures in the elderly populace – a cross sectional study from rural India. Epilepsy Res. 2021;171:106564.
56. Verma A, Kumar A, Sachan D. Comparison of clinical profile and outcome of de novo convulsive status epilepticus with those with a past history of epilepsy in the elderly populace. Acta Neurol Taiwanica. 2022;31(3):131–6.
57. Fiest KM, Sauro KM, Wiebe S, et al. Prevalence and incidence of epilepsy: a systematic review and meta-analysis of international studies. Neurology. 2017;88(3):296–303.
58. Pennell PB. Hormonal aspects of epilepsy. Neurol Clin. 2009;27(4):941–65.
59. Harden CL, Pennell PB. Neuroendocrine considerations in the treatment of men and women with epilepsy. Lancet Neurol. 2013;12(1):72–83.
60. Herzog AG, Fowler KM. Sexual hormones and epilepsy: threat and opportunities. Curr Opin Neurol. 2005;18(2):167–72.
61. Isojärvi JI, Taubøll E, Herzog AG. Effect of antiepileptic drugs on reproductive endocrine function in individuals with epilepsy. CNS Drugs. 2005;19(3):207–23.
62. Morrell MJ. Reproductive and metabolic disorders in women with epilepsy. Epilepsia. 2003;44(Suppl 4):11–20.
63. Morrell MJ, Flynn KL, Seale CG, et al. Reproductive dysfunction in women with epilepsy: antiepileptic drug effects on sex-steroid hormones. CNS Spectr 2001;6(9):771–2, 83–86.
64. Svalheim S, Sveberg L, Mochol M, et al. Interactions between antiepileptic drugs and hormones. Seizure. 2015;28:12–7.
65. Isojärvi JI, Laatikainen TJ, Pakarinen AJ, et al. Polycystic ovaries and hyperandrogenism in women taking valproate for epilepsy. N Engl J Med. 1993;329(19):1383–8.
66. Harden CL. Sexual dysfunction in women with epilepsy. Seizure. 2008;17(2):131–5.
67. Zelená V, Kuba R, Soška V, et al. Depression as a prominent cause of sexual dysfunction in women with epilepsy. Epilepsy Behav. 2011;20(3):539–44.

68. Harden CL, Koppel BS, Herzog AG, et al. Seizure frequency is associated with age at menopause in women with epilepsy. Neurology. 2003;61(4):451–5.
69. Dutton C, Foldvary-Schaefer N. Contraception in women with epilepsy: pharmacokinetic interactions, contraceptive options, and management. Int Rev Neurobiol. 2008;83:113–34.
70. Crawford P. Interactions between antiepileptic drugs and hormonal contraception. CNS Drugs. 2002;16(4):263–72.
71. Crawford P, Chadwick DJ, Martin C, et al. The interaction of phenytoin and carbamazepine with combined oral contraceptive steroids. Br J Clin Pharmacol. 1990;30(6):892–6.
72. Dickins M, Chen C. Chemistry, biotransformation, and pharmacokinetics. Antiepileptic drugs. Philadelphia: Lippincott Williams & Wilkins; 2002. p. 370–9.
73. Battino D, Tomson T, Bonizzoni E, et al. Seizure control and treatment changes in pregnancy: observations from the EURAP epilepsy pregnancy registry. Epilepsia. 2013;54(9):1621–7.
74. King A, Gerard EE. Contraception, fecundity, and pregnancy in women with epilepsy: an update on recent literature. Curr Opin Neurol. 2022;35(2):161–8.
75. Bhatia M, Adcock JE, Mackillop L. The management of pregnant women with epilepsy: a multidisciplinary collaborative approach to care. Obstetr Gynaecol. 2017;19(4):279–88.
76. Morrow J, Russell A, Guthrie E, et al. Malformation risks of antiepileptic drugs in pregnancy: a prospective study from the UK epilepsy and pregnancy register. J Neurol Neurosurg Psychiatry. 2006;77(2):193–8.
77. Tomson T, Battino D, Bonizzoni E, et al. Declining malformation rates with changed antiepileptic drug prescribing: an observational study. Neurology. 2019;93(9):e831–e40.
78. Vajda FJE, O'Brien TJ, Graham JE, et al. The contribution of non-drug factors to fetal malformation in anti-seizure-medication-treated pregnancy. Epilepsy Behav. 2021;118:107941.
79. Meador KJ, Baker GA, Browning N, et al. Fetal antiepileptic drug exposure and cognitive outcomes at age 6 years (NEAD study): a prospective observational study. Lancet Neurol. 2013;12(3):244–52.
80. Knight R, Wittkowski A, Bromley RL. Neurodevelopmental outcomes in children exposed to newer antiseizure medications: a systematic review. Epilepsia. 2021;62(8):1765–79.
81. Spiegel R, Merius H. Principles of epilepsy Management for Women in their reproductive years. Front Neurol. 2020;11:322.
82. Hernández-Díaz S, Werler MM, Walker AM, et al. Folic acid antagonists during pregnancy and the risk of birth defects. N Engl J Med. 2000;343(22):1608–14.
83. Voinescu PE, Park S, Chen LQ, et al. Antiepileptic drug clearances during pregnancy and clinical implications for women with epilepsy. Neurology. 2018;91(13):e1228–e36.
84. Pennell PB, Newport DJ, Stowe ZN, et al. The impact of pregnancy and childbirth on the metabolism of lamotrigine. Neurology. 2004;62(2):292–5.
85. Harden CL, Pennell PB, Koppel BS, et al. Management issues for women with epilepsy—focus on pregnancy (an evidence-based review): III. Vitamin K, folic acid, blood levels, and breast-feeding: report of the Quality Standards Subcommittee and Therapeutics and Technology Assessment Subcommittee of the American Academy of Neurology and the American Epilepsy Society. Epilepsia. 2009;50(5):1247–55.
86. Knight MKS, Brocklehurst P, et al. Epilepsy in pregnancy. Royal College Obstetr Gynaecol. 2016;
87. Breastfeeding and the use of human milk. Pediatrics. 2012;129(3):e827–41.
88. Davanzo R, Dal Bo S, Bua J, et al. Antiepileptic drugs and breastfeeding. Ital J Pediatr. 2013;39:50.
89. Ito S. Drug therapy for breast-feeding women. N Engl J Med. 2000;343(2):118–26.
90. Ip S, Chung M, Raman G, et al. A summary of the Agency for Healthcare Research and Quality's evidence report on breastfeeding in developed countries. Breastfeed Med. 2009;4(Suppl 1):S17–30.
91. HALE T HTW. Medications and mothers' Milk. Hale Pub; 2012.
92. Veiby G, Bjørk M, Engelsen BA, et al. Epilepsy and recommendations for breastfeeding. Seizure. 2015;28:57–65.

93. Wilner AN, Sharma BK, Soucy A, et al. Common comorbidities in women and men with epilepsy and the relationship between number of comorbidities and health plan paid costs in 2010. Epilepsy Behav. 2014;32:15–20.
94. Ruiz-Giménez J, Sánchez-Alvarez JC, Cañadillas-Hidalgo F, et al. Antiepileptic treatment in patients with epilepsy and other comorbidities. Seizure. 2010;19(7):375–82.
95. Meier C, Kraenzlin ME. Antiepileptics and bone health. Ther Adv Musculoskelet Dis. 2011;3(5):235–43.
96. WHO. Epilepsy: a public health imperative. Geneva: World Health Organization; 2019. Contract No.: Licence: CC BY-NC-SA 3.0 IGO
97. Keezer MR, Sisodiya SM, Sander JW. Comorbidities of epilepsy: current concepts and future perspectives. Lancet Neurol. 2016;15(1):106–15.
98. Asadi-Pooya AA, Barzegar Z. Marital status in young adult patients with seizures: epilepsy vs. functional seizures. Epilepsy Behav. 2021;121(Pt A):108066.
99. Jacoby A, Austin JK. Social stigma for adults and children with epilepsy. Epilepsia. 2007;48(Suppl 9):6–9.
100. Lim KS, Wo SW, Wong MH, et al. Impact of epilepsy on employment in Malaysia. Epilepsy Behav. 2013;27(1):130–4.
101. Begley C, Wagner RG, Abraham A, et al. The global cost of epilepsy: a systematic review and extrapolation. Epilepsia. 2022;63(4):892–903.
102. Hakami T. Neuropharmacology of Antiseizure drugs. Neuropsychopharmacol Rep. 2021;41(3):336–51.
103. Chen Z, Brodie MJ, Kwan P. What has been the impact of new drug treatments on epilepsy? Curr Opin Neurol. 2020;33(2):185–90.
104. Perucca E, Brodie MJ, Kwan P, et al. 30 years of second-generation antiseizure medications: impact and future perspectives. Lancet Neurol. 2020;19(6):544–56.
105. Kwan P, Arzimanoglou A, Berg AT, et al. Definition of drug resistant epilepsy: consensus proposal by the ad hoc task force of the ILAE commission on therapeutic strategies. Epilepsia. 2010;51(6):1069–77.
106. Chen Z, Brodie MJ, Liew D, et al. Treatment outcomes in patients with newly diagnosed epilepsy treated with established and new antiepileptic drugs: a 30-year longitudinal cohort study. JAMA Neurol. 2018;75(3):279–86.
107. Chen Z, Rollo B, Antonic-Baker A, et al. New era of personalised epilepsy management. BMJ. 2020;371:m3658.
108. Nabbout R, Kuchenbuch M. Impact of predictive, preventive and precision medicine strategies in epilepsy. Nat Rev Neurol. 2020;16(12):674–88.
109. Walker LE, Mirza N, Yip VLM, et al. Personalized medicine approaches in epilepsy. J Intern Med. 2015;277(2):218–34.
110. Chung WH, Hung SI, Hong HS, et al. Medical genetics: a marker for Stevens-Johnson syndrome. Nature. 2004;428(6982):486.
111. Bernasconi A, Antel SB, Collins DL, et al. Texture analysis and morphological processing of magnetic resonance imaging assist detection of focal cortical dysplasia in extra-temporal partial epilepsy. Ann Neurol. 2001;49(6):770–5.
112. Liu G, Xiao R, Xu L, et al. Minireview of epilepsy detection techniques based on electroencephalogram signals. Front Syst Neurosci. 2021;15:685387.
113. Mintz Y, Brodie R. Introduction to artificial intelligence in medicine. Minim Invasive Ther Allied Technol. 2019;28(2):73–81.
114. Falagario U, Veccia A, Weprin S, et al. Robotic-assisted surgery for the treatment of urologic cancers: recent advances. Expert Rev Med Devices. 2020;17(6):579–90.
115. Barba P, Stramiello J, Funk EK, et al. Remote telesurgery in humans: a systematic review. Surg Endosc. 2022;36(5):2771–7.
116. Najafabadipour M, Zanin M, Rodriguez-Gonzalez A, et al. Reconstructing the patient's natural history from electronic health records. Artif Intell Med. 2020;105:101860.

117. Middleton B, Sittig DF, Wright A. Clinical decision support: a 25 year retrospective and a 25 year vision. Yearb Med Inform. 2016;Suppl 1(Suppl 1):S103–16.
118. Shortliffe EH, Davis R, Axline SG, et al. Computer-based consultations in clinical therapeutics: explanation and rule acquisition capabilities of the MYCIN system. Comput Biomed Res. 1975;8(4):303–20.
119. Abbasi MU, Rashad A, Basalamah A, et al. Detection of epilepsy seizures in neo-Natal EEG using LSTM architecture. IEEE Access. 2019;7:179074–85.
120. Bzdok D, Krzywinski M, Altman N. Machine learning: supervised methods. Nat Methods. 2018;15(1):5–6.
121. Fix E, Hodges JL. Discriminatory analysis – nonparametric discrimination: consistency properties. Int Stat Rev. 1989;57(3):238–47.
122. Hearst MA, Dumais ST, Osuna E, et al. Support vector machines. IEEE Intellig Syst Appl. 1998;13(4):18–28.
123. Chen T, Guestrin C, editors. XGBoost: a scalable tree boosting system2016: Association for Computing Machinery.
124. Steyerberg E. Clinical prediction models: a practical approach to development, validation, and updating. 2nd ed. New York: Springer International Publishing; 2019.
125. Devinsky O, Dilley C, Ozery-Flato M, et al. Changing the approach to treatment choice in epilepsy using big data. Epilepsy Behav. 2016;56:32–7.
126. Ouyang CS, Chiang CT, Yang RC, et al. Quantitative EEG findings and response to treatment with antiepileptic medications in children with epilepsy. Brain Dev. 2018;40(1):26–35.
127. Zhang JH, Han X, Zhao HW, et al. Personalized prediction model for seizure-free epilepsy with levetiracetam therapy: a retrospective data analysis using support vector machine. Br J Clin Pharmacol. 2018;84(11):2615–24.
128. Jia Y, Gu H, Luo Q. Sample entropy reveals an age-related reduction in the complexity of dynamic brain. Sci Rep. 2017;7(1):7990.
129. Jiang JL, Su X, Zhang H, et al. A novel approach to active compounds identification based on support vector regression model and mean impact value. Chem Biol Drug Des. 2013;81(5):650–7.
130. Yao L, Cai M, Chen Y, et al. Prediction of antiepileptic drug treatment outcomes of patients with newly diagnosed epilepsy by machine learning. Epilepsy Behav. 2019;96:92–7.
131. Petrovski S, Szoeke CE, Sheffield LJ, et al. Multi-SNP pharmacogenomic classifier is superior to single-SNP models for predicting drug outcome in complex diseases. Pharmacogenet Genomics. 2009;19(2):147–52.
132. Shazadi K, Petrovski S, Roten A, et al. Validation of a multigenic model to predict seizure control in newly treated epilepsy. Epilepsy Res. 2014;108(10):1797–805.
133. Marson AG, Al-Kharusi AM, Alwaidh M, et al. The SANAD study of effectiveness of valproate, lamotrigine, or topiramate for generalised and unclassifiable epilepsy: an unblinded randomised controlled trial. Lancet. 2007;369(9566):1016–26.
134. de Jong J, Cutcutache I, Page M, et al. Towards realizing the vision of precision medicine: AI based prediction of clinical drug response. Brain. 2021;144(6):1738–50.
135. Terman SW. Rise of the machines? Predicting Brivaracetam response using machine learning. Epilepsy Curr. 2022;22(2):111–3.
136. Hakeem H, Feng W, Chen Z, et al. Development and validation of a deep learning model for predicting treatment response in patients with newly diagnosed epilepsy. JAMA Neurol. 2022;79(10):986–96.
137. Ashish V, Noam S, Niki P, et al. Attention Is All You Need. Available from: https://arxiv.org/abs/1706.03762
138. Lawn N, Chan J, Lee J, et al. Is the first seizure epilepsy--and when? Epilepsia. 2015;56(9):1425–31.
139. Chiang S, Rao VR. Choosing the best Antiseizure medication – can artificial intelligence help? JAMA Neurol. 2022;79(10):970–2.

140. Terman SW. Deep thoughts-predicting initial treatment response in newly diagnosed epilepsy. Epilepsy Curr. 2023;23(2):90–2.
141. Silva-Alves MS, Secolin R, Carvalho BS, et al. A prediction algorithm for drug response in patients with mesial temporal lobe epilepsy based on clinical and genetic information. PLoS One. 2017;12(1):e0169214.
142. Hastie T, Tibshirani R, Friedman J. The elements of statistical learning: data mining, inference, and prediction. 2nd ed. New York: Springer; 2009.
143. An S, Malhotra K, Dilley C, et al. Predicting drug-resistant epilepsy – a machine learning approach based on administrative claims data. Epilepsy Behav. 2018;89:118–25.
144. Michalski R, Carbonell J, Mitchell T. Machine learning: an artificial intelligence approach. Springer Science & Business Media; 2013.
145. Brier G. Verification of forecasts expressed in terms of probability. Mon Weather Rev. 1950;78:1–3.
146. Niculescu-Mizil A, Caruana R, editors. Predicting good probabilities with supervised learning. The 22nd international conference on machine learning. Bonn, Germany; 2005.
147. Smolyansky ED, Hakeem H, Ge Z, et al. Machine learning models for decision support in epilepsy management: a critical review. Epilepsy Behav. 2021;123:108273.
148. Delen D, Davazdahemami B, Eryarsoy E, et al. Using predictive analytics to identify drug-resistant epilepsy patients. Health Informatics J. 2020;26(1):449–60.
149. Hirsch LJ, Gaspard N, van Baalen A, et al. Proposed consensus definitions for new-onset refractory status epilepticus (NORSE), febrile infection-related epilepsy syndrome (FIRES), and related conditions. Epilepsia. 2018;59(4):739–44.
150. Feikes H, Smith LL, Hinshaw DB. Acute symptomatic postoperative hyponatremia. Am Surg. 1964;30:505–10.
151. Varavithya W, Hellerstein S. Acute symptomatic hyponatremia. J Pediatr. 1967;71(2):269–83.
152. Pilke A, Partinen M, Kovanen J. Status epilepticus and alcohol abuse: an analysis of 82 status epilepticus admissions. Acta Neurol Scand. 1984;70(6):443–50.
153. Hauser WA. Seizure disorders: the changes with age. Epilepsia. 1992;33 Suppl 4(s4):S6–14.
154. Grau-Lopez L, Flores-Pina B, Jimenez M, et al. Epileptiform electroencephalogram discharges increase seizure recurrence risk in patients with acute symptomatic seizure due to a structural brain lesion. Seizure. 2024;117:56–9.
155. Pais-Cunha I, Almeida AI, Curval AR, et al. Cerebral venous thrombosis in pediatric age: risk factors and prognosis. Neuropediatrics. 2024;55(3):183–90.
156. Hernandez-Prieto A, Garrido-Martin M, Gomez-Martin H, et al. Neonatal seizures and progression to epilepsy in a tertiary hospital. Rev Neurol. 2023;77(10):249–52.
157. Lekoubou A, Ssentongo P, Maffie J, et al. Associations of small vessel disease and acute symptomatic seizures in ischemic stroke patients. Epilepsy Behav. 2023;145:109233.
158. Karan AA, Spivak YS, Suleymanova EM, et al. Distant neuroinflammation acutely induced by focal brain injury and its control by endocannabinoid system. Exp Neurol. 2024;373:114679.
159. Tsur A, Spierer R, Cohen R, et al. First unprovoked seizures among soldiers recruited to the Israeli defense forces during 10 consecutive years: a population-based study. Epilepsia. 2024;65(1):127–37.
160. De Stefano P, Menetre E, Stancu P, et al. Added value of advanced workup after the first seizure: a 7-year cohort study. Epilepsia. 2023;64(12):3246–56.
161. Sinka L, Abraira L, Imbach LL, et al. Association of Mortality and Risk of epilepsy with type of acute symptomatic seizure after ischemic stroke and an updated prognostic model. JAMA Neurol. 2023;80(6):605–13.
162. Hersh N, Ben Zvi H, Goldstein L, et al. Epilepsy following herpes simplex encephalitis – a case series. Epilepsy Res. 2023;192:107137.
163. Lopez-Espejo M, Skorin I, Mesa T, et al. Three-year incidence and acute setting predictors of epilepsy after neonatal and childhood arterial ischaemic stroke: a disease-based cohort study. Eur J Pediatr. 2024;183(3):1415–23.

164. Meletti S, Turchi G, Orlandi N, et al. Electrographic seizure duration and inter-seizure intervals in focal status epilepticus. Epileptic Disord. 2023;25(4):519–27.
165. Kim JW, Stetefeld HR, Fink GR, et al. Seizures at stroke onset: a case-control study. Seizure. 2023;113:28–33.
166. Agircan D, Bal M, Demir TG, et al. Multi-inflammatory index as a new predictive and prognostic marker of acute symptomatic seizures in patients with cerebral venous sinus thrombosis. J Stroke Cerebrovasc Dis. 2023;32(12):107453.
167. Rodrigo-Gisbert M, Abraira L, Quintana M, et al. Risk assessment of long-term epilepsy after de novo status epilepticus with clinical and electroencephalographic biomarkers: the AFTER score. Epilepsy Behav. 2023;149:109531.
168. Rodrigo-Gisbert M, Gomez-Dabo L, Quintana M, et al. Prediction of long-term unprovoked seizures after status epilepticus. Epilepsia. 2023;64(9):2399–408.
169. Tatillo C, Legros B, Depondt C, et al. Prognostic value of early electrographic biomarkers of epileptogenesis in high-risk ischaemic stroke patients. Eur J Neurol. 2024;31(1):e16074.
170. Byrnes M, Thompson NR, Hantus ST, et al. Characteristics and attendance of patients eligible for the PASS clinic: a transition of care model after acute symptomatic seizures. Neurol Clin Pract. 2024;14(1):e200232.
171. Tyvaert L. How autoimmunity changed our diagnostic practice in epileptology? Rev Neurol (Paris). 2023;179(4):316–29.
172. Rada A, Bien CG. What is autoimmune encephalitis-associated epilepsy? Proposal of a practical definition Epilepsia. 2023;64(9):2249–55.
173. Byrnes M, Chandan P, Newey C, et al. Acute symptomatic seizure associated with chronic Antiseizure medication use after stroke. Neurol Clin Pract. 2022;12(6):e154–e61.
174. Sortino V, Pratico A, Marino S, et al. Efficacy of the anti-seizure medications in acute symptomatic neonatal seizures caused by stroke. A systematic review. Acta bio-medica: Atenei Parmensis. 2022;93(6):e2022328.
175. Zaccara G, Lattanzi S, Brigo F. Acute symptomatic seizures after stroke: a scoping review on primary prevention, treatment with antiseizure medications and drug discontinuation. Epilepsy Behav. 2023;149:109499.
176. Qiang J, Wang Y, Zhai Q, et al. Predictors of unprovoked seizures in intracerebral hemorrhages. Acta Neurol Belg. 2023;123(6):2195–200.
177. Herzig-Nichtweiss J, Salih F, Berning S, et al. Prognosis and management of acute symptomatic seizures: a prospective, multicenter, observational study. Ann Intensive Care. 2023;13(1):85.
178. Dalla Corte A, Pinzetta G, Ruwel AG, et al. Anatomical Organization of the Amygdala: a brief visual review. Cogn Behav Neurol. 2024;37(1):13–22.
179. Shakhatreh L, Sinclair B, McLean C, et al. Amygdala enlargement in temporal lobe epilepsy: histopathology and surgical outcomes. Epilepsia. 2024;65(6):1709–19.
180. Kaada BR, Andersen P, Jansen J Jr. Stimulation of the amygdaloid nuclear complex in unanesthetized cats. Neurology. 1954;4(1):48–64.
181. Sawa M, Aida S, Hirasawa R, et al. Experimentally induced epilepsy by the local application of alumina cream into the amygdaloid nuclei in dogs. Folia Psychiatr Neurol Jpn. 1954;8(2):189.
182. Morris AA. Temporal lobectomy with removal of uncus, hippocampus, and amygdala; results for psychomotor epilepsy three to nine years after operation. AMA Arch Neurol Psychiatry. 1956;76(5):479–96.
183. De Giacomo P. A hypothesis based on histochemical data regarding the site from which originate the automatic movements present in rhinencephalic epilepsy and an added note concerning the distribution of cholinesterase activity in the amygdaloid complex of man. Riv Neurol. 1961;31:286–9.
184. Pagni CA. Electroclinical study of Amygdalo-Hippocampic after-discharges in man using depth electrodes implanted by the stereotactic method. Confin Neurol. 1963;23:477–99.

185. Yang YC, Wang GH, Chou P, et al. Dynamic electrical synapses rewire brain networks for persistent oscillations and epileptogenesis. Proc Natl Acad Sci USA. 2024;121(8):e2313042121.
186. Rhone AE, Kovach CK, Harmata GIS, et al. A human amygdala site that inhibits respiration and elicits apnea in pediatric epilepsy. JCI Insight. 2020;5(6):e134852.
187. Nobis WP, Otárula KAG, Templer JW, et al. The effect of seizure spread to the amygdala on respiration and onset of ictal central apnea. J Neurosurg. 2020;132(5):1313–23.
188. Dlouhy BJ, Gehlbach BK, Kreple CJ, et al. Breathing inhibited when seizures spread to the amygdala and upon amygdala stimulation. J Neurosci. 2015;35(28):10281–9.
189. Maguire MJ, Jackson CF, Marson AG, et al. Treatments for the prevention of sudden unexpected death in epilepsy (SUDEP). Cochrane Database Syst Rev. 2020;2020(4):CD011792.
190. Legouhy A, Allen LA, Vos SB, et al. Volumetric and microstructural abnormalities of the amygdala in focal epilepsy with varied levels of SUDEP risk. Epilepsy Res. 2023;192:107139.
191. Zeicu C, Legouhy A, Scott CA, et al. Altered amygdala volumes and microstructure in focal epilepsy patients with tonic-Clonic seizures, Ictal and Post-Ictal Central Apnea. Cold Spring Harbor Laboratory; 2023.
192. Ghazale PP, dos Santos Borges K, Gomes KP, et al. Alterations in aortic vasorelaxation in rats with epilepsy induced by the electrical amygdala kindling model. Epilepsy Res. 2022;182:106920.
193. Marincovich A, Bravo E, Dlouhy B, et al. Amygdala lesions reduce seizure-induced respiratory arrest in DBA/1 mice. Epilepsy Behav. 2021;121:106440.
194. Bhasin H, Sharma S, Ramachandrannair R. Can we prevent sudden unexpected death in epilepsy (SUDEP)? Can J Neurol Sci. 2021;48(4):464–8.
195. Faingold CL, Feng HJ. A unified hypothesis of SUDEP: seizure-induced respiratory depression induced by adenosine may lead to SUDEP but can be prevented by autoresuscitation and other restorative respiratory response mechanisms mediated by the action of serotonin on the periaqueductal gray. Epilepsia. 2023;64(4):779–96.
196. Somani A, Perry C, Patodia S, et al. Neuropeptide depletion in the amygdala in sudden unexpected death in epilepsy: a postmortem study. Epilepsia. 2020;61(2):310–8.
197. Campbell JM, Yost S, Gautam D, et al. Delays in the diagnosis and surgical treatment of drug-resistant epilepsy: a cohort study. Epilepsia. 2024;65(5):1314–21.
198. Collard R, Aziz MC, Rapp K, et al. Galanin analogs prevent mortality from seizure-induced respiratory arrest in mice. Front Neural Circ. 2022;16
199. Lacuey N, Hampson JP, Harper RM, et al. Limbic and paralimbic structures driving ictal central apnea. Neurology. 2019;92(7):e655.
200. Tio E, Culler GW, Bachman EM, et al. Ictal central apneas in temporal lobe epilepsies. Epilepsy Behav. 2020;112:107434.
201. Walker F, Fish DR. Recording respiratory parameters in patients with epilepsy. Epilepsia. 1997;38(11 Suppl):S41–2.
202. Schuele SU, Afshari M, Afshari ZS, et al. Ictal central apnea as a predictor for sudden unexpected death in epilepsy. Epilepsy Behav. 2011;22(2):401–3.
203. So EL, Sam MC, Lagerlund TL. Postictal central apnea as a cause of SUDEP: evidence from near-SUDEP incident. Epilepsia. 2000;41(11):1494–7.
204. Vilella L, Lacuey N, Hampson JP, et al. Postconvulsive central apnea as a biomarker for sudden unexpected death in epilepsy (SUDEP). Neurology. 2019;92(3):e171–e82.
205. Joyal KG, Kreitlow BL, Buchanan GF. The role of sleep state and time of day in modulating breathing in epilepsy: implications for sudden unexpected death in epilepsy. Front Neural Circ. 2022;16:983211.
206. Micalizzi E, Ballerini A, Giovannini G, et al. The role of the amygdala in ictal central apnea: insights from brain MRI morphometry. Ann Clin Translat Neurol. 2024;11(1):121–32.
207. Teran FA, Bravo E, Richerson GB. Sudden unexpected death in epilepsy: respiratory mechanisms. Handbook of clinical neurology: Elsevier; 2022. p. 153–76.

208. Kim W, Lee H, Lee KW, et al. The Association of Nocturnal Seizures and Interictal Cardiac/central autonomic function in frontal lobe epilepsy: heart rate variability and central autonomic network analysis. Neuropsychiatr Dis Treat. 2023;19:2081–91.
209. Zhao H, Long L, Xiao B. Advances in sudden unexpected death in epilepsy. Acta Neurol Scand. 2022;146(6):716–22.
210. O'Neal TB, Shrestha S, Singh H, et al. Sudden unexpected death in epilepsy. Neurol Int. 2022;14(3):600–13.
211. Bosco F, Guarnieri L, Leo A, et al. Audiogenic epileptic DBA/2 mice strain as a model of genetic reflex seizures and SUDEP. Front Neurol. 2023:14.
212. Petrucci AN, Joyal KG, Chou JW, et al. Post-ictal generalized EEG suppression is reduced by enhancing dorsal raphe serotonergic neurotransmission. Neuroscience. 2021;453:206–21.
213. Lacuey N, Martins R, Vilella L, et al. The association of serotonin reuptake inhibitors and benzodiazepines with ictal central apnea. Epilepsy Behav. 2019;98:73–9.
214. Ito Y, Hata N, Maesawa S, et al. Characteristics of deceased subjects transported to a postmortem imaging center due to unusual death related to epilepsy. Epilepsia Open. 2024;9(2):592–601.

Chapter 4
Clinical Application of Anti-seizure Medication as Drug Therapy

Liemin Zhou and Ziyi Chen

4.1 Pharmacological Treatment of Different Types of Epileptic Seizures

4.1.1 Classification of Epileptic Seizures

The International League Against Epilepsy (ILAE) established its classification system for epileptic seizures, which is currently the most widely used classification system worldwide, in 1981 [1]. In 2017, the ILAE introduced the latest version of the classification system based on accumulating clinical evidence over the past 30 years, in an effort to revise and supplement the types of seizures and terms used [2]. This chapter discusses the selection of anti-seizure medications (ASMs) according to the latest classifications of seizures, with some evidence-based medical references comparing the two sets of classifications from 1981 and 2017.

Seizures are classified based on initial clinical manifestations and electroencephalogram (EEG) changes. In addition to symptomatic descriptions, the use of seizure recordings is encouraged. The latest classification emphasizes the practicality of clinical use and allows for specific refinement of classification based on clinical needs.

L. Zhou (✉)
Department of Neurology, The Seven Affiliated Hospital of Sun Yat-sen University, Shenzhen, China

Z. Chen
Department of Neurology, The Seven Affiliated Hospital of Sun Yat-sen University, Shenzhen, China

X. Wang, L. Zhou (eds.), *Pharmacological Treatment of Epileptic Seizures*,
https://doi.org/10.1007/978-981-96-8520-2_4

4.1.1.1 Focal Onset Seizures

Seizures consistently originate from a localized or more widely distributed epileptogenic network within one cerebral hemisphere, with predominant conduction pathways of discharge, and can subsequently involve the opposite cerebral hemisphere. Focal-onset seizures may originate from subcortical gray matter structures. Some patients may have multiple epileptogenic networks and various types of seizures, but the initiating brain region for each seizure type is consistent. The EEG manifestations of various focal seizures during the seizure period show evolving features of epileptic activity, with specific manifestations varying due to differences in the starting site, propagation speed, and range of discharge. Focal-onset seizures are classified into three levels. The first level is based on whether the patient perceives themselves and the environment throughout the entire seizure process; seizures are thus classified into preserved awareness and impaired awareness. The second level is based on the initial symptoms, including motor symptom onset, such as automatisms, atonia, clonic, tonic, hyperkinetic, myoclonic, and tonic–clonic seizures; and nonmotor symptom onset, such as autonomic, behavioral arrest, and cognitive, emotional, and sensory symptoms. The third level includes progression to bilateral tonic–clonic seizures.

4.1.1.2 Generalized-Onset Seizures

Seizures originate from a point in the epileptogenic network formed by the bilateral cerebral cortex and subcortical structures and rapidly spread throughout the entire network. The origin point of each seizure varies within the network. Generalized-onset seizures may not necessarily involve all cortices and can be asymmetric. Generalized onset seizures include tonic–clonic seizures, tonic seizures, clonic seizures, myoclonic seizures, myoclonic-tonic–clonic seizures, atonic seizures, myoclonic-atonic seizures, epileptic spasms, typical absence seizures, atypical absence seizures, myoclonic absence seizures, and eyelid myoclonic absence seizures.

4.1.1.3 Seizures of Unknown Onset

Patients with insufficient information about seizure onset may be temporarily classified into this category until further information is available to determine focal or generalized onset.

4.1.1.4 Unclassifiable Seizures

Patients with insufficient information about seizures may be temporarily classified into this category until further information is available for seizure type diagnosis.

4.1.2 *Principles of Selecting Anti-seizure Medications*

Selecting medications based on seizure types and syndromes is the fundamental principle of epilepsy treatment, and takes into consideration the patient's age, sex, adverse drug reactions, comorbidities, concomitant medications, and patient or caregiver preferences.

4.1.2.1 Medication Selection for Focal-Onset Seizures

Carbamazepine, lamotrigine, and levetiracetam are first-line drugs for patients with newly diagnosed focal-onset seizures [3, 4]. The Standard and New Antiepileptic Drugs (SANAD) study compared the effects of extended-release carbamazepine tablets with those of lamotrigine and gabapentin, while the SANADII study compared the effects of lamotrigine with levetiracetam and zonisamide. Both studies showed that lamotrigine had better efficacy and safety, and recommended it as the first choice for focal-onset seizures [3, 4]. A meta-analysis of monotherapy for focal epilepsy included ten ASMs—carbamazepine, lamotrigine, levetiracetam, oxcarbazepine, valproic acid, zonisamide, topiramate, phenytoin, phenobarbital, and gabapentin—with the highest retention rates observed for lamotrigine and levetiracetam [5]. Oxcarbazepine is the first-line treatment for newly diagnosed focal-onset seizures in children. If carbamazepine, oxcarbazepine, or lamotrigine is not suitable or is not tolerated, valproic acid, primidone, or lacosamide may be considered. If the first-selected drug among these seven ASMs is ineffective, another drug can be selected from them. If a second ASM agent with good tolerability is ineffective, combination therapy may be considered [5].

When first-line treatment is ineffective or intolerable, carbamazepine, oxcarbazepine, lamotrigine, levetiracetam, valproic acid, topiramate, clobazam, gabapentin, zonisamide, primidone, pregabalin, and lacosamide can be added for focal-onset seizures. If additional treatment is ineffective or intolerable, other ASMs to consider include phenobarbital and phenytoin. The difference in the efficacy of these drugs for focal-onset seizures is not significant, and the choice should take into consideration the patient's age, comorbidities, accompanying diseases, potential adverse reactions, economic burden, drug accessibility, and expectations for quality of life.

There is a lack of evidence-based medicine for drug selection in focal-onset myoclonic seizures and atonic seizures. Focal-onset myoclonic and atonic seizures often present with drug resistance and have poorer drug responsiveness than focal-onset tonic–clonic seizures or sensory seizures. Currently preferred drug spectra for focal-onset seizures and for worsening of generalized-onset myoclonic or atonic seizures are exactly the same. Therefore, broad-spectrum ASMs such as valproic acid, levetiracetam, and clonazepam are often used in clinical practice [6]. Occasional reports of the effectiveness of carbamazepine and phenobarbital, as well as reports of worsening seizures, have emerged [7].

4.1.2.2 Medication Selection for Generalized Onset Seizures

Tonic–Clonic Seizures and Myoclonic-Tonic–Clonic Seizures

Valproic acid has been a first-line drug for newly diagnosed generalized-onset tonic–clonic seizures for nearly half a century [5, 8, 9]. If valproic acid is not suitable, lamotrigine or levetiracetam may be used [9]. Carbamazepine and oxcarbazepine can be used only for patients with generalized tonic–clonic seizures. When the first-line drug therapy is ineffective or intolerable, lamotrigine, clobazam, levetiracetam, valproic acid, topiramate, perampanel, and lacosamide can be added as adjunctive therapies [10]. If patients with generalized-onset tonic–clonic seizures also have absences or myoclonic seizures, carbamazepine, oxcarbazepine, gabapentin, phenytoin, pregabalin, tiagabine, and vigabatrin cannot be used [11]. In patients who have myoclonic seizures or suspected juvenile myoclonic epilepsy, lamotrigine may exacerbate myoclonic seizures. There are no targeted clinical trials for myoclonic-tonic–clonic seizures, and drug selection is generally based on principles for tonic–clonic seizures.

Generalized-Onset Tonic, Clonic, or Atonic Seizures

Valproic acid is the first-line drug treatment for patients with generalized-onset tonic, clonic, or atonic seizures. If valproic acid is ineffective or not tolerated, lamotrigine or rufinamide may be added. If adjunctive therapy is still ineffective or intolerable, topiramate may be considered. Carbamazepine, oxcarbazepine, gabapentin, pregabalin, vigabatrin, and tiagabine are not recommended [11].

Generalized-Onset Myoclonic Seizures

Valproic acid is the first-line treatment for newly diagnosed myoclonic seizures. If valproic acid is not suitable or tolerable, use of levetiracetam [12] or topiramate [13] may be considered; however, compared to levetiracetam and valproic acid, topiramate has more side effects. When the first-line treatment is ineffective or intolerable, levetiracetam, valproic acid, or topiramate may be added for patients with myoclonic seizures. If adjunctive therapy is ineffective or intolerable, options may include clonazepam, clorazepate, lorazepam, or zonisamide. Carbamazepine, gabapentin, oxcarbazepine, phenytoin, pregabalin, vigabatrin, and tiagabine cannot be used [11].

Myoclonic-Atonic Seizures

This seizure type is common in Doose syndrome patients. The first-line drugs for treating seizures are valproic acid, levetiracetam, and zonisamide. If drug tolerance is needed, a ketogenic diet may be considered [14].

Epileptic Spasms

The UKISS and PERC studies recommend the use of ACTH and aminohexenoic acid for the treatment of epileptic spasms [15–18]. The International Collaborative Infantile Spasms Study (ICISS) further recommends early combination therapy with ACTH and vigabatrin [19].

Absence Seizures

① *Typical absence seizures and myoclonic absence seizures*: Ethosuximide or valproic acid is the first-line drug for treating typical absence seizures [20]. If there is a high risk of generalized tonic–clonic seizures, valproic acid should be considered first if there are no contraindications [21]. When ethosuximide and valproic acid are not suitable, ineffective, or not tolerated, lamotrigine use may be considered [22]. If two first-line anti-seizure medications are ineffective, a combination of ethosuximide, valproic acid, and lamotrigine may be considered. If combination therapy is ineffective or not tolerated, clinical data should be reviewed to re-evaluate the diagnosis, and if accurate, clorazepate, clonazepam, levetiracetam, topiramate, lorazepam, or zonisamide use may be considered. Carbamazepine, gabapentin, oxcarbazepine, phenytoin, pregabalin, vigabatrin, and aminohexenoic acid cannot be used. The treatment of myoclonic absence seizures requires robust evidence-based medicine, and currently, clinical practice remains consistent with the principles of treating typical absence seizures.

② *Atypical Absence Seizures*: Broad-spectrum anti-seizure medications such as valproic acid, levetiracetam, topiramate, clonazepam, and clobazam are routinely used for atypical absence seizures. Stiripentol can also be used for monotherapy in refractory patients [23].

③ *Eyelid Myoclonic Absence Seizures*: Traditional anti-seizure medications for treating eyelid myoclonic absence seizures include ethosuximide, valproic acid, benzodiazepines, and phenobarbital. Levetiracetam has been shown to be effective for treating this seizure type in multicenter placebo-controlled studies [24]. In clinical practice, lamotrigine is as effective as the aforementioned drugs [25, 26].

4.1.2.3 Medication Selection for Unclassifiable Seizures

For unclassifiable seizures, it is recommended in clinical practice to collect as much data as possible and to improve seizure classification. This may include telephone inquiries with witnesses who were not present at the outpatient clinic, asking family members to search for surveillance footage around the time of the seizure, or exporting data from motion bracelets or watches worn by the patient at the time of the seizure. If these methods do not provide sufficient information, long-term video electroencephalographic monitoring should be conducted to capture clinical seizures and obtain more accurate clinical-electrophysiological evidence for newly diagnosed epilepsy patients.

There is limited evidence-based treatment for unclassifiable seizures. The SANAD study suggested the use of phenytoin as a preferred option due to its low rate of adverse reactions and high retention rate, with lamotrigine and topiramate as alternative options for patients of childbearing age or those with contraindications to valproic acid [8]. The SANADII study compared the effects of valproic acid with those of levetiracetam and found no significant advantage of the latter; thus, levetiracetam is recommended as an alternative when valproic acid cannot be used.

4.2 Pharmacologic Treatment of Refractory Epilepsy

Epilepsy is a chronic brain disorder caused by a variety of etiologies, characterized by recurrent, seizure-inducing, and transient central nervous system malfunctions due to excessive neuronal discharge, affecting more than 70 million people worldwide. Despite the continuous introduction of new ASMs, approximately one-third of patients with epilepsy have seizures for which pharmacological treatment is ineffective. In 2010, the International League Against Epilepsy defined drug-refractory epilepsy (DRE) as a condition in which a sustained seizure-free status has not been achieved with the application of two correctly selected and tolerated ASMs (monotherapy or combinations), assessed over a period of time that can be 1 year or at least three times the previous longest seizure-free interval [27]. DRE is associated with the emergence of multiple comorbidities, mood disorders, and personality changes, severe psychosocial problems, increased risk of sudden death, increased mortality, cognitive problems, and decreased quality of life [28–31]. One study reported that in 2016, epilepsy accounted for the loss of more than 13 million disease-adjusted life years [32]. Between 30% and 40% of pediatric patients with epilepsy also suffer from intellectual disability, making it the most burdensome disease across the spectrum of neurological disorders in children and young adults [33, 34]. When assessing direct and indirect costs, the wage-based productivity losses associated with epilepsy are nearly equal to the combined wage losses due to anxiety, asthma, and depression [35].

Therefore, there is an urgent need to explore and study the treatment of DRE. Identifying which epilepsies can develop into DRE at an early stage is important for determining the prognoses of patients, and understanding the causes or mechanisms of DRE resistance is crucial for determining the exact treatment strategy and precise treatment. Current therapeutic strategies for DRE include pharmacologic therapy, epilepsy surgery, neuromodulation, a ketogenic diet, and lifestyle modification [28]. Among these options, anti-seizure medication is still the main treatment for DRE [36]. This section discusses in detail the strategies used for the pharmacologic treatment of refractory epilepsy.

4.2.1 Risk Factor Prediction for Drug-Refractory Epilepsy

It is important to assess the timing of treatment for DRE, and if DRE can be identified at an early stage during clinical diagnosis and treatment, early standardized management can help to improve patient prognosis. At present, an increasing number of scholars have conducted studies on the risk factors or predictors of DRE. Wang et al. [37] published a meta-analysis on the risk factors for refractory epilepsy in 2019, summarizing the studies that retained patients for the longest follow-up period or the largest sample size among 8397 studies between 1993 and 2018. Ultimately, 16 studies were included in the final meta-analysis, including 9 prospective analyses and 7 retrospective analyses. The prevalence of DRE was approximately 27%, according to the criteria of DRE defined by the International League Against Epilepsy in 2010, in which electroencephalogram (EEG) abnormalities (including slow waves and epileptiform discharges), status epilepticus (SE), symptomatic etiology, febrile convulsions, and multiple seizure types are strong risk factors for refractory epilepsy, while poor short-term treatment outcomes, neurodevelopmental delay, and high seizure frequency in the initial stages of epilepsy are not definite risk factors for DRE; however, the predictive effect of focal seizures is erratic.

In 2022, by summarizing and comparing the results of national and international studies, Li et al. [38] classified the levels of evidence of association found in the studies into four levels: (a) very little evidence: ≤1 available study; (b) insufficient (weak) evidence: two available studies reported significant associations in the same direction or three available studies, two of which reported significant associations in the same direction, and the third reported no significant associations; (c) strong evidence: three available studies reporting significant associations in the same direction or ≥4 available studies, of which >66% reported significant associations in the same direction and < 25% reported opposite associations; and (d) inconsistent evidence: remaining cases. However, the level of evidence for no association was as follows: (a) strong evidence: > four available studies, > 85% of which reported no association; (b) insufficient (weak) evidence: > four available studies, > 75% of which reported no association. Evidence was obtained on the basis of available univariate associations or on the basis of multivariate associations when univariate associations were unavailable. Clinical predictors of participation in the studies included ① age at onset, ② abnormal EEG (abnormal EEG (not refined), focal slowing, epileptiform discharges, generalized discharges), ③ type of seizure not refined (focal seizures, generalized seizures, mixed seizures), ④ status epilepticus, ⑤ febrile convulsions, ⑥ initial frequency of seizures not refined (at any time of the day, >1 seizure per month, >10 seizures prior to treatment), ⑦ symptomatic etiology (cortical dysplasia, asphyxia, perinatal hypoxic ischemic encephalopathy, temporal lobe medial sclerosis, neoplastic etiology, infectious etiology, vascular etiology, traumatic etiology, history of brain surgery, history of brain injury), ⑧ developmental delay, ⑨ comorbidities not subdivided (psychiatric disorders, depression, obesity), ⑩ failure to respond or poor response to the first ASM, ⑪ epileptic duration, ⑫ male sex, ⑬ neonatal epilepsy, ⑭ family history of epilepsy, ⑮ abnormalities in neuroimaging, and ⑯ abnormal neurological examination (remarks: not refined: a specific determinant or type not clearly identified in the study; EEG). Results: In the clinical predictor analysis, mixed seizure types, status epilepticus, no or poor response to first ASM, neonatal seizures, abnormal neuroimaging findings, and abnormal neurologic examination findings were strong predictors of DRE, whereas the grade of unassociated evidence showed that male sex and family history of epilepsy were strongly unassociated with DRE [38].

In the biochemical predictor analysis, the biochemical predictors involved in the analysis included ① inflammation-related predictors: high mobility group protein 1 (HMGB1), soluble vascular cell adhesion molecule 1 (sVCAM-1), activation- regulated chemokine (TARC)/soluble intercellular adhesion molecule 5 (sICAM5), neural cell adhesion molecule 1 (NCAM-1), human chitin 40 (YKL-40), programmed death receptor 1 (PD-1), zinc transporter 3 (ZnT3) and glial cell protofibrillary acidic protein (GFAP), ② epigenetic predictors (miR-4521, miR-139-5p, miR-34c-5p, miR-145-5p, miR-146a and miR-134, miR-146a and miR-134, miR-142 and miR-223, miR-342-5p, miR-584-5p, miR-150-5p, miR-125b-5p, miR-199a-3p, miR-199a-5p, miR 194-5p, miR-301a-3p, miR-30b-5p, miR-342-5p, miR-4446-3p), ③ genetic predictors (ABCB1, ABCC2, SCN1A, CACNA1A, CCL2), resulting in studies that found strong evidence that the inflammation-related marker HMGB1 and the genetic marker SCN1A are associated with DRE [38].

4.2.2 Mechanisms of Drug-Resistant Epilepsy

Bazhanova ED et al. [39] reviewed the global literature on the causes and mechanisms of drug resistance in epilepsy in 2021 and proposed eight current hypotheses regarding the causes of drug resistance in epilepsy (Table 4.1): the pharmacokinetic hypothesis, the transporter protein hypothesis, the neural network hypothesis, the intrinsic severity hypothesis, the genetic variation hypothesis, the epigenetic hypothesis, the target site hypothesis, and the neuroinflammatory hypothesis. The following describes the specific meanings of the eight hypotheses and the evidence supporting and not supporting the hypotheses. ① The pharmacokinetic hypothesis refers to the fact that the overexpression of drug efflux carriers in peripheral organs reduces anticonvulsant drug levels and that the overexpression of transporters in the blood–brain

Table 4.1 Eight hypotheses of drug-resistant epilepsy mechanisms

Hypotheses of epilepsy drug resistance
Target hypothesis
Genetic variants hypothesis
Transport hypothesis
Epigenetic hypothesis
Neural network hypothesis
Pharmacokinetic hypothesis
Hypothesis of neuroinflammation
Intrinsic severity hypothesis

barrier and neurons does not account for the clinically observed decrease in drug concentrations [28]. There are also animal studies that do not support the pharmacokinetic hypothesis [40]. ② The transporter protein hypothesis states that the overexpression of drug efflux carriers in the blood–brain barrier reduces anticonvulsant drug levels and that multidrug resistance proteins are overexpressed in cerebral capillary endothelial cells and astrocytes of patients with drug-resistant epilepsy [41]. This hypothesis is supported only by animal studies and not in human tissues [42]. ③ The neural network hypothesis refers to neuronal degeneration and synaptic network remodeling leading to the inhibition of the brain's seizure control system and the limitation of drug access to targets. Cortical dysplasia is often associated with drug-resistant epilepsy. The basis of pathological neural networks in focal drug-resistant epilepsy [43] supports this hypothesis, while some patients with cortical dysplasia and altered neural networks are not drug resistant. The finding that some patients do not respond to anti-seizure medications after temporal lobectomy [44] does not support this hypothesis. ④ The intrinsic severity hypothesis refers to neurobiological factors that influence both the severity of epilepsy and drug resistance, a hypothesis supported by clinical reports and transcriptomic analysis of human hippocampal tissue. However, the results of these studies, suggesting that drug resistance does not depend on the number and severity of pretreatment seizures [28], do not support this hypothesis. ⑤ The genetic variation hypothesis refers to genetic polymorphisms that are associated with pharmacodynamics, metabolic pathways, enzymes, ion channels, and neurotransmitter receptors, and the blockage of drug binding, metabolism, and transport leads to the development of resistance. It has been found that polymorphisms are associated with various types of epilepsy, and that genetic changes occur in patients with untreatable epilepsy [45], supporting this hypothesis. ⑥ The epigenetic hypothesis refers to the idea that changes in the epigenome can play a role in the pattern of drug resistance, and manipulation of microRNAs can influence the course of seizures and epileptic episodes in experiments using laboratory animals [40, 43, 46], supporting this hypothesis. However, it is difficult to separate cause from effect and significance from collateral phenomena, especially in humans, where no favorable evidence can be provided. ⑦ The target hypothesis refers to potentially dependent quantitative and qualitative changes in ion channels and neurotransmitter receptors leading to a reduction in drug susceptibility and development of drug resistance, which is supported by studies of Dravet syndrome and by studies of the effectiveness of carbamazepine and phenytoin [28, 40, 47], whereas patients with drug-resistant epilepsy are usually unresponsive to different classes of drugs with different mechanisms of action. ⑧ The neuroinflammatory hypothesis refers to the fact that neuroinflammation can induce blood–brain barrier dysfunction and upregulate Pgp expression in drug-resistant epilepsy, which has been found experimentally and clinically to increase blood–brain barrier permeability in patients with chronic epileptic foci. Many studies have shown increased cytokine levels in the brains and plasma of patients with drug-resistant epilepsy and in animal models [48], supporting this hypothesis.

4.2.3 Pharmacologic Strategies for Treating Drug-Resistant Epilepsy

It is undeniable that drug treatment of DRE still serves as the main strategy, and many domestic and international scholars are now investing in research on anti-seizure medications; almost one drug is developed every year. The three generations of anti-seizure medications used are listed in Table 4.2 [49]. The selection of effective ASMs and the formulation of effective combination drug regimens are crucial for the treatment of DRE, which will be explained in detail in the following sections.

4.2.3.1 Pretreatment Assessment

Many epileptologists believe that a careful evaluation is needed before proceeding with medicating DRE patients and that medication decisions are made after the evaluation has once again clarified the circumstances under which DRE was achieved. The pretreatment assessment includes the following: first, the diagnosis of DRE needs to be reviewed for errors based on medical history; second, whether the clarification of seizure types and syndromes is correct and complete; third, whether

Table 4.2 Three generations of anti-seizure medications

First-generation ASMs	Second-generation ASMs	Third-generation ASMs
Bromide, Phenobarbital, Mephobarbital, Phenytoin, Acetazolamide, Trimethadione, Mephenytoin, Paramethadione, Corticosteroids/ACTH, Phenacemide, Phensuximide, Primidone, Methsuximide, Ethotoin, Ethsuximide	Chlordiazepoxide, Sulthiame, Diazepam, Carbamazepine, Valproate, Clonazepam, Clobazam	Progabide, Vigabatrin, Zonisamide, Lamotrigine, Oxcarbazepine, Felbamate, Gabapentin, Topiramate, Tiagabine, Levetiracetam, Pregabalin, Stiripentol, Rufinamide, Lacosamide, Eslicarbazepine acetate, Retigabine (ezogabine), Perampanel, Imepitoin (dogs), Brivaracetam, Everolimus

the ASM is adequately dosed; fourth, how well the patient adheres to the medication and whether the medications are being taken as prescribed; and fifth, whether the patient has a poor lifestyle (substance abuse, addiction to sensory stimuli such as games) that can easily induce seizures [50–56].

4.2.3.2 Objectives of Treatment

Studies have shown that patients with DRE have significant neuropsychological, psychiatric, and social impairments, and they are also affected in terms of their employment, decreased marriage rates, increased divorce rates, and decreased quality of life [57]. The primary goal pursued by domestic and international epileptologists is to completely control seizures, improve the quality of life of patients, and enable them to return to normal life. However, drug-refractory epilepsy has a complex mechanism and etiology, and it is often difficult to achieve complete seizure control; therefore, the goal is to minimize seizures and to improve quality of life so that patients can adapt to a normal social life [58].

4.2.3.3 Principles and Methods of Treatment

The current principles for the selection of ASMs are based on the type of seizure and epileptic syndrome, as well as the etiologic profile; the efficacy, tolerability, half-life, and potential drug–drug interactions, as well as the individual-specific adverse effects of the ASMs; and the impact on comorbidities and the pharmacoeconomic cost of the medication. Issues to consider when replacing or combining drugs with a second drug when the first drug is poorly controlled or when intolerable side effects occur include proper drug selection, failure to titrate the drug to the individual's optimal dose, poor timing of dosing, too rapid a dose increase, and poor control of the cause of the seizure. If seizure control is not achieved with an adequate dose of the second ASM, a combination of drugs should be considered [59]. The most famous study on how patients respond to combination medication was published by Brodie MJ et al. [60] in 2012, patients who were newly diagnosed with epilepsy and prescribed their first ASM between July 1, 1982 and April 1, 2006, were followed up with gradual adjustments of the ASM regimen as seizures progressed, up to March 31, 2008. This study had a total enrollment of 1098 patients, and at the time of the last outpatient visit, 749 (68%) patients were seizure-free. The maximum number of drugs used was nine. In terms of progressively added ASMs versus seizure-free status, the use of two ASMs resulted in a seizure-free rate in the cohort of up to 62.8%, whereas the cohort was only 5.5% seizure-free when the total number of additional medications was increased from 3 to 9 (Table 4.3) [60].

The pharmacological treatment of DRE is mainly a combination therapy, and many epileptologists have different opinions about combination therapy. However, the most important point is that a combination of ASMs based on different mechanisms of action is more effective and has fewer side effects than a combination of

Table 4.3 Seizure-free rates with continuous use of anti-seizure medications

Order of addition of drugs	Number of patients	Seizure-free rate of the cohort (%)	Seizure-free rate (%) of the additive drug order present
First drug	1098	49.5	49.5
Second drug	398	13.3	36.7
Third drug	168	3.7	24.4
Fourth drug	68	1.0	16.2
Fifth drug	32	0.4	12.5
Sixth drug	16	0.2	12.5
Seventh drug	9	0.2	22.2
Eighth drug	3	0.0	0.0
Ninth drug	2	0.0	0.0

drugs with the same mechanism; this is understood by most people [61]. The mechanisms of common ASMs are summarized in Table 4.4 [62]. The metabolic effects of combining ASMs should also be taken into account, e.g., sodium valproate is a selective hepatic enzyme inhibitor that increases the blood levels of other medications; while carbamazepine, phenytoin, phenobarbital, and pramipexole are broad-spectrum hepatic enzyme inducers that decrease the blood levels of other medications metabolized by the liver. The prevalence of comorbidities in patients with epilepsy is two to eight times greater than that in the general population. Approximately half of patients with epilepsy have at least one comorbidity, and it is even more common in patients with DRE [62]. Drug combinations should also focus on comorbidities, and the selection of ASMs for epilepsy with concomitant comorbidities is summarized as follows: ① Obesity ± diabetes mellitus: choose topiramate (TPM), zonisamide(ZNS); avoid VPA, pregabalin (PGB), gabapentin (GBP), pirempanel (PER). ② Migraine: choose TPM, VPA, ZNS, PBG, GBP. ③ Rash: choose levetiracetam (LEV), GBP, PGB, TPM, VPA, PER, lacosamide (LCM), avoid lamotrigine (LTG), oxcarbazepine (OXC), carbamazepine (CBZ), phenytoin (PHT), PB. ④ Neuropathic pain: choose PGB, GBP, CBZ, OXC, PHT. ⑤ Depression ± behavioral/psychological problems: choose LTG, CBZ, OXC, VPA, PGB; avoid LEV, PB, pramipexole (PRM), TPM, ZNS. ⑥ Cognitive dysfunction: choose LTG, LEV, OXC; avoid phenobarbital (PB), TPM, ZNS. ⑦ Concomitant drug use: choose GBP, LEV, PGB, VPA; avoid enzyme-inducing drugs. ⑧ Restless legs syndrome: choose GBP, PGB, clonazepam (CZP). ⑨ Kidney stones: avoid TPM, ZNS. ⑩ Glaucoma: avoid TPM. ⑪ Hematological diseases: avoid CBZ, VPA. ⑫ Hyponatremia: avoid OXC, escrivastigmine (ESL), CBZ. ⑬: choose new ASMs (nonhepatotoxic, renal excretion), avoid VPA. ⑭ Kidney disease: choose obsolete ASMs (excretion through hepatic metabolism). ⑮ Osteoporosis: choose LTG, LEV; avoid enzyme-inducing drugs, TPM, VPA, ZNS. ⑯ Gait disorders: avoid CBZ, PHT, PER. ⑰ Tremor: choose TPM, PER; avoid VPA. ⑱ Parkinson's syndrome: choose ZNS. ⑲ Arrhythmia: avoid CBZ, LTG, LCM, and other sodium channel blockers. ⑳ Cancer: choose VPA, LEV, PER; avoid enzyme-inducing drugs. ㉑ Heat stroke: avoid TPM, ZNS. ㉒ Atherosclerosis: avoid enzyme-inducing drugs [63]. Lee BI et al. also proposed steps for drug combination therapy (Table 4.5) [63].

Table 4.4 Mechanisms of anti-seizure medications

Veterinary drug/machine	BZDs	PB	CBZ	PHT	VPA	ETV	FBM	GBP	LCM	LTG	LEV	OXC	PGB	RUF	TGB	TPM	ZNS
Sodium channel			+++	+++	+++		++	+		+++		+++		++		++	+++
Calcium channel/ current			+		+	+++	++	++		+		+	++			++	++
GABAergic Transmission effects of	+++	+++	+		+		++	+							+++	++	
Glutamate receptor (Glu), an amino acid							++									++	
Other mechanisms									Binds to CRMP-2 receptor		Regulation of presynaptic neurotransmitter release through SV2A receptor binding					Weak carbonic anhydrase inhibitor	Weak carbonic anhydrase inhibitor

Abbreviations: *GABA* gamma-aminobutyric acid, ϒ-aminobutyric acid type B, *SV2A* synaptic vesicle glycoprotein 2A
++ likely target; +++ very likely target

Table 4.5 In the second drug selection process, the therapeutic index was defined as the ratio of the effective dose (ED50) to the toxic dose (TD50)

Comprehensive drug selection
Step 1: Preferred drug candidate
Medications that have not been used before
Previously used drugs have proven at least partially effective
Drugs with the high therapeutic index or good tolerability
Drugs with no or low risk of pharmacokinetic interactions with concomitant drugs
Drugs with ideal mechanisms of action
Effective for patients with comorbidities
Step 2: Medications that match partner medications
Drugs known to interact synergistically
Drugs showing different side effects
Drugs with no or minimal potential for pharmacokinetic interactions

Charyyeva G et al. [64] summarized the drug preferences for monotherapy and combination therapy for different seizure types and syndromes as follows: ① Focal seizures (structural and metabolic): The preferred single drugs include CBZ, LEV, PHT, ZNS, VPA, GBP, LTG, OXC, EST, LCM, PB, TPM, and CZP [65]. Preferred drugs for combination therapy or multidrug therapy include CBZ, LEV, ZNS, TPM, VPA, LTG, OXC, EST, LCM, BRV, PER, GBP, PGB, PB, CZP, and PHT. ② Isolated generalized epileptic seizures: The preferred drugs for monotherapy include VPA, PB, PHT, LEV, LTG, and TPM [66]. The preferred drugs for combination or multiple drugs include LTG, OXC, TPM, VPA, LEV, PER, PB, CZP, and PHT. ③ Myoclonic seizures: monotherapy preferred drugs include VPA, TPM, ZNS, and LEV; combination or polypharmacy preferred drugs include VPA, TPM, LEV, ZNS, CZP, PB, ESM [67]. ④ Aphasic seizures (juvenile aphasic epilepsy): single-agent preferences include valproate; combination or multidrug preferences include LEV, ZNS, TPM, ESM, or LTG [68]. ⑤ Unspecified seizure type: single-agent preferred drugs include broad-spectrum ASMs. The World Health Organization has developed initial doses of ASM and maintenance therapy for adults (Table 4.6).

4.2.3.4 First-Line Anti-seizure Medications

Currently, old and new ASMs are divided into three generations. Generation I ASMs include PB, PHT, ESM, CZP, CBZ, and VPA; generation II ASMs include LTG, GBP, TPM, PGB, OXC, LEV, ZNS, and aminocaproic acid; and generation III ASMs include LCM, ESM, lufenamide, piracetam, and BRV [66, 69]. The advantages, disadvantages, and major side effects of current first-line ASMs are summarized in Table 4.7 [70].

Table 4.6 Initial target dose and maintenance dose of anti-seizure medications in adults

Medications	ITD (mg/day)	MD (mg/day)	DDD(mg)
Carbamazepine	400–600	400–1200	1000
Chlorpazan	10	10–40	8
Eslicarbazepine	800	800–1200	800
Ethosuximide	500	500–1500	1250
Gabapentin	900	900–3600	1800
Lacosamide	200	200–400	300
Lamotrigine	150 (single drug)	200–400	300
Lamotrigine	75 (combined with valproic acid)	75–200	
Lamotrigine	300 (coenzyme inducer)	200–500	
Levetiracetam	1000	1000-3000	1500
Oxcarbazepine	600	600–2400	1000
Perampanel	4	4–12	8
Phenobarbital	60	60–120	100
Phenytoin sodium (a sedative)	200	200–400	300
Pregabalin	300	300–600	300
Povidone	500	500–1500	1250
Lufenamide	1200	1200–3200	1400
Topiramate	100	100–400	300
Valproic acid	500	500–2000	1500
Chlordiazepoxide	1000	1000–3000	2000
Zonisamide	200	200–600	200

Abbreviations: *ITD* initial target dose, *MD* maintenance dose, *DDD* defined daily mean dose

Table 4.7 Advantages and disadvantages of first-line anti-seizure medications

Name of drug	Advantages	Disadvantages	Important adverse reactions
Carbamazepine	Efficacy in focal seizures, widespread use, and clinical experience, mood stabilizer, low cost	Enzyme inducer; can exacerbate catatonic and myoclonic seizures	Hypersensitivity reactions, cardiac conduction abnormalities, hyponatremia
Ethosuximide	Effective in disorienting seizures; May not have enzyme-inducing properties; low cost	No therapeutic effect on generalized tonic–clonic seizures, can coexist with catatonic seizures in some syndromes	Allergic reactions, gastrointestinal side effects
Gabapentin	Virtually no drug interactions; Better-tolerated and effective for neuropathic pain	Relatively mild, limited to focal seizures; may induce myoclonic seizures	Weight gain

(continued)

Table 4.7 (continued)

Name of drug	Advantages	Disadvantages	Important adverse reactions
Lamotrigine	Effective in focal and most generalized seizure types, lacks enzyme-inducing properties, effective in bipolar depression	Requires slow titration; is required for administration of drugs that interact with valproate, enzyme inducers, and estrogens; can exacerbate infantile heavy myoclonic epilepsy	Rash and other severe allergic reactions
Levetiracetam	Effects on focal, myoclonic, and predominantly generalized tonic–clonic seizures; few drug interactions; relatively well tolerated	Costs more than most other anti-seizure medications	Irritability, mood changes
Oxcarbazepine	Similar to carbamazepine, it has a lower risk of rash and lower enzyme induction potential	Reduces blood levels of oral contraceptives; can exacerbate catatonic and myoclonic seizures	Rash and other hypersensitivity reactions; hyponatremia more common than carbamazepine
Phenobarbital	Effective for focal and most generalized seizure types, well-understood and studied, once-daily dosing, low cost	Enzyme inducer; can exacerbate catatonic seizures	Adverse cognitive and behavioral effects
Phenytoin	Anti-focal seizures, experienced and cost effective	Enzyme inducer, variable and dose-dependent kinetics; may exacerbate catatonic and myoclonic seizures	Rash and other allergic reactions; connective tissue and surface adverse effects
Topiramate	Treatment of focal and generalized attacks; effective in migraine prevention	Slow titration	Adverse effects of cognitive decline, weight loss, sensory abnormalities, kidney stones, glaucoma
Valproic acid	Very effective in most generalized seizure types; also effective in focal seizures; effective in migraine prevention; mood stabilizer	Selective enzyme inhibitors; caution should be taken in women with epilepsy of childbearing age	Weight gain, adverse endocrine effects, alopecia, hepatotoxicity, pancreatitis, greater teratogenic potential than other anti-seizure medications, postnatal cognitive effects after fetal exposure

(continued)

Table 4.7 (continued)

Name of drug	Advantages	Disadvantages	Important adverse reactions
Aminohexenoic acid	Effective in treating infantile spasms	Unfavorable risk-benefit ratio for external use in patients with infantile spasms	Irreversible visual field defects, weight gain
Zonisamide	Effective against focal and probably the other most prevalent type of seizures; lacks enzyme-inducing properties; once-daily dose	Limited experience outside Japan and some Pacific Rim countries	Rash and other allergic reactions, weight loss, kidney stones, low amniotic fluid

4.2.3.5 Third-Generation Anti-seizure Medications and New-Generation ASMs

Due to the difficulty of treating DRE, an increasing number of researchers are investigating new ASMs, and the following summarizes the chemical structures, main mechanisms of action, indications, maintenance doses, precautions, and side effects of new-generation ASMs used in the clinic since 2006 (Table 4.8) [71–81].

4.2.3.6 Assessment and Monitoring of Treatment Effects

Assessing the efficacy of ASMs and monitoring the side effects are critical components of DRE management and should result in timely adjustments to medication regimens and the mitigation of adverse factors. Three specific aspects of treatment outcome are usually assessed. First, seizure frequency and severity: monitoring changes in seizure frequency and severity are primary indicators of treatment response. Accurate seizure diaries and detailed descriptions of patients and their caregivers are valuable sources of information. EEG can also be reviewed regularly. Some studies recommend rechecking once every 4–6 months [64]. It is now also possible to accurately assess the frequency and extent of seizures by wearing artificial intelligence seizure monitoring equipment. Assessing the impact of treatment on an individual's quality of life can provide a comprehensive picture of the overall benefit of treatment in patients with DRE. Validated questionnaires and scales, such as the Quality of Life in Epilepsy (QOLIE) measure, can be used to assess the subjective experience of treatment outcome. Neuropsychological assessment, cognitive functioning, behavior, and emotional well-being can be affected by the epilepsy itself and its treatments; therefore, neuropsychological assessments can help to identify any cognitive or behavioral changes in the disease itself related to the intervention.

Table 4.8 Main anti-seizure medications since 2006

Veterinary drug	Chemical structure (2D)	Main mechanism of action	Approved indications	Effective daily maintenance dose	Comments[a]
Eslicarbazepine acetate	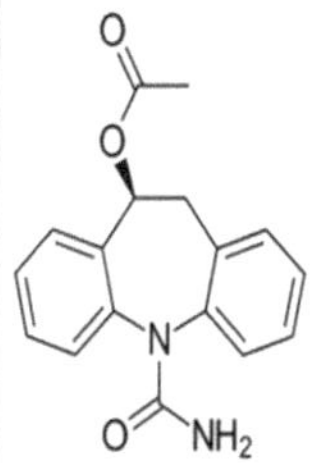	Blocking voltage-dependent sodium channels	EU approval: adult focal epilepsy with or without secondary generalization	800–1200 mg/d	Precursor drug of eslicarbazepine, the main active metabolite of oxcarbazepine
Lacosamide	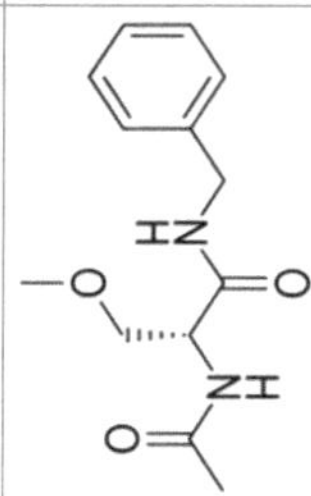	Enhanced voltage-dependent slow inactivation of sodium channels	EU approval: adjunctive treatment of focal seizures with or without secondary generalization in patients aged > = 16 years	200–400 mg/day administered twice daily	Low drug–drug interactions; preliminary data suggest improved tolerability when combined with nonsodium channel blockers; also available as a parenteral formulation
Perampanel	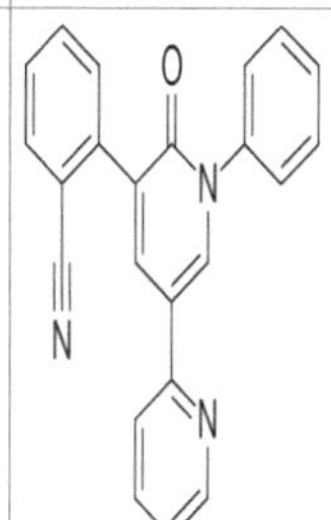	Noncompetitive antagonists of glutamatergic AMPA receptors	EU approval: adjunctive treatment of focal epilepsy with or without secondary generalization in patients aged >12 years	4–12 mg once daily	Carbamazepine, phenytoin, and oxcarbazepine reduce perampanel serum concentrations two- to threefold; approved for once-daily administration

Regabine (also known as egabine)	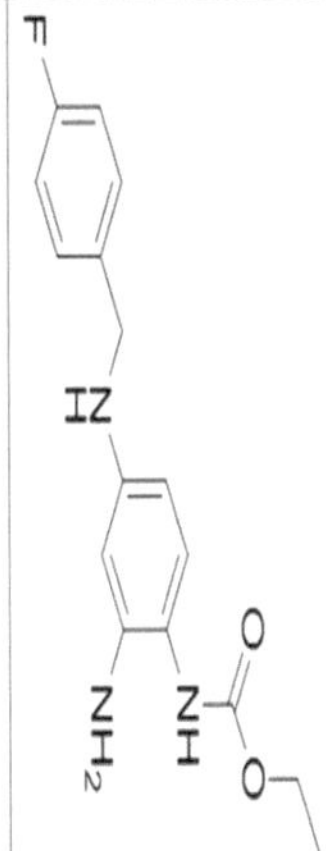	Kv7 channel-mediated enhancement of neuronal M-type potassium currents	EU approval: adjunctive therapy for drug-resistant focal seizures with or without secondary promotion in patients aged greater than or equal to 18 years when other appropriate drug combinations have proved inadequate or are not tolerated	600–1200 mg/day, three doses per day	High rates of discoloration of ocular tissues (including the retina), skin, lips, and nails in long-term studies; therefore, regabine should be considered an orphan drug requiring ophthalmologic examination prior to and during use
Lufenamide	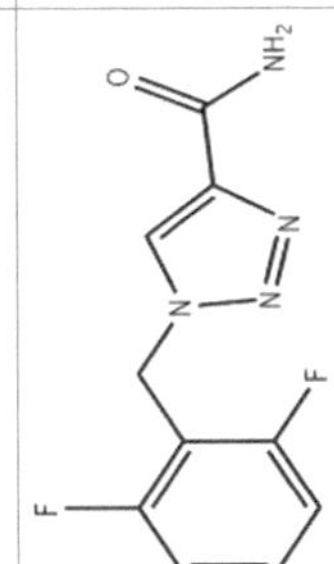	Blocking voltage-dependent sodium channels	EU approval: for age ≥4 years Lennox-Gastaut Adjunctive therapy for syndrome-associated seizures	Depending on age and age variations; twice daily	Valproic acid increases serum lufenamide concentrations, especially in younger children; lufenamide is an inducer of cytochrome CYP3A4

(continued)

Table 4.8 (continued)

Veterinary drug	Chemical structure (2D)	Main mechanism of action	Approved indications	Effective daily maintenance dose	Comments[a]
Stavudine	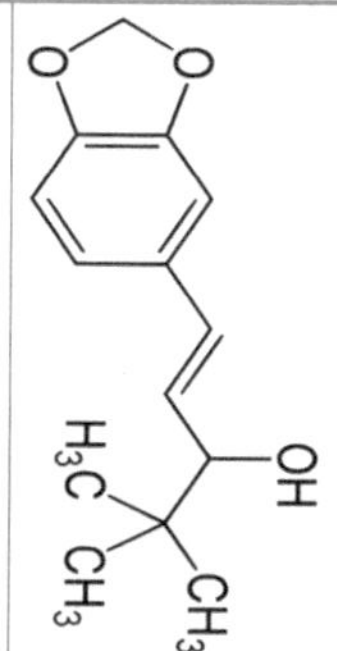	Enhanced GABAergic transmission	EU approval: adjunctive therapy, combined with clobazam and valproate, refractory generalized tonic clonic seizures in patients with severe myoclonic epilepsy in infancy	50 mg/day two or three times daily	Stavudine inhibits the metabolism of many coadministered anti-seizure medications and requires dose adjustment when coadministered
Phenobarbital	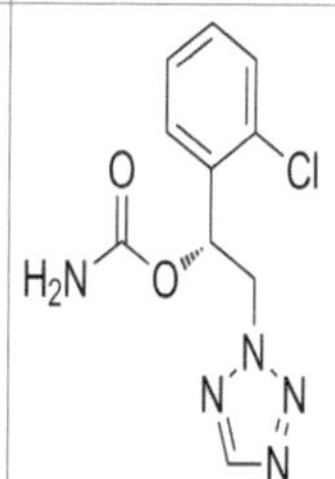	Binding site different from conventional sodium channel blockers blocks sodium channels and enhances GABAergic transmission	Approved by the U.S. Food and Drug Administration (FDA): drugs for the treatment of partial (localized) seizures in adults as further combination therapy for medically refractory partial epilepsy in adults	25–400 mg/day	Slow titration is recommended and the most common side effects are drowsiness, dizziness, headache and fatigue;

Boissetin	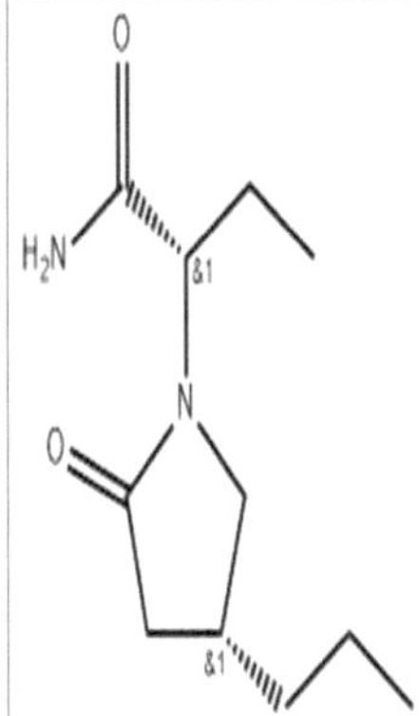	Controls seizures by modulating the release of SV2A receptor-bound presynaptic neurotransmitters, but with 15–30 times the affinity of levetiracetam, a fast-acting drug	Adjunctive treatment of partial seizures with or without secondary generalized seizures in patients 16 years of age and older	100–200 mg/day	May be added as an add-on therapy for patients with drug-refractory adult partial epilepsy who have failed five or more treatments; most frequent side effects are drowsiness, dizziness, headache, and fatigue.
Cannabidiol	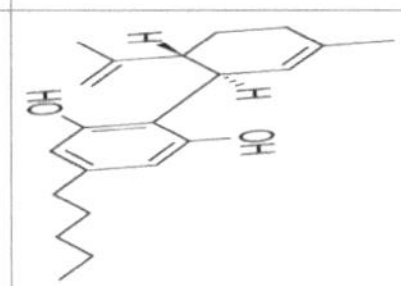	Cannabidiol, whose mechanism of action is unknown, binds to both cannabinoid receptors 1 and 2; some clinical studies have found that it effectively increases the concentration of the clobazam metabolite, N-desmethylclobazam, to enhance antiepileptic effects	May be used as adjunctive therapy for seizures associated with Dravet syndrome and Lennox-Gastaut syndrome in children	20 mg/day	The most common side effects are drowsiness, loss of appetite and diarrhea, and increased liver enzymes

Abbreviations: *AMPA* alpha-amino-3-hydroxy-5-methyl-4-isoxazolepropionic acid
[a]More information, including side effects

Second, monitoring the side effects of medicines is essential to minimize their impact on patients and to ensure patient safety and health. Regular monitoring should include the following: a. Adverse event reporting: primarily through regular follow-up revisits, specialists should proactively ask individuals and their caregivers about any potential side effects. b. Clinical examination: regular clinical examinations, including physical and neurological assessments, can help to detect any adverse physical reactions or neurological abnormalities associated with treatment; c. Laboratory tests: depending on the specific medication used, blood tests, such as liver function tests and complete blood count, follow-up check of abdominal organs (ultrasound once a year), electrocardiogram (once every 6 months), complete blood count and urinalysis once every 3 months, and biochemical blood tests once every 6 months [65], may be required to monitor potential drug-related side effects.

4.2.3.7 Future Prospects and Research Directions in Drug Therapy

Following the intensive study of the genetics of epilepsy, a foundation has been laid for the early realization of individualized and precision therapy [82, 83]. In terms of drug research and development, through the study of DRE mechanisms, we can transform the current epilepsy animal models for anti-seizure medication screening to make their manifestations more similar to those of real patients and to more effectively screen effective anti-seizure medications with different mechanisms [84, 85]. In the future, more attention should be given to understanding the etiology of DRE, such as immunity, genetics, the development of immunosuppressive drugs targeting brain (and peripheral) inflammation, and inhibitors of the mTOR pathway, and exploring more options for refractory epilepsy pharmacotherapy from different approaches [86–88].

4.3 Drug Therapy for Seizures of Different Etiologies

4.3.1 Selection of Anti-seizure Medications for Epileptic Seizures and Epilepsy After Cerebrovascular Disease

Cerebrovascular diseases encompass a spectrum of conditions characterized by functional impairment of the brain due to vascular alterations, including ischemic and hemorrhagic types, which predominantly affect middle-aged and elderly individuals. Common manifestations include motor, language, sensory, and consciousness impairments. According to the 2019 Global Burden of Diseases (GBD) report, stroke remains a leading cause of disability and mortality globally. In China, there were 39.4 million new stroke cases in 2019, indicating a significant disease burden. Ischemic stroke/cerebral infarction accounts for 83% of hospitalized cerebrovascular disease patients. Acute cerebral infarction is associated with numerous complications, among which poststroke seizures significantly increase mortality and disability rates, prolong hospitalization [89], and exacerbate the burden of stroke [90].

4.3.1.1 Definition of Epilepsy and Epileptic Attacks in Cerebrovascular Diseases

Cerebrovascular diseases can be classified into ischemic and hemorrhagic types, with the former comprising approximately 80%, including conditions such as cerebral infarction, cerebral embolism, and transient ischemic attacks, and the latter constituting approximately 20%, including conditions such as cerebral hemorrhage, subarachnoid hemorrhage, epidural hemorrhage, and subdural hemorrhage. Disease progression can be acute or chronic, with the former encompassing ischemic and hemorrhagic cerebrovascular diseases and the latter, including cerebral small vessel disease, atherosclerosis, aneurysms, cerebral vascular malformations, and Moyamoya disease.

Epilepsy in cerebrovascular diseases primarily refers to seizures arising from acute stroke events. The ILAE proposed a clinical practical definition of epilepsy in 2017 [91], which specifies that epilepsy comprises at least two nonprovoked seizures occurring more than 24 h apart within 1 year, with a risk of more than 60% for two unprovoked seizures to recur within 10 years after a single seizure and a diagnosis of epilepsy syndrome. The risk of epilepsy recurrence is even greater if a single seizure occurs after 1 month of acute cerebral infarction [92]. Therefore, according to this practical definition, patients who experience a single unprovoked seizure within 30 days after a stroke and have a subsequent risk of more than 60% for another seizure may be considered for a diagnosis of poststroke epilepsy (PSE).

In 2010, the ILAE Working Group proposed a definition for acute symptomatic seizures, specifying them as seizures closely related to acute central nervous system damage, with the time interval between injury and seizure varying depending on different clinical circumstances [93]. This literature explicitly states that seizures induced by structural or metabolic changes within 7 days after a stroke should be classified as acute symptomatic seizures, since seizures during this period do not represent changes in neural networks and do not necessarily indicate the occurrence of poststroke epilepsy [92].

The time boundaries for early-onset seizures (ESs) and late-onset seizures (LSs) after stroke remain controversial in the literature. Recent meta-analyses have indicated that the longer the time after a stroke event, the lower the incidence of seizure events. Considering the epidemiological characteristics of early-onset and late-onset seizures, 14 days has been proposed as the ideal boundary between the two. A 2021 retrospective study revealed a significantly greater proportion of subsequent PSEs in ischemic stroke patients who experienced seizures 4–7 days after stroke than in those who experienced seizures 1–3 days after stroke (35.5% vs. 10.0%, $p = 0.002$). Cox risk modeling confirmed the association between seizures occurring 4–7 days after stroke and PSE (HR 3.84, 95% CI 1.77–8.31; $p = 0.001$) [94].

Moreover, more than 70% of poststroke seizures following endovascular treatment occur within 1–3 days after stroke. Thus, a second perspective suggests that the boundary between ESs and LSs is 3 days. Additionally, multiple studies have shown that the initial 24 h after ischemic stroke represent the peak period for seizure occurrence [95, 96]. Therefore, there is currently no consensus on the classification of ES and LS, but a trend has been observed indicating that the longer the time after a stroke event is, the lower the incidence of acute symptomatic seizures and the greater the likelihood of subsequent PSE.

Reperfusion therapy for ischemic stroke, including intravenous thrombolysis and endovascular treatment, is currently the only clearly effective rescue strategy. In 1995, the National Institute of Neurological Disorders and Stroke (NINDS) first proposed the efficacy of intravenous infusion of recombinant tissue plasminogen activator (rtPA) within 3 h of onset for acute ischemic stroke [97]. Three consecutive 2015 articles in the New England Journal of Medicine confirmed that bridging intravenous thrombolysis with endovascular treatment significantly improved the prognoses of patients with ischemic stroke. Endovascular treatment can be performed within 6 h of anterior circulation occlusion onset and within 24 h of posterior circulation occlusion onset. There is currently no unified international guideline or consensus regarding poststroke seizures after reperfusion therapy. The definition of thrombolysis-related poststroke seizures still needs to be refined in conjunction with factors such as stroke type, responsible vascular location, etiology, and reperfusion intervention time. Based on the integration of the above definitions and the literature in this field, poststroke seizures following reperfusion therapy are limited to patients with cerebral infarction who have received intravenous thrombolysis and/or endovascular treatment, without any other obvious causes or a history of seizures before stroke, who experienced two or more seizures within 7 days after the stroke event, or who experienced one or more seizures within 30 days after the stroke event.

4.3.1.2 Epidemiology

The incidence of epilepsy varies greatly among different populations with cerebrovascular diseases. The incidence of epileptic seizures associated with ischemic cerebrovascular disease ranges from 1.5% to 12.4%, while that following cerebral hemorrhage ranges from 6.6% to 15%, and after subarachnoid hemorrhage, it is 11%. The incidence of seizures caused by cerebral venous sinus thrombosis is as high as 50%. The incidence of seizures after thrombolysis ranges from 5% to 13.5%, similar to that of stroke-related seizures; early seizures occur at a rate of 2–5.5%, and late seizures occur at a rate of 3–12%. Due to differences in the stroke types included, follow-up times, and definitions of early and late seizures in different studies, the incidence rates vary. Currently, most studies lack neurophysiological assessments, and the frequency of acute symptomatic seizures may be underestimated.

Stroke and epilepsy have a bidirectional and inseparable relationship and influence each other. Stroke is a major cause of epilepsy in middle-aged and elderly people. Due to the trend toward an increase in the global aging population and the high incidence of cerebrovascular diseases, the number of patients with epilepsy caused by stroke is expected to continue to increase in the coming decades. A 2018 report from the International League Against Epilepsy Prevention Task Force mentioned that stroke is the most common preventable cause of epilepsy in elderly people in both high-income and low-income countries. A 25-year prospective study based on a community population revealed that premature death in epilepsy patients is mainly associated with three major causes, including stroke, with very few deaths related directly to epilepsy. Patients with epilepsy, especially young patients or those taking high doses of anti-seizure medications, have a greater risk of cerebrovascular disease than does the general population [98]. The risk is highest in the first year after epilepsy diagnosis [99]. A retrospective 2019 study in Sweden analyzed the number of seizures patients experienced before stroke and the expected number of seizures in Sweden over the past 10 years and revealed that approximately 5–20% of cases of epilepsy onset after age 60 are indicative of stroke occurrence [100].

Early clinical trials proposed that epilepsy is a contraindication for thrombolysis in patients with acute ischemic stroke [97]. In current clinical practice, a case-by-case analysis is needed: if a patient has a history of epilepsy and experiences an acute stroke, a thrombolysis assessment should be initiated; if acute symptomatic seizure is the initial symptom of stroke and Todd's paralysis is confirmed through clinical and imaging examinations, immediate consideration of vascular reperfusion therapy is warranted; if the patient is in status epilepticus and limb muscle strength cannot recover to the preonset level between seizures, the possibility of Todd's paralysis should be taken into consideration, although CT perfusion (CTP) and magnetic resonance imaging (MRI) with arterial spin labeling (ASL), diffusion-weighted imaging (DWI), or perfusion-weighted imaging (PWI) often show increased perfusion due to status epilepticus. Further, the quality of imaging results may be compromised due to interference from status epilepticus, requiring careful consideration of thrombolysis feasibility.

4.3.1.3 Pathogenetic Mechanisms of Epilepsy Related to Etiology

The pathogenetic mechanisms of epilepsy related to cerebrovascular diseases are complex and varied, and are temporally associated with the occurrence of stroke and epileptic seizures. Early poststroke seizures are mainly caused by hypoperfusion with or without reperfusion, leading to increased excitability mediated by glutamate due to cerebral tissue hypoxia and reduced inhibition by GABA. After the stroke, blood–brain barrier disruption activates astrocytes, releasing inflammatory factors such as transforming growth factor-β (TGF-β), tumor necrosis factor-α (TNF-α), and interleukin-6 (IL-6), while proteinase-activated receptor-1 (PAR-1) expression is upregulated. Ion channel dysfunction occurs following stroke, particularly in the ischemic penumbra, leading to intracellular sodium and calcium efflux and extracellular potassium influx, resulting in cellular depolarization. Thrombin can induce increased depolarization. Immediate changes in gene expression are observed, with upregulation of the expression of factors related to verification and cell death and alterations in the expression of neuroplasticity-related factors. During reperfusion, some blood leaks into ischemic necrotic vascular neuronal units, leading to hemosiderin deposition. These factors all contribute to the occurrence of early poststroke seizures.

The pathophysiological mechanisms of late poststroke seizures involve several factors, such as chronic inflammatory responses, glial scar formation, hemosiderin deposition, increased neuronal excitability, and neural network formation. White matter rarefaction, vascular regeneration, neural regeneration, and selective neuronal loss occur in glial scar lesions. A series of subtle changes result in increased excitability and neuronal synchrony, including changes in synaptic plasticity, afferent nerve tissue, and collateral sprouting. Stroke comorbidities, such as hyperglycemia, dementia, hypertension, depression, antidepressant treatment, and alcohol abuse, also influence the occurrence of poststroke epilepsy.

The mechanisms of epilepsy formation after reperfusion therapy for stroke are more complex than the pathological mechanisms of poststroke epilepsy. A research team from the University of São Paulo first discovered that seizures may occur after intravenous thrombolysis in patients with acute myocardial infarction. The study included 348 patients with acute myocardial infarction and used three different thrombolysis regimens: t-PA plus urokinase (43 patients), t-PA alone (142 patients), and streptokinase (163 patients). Two patients experienced seizures while receiving t-PA combined with urokinase, and neither patient had a history of stroke [101]. Chronic alcohol abuse can upregulate the expression of NMDA receptors, leading to seizures after ethanol withdrawal (EW). A 2005 animal experiment revealed increased expression levels and activity of tPA in brain slices during ethanol intoxication and EW in wild-type mice, consistent with the upregulation of NMDA receptor expression, while no such changes were found in tPA-deficient mice. Upregulation of expression of the NR2B subunit of NMDA receptors during the ethanol response requires tPA expression mediation, and tPA-deficient mice or specific antagonists of NR2B subunits can eliminate the expression-promoting effect of tPA-mediated EW seizures [102]. Tissue plasminogen activator (tPA) is one of the immediate early genes (IEGs) whose expression is induced by neuronal activity in rat hippocampal neurons, with significantly increased tPA mRNA expression levels observed throughout the brain 1–4 h after seizures [103]. tPA-deficient mice are resistant to neuronal degeneration and seizures induced by excitotoxicity in the hippocampus [104]. Neuroserpin is a serine protease inhibitor that is mainly expressed in the central nervous system and inhibits tPA activity. Increased expression levels of neuroserpin antigen and tPA antigen are observed early after seizures, and inhibiting the increase in tPA activity by injecting neuroserpin or knocking out expression of the tPA gene in mice significantly reduces seizure activity [105].

Vascular reperfusion leading to cortical reperfusion and hyperperfusion in some regions can result in acute symptomatic seizures. In 2004, an animal model of acute occlusion and reperfusion injury of the middle cerebral artery (MCA) was established by transient occlusion of the middle cerebral artery using microvascular clamps in cats for 1 h. Subsequent observations on FLAIR, DWI, and PWI revealed prolonged hyperperfusion lasting up to 48 h (including certain noninfarcted areas), leading to delayed cellular perfusion injury [106]. Both hypertensive encephalopathy (HTE) [107] and postcarotid endarterectomy [108] can cause seizures due to cerebral hyperperfusion. The occurrence of acute symptomatic seizures indicates effective improvement in cortical perfusion in the corresponding area; therefore, seizures during thrombolysis may be a favorable indicator of intracranial artery reperfusion during thrombolysis [109].

4.3.1.4 Risk Factors for Poststroke Epilepsy

More precise predictors of poststroke epilepsy include cortical involvement, hemorrhagic transformation, disease severity, and etiology, such as large artery atherosclerosis [96, 110, 111]. In 2018, a study proposed using the SeLECT score (including stroke severity, etiology of large artery atherosclerosis, early seizure onset, cortical involvement, and affected area of the middle cerebral artery) to identify individuals at high risk for late-onset poststroke epilepsy for early prevention [112]. A retrospective study in 2021 developed a nomogram to predict the individual risk of poststroke epilepsy after early seizures (the nomogram showed a c-index of 0.73), suggesting that an NIHSS score >14, early seizures 4–7 days after stroke, the involvement of multiple brain lobes, and multiple early seizures within the first week after stroke are independently associated with the occurrence of poststroke epilepsy [94].

The predictive value of EEG for poststroke epilepsy is currently inconsistent. A 2020 study published in JAMA Neurology proposed the 2HELPS2B score to assist in monitoring seizures in hospitalized patients. For patients with any highly epileptiform EEG patterns within the first hour of EEG examination (i.e., a 2HELPS2B score of 2), recording for at least 24 h is recommended [113]. A prospective study revealed that poststroke epilepsy can be predicted by EEG, with the first EEG showing asymmetric background activity or interictal epileptiform activity being potential predictors of poststroke epilepsy, and periodic discharges on the first EEG being an independent predictor of seizure-like activity during hospitalization [114]. A 2021 multicenter study reported negative results: EEG abnormalities observed within 7 days of stroke onset did not predict the risk of poststroke epilepsy after multivariate correction [110].

There is currently no consensus on whether reperfusion therapy leads to more seizures. A 2013 single-center cohort study revealed a significant association between rt-PA thrombolysis and seizures, with up to 12 of 28 thrombolysis patients experiencing early seizures [115]. Thrombolysis is an independent risk factor for early seizures [116]. Endovascular treatment, including arterial thrombolysis and mechanical thrombectomy, has been reported to increase the risk of seizures in patients [117], but there are also contradictory research findings suggesting that endovascular treatment does not lead to more seizures [110, 118]. More high-quality

RCTs or prospective studies are needed to explore their correlation. The predictors of epilepsy in patients undergoing reperfusion therapy, including high NIHSS score, hemorrhage, younger age, and large artery atherosclerotic stroke, are similar to those of poststroke epilepsy [119, 120]. The Code Stroke system is an effective measure used to shorten reperfusion time, enabling rapid identification and timely intervention of acute stroke patients regarding blood pressure, temperature, and blood glucose levels, thereby preventing poststroke epilepsy [119]. The relationship between risk factors for stroke and poststroke epilepsy is not yet clear, but high blood glucose levels on admission may be associated with seizure occurrence [121], and both high and low cholesterol levels may have an impact [115]. However, some studies have suggested that baseline characteristics such as blood glucose and lipid levels are not associated with early or late poststroke epilepsy [112]. Currently, there is a lack of research on predictors related to changes in the internal environment during reperfusion therapy.

4.3.1.5 Drug Selection

(1) Based on clinical evidence, expert consensus, guidelines, etc.

There is limited clinical research on drug treatment for poststroke epilepsy. Long-term follow-up has shown favorable efficacy, safety, and retention rates in patients with single late-onset epileptic seizures after stroke who are treated with gabapentin [122]. A meta-analysis revealed that levetiracetam and lamotrigine are more effective than carbamazepine, with the fewest side effects associated with lamotrigine [123]. However, due to the small number of patients included in these studies, more definitive conclusions cannot be drawn. In recent years, randomized double-blind clinical trials have been conducted on cohorts of patients with cerebrovascular disease-related seizures. The results have indicated that lacosamide is safer and more effective than carbamazepine for controlling poststroke epilepsy, and it is a candidate drug [124].

(2) Limitations of etiology on drug selection and interactions between concomitant medications and anti-seizure medications.

Age, cerebrovascular disease status, and underlying disease status, as well as interactions between concomitant medications and anti-seizure drugs, need to be considered in the treatment of seizures caused by cerebrovascular disease. These patients often have concurrent conditions such as hypertension, diabetes, dyslipidemia, coronary artery disease, arrhythmia, chronic bronchitis, and osteoporosis, and may require long-term intervention with two or more anti-seizure drugs in addition to other medications. Drug treatment is also influenced by factors such as aging, pharmacokinetic and pharmacodynamic changes, poor compliance, and the level of caregiver support.

Among anti-seizure drugs, voltage-gated sodium channel blockers can interfere with action potentials, leading to arrhythmias. Drugs such as carbamazepine and lamotrigine can cause electrocardiographic abnormalities, such as mild prolongation of the PQ interval and bradycardia, and severe cases may present with

Brugada syndrome. The use of carbamazepine and oxcarbazepine in combination with drugs for treating ventricular arrhythmias should be avoided. Additionally, carbamazepine and oxcarbazepine may cause asymptomatic hyponatremia, which can become severe in patients using diuretics or consuming low-sodium diets due to hypertension or congestive heart failure [125]. Carbamazepine can increase total cholesterol and low-density lipoprotein cholesterol levels and may reduce the efficacy of warfarin. In combination with antiplatelet drugs, valproate may increase the hepatotoxicity of statins and increase the risk of bleeding. Levetiracetam may reduce the efficacy of the novel anticoagulants dabigatran and rivaroxaban by inducing p-glycoprotein expression. Furthermore, continuous anti-seizure medication use is significantly associated with accelerated atherosclerosis and increased intima-media thickness of the carotid artery in patients with epilepsy [125]. Balancing the efficacy of anti-seizure medication and the risk of stroke-related adverse effects remains a challenge.

In summary, the treatment of cerebrovascular disease-related epilepsy requires consideration of etiology and disease resolution, whether the epileptic seizures caused by these factors meet the diagnosis of epilepsy, and the effects of underlying diseases, comorbidities, and medication use.

4.3.2 Selection of Anti-seizure Medications for Posttraumatic Seizures and Epilepsy

Traumatic brain injury (TBI) refers to damage to the brain caused by external mechanical forces, including impacts, collisions, acceleration–deceleration forces, penetrating injuries, or diffuse axonal injuries [126]. TBI can lead to a range of sequelae in patients, including seizures and epilepsy.

4.3.2.1 Classification and Definition of Posttraumatic Seizures (PTS)

Posttraumatic seizures occurring after TBI are classified based on the time elapsed since the initial seizure following the injury: those occurring within 24 h are termed immediate posttraumatic seizures, those occurring between 24 h and 1 week are classified as early posttraumatic seizures, and those occurring more than 1 week after the injury are categorized as late posttraumatic seizures [127]. Currently, international terminology predominantly employs the concepts of PTS and posttraumatic epilepsy (PTE). Specifically, PTS refers to seizures occurring within 1 week after TBI, encompassing both immediate and early posttraumatic seizures [128]. PTE, in line with the latest ILAE definition of epilepsy, refers to the occurrence of nonprovoked seizures for the first time 1 week after TBI, with a minimum interval of 24 h between the first and second nonprovoked seizures, and a causal relationship with prior TBI [128].

4.3.2.2 Epidemiology

Approximately 69 million individuals suffer from TBI annually worldwide. The incidence rates in the United States and Europe are 1299/100,000 and 1012/100,000 individuals, respectively [129]. Epidemiological data on TBI in China are incomplete, with the latest available data from 1983 to 1985 indicating incidence rates ranging from 118 to 1419/100,000 individuals across 23 provinces and municipalities, showing significant regional disparities in TBI occurrence. The annual incidence rate of posttraumatic seizures is approximately 200 cases per 100,000 people [130, 131], making it the most common etiology of acquired epilepsy, accounting for 20% of all epilepsy cases and representing the most frequent cause among adult patients [132, 133]. Data from some epilepsy centers indicate that seizures due to TBI represent 20% of cases [127, 134]. A multicenter study from western China reported posttraumatic epilepsy rates of 6.2% within 1 year and 10.6% within 8 years after TBI [135]. Early posttraumatic seizures occurring within 1 month after TBI are observed within the first week in 90% of patients, with more than half occurring within 24 h [136]. Approximately 10% of patients who experience early posttraumatic seizures progress to posttraumatic epilepsy. Approximately 40% of posttraumatic epilepsy patients experience seizures within 6 months of TBI, approximately 50–80% experience seizures within 1 year, and approximately 75–90% experience seizures within 2 years after TBI [127, 137, 138]. Although the risk of PTE decreases as the interval between injury and seizure onset lengthens, late-onset seizures can occur up to 15 years after the initial injury [139–141]. TBI severity is associated with the likelihood of developing posttraumatic epilepsy, with 5-year risk estimates of 0.7%, 1.2%, and 10% for mild, moderate, and severe TBI, respectively [140, 142]. In patients with different severity levels of TBI and follow-up periods exceeding 30 years, the 5-year risk estimates for posttraumatic epilepsy are 2.1%, 4.2%, and 16.7% [142, 143]. Data from a population of military veterans with penetrating head injuries indicate a high incidence (50%) of late-onset nonprovoked posttraumatic epilepsy, with a greater proportion of clinical and subclinical seizures in these patients than in nonpenetrating head injury patients [144].

4.3.2.3 Pathophysiological Mechanisms of Posttraumatic Seizures and Epilepsy

Pathophysiological Mechanisms of Posttraumatic Seizures

Seizures occurring within 1 week after injury are predominantly attributed to acute trauma or subsequent complications [140]. The underlying mechanisms include acute brain injury resulting from shearing forces, direct cranial impact, diffuse axonal injury, brain tissue displacement, or contusion [145]. Damaged axons swell and retract, leading to secondary axonal injury and distal Wallerian degeneration [146]. Subsequent brain tissue death may result from cytotoxic processes such as the release of oxygen free radicals and cytokines, as well as intracellular calcium influx

[145]. Complications following cranial trauma, such as hypoxia, increased intracranial pressure, hypotension, ischemia, brain edema, intracranial hemorrhage, electrolyte imbalances, or infections, can precipitate symptomatic seizures, mostly occurring within weeks after trauma [137, 140]. Additionally, alterations in inflammatory markers, blood–brain barrier integrity, astrocytes, glucose metabolism, and metabolic dysregulation have been implicated in the pathogenesis of posttraumatic seizures [147–150]. For example, posttraumatic inflammation triggers toll-like receptor-1 (TLR-1) expression elevation in the hippocampi of rodent models, leading to protein kinase B (Akt) phosphorylation and activation of the nuclear factor κB (NF-κB) and mammalian target of rapamycin (mTOR) pathways [151]; HMBP-1 protein expression activates the MAPK/ERK 1/2 pathway [152]; and NMDA receptor activation increases neuronal excitability [153], among others.

Pathophysiological Mechanisms of Posttraumatic Epilepsy

Research has suggested that an increased risk of delayed-onset seizures is associated with early-onset seizures; however, an increased risk of PTE is not a direct consequence of early seizure activity [137, 140, 154]. Population-based studies analyzing large samples have shown that the increased risk of PTE following TBI may be attributed to various factors, including the occurrence of cerebral contusion or hematoma, particularly subdural hematomas and skull fractures, or age [140]. Cerebral contusions, lacerations resulting from direct or indirect traumatic brain injury, and compression-induced brain trauma can evolve into epilepsy after a period of asymptomatic latency, which can range from months to years and is dependent on the individual [128]. Studies have indicated that following TBI, injured brain tissue undergoes cellular apoptosis and long-term remodeling of neural circuits over time, including inhibition and apoptosis of GABAergic neurons and enhanced excitability of glutamatergic neurons. Ultimately, these changes lead to an imbalance between excitatory and inhibitory neurotransmitters, increasing the risk of spontaneous epileptic seizures [155–157]. There is also evidence suggesting that the deposition of iron-containing hemosiderin, the formation of iron-free radicals, and iron-related necrosis are involved in epileptogenesis [158]. Following the advancement of genetic testing technologies, the role of genetics in PTE is gradually gaining attention, especially with the discovery of certain genes that serve as biomarkers for predicting the occurrence of PTE following TBI. Genes such as SLC1A3, SLC1A1, ADK, NT5E, IL1B, GAD1, MTHFR, ADORA1, and APOE have been extensively reported to influence various pathological and physiological processes, including stress response, regulation of biomass, metabolic processes, signaling pathways, responses to external stimuli and their regulation, and cellular localization, among others, thus facilitating the onset of epilepsy [159]. The relationship between the gamma-aminobutyric acid (GABA) signaling pathway and PTE is significant. Changes of decreased GABAergic activity and increased glutamate content may be associated with microRNA regulation, indicating the involvement of epigenetic regulation in PTE [160]. Currently, mechanistic studies on epilepsy are primarily based on animal experiments rather than specifically targeting traumatic epilepsy. Animal models for studying PTE mainly include fluid percussion models, controlled cortical impact models, liquid impact models, cortical undercut models, impact acceleration models, penetrating brain injury models, and canine models of PTE [157, 161–164]. Based on fluid percussion model studies, selective apoptosis of interneurons in the dentate gyrus and partial survival of mossy fibers may lead to sustained granule cell hyperexcitability [165]. Recent studies have increasingly shown that a severe fluid impact leading to focal TBI can trigger spontaneous epileptic seizures [157, 166]. Seizures originate from the lesion site and progress over time with worsening clinical and electrophysiological symptoms [167, 168]. Controlled cortical impact models involve creating a focal brain contusion using an impactor controller, allowing for sustained or reproducible outcomes without diffuse brain injury. Studies have shown that damage to the dentate gyrus leads to mossy fiber sprouting and structural reorganization, resulting in increased spontaneous excitability [169, 170]. Rat models of penetrating brain injury better simulate the conditions of TBI, but whether this model can produce delayed-onset epileptic seizures remains uncertain [157]. The cortical undercut model involves transverse transection of the white matter with a needle, resulting in isolation of a small portion of the cortex, and monitoring seizure-like activity in brain slices. Increased axonal sprouting adjacent to pyramidal cells is associated with increased excitatory connections [171]. Recent studies have shown reduced GABA output from fast-spiking neurons in the cortex [172]. Early application of tetrodotoxin after trauma delays action potentials and prevents induced or noninduced epileptoid activity in brain slices, suggesting that posttraumatic epilepsy can be an event-dependent process [173]. Administration of tetrodotoxin within 3 days of trauma can prevent delayed epilepsy in PTE animal models [174]. The occurrence of epileptogenesis overlaps with the recovery process after injury, suggesting common underlying mechanisms, including neuroregeneration, axonal sprouting, and event dependence [155]. Therefore, disease-modifying agents and anti-seizure drugs may have both positive and negative effects on recovery and epileptogenicity. Limited research suggests that anti-seizure drugs, including ramacemide, topiramate, piracetam, and levetiracetam, have no beneficial or harmful effects on recovery following TBI [155].

Risk Factors for Posttraumatic Seizures

Posttraumatic epilepsy has a significant impact on quality of life due to its tendency to occur following brain injury. Therefore, it is crucial to predict whether patients will develop PTE after TBI. Current research indicates that several factors can serve as risk factors for PTE, including TBI severity, intracranial hemorrhage, early post-traumatic seizures, age, and genetics [175].

① *Severity of Traumatic Brain Injury*: Studies have suggested that the risk of PTE increases with TBI severity. TBI severity primarily depends on the duration of consciousness loss or amnesia and structural brain damage [137]. Mild TBI refers to a lack of skull fractures or consciousness loss, or amnesia lasting ≤5 minutes; moderate TBI involves skull fractures or other injuries, consciousness loss, or amnesia lasting 30 min to 24 h without meeting the criteria for severe TBI; severe TBI indicates evidence of cerebral contusion, intracerebral hematoma, or consciousness loss or amnesia lasting more than 24 h [137]. The risks of developing PTE after mild, moderate, and severe TBI increase by 1.5, 2.9, and 17.2 times, respectively [137]. In 2017, the US Defense and Veterans Brain Injury Center introduced new grading criteria for TBI severity, emphasizing the importance of imaging examinations while defining the duration of consciousness loss and posttraumatic amnesia [176].

② *Intracranial Hemorrhage*: Studies have indicated that traumatic intracranial hemorrhage increases the risk of posttraumatic epilepsy by 30% [128].

③ *Early Posttraumatic Seizures*: Early posttraumatic seizures are associated with PTE. After experiencing the first delayed-onset nonprovoked seizure, 86% of patients experience a second seizure within 2 years, with the highest probability observed in patients who have undergone focal brain trauma or coma for more than 7 days [140]. Studies have suggested that the correlation between them is related to TBI severity. In mild TBI, early posttraumatic seizures do not increase the risk of PTE, but in moderate and severe TBI, early posttraumatic seizures increase the risk of PTE by 25% [128].

④ *Age*: Research has indicated that although children under 5 years of age are more likely to experience seizures within 1 h of mild TBI, age cannot be used as a predictor of delayed-onset seizures in children with TBI. Additionally, individuals over 65 years of age are more likely to experience severe TBI, which is correlated with delayed-onset seizures [128].

⑤ *Genetics*: The role of genetics as a hereditary biomarker for posttraumatic epilepsy has garnered considerable attention in recent years, leading to conflicting conclusions [159, 177]. However, with the continuous advancement of genetic technologies and their gradual integration into clinical practice, genetic polymorphisms are promising biological markers.

4.3.2.4 Selection of Anti-seizure Medications for Posttraumatic Seizures and Epilepsy

① *Drug Selection for Posttraumatic Seizures*: Seizures following TBI are presumed to be predominantly focal in nature, but seizures can easily generalize, presenting early as symptoms of generalized seizures within the first week after TBI, and early clinical seizures (electrical seizures) within the first week are also very common [127]. Studies have shown that 20% of posttraumatic seizures can progress to status epilepticus, especially in pediatric patients. Continuous EEG monitoring of patients with severe TBI has revealed that 22% of patients experience seizures within the first week, presenting as generalized tonic–clonic seizures or myoclonus, with over 50% of patients having only EEG-detected electrical seizures [127].

Following the occurrence of the first posttraumatic seizure, consideration should be given to whether seizure prophylaxis should be initiated during the acute phase. Because patients remain in the acute phase of TBI within the first week after TBI, management of the patient's overall internal environment and treatment of syndromes such as brain edema and brain contusion take precedence, while the use of ASMs for prophylaxis of acute-phase seizures following TBI is controversial. The controversy revolves around whether ASMs can effectively prevent seizures during the acute phase and whether the side effects of ASMs interfere with recovery after TBI. Meta-analyses have shown that phenytoin and carbamazepine have a preventive effect on early posttraumatic seizures. The Cochrane Database includes six studies demonstrating the prophylactic effect of ASMs on early posttraumatic seizures. Among 100 TBI patients, 10 patients may not experience early posttraumatic seizures within 1 week [178, 179]. However, studies have shown that controlling seizures is not associated with reduced mortality or neurological disability, nor does it reduce the risk of delayed-onset seizures.

Based on prospective research results, the American Neurological Association has issued recommendations for the prophylactic use of ASMs in adult TBI patients [180, 181]. The current recommendation is short-term use of phenytoin sodium for prophylaxis in adult patients with severe TBI to prevent early posttraumatic seizures, while no recommendations are available for pediatric patients with severe TBI. Phenytoin can be administered intravenously as early as possible after TBI, but data on this topic are limited. Levetiracetam can also be used in similar circumstances, with several studies showing similar efficacy to that of phenytoin and fewer side effects [171, 179, 182]. Although there are no guideline recommendations, level-three evidence suggests that prophylactic use of phenytoin sodium reduces the risk of early posttraumatic seizures in pediatric patients with severe TBI [183–185]. However, there is currently no evidence to support the benefit of using ASMs after 7 days posttrauma [181]. Steroids used after TBI do not prevent delayed-onset posttraumatic seizures, and early steroid use has been shown to increase epileptic activity [186]. In 2017, the Chinese Neurosurgical Society's Neurotrauma Professional Group published the Expert Consensus on the Prevention and Treatment of Post-Traumatic Epilepsy in China, which also recommended anti-seizure prophylaxis for early seizure-like events in high-risk populations after trauma. This expert consensus has been controversial; the controversy centers on whether the 7-day prophylactic use of ASMs is intended to prevent seizures within 7 days after trauma rather than preventing delayed-onset seizures after 7 days, although its target population includes both early- and late-stage high-risk populations for posttraumatic seizures [187].

② *Drug Selection for Posttraumatic Seizures*: Currently, there are no international guidelines recommending prophylactic drug treatment for delayed-onset posttraumatic seizures. Previous studies have shown that phenytoin and barbiturates are effective in preventing delayed-onset seizures after trauma [188]. Therefore, it is common in clinical practice to prescribe medications to patients with severe TBI or those who experienced posttraumatic seizures within 1 week, with a medication duration of 6 months or longer [189]. However, subsequent randomized, double-blind, prospective evaluations of anti-seizure drugs, such as phenytoin, phenobarbital, carbamazepine, and sodium valproate, have been shown to be ineffective for preventing seizures [180, 190, 191].

Compared to patients who develop seizures more than a year after TBI, patients who develop seizures within 1 year after injury are more likely to achieve seizure remission after medication [192]. However, studies have not demonstrated a relationship between the occurrence of the first seizure and medication efficacy [141]. Research has shown that a high seizure frequency in the first year can predict the severity of future seizures and the intractability to medication, similar to other symptomatic seizures [141, 193]. Seizures that occur secondary to severe traumatic brain injury and seizures subject to ineffective early treatment tend to be refractory to medication [194]. The probability of spontaneous seizure remission is low, but for some selected patients (normal EEG, no imaging lesions, good initial treatment response, no seizures for at least 2 years), dose reduction is feasible.

③ *Development of New Anti-seizure Medications for Posttraumatic Seizures*: In recent years, with the deepening understanding of the mechanisms of PTE and the use of animal models of PTE, there have been growing advancements in the development of new anti-seizure drugs for the treatment of PTE.

Studies have shown that atipamezole, a selective α2-adrenergic receptor antagonist, or the cannabinoid receptor 1 antagonist SR141716A has anti-seizure effects on a lateral fluid percussion brain injury seizure model in animals. Treatment with atipamezole starting 7 days after traumatic brain injury reduced the susceptibility of pentylentetrazol-exposed rats to seizures in 14 weeks after treatment, but it did not prevent the development of seizures. SR141716A administered as a single dose 2 minutes after traumatic brain injury or starting 30 minutes after traumatic brain injury and continuing for 9 weeks, did not have anti-seizure effects. Mechanistic studies have shown that the anti-seizure effect of atipamezole is mainly mediated through its effects on α2-adrenergic receptor subtypes, and animals carrying the Adra2A gene mutation encoding the N79P amino acid substitution exhibit anti-seizure effects following traumatic brain injury. On the other hand, the use of the receptor subtype-specific antagonist ORM-12741 to block α2c-adrenergic receptors did not improve the prognoses of traumatic brain injury patients [195].

Studies have shown that Minozac, an anti-inflammatory agent, can prevent increased susceptibility to seizures in a "double hit" mouse model of closed skull traumatic brain injury and electroshock-induced seizures, mainly by inhibiting the upregulation of proinflammatory cytokines [196].

Another study used an rpFPI rat model of lateral fluid percussion injury to investigate whether brivaracetam could prevent and treat posttraumatic epilepsy. Three months later, rats treated with brivaracetam starting 30 minutes, 4 h, and 8 h after traumatic brain injury showed a 38% reduction in the overall seizure occurrence rate, a 59% reduction in seizure frequency, a 67% reduction in seizure duration, and a 45% reduction in the proportion of spreading seizures, demonstrating good anti-seizure properties and providing support for clinical trials of brivaracetam and other SV2A-targeting drugs for the prevention of posttraumatic epilepsy in humans [197].

4.3.3 Selection of Anti-seizure Medication for Brain Tumor-Associated Epilepsy

Brain tumor-related epilepsy (BTRE) is a group of clinical symptoms caused by the abnormal firing of neuronal cells around a lesion due to an intracranial tumor itself or its occupying effect; these symptoms include changes in seizure consciousness level, limb movements, limb sensations, autonomic nervous system functions, and other disorders. According to the ILAE International Epilepsy Cause Classification System updated by the ILAE in 2017, it is a structural cause. BTRE is a clinical symptom of disease progression in patients with brain tumors and can appear either at the beginning of the disease or after surgery, chemoradiotherapy, or other treatments.

4.3.3.1 Epidemiology

The epidemiology, histological subtypes, clinical features, treatment, and outcomes of malignant and nonmalignant CNS tumors are diverse and vary widely. The incidence of primary brain and other central nervous system tumors is estimated to be 23.8 per 100,000 people [198]. Malignant tumors account for 30% of central nervous system tumors. Glioma is the most common primary brain tumor in adults, accounting for approximately 25% of the total incidence of tumors and approximately 80% of the incidence of malignant tumors of the central nervous system [199].

Epileptic seizures often occur in patients with brain tumors, usually reaching a prevalence of 20–60%, and epileptic seizures can be the first clinical symptom in patients with low-grade gliomas [200]. Glioma is the most common primary brain tumor in adults, and 40–70% of patients with glioma have one or more seizures during the course of the disease. When epilepsy recurs or even worsens in patients whose brain tumors are actively treated, this may indicate that the tumor has progressed or relapsed, and it is also an important clinical indicator for determining whether the survival and prognoses of brain tumor patients are optimistic.

4.3.3.2 Pathophysiological Mechanism

The underlying pathophysiological mechanisms of BTRE are not well understood. Mechanical compression, tumor vascularization, oxygen demand imbalance, inflammatory processes and neurotransmitter imbalance play major roles in the development of epilepsy in brain tumor patients [201].

Mechanical compression may cause ischemia and metabolic changes, followed by disruption of the blood–brain barrier, leading to a greater risk of seizures. The blood vessel supply of brain tumors is often unbalanced and unable to meet the oxygen needs of the tumor and the peri-tumor area, resulting in tissue hypoxia; this, in turn, leads to acidosis, glial swelling, and tissue damage. High-grade gliomas cause hemorrhage, necrosis, and gliosis of the surrounding cortex due to their rapid growth. These factors contribute to epilepsy in patients with brain tumors [202].

The incidence of seizures is inversely related to the rate of tumor growth, possibly because slow-growing tumors are more likely to present with epilepsy as the first symptom [203]. In low-grade gliomas, their slow growth into the surrounding brain tissue can separate and invade the cortical–subcortical local and distal networks, leading to epileptogenesis. Changes in the balance of neurotransmitters lead to epileptogenic generation of the tumor itself and tissues near the lesion, which means that the "epileptogenic region" includes peritumoral tissues [204]. Therefore, even complete removal of the brain tumor does not necessarily mean that the epileptogenic area is also removed, as BTRE may be produced by surrounding tissue.

The effect of neurotransmitter imbalance on the development of epilepsy in BTRE patients, particularly a reduction in inhibitory GABAergic neurotransmission and an increase in excitatory glutamatergic synaptic input, has been demonstrated in multiple preclinical and clinical studies [205]. Studies have shown that glioma and breast cancer BMSs can integrate into neuronal circuits. Gliomas can form microtubules, which are thin tubes with membranes that resemble the axons and dendritic growth of developing neurons. On the surfaces of these microtubules, functional synapses (glial synapses) between neurons and glioma cells signal via postsynaptic currents mediated by alpha-amino-3-hydroxy-5-methylisoxazol.

−4-propionic acid (AMPA) glutamate receptors [206, 207]. The interaction between neurons and brain tumor cells implies that seizures may promote brain tumor progression and, conversely, that AMPA glutamate receptors are a potential therapeutic target for treating tumors and BTRE [208]. AMPA receptor antagonist drugs may have dual effects on reducing seizures and tumor growth.

It has been reported that the risk of seizures is greater for brain tumors located in the frontal, parietal, and temporal lobes [209] than for those located in the occipital lobe. More than four brain metastatic sites; high-risk sites for metastasis, such as the frontal, parietal, temporal, or occipital cortices; or melanoma as the primary tumor, are risk factors for BTRE [210]. In low-grade gliomas, lesions involving the left premotor area are more likely to develop into bilateral tonic–clonic seizures [203].

Among the molecular markers of great importance for treatment decisions in brain glioma patients, isocitrate dehydrogenase isoenzyme 1 or 2 (IDH 1/2) is the only known marker that has been reported to be associated with increased seizure rates. Several clinical studies have shown that IDH 1/2 mutations increase the risk of seizures before and around brain tumors [201]. IDH 1/2 mutation leads to a loss of the ability of IDH to catalyze the conversion of isocitric acid to α-ketoglutaric acid and further leads to an increase in the ability of IDH to catalyze the reduction of α-ketoglutaric acid to 2-hydroxyglutaric acid. This mechanism leads to the accumulation of 2-hydroxyglutaric acid, which has structural similarities to glutamate and is able to activate the NMDA receptor, thus acting as a glutamate agonist. Higher glutamate levels lead to a greater probability of seizures. This activation mechanism may explain the epileptogenic potential of IDH mutations.

4.3.3.3 Anti-seizure Medication Therapy for Brain Tumor-Associated Epilepsy

① *Primary Prevention of Epilepsy*: Recent studies have shown that patients with newly diagnosed brain tumors who have not experienced seizures do not benefit from anti-seizure medications [211]. Primary prevention is unlikely to be effective in improving progression-free survival or reducing the incidence of a first seizure within 6 months of diagnosis. Therefore, prophylactic use of anti-seizure medication is not recommended for patients with brain tumors who do not experience concomitant seizures [212].

② *Secondary Prevention of Epilepsy*: In patients with brain tumors, the occurrence of the first seizure indicates a diagnosis of epilepsy. Therefore, according to the general recommendations of the ILAE, ASM treatment usually starts after the first seizure.

Currently, tumor histology, grade, location, and molecular markers have no influence on ASM selection [213]. Several clinical studies have shown the antitumor effects of valproic acid (VPA) and levetiracetam in patients with glioblastoma [201]; however, a comprehensive meta-analysis of four prospective trials did not confirm this effect [214]. In vitro studies have shown that perampanel has good antitumor activity, but it has not been found to slow tumor progression in rat models. There are few clinical data on the potential antitumor activity of perampanel [215]. Currently, therefore, ASMs for treatment of BTRE should be selected based on their pharmacokinetic and pharmacodynamic properties, tolerability, and side effects rather than considering their possible antitumor effects. It is agreed that non-enzyme-induced ASMs are superior to enzyme-induced ASMs to avoid changes that interfere with the pharmacokinetics of antitumor drugs and other drugs (e.g., dexamethasone).

Patients with brain tumors are susceptible to the neurological side effects of ASM, particularly cognitive decline, depression, and anxiety, although other factors have a considerable impact on this population. Cognitive decline is most common with the use of first-generation ASMs. Therefore, first-generation ASMs are rarely used in patients with brain tumors. Valproic acid is effective, but because it can cause blood-related side effects, these side effects may be compounded in patients receiving chemotherapy.

In general, current recommendations for ASM selection in BTRE patients are based on treatment recommendations for focal epilepsy. LEV or LTG are important treatment options for focal epilepsy. Although LTG itself is not an enzyme-inducing drug, its metabolism is affected by drugs that induce activity of the cytochrome P450-3A4 system. In addition to potential interactions with antitumor drugs, another disadvantage of LTG is that it can only be used as an oral formulation and can only be titrated slowly at the beginning of drug treatment. These two aspects are particularly relevant for patients with brain tumors in cases of decreased consciousness, difficulty swallowing, and/or the need for immediate control of seizures. Levetiracetam and lacosamide (LCM) have advantages because they are widely used in oral liquid form and can be quickly titrated by intravenous injection.

Levetiracetam is currently the first-line anti-seizure medication for many neuro-oncologists. In a recent article, levetiracetam was shown to be more effective than valproic acid despite some similar side effects [216]. However, levetiracetam carries an increased risk of psychiatric side effects. Conversely, some ASMs have beneficial side effects, such as mood stabilization and anti-anxiety effects. Therefore, clinicians should carefully evaluate the psychological aspects before deciding on the most appropriate ASMs.

Lacosamide can be used as another anti-seizure medication option for the treatment of BTRE; it can be administered intravenously and has a fast titration rate, a low incidence of neuropsychiatric side effects, and few interactions with other drugs. Lacosamide has been shown to be effective in several trials of BTRE and can be used as a primary drug treatment [201]. A recent retrospective analysis of LCM monotherapy in 132 patients with primary brain tumors revealed that 64.4% of patients were seizure-free at 3 months, and 55% were seizure-free at 6 months [217]. It is important to note that second-degree or higher atrioventricular block must be ruled out by electrocardiogram before starting LCM treatment.

The current study did not show that monotherapy is better than other additive treatments. In a small retrospective study, 33 patients with primary brain tumors received brivaracetam addition therapy, which reduced the number of monthly seizures from 7 to 2 [218]. Perampanel, a noncompetitive AMPA receptor antagonist, is of particular value due to its potential antitumor benefits. In several small studies, 57% of patients receiving additive therapy achieved seizure control [219].

Current evidence suggests that PER is an effective and generally well-tolerated treatment option for patients with BTRE. A retrospective analysis of the efficacy and safety of PER in BTRE included seven studies and six clinical trials of patients with varying tumor pathologies and study numbers. Eight to 36 patients with BTRE were enrolled and received PER addition therapy (mean dose 4–7 mg/day). After 6–12 months of follow-up, the response rate (≥50% reduction in seizure frequency) reached 75% in one study, and the seizure-free rate reached 94% in the other study. In terms of tolerability, 11–52% of patients experienced nonserious adverse events (most commonly dizziness, vertigo, anxiety, and irritability). Retention rates ranged from 56–83%, with only 12.5% of patients discontinuing medication due to adverse events [127]. Studies with larger sample sizes should be conducted for the same tumor pathologies while evaluating the effects of PER on tumor progression, overall survival, and progression-free survival.

Approximately 60% of patients with brain tumors fail to achieve seizure-free status at the time of initial ASM therapy, and of these patients, only 40% eventually achieve seizure-free status after second-line monotherapy or multidrug therapy [220]. As a practical approach, if the first ASM reduces seizure frequency but fails to completely control epilepsy, combination therapy is the preferred treatment option. If the first ASM does not have any effect on seizure frequency, a second monotherapy should be started. Nonhepatic enzyme-induced anti-seizure medication is preferred whenever possible. The combination of two ASMs with the same mechanism of action usually increases side effects.

③ *Status Epilepticus*: Among all adults with status epilepticus, 3–12% of cases are caused by brain tumors. Patients with brain tumors are nearly three times more likely to die from epilepsy than are those with general epilepsy. The appearance of tumor-associated status epilepticus indicates tumor progression. A 2021 study showed that the clinical manifestations of TASE were most common with focal attacks (74%) and less common with generalized attacks (17%) [221]. First-line therapies (diazepam, midazolam) and second-line therapies (levetiracetam, phenytoin, valproic acid) should be used immediately for epileptic status in patients with brain tumors.

④ *Withdrawal of ASM*: There are limited data on the ability to withdraw/stop ASM use in patients with brain tumors associated with epilepsy. To assess the risk of recurrent seizures and to guide patients who wish to taper ASM use, risk calculators may be a valuable option; however, these calculators are not specifically designed for epilepsy patients with brain tumors [222]. These tools help physicians determine the risk of relapse for individual patients; conversely, visualization of specific percentages of seizure recurrence risk can sometimes help convince patients for whom medication withdrawal is not appropriate to continue taking it.

Discontinuing ASM use in patients with gliomas is a controversial issue for which guidelines and expert consensus have not yet been reached. One study revealed that 71% of glioma patients with recurrent seizures within 6 months after drug withdrawal [223].

ASMs should not be discontinued in patients who have experienced tumor progression, who have highly malignant tumors, who have a short life expectancy, or who have had past seizures that were difficult to control. Discontinuation of ASM use is problematic for patients with few or no side effects, who may be well integrated into society and careers after brain tumor treatment, but who will have a heavy social burden if seizures relapse.

Discontinuation of ASM use is not recommended for patients at high risk of recurrent seizures, regardless of their duration; however, determining the risk of recurrent seizures is difficult because it is affected by a number of factors (such as tumor grade, location, and type of treatment). Molecular pathologic features with an IDH 1/2 gene negative for mutations may predict a good prognosis in patients with grade 2 or 3 glioma, who generally have stable brain tumor disease and can achieve long-term seizure-free status. However, phasing out ASM use has to be considered for patients who develop serious side effects (which cannot be resolved by changing medication), or in patients who still have a clear will even after a detailed understanding of the risk of recurrent seizures and the impact on daily life (e.g., whether they are fit to drive).

4.3.4 Pharmacologic Treatment of Focal Cortical Dysplasia-Associated Epilepsy

Focal cortical dysplasia (FCD) is a common cause of focal epilepsy, and it occurs in a majority of patients with drug-resistant epilepsy. Despite the increasing predominance of surgery, medication use remains fundamental for treating FCD. This section focuses on the pharmacologic treatment of FCD-related epilepsy.

4.3.4.1 Definition

Focal cortical dysplasia refers to alterations in cortical cells and lamina structures resulting from abnormal cell proliferation, differentiation, migration, synaptogenesis, and reorganization during brain development [224]. Focal cortical dysplasia occurs mainly during in utero brain development and is also associated with perinatal and early postnatal injuries. It is a subtype of malformation of cortical development (MCD) and can be categorized into different pathological subtypes based on different pathological, imaging, and electrophysiological features [225].

4.3.4.2 Pathologic Typing

Historical Evolution

In 1957, Crome [226] first identified and described giant, morphologically abnormal neurons in brain specimens from three patients with drug-refractory epilepsy (DRE). In 1971, Taylor et al. [227] first coined the term "focal cortical dysplasia," based on irregular dysmorphic neurons and enlarged, ballooned cells in the cortex outside of the first layer, by analyzing the histopathology of surgical specimens from 10 patients with DRE who underwent surgery. In 2004, Palmini et al. [228] categorized FCDs into two types based on the presence (FCD type II) or absence (FCD type I) of dysmorphic neurons. In 2011, the ILAE proposed a more detailed classification system [229], namely, FCD type I (including Ia [abnormal radial lamination], Ib [abnormal tangential lamination] and Ic [abnormal radial and tangential lamination]), FCD type II (including IIa [dyslamination with dysmorphic neurons] and IIb [dyslamination with dysmorphic neurons and balloon cells]), and FCD type III (including IIIa [cortical lamination abnormalities in the temporal lobe associated with hippocampal sclerosis], IIIb [cortical lamination abnormalities adjacent to a glial or glioneuronal tumor], IIIc [cortical lamination abnormalities adjacent to vascular malformation], and IIId [cortical lamination abnormalities adjacent to any other lesion acquired during early life, e.g., trauma, ischemic injury, encephalitis]). In 2018, Najm IM et al. [230] introduced the challenges in distinguishing FCD I and FCD III and discussed the possibility of classifying FCDs in the context of molecular/genetic mechanisms and clinical practice. In 2021, Blümcke et al. [231] proposed the use of genetic analysis of somatic brain mutations in neurosurgically resected brain specimens to better categorize FCDs.

Updated Classification for Focal Cortical Dysplasia

In 2022, the ILAE developed an updated histopathology-based FCD classification for FCD [232]:

(1) FCD type I: FCD type Ia (abundant microcolumns); FCD type Ib (abnormal layering); and FCD type Ic (vertical and horizontal abnormalities).
(2) FCD type II: FCD IIa (dysmorphic neurons); FCDIIb (dysmorphic neurons and balloon cells).
(3) FCD type III: FCD IIIa (cortical dyslamination associated with hippocampal sclerosis); FCD IIIb (cortical dyslamination adjacent to brain tumor); FCD IIIc (cortical dyslamination adjacent to vascular malformation); FCD IIId (cortical dyslamination adjacent to lesion acquired during early life, e.g., stroke).
(4) White matter: mild malformations of cortical development (mMCD) with excessive heterotopic neurons; mMCD with oligodendroglial hyperplasia in epilepsy (MOGHE).
(5) No definite FCD on histopathology: abnormalities in cortical organization remain ambiguous, and histopathological findings are not compatible with FCD I, II, or III.

Molecular Pathological Characterization

The presence of cells expressing immature markers such as microtubule-associated protein 1B (MAP 1B), neuronal nuclei (NeuN), vimentin, nestin, and α-internexin is a marked characteristic of FCD type II, in contrast to FCD type I, in which cells hardly express progenitor proteins [233, 234]. In addition, balloon cells in FCD type II also express stem cell markers such as Sox2, Oct4, c-Myc, and Klf4, a feature that has been associated with enhancement of the mammalian target of rapamycin (mTOR) signaling pathway [233].

4.3.4.3 Clinical Features and Epidemiology

Seizures are the predominant clinical manifestation in patients with FCD. Nathan T Cohen et al. [235] investigated the prevalence of seizures in 143 patients with 3 T-MRI-confirmed FCD from the Children's Hospital of George Washington University and found that 124 (87%) of them had recurrent noninduced seizures (i.e., epilepsy), 12 (8.5%) had only one seizure or multiple induced seizures, and only 7 (4.9%) had no seizures. Moreover, FCD accounts for approximately 25% of patients with focal epilepsy [236]. In patients who have undergone epilepsy surgery, approximately 40–50% of children and 20% of adults experience FCD [237]. FCD type I is most often located in the temporal lobe and is usually negative for, or has only slight, gray–white matter border blurring on brain MRI [238, 239]. FCD type II occurs predominantly outside the temporal lobe, especially in the frontal lobe, and MRI frequently reveals abnormal changes, such as focal thickened cortex, blurring of gray–white matter boundaries, and the "transmantle sign" (i.e., a funnel-shaped high signal from the gyrus pointing to the ventricles on the T2/T2-Flair sequence of MRI; in other words, a "penetration sign," which is a characteristic sign of FCD type IIb) [240, 241].

4.3.4.4 Pathogenic Mechanisms

The mechanisms of epileptogenicity in FCD have been extensively studied over the past two decades. There may be three main mechanisms involved: altered synaptic function, glial cell dysfunction, and dysregulation of extrasynaptic regulation [225].

Alterations in Synaptic Function

Some researchers have compared the pathological alterations between FCD type I/II and non-FCD patients and discovered that in FCD type I patients, the postsynaptic function of GABAA receptors remains unchanged or mildly decreased, in contrast to that in FCD type II patients [242]. Moreover, in FCD type II patients, the most pronounced postsynaptic changes were observed in the areas with the greatest morphological abnormalities, which were characterized by loss of inhibitory neurons and reorganization of GABAergic and glutamatergic neurons. The most predominant synaptic changes were GABAergic rather than glutamatergic and were accompanied by an increase in the function of pre- and postsynaptic GABA. It is unclear whether the increase in GABA synaptic activity is a compensatory mechanism to control hyperexcitability or is a component of epileptic triggering.

In specimens of FCD from patients with drug-resistant epilepsy, the expression of α4-containing GABAA receptors was greater than that of α1-containing GABAA receptors. The expression of the α4 and γ2 subunits of the GABAA receptor is increased in patients with FCD type I and FCD type II compared to controls, while the alterations are more severe in patients with FCD type II [243]. Patients not taking benzodiazepines also showed increased expression of α4-containing GABAA receptors, suggesting that altered GABAA receptor expression may be responsible for resistance to benzodiazepines.

The effects of GABAA receptor activators are dependent on the intra- and extracellular concentration differences of Cl- ions. In healthy human neonatal cortical neurons, the efflux of Cl- ions via KCC2 is more potent than the uptake of Cl ions by NKCC1, and GABAergic signaling triggers an inward flow of Cl ions, resulting in the emergence of a postsynaptic hyperpolarizing current. However, under conditions of neuronal injury, NKCC1 expression is functionally upregulated more than that of KCC2, and GABAergic signaling triggers a reversal of the Cl ion current, leading to depolarization of the GABA response. Under these conditions, the administration of GABAA receptor activators (phenobarbital or benzodiazepines) may lead to depolarization of the Cl ion current and exacerbate seizures [244].

The NMDA receptor 1 subunit (NR1) protein and NMDA receptor 2B (NR2B) mRNA/protein subunits are selectively expressed on dysplastic neurons in resected tissues of FCD patients [245]. Changes in the expression of AMPA receptors have also been observed. Immunocytochemical assays have revealed significantly increased expression of GluR2/3 subunits in dysplastic and giant neurons [246].

Glial Cell Dysfunction

Impaired glial buffering mechanisms to glutamate and potassium have been identified in animal models of tuberous sclerosis complex (TSC) and human tissues and may increase neuronal excitability in TSC and thus cause seizures. A large number of balloon cells express glial biomarkers. A recent study revealed differential expression of the glial glutamate transporter (GLT1) and glutamine synthase (GS) in balloon cells but not in aberrant or normal neurons. This differential expression of GLT1 and GS may be responsible for the hyperexcitability observed in balloon cells [247].

Extrasynaptic Mechanisms

Recent studies of a large number of FCD type I and type II samples have shown increased astrocyte proliferation and diffusion disorders in abnormally hyperplastic tissues. In addition, the same studies have shown increased extracellular space in FCD type II lesions (but not FCD type I lesions). These observations suggest altered diffusion of neuroactive substances through the extracellular space, but the exact significance is unclear [225].

4.3.4.5 Treatment

Risk of Drug Resistance in Focal Cortical Dysplasia

The study by Nathan T Cohen et al. [235] reported that up to 74% of patients with FCD-related epilepsy were medically refractory, and failure of the first ASM was strongly associated with early development of medically refractory epilepsy (OR 346; 95% CI 19.6–6100). Cox regression analysis suggested that the location or pathologic subtype of FCD and age at onset of epilepsy were not risk factors. Another study showed that up to 94.2% of patients with FCD-related epilepsy were drug resistant, while 59.8% of those who received surgery were seizure free for at least 1 year after surgery [248]. This study also revealed that concordance between the location of the FCD on MRI and ictal EEG and an older age of seizure onset were two factors associated with a favorable surgical outcome after 1 year. In addition, a meta-analysis showed that the shorter the interval between surgical treatment and the onset of epilepsy was, the greater the proportion of patients who were seizure free after surgery [249].

Mechanisms of Drug Resistance

The mechanisms of drug resistance in FCD are still unclear. Apart from its epileptogenic nature, another mechanism that explains the drug resistance of FCD may be the overexpression of multidrug resistance gene-1 p-glycoprotein (MDR1) and multidrug resistance-associated protein-1 (MRP1) [250] which can remove ASMs from the nervous system, thereby reducing the concentration of effective drugs in the brain. However, whether the overexpression of these transporters in epileptogenic tissues is the cause of drug resistance or is secondary to chronic seizures as well as the use of ASMs is unclear. Moreover, whether it can be used as a therapeutic target has not been determined.

Selection of Anti-seizure Medications

None of the ASMs have been shown to be more effective than others in patients with FCD. The selection of ASMs depends on the type of seizure (focal seizures or spasms) and the age of the patient. In the majority of patients, there is a trend toward drug resistance, with only approximately 17% of patients treated with ASMs maintaining a brief seizure-free period of at least 1 year [224].

In a recent retrospective study [251], the authors analyzed the efficacy of ASMs in 164 patients with epilepsy due to MCD, 87 of whom had FCD or giant gyrus. In the initial regimen during which most patients received monotherapy, the therapeutic response rate (reduction in seizure frequency ≥50%) was 50% for lamotrigine, 31.6% for carbamazepine, 30% for oxcarbazepine, 20.5% for valproic acid, and only 4.5% for levetiracetam. The difference in drug responsiveness between levetiracetam and sodium channel blockers (carbamazepine, oxcarbazepine, and lamotrigine) was statistically significant.

Levetiracetam (LEV) monotherapy may lead to the exacerbation of seizures in FCD-related epilepsy patients. In a case report [252], the paradoxical effect of ASMs was defined as an increase in seizure frequency (by at least 25%) and/or the development of a more severe degree of seizure shortly after the administration of a medication considered effective in this type of epilepsy; further, the patient experienced a significant worsening of the baseline seizures closely related to dose titration after intake of a low-dose LEV, accompanied by a rapid improvement in seizure frequency shortly after LEV discontinuation. In another study [253], the authors retrospectively analyzed the data of 139 patients treated with LEV. Seizure exacerbation was defined as a 100% or greater increase in seizure frequency within 1 month of drug introduction. Five of these patients met the criteria and were treated with LEV in addition to the original therapy with sodium channel blockers (carbamazepine, oxcarbazepine or lamotrigine). Low-dose (500–1000 mg) LEV administration resulted in seizure exacerbation. In addition to increased frequency and duration, two patients developed new seizure types. The seizure frequency returned to baseline after the discontinuation of LEV. Four out of the five patients were considered to have FCD on MRI. No paradoxical effect of LEV was found in the idiopathic epilepsy group or in the group with symptomatic epilepsy other than FCD.

Potential Therapeutic Roles of mTOR Inhibitors

Tuberous sclerosis complex (TSC) is a genetic disease involving multiple organ systems caused by abnormalities in the mTOR signaling pathway and is characterized by cortical malformations and migratory abnormalities in the brain. The histopathological, molecular, and physiologic features of the nodules and radial migration lines of TSC patients are similar to those of FCD type IIb patients [254]. Chimeric mutations in various genes, such as TSC1/TSC2, PTEN, STRADα, AMPK, NPRL3, MTOR, and PIK3CA [255], all of which are associated with the mTOR pathway, are detected in FCD IIb tissues; therefore, both FCD IIb and TSC are thought to be mTOR signaling-related diseases caused by a series of pathogenic variants in mTOR pathway protein-encoding genes leading to differential activation of the mTOR signaling pathway.

In electrophysiological studies performed on brain slices of resected brain tissues from patients with TSC, rapamycin (an inhibitor of the mTOR pathway) was found to reduce the amplitude and frequency of 4-AP-induced paroxysmal discharges and spontaneous excitatory postsynaptic potentials, as well as the bursts of discharges induced by blockade of the anti-gamma-aminobutyric acid type A receptor (GABAAR) [85, 256]. In a large, randomized, double-blind, placebo-controlled clinical trial of adjunctive everolimus for treating TSC, the overall efficacy rate (more than 50% reduction in seizure frequency) was 40% in the group receiving adjunctive everolimus (vs. 15.1% in the placebo group) [257]. A post hoc analysis of this clinical trial revealed an efficacy rate of up to 60% in the subgroup of patients younger than 6 years old, compared to 30% in the older subgroup [258]. This suggests that the earlier everolimus is administered, the better the outcome may be.

Jae Seok Lim et al. [259] identified a mutation (p.Leu2427Pro) in a protein related to the mTOR signaling pathway in surgical specimens of patients with FCD type II, and focal cortical expression of this mutation by in utero electroporation of mice disrupted neuronal migration and caused cytomegalic neurons as well as spontaneous seizures. Furthermore, inhibition of mTOR with rapamycin successfully suppressed the development of cytomegalic neurons and reduced seizure symptoms. Mitsuhiro Kato et al. [260] conducted a single-arm, open-label, multicenter clinical trial evaluating the efficacy and safety of adjunctive sirolimus administration in patients with FCD type IIwith an observation period of 3 months. They reported a 25% reduction in seizure frequency in the adjunctive sirolimus administration group (vs. 0.5% in the control group). However, because of the inconsistency of baseline data between the two groups, the statistical requirements for comparison could not be met.

In conclusion, mTOR could be a therapeutic target for intractable epilepsy associated with FCD, and inhibitors of the mTOR pathway, such as everolimus, sirolimus, or rapamycin, offer new therapeutic options.

Other Medications

A meta-analysis showed that intravenous gammaglobulin administration in patients with FCD-related refractory epilepsy can significantly reduce seizure frequency [261]. However, due to the small number of patients receiving gamma globulin, its effectiveness still needs further validation.

4.3.5 Pharmacological Treatment of Epileptic Seizures in Autoimmune Encephalitis

Autoimmune encephalitis (AE) is a rapidly progressing inflammatory disease of the brain characterized by a range of clinical symptoms, such as mental abnormalities, cognitive impairment, seizures, involuntary movements, language disorders, and decreased levels of consciousness. AE is categorized into two main types based on the location of the antibody-binding antigen. One type targets the neuronal cell membrane or synaptic antigens and is exemplified by anti-N-methyl-D-aspartate receptor (NMDAR) encephalitis. The other type targets cytoplasmic or cytosolic antigens and is represented by anti-glutamic acid decarboxylase isotype 65 (GAD65) encephalitis [262].

Clinically, seizures are one of the core symptoms of AE and are often the first symptom of AE. The 2020 International League Against Epilepsy Working Group on Autoimmunity and Inflammation clarified the concept of acute symptomatic seizures secondary to autoimmune encephalitis (ASSAEs). ASSAEs refer to seizures that occur during the acute phase of AE and are a symptomatic concept [263]. In addition to the manifestation of seizures, the acute phase of AE can also cause new-onset refractory status epilepticus (NORSE), which is defined as the new onset of refractory status epilepticus in patients without a history of active epilepsy or neurologic dysfunction and without obvious acute or active structural, toxic, or metabolic etiology. Febrile infection-related epilepsy syndrome (FIRES) was defined as the presence of antecedent febrile symptoms during the 2-week-to-24-h period prior to onset [264].

4.3.5.1 Epidemiological Information.

International epidemiological data reveal that the annual incidence of AE is 0.8/100,000, a rate comparable to that of viral encephalitis (0.6/100,000). The incidence of AE is 13.7/100,000, which is slightly greater than that of viral encephalitis (8.3/100,000) [265]. There is a lack of epidemiologic information on AE in China.

Seizures are a common clinical symptom during the acute phase of AE, with 79.5% of patients experiencing seizures during this period. Of these, 73.5% originate in the temporal lobe, and the most common type of seizure is focal progression to bilateral tonic–clonic seizures. Additionally, 28.9% of cases may manifest as status epilepticus [266]. A multicenter study conducted abroad revealed that 37% of patients with NORSE had AE as the underlying etiology [267].

4.3.5.2 Pathogenesis

The current understanding suggests that persistent neuroinflammatory responses and altered neuronal excitability caused by antibodies acting on synaptic receptors are responsible for seizures secondary to AE [268]. The binding of NMDAR antibodies to the GluN1 subunit of NMDARs on the postsynaptic membrane of neurons leads to the internalization of the receptor, thereby affecting the normal electrical activity of the neuron and resulting in seizures [269]. The pathogenic mechanism of intracellular antibodies is not clear, but it may be associated with T lymphocyte-mediated immune responses. In summary, disruption of the neuronal excitatory/inhibitory balance in vivo, due to antibody-mediated immune responses, cytokines, and T lymphocyte-mediated immune responses, is considered the primary cause of seizures or status epilepticus in patients with AE.

4.3.5.3 Clinical Manifestations

Clinical AE against neuronal surface antigens is the primary cause of ASSAEs and NORSE. The most common AE is anti-N-methyl-D-aspartate receptor (NMDAR) encephalitis, followed by anti-gamma-aminobutyric acid type B receptor

(GABABR) encephalitis, anti-leucine-rich glioma-inactivated protein-1 (LGI-1) encephalitis, and anti-contactin-associated protein-like 2 (CASPR2) encephalitis.

① Anti-NMDAR encephalitis, which targets neuronal cell membrane surface antigens, is the most prevalent clinical AE, accounting for approximately 80% of ASSAE cases in the acute phase of encephalitis [270]. The most common seizure type is focal progression to bilateral tonic–clonic seizures, with approximately 33.1% of patients experiencing persistent status epilepticus in the acute phase. Aggressive immunotherapy combined with ASMs yields a favorable overall prognosis, and chronic epilepsy is less common. As a result, the majority of patients do not require long-term ASM treatment [271, 272]. In most cases, ASMs can be administered during the acute phase of anti-NMDAR encephalitis, and the decision to taper ASM use over a year depends on the patient's seizure profile [273].

Anti-GABABR encephalitis is another prevalent clinical AE caused by the presence of neuronal cell membrane surface antigens. This type of AE is associated with a high likelihood of seizures and persistent epileptic status in the acute phase, with ASSAEs occurring in up to 90% or more of patients. The common seizure types include focal seizures and focal progression to bilateral tonic–clonic seizures [274]. In addition to seizures, patients with anti-GABABR encephalitis often present with other limbic system symptoms, such as mental abnormalities and cognitive decline. Due to the high comorbidity rate with small cell lung cancer, tumor screening and long-term follow-up are recommended. Adequate immunotherapy for encephalitis typically leads to the resolution of seizures in patients with anti-GABABR encephalitis, and only a small proportion of patients require long-term administration of ASMs [272].

The most frequent manifestation of ASSAEs in patients with anti-LGI-1 encephalitis is focal seizures, in which rapid cognitive decline and intractable hyponatremia are the main clinical features. Faciobrachial dystonic seizures (FBDSs) and hair-raising seizures are characteristic seizure types of anti-LGI-1 encephalitis, and FBDSs are characterized by recurrent, rapid twitching of the muscles of one side of the upper limb, face, and neck, with multiple frequent seizures during the day [275]. Immunotherapy is significantly more effective for controlling FBDS symptoms than treatment with ASMs alone [276].

Hormone therapy during immunotherapy may also be more effective than intravenous gamma globulin infusion in controlling FBDS symptoms in patients with anti-LGI-1 encephalitis [277]. ASSAEs in the acute phase of anti-LGI-1 encephalitis typically resolve after early and adequate immunotherapy. However, there is a risk of recurrence, reaching up to 35% over the subsequent 8 years of follow-up [278].

② In anti-contactin-associated protein-like 2 (CASPR2) encephalitis, approximately 38% of patients develop ASSAEs in the acute phase. The most common type of seizure observed was focal onset seizures with perceptual deficits, followed by bilateral tonic–clonic seizures. Seizures in this condition are often accompanied by cognitive impairment and mood disorders, in addition to epileptic seizures.

Table 4.9 Common secondary epileptic seizures caused by anti-neuronal surface antigens

Neuronal surface antigen	Incidence of seizure	Incidence of epilepsy	Tumor incidence rate	Main tumor types
NMDAR	70–80%	<5%	30–40%	Teratoma
GABAbR	90–95%	20–30%	50–60%	Small-cell lung carcinoma
LGI-1	80%	15%	<5%	Thymoma
CASPR2	40–50%	<10%	<20%	Thymoma

After first- and second-line immunotherapy combined with ASMs, seizures are controlled in some patients. However, a subset of patients still requires continued treatment with ASMs at 1-year follow-up [279] (Table 4.9).

4.3.5.4 Anti-seizure Medications

Immunotherapy is instrumental in controlling ASSAEs. Findings from international studies indicate that, following treatment with immunization and ASMs, approximately 89% of patients with antineuronal surface antigen AE can achieve seizure-free status [280]. Importantly, individuals who undergo immunotherapy tend to achieve seizure remission earlier than those treated solely with ASMs. On average, the time from the initiation of immunotherapy to achieving a seizure-free status is reported to be 28 days [281]. The RITE (Rapid Intervention and Treatment Effectiveness) score, specifically a score of ≥7, can serve as a clinical predictor for a favorable outcome in terms of seizure control after individuals receive immunotherapy for AE [282]. In the realm of immunotherapeutic approaches, traditional first-line strategies include intravenous glucocorticoids, intravenous gamma globulin, and plasma exchange. In cases where first-line immunotherapy is ineffective, second-line interventions, such as rituximab and cyclophosphamide, may be considered.

For patients with AE-induced NORSE, first-line immunotherapy should be initiated within 72 h of disease onset. Additionally, second-line immunotherapy and a ketogenic diet should be initiated within 1 week in instances of a poor outcome. Rituximab is the preferred second-line immunotherapy for antibody-positive AE-induced NORSE, while blockers of the interleukin receptor (e.g., anabolic acid and tocilizumab) are recommended for the treatment of cryptogenic NORSE [283]. These comprehensive strategies underscore the importance of timely and targeted immunotherapeutic interventions for managing AEs and associated complications.

Achieving clinical control of ASSAEs with ASMs alone is often challenging, with a success rate of only 15%. Compared with levetiracetam, sodium channel blockers, including carbamazepine, oxcarbazepine, and lacosamide, demonstrate greater efficacy in controlling seizures [284]. Notably, in the case of anti-LGI-1 encephalitis, the use of carbamazepine, an aromatic ASM, is associated with an elevated risk of skin sensitization, necessitating close monitoring [281, 285].

Patients with anti-LGI-1 encephalitis commonly experience intractable hyponatremia. Therefore, when using oxcarbazepine to control seizures caused by anti-LGI-1 encephalitis, careful monitoring of blood sodium levels is essential to prevent exacerbation of hyponatremia [286]. In contrast, patients with anti-NMDAR encephalitis who have undergone sufficient immunotherapy generally do not require long-term ASM treatment. Several factors, including the use of multiple ASMs during the acute phase, the presence of epileptiform discharges in electroencephalography (EEG) monitoring, and delayed initiation of immunotherapy, are identified as the primary risk factors for the development of chronic epilepsy in the later phase [287]. The intricacies of ASM management highlight the importance of tailored therapeutic approaches based on the specific characteristics of each AE subtype.

Early recognition of ASSAEs is crucial for effective management. An APE2 score ≥4 is indicative of an ASSAE, necessitating early initiation of immunotherapy. Early intervention with immunotherapy is closely linked to successful ASSAE control and favorable long-term outcomes in AE patients [288]. In the context of ASMs, the preference is for selecting appropriate agents based on the adequacy of immunotherapy. Sodium channel blockers are not the first choice, and caution is advised when using them in patients with anti-LGI-1 encephalitis due to the potential for adverse effects such as skin irritation and severe hyponatremia. This underscores the importance of tailoring treatment approaches to the specific characteristics of the autoimmune subtype to optimize therapeutic outcomes.

4.3.6 Medication for Seizures Caused by Other Immune Factors

The role of autoimmunity in the development of epilepsy has long been recognized, dating back to the identification of immune inflammation in Rasmussen's encephalitis in 1958 [289]. Subsequent findings included the infiltration of inflammatory cells in pathologic specimens from patients with temporal lobe epilepsy. In the 1980s and 1990s, clinical evidence demonstrated the effectiveness of glucocorticoid and adrenocorticotropic hormone therapy in treating clinical infantile spasms, and paraneoplastic antibodies were found to be associated with epilepsy due to limbic encephalitis. These observations have led to an increased understanding of the significant role of immunity in epilepsy development [290].

The term "autoimmune epilepsy" was first introduced at the International Congress of Immunology in Geneva in 2002 [291]. In 2017, the ILAE identified autoimmunity as one of the six major causes of epilepsy [292]. The 2020 ILAE Autoimmunity and Inflammation Working Group clarified the concept of autoimmune-associated epilepsy (AAE), defined as chronic epileptic seizures caused by autoimmune encephalitis (AE) occurring due to persistent immune responses or structural changes in the brain resulting from the acute phase of encephalitis [263]. In 2023, Rada et al. proposed the term autoimmune encephalopathy-associated epilepsy (AEAE), encompassing conditions such as Rasmussen's encephalitis, glutamic acid decarboxylase 65 (GAD65) antibody-associated epilepsy, and paraneoplastic antibody-associated epilepsy. For autoimmune encephalitis patients receiving anti-neuronal surface antigen immunotherapy, seizures persisting for at least 2 years after immunotherapy, with no apparent signs of encephalitis on cranial magnetic resonance imaging (MRI), normal cerebrospinal fluid (CSF) cell counts, or a substantial decrease in antibody titer, are categorized as AEAE in the chronic phase of AE [293].

4.3.6.1 Rasmussen Encephalitis

(1) *Definitions*: Rasmussen encephalitis (RE) is a rare chronic disease of the nervous system that was first described by the neurosurgeon Theodore Rasmussen in 1958. It is characterized by chronic inflammation leading to progressive cortical atrophy in one cerebral hemisphere, with clinical manifestations of drug-refractory epilepsy, progressive neurological deficits, and persistent cognitive decline.
(2) *Epidemiological Information*: RE is uncommon clinically and primarily affects children, with onset typically occurring at approximately 6 years of age. An epidemiologic survey in Germany indicated an annual incidence of RE of 2.4 per ten million individuals under 18 years of age [292].
(3) *Pathologic Mechanisms*: The typical histopathological changes in RE are persistent inflammatory stimulation of the cortex of one cerebral hemisphere leading to loss of neurons and proliferation of glial cells [289]. Microglia and lymphocyte infiltration, the appearance of perivascular cuffs composed of lymphocytes and phagocytes, and neuronal death and phagocytosis are the most common pathological changes seen in RE; as the disease progresses, end-stage pathological changes include spongy cortical cavitation, marked astrocyte proliferation, and neuronal cell loss [294].
(4) *Clinical Manifestations*: The clinical manifestations of RE progress through the prodromal, acute, and chronic phases. The prodromal phase involves less frequent seizures and mild hemiparesis symptoms. The acute phase is characterized by frequent focal seizures, with 50% of patients developing partial epilepsy continua (PEC). Without intervention, PEC can lead to hemiparesis, hemianopsia, and cognitive decline within a year. In the chronic phase, seizure frequency is stabilized with severe neurological deficits, cognitive decline, and drug-refractory focal epilepsy [295].
(5) *Medication*: The therapeutic goals for RE are to minimize seizure severity and frequency and to greatly improve motor and cognitive function. The efficacy of ASMs against RE is generally poor, and their primary role is to prevent the occurrence of severe seizures and PEC.

Case reports and uncontrolled studies have suggested that glucocorticoids, gamma globulin, and immunomodulatory drugs such as tacrolimus, rituximab, and anabolic acid can improve cognitive function and seizure control in patients with RE, thereby improving the overall prognosis [296–298]. The results are summarized in the following table.

In pediatric patients with RE, hemispheric dissociation surgery is an important treatment modality that not only provides effective seizure control but also improves motor function [299].

4.3.6.2 Anti-GAD65-Associated Epilepsy

(1) *Definitions*: Gamma-aminobutyric acid (GABA) is an enzyme present in neurons and pancreatic islet β cells that plays a role in converting glutamate to gamma-aminobutyric acid through decarboxylation. There are two isoforms of GABA, namely, GAD65 and GAD67. Antibodies against GAD65 have not only been linked to type 1 diabetes mellitus but also to various neurological disorders, such as stiff-man syndrome, cerebellar ataxia, and limbic encephalitis. In the case of anti-GAD65 encephalitis, recurrent poorly controlled seizures can be the primary or sole clinical manifestation, leading to the term "anti-GAD65-associated epilepsy" [300].

(2) *Epidemiological Information*: Clinical anti-GAD65-associated epilepsy is considered uncommon, with an estimated prevalence of approximately 1.9 cases per 100,000 individuals with limbic encephalitis [265].

(3) *Pathogenesis*: Surgical resection specimens from patients with anti-GAD65-associated epilepsy have revealed the presence of cytotoxic T lymphocytes. It is currently understood that tissue damage mediated by cytotoxic T lymphocytes is a major contributing factor to the pathogenesis of this condition, particularly related to anti-neuronal intracellular antigens [301].

(4) *Clinical Manifestations*: Patients with anti-GAD65-associated epilepsy can present with acute or subacute onset, exhibiting clinical features reminiscent of limbic encephalitis. These manifestations may include seizures, mental and behavioral abnormalities, and cognitive decline. However, a more common presentation involves a chronic, insidious onset of recurrent seizures without evident clinical or imaging signs of active inflammatory changes in the brain [302].

Cranial magnetic resonance imaging (MRI) during the acute phase may reveal swelling and abnormal signals in the limbic system. In the chronic phase, there may be high signal in the hippocampus accompanied by reduced hippocampal volume on fluid-attenuated inversion recovery (FLAIR) sequences. These imaging findings contribute to the diagnostic evaluation of anti-GAD65-associated epilepsy.

(5) *Medication*: Anti-GAD65-associated epilepsy is predominantly characterized by drug-refractory seizures, and the limited number of cases contributes to a scarcity of high-quality studies. Research has indicated that this form of epi-

lepsy is not only unresponsive to ASMs but also shows reduced response to first-line immunotherapy interventions [303]. A recent study demonstrated that a combination of phenobarbital and clobazam therapy was effective in reducing seizure frequency in patients with anti-GAD65-associated epilepsy when administration of multiple ASMs failed to produce the desired outcome [304].

Although surgical outcomes for patients with anti-GAD65-related epilepsy are reportedly less favorable than those for patients with other causes of medial temporal lobe epilepsy, surgical intervention may be considered following a thorough surgical evaluation when ASMs and immunotherapy are shown to be ineffective [301]. The decision for surgical intervention should involve careful weighing of potential benefits and risks.

4.3.6.3 Paraneoplastic Antibody-Associated Epilepsy

(1) *Definitions*: Paraneoplastic antibody (intracellular antibody)-mediated encephalitis predominantly affects the limbic system and cerebral cortex, resulting in seizures that are often poorly responsive to drugs. This tendency to resist treatment by medications can lead to the development of chronic epilepsy, termed paraneoplastic antibody-associated epilepsy [305].
(2) *Epidemiological Information*: Information on paraneoplastic antibody-associated epilepsy is primarily derived from case reports or analyses of small sample sizes, and comprehensive epidemiological data are currently lacking.
(3) *Pathogenesis*: The pathogenesis of paraneoplastic antibody-associated epilepsy is similar to that of anti-GAD65-associated epilepsy. Both conditions lead to pathophysiological alterations through T lymphocyte-mediated immune responses and the release of inflammatory factors.
(4) *Clinical Manifestations*: The clinical manifestations of paraneoplastic antibody-associated epilepsy closely resemble those of anti-GAD65-associated epilepsy, often presenting with symptoms indicative of temporal lobe epilepsy. Focal onset seizures with perceptual deficits and focal progression to bilateral tonic–clonic seizures are the most commonly observed seizure types. Seizures tend to be more frequent in this context and, in severe cases, may progress to status epilepticus. Recent studies have identified Hu antibody-associated epilepsy as the most common type, primarily associated with small cell lung cancer, followed by Ma2 antibody-associated epilepsy, which is predominantly linked to germ cell tumors [306].
(5) *Medication*: Patients with paraneoplastic antibody-associated epilepsy generally exhibit a poor response to ASMs. Early detection of tumors provides an opportunity for tumor-specific therapy, potentially improving the overall prognosis [307]. First- and second-line immunotherapies are options for treating paraneoplastic antibody-associated epilepsy. Surgical interventions can also be considered if tumor-specific and immunotherapeutic approaches are shown to be ineffective [301].

4.3.7 *Medication for Seizures Associated with Different Types of Encephalopathies*

Encephalopathy is a brain dysfunction characterized by altered consciousness due to a variety of causes, which can result from total brain damage or focal lesions [308]. It describes a clinical state rather than a stand-alone disease diagnosis, and its etiology is very diverse. Epileptic seizures are among the most common clinical manifestations in patients with encephalopathy. This section focuses on the pharmacological management of seizures caused by different encephalopathies, such as hypoxic-ischemic encephalopathy, metabolic encephalopathy, autoimmune-related encephalopathy, toxic encephalopathy, and radiation encephalopathy.

4.3.7.1 Hypoxic-Ischemic Encephalopathy

Definition

Hypoxic-ischemic encephalopathy (HIE) refers to severe brain dysfunction caused by cerebral ischemia and/or hypoxia. Neonatal HIE is usually caused by intrauterine fetal distress, asphyxia, or neonatal pneumonia [309], while HIE in adults is most likely caused by cardiac arrest and, occasionally, by drowning, hanging, carbon monoxide poisoning, altitude sickness, respiratory failure, severe sleep apnea-hypopnea syndrome, etc.

Clinical Features and Epidemiology

Posthypoxic myoclonus is the main seizure manifestation of hypoxic-ischemic encephalopathy and can be divided into acute and delayed forms. Acute myoclonus occurs within 24 h after cerebral hypoxia-ischemia and manifests as coma with myoclonic status epilepticus. Myoclonus is usually systemic, mainly in the face, upper limbs, and diaphragm, and lasts for 1–31 days, often suggesting a poor prognosis. Late-onset myoclonus occurs days to weeks after hypoxia and ischemia when the patient's consciousness is restored, manifests as intentional or action myoclonus, and may be accompanied by cognitive impairment, ataxia, dysarthria and other symptoms. Delayed myoclonus after cerebral hypoxia, also known as Lance–Adams syndrome, was first described by Lance and Adams in 1963 [310]. Acute myoclonus is more common after cerebral ischemia and hypoxia, accounting for approximately 16–37% of HIE cases, while the incidence of delayed myoclonus after recovery of consciousness is much lower (less than 0.5%).

There is still some controversy about whether myoclonus after cerebral hypoxia is caused by epileptic seizures. Jonathan Elmer et al. analyzed the scalp electroencephalography (EEG) patterns of 401 patients who were in a coma after cardiac arrest, 69 of whom (16%) had acute early myoclonus [311]. EEG changes in these 69 patients can be categorized in four patterns: (1) burst-suppression background with high-amplitude polyspikes in lockstep with myoclonic jerks; (2) continuous background with narrow sharp waves distributed in the vertex in lockstep with myoclonic jerks; (3) subcortical myoclonus (no epileptiform discharge associated with myoclonic jerks); and (4) an unclassifiable pattern. Pattern 1 was most common, occurring in 48 patients (74%); followed by pattern 2 in 8 patients (12%); and the remaining patients had subcortical myoclonus ($n = 2$, 3%) or other types ($n = 7$, 11%). Of the 69 patients, 4 out of 8 (50%) with EEG pattern 2 survived and subsequently developed classic Lance-Adams syndrome, while the remaining 61 patients with EEG patterns 1, 3, and 4 did not survive. Although there was a lockstep relationship between myoclonic jerks and EEG discharges in the majority of patients, there were also a number of patients whose myoclonus was not clearly related to EEG epileptic changes and whose seizure characteristics were different from those of traditional "myoclonic epilepsies" and "status epilepticus" [312]. Therefore, many scholars suggest that post-hypoxic myoclonus is of cortical/subcortical origin and does not fit the traditional definition of epileptic seizures.

In addition to myoclonus, some patients may experience generalized tonic–clonic seizures after cerebral ischemia. If cerebral ischemia-hypoxia is not severe or resuscitation is timely, only localized brain injury may persist. For example, hippocampal injury can cause hippocampal sclerosis, resulting in medial temporal lobe epilepsy several years later. In addition, injury to the occipital lobe evolves into encephalomalacia and gliosis, which might subsequently cause focal occipital lobe epilepsy.

Pathogenic Mechanisms

The brain consumes the most oxygen of all organs in the human body, and the cerebral cortex, hippocampus, basal ganglia region, brainstem, and cerebellum are less tolerant to hypoxia than other regions. Ischemia and hypoxia lead to a lack of oxygen and glucose in the brain, which causes anaerobic metabolism, leading to a decrease in adenosine triphosphate (ATP) levels and an accumulation of lactic acid. When the cell membrane depolarizes, the cell releases the excitatory amino acid glutamate, which binds to the ligand-gated N-methyl-D-aspartate (NMDA) receptor to open channels for a large amount of transmembrane calcium ions and sodium ions to flow into the cell. However, when the cell membrane repolarizes, the depletion of ATP reduces the ionic transmembrane translocation of ions, leading to the buildup of intracellular sodium, calcium, and water, in turn causing cellular excitotoxicity. Peroxidation of free fatty acids by oxygen radicals causes additional cellular damage. Energy depletion, acidosis, glutamate release, lipid peroxidation, and the toxic effects of nitric oxide led to cell necrosis and the activation of apoptotic cascades [309, 313].

There are three phases of recovery based on the timing of injury and resuscitation. The first phase is 30–60 minutes after acute hypoxia-ischemia, during which the main injuries are oxidative damage, inflammation, and activation of the apoptotic cascade. In some patients, this phase can last up to 1–6 h due to medical interventions such as cardiopulmonary resuscitation. The second phase of injury occurs after approximately 6–15 h. Cytotoxic edema, excitotoxicity, secondary energy failure, and loss of mitochondrial function characterize this phase. Seizures usually occur during the second phase. The third phase occurs within months after acute injury and is characterized by delayed cell death, brain remodeling, and astrocyte proliferation [309, 314]. The pathogenesis of post-hypoxic myoclonus is unclear. It may be due to abnormal cortical firing, abnormalities in the cerebellar-brainstem and thalamocortical circuits, and impaired metabolism of the neurotransmitter 5-hydroxytryptamine (5-HT) [315].

Treatment

During the acute phase of cerebral hypoxia-ischemia, the administration of hypothermia therapy can reduce the extent of cerebral damage and the severity of seizures in the acute phase, increase the chances of resuscitation, and reduce the risk of late-onset epilepsy [316]. A retrospective study that included 56 neonates with HIE revealed that hypothermia therapy applied in the acute phase significantly reduced the incidence of seizures after 6 months [317]. In neonates with focal cerebral ischemic-hypoxic lesions, hypothermia therapy also significantly reduced the risk of seizures [318]. In addition, phenobarbital is thought to have potential neuroprotective effects during the acute phase of cerebral hypoxia-ischemia and could enhance the beneficial effects of hypothermia; it should be initiated at the latent stage before seizure onset [316]. In animal models of hypoxic-ischemic injury, phenobarbital plus hypothermia had significantly better outcomes than hypothermia or normothermia alone [319], but the results of this study need to be confirmed by large clinical studies.

For the treatment of post-hypoxic myoclonus, the combination of clonazepam, sodium valproate, piracetam and levetiracetam has a significant effect on more than 50% of patients, and clonazepam is considered to be the most effective [320]. Moreover, these drugs are also effective in patients with generalized tonic clonic seizures.

In addition, based on the doctrine of impaired 5-HT metabolism, some studies have attempted to apply L-5-hydroxytryptophan (L-5-HTP), a direct precursor of 5-HT, in the treatment of myoclonus after cerebral hypoxia [321], and myoclonus improved in some patients after the administration of L-5-HTP. The side effects of L-5-HTP, such as nausea, vomiting, and diarrhea, can be reduced by combining it with carbidopa, an aromatic L-amino acid decarboxylase inhibitor.

In recent years, there have been case reports of perampanel use improving post-hypoxic myoclonus [322, 323]. Perampanel is a selective A-amino-3-hydroxy-5--methyl-4-isoxazolepropionic acid (AMPA) receptor antagonist, and the mechanism underlying its effect on myoclonus is still unclear. More therapeutic experience is needed in the future to elucidate its mechanisms.

For medial temporal lobe epilepsy caused by hippocampal sclerosis after ischemia and hypoxia, sodium channel blockers such as oxcarbazepine, carbamazepine, and lamotrigine, or a combination of drugs with other mechanisms, can be used, but such patients tend to be medically refractory as well. Treatment for epilepsy caused by encephalomalacia in the occipital lobe is consistent with that for focal epilepsy.

4.3.7.2 Metabolic Encephalopathy

Hepatic Encephalopathy

(1) *Definition*: Hepatic encephalopathy (HE) is a disorder in which the central nervous system is dysfunctional due to chronic liver disease. The liver is responsible for metabolism and detoxification under normal conditions, but when its function is impaired due to a variety of liver diseases, toxins accumulate in the blood, which in turn affects the normal function of the nervous system [324].

(2) *Clinical Features and Epidemiology*: There is a correlation between liver disease and the risk of epilepsy. A large population-based cohort study revealed that the proportion of people with liver disorders who experienced seizures was approximately 2.5%, and the risk of status epilepticus in patients with cirrhosis was 1.3–2.8 times greater than that in patients without cirrhosis [325]. In 2020, the New York State Inpatient Database showed that patients with worsening liver disease had a two- to threefold increased risk of rehospitalization for seizures within 6 months of discharge and a three- to fivefold increased risk of rehospitalization for status epilepticus [326].

    The seizures of patients with HE can manifest as GTCSs or convulsive or nonconvulsive status epilepticus. Marco Olivero et al. [327] described a case of HE with nonconvulsive status epilepticus as the first symptom, in which the patient presented with persistent confusion and a decreased level of consciousness, and the EEG showed paroxysmal sharp wave rhythms superimposed on a background of widespread slow waves. In stages III and IV of HE, EEG may reveal typical triphasic waves.

    Typical brain imaging changes in HE include symmetrical high signals in the bilateral pallidum on magnetic resonance T1W sequences, accompanied by high signals in the bilateral pyramidal tracts and the white matter of the subcortical hemispheres on T2-FLAIR sequences [328].

(3) *Pathogenic Mechanisms*: The mechanisms by which HE causes seizures can be explained as follows [329–332]:

    ① *Ammonia Toxicity*: Chronic liver disease results in the inability of the liver to metabolize ammonia effectively, leading to elevated blood ammonia concentrations. A high concentration of blood ammonia enters brain tissue through the blood–brain barrier, and its inherent excitotoxicity affects the normal function of neurotransmitters and interferes with neuronal excitability, thus triggering seizures.

② *Neurotransmitter Disorders*: HE interferes with the synthesis, release, and metabolism of a variety of neurotransmitters, such as glutamate and gamma-aminobutyric acid (GABA), among which an increase in synaptic glutamate is more closely associated with hyperammonemia. These abnormal changes may lead to abnormal neuronal discharges and seizures.

③ *Cerebral Edema*: HE can lead to the development of cerebral edema. Cerebral edema increases pressure in the brain, compresses nerve tissue, and interferes with the normal function of neurons, which can lead to seizures.

④ *Inflammatory Response*: Liver disease can lead to an inflammatory response and abnormal activation of the immune system. The inflammatory response can cause inflammatory damage to neurons, affecting their normal function and thus promoting seizures.

⑤ *Treatment*: For patients with HE and epileptic seizures, treating the primary liver disease is the first task, and it is also important to remove the HE-inducing factors (e.g., infections, gastrointestinal hemorrhage, volume-deficient alkalosis, and electrolyte disorders) as soon as possible [333]. Lowering blood ammonia is an essential symptomatic treatment. Laxatives such as lactulose and lactitol, antimicrobial agents that can inhibit the growth of ammonia-producing bacteria (e.g., neomycin), and drugs that can promote the clearance of ammonia, such as L-ornithine, L-methionine, arginine and glutamine, can all be used to reduce blood ammonia levels. Status epilepticus caused by HE is sometimes difficult to control with intravenous phenytoin or benzodiazepines, but lowering blood ammonia levels can dramatically stop it.

The use of ASMs should be individualized, and the use of hepatotoxic drugs such as valproic acid needs to be avoided. Loss of hepatocytes and disturbances in hepatic blood flow can decrease the metabolism of ASMs, and hypoproteinemia, decreased albumin binding, and impaired metabolism of cytochrome P450 (CYP450) and glucosyltransferase can lead to increased serum levels of ASMs [334]. Therefore, the doses of relevant drugs metabolized by the liver need to be adjusted. In addition, phenobarbital and benzodiazepines have sedative effects and may aggravate impaired consciousness in patients with HE and should be used with caution.

Low protein-binding ASMs, such as gabapentin, topiramate, aminocaproic acid, and levetiracetam, induce very little hepatic metabolism and are therefore relatively suitable. Topiramate is a selective enzyme inducer/inhibitor, whereas gabapentin, levetiracetam, and aminoglutethimide have no significant effects on CYP450. Levetiracetam is predominantly metabolized by the kidneys with linear pharmacokinetics and reaches a steady state after 2 days of twice-daily dosing [335].

Hepatolenticular degeneration (Wilson's disease) rarely causes seizures, but D-penicillamine treatment can lead to pyridoxine deficiency, which can cause seizures, and treatment with pyridoxine or other copper chelators is recommended [336].

4.3.7.3 Uremic Encephalopathy

Definition

Uremic encephalopathy (UE) is a disorder of the central nervous system caused by chronic kidney disease [337]. One of the main functions of the kidneys is the elimination of metabolites from the body and the regulation of fluid balance. Chronic kidney disease may lead to uremia (i.e., the accumulation of toxins and metabolites in the body), which in turn affects the normal functioning of the nervous system.

Clinical Features and Epidemiology

The incidence of symptomatic seizures in patients with chronic kidney disease has been reported to be approximately 10% [338]. Seizures may also be associated with dialysis. Acute dialysis disequilibrium syndrome (DDS) is reversible and occurs mainly in patients with severe hyperazotemia at the start of dialysis treatment. During hemodialysis, urea is removed from the blood faster than from the brain, leading to osmotic pressure gradients and cerebral edema, which can cause reversible posterior encephalopathy (PRES) with clinical manifestations of irritability, headache, vomiting, blurred vision, seizures, and impaired consciousness. The seizures are mainly manifested as GTCSs and sometimes even status epilepticus. Uncontrolled hypertension, electrolyte disturbances, erythropoietin, cytotoxic drugs, and the use of immunosuppressants are risk factors for PRES [339–341]. In addition, the high aluminum concentration in dialysis fluids was once considered a cause of seizures, so aluminum-free water is now routinely used [342].

Pathogenic Mechanisms

The mechanisms by which renal encephalopathy causes seizures may be related to the following factors [337, 343]:

(1) *Accumulation of Nitrogenous Substances*: In chronic kidney disease, the kidneys are unable to effectively eliminate nitrogenous substances, such as urea and creatinine, from the body. The accumulation of these substances in the body can lead to nitrogen toxicity, which affects the normal function of the nervous system, including the triggering of seizures.
(2) *Electrolyte disorders*: Kidney dysfunction can lead to disturbances in fluid and electrolyte balance. Abnormal changes in the concentrations of electrolytes such as serum sodium, potassium, and calcium may affect the electrical activities of neurons, leading to abnormal discharges and the occurrence of seizures.

(3) *Neurotransmitter abnormalities*: The accumulation of metabolites such as ammonia and phenylpyruvic acid in the serum may affect the normal synthesis, release and transport of neurotransmitters, leading to abnormal neurotransmitter function, which in turn affects neuronal excitability and contributes to the occurrence of seizures.
(4) *Neuroinflammatory Response*: In the uremic state, inflammation may increase in the body, leading to inflammatory reactions and damage to the nervous system. These inflammatory responses can activate neuronal excitability and cause seizures.

Treatment

Etiology is not a determining factor in the selection of ASMs in patients with renal disease. Age, type of epilepsy (focal or generalized), drug interactions and creatinine clearance rate are determining factors in selecting medications.

It is important for patients with renal disease to consider the pharmacokinetics, metabolites, renal excretion rate, protein binding rate, and additional postdialysis supplemental dosage requirements of each ASM. During hemodialysis, drugs with high water solubility and low protein binding rates are readily cleared by dialysis. Therefore, gabapentin, topiramate, phenobarbital, and levetiracetam require supplemental dosing after hemodialysis. In contrast, drugs with high protein binding rates, such as phenytoin sodium, carbamazepine, and valproate, are less likely to require supplemental dosing after dialysis.

Phenytoin is one of the oldest ASMs, and its main action is to inhibit voltage-gated sodium channels, thereby stabilizing the inactivated state of these channels, decreasing the release of glutamate and enhancing the release of GABA [344]. The drug is excreted directly from the urine in less than 5% of patients, so it is safe for use in patients with UE. The mechanism of action of carbamazepine is similar to that of phenytoin, and carbamazepine is metabolized primarily in the liver and does not require dose adjustments in cases of renal failure [345]. The mechanisms of VPA include blockade of voltage-gated sodium and calcium channels and enhancement of the GABAergic system, and less than 3% of this drug is excreted in the urine; therefore, no dose adjustment is needed in patients with UE [346].

In recent years, levetiracetam has become one of the most commonly used drugs for partial and generalized seizures. Its anti-seizure effect is exerted by inhibiting the release of synaptic vesicle protein SV2A. A small portion of the drug is bound to plasma proteins, and 2/3 is excreted directly by the kidney [345]. Therefore, the drug requires dose adjustment in patients with renal insufficiency.

The dosage adjustment regimens of commonly used ASM agents in different renal function states and after dialysis are detailed in Table 4.10 [345].

Table 4.10 Dose adjustment regimens for commonly used ASMs in patients with different renal function states and after dialysis [257]

ASM	Protein binding ratio	Main metabolic pathways	Renal excretion rate	Glomerular filtration rate > 60	Glomerular filtration rate 30–59	Glomerular filtration rate 15–29	Glomerular filtration rate <15	Postdialysis
Carbamazepine	70–80%	Liver (CYP450)	Trace (element)	200–800 mg, 2×/day	No adjustment required	No adjustment required	No adjustment required	No supplemental dosage required
Phenytoin	90%	Liver (CYP450)	<5%	150–200 mg, 2–3 times/day	No adjustment required	No adjustment required	No adjustment required	No supplemental dosage required
Valproic acid	90%	Liver (CYP450)	1%–3%	30–60 mg/kg/day, 2–3 times/day	No adjustment required	No adjustment required	No adjustment required	No supplemental dosage required
Perampanel	95%	Liver (CYP3A4)	2%	4–12 mg per day	Insufficient data, no adjustment may be required	Insufficient data, no adjustment may be required	Insufficient data, no adjustment may be required	Insufficient data, no adjustment may be required
Chlorbazam	86%	Liver (CYP3A4)	94%	20–40 mg per day	No adjustment required	No adjustment required	No adjustment required	No supplemental dosage required
Zonisamide	40%–60%	Liver (CYP450)	30%–35%	100–600 mg per day	No adjustment required	No adjustment required	No adjustment required	If postdialysis seizures occur, 50% of the daily dose needs to be supplemented
Lacosamide	<15%	Liver (CYP450)	40%	50–200 mg, 2×/day	No adjustment required	Slow titration, maximum 300 mg/day	Slow titration, maximum 300 mg/day	50% daily dose supplementation
Lamotrigine	50–55%	Liver	10%	50–250 mg, 2×/day	May need to be reduced	May need to be reduced	May need to be reduced	Appropriate amount

Levetiracetam	<10%	Hydrolysis	66%	500–1500 mg, 2 times/day	50% daily dose reduction	50% daily dose reduction	50% daily dose reduction	500–1000 mg/day, supplemented with 50% of the daily dose after dialysis
Oxcarbazepine	40%	Liver	50%	300–1200 mg, 2×/day	No adjustment required	Halve regular dose at start	Halve regular dose at start	Insufficient data, need to monitor blood levels
Phenobarbital	55%	Liver (CYP450)	25%	60–100 mg, 2–3 times/day	May need to be reduced	May need to be reduced	May need to be reduced	50% daily dose supplementation
Topiramate	20%	Hydrolysis	60–70%	100–200 mg, 2 times/day	50% daily dose reduction	50% daily dose reduction	50% daily dose reduction	50% daily dose supplementation
Aminohexenoic acid	0%	Excretion in the original form	70–80%	1000–3000 mg per day	25% daily dose reduction	50% daily dose reduction	75% daily dose reduction	50% daily dose supplementation

4.3.7.4 Pulmonary Encephalopathy

Definition

Pulmonary encephalopathy (PE) is a pathological state of brain dysfunction caused by severe pulmonary disease [346]. It usually results from hypoxemia and carbon dioxide retention due to lung diseases such as chronic obstructive pulmonary disease (COPD), pulmonary fibrosis, pulmonary hypertension, or pulmonary thromboembolism.

Clinical Features and Epidemiology

The main manifestation is diffuse cerebral dysfunction, which is usually characterized by impaired consciousness, such as confusion, delirium, and even deep coma. A minority of patients may have other clinical manifestations, such as seizures, headache, or extrapyramidal symptoms [258]. However, the proportion of patients with PE presenting with seizures has not been clearly reported. Nevertheless, there appears to be a link between COPD and epilepsy. Large cohort studies in several countries have revealed that COPD is a common comorbidity in patients with epilepsy [347–349]. Smoking may be a risk factor for this comorbidity, but the exact mechanism is unclear. Prolonged chronic hypoxic states, in turn, may also increase the risk of epilepsy [350].

Pathogenic Mechanisms

The mechanisms by which PE causes seizures may be related to the following factors [346, 351, 352]:

(1) *Hypoxemia*: Patients with PE suffer from insufficient oxygen supply due to lung disease, which can cause hypoxemia. Hypoxemia can lead to neuronal damage and metabolic abnormalities in the brain, thus promoting seizures.
(2) *Acid–Base Imbalance*: Patients with PE often experience respiratory acidosis and metabolic alkalosis. An acid-base imbalance may interfere with the normal function of neurons, leading to seizures.
(3) *Chronic Carbon Dioxide Retention*: Patients with PE often suffer from chronic carbon dioxide retention, known as chronic respiratory acidosis. The accumulation of carbon dioxide can lead to cerebral vasodilation and increased blood flow, further impairing neuronal function and contributing to the occurrence of seizures.
(4) *Inflammatory Response*: Lung diseases are often accompanied by an inflammatory response that leads to the release of inflammatory mediators and cytokines. These inflammatory factors may affect the normal function of neurons through a variety of pathways, including the regulation of neurotransmission, ion channel activity, and neuronal excitability.

Treatment

The treatment of seizures in patients with PE usually follows the conventional principles of drug selection, but care should be taken to avoid the use of benzodiazepines, which can cause respiratory depression and respiratory muscle weakness and exacerbate hypoxia and carbon dioxide retention, leading to worsening of the condition [353].

4.3.7.5 Autoimmune-Related Encephalopathy

Hashimoto's Encephalopathy

Definition

Hashimoto's encephalopathy is an encephalopathic syndrome characterized by elevated levels of serum and/or cerebrospinal fluid antithyroid-associated antibodies with symptoms such as altered consciousness, psychosis, hallucinations, and seizures and, in most cases, sensitivity to glucocorticoid therapy.

Clinical Features and Epidemiology

The disease was first described in 1966 by Lord Brain et al. [354]. To date, the disease is relatively rare, with a prevalence of approximately 2.1/100,000 adults [355]. The male-to-female ratio of patients is 1:4 [356]. It can occur in all age groups, with a median age of onset of 12–14 years for adolescents and 45–48 years for adults [355, 357]. Older adults are more vulnerable, and the overall median age of onset is 41–48 years [358].

The clinical symptoms of Hashimoto's encephalopathy can vary but are predominantly encephalopathic. In a systematic review of 251 patients described in the literature, Charlotte Laurent et al. [359] summarized the clinical presentations as follows: tics (n = 117, 47%), confusion (n = 115, 46%), speech disorders (n = 91, 37%), memory impairments (n = 107, 43%), gait disorders (n = 67, 27%), and persecutory delusions (n = 61, 25%). Of these, 28 patients (11%) had progressive memory impairment, and 26 (10%) had only isolated mental disorders. Kothbauer-Magreiter et al. [360] classified symptoms of Hashimoto's encephalopathy into two categories: (1) the vascular type, which is characterized by recurrent stroke-like symptoms (e.g., hemiparesis, aphasia, and gait abnormalities) with less severe cognitive impairment, and (2) the slowly progressive type, which is characterized by insidiously worsening dementia, impaired consciousness, psychotic disorders, hallucinations, and epileptic seizures.

Seizures are common in patients with Hashimoto's encephalopathy, accounting for approximately 2/3 of cases [361]. The most common type of seizure is focal to generalized seizure [362]. In addition, it can also present as status epilepticus, including epilepsia partialis continua (EPC) and nonconvulsive status epilepticus

(NCSE), in approximately 12% of cases [363]. Presentation with progressive myoclonic epilepsy has also been reported [364]. Therefore, patients with unexplained focal or generalized seizures accompanied by encephalopathic symptoms should be screened for the possibility of Hashimoto's encephalopathy [365].

Imaging in patients with Hashimoto's encephalopathy is usually normal, or these patients present with nonspecific changes, such as ischemic foci, white matter demyelination, and focal vasogenic edema [366]. More than 90–98% of patients present with nonspecific EEG abnormalities, usually characterized by background slowing, and other abnormalities, such as focal spikes or sharp waves, biphasic or triphasic waves, frontal intermittent rhythmic delta activity (FIRDA), and periodic synchronous discharge (PSD) [361, 367]. Nonspecific EEG abnormalities are not associated with the diagnosis of Hashimoto's encephalopathy but can improve rapidly after hormone therapy, which may play a role in monitoring the response to treatment [368]. Mild abnormalities of the cerebrospinal fluid are observed in approximately 80% of patients, mainly presenting as mild protein level elevation and an elevated lymphocyte ratio [369]. Elevated levels of serum thyroid-associated antibodies, such as thyroperoxidase antibody (TPOAb) and thyroglobulin antibody (TgAb), are essential for diagnosis, and TPOAb levels, in particular, may be markedly elevated, but their titers are not necessarily related to the severity of the disease [369].

Pathogenic Mechanisms

The pathogenesis of Hashimoto's encephalopathy and its relationship to Hashimoto's thyroiditis and thyroid-associated antibodies are not clear. Currently, there are two possible pathogenic mechanisms:

(1) Autoimmune vasculitis in the central nervous system (CNS).

Autoimmune vasculitis in the central nervous system mainly presents with perivascular lymphoid infiltration of small and medium vessels, with or without immune complex deposits. The infiltrating immune cells are mainly T lymphocytes [370]. The infiltration involves the areas around small veins and arterioles of the entire brain, including the perichondrium, cortex, white matter, basal ganglia, and brainstem [371]. Nolte et al. [372] described the case of a patient with Hashimoto's encephalopathy who died of heart failure, whose vasculitis only occurred in the veins and small veins of the brainstem, suggesting that there may be some specific brain regions in which this vasculitis is prevalent. Vasculitis can cause cerebral microcirculatory disorders, decreased cerebral perfusion, and inflammatory edema, resulting in cerebral neuronal dysfunction and excitation/inhibition imbalance, which in turn may cause corresponding neurologic deficits and seizures.

(2) Autoimmune response to antigens of both the thyroid gland and the central nervous system.

The main support for this hypothesis lies in the presence of thyroid-related antibodies in the cerebrospinal fluid or brain tissue of some patients with Hashimoto's encephalopathy. It is possible that thyroid-related antibodies produced outside the brain can enter the CNS through the blood–brain barrier and attack the target tissue of the brain. For example, Moodley et al. [373] confirmed the presence of thyroid-related antibody targets in the brain by analyzing brain tissues from five adult patients who died after trauma, with thyrotropin receptor antibody targets located on cortical neurons and soft meningeal blood vessels, whereas thyroglobulin antibody targets localized only in vascular smooth muscle in the brain. Interestingly, however, Ferracci et al. [369] described the presence of thyroid antibodies in the cerebrospinal fluid of five patients, but their blood–brain barrier was intact, suggesting possible intrathecal synthesis. Attack by relevant antibodies can directly cause neuronal dysfunction, leading to encephalopathy.

Treatment

The application of ASMs alone, such as valproic acid, levetiracetam, carbamazepine, and oxcarbazepine, may be ineffective for treating seizures in these patients, and only by effective immunotherapy can the seizures be fully controlled [374].

Once the disease is diagnosed or suspected, early initiation of glucocorticoid therapy is usually recommended. There is no standardized dose or course for this therapy. A common regimen for adult patients is intravenous injection of 500–1000 mg/day methylprednisolone for 5 days, with a sequential oral dosage of 60 mg/day and a reduction of 10 mg every 2 weeks, followed by maintenance at the lowest dose for 1–2 years [375]. More than 90% of patients experience complete or partial remission with hormone therapy [359]. Because of its sensitivity to glucocorticoids, this disease has been named steroid-responsive encephalopathy associated with autoimmune thyroiditis (SREAT). However, glucocorticoid therapy is not effective in all patients. In the acute phase, if glucocorticoid therapy is not effective, immunoglobulin therapy (a total dosage of 2 g/kg) [376] or plasma exchange therapy [377] may be therapeutic options.

Other immunomodulators, such as azathioprine, methotrexate, cyclophosphamide, mycophenolate mofetil, hydroxychloroquine sulfate, and rituximab, may be given if glucocorticoid monotherapy fails or glucocorticoid-related side effects need to be prevented [378].

Hashimoto's encephalopathy relapse occurs in approximately 16% of patients, especially those who are comatose at onset. However, TgAb(+) alone without other antibody positivity is associated with a favorable outcome [359].

Lupus Encephalopathy

Definition

Lupus encephalopathy (LE) refers to a series of brain dysfunctions caused by systemic lupus erythematosus (SLE) involving the central nervous system and is a relatively serious complication of SLE.

Clinical Features and Epidemiology

In 1999, the American College of Rheumatology listed 19 complications of SLE involving the nervous system and categorized them as neuropsychiatric systemic lupus erythematosus (NPSLE) [379], including 12 CNS symptoms and 7 peripheral nervous system (PNS) symptoms, as shown in Table 4.11.

Approximately 37–95% of patients present with at least one symptom of NPSLE [380]. The prevalence of different symptoms varies, with the most common being headache, mild cognitive dysfunction and mood disorders. Seizures, stroke, and anxiety disorders are also prevalent, as shown in Table 4.12 [381].

Seizures in patients with SLE can include generalized tonic–clonic seizures or partial seizures (complex partial seizures or simple partial seizures). Most seizures are isolated, but recurrences can occur in 12–43% of patients, especially within the first year after onset [382]. Seizures may result from the direct toxic effects of

Table 4.11 Neurologic complications of SLE

	Symptoms
CNS	Aseptic meningitis
	Cerebrovascular disease
	Demyelination syndrome (medicine)
	Headache (including migraine and benign intracranial pressure elevation)
	Movement disorders (chorea)
	Myelopathy
	Seizures
	Delirium
	Neurosis
	Cognitive impairment
	Emotional disorder
	Mental disorder
PNS	Acute inflammatory demyelinating polyneuropathy/neuropathy (Guillain–Barre syndrome)
	Autonomic disorder
	Mononeuritis simplex/multiple mononeuritis
	Myasthenia gravis
	Cranial neuropathy
	Plexopathy
	Polyneuropathy

Table 4.12 Frequency of different symptoms of NPSLE

Frequency	Symptoms
Common, >10–20%	Headaches, mild cognitive dysfunction, mood disorders
Frequent, 5–10%	Seizures, stroke, anxiety
Uncommon, 3–5%	Psychosis, peripheral neuropathy, delirium, severe cognitive impairment
Rare, <1–2%	Chorea, movement disorders, myelopathy, aseptic meningitis, cranial neuropathy, mononeuropathy, demyelination syndrome, Guillain–Barre syndrome, autonomic disorders, myasthenia gravis, plexopathy

autoantibodies related to SLE or may be a symptom of other complications associated with the disease, such as cerebral infarction/hemorrhage, posterior reversible encephalopathy syndrome (PRES), cerebral venous sinus thrombosis, and meningeal hemosiderin deposits. Usually, seizures are more common in adolescents [382]. Approximately 25% of patients with SLE show abnormalities in brain imaging, mainly cerebral atrophy, ischemic/hemorrhagic lesions, and demyelinating lesions [383].

Pathogenic Mechanisms

The pathogenic and epileptogenic mechanisms of NPSLE are complex and involve multiple mechanisms and interactions.

(1) Genetic susceptibility: To date, several genes associated with SLE, including HLADRB1, IRF5, STAT4, BLK, TNFAIP3, TNIP1, FCGR2B, and TNFSF13, have been identified. A Japanese study revealed that the greater the number of gene variants one carries that are related to SLE, the greater the probability of developing NPSLE [384]. In addition, variants in TREX1, the causative gene for Aicardi-Goutieres syndrome, have also been found to be associated with SLE, and variants in TREX1 are especially common in patients with manifestations of CNS involvement, such as seizures [385].
(2) Autoantibodies: Antiphospholipid (aPL) antibody levels are elevated in the majority of SLE patients with seizures, strokes, and headaches [386]. However, in epilepsy patients without SLE, those patients who had seizures for the past month were more likely to be aPL antibody-positive than those who were seizure free for the past year [387]. This can be explained by the fact that aPL antibodies themselves are neuropathogenic in nature and can cause seizures through direct neurotoxic effects [388]. Anti-ribosomal protein (anti-Rib-P) antibodies are also common in patients with SLE, and a large cohort study revealed that patients with elevated levels of this antibody early in the course of the disease had a significantly greater risk of developing lupus psychosis during the next 3 years of follow-up [389]. Anti-glutamate receptor (anti-NMDA or anti-NR2) antibodies can be found in 30–40% of patients with SLE, and they

are double-stranded DNA antibodies. The NMDA receptor is widely distributed in the brain, especially in the amygdala and hippocampus, and is strongly correlated with memory and affective functions [390]. Elevated levels of this antibody can be used as a marker to distinguish lupus encephalopathy from lupus peripheral neuropathy [391].

(3) Vasculopathy: Deposition of lupus-associated immune complexes in the vascular wall can cause vascular damage, resulting in multiple small vessel inflammatory lesions, microemboli, microinfarcts, and microhemorrhages [392]. Antiphospholipid antibodies may cause hypercoagulability and contribute to the formation of cerebral thrombi.

(4) Inflammatory factors: The expression of several cytokines and chemokines is upregulated during the active period of disease and downregulated after effective treatment [393]. These cytokines and inflammatory mediators disrupt the blood–brain barrier, causing neuroinflammation and interfering with the normal functioning of neurons.

Treatment

There is no uniform expert consensus on the treatment of seizures in patients with NPSLE. The European League Against Rheumatism (EULAR) does not recommend the use of ASMs in patients with only a single seizure and a low risk of recurrence, but treatment should be initiated promptly if there is a high risk of seizure recurrence (i.e., recurrent seizures, the presence of an abnormal brain lesion, or abnormal epileptiform discharges on the EEG) [394]. The selection of ASMs is usually based on the seizure type (generalized or partial). In most patients, seizures are easily controlled, and medications can be successfully tapered [389].

Two large cohort studies suggested that antimalarial drugs, such as hydroxychloroquine, had a protective role in preventing seizures in patients with SLE [389, 394], but the exact mechanism is unclear. In addition, because hydroxychloroquine has antithrombotic effects, it may be used in combination with aspirin to treat seizures caused by thrombotic events due to aPL antibodies [395]. If aPL antibody levels are markedly elevated (moderate to high titers) or accompanied by a hypercoagulable state, anticoagulative therapy may be considered [393].

If the seizures, or sometimes status epilepticus, are due to an acute inflammatory response, immunotherapy should be initiated in addition to ASMs [381]. In 2010, the EULAR recommended the use of glucocorticoids as a first-line treatment, and if this treatment is not effective, the addition of another immunosuppressive agent, such as intravenous cyclophosphamide therapy, may be considered [396]. It was reported that in some patients with refractory epilepsy, the combination of intravenous high-dose methylprednisolone and cyclophosphamide is effective in reducing the frequency of seizures [397].

4.3.7.6 Toxic Encephalopathy

Carbon Monoxide Poisoning

Definition

Delayed encephalopathy after acute carbon monoxide poisoning (DEACMP) refers to a cerebral disorder characterized by a sudden recurrence of dementia, psychiatric symptoms, or extrapyramidal symptoms in patients with acute carbon monoxide poisoning (ACMP) 2–60 days after recovery of consciousness and normal or almost-normal neurological function [398].

Clinical Features and Epidemiology

Common neurological manifestations of DEACMP include disorders such as decreased numeracy and memory, language disorders, dystonia, disorientation, dementia, Parkinson's syndrome, and action myoclonus and seizures [187]. The incidence of concomitant epilepsy in patients with carbon monoxide poisoning is approximately 20% [399], with a small percentage occurring during the ACMP phase and the majority occurring during the DEACMP phase. Seizures can be generalized tonic–clonic and/or partial.

The brain images of patients with DEACMP are often abnormal. Computerized tomographic (CT) scanning mainly shows diffuse abnormalities, such as low-density changes in the bilateral globus pallidus, frontal, dorsal occipital, subcortical white matter, and bilateral basal nuclei; lateral ventricle dilatation; cerebral sulcus widening; and brain tissue atrophy. The main MRI manifestations are as follows: (1) subcortical white matter abnormalities, mainly in the cortical points of the subcortex, plaque or fusion lesions with low T1WI signals and high T2WI signals; (2) deep white matter lesions, in the periventricular white matter and semiovoid centers with extensive T2WI low signals and T2WI high signals; and (3) basal ganglia lesions, bilateral symmetrical T1WI low signals and T2WI high signals in the basal ganglia [400].

Pathogenic Mechanisms

The pathogenesis of DEACMP is unclear. Some studies have shown that hypoxemia caused by carbon monoxide inhalation does not necessarily injure the cerebral cortex. The following points are thought to contribute to the development of DEACMP [401]:

(1) Vascular wall degeneration, vasomotor nerve palsy, vasodilatation, congestion, vascular rupture, and occlusive endarteritis can lead to necrosis, softening, and degeneration of brain cells.
(2) Oligodendrocytes are susceptible to hypoxia, which triggers extensive demyelination.

(3) Immune dysfunction, abnormalities in dopamine, 5-hydroxytryptamine, acetylcholine and other neurotransmitters, and lipid peroxidation due to free radicals can cause cerebral dysfunction.

Treatment

Hyperbaric oxygen therapy (HOT) is usually considered to be effective when initiated within 24 h of the acute phase of CMP, and the initiation of treatment within 6 h can further improve neurologic outcomes at 6 months [402]. For those with DEACMP, there seems to be no effective treatment. Leucine-rich repeat and immunoglobulin-like domain-containing protein-1 (LINGO-1), a nerve growth inhibitory factor expressed in the regeneration microenvironment of the CNS, is also highly expressed in a rat model of DEACMP, whereas intraperitoneal injection of retinoic acid (10 mg/kg) can suppress the expression of LINGO-1 and ameliorate the clinical symptoms of these rats [403]. ASMs are usually selected for epileptic seizures according to seizure type, according to principles similar to those used for patients with HIE.

Chronic Alcoholic Encephalopathy

Definition

Chronic alcoholic encephalopathy (CAE) is a chronic, relapsing brain dysfunction resulting from severe damage caused by alcohol toxicity to the CNS in patients with prolonged excessive alcohol consumption. The National Institute on Alcohol Abuse and Alcoholism (NIAAA) notes that one standard unit of alcohol is equivalent to 14 g of pure alcohol and suggests that the lower limit for the risk of alcohol poisoning is 14 units of alcohol per week for men and 7 units of alcohol per week for women. People with CAE usually have a long history of chronic alcohol use and consume more than this limit.

Clinical Features and Epidemiology

CAE can manifest as one of six syndromes: Wernicke's encephalopathy, Korsakoff's syndrome, chronic alcoholic dementia, alcoholic tremens-delirium, alcoholic epilepsy, and alcoholic mental and behavioral disorders. Seizures are predominantly generalized tonic–clonic, and partial seizures may be due to concurrent metabolic, toxic, infectious, traumatic, neoplastic, or cerebrovascular disorders. Alcoholism is a major trigger for status epilepticus (9–25% of cases) [403].

MRI is a preferred imaging method for patients with CAE; it usually shows symmetrical abnormal signals on T2W images in the bilateral thalamus and brainstem, and it is characterized by symmetrical long T2 signals around the third ventricle and aqueduct and atrophy of the papillary bodies [404, 405].

Pathogenic Mechanisms

The relationship between alcohol consumption and seizures is complex and multifaceted. The most important risk factor for seizures associated with alcohol consumption is withdrawal [406]. Ethanol exerts its neuromodulatory effects primarily through the perturbation of receptor-governed ion channel functions on neuronal membranes. It acts as an antagonist of the N-methyl-D-aspartate (NMDA) receptor, a key receptor for glutamate, thus attenuating excitatory glutamatergic synaptic signaling. Ethanol also impedes calcium ion translocation across the NMDA receptor, a process that is dependent on the ethanol concentration. Notably, sustained ethanol exposure precipitates an increase in NMDA receptor activity, a condition posited to underpin the clinical phenomena associated with alcohol withdrawal syndrome. Furthermore, ethanol has been shown to potentiate chloride ion flow through the gamma-aminobutyric acid type A (GABAA) receptor, mimicking the pharmacological effects of benzodiazepines. Adaptations within the CNS to chronic ethanol exposure manifest as tolerance, characterized by quantitative alterations in GABAA and NMDA receptor populations. These adaptations include a decrease in GABAA receptor numbers and an increase in NMDA receptor numbers, coupled with decreased GABAA receptor sensitivity to GABA and increased NMDA receptor sensitivity to glutamate. Additional mechanisms, such as the desensitization of adenosine receptor responses during alcohol withdrawal and genetic polymorphisms in the neuropeptide Y-encoding gene, have been proposed to contribute to the pathophysiology of alcohol withdrawal seizures. Evidence supporting a genetic predisposition includes studies demonstrating familial aggregation of seizure susceptibility associated with alcohol use.

Treatment

Benzodiazepines can significantly reduce the risk of seizures during withdrawal, whereas the use of antipsychotics may increase this risk. Among benzodiazepines, clonazepam is the most effective in preventing seizures, and lorazepam is also effective [407]. Sodium channel blockers such as carbamazepine and phenytoin are not effective for preventing seizures in rodent models of alcohol withdrawal, since clinical evidence is lacking. Sodium valproate, gabapentin, and topiramate have been shown to be effective in animal models. After the first seizure triggered by alcohol withdrawal, benzodiazepines need to be used for 7 days. Patients who experience a single seizure do not need long-term ASM treatment, and the best treatment is prevention, i.e., avoidance of long-term alcohol abuse [408].

4.3.7.7 Heroin-Induced Spongiform Leukoencephalopathy

Definition

Heroin-induced spongiform leukoencephalopathy (HSLE) is a toxic encephalopathy caused by dermabrasion or intravenous injection of heroin and is characterized by vacuolated spongy degeneration of the cerebral white matter.

Clinical Features and Epidemiology

The disease was first described in Amsterdam in 1982 by Woltes et al. [409]. With acute or subacute onset, symptoms of cerebellar injury are usually the first clinical manifestation. Further aggravation of the disease may result in damage to the pyramidal and extrapyramidal systems or even coma and decortication, while sensation is often normal. There have been reports of epileptic seizures in patients with HSLE, which are associated with cortical necrosis of the hippocampus [410]. The imaging changes in HSLE are located in the white matter region of the brain, especially the cerebellum, showing extensive and symmetrical alterations. The most characteristic features are symmetrical, round-like or butterfly-like lesions on both sides of the cerebellar midline with clear borders, which often show low signals on T1WI and high signals on T2WI, the pathology of which reveals white matter vacuolization [411].

Pathogenic Mechanisms

The exact pathogenesis of HSLE is not yet completely clear. When heated, heroin and its additives become more toxic to neural tissues, and the harmful components, along with their metabolites, may have direct toxic effects on the structure and function of cerebral white matter. In addition, cerebral vasospasm, hypoxia, and ischemia caused by heroin may also be related to the development of HSLE [412].

Treatment

Lacking appropriate research evidence, the treatment of seizures due to HSLE usually follows the principles of conventional ASM selection, but attention should be given to liver and kidney function, as these patients often have impaired functions due to drug and toxic substance abuse.

4.3.7.8 Radiation Encephalopathy

Definition

Radiation encephalopathy (RE) refers to cerebral injury and dysfunction caused by radiation exposure [413] and was first described by Fisher et al. in 1930. It can occur in patients with tumors that are being treated with radiation (commonly head and neck tumors, such as nasopharyngeal carcinoma) or in people exposed to radioactive contamination. The manifestations and severity of RE depend on the dose of irradiation, the mode of irradiation, the site of irradiation, and the sensitivity of the individuals. The time of onset after radiotherapy can be categorized into acute and delayed RE, and the latter can be further divided into early delayed and late delayed RE.

Clinical features and epidemiology

Acute RE occurs within 1–4 weeks after the start of radiation therapy. Clinical manifestations include headache, nausea, vomiting, and other symptoms of cranial hypertension, and death may even occur due to brain herniation caused by a rapid increase in intracranial pressure. Large lesions with low T1W and high T2W signals accompanied by enhancement can be seen on brain MRI. Pathologic changes are mainly coagulative necrosis, also known as radioactive brain necrosis, which manifests as degenerative necrosis of neurons, gliosis, and perivascular lymphocytic infiltration under the microscope. Early delayed RE occurs within 1–6 months after the start of radiation therapy, while late delayed RE occurs after 6 months. Clinical manifestations include the slow onset of headache, limb dysfunction, seizures, impaired consciousness, and memory impairment [413]. Brain MRI usually shows irregularly shaped lesions with low T1W and high T2W signals, often with surrounding enhanced cystic degeneration in the middle of the lesion. Pathologic changes include vasculitis, capillary proliferation, white matter demyelination, and cerebral white matter necrosis [414]. Currently, it is speculated that acute and early delayed RE are reversible, whereas late delayed RE is progressive and irreversible.

Approximately 15.8% of patients with RE may experience seizures, with generalized tonic–clonic seizures being predominant and focal status epilepticus occurring in a minority of patients [415].

Pathogenic Mechanisms

There are two main hypotheses for the mechanism of injury in RE: vascular endothelial cell damage and loss of the regenerative capacity of brain glial cells. Together, these two mechanisms can cause cerebral ischemia and/or hemorrhage, cerebral edema, and cerebral white matter demyelination as well as necrosis. The epileptogenic mechanism of RE may be related to alterations in ion channels, excitatory/inhibitory neurotransmitter imbalances, and abnormalities in neural networks caused by the abovementioned brain injuries [413].

Treatment

Glucocorticoid therapy, such as dexamethasone, should be used for seizures occurring in the early stage of RE (within 6 months) [416]. In the majority of patients, remission can be achieved after treatment, and long-term use of ASMs is not necessary. Late-onset seizures often require long-term medications. Most patients can be treated by monotherapy with sodium channel blockers such as carbamazepine, oxcarbazepine, and lamotrigine or broad-spectrum ASMs such as valproic acid, levetiracetam, and topiramate. Specifically, valproic acid, a histone deacetylase inhibitor, can enhance radiosensitivity in esophageal squamous cell carcinoma [417], and thus, it can not only control seizures but also improve the efficacy of radiation therapy for tumors in such patients.

4.3.8 Seizures and the Selection of Anti-seizure Medications After Organ Transplantation

Organ transplantation is a surgical procedure in which a healthy organ (e.g., kidney, liver, heart, or lungs) is transferred from one person to another, who requires the organ to replace their unhealthy or damaged organ. Kidney transplantation is the most common type, followed by liver, heart, lung, and hematopoietic stem cell transplantation. Approximately one-third of patients who undergo solid organ transplants develop neurological symptoms. Epidemiological studies have shown that 2–24% of solid organ transplant recipients experience seizures, compared to 7–27% of hematopoietic stem cell transplant recipients [418]. This makes epilepsy the second most common central nervous system complication after organ transplantation, following neurotoxicity [419].

Organ transplantation can be categorized into two types based on the transplanted organ: solid organ transplantation (including kidney, liver, heart, and lung.) and nonsolid organ transplantation (including bone marrow, pancreatic islet, and cornea). Solid organ transplants, such as those involving the kidney, liver, heart, and lung, constitute the majority. According to the World Health Organization, kidney transplants are the most common, followed by liver, heart, and lung transplants. Nonsolid organ transplants make up a relatively small proportion of total organ transplants [420].

Epilepsy after organ transplantation is primarily defined as seizures that develop following the transplantation of a solid or nonsolid organ from a donor. While there is no precise definition for epilepsy after organ transplantation, one can refer to the clinically useful epilepsy definition proposed by the ILAE in 2017. This definition emphasizes the necessity to focus on prerequisites such as the occurrence of seizures in patients after undergoing organ transplantation, attributed to the side effects of immunosuppressive medications or other reasons. It is crucial to distinguish post-transplant seizures, as many epileptic events occur postoperatively due to preexisting organ dysfunction or acute symptoms related to the surgery. This subset of seizures rarely recurs after eliminating the causative factor, underscoring the importance of determining the etiology of the seizures. Common causative factors include postoperative malignant hypertension, disorders of ion metabolism, blood glucose abnormalities, high blood concentrations of antirejection drugs, abnormal metabolism, and central nervous system infections. These seizures do not meet the 2017 definition of epilepsy of the ILAE and are considered episodic seizure events after organ transplantation.

4.3.8.1 Epidemiology

The incidence of seizures varies after different types of organ transplantation. Seizures following liver transplantation may be primarily related to neurotoxicity caused by cyclosporine or tacrolimus, with an incidence typically ranging from 1% to 42% [421]. Studies have shown that the incidence of epilepsy after liver transplantation is related to the status of the donor organ, and the incidence of epilepsy is lower in patients receiving living liver transplants than in those receiving cadaveric donor livers [422]. The predominant form of epilepsy in adults after liver transplantation is generalized forced clonic seizures, whereas in children, there appears to be a greater prevalence of focal seizures.

Postrenal transplantation epilepsy may be associated with neurotoxicity of CNI-like drugs and hormones, hydroelectrolyte disturbances, intracranial infections, ischemic-hypoxic brain damage, and uremic encephalopathy, side effects of other drugs such as levofloxacin, with a prevalence rate of approximately 2.2% in adults and the highest incidence rate of approximately 20% in children. The most commonly reported type of epilepsy after renal transplantation is generalized epilepsy, especially generalized forced clonus. Focal epilepsy is relatively rare [423, 424]. The duration of seizures after renal transplantation varies, ranging from 24 h to 1 month after surgery, and some patients may develop seizures many years after transplantation [425].

Early seizures after heart transplantation are associated with immunosuppressant-induced stroke and reversible posterior encephalopathy (PRES), with relatively few non-immunosuppressant-related factors. Other potential etiologies may include tumors, a history of preoperative seizures, diabetes mellitus, and renal insufficiency. Additionally, hypoxic encephalopathy due to cardiac arrest can also induce seizures.

The incidence of postoperative seizures after heart transplantation is approximately 2–20%. The most commonly reported seizures are generalized forced clonic seizures, followed by myoclonic seizures. Status epilepticus and generalized myoclonic epilepsy usually manifest early in the postoperative period (approximately 2 months posttransplantation), while generalized forced clonic and focal motor seizures are more likely to appear later [426].

In addition to solid organ transplants causing epilepsy, nonsolid organ transplants can also lead to the development of epilepsy. The most common scenario is observed in hematopoietic stem cell transplantation. A retrospective study involving over 1400 hematopoietic stem cell transplant recipients revealed that 7% of patients developed seizures postoperatively, and 40% of these seizures were related to medication administration [427]. The proportion of generalized versus focal seizures in the context of seizures after hematopoietic stem cell transplantation appears to be similar, with the first seizure after transplantation typically characterized by a focal nonconvulsive seizure.

4.3.8.2 Mechanisms of Epilepsy Development After Organ Transplantation

(1) *Immunosuppressants*: Immunosuppressive drugs administered after organ transplantation are utilized to prevent the immune system of the recipient from attacking the newly transplanted organ. The main immunosuppressive drugs include the following:

① Glucocorticoid drugs, such as prednisone and methylprednisolone, inhibit the activity of T and B lymphocytes.

② Calcineurin inhibitors, such as cyclosporine and tacrolimus, inhibit the immune response by blocking calcineurin signaling.

③ Antimetabolites, e.g., propylthiouracil, pyrrolidone acid, and mycophenolic acid, interfere with DNA synthesis or RNA transcription, thereby inhibiting the proliferation of immune cells.

④ Antibody agents, e.g., rituximab and belistat.

The immediate cause of seizures due to immunosuppressive drug administration is considered to be the neurotoxic effects of these drugs, including cyclosporine and tacrolimus. Although rapamycin and mycophenolate mofetil have rarely been reported to have significant neurotoxic effects, the neurotoxicity of tacrolimus has rarely been reported [428]. The incidence of tacrolimus-associated epilepsy has been shown to be 5–11% [429]. Cyclosporine, a calmodulin neurotransmitter inhibitor commonly used in immunosuppressive therapy after organ transplantation, has been found to decrease the GABA concentration, affecting neuronal excitability. Cyclosporine has also been reported to be associated with the occurrence of reversible posterior encephalopathy syndrome [430, 431]. OKT3, a monoclonal antibody that inhibits the function of human T lymphocytes, reduces the activity of the immune system, leading to the systemic release of proinflammatory cytokines involved in the pathogenesis of cerebral edema, potentially contributing to the development of meningitis and seizures [432].

(2) *Central Nervous System Infections*: Central nervous system (CNS) infections may occur in 5–10% of patients after organ transplantation and can manifest at any time after solid organ transplantation. The onset of CNS aspergillosis typically occurs 21–24 days after transplantation, bacterial infections usually occur 2 months after transplantation, and viral and opportunistic infections often present approximately 6 months after transplantation. Clinical manifestations include acute encephalitis, acute meningitis, chronic meningitis, and leukoencephalopathy [433]. Studies have indicated that patients with solid organ transplants are at a greater risk of developing community-acquired bacterial meningitis, with a Dutch study showing a 5.4-fold increase in incidence compared to that of the general population [434]. After organ transplantation, patients are at heightened risk of developing listeriosis, with clinical manifestations of neurologic listeriosis including meningoencephalitis (85%), meningitis (13%), and brain abscess (2%) [435]. Other sources of infection include West Nile virus, lymphocytic choroid plexus meningitis virus, human herpesvirus-6, varicella-zoster virus, *Cryptococcus*, and fungi, which are more prevalent in patients after organ transplantation [433].

(3) *Reversible Encephalopathy Syndrome*: A cluster of clinical imaging syndromes, initially described by Hinchey et al. in 1996 as reversible posterior leukoencephalopathy syndrome, was later designated posterior reversible encephalopathy syndrome (PRES) by Casey et al. in 2000. PRES is a reversible encephalopathy syndrome characterized by symptoms such as headache, visual impairment, impaired consciousness, and epilepsy. It is often associated with conditions such as hypertension, renal insufficiency, and immunosuppression. The incidence of epilepsy in PRES patients is reported to be 60–75%, with a higher frequency observed after hematopoietic stem cell transplantation (1.1–20%). This increased incidence posttransplantation may be linked to the release of inflammatory factors induced by systemic irradiation before the operation and the use of high-dose antirejection drugs [436]. The reported incidence of PRES after solid organ transplantation ranges from 1.1% to 20%, with calcineurin inhibitor (CNI) drugs being identified as the primary risk factors for PRES in posttransplant recipients [437]. Cyclosporine A and tacrolimus administration disrupt tight junctions between cerebral capillary endothelial cells, potentially contributing to PRES development through mechanisms such as inward endoplasmic reticulum calcium flow, reduced claudin-5 expression and phosphorylation, and inhibition of P-glycoprotein expression, thereby enhancing blood–brain barrier permeability [438].

(4) *Cerebrovascular disease*: Another risk factor associated with epilepsy development after organ transplantation is cerebrovascular events, including stroke, cerebral hemorrhage, and subdural hematoma, which often occur within 30 days after surgery [439]. The relationship between organ transplantation and cerebrovascular disease is complex and influenced by factors such as bacterial endocarditis, hypercoagulable states, atherosclerosis, vasculitis, and arrhythmias [440–442]. Stroke may result from perioperative arterial embolism detaching from the carotid or intracranial arteries. In the early stages of stroke, seizures

are associated with massive glutamate release and focal metabolic imbalances, while in the late stages, seizures may be caused by scarring and glioblast proliferation [443].

4.3.8.3 Anti-seizure Medication Selection

For acute seizures following organ transplantation, such as status epilepticus, intravenous lorazepam and, if necessary, fosphenytoin may be administered. After achieving seizure control, it is crucial to identify and correct factors associated with toxic calcineurin inhibitor (CNI) levels, electrolyte or glucose abnormalities, and hypertension. When selecting an anti-seizure medication for a solid organ transplant patient, considerations should include the type of seizure, patient safety and tolerability, and organ dysfunction, particularly of the liver and kidneys.

In general, anti-seizure medications with extensive hepatic metabolism, hepatic enzyme induction, significant protein affinity, and substantial interactions should be avoided for posttransplant patients. First-generation anti-seizure medications, such as phenytoin, phenobarbital, and carbamazepine, have significant interactions with immunosuppressive drugs, potentially increasing the metabolism of CNIs and corticosteroids by inducing activity of hepatic cytochrome P450 enzymes. Therefore, these drugs should generally be avoided for treating seizures after organ transplantation [444]. Valproate, a broad-spectrum anti-seizure medication effective in treating various types of epilepsy, is contraindicated in organ transplant patients, especially liver transplant recipients. This is due to its primary metabolism by the liver and its association with liver failure [127, 445].

Levetiracetam is currently considered the drug of choice for anti-seizure medication selection after solid organ transplantation. It is widely used in infants, children, and adults and is available in various forms, such as tablets, oral solutions, and injections. Levetiracetam is primarily metabolized in the blood and excreted by the kidneys, making it less likely to induce hepatic metabolism and drug–drug interactions [446, 447]. The recommended dosage for levetiracetam is considered to be 1000 mg/day, with incremental increases of 1000 mg every 1–2 weeks, up to a maximum of 3000 mg/day. If administered intravenously, a single injection of 1000 mg is typically given, and the effect is generally achieved within 15–60 minutes. No interactions have been identified between levetiracetam and various drug-metabolizing enzymes [448–450]. Furthermore, the impact of levetiracetam on metabolic enzymes has not been observed. Notably, levetiracetam does not affect cyclosporine metabolism [451].

In a study conducted by Chih-Hsiang Lin et al., 15 patients who received levetiracetam, either intravenously or orally, as a single agent for seizure control after liver transplantation were seizure free during the treatment period. Unfortunately, two patients died during the follow-up period due to severe infection and cancer. Importantly, there were no neurological sequelae that interfered with the patients' daily activities throughout the course of drug administration. This lack of interference was not attributed to the inefficacy of immunosuppressant drugs or hepatic failure, nor was it due to donor liver rejection as a result of ineffective immunosuppressive drugs [452].

Known major side effects of levetiracetam, such as somnolence, weakness, infection, and dizziness, are commonly observed. Behavioral abnormalities, including irritability, personality changes, psychotic-like episodes, and mild leukopenia, are relatively infrequent. In addition to levetiracetam, lacosamide is also considered an alternative drug, and it may be beneficial for patients with drug-resistant post-transplant epilepsy. The recommended initial dose is typically 50 mg twice daily, with an incremental increase of 100 mg per week to reach a therapeutic dose range of 200–400 mg/day. No dose adjustment is required for patients with mild to moderate renal impairment. However, a 25% reduction in the maximum dose is recommended for patients with mild or moderate hepatic impairment. Dose adjustments in patients with hepatic impairment should be approached with caution, and lacosamide is not recommended for use in patients with severe hepatic impairment. Common adverse reactions include dizziness, headache, nausea, and diplopia, which are typically mild to moderate in severity. Some reactions are dose-related and can be resolved by dose reduction. Other side effects may include immune system abnormalities and psychiatric abnormalities. Notably, no clinically relevant drug–drug interactions are currently known.

The selection of anti-seizure medications can vary based on the type of organ transplantation. For patients after liver transplantation, careful consideration should be given to avoiding the use of anti-seizure medications metabolized by the liver. The new generation of anti-seizure medications, which undergo minimal or no liver metabolism, exhibit limited drug–drug interactions and have low protein-binding capacity, making them a preferred choice. Benzodiazepines are typically used as first-line therapeutic agents for status epilepticus. However, in the management of acute seizures after liver transplantation, benzodiazepines, such as diazepam, lorazepam, and midazolam, which are primarily metabolized by the liver, are not utilized as first-line agents. Levetiracetam is the preferred option, and lorazepam metabolism is minimally affected by liver disease, reducing the likelihood of drug–drug interactions [453, 454]. While a broader range of choices is available for the treatment of seizures after renal transplantation, given that most anti-seizure medications are metabolized by the liver, attention must be given to the interaction of these medications with immunosuppressants to avoid potential drug interactions. In addition to levetiracetam, lamotrigine and the combination of clonazepam and levetiracetam appear to be viable options [423]. The selection of drugs for treating seizures after heart transplantation must be individualized and take into consideration the overall health of the patient, as most patients typically do not exhibit abnormalities in liver and kidney function. The primary concern in this context is often focused on potential drug–drug interactions. Currently, there is no consensus on the standardized choice of anti-seizure medications after heart transplantation. In a study by Ocal et al., levetiracetam demonstrated efficacy in controlling 80% of seizures in pediatric patients and some seizures in adult patients. Additionally, the combination of levetiracetam with phenytoin sodium was effective in controlling persistent status epilepticus [426]. Other studies have indicated that gabapentin and valproic acid can also be effective in managing seizures after heart transplantation [455]. Some studies recommend benzodiazepines, such as valium or midazolam, as first-line anti-seizure medications for patients with seizures after hematopoietic stem cell transplantation [456]. Levetiracetam, commonly recommended for solid organ transplantation, is not recommended in this context. A study described instances of secondary graft failure after levetiracetam use, suggesting a potential association with levetiracetam-induced myelodysplastic syndrome [457].

In summary, the treatment approach for epilepsy after organ transplantation aligns with conventional epilepsy management. The primary goal is to control seizures and prevent their recurrence, with drug therapy being the initial choice. However, a key difference lies in the need to be vigilant about potential adverse effects on the transplanted organ resulting from anti-seizure medication use, as well as interactions with immunosuppressants, hormones, and other medications.

When selecting anti-seizure medications after organ transplantation, levetiracetam is the preferred treatment option. Its safety and efficacy have been confirmed in various studies. Other anti-seizure medications, including lacosamide and lamotrigine, should be chosen based on the specific characteristics of the organ transplantation and individual patient considerations. Careful consideration of potential interactions with immunosuppressants, hormones, and other drugs is essential during the selection process.

4.4 Seizures in Neurodegenerative Diseases

4.4.1 Seizures in Multiple Sclerosis

Many neurodegenerative diseases can involve seizures. Since the courses of these degenerative diseases and epilepsy are relatively long, it is not clear whether the relationship between degenerative diseases and epilepsy is causal or only a comorbidity. In 2024, Ouyang J [458] used Mendelian randomization to analyze single-nucleotide polymorphisms in patients with a variety of neurodegenerative diseases based on genome-wide association studies and found that only MS and epilepsy had a causal relationship. The causal relationships between Alzheimer's disease (AD), Parkinson's disease (PD), amyotrophic lateral sclerosis (ALS), and epilepsy were not supported, suggesting that the causal relationship between MS and epilepsy is supported by genetic prediction.

4.4.1.1 Historical Evolution

The literature described the occurrence of epileptic seizures in multiple sclerosis patients in the 1930s. In 1947, BRONISCH FW [459] studied the possible mechanism of epileptic seizures in multiple sclerosis; in 1955, HAMLIN PG [460] reported that status epileptic persists in multiple sclerosis patients. In 1962, Rafalowska J [461] described the epidemiological data of epileptic seizures in patients with multiple sclerosis; in 1965, Boudin G [462] described two anatomic clinical cases of multiple sclerosis with epileptic seizures; and in 2023, Van Klink N [463] described cases in which surgery did not induce multiple sclerosis in patients with epilepsy. In recent years, researchers have begun to study the novel mechanism of epilepsy in multiple sclerosis, and representative research results on the relationships among brain networks, epilepsy, and multiple sclerosis have been described by Ciolac D et al. [464]. In 2023, Drulovic J et al. [465] reported that epileptic seizures had a significant impact on multiple sclerosis patients, and these findings contributed to a deeper understanding of epileptic seizures in multiple sclerosis patients.

4.4.1.2 Epidemiology

The prevalence of epilepsy in multiple sclerosis patients varies widely. Drulovic J [465] studied 326 patients with multiple sclerosis and reported that 127 of them (38.0%) had seizures. Among the 361 patients with multiple sclerosis described by Nurre ER [466], 74 (20.4%) had seizures. Sanchez M [467] reported that only 1.95% of patients with multiple sclerosis had epilepsy. A Ghezzi [468] described 2353 patients with multiple sclerosis, 40 of whom had seizures. The overall prevalence of epilepsy in multiple sclerosis patients is approximately 1.7% to 20%.

4.4.1.3 Relationship Between Multiple Sclerosis and Epilepsy

The prevalence of epilepsy in people with multiple sclerosis is 3–6 times greater than that in the general population, but the relationship between the two is unclear. To understand whether there is a causal relationship between multiple sclerosis and epilepsy, Zuo H and Peng [469] used Mendelian randomization analysis and inverse variance weighting as the main methods to study the relationship between multiple sclerosis and epilepsy and found that there was an obvious causal relationship between the two, which is consistent with the results of Ouyang J et al. [458] supporting a causal relationship between multiple sclerosis and epilepsy.

4.4.1.4 Clinical Features of Epilepsy in Multiple Sclerosis Patients

Seizures in Multiple Sclerosis

The main characteristics of multiple sclerosis are the presence of multiple lesions in the brain and the remission of recurrent disease, which are often accompanied by paroxysmal symptoms, such as trigeminal neuralgia, paroxysmal dysarthria, and seizures. To understand the characteristics of epilepsy in patients with multiple sclerosis, Nurre ER [466] described the results of a single-center retrospective study, which revealed a high incidence of epilepsy in patients with multiple sclerosis. At the time of the seizure, most imaging studies can find multiple focal points, and EEG data also show that the patient has cortical dysfunction, mainly in the temporal lobe. The authors suggested that the timing of seizures in multiple sclerosis varies according to the type of multiple sclerosis, and epilepsy is more likely to occur in patients with progressive multiple sclerosis. Sanchez M [467] also conducted an observational retrospective study of multiple sclerosis patients and found that 25 patients (18 women) had epilepsy, and most of these patients had brain atrophy and cortical or paracortical lesions. There were no significant differences in disease activity, level of disability, or response to disease treatment between MS patients with epilepsy and those without epilepsy, suggesting that the epilepsy course in MS patients is benign.

Characteristics of Seizures

① The time of seizure: Sokic DV [469] described 20 patients with multiple sclerosis who had seizures. Among these patients, 4 had seizures 1–5 years before the diagnosis of multiple sclerosis, 8 had seizures during the relapse period of multiple sclerosis, 2 of whom had seizures as the only manifestation of recurrence, and 12 had seizures throughout the whole process. Among the 40 patients described by A Ghezzi [468], 13 had epilepsy occurring before MS, 4 had both diseases occurring simultaneously, and 23 had epilepsy occurring after MS onset. P Striano [471] reported that 4.8% of 270 patients diagnosed with MS had seizures, 4 of whom had seizures 1–2 years after the MS diagnosis and 6 of whom had seizures 8–23 years after the MS diagnosis. Gurtubay [472] analyzed the clinical, EEG and neuroimaging results of epileptic seizures in 7 patients with multiple sclerosis and found that epilepsy was the first symptom in 2 patients. ② Seizure type: Among the 74 patients described by Nurre ER [466], 12% had general tonic–clonic seizures, 68% had focal seizures, and 13% had unclassified epileptic seizures. Most of the cases described by Sokic DV [470] involved focal secondary generalized seizures, and 5 patients had status epilepticus. Striano [471] reported that most of the patients had focal or focal secondary generalized seizures. Among the 7 patients described by G Gurtubay [472], 2 had general seizures, 3 had partial sensory and/or motor seizures and secondary general seizures, 1 had simple partial motor seizures, 2 had partially complex seizures, and 1 had multiple seizure types. ③ EEG and magnetic resonance findings: Among the patients described by Sokic DV [470], 11 had abnormal EEG; among the patients described by A Ghezzi [468], 11 had episodic discharge on EEG, 15 showed theta and/or delta activity on EEG, and 14 had normal EEG. Magnetic resonance imaging (MRI) was performed for 12 patients: 3 patients had lesions adjacent to the cerebral cortex.

4.4.1.5 Treatment

In addition to the treatment of the primary disease, antiepileptic drugs should be used in patients with seizures to control the seizures. Nurre ER et al. [466] suggest that early use of antiepileptic drugs is beneficial to patients, the specific drug selection is no different from general seizures, and that ASM selection can be determined based on other symptomatic epilepsies.

4.4.1.6 Prognosis

Recent research indicates that seizures do not affect the prognoses of MS patients.

4.4.2 Seizures in Alzheimer's Disease

Alzheimer's disease and epilepsy are common neurological disorders in elderly people. Neurodegenerative diseases, mostly Alzheimer's disease, account for approximately 10% of late-onset epilepsy patients over the age of 65. There is a bidirectional association between Alzheimer's disease and epilepsy. Epilepsy is a risk factor for Alzheimer's disease, and Alzheimer's disease is also an independent risk factor for epilepsy in elderly people [473].

4.4.2.1 Historical Evolution

AD was described very early. However, the relationship between AD and epilepsy was described later. NAVILLE [474] first noted the relationship between epileptic seizures and AD in 1946. Dascalov D et al. [475] described epileptiform discharge on the EEG of AD patients in 1969. In 1986, Gimenez-Roldan S [476] reported that patients with AD had myoclonic and photosensitive seizures, suggesting that epilepsy might be an early manifestation of AD. Later, Paul LA [477] reported that AD and epilepsy might share a common brain structure. In 1994, Mendez MF [478] described a clinicopathological study of epileptic seizures in AD patients. In 2019, Paudel YN [479] reported that the Tau protein may represent a common pathway connecting AD and epilepsy. In 2023, Hautecloque-Raysz G [480] reported that anti-seizure drugs may improve cognitive function in AD patients. Tombini M et al. [481] reported that there may be a bidirectional relationship between epilepsy and AD. Patients with AD are more likely to suffer from epilepsy, and patients with late-onset epilepsy also have a significantly increased risk of suffering from AD, further revealing the relationship between the two.

4.4.2.2 Epidemiological Investigation

To understand the prevalence of epilepsy in AD patients, Xu Y et al. [482] conducted a study of 380,777 AD patients and 727,446 epilepsy patients and reported that the seizure rate in AD patients was 4.2–31.5 times/1000 people/year and that the prevalence of epilepsy in clinically diagnosed AD patients was 1.5–12.7%. The prevalence of epilepsy in pathologically confirmed AD patients was 16%, and the younger the age of the patient, the greater the risk of seizures. Haoudy S et al. [483] conducted a study on patients diagnosed with AD whose cerebrospinal fluid examination showed positive AD markers and found that 40% of the patients had seizures. Mendez M [484] found that the incidence of epilepsy in dementia patients varied according to the cause of dementia. In Alzheimer's disease, approximately 10–22% of patients have had at least one seizure. In a cohort of 177 newly diagnosed AD patients, Lozsadi DA [485] reported that 12 (6.8%) had a history of epilepsy and/or were using antiepileptic drugs at the time of diagnosis. In his study on 937 AD patients, Cheng CH [486] reported that 44 (4.7%) had seizures. Hommet C et al. [487] conducted a study on hospitalized AD patients and reported for the first time that 2.5% of AD patients were admitted to a hospital with epilepsy. Accordingly, the prevalence of epilepsy in patients with AD ranges from 1.5% to 41.7%.

4.4.2.3 The Tau Hypothesis in AD and Epilepsy

Multiple studies have suggested a bidirectional link between these two common neurodegenerative diseases. Compared with healthy subjects, patients with either disease had almost twice the risk of contracting the other, suggesting a common underlying mechanism between seizures and AD [488]. The bridge between them is the tau protein. Tau is a microtubule-associated protein that binds and promotes the assembly of microtubules in neurons under physiological conditions. However, under pathological conditions, the accumulation of overphosphorylated tau proteins can produce neurotoxicity, cause neurodegeneration, and lead to the occurrence of Tau disease [489].

Tau protein is generally present in cells, but there is tau phosphorylation and hyperphosphorylation in patients with AD. This phosphorylated tau protein is released from the cell, leading to decreased neuronal stability and the formation of AD in neurofibrillary tangles. However, increased or excessive phosphorylation of the tau protein can cause neuronal excitatory toxicity and cascade reactions, thus destroying the balance between neuronal excitation and inhibition and leading to epilepsy [481, 490]. Zawar I et al. [491] also suggested that gene mutation in AD patients could increase the accumulation of tau protein, thus increasing the overexcitability of neurons, and that the overexcitability of neurons could increase the secretion of tau and trigger epileptic seizures, which are speculated to be manifestations of AD. Alves SS [492] used animal experiments to support this view. This group established an AD model by streptozotocin (STZ) induction and then stimulated it with high-frequency sound, resulting in seizures, and determined that AD was the cause of the seizures. However, some people speculate that epilepsy itself is a type of tau protein disease, and an increase in tau protein levels, especially of excessive phosphorylation, can cause neuronal excitotoxicity and brain tissue damage through cascade reactions, thus causing the occurrence of AD. It is suggested that AD is consistent with the cognitive function damage caused by repeated seizures in patients with epilepsy. Inhibition of neuronal excitotoxicity with antiepileptic drugs can improve the cognitive function of AD patients [490], and Rizzello E [493] confirmed the hypothesis that epilepsy causes AD through animal experiments. They found that repeated seizures can selectively lead to memory deficits and an increase in oligaβ42 expression and fibril types, which are important links in the formation of AD. However, Ouyang J [458] used a Mendelian randomization method to analyze the single nucleotide polymorphisms of AD and found no causal relationship between AD and epilepsy, suggesting that epilepsy is more likely to be a comorbidity of AD. This view is supported by the study of Haoudy S et al. [483], who suggest that epilepsy is a comorbidity of AD, accounting for 40% of AD patients. This view is also supported by Cretin B [494], who speculates that epilepsy is an increasingly recognized comorbidity in AD. These studies support a bidirectional association between AD and epilepsy, as epilepsy is a risk factor for Alzheimer's disease, and in turn, Alzheimer's disease is an independent risk factor for epilepsy in older adults [494].

4.4.2.4 Clinical Characteristics of Seizures in AD Patients

Types of Seizures

Although the study by Haoudy S [483] on patients diagnosed with AD accompanied by seizures showed that the main seizure types of patients were tonic clonus (25%), temporal lobe epilepsy (25%), myoclonus (25%), focal extratemporal lobe epilepsy (8%), and 17% unclassified epilepsy, Andras Horvath [495] monitored 42 patients with AD accompanied by seizures with 24-h ambulatory EEG and found that most patients' seizures manifested as focal seizures without motor symptoms, 24% of which needed to be confirmed by EEG. Seventy-two percent of patients presented with focal seizures of unconsciousness disturbance, 55% did not have any motor activity, and 28% had epileptiform discharges but no clinical seizures. Samudra N et al. [496] also reported that this "subclinical epileptiform activity" is common in AD patients, with prevalence estimates ranging from 22% to 54%, and Yang F et al. [497] supported this view, suggesting that it is challenging to identify seizures in AD patients. This type of seizure is usually clinically nonmotor and may overlap with some AD symptoms. In addition to seizures, epileptiform discharges may also exacerbate cognitive decline in people with AD, highlighting the importance of early identification and treatment.

In addition, there are several special types of seizures in AD. In 2023, Lee HC [498] described two cases of seizures in which aphasia status epileptica was the only manifestation. Both patients had atypical epileptic EEGs, which improved after taking antiepileptic drugs. It is suggested that this type of seizure can occur at any stage of AD, and significant improvement in clinical symptoms and EEG after treatment with antiepileptic drugs is the key to diagnosis.

Time of Onset of Epileptic Seizures in AD

Romanelli MF et al. [499] suggested that epileptic seizures generally occur in the late stage of AD. Among the 44 AD patients described, 7 had at least one documented seizure, and all 7 AD patients had progressed to the severe stage of dementia when the first seizure occurred. Mendez M et al. [484] also reported that 10–22% of AD patients experienced seizures, but most of these seizures occurred in the late stage of the disease, and the average course of epilepsy was 6 years. Among the 937 AD patients described by Cheng CH [485], 44 had seizures, most of which occurred in the late stage of the disease. The average time from the diagnosis of AD to the occurrence of seizures was 3.6 years. However, the results of a study by Lozsadi DA [485] do not support this view. They reported that 12 of the 177 newly diagnosed AD patients in their cohort developed seizures, six of which occurred at approximately the same time as cognitive decline, suggesting that while seizures are more common later in the course of AD, they can also occur along with and are symptoms of the disease and may reflect a common pathogenesis. A study by Cretin B [494] also revealed that epileptic seizures can occur in the early stage of AD. When AD patients have only mild or subjective cognitive impairment, they may have generalized or focal epileptic seizures (usually located in the frontal or temporal lobes). It has also been found that the first symptom of AD is epilepsy, and these patients do not develop cognitive dysfunction until many years after the seizure and are ultimately diagnosed with AD. These studies suggest that seizures in patients with AD may accompany the full course of AD.

Other Manifestations

Seizures in AD patients may manifest as subclinical electrical activity that may cause neuronal necrosis and cognitive dysfunction. Hautecloque-Raysz G [480] compared the cognitive function of AD patients with seizures and AD patients without seizures and found that AD patients with seizures had more obvious cognitive dysfunction.

4.4.2.5 Diagnosis of Seizures in AD

AD and epilepsy are common neurological disorders that are linked to and adversely affect the quality of life of patients, making them serious public health problems. The diagnosis of epilepsy in AD patients is a major challenge because seizures in

AD patients can manifest as subclinical electrical activity with no significant motor symptoms, and many of the manifestations overlap with the manifestations of AD.

Epileptic seizures in AD patients can manifest as focal seizures with no motor symptoms or only subclinical electrical activity, so examination via electroencephalography, especially long-range electroencephalogram monitoring, is necessary. Because seizures in AD patients are sensitive to anti-seizure drugs regardless of whether they occur early or late in the disease, observing their response to anti-seizure drugs can also aid in diagnosis.

4.4.2.6 Treatment

AD is a lifelong disease that cannot presently be treated, but seizure control can effectively reduce impairment of cognitive function. Therefore, when AD patients have seizures, the use of antiepileptic drugs is necessary, and antiepileptic drugs targeting abnormal network overexcitation may also change the natural progression of AD [488]. However, until now, there have been no guidelines for treating seizures in people with AD due to a lack of randomized clinical trials sufficient to answer relevant questions. Eduardo Cumbo et al. [500] conducted a prospective, randomized, three-group parallel case–control study to evaluate the effect of antiepileptic drugs on epilepsy in AD patients. Among the patients, 38 took levetiracetam, 28 took phenobarbital, and 29 took lamotrigine; the results showed that there was no significant difference in the efficacy of the three AEDs. Levetiracetam causes fewer adverse events than other AEDs and is associated with improved cognitive function, which can be used to control seizures in patients with AD [501]. Moreover, animal experiments have revealed that levetiracetam can reduce abnormal cortical discharge and reverse memory deficits in Alzheimer's disease mouse models and improve memory difficulties in patients with mild cognitive impairment; therefore, levetiracetam is recommended for the first time [502]. Filippo Sean Giorgi [503] also suggested that newer antiepileptic drugs such as levetiracetam and lamotrigine are good choices.

References

1. Commission on Classification and Terminology of the ILAE. Proposal for revised clinical and electroencephalographic classification of epileptic seizures. From the Commission on Classification and Terminology of the International League Against Epilepsy. Epilepsia. 1981;22(4):489–501.
2. Fisher RS, Cross JH, French JA, et al. Operational classification of seizure types by the international league against epilepsy: position paper of the ILAE Commission for Classification and Terminology. Epilepsia. 2017;58(4):522–30.
3. Marson AG, Al-Kharusi AM, Alwaidh M, et al. The SANAD study of effectiveness of carbamazepine, gabapentin, lamotrigine, oxcarbazepine, or topiramate for treatment of partial epilepsy: an unblinded randomised controlled. Lancet. 2007;369(9566):1000–15.

4. Marson A, Burnside G, Appleton R, et al. The SANAD II study of the effectiveness and cost-effectiveness of levetiracetam, zonisamide, or lamotrigine for newly diagnosed focal epilepsy: an open-label, non-inferiority, multicentre, phase 4, randomised controlled. Lancet. 2021;397(10282):1363–74.
5. Nevitt SJ, Sudell M, Cividini S, et al. Antiepileptic drug monotherapy for epilepsy: a network meta-analysis of individual participant data. Cochrane Database Syst. 2022;4(4):CD011412.
6. Kalita J, Chaudhary SK, Kumar B, et al. Case report: focal myoclonus with a striatal lesion as a presentation of subacute Sclerosing Panencephalitis. Am J Trop Med Hyg. 2022;106(6):1729–31.
7. Gasca-Salas C, Lang AE. Focal predominant forms of Posthypoxic action myoclonus. Mov Disord Clin Pract. 2016;3(4):417–20.
8. Marson AG, Al-Kharusi AM, Alwaidh M, et al. The SANAD study of effectiveness of valproate, lamotrigine, or topiramate for generalised and unclassifiable epilepsy: an unblinded randomised controlled trial. Lancet. 2007;369(9566):1016–26.
9. Marson A, Burnside G, Appleton R, et al. The SANAD II study of the effectiveness and cost-effectiveness of valproate versus levetiracetam for newly diagnosed generalised and unclassifiable epilepsy: an open-label, non-inferiority, multicentre, phase 4, randomised controlled trial. Lancet. 2021;397(10282):1375–86.
10. Vossler DG, Knake S, O'Brien TJ, et al. Efficacy and safety of adjunctive lacosamide in the treatment of primary generalised tonic-clonic seizures: a double-blind, randomised, placebo-controlled trial. J Neurol Neurosurg Psychiatry. 2020;91(10):1067–75.
11. Brodie MJ, Besag F, Ettinger AB, et al. Epilepsy, antiepileptic drugs, and aggression: an evidence-based review. Pharmacol Rev. 2016;68(3):563–602.
12. Noachtar S, Andermann E, Meyvisch P, et al. Levetiracetam for the treatment of idiopathic generalized epilepsy with myoclonic seizures. Neurology. 2008;70(8):607–16.
13. Biton V, Bourgeois BF, Investigators YYS. Topiramate in patients with juvenile myoclonic epilepsy. Arch Neurol. 2005;62(11):1705–8.
14. Nickels K, Kossoff EH, Eschbach K, et al. Epilepsy with myoclonic-atonic seizures (Doose syndrome): clarification of diagnosis and treatment options through a large retrospective multicenter cohort. Epilepsia. 2021;62(1):120–7.
15. Lux AL, Edwards SW, Hancock E, et al. The United Kingdom Infantile Spasms Study comparing vigabatrin with prednisolone or tetracosactide at 14 days: a multicentre, randomised controlled trial. Lancet. 2004;364(9447):1773–8.
16. Knupp KG, Coryell J, Nickels KC, et al. Response to treatment in a prospective national infantile spasms cohort. Ann Neurol. 2016;79(3):475–84.
17. Lux AL, Edwards SW, Hancock E, et al. The United Kingdom Infantile Spasms Study (UKISS) comparing hormone treatment with vigabatrin on developmental and epilepsy outcomes to age 14 months: a multicentre randomised trial. Lancet Neurol. 2005;4(11):712–7.
18. Knupp KG, Leister E, Coryell J, et al. Response to second treatment after initial failed treatment in a multicenter prospective infantile spasms cohort. Epilepsia. 2016;57(11):1834–42.
19. O'Callaghan FJ, Edwards SW, Alber FD, et al. Safety and effectiveness of hormonal treatment versus hormonal treatment with vigabatrin for infantile spasms (ICISS): a randomised, multicentre, open-label trial. Lancet Neurol. 2017;16(1):33–42.
20. Brigo F, Igwe SC, Lattanzi S. Ethosuximide, sodium valproate or lamotrigine for absence seizures in children and adolescents. Cochrane Database Syst Rev. 2019;2(2):CD003032.
21. Glauser T, Ben-Menachem E, Bourgeois B, et al. Updated ILAE evidence review of antiepileptic drug efficacy and effectiveness as initial monotherapy for epileptic seizures and syndromes. Epilepsia. 2013;54(3):551–63.
22. Pearl PL. Epilepsy syndromes in childhood. Continuum (Minneap Minn). 2018;24(1, Child Neurology):186–209.
23. Balestrini S, Doccini V, Boncristiano A, et al. Efficacy and safety of long-term treatment with Stiripentol in children and adults with drug-resistant epilepsies: a retrospective cohort study of 196 patients. Drugs Real World Outcomes. 2022;9(3):451–61.

24. Striano P, Sofia V, Capovilla G, et al. A pilot trial of levetiracetam in eyelid myoclonia with absences (Jeavons syndrome). Epilepsia. 2008;49(3):425–30.
25. Smith KM, Youssef PE, Wirrell EC, et al. Jeavons syndrome: clinical features and response to treatment. Pediatr Neurol. 2018;86:46–51.
26. Baumer FM, Porter BE. Clinical and electrographic features of sunflower syndrome. Epilepsy Res. 2018;142:58–63.
27. Kwan P, Arzimanoglou A, Berg AT, et al. Definition of drug resistant epilepsy: consensus proposal by the ad hoc Task Force of the ILAE Commission on Therapeutic Strategies. Epilepsia. 2010;51(6):1069–77.
28. Tang F, Hartz AMS, Bauer B. Drug-resistant epilepsy: multiple hypotheses, few answers. Front Neurol. 2017;8:301.
29. Siddiqui A, Kerb R, Weale ME, et al. Association of multidrug resistance in epilepsy with a polymorphism in the drug-transporter gene ABCB1. N Engl J Med. 2003;348(15):1442–8.
30. Loscher W, Potschka H. Drug resistance in brain diseases and the role of drug efflux transporters. Nat Rev Neurosci. 2005;6(8):591–602.
31. French JA. Refractory epilepsy: clinical overview. Epilepsia. 2007;48(Suppl 1):3–7.
32. World Health Organization. Epilepsy: a public health imperative. World Health Organization; 2019.
33. Group GBDNDC. Global, regional, and national burden of neurological disorders during 1990-2015: a systematic analysis for the Global Burden of Disease Study 2015. Lancet Neurol. 2017;16(11):877–97.
34. Wei SH, Lee WT. Comorbidity of childhood epilepsy. J Formos Med Assoc. 2015;114(11):1031–8.
35. Libby AM, Ghushchyan V, McQueen RB, et al. Economic differences in direct and indirect costs between people with epilepsy and without epilepsy. Med Care. 2012;50(11):928–33.
36. Kwan P, Brodie MJ. Early identification of refractory epilepsy. N Engl J Med. 2000;342(5):314–9.
37. Xue-Ping W, Hai-Jiao W, Li-Na Z, et al. Risk factors for drug-resistant epilepsy: a systematic review and meta-analysis. Medicine (Baltimore). 2019;98(30):e16402.
38. Li Z, Cao W, Sun H, et al. Potential clinical and biochemical markers for the prediction of drug-resistant epilepsy: a literature review. Neurobiol Dis. 2022;174:105872.
39. Bazhanova ED, Kozlov AA, Litovchenko AV. Mechanisms of drug resistance in the pathogenesis of epilepsy: role of Neuroinflammation. A literature review. Brain Sci. 2021;11(5)
40. Loscher W, Potschka H, Sisodiya SM, et al. Drug resistance in epilepsy: clinical impact, potential mechanisms, and new innovative treatment options. Pharmacol Rev. 2020;72(3):606–38.
41. Tishler DM, Weinberg KI, Hinton DR, et al. MDR1 gene expression in brain of patients with medically intractable epilepsy. Epilepsia. 1995;36(1):1–6.
42. Weidner LD, Kannan P, Mitsios N, et al. The expression of inflammatory markers and their potential influence on efflux transporters in drug-resistant mesial temporal lobe epilepsy tissue. Epilepsia. 2018;59(8):1507–17.
43. Barkovich AJ, Dobyns WB, Guerrini R. Malformations of cortical development and epilepsy. Cold Spring Harb Perspect Med. 2015;5(5):a022392.
44. Fang M, Xi ZQ, Wu Y, et al. A new hypothesis of drug refractory epilepsy: neural network hypothesis. Med Hypotheses. 2011;76(6):871–6.
45. Liu X, Ou S, Xu T, et al. New differentially expressed genes and differential DNA methylation underlying refractory epilepsy. Oncotarget. 2016;7(52):87402–16.
46. Morris G, Reschke CR, Henshall DC. Targeting microRNA-134 for seizure control and disease modification in epilepsy. EBioMedicine. 2019;45:646–54.
47. Kwan P, Poon WS, Ng HK, et al. Multidrug resistance in epilepsy and polymorphisms in the voltage-gated sodium channel genes SCN1A, SCN2A, and SCN3A: correlation among phenotype, genotype, and mRNA expression. Pharmacogenet Genomics. 2008;18(11):989–98.

48. Friedman A, Heinemann U. Role of blood-brain barrier dysfunction in epileptogenesis. In: Noebels JL, Avoli M, Rogawski MA, et al., editors. Jasper's basic mechanisms of the epilepsies. 4th ed. Bethesda; 2012.
49. Porter RJ, Kupferberg HJ. The anticonvulsant screening program of the National Institute of Neurological Disorders and Stroke, NIH: history and contributions to clinical Care in the Twentieth Century and beyond. Neurochem Res. 2017;42(7):1889–93.
50. Kwan P, Schachter SC, Brodie MJ. Drug-resistant epilepsy. N Engl J Med. 2011;365(10):919–26.
51. Livingston JH. Management of intractable epilepsy. Arch Dis Child. 1991;66(12):1454–6.
52. French J. Pseudoseizures in the era of video-electroencephalogram monitoring. Curr Opin Neurol. 1995;8(2):117–20.
53. Tabarki B, Thabet F. Vitamin-responsive epilepsies: an update. Arch Pediatr. 2013;20(11):1236–41.
54. Commission on Classification and Terminology of the International League Against Epilepsy. Proposal for revised classification of epilepsies and epileptic syndromes. Epilepsia. 1989;30(4):389–99.
55. Sazgar M, Bourgeois BF. Aggravation of epilepsy by antiepileptic drugs. Pediatr Neurol. 2005;33(4):227–34.
56. Smith D, Chadwick D. The management of epilepsy. J Neurol Neurosurg Psychiatry. 2001;70(Suppl 2):II15–21.
57. Brodie MJ. Diagnosing and predicting refractory epilepsy. Acta Neurol Scand Suppl. 2005;181:36–9.
58. Wang XF, Sun HB. Refractory epilepsy. Shanghai Science and Technology Press; 2002.
59. Singh RCK, Baishya J, et al. Management of Refractory Epilepsy. Int J Epidemiol. 2020;6:15–23.
60. Brodie MJ, Barry SJ, Bamagous GA, et al. Patterns of treatment response in newly diagnosed epilepsy. Neurology. 2012;78(20):1548–54.
61. Schmidt D. Modern management of epilepsy: rational polytherapy. Baillieres Clin Neurol. 1996;5(4):757–63.
62. Keezer MR, Sisodiya SM, Sander JW. Comorbidities of epilepsy: current concepts and future perspectives. Lancet Neurol. 2016;15(1):106–15.
63. Lee BI, Park KM, Kim SE, et al. Clinical opinion: earlier employment of polytherapy in sequential pharmacotherapy of epilepsy. Epilepsy Res. 2019;156:106165.
64. Charyyeva GTL, Subbotina O. Pharmacoresistance in epilepsy and ways for overcoming it. Vestnik Saint Petersburg Univ Med. 2020;15(3):184–97.
65. Panayiotopoulos CP. A Clinical guide to epileptic syndromes and their treatment. In: Epileptic encephalopathies in infancy and early childhood; 2010. p. 275–326.
66. Karpova VIPOA, Mukhin K, Yu PAC. Valproic acid and its salts-from the history of discovery to clinical practice. Russkiy Zhurnal Detskoy Nevrologii. 2011;6(3):36–46.
67. Pylaeva OAMKY, Mironov MB. Efficacy and tolerability of lacosamide (vimpat) for treatment of epilepsy in adults. Russ J Child Neurol. 2014;9(4):59–68.
68. Mukhin KYFNV, Glukhova LY, et al. Juvenile myoclonic epilepsy: a focus on the efficacy of therapy and the rate of relapses according to long long-term follow-up data. Russ J Child Neurol. 2016;10(4):7–16.
69. N VP. Prospects of application of new antiepileptic drugs. Epilepsy Paroxysmal Conditions. 2015;7(4):40–9.
70. Perucca E, Tomson T. The pharmacological treatment of epilepsy in adults. Lancet Neurol. 2011;10(5):446–56.
71. Fattore C, Perucca E. Novel medications for epilepsy. Drugs. 2011;71(16):2151–78.
72. Prunetti P, Perucca E. New and forthcoming anti-epileptic drugs. Curr Opin Neurol. 2011;24(2):159–64.
73. Plosker GL. Perampanel: as adjunctive therapy in patients with partial-onset seizures. CNS Drugs. 2012;26(12):1085–96.

74. Moshe SL, Perucca E, Ryvlin P, et al. Epilepsy: new advances. Lancet. 2015;385(9971):884–98.
75. Abou-Khalil BW. Update on antiepileptic drugs 2019. Continuum (Minneap Minn). 2019;25(2):508–36.
76. Board KESE. Clinical Epileptology. 3rd ed. Seoul: Panmunedu; 2018. p. 353–87.
77. Sperling MR, Klein P, Aboumatar S, et al. Cenobamate (YKP3089) as adjunctive treatment for uncontrolled focal seizures in a large, phase 3, multicenter, open-label safety study. Epilepsia. 2020;61(6):1099–108.
78. Klein P, Schiemann J, Sperling MR, et al. A randomized, double-blind, placebo-controlled, multicenter, parallel-group study to evaluate the efficacy and safety of adjunctive brivaracetam in adult patients with uncontrolled partial-onset seizures. Epilepsia. 2015;56(12):1890–8.
79. Shin DJSYM, Jung KY, et al. Practical Drug Treatment Recommendations on the Drug Refractory Epilepsy Patients: 2021 Clinical Guideline Subcommittee for Epilepsy in the Korean Neurological Association. J Korean Neurol Assoc. 2021;39(4):255–69.
80. Devinsky O, Patel AD, Cross JH, et al. Effect of Cannabidiol on drop seizures in the Lennox-Gastaut syndrome. N Engl J Med. 2018;378(20):1888–97.
81. Thiele EA, Marsh ED, French JA, et al. Cannabidiol in patients with seizures associated with Lennox-Gastaut syndrome (GWPCARE4): a randomised, double-blind, placebo-controlled phase 3 trial. Lancet. 2018;391(10125):1085–96.
82. Galanopoulou AS, Moshe SL. In search of epilepsy biomarkers in the immature brain: goals, challenges and strategies. Biomark Med. 2011;5(5):615–28.
83. Engel J Jr, Pitkanen A, Loeb JA, et al. Epilepsy biomarkers. Epilepsia. 2013;54(Suppl 4):61–9.
84. Galanopoulou AS, Buckmaster PS, Staley KJ, et al. Identification of new epilepsy treatments: issues in preclinical methodology. Epilepsia. 2012;53(3):571–82.
85. Galanopoulou AS, Gorter JA, Cepeda C. Finding a better drug for epilepsy: the mTOR pathway as an antiepileptogenic target. Epilepsia. 2012;53(7):1119–30.
86. Galanopoulou AS. Developmental patterns in the regulation of chloride homeostasis and GABA(A) receptor signaling by seizures. Epilepsia. 2007;48(Suppl 5):14–8.
87. Pitkanen A. Therapeutic approaches to epileptogenesis–hope on the horizon. Epilepsia. 2010;51(Suppl 3):2–17.
88. D'Ambrosio R, Eastman CL, Fattore C, et al. Novel frontiers in epilepsy treatments: preventing epileptogenesis by targeting inflammation. Expert Rev Neurother. 2013;13(6):615–25.
89. Burneo JG, Fang J, Saposnik G, et al. Impact of seizures on morbidity and mortality after stroke: a Canadian multi-centre cohort study. Eur J Neurol. 2010;17(1):52–8.
90. Huang CW, Saposnik G, Fang J, et al. Influence of seizures on stroke outcomes: a large multicenter study. Neurology. 2014;82(9):768–76.
91. Fisher RS, Acevedo C, Arzimanoglou A, et al. ILAE official report: a practical clinical definition of epilepsy. Epilepsia. 2014;55(4):475–82.
92. Hesdorffer DC, Benn EK, Cascino GD, et al. Is a first acute symptomatic seizure epilepsy? Mortality and risk for recurrent seizure. Epilepsia. 2009;50(5):1102–8.
93. Beghi E, Carpio A, Forsgren L, et al. Recommendation for a definition of acute symptomatic seizure. Epilepsia. 2010;51(4):671–5.
94. Lin R, Yu Y, Wang Y, et al. Risk of post-stroke epilepsy following stroke-associated acute symptomatic seizures. Front Aging Neurosci. 2021;13:707732.
95. Bladin CF, Alexandrov AV, Bellavance A, et al. Seizures after stroke: a prospective multicenter study. Arch Neurol. 2000;57(11):1617–22.
96. Beghi E, D'Alessandro R, Beretta S, et al. Incidence and predictors of acute symptomatic seizures after stroke. Neurology. 2011;77(20):1785–93.
97. The National Institute of Neurological Disorders and Stroke rt-PA Stroke Study Group. Tissue plasminogen activator for acute ischemic stroke. N Engl J Med. 1995;333(24):1581–7.
98. Chang CS, Liao CH, Lin CC, et al. Patients with epilepsy are at an increased risk of subsequent stroke: a population-based cohort study. Seizure. 2014;23(5):377–81.

99. Larsson D, Farahmand B, Asberg S, et al. Risk of stroke after new-onset seizures. Seizure. 2020;83:76–82.
100. Zelano J, Larsson D, Kumlien E, et al. Pre-stroke seizures: a nationwide register-based investigation. Seizure. 2017;49:25–9.
101. Caramelli P, Mutarelli EG, Caramelli B, et al. Neurological complications after thrombolytic treatment for acute myocardial infarction: emphasis on unprecedented manifestations. Acta Neurol Scand. 1992;85(5):331–3.
102. Pawlak R, Melchor JP, Matys T, et al. Ethanol-withdrawal seizures are controlled by tissue plasminogen activator via modulation of NR2B-containing NMDA receptors. Proc Natl Acad Sci USA. 2005;102(2):443–8.
103. Qian Z, Gilbert ME, Colicos MA, et al. Tissue-plasminogen activator is induced as an immediate-early gene during seizure, kindling and long-term potentiation. Nature. 1993;361(6411):453–7.
104. Tsirka SE, Gualandris A, Amaral DG, et al. Excitotoxin-induced neuronal degeneration and seizure are mediated by tissue plasminogen activator. Nature. 1995;377(6547):340–4.
105. Yepes M, Sandkvist M, Coleman TA, et al. Regulation of seizure spreading by neuroserpin and tissue-type plasminogen activator is plasminogen-independent. J Clin Investig. 2002;109(12):1571–8.
106. Lee SK, Kim DI, Kim SY, et al. Reperfusion cellular injury in an animal model of transient ischemia. AJNR Am J Neuroradiol. 2004;25(8):1342–7.
107. Schwartz RB. Hyperperfusion encephalopathies: hypertensive encephalopathy and related conditions. The Neurologist. 2002;8(1):22–34.
108. Karapanayiotides T, Meuli R, Devuyst G, et al. Postcarotid endarterectomy hyperperfusion or reperfusion syndrome. Stroke. 2005;36(1):21–6.
109. Seeck M, Vulliemoz S. Seizures during stroke thrombolysis heralding dramatic neurologic recovery. Neurology. 2007;69(4):409–10.
110. Ferreira-Atuesta C, Dohler N, Erdelyi-Canavese B, et al. Seizures after Ischemic Stroke: A Matched Multicenter Study. Ann Neurol. 2021;90(5):808–20.
111. Burneo JG, Antaya TC, Allen BN, et al. The risk of new-onset epilepsy and refractory epilepsy in older adult stroke survivors. Neurology. 2019;93(6):e568–77.
112. Galovic M, Dohler N, Erdelyi-Canavese B, et al. Prediction of late seizures after ischaemic stroke with a novel prognostic model (the SeLECT score): a multivariable prediction model development and validation study. Lancet Neurol. 2018;17(2):143–52.
113. Struck AF, Tabaeizadeh M, Schmitt SE, et al. Assessment of the validity of the 2HELPS2B score for inpatient seizure risk prediction. JAMA Neurol. 2020;77(4):500–7.
114. Bentes C, Martins H, Peralta AR, et al. Early EEG predicts poststroke epilepsy. Epilepsia Open. 2018;3(2):203–12.
115. Alvarez V, Rossetti AO, Papavasileiou V, et al. Acute seizures in acute ischemic stroke: does thrombolysis have a role to play? J Neurol. 2013;260(1):55–61.
116. Brigo F, Schneider M, Wagenpfeil G, et al. Intravenous thrombolysis with tPA and cortical involvement increase the risk of early poststroke seizures: results of a case-control study. Epilepsy Behav. 2020;104(Pt B):106312.
117. Naylor J, Thevathasan A, Churilov L, et al. Association between different acute stroke therapies and development of post stroke seizures. BMC Neurol. 2018;18(1):61.
118. De Reuck J, Van Maele G. Acute ischemic stroke treatment and the occurrence of seizures. Clin Neurol Neurosurg. 2010;112(4):328–31.
119. Chen Z, Churilov L, Chen Z, et al. Association between implementation of a code stroke system and poststroke epilepsy. Neurology. 2018;90(13):e1126–33.
120. Brigo F, Schneider M, Wagenpfeil G, et al. Early poststroke seizures following thrombolysis and/or thrombectomy for acute stroke: Clinical and stroke characteristics. Epilepsy Behav. 2020;104(Pt B):106353.

121. Hamidou B, Aboa-Eboule C, Durier J, et al. Prognostic value of early epileptic seizures on mortality and functional disability in acute stroke: the Dijon Stroke Registry (1985–2010). J Neurol. 2013;260(4):1043–51.
122. Alvarez-Sabin J, Montaner J, Padro L, et al. Gabapentin in late-onset poststroke seizures. Neurology. 2002;59(12):1991–3.
123. Brigo F, Lattanzi S, Zelano J, et al. Randomized controlled trials of antiepileptic drugs for the treatment of post-stroke seizures: a systematic review with network meta-analysis. Seizure. 2018;61:57–62.
124. Rosenow F, Brandt C, Bozorg A, et al. Lacosamide in patients with epilepsy of cerebrovascular etiology. Acta Neurol Scand. 2020;141(6):473–82.
125. Berghuis B, van der Palen J, de Haan GJ, et al. Carbamazepine- and oxcarbazepine-induced hyponatremia in people with epilepsy. Epilepsia. 2017;58(7):1227–33.
126. Pickelsimer EE, Selassie AW, Gu JK, et al. A population-based outcomes study of persons hospitalized with traumatic brain injury: operations of the South Carolina Traumatic Brain Injury Follow-up Registry. J Head Trauma Rehabil. 2006;21(6):491–504.
127. Agrawal A, Timothy J, Pandit L, et al. Post-traumatic epilepsy: an overview. Clin Neurol Neurosurg. 2006;108(5):433–9.
128. Frey LC. Epidemiology of posttraumatic epilepsy: a critical review. Epilepsia. 2003;44(s10):11–7.
129. Dewan MC, Rattani A, Gupta S, et al. Estimating the global incidence of traumatic brain injury. J Neurosurg. 2018;130(4):1080–97.
130. Bruns J Jr, Hauser WA. The epidemiology of traumatic brain injury: a review. Epilepsia. 2003;44(s10):2–10.
131. Annegers JF, Grabow JD, Kurland LT, et al. The incidence, causes, and secular trends of head trauma in Olmsted County, Minnesota, 1935–1974. Neurology. 1980;30(9):912–9.
132. Annegers JF, Rocca WA, Hauser WA. Causes of epilepsy: contributions of the Rochester epidemiology project. Mayo Clin Proc. 1996;71(6):570–5.
133. Hauser WA, Annegers JF, Rocca WA. Descriptive epidemiology of epilepsy: contributions of population-based studies from Rochester, Minnesota. Mayo Clin Proc. 1996;71(6):576–86.
134. Hauser WA, Annegers JF, Kurland LT. Incidence of epilepsy and unprovoked seizures in Rochester, Minnesota: 1935–1984. Epilepsia. 1993;34(3):453–68.
135. Wang XP, Zhong J, Lei T, et al. Epidemiology of traumatic brain injury-associated epilepsy in western China: an analysis of multicenter data. Epilepsy Res. 2020;164:106354.
136. Kuhl DA, Boucher BA, Muhlbauer MS. Prophylaxis of posttraumatic seizures. DICP. 1990;24(3):277–85.
137. Annegers JF, Grabow JD, Groover RV, et al. Seizures after head trauma: a population study. Neurology. 1980;30(7 Pt 1):683–9.
138. Bushnik T, Englander J, Wright J, et al. Traumatic brain injury with and without late posttraumatic seizures: what are the impacts in the post-acute phase: a NIDRR Traumatic Brain Injury Model Systems study. J Head Trauma Rehabil. 2012;27(6):E36–44.
139. Walker AE, Erculei F. Post-traumatic epilepsy 15 years later. Epilepsia. 1970;11(1):17–26.
140. Annegers JF, Hauser WA, Coan SP, et al. A population-based study of seizures after traumatic brain injuries. N Engl J Med. 1998;338(1):20–4.
141. Salazar AM, Jabbari B, Vance SC, et al. Epilepsy after penetrating head injury. I. Clinical correlates: a report of the Vietnam Head Injury Study. Neurology. 1985;35(10):1406–14.
142. Shekh-Ahmad T, Lieb A, Kovac S, et al. Combination antioxidant therapy prevents epileptogenesis and modifies chronic epilepsy. Redox Biol. 2019;26:101278.
143. Christensen J, Pedersen MG, Pedersen CB, et al. Long-term risk of epilepsy after traumatic brain injury in children and young adults: a population-based cohort study. Lancet. 2009;373(9669):1105–10.
144. Olson S. Review of the role of anticonvulsant prophylaxis following brain injury. J Clin Neurosci. 2004;11(1):1–3.
145. Miller JD. Head injury. J Neurol Neurosurg Psychiatry. 1993;56(5):440–7.

146. Povlishock JT. Traumatically induced axonal injury: pathogenesis and pathobiological implications. Brain Pathol. 1992;2(1):1–12.
147. Sharma R, Leung WL, Zamani A, et al. Neuroinflammation in post-traumatic epilepsy: pathophysiology and tractable therapeutic targets. Brain Sci. 2019;9(11)
148. Xu S, Sun Q, Fan J, et al. Role of astrocytes in post-traumatic epilepsy. Front Neurol. 2019;10:1149.
149. Dadas A, Janigro D. Breakdown of blood brain barrier as a mechanism of post-traumatic epilepsy. Neurobiol Dis. 2019;123:20–6.
150. Koenig JB, Dulla CG. Dysregulated glucose metabolism as a therapeutic target to reduce post-traumatic epilepsy. Front Cell Neurosci. 2018;12:350.
151. Ye Y, Mauro M, Bovenzi M, et al. Association between vasoconstriction during and following exposure to hand-transmitted vibration. Int Arch Occup Environ Health. 2014;87(1):41–9.
152. Pedrazzi M, Patrone M, Passalacqua M, et al. Selective proinflammatory activation of astrocytes by high-mobility group box 1 protein signaling. J Immunol. 2007;179(12):8525–32.
153. Viviani B, Bartesaghi S, Gardoni F, et al. Interleukin-1beta enhances NMDA receptor-mediated intracellular calcium increase through activation of the Src family of kinases. J Neurosci. 2003;23(25):8692–700.
154. Asikainen I, Kaste M, Sarna S. Early and late posttraumatic seizures in traumatic brain injury rehabilitation patients: brain injury factors causing late seizures and influence of seizures on long-term outcome. Epilepsia. 1999;40(5):584–9.
155. Pitkanen A, Immonen RJ, Grohn OH, et al. From traumatic brain injury to posttraumatic epilepsy: what animal models tell us about the process and treatment options. Epilepsia. 2009;50(Suppl 2):21–9.
156. Prince DA, Parada I, Scalise K, et al. Epilepsy following cortical injury: cellular and molecular mechanisms as targets for potential prophylaxis. Epilepsia. 2009;50(Suppl 2):30–40.
157. Hunt RF, Boychuk JA, Smith BN. Neural circuit mechanisms of post-traumatic epilepsy. Front Cell Neurosci. 2013;7:89.
158. Willmore LJ, Ueda Y. Posttraumatic epilepsy: hemorrhage, free radicals and the molecular regulation of glutamate. Neurochem Res. 2009;34(4):688–97.
159. Pitkanen A, Paananen T, Kyyriainen J, et al. Biomarkers for posttraumatic epilepsy. Epilepsy Behav. 2021;121(Pt B):107080.
160. Henshall DC, Hamer HM, Pasterkamp RJ, et al. MicroRNAs in epilepsy: pathophysiology and clinical utility. Lancet Neurol. 2016;15(13):1368–76.
161. McIntosh TK, Vink R, Noble L, et al. Traumatic brain injury in the rat: characterization of a lateral fluid-percussion model. Neuroscience. 1989;28(1):233–44.
162. Hicks RR, Li C, Zhang L, et al. Alterations in BDNF and trkB mRNA levels in the cerebral cortex following experimental brain trauma in rats. J Neurotrauma. 1999;16(6):501–10.
163. Keith KA, Huang JH. Animal models of post-traumatic epilepsy. Diagnostics (Basel). 2019;10(1):4.
164. Shandra O, Robel S. Inducing post-traumatic epilepsy in a mouse model of repetitive diffuse traumatic brain injury. J Vis Exp. 2020;156
165. Santhakumar V, Bender R, Frotscher M, et al. Granule cell hyperexcitability in the early post-traumatic rat dentate gyrus: the 'irritable mossy cell' hypothesis. J Physiol. 2000;524(Pt 1):117–34.
166. D'Ambrosio R, Fairbanks JP, Fender JS, et al. Post-traumatic epilepsy following fluid percussion injury in the rat. Brain. 2004;127(Pt 2):304–14.
167. D'Ambrosio R, Fender JS, Fairbanks JP, et al. Progression from frontal-parietal to mesial-temporal epilepsy after fluid percussion injury in the rat. Brain. 2005;128(Pt 1):174–88.
168. Kharatishvili I, Nissinen JP, McIntosh TK, et al. A model of posttraumatic epilepsy induced by lateral fluid-percussion brain injury in rats. Neuroscience. 2006;140(2):685–97.
169. Bolkvadze T, Pitkanen A. Development of post-traumatic epilepsy after controlled cortical impact and lateral fluid-percussion-induced brain injury in the mouse. J Neurotrauma. 2012;29(5):789–812.

170. Hunt RF, Scheff SW, Smith BN. Posttraumatic epilepsy after controlled cortical impact injury in mice. Exp Neurol. 2009;215(2):243–52.
171. Salin P, Tseng GF, Hoffman S, et al. Axonal sprouting in layer V pyramidal neurons of chronically injured cerebral cortex. J Neurosci. 1995;15(12):8234–45.
172. Ma Y, Prince DA. Functional alterations in GABAergic fast-spiking interneurons in chronically injured epileptogenic neocortex. Neurobiol Dis. 2012;47(1):102–13.
173. Graber KD, Prince DA. Tetrodotoxin prevents posttraumatic epileptogenesis in rats. Ann Neurol. 1999;46(2):234–42.
174. Graber KD, Prince DA. A critical period for prevention of posttraumatic neocortical hyperexcitability in rats. Ann Neurol. 2004;55(6):860–70.
175. Xu T, Yu X, Ou S, et al. Risk factors for posttraumatic epilepsy: a systematic review and meta-analysis. Epilepsy Behav. 2017;67:1–6.
176. Suri P, Stolzmann K, Iverson KM, et al. Associations between traumatic Brain injury history and future headache severity in veterans: a longitudinal study. Arch Phys Med Rehabil. 2017;98(11):2118–2125 e2111.
177. Cotter D, Kelso A, Neligan A. Genetic biomarkers of posttraumatic epilepsy: a systematic review. Seizure. 2017;46:53–8.
178. Schierhout G, Roberts I. Anti-epileptic drugs for preventing seizures following acute traumatic brain injury. Cochrane Database Syst Rev. 2001;4:CD000173.
179. Haltiner AM, Newell DW, Temkin NR, et al. Side effects and mortality associated with use of phenytoin for early posttraumatic seizure prophylaxis. J Neurosurg. 1999;91(4):588–92.
180. Chang BS, Lowenstein DH, Quality Standards Subcommittee of the American Academy of N. Practice parameter: antiepileptic drug prophylaxis in severe traumatic brain injury: report of the Quality Standards Subcommittee of the American Academy of Neurology. Neurology. 2003;60(1):10–6.
181. Hung C, Chen JW. Treatment of post-traumatic epilepsy. Curr Treat Options Neurol. 2012;14(4):293–306.
182. Jones KE, Puccio AM, Harshman KJ, et al. Levetiracetam versus phenytoin for seizure prophylaxis in severe traumatic brain injury. Neurosurg Focus. 2008;25(4):E3.
183. Young B, Rapp RP, Norton JA, et al. Failure of prophylactically administered phenytoin to prevent early posttraumatic seizures. J Neurosurg. 1983;58(2):231–5.
184. Lewis RJ, Yee L, Inkelis SH, et al. Clinical predictors of post-traumatic seizures in children with head trauma. Ann Emerg Med. 1993;22(7):1114–8.
185. Tilford JM, Simpson PM, Yeh TS, et al. Variation in therapy and outcome for pediatric head trauma patients. Crit Care Med. 2001;29(5):1056–61.
186. Watson NF, Barber JK, Doherty MJ, et al. Does glucocorticoid administration prevent late seizures after head injury? Epilepsia. 2004;45(6):690–4.
187. 李敏;李立宏;江基尧.颅脑创伤后癫痫防治中国专家共识. 中华神经外科杂志. 2017;33(07):652–54.
188. Servit Z, Musil F. Prophylactic treatment of posttraumatic epilepsy: results of a long-term follow-up in Czechoslovakia. Epilepsia. 1981;22(3):315–20.
189. Rapport RL 2nd, Penry JK. A survey of attitudes toward the pharmacological prophylaxis of posttraumatic epilepsy. J Neurosurg. 1973;38(2):159–66.
190. McQueen JK, Blackwood DH, Harris P, et al. Low risk of late post-traumatic seizures following severe head injury: implications for clinical trials of prophylaxis. J Neurol Neurosurg Psychiatry. 1983;46(10):899–904.
191. Temkin NR, Dikmen SS, Anderson GD, et al. Valproate therapy for prevention of posttraumatic seizures: a randomized trial. J Neurosurg. 1999;91(4):593–600.
192. Jennett B. Epilepsy and acute traumatic intracranial haematoma. J Neurol Neurosurg Psychiatry. 1975;38(4):378–81.
193. MacDonald BK, Cockerell OC, Sander JW, et al. The incidence and lifetime prevalence of neurological disorders in a prospective community-based study in the UK. Brain. 2000;123(Pt 4):665–76.

194. Haltiner AM, Temkin NR, Dikmen SS. Risk of seizure recurrence after the first late posttraumatic seizure. Arch Phys Med Rehabil. 1997;78(8):835–40.
195. Nissinen J, Andrade P, Natunen T, et al. Disease-modifying effect of atipamezole in a model of post-traumatic epilepsy. Epilepsy Res. 2017;136:18–34.
196. Chrzaszcz M, Venkatesan C, Dragisic T, et al. Minozac treatment prevents increased seizure susceptibility in a mouse “two-hit” model of closed skull traumatic brain injury and electroconvulsive shock-induced seizures. J Neurotrauma. 2010;27(7):1283–95.
197. Eastman CL, Fender JS, Klein P, et al. Therapeutic effects of time-limited treatment with Brivaracetam on posttraumatic epilepsy after fluid percussion injury in the rat. J Pharmacol Exp Ther. 2021;379(3):310–23.
198. Ostrom QT, Patil N, Cioffi G, et al. Corrigendum to: CBTRUS statistical report: primary Brain and other central nervous system tumors diagnosed in the United States in 2013–2017. Neuro-Oncology. 2022;24(7):1214.
199. Miller KD, Ostrom QT, Kruchko C, et al. Brain and other central nervous system tumor statistics, 2021. CA Cancer J Clin. 2021;71(5):381–406.
200. Vecht CJ, Kerkhof M, Duran-Pena A. Seizure prognosis in brain tumors: new insights and evidence-based management. Oncologist. 2014;19(7):751–9.
201. Seidel S, Wehner T, Miller D, et al. Brain tumor related epilepsy: pathophysiological approaches and rational management of antiseizure medication. Neurol Res Pract. 2022;4(1):45.
202. Shamji MF, Fric-Shamji EC, Benoit BG. Brain tumors and epilepsy: pathophysiology of peritumoral changes. Neurosurg Rev. 2009;32(3):275–84; discussion 284-276.
203. Chen DY, Chen CC, Crawford JR, et al. Tumor-related epilepsy: epidemiology, pathogenesis and management. J Neuro-Oncol. 2018;139(1):13–21.
204. McGonigal A, Bartolomei F, Chauvel P. On seizure semiology. Epilepsia. 2021;62(9):2019–35.
205. Pallud J, Capelle L, Huberfeld G. Tumoral epileptogenicity: how does it happen? Epilepsia. 2013;54(Suppl 9):30–4.
206. Venkataramani V, Tanev DI, Strahle C, et al. Glutamatergic synaptic input to glioma cells drives brain tumour progression. Nature. 2019;573(7775):532–8.
207. Venkatesh HS, Morishita W, Geraghty AC, et al. Electrical and synaptic integration of glioma into neural circuits. Nature. 2019;573(7775):539–45.
208. Venkataramani V, Tanev DI, Kuner T, et al. Synaptic input to brain tumors: clinical implications. Neuro-Oncology. 2021;23(1):23–33.
209. Zhang J, Yao L, Peng S, et al. Correlation between glioma location and preoperative seizures: a systematic review and meta-analysis. Neurosurg Rev. 2019;42(3):603–18.
210. Lamba N, Catalano PJ, Cagney DN, et al. Seizures among patients with Brain metastases: a population- and institutional-level analysis. Neurology. 2021;96(8):e1237–50.
211. van Opijnen MP, Tesileanu CMS, Dirven L, et al. IDH1/2 wildtype gliomas grade 2 and 3 with molecular glioblastoma-like profile have a distinct course of epilepsy compared to IDH1/2 wildtype glioblastomas. Neuro-Oncology. 2023;25(4):701–9.
212. Walbert T, Harrison RA, Schiff D, et al. SNO and EANO practice guideline update: anticonvulsant prophylaxis in patients with newly diagnosed brain tumors. Neuro-Oncology. 2021;23(11):1835–44.
213. Maschio M, Aguglia U, Avanzini G, et al. Management of epilepsy in brain tumors. Neurol Sci. 2019;40(10):2217–34.
214. Happold C, Gorlia T, Chinot O, et al. Does Valproic acid or Levetiracetam improve survival in glioblastoma? A pooled analysis of prospective clinical trials in newly diagnosed glioblastoma. J Clin Oncol. 2016;34(7):731–9.
215. Tabaee Damavandi P, Pasini F, Fanella G, et al. Perampanel in Brain tumor-related epilepsy: a systematic review. Brain Sci. 2023;13(2)
216. van der Meer PB, Dirven L, Fiocco M, et al. First-line antiepileptic drug treatment in glioma patients with epilepsy: Levetiracetam vs valproic acid. Epilepsia. 2021;62(5):1119–29.

217. Mo F, Meletti S, Belcastro V, et al. Lacosamide in monotherapy in BTRE (brain tumor-related epilepsy): results from an Italian multicenter retrospective study. J Neuro-Oncol. 2022;157(3):551–9.
218. Maschio M, Maialetti A, Mocellini C, et al. Effect of Brivaracetam on efficacy and tolerability in patients with Brain tumor-related epilepsy: a retrospective multicenter study. Front Neurol. 2020;11:813.
219. Lange F, Hornschemeyer J, Kirschstein T. Glutamatergic mechanisms in glioblastoma and tumor-associated epilepsy. Cells. 2021;10(5)
220. Vecht CJ, van Breemen M. Optimizing therapy of seizures in patients with brain tumors. Neurology. 2006;67(12 Suppl 4):S10–3.
221. Mastall M, Wolpert F, Gramatzki D, et al. Survival of brain tumour patients with epilepsy. Brain. 2021;144(11):3322–7.
222. Lamberink HJ, Otte WM, Geerts AT, et al. Individualised prediction model of seizure recurrence and long-term outcomes after withdrawal of antiepileptic drugs in seizure-free patients: a systematic review and individual participant data meta-analysis. Lancet Neurol. 2017;16(7):523–31.
223. Jiang H, Deng G, Liu B, et al. Analysis of the short-term outcomes and risk factors of seizure relapse in patients with gliomas after antiepileptic drugs withdrawal. J Clin Neurosci. 2020;82(Pt A):20–5.
224. Guerrini R, Barba C. Focal cortical dysplasia: an update on diagnosis and treatment. J Expert Rev Neurother. 2021;21(11):1213–24.
225. Najm IM, Tassi L, Sarnat HB, et al. Epilepsies associated with focal cortical dysplasias (FCDs). J Acta Neuropathol. 2014;128(1):5–19.
226. Crome L. Infantile cerebral gliosis with giant nerve cells. J Neurol Neurosurg Psychiatry. 1957;20(2):117–24.
227. Taylor DC, Falconer MA, Bruton CJ, et al. Focal dysplasia of the cerebral cortex in epilepsy. J Neurol Neurosurg Psychiatry. 1971;34(4):369–87.
228. Palmini A, Najm I, Avanzini G, et al. Terminology and classification of the cortical dysplasias. Neurology. 2004;62(6 Suppl 3):S2–8.
229. Blumcke I, Thom M, Aronica E, et al. The clinicopathologic spectrum of focal cortical dysplasias: a consensus classification proposed by an ad hoc Task Force of the ILAE Diagnostic Methods Commission. Epilepsia. 2011;52(1):158–74.
230. Najm IM, Sarnat HB, Blumcke I. Review: the international consensus classification of focal cortical dysplasia – a critical update 2018. Neuropathol Appl Neurobiol. 2018;44(1):18–31.
231. Blumcke I, Cendes F, Miyata H, et al. Toward a refined genotype-phenotype classification scheme for the international consensus classification of Focal Cortical Dysplasia. Brain Pathol. 2021;31(4):e12956.
232. Najm I, Lal D, Alonso VM, et al. The ILAE consensus classification of focal cortical dysplasia: an update proposed by an ad hoc task force of the ILAE diagnostic methods commission. Epilepsia. 2022;63(8):1899–919.
233. Orlova KA, Tsai V, Baybis M, et al. Early progenitor cell marker expression distinguishes type II from type I focal cortical dysplasias. J Neuropathol Exp Neurol. 2010;69(8):850–63.
234. Crino PB, Trojanowski JQ, Eberwine J. Internexin, MAP1B, and nestin in cortical dysplasia as markers of developmental maturity. Acta Neuropathol. 1997;93(6):619–27.
235. Cohen NT, Chang P, You X, et al. Prevalence and risk factors for Pharmacoresistance in children with focal cortical dysplasia-related epilepsy. Neurology. 2022;99(18):e2006–13.
236. Bast T, Ramantani G, Seitz A, et al. Focal cortical dysplasia: prevalence, clinical presentation and epilepsy in children and adults. Acta Neurol Scand. 2006;113(2):72–81.
237. Blumcke I, Spreafico R, Haaker G, et al. Histopathological findings in Brain tissue obtained during epilepsy surgery. N Engl J Med. 2017;377(17):1648–56.
238. Widdess-Walsh P, Kellinghaus C, Jeha L, et al. Electro-clinical and imaging characteristics of focal cortical dysplasia: correlation with pathological subtypes. Epilepsy Res. 2005;67(1–2):25–33.

239. Krsek P, Pieper T, Karlmeier A, et al. Different presurgical characteristics and seizure outcomes in children with focal cortical dysplasia type I or II. Epilepsia. 2009;50(1):125–37.
240. Chassoux F, Landre E, Mellerio C, et al. Type II focal cortical dysplasia: electroclinical phenotype and surgical outcome related to imaging. Epilepsia. 2012;53(2):349–58.
241. Crino PB. Focal cortical dysplasia. Semin Neurol. 2015;35(3):201–8.
242. Guerrini R, Duchowny M, Jayakar P, et al. Diagnostic methods and treatment options for focal cortical dysplasia. Epilepsia. 2015;56(11):1669–86.
243. Sharma D, Dixit AB, Dey S, et al. Increased levels of alpha4-containing GABA(A) receptors in focal cortical dysplasia: a possible cause of benzodiazepine resistance. Neurochem Int. 2021;148:105084.
244. Puskarjov M, Kahle KT, Ruusuvuori E, et al. Pharmacotherapeutic targeting of cation-chloride cotransporters in neonatal seizures. Epilepsia. 2014;55(6):806–18.
245. Finardi A, Colciaghi F, Castana L, et al. Long-duration epilepsy affects cell morphology and glutamatergic synapses in type IIB focal cortical dysplasia. Acta Neuropathol. 2013;126(2):219–35.
246. Moddel G, Jacobson B, Ying Z, et al. The NMDA receptor NR2B subunit contributes to epileptogenesis in human cortical dysplasia. Brain Res. 2005;1046(1–2):10–23.
247. Wong M, Crino PB. Tuberous sclerosis and epilepsy: role of astrocytes. Glia. 2012;60(8):1244–50.
248. Zvi IB, Enright N, D'Arco F, et al. Children with seizures and radiological diagnosis of focal cortical dysplasia: can drug-resistant epilepsy be predicted earlier? Epileptic Disord. 2022;24(1):111–22.
249. Bjellvi J, Olsson I, Malmgren K, et al. Epilepsy duration and seizure outcome in epilepsy surgery: a systematic review and meta-analysis. Neurology. 2019;93(2):e159–66.
250. Ak H, Ay B, Tanriverdi T, et al. Expression and cellular distribution of multidrug resistance-related proteins in patients with focal cortical dysplasia. Seizure. 2007;16(6):493–503.
251. Chen W, Jin B, Aung T, et al. Response to antiseizure medications in epileptic patients with malformation of cortical development. Ther Adv Neurol Disord. 2021;14:17562864211050027.
252. Fois C, Rassu AL, Mandia D, et al. Paradoxical effect of Levetiracetam in newly diagnosed type II focal cortical dysplasia. Clin Neuropharmacol. 2016;39(5):265–8.
253. Cvetkovska E, Kuzmanovski I, Babunovska M, et al. Levetiracetam-induced seizure aggravation in patients with focal cortical dysplasia. Clin Neuropharmacol. 2018;41(6):218–21.
254. Nguyen LH, Mahadeo T, Bordey A. mTOR hyperactivity levels influence the severity of epilepsy and associated neuropathology in an experimental model of tuberous sclerosis complex and focal cortical dysplasia. J Neurosci. 2019;39(14):2762–73.
255. Marsan E, Baulac S. Review: mechanistic target of rapamycin (mTOR) pathway, focal cortical dysplasia and epilepsy. Neuropathol Appl Neurobiol. 2018;44(1):6–17.
256. Cepeda C, Levinson S, Yazon VW, et al. Cellular antiseizure mechanisms of everolimus in pediatric tuberous sclerosis complex, cortical dysplasia, and non-mTOR-mediated etiologies. Epilepsia Open. 2018;3(Suppl 2):180–90.
257. French JA, Lawson JA, Yapici Z, et al. Adjunctive everolimus therapy for treatment-resistant focal-onset seizures associated with tuberous sclerosis (EXIST-3): a phase 3, randomised, double-blind, placebo-controlled study. J Lancet. 2016;388(10056):2153–63.
258. Curatolo P, Franz DN, Lawson JA, et al. Adjunctive everolimus for children and adolescents with treatment-refractory seizures associated with tuberous sclerosis complex: post-hoc analysis of the phase 3 EXIST-3 trial. Lancet Child Adolesc Health. 2018;2(7):495–504.
259. Lim JS, Kim WI, Kang HC, et al. Brain somatic mutations in MTOR cause focal cortical dysplasia type II leading to intractable epilepsy. J Nat Med. 2015;21(4):395–400.
260. Kato M, Kada A, Shiraishi H, et al. Sirolimus for epileptic seizures associated with focal cortical dysplasia type II. Ann Clin Transl Neurol. 2022;9(2):181–92.
261. Al AF, Dudley R, Bello-Espinosa LE, et al. Intravenous immunoglobulin as a treatment for intractable epilepsy secondary to focal cortical dysplasia: a meta-analysis. J Pediatr Neurol. 2017;76:79–81.

262. Graus F, Titulaer MJ, Balu R, et al. A clinical approach to diagnosis of autoimmune encephalitis. Lancet Neurol. 2016;15(4):391–404.
263. Steriade C, Britton J, Dale RC, et al. Acute symptomatic seizures secondary to autoimmune encephalitis and autoimmune-associated epilepsy: conceptual definitions. Epilepsia. 2020;61(7):1341–51.
264. Hirsch LJ, Gaspard N, van Baalen A, et al. Proposed consensus definitions for new-onset refractory status epilepticus (NORSE), febrile infection-related epilepsy syndrome (FIRES), and related conditions. Epilepsia. 2018;59(4):739–44.
265. Dubey D, Pittock SJ, Kelly CR, et al. Autoimmune encephalitis epidemiology and a comparison to infectious encephalitis. Ann Neurol. 2018;83(1):166–77.
266. Zhang W, Wang X, Shao N, et al. Seizure characteristics, treatment, and outcome in autoimmune synaptic encephalitis: a long-term study. Epilepsy Behav. 2019;94:198–203.
267. Gaspard N, Foreman BP, Alvarez V, et al. New-onset refractory status epilepticus: etiology, clinical features, and outcome. Neurology. 2015;85(18):1604–13.
268. Wesselingh R, Butzkueven H, Buzzard K, et al. Seizures in autoimmune encephalitis: kindling the fire. Epilepsia. 2020;61(6):1033–44.
269. Venkatesan A, Adatia K. Anti-NMDA-receptor encephalitis: from bench to clinic. ACS Chem Neurosci. 2017;8(12):2586–95.
270. Ni G, Lin W, Cai X, et al. Associations between seizures and MRI in patients with anti-NMDAR encephalitis. Acta Neurol Scand. 2020;142(5):460–5.
271. Liu X, Yan B, Wang R, et al. Seizure outcomes in patients with anti-NMDAR encephalitis: a follow-up study. Epilepsia. 2017;58(12):2104–11.
272. Liu X, Guo K, Lin J, et al. Long-term seizure outcomes in patients with autoimmune encephalitis: a prospective observational registry study update. Epilepsia. 2022;63(7):1812–21.
273. Du J, Guo Y, Zhu Q. Use of anti-seizure medications in different types of autoimmune encephalitis: a narrative review. Front Neurol. 2023;14:1111384.
274. Zhu F, Shan W, Lv R, et al. Clinical characteristics of anti-GABA-B receptor encephalitis. Front Neurol. 2020;11:403.
275. Irani SR, Michell AW, Lang B, et al. Faciobrachial dystonic seizures precede Lgi1 antibody limbic encephalitis. Ann Neurol. 2011;69(5):892–900.
276. Feyissa AM, Lamb C, Pittock SJ, et al. Antiepileptic drug therapy in autoimmune epilepsy associated with antibodies targeting the leucine-rich glioma-inactivated protein 1. Epilepsia Open. 2018;3(3):348–56.
277. Rodriguez A, Klein CJ, Sechi E, et al. LGI1 antibody encephalitis: acute treatment comparisons and outcome. J Neurol Neurosurg Psychiatry. 2022;93(3):309–15.
278. van Sonderen A, Thijs RD, Coenders EC, et al. Anti-LGI1 encephalitis: clinical syndrome and long-term follow-up. Neurology. 2016;87(14):1449–56.
279. Garrido Sanabria ER, Zahid A, Britton J, et al. CASPR2-IgG-associated autoimmune seizures. Epilepsia. 2022;63(3):709–22.
280. Chen B, Lopez Chiriboga AS, Sirven JI, et al. Autoimmune encephalitis-related seizures and epilepsy: diagnostic and therapeutic approaches. Mayo Clin Proc. 2021;96(8):2029–39.
281. de Bruijn M, van Sonderen A, van Coevorden-Hameete MH, et al. Evaluation of seizure treatment in anti-LGI1, anti-NMDAR, and anti-GABA(B)R encephalitis. Neurology. 2019;92(19):e2185–96.
282. Dubey D, Singh J, Britton JW, et al. Predictive models in the diagnosis and treatment of autoimmune epilepsy. Epilepsia. 2017;58(7):1181–9.
283. Wickstrom R, Taraschenko O, Dilena R, et al. International consensus recommendations for management of new onset refractory status epilepticus (NORSE) incl. Febrile infection-related epilepsy syndrome (FIRES): statements and supporting evidence. Epilepsia. 2022;63(11):2840–64.
284. Wagner JN. Anticonvulsive treatment in autoimmune encephalitis: a systematic literature review. Wien Med Wochenschr. 2023;174:22.

285. Shin YW, Ahn SJ, Moon J, et al. Increased adverse events associated with antiepileptic drugs in anti-leucine-rich glioma-inactivated protein 1 encephalitis. Epilepsia. 2018;59(Suppl 2):108–12.
286. Feyissa AM, Lopez Chiriboga AS, Britton JW. Antiepileptic drug therapy in patients with autoimmune epilepsy. Neurol Neuroimmunol Neuroinflamm. 2017;4(4):e353.
287. Zhong R, Zhang X, Chen Q, et al. Acute symptomatic seizures and risk of epilepsy in autoimmune encephalitis: a retrospective cohort study. Front Immunol. 2022;13:813174.
288. Dubey D, Kothapalli N, McKeon A, et al. Predictors of neural-specific autoantibodies and immunotherapy response in patients with cognitive dysfunction. J Neuroimmunol. 2018;323:62–72.
289. Rasmussen T, Olszewski J, Lloydsmith D. Focal seizures due to chronic localized encephalitis. Neurology. 1958;8(6):435–45.
290. Geis C, Planaguma J, Carreno M, et al. Autoimmune seizures and epilepsy. J Clin Invest. 2019;129(3):926–40.
291. Levite M. Autoimmune epilepsy. Nat Immunol. 2002;3(6):500.
292. Jansweijer JA, Nieuwhof K, Russo F, et al. Truncating titin mutations are associated with a mild and treatable form of dilated cardiomyopathy. Eur J Heart Fail. 2017;19(4):512–21.
293. Rada A, Bien CG. What is autoimmune encephalitis-associated epilepsy? Proposal of a practical definition. Epilepsia. 2023;64(9):2249–55.
294. Pardo CA, Vining EP, Guo L, et al. The pathology of Rasmussen syndrome: stages of cortical involvement and neuropathological studies in 45 hemispherectomies. Epilepsia. 2004;45(5):516–26.
295. Varadkar S, Bien CG, Kruse CA, et al. Rasmussen's encephalitis: clinical features, pathobiology, and treatment advances. Lancet Neurol. 2014;13(2):195–205.
296. Mochol M, Tauboll E, Sveberg L, et al. Seizure control after late introduction of anakinra in a patient with adult onset Rasmussen's encephalitis. Epilepsy Behav Rep. 2021;16:100462.
297. Takahashi Y, Yamazaki E, Mine J, et al. Immunomodulatory therapy versus surgery for Rasmussen syndrome in early childhood. Brain Dev. 2013;35(8):778–85.
298. Thilo B, Stingele R, Knudsen K, et al. A case of Rasmussen encephalitis treated with rituximab. Nat Rev Neurol. 2009;5(8):458–62.
299. Nava BC, Costa UT, Hamad APA, et al. Long-term seizure outcome and mobility after surgical treatment for Rasmussen encephalitis in children: a single-center experience. Epileptic Disord. 2023;25(5):749–57.
300. Dade M, Berzero G, Izquierdo C, et al. Neurological syndromes associated with anti-GAD antibodies. Int J Mol Sci. 2020;21(10)
301. Carreno M, Bien CG, Asadi-Pooya AA, et al. Epilepsy surgery in drug resistant temporal lobe epilepsy associated with neuronal antibodies. Epilepsy Res. 2017;129:101–5.
302. Errichiello L, Perruolo G, Pascarella A, et al. Autoantibodies to glutamic acid decarboxylase (GAD) in focal and generalized epilepsy: a study on 233 patients. J Neuroimmunol. 2009;211(1–2):120–3.
303. Malter MP, Frisch C, Zeitler H, et al. Treatment of immune-mediated temporal lobe epilepsy with GAD antibodies. Seizure. 2015;30:57–63.
304. Serrano-Castro PJ, Rodriguez-Uranga JJ, Cabezudo-Garcia P, et al. Cenobamate and Clobazam combination as personalized medicine in autoimmune-associated epilepsy with anti-Gad65 antibodies. Neurol Neuroimmunol Neuroinflamm. 2023;10(6)
305. Vincent A, Crino PB. Systemic and neurologic autoimmune disorders associated with seizures or epilepsy. Epilepsia. 2011;52(Suppl 3):12–7.
306. Smith KM, Britton JW, Thakolwiboon S, et al. Seizure characteristics and outcomes in patients with neurological conditions related to high-risk paraneoplastic antibodies. Epilepsia. 2023;64(9):2385–98.
307. Toledano M, Britton JW, McKeon A, et al. Utility of an immunotherapy trial in evaluating patients with presumed autoimmune epilepsy. Neurology. 2014;82(18):1578–86.

308. Erkkinen MG, Berkowitz AL. A clinical approach to diagnosing encephalopathy. Am J Med. 2019;132(10):1142–7.
309. Douglas-Escobar M, Weiss MD. Hypoxic-ischemic encephalopathy: a review for the clinician. JAMA Pediatr. 2015;169(4):397–403.
310. Lance JW, Adams RD. The syndrome of intention or action myoclonus as a sequel to hypoxic encephalopathy. Brain. 1963;86:111–36.
311. Elmer J, Rittenberger JC, Faro J, et al. Clinically distinct electroencephalographic phenotypes of early myoclonus after cardiac arrest. Ann Neurol. 2016;80(2):175–84.
312. Wijdicks E. Looking back at the Lance-Adams syndrome: uncommon and unalike. Neurocrit Care. 2022;41:695.
313. Zhao M, Zhu P, Fujino M, et al. Oxidative stress in hypoxic-ischemic encephalopathy: molecular mechanisms and therapeutic strategies. Int J Mol Sci. 2016;17(12)
314. Bennet L, Roelfsema V, Pathipati P, et al. Relationship between evolving epileptiform activity and delayed loss of mitochondrial activity after asphyxia measured by near-infrared spectroscopy in preterm fetal sheep. J Physiol. 2006;572(Pt 1):141–54.
315. Gupta HV, Caviness JN. Post-hypoxic myoclonus: current concepts, neurophysiology, and treatment. J Tremor Other Hyperkinet Mov (NY). 2016;6:409.
316. Zhou KQ, McDouall A, Drury PP, et al. Treating seizures after hypoxic-ischemic encephalopathy-current controversies and future directions. Int J Mol Sci. 2021;22(13)
317. Ghosh S, Tran L, Shuster JJ, et al. Therapeutic hypothermia for neonatal hypoxic ischemic encephalopathy is associated with short-term reduction of seizures after discharge from the neonatal intensive care unit. Childs Nerv Syst. 2017;33(2):329–35.
318. Harbert MJ, Tam EW, Glass HC, et al. Hypothermia is correlated with seizure absence in perinatal stroke. J Child Neurol. 2011;26(9):1126–30.
319. Krishna S, Hutton A, Aronowitz E, et al. The effects of adding prophylactic phenobarbital to therapeutic hypothermia in the term-equivalent hypoxic-ischemic rat. Pediatr Res. 2018;83(2):506–13.
320. Frucht S, Fahn S. The clinical spectrum of posthypoxic myoclonus. Mov Disord. 2000;15(Suppl 1):2–7.
321. Tai KK, Bhidayasiri R, Truong DD. Post-hypoxic animal model of myoclonus. Parkinsonism Relat Disord. 2007;13(7):377–81.
322. Katsuki M, Narita N, Yasuda I, et al. Lance-Adams syndrome treated by Perampanel in the acute term. Cureus. 2021;13(3):e13761.
323. Kamel WA, Al-Hashel JY, Abdulsalam AJ, et al. Perampanel in refractory post-hypoxic myoclonus: see the difference! Acta Neurol Belgica. 2020;120(3):741–2.
324. Wijdicks EF. Hepatic encephalopathy. N Engl J Med. 2016;375(17):1660–70.
325. Alkhachroum AM, Rubinos C, Kummer BR, et al. Risk of seizures and status epilepticus in older patients with liver disease. Epilepsia. 2018;59(7):1392–7.
326. Gursky JM, Rossi KC, Jette N, et al. Exacerbation of hepatic cirrhosis may trigger admission for epilepsy and status epilepticus. Epilepsia. 2020;61(3):400–7.
327. Olivero M, Gagliardi D, Costamagna G, et al. Newly diagnosed hepatic encephalopathy presenting as non-convulsive status epilepticus: a case report and literature review. Front Neurol. 2022;13:880068.
328. Rovira A, Alonso J, Cordoba J. MR imaging findings in hepatic encephalopathy. Am J Neuroradiol. 2008;29(9):1612–21.
329. Butterworth RF. Pathogenesis of hepatic encephalopathy: new insights from neuroimaging and molecular studies. J Hepatol. 2003;39(2):278–85.
330. Felipo V, Hermenegildo C, Montoliu C, et al. Neurotoxicity of ammonia and glutamate: molecular mechanisms and prevention. J Neuro-Oncol. 1998;19(4–5):675–81.
331. Rose CF, Amodio P, Bajaj JS, et al. Hepatic encephalopathy: novel insights into classification, pathophysiology and therapy. J Hepatol. 2020;73(6):1526–47.
332. Haussinger D, Dhiman RK, Felipo V, et al. Hepatic encephalopathy. Nat Rev Dis Primers. 2022;8(1):43.

333. Krasko A, Deshpande K, Bonvino S. Liver failure, transplantation, and critical care. J Crit Care Clin. 2003;19(2):155–83.
334. Sheth RD. Metabolic concerns associated with antiepileptic medications. Neurology. 2004;63(10 Suppl 4):S24–9.
335. Kanner AM, Ashman E, Gloss D, et al. Practice guideline update summary: efficacy and tolerability of the new antiepileptic drugs I: treatment of new-onset epilepsy: report of the Guideline Development, Dissemination, and Implementation Subcommittee of the American Academy of Neurology and the American Epilepsy Society. Neurology. 2018;91(2):74–81.
336. Berger B, Mader I, Damjanovic K, et al. Epileptic status immediately after initiation of D-penicillamine therapy in a patient with Wilson's disease. Clin Neurol Neurosurg. 2014;127:122–4.
337. Rosner MH, Husain-Syed F, Reis T, et al. Uremic encephalopathy. Kidney Int. 2022;101(2):227–41.
338. Titoff V, Moury HN, Titoff IB, et al. Seizures, antiepileptic drugs, and CKD. Am J Kidney Dis. 2019;73(1):90–101.
339. Alhilali LM, Reynolds AR, Fakhran S. A multi-disciplinary model of risk factors for fatal outcome in posterior reversible encephalopathy syndrome. J Neurol Sci. 2014;347(1–2):59–65.
340. Li R, Mitchell P, Dowling R, et al. Is hypertension predictive of clinical recurrence in posterior reversible encephalopathy syndrome? J Clin Neurosci. 2013;20(2):248–52.
341. Fugate JE, Rabinstein AA. Posterior reversible encephalopathy syndrome: clinical and radiological manifestations, pathophysiology, and outstanding questions. Lancet Neurol. 2015;14(9):914–25.
342. Lacerda G, Krummel T, Sabourdy C, et al. Optimizing therapy of seizures in patients with renal or hepatic dysfunction. Neurology. 2006;67(12 Suppl 4):S28–33.
343. Seifter JL, Samuels MA. Uremic encephalopathy and other brain disorders associated with renal failure. Semin Neurol. 2011;31(2):139–43.
344. Keppel HJ, Kopsky DJ. Phenytoin: 80 years young, from epilepsy to breast cancer, a remarkable molecule with multiple modes of action. J Neurol. 2017;264(8):1617–21.
345. Bansal AD, Hill CE, Berns JS. Use of antiepileptic drugs in patients with chronic kidney disease and end stage renal disease. Semin Dial. 2015;28(4):404–12.
346. Angel MJ, Young GB. Metabolic encephalopathies. Neurol Clin. 2011;29(4):837–82.
347. Kadima NT, Kobau R, Zack MM, Helmers S. Comorbidity in adults with epilepsy–United States, 2010. MMWR Morb Mortal Wkly Rep. 2013;62(43):849–53.
348. Tellez-Zenteno JF, Matijevic S, Wiebe S. Somatic comorbidity of epilepsy in the general population in Canada. J Epilepsia. 2005;46(12):1955–62.
349. Gaitatzis A, Carroll K, Majeed A, et al. The epidemiology of the comorbidity of epilepsy in the general population. Epilepsia. 2004;45(12):1613–22.
350. Oliveira AJ, Zamagni M, Dolso P, et al. Respiratory disorders during sleep in patients with epilepsy: effect of ventilatory therapy on EEG interictal epileptiform discharges. J Clin Neurophysiol. 2000;111(Suppl 2):S141–5.
351. Camp B, Stegemann-Koniszewski S, Schreiber J. Infection-associated mechanisms of neuro-inflammation and neuro-immune crosstalk in chronic respiratory diseases. J Int J Mol Sci. 2021;22(11)
352. Caldwell HG, Carr J, Minhas JS, et al. Acid-base balance and cerebrovascular regulation. J Physiol. 2021;599(24):5337–59.
353. Vozoris NT, Fischer HD, Wang X, et al. Benzodiazepine drug use and adverse respiratory outcomes among older adults with COPD. Eur Respir J. 2014;44(2):332–40.
354. Brain L, Jellinek EH, Ball K. Hashimoto's disease and encephalopathy. J Lancet. 1966;2(7462):512–4.
355. Ferracci F, Bertiato G, Moretto G. Hashimoto's encephalopathy: epidemiologic data and pathogenetic considerations. J Neurol Sci. 2004;217(2):165–8.
356. Ferracci F, Carnevale A. The neurological disorder associated with thyroid autoimmunity. J Neurol. 2006;253(8):975–84.

357. Hilberath JM, Schmidt H, Wolf GK. Steroid-responsive encephalopathy associated with autoimmune thyroiditis (SREAT): case report of reversible coma and status epilepticus in an adolescent patient and review of the literature. Eur J Pediatr. 2014;173(10):1263–73.
358. Tamagno G, Federspil G, Murialdo G. Clinical and diagnostic aspects of encephalopathy associated with autoimmune thyroid disease (or Hashimoto's encephalopathy). Intern Emerg Med. 2006;1(1):15–23.
359. Laurent C, Capron J, Quillerou B, et al. Steroid-responsive encephalopathy associated with autoimmune thyroiditis (SREAT): characteristics, treatment and outcome in 251 cases from the literature. J Autoimmun Rev. 2016;15(12):1129–33.
360. Kothbauer-Margreiter I, Sturzenegger M, Komor J, et al. Encephalopathy associated with Hashimoto thyroiditis: diagnosis and treatment. J Neurol. 1996;243(8):585–93.
361. Chaudhuri J, Mukherjee A, Chakravarty A. Hashimoto's encephalopathy: case series and literature review. Curr Neurol Neurosci Rep. 2023;23(4):167–75.
362. Li J, Li F. Hashimoto's encephalopathy and seizure disorders. Front Neurol. 2019;10:440.
363. Chaigne B, Mercier E, Garot D, et al. Hashimoto's encephalopathy in the intensive care unit. Neurocrit Care. 2013;18(3):386–90.
364. Arya R, Anand V, Chansoria M. Hashimoto encephalopathy presenting as progressive myoclonus epilepsy syndrome. Eur J Paediatr Neurol. 2013;17(1):102–4.
365. Alink J, de Vries TW. Unexplained seizures, confusion or hallucinations: think Hashimoto encephalopathy. Acta Paediatr. 2008;97(4):451–3.
366. Kelley BP, Patel SC, Marin HL, et al. Autoimmune encephalitis: pathophysiology and imaging review of an overlooked diagnosis. AJNR Am J Neuroradiol. 2017;38(6):1070–8.
367. Muramatsu T, Hamano T, Shirafuji N, et al. Hashimoto's encephalopathy presenting periodic synchronous discharge, as a differential diagnosis for Creutzfeldt-Jakob disease. Rinsho Shinkeigaku. 2013;53(9):716–20.
368. Waliszewska-Prosol M, Ejma M. Assessment of visual and brainstem auditory evoked potentials in patients with Hashimoto's thyroiditis. J Immunol Res. 2021;2021:3258942.
369. Ferracci F, Moretto G, Candeago RM, et al. Antithyroid antibodies in the CSF: their role in the pathogenesis of Hashimoto's encephalopathy. Neurology. 2003;60(4):712–4.
370. Tsai SL, Lewis EC, Sell E, et al. Central nervous system vasculitis with positive antithyroid antibodies in an adolescent boy. J Pediatr Neurol. 2011;45(3):189–92.
371. Duffey P, Yee S, Reid IN, et al. Hashimoto's encephalopathy: postmortem findings after fatal status epilepticus. Neurology. 2003;61(8):1124–6.
372. Nolte KW, Unbehaun A, Sieker H, et al. Hashimoto encephalopathy: a brainstem vasculitis? Neurology. 2000;54(3):769–70.
373. Moodley K, Botha J, Raidoo DM, et al. Immuno-localisation of anti-thyroid antibodies in adult human cerebral cortex. J Neurol Sci. 2011;302(1–2):114–7.
374. Varrasi C, Vecchio D, Magistrelli L, et al. Auditory seizures in autoimmune epilepsy: a case with anti-thyroid antibodies. Epileptic Disord. 2017;19(1):99–103.
375. Watemberg N, Greenstein D, Levine A. Encephalopathy associated with Hashimoto thyroiditis: pediatric perspective. J Child Neurol. 2006;21(1):1–5.
376. Cornejo R, Venegas P, Goni D, et al. Successful response to intravenous immunoglobulin as rescue therapy in a patient with Hashimoto's encephalopathy. BMJ Case Rep. 2010;2010:bcr0920103332.
377. Boers PM, Colebatch JG. Hashimoto's encephalopathy responding to plasmapheresis. J Neurol Neurosurg Psychiatry. 2001;70(1):132.
378. Marshall GA, Doyle JJ. Long-term treatment of Hashimoto's encephalopathy. J Neuropsychiatry Clin Neurosci. 2006;18(1):14–20.
379. Liang MH, et al. The American College of Rheumatology nomenclature and case definitions for neuropsychiatric lupus syndromes. Arthritis Rheum. 1999;42(4):599–608.
380. Govoni M, Bortoluzzi A, Padovan M, et al. The diagnosis and clinical management of the neuropsychiatric manifestations of lupus. J Autoimmun. 2016;74:41–72.

381. Appenzeller S, Cendes F, Costallat LT. Epileptic seizures in systemic lupus erythematosus. Neurology. 2004;63(10):1808–12.
382. Devinsky O, Schein A, Najjar S. Epilepsy associated with systemic autoimmune disorders. Epilepsy Curr. 2013;13(2):62–8.
383. Petri M, Naqibuddin M, Carson KA, et al. Brain magnetic resonance imaging in newly diagnosed systemic lupus erythematosus. J Rheumatol. 2008;35(12):2348–54.
384. Koga M, Kawasaki A, Ito I, et al. Cumulative association of eight susceptibility genes with systemic lupus erythematosus in a Japanese female population. J Hum Genet. 2011;56(7):503–7.
385. de Vries B, Steup-Beekman GM, Haan J, et al. TREX1 gene variant in neuropsychiatric systemic lupus erythematosus. Ann Rheum Dis. 2010;69(10):1886–7.
386. Postal M, Costallat LT, Appenzeller S. Neuropsychiatric manifestations in systemic lupus erythematosus: epidemiology, pathophysiology and management. CNS Drugs. 2011;25(9):721–36.
387. Liimatainen S, Peltola M, Fallah M, et al. The high prevalence of antiphospholipid antibodies in refractory focal epilepsy is related to recurrent seizures. Eur J Neurol. 2009;16(1):134–41.
388. Cimaz R, Meroni PL, Shoenfeld Y. Epilepsy as part of systemic lupus erythematosus and systemic antiphospholipid syndrome (Hughes syndrome). Lupus. 2006;15(4):191–7.
389. Hanly JG, Urowitz MB, Su L, et al. Seizure disorders in systemic lupus erythematosus results from an international, prospective, inception cohort study. Ann Rheum Dis. 2012;71(9):1502–9.
390. Kowal C, Degiorgio LA, Lee JY, et al. Human lupus autoantibodies against NMDA receptors mediate cognitive impairment. Proc Natl Acad Sci USA. 2006;103(52):19854–9.
391. Kozora E, West SG, Maier SF, et al. Antibodies against N-methyl-D-aspartate receptors in patients with systemic lupus erythematosus without major neuropsychiatric syndromes. J Neurol Sci. 2010;295(1–2):87–91.
392. Wang JB, Li H, Wang LL, et al. Role of IL-1beta, IL-6, IL-8 and IFN-gamma in pathogenesis of central nervous system neuropsychiatric systemic lupus erythematous. Int J Clin Exp Med. 2015;8(9):16658–63.
393. Bertsias GK, Ioannidis JP, Aringer M, et al. EULAR recommendations for the management of systemic lupus erythematosus with neuropsychiatric manifestations: report of a task force of the EULAR standing committee for clinical affairs. Ann Rheum Dis. 2010;69(12):2074–82.
394. Andrade RM, Alarcon GS, Gonzalez LA, et al. Seizures in patients with systemic lupus erythematosus: data from LUMINA, a multiethnic cohort (LUMINA LIV). Ann Rheum Dis. 2008;67(6):829–34.
395. Popescu A, Kao AH. Neuropsychiatric systemic lupus erythematosus. Curr Neuropharmacol. 2011;9(3):449–57.
396. Bertsias GK, Boumpas DT. Pathogenesis, diagnosis and management of neuropsychiatric SLE manifestations. Nat Rev Rheumatol. 2010;6(6):358–67.
397. Bujan S, Ordi-Ros J, Paredes J, et al. Contribution of the initial features of systemic lupus erythematosus to the clinical evolution and survival of a cohort of Mediterranean patients. Ann Rheum Dis. 2003;62(9):859–65.
398. Weaver LK. Clinical practice. Carbon monoxide poisoning. N Engl J Med. 2009;360(12):1217–25.
399. Liu J, Si Z, Liu J, et al. Clinical and imaging prognosis in patients with delayed encephalopathy after acute carbon monoxide poisoning. Behav Neurol. 2020;2020:1719360.
400. Jeon SB, Sohn CH, Seo DW, et al. Acute Brain lesions on magnetic resonance imaging and delayed neurological sequelae in carbon monoxide poisoning. JAMA Neurol. 2018;75(4):436–43.
401. Rose JJ, Wang L, Xu Q, et al. Carbon monoxide poisoning: pathogenesis, management, and future directions of therapy. Am J Respir Crit Care Med. 2017;195(5):596–606.
402. Lee Y, Cha YS, Kim SH, et al. Effect of hyperbaric oxygen therapy initiation time in acute carbon monoxide poisoning. Crit Care Med. 2021;49(10):e910–9.

403. Huang YQ, Peng ZR, Huang FL, et al. Mechanism of delayed encephalopathy after acute carbon monoxide poisoning. Neural Regen Res. 2020;15(12):2286–95.
404. Cerase A, Rubenni E, Rufa A, et al. CT and MRI of Wernicke's encephalopathy. Radiol Med. 2011;116(2):319–33.
405. Geibprasert S, Gallucci M, Krings T. Alcohol-induced changes in the brain as assessed by MRI and CT. Eur Radiol. 2010;20(6):1492–501.
406. Gordon E, Devinsky O. Alcohol and marijuana: effects on epilepsy and use by patients with epilepsy. Epilepsia. 2001;42(10):1266–72.
407. Matz R. Lorazepam for the prevention of recurrent seizures related to alcohol. N Engl J Med. 1999;341(8):609–10.
408. Leach JP, Mohanraj R, Borland W. Alcohol and drugs in epilepsy: pathophysiology, presentation, possibilities, and prevention. Epilepsia. 2012;53(Suppl 4):48–57.
409. Wolters EC, van Wijngaarden GK, Stam FC, et al. Leucoencephalopathy after inhaling "heroin" pyrolysate. J Lancet. 1982;2(8310):1233–7.
410. Benoilid A, Collongues N, de Seze J, et al. Heroin inhalation-induced unilateral complete hippocampal stroke. J Neuro-Oncol. 2013;19(4):313–5.
411. Buttner A, Mall G, Penning R, et al. The neuropathology of heroin abuse. Forensic Sci Int. 2000;113(1–3):435–42.
412. Alambyan V, Pace J, Miller B, et al. The emerging role of inhaled heroin in the opioid epidemic: a review. JAMA Neurol. 2018;75(11):1423–34.
413. Greene-Schloesser D, Robbins ME, Peiffer AM, et al. Radiation-induced brain injury: a review. Front Oncol. 2012;2:73.
414. Aoki S, Hayashi N, Abe O, et al. Radiation-induced arteritis: thickened wall with prominent enhancement on cranial MR images report of five cases and comparison with 18 cases of Moyamoya disease. Radiology. 2002;223(3):683–8.
415. Tang Y, Li Y, Luo D, et al. Epilepsy related to radiotherapy in patients with nasopharyngeal carcinoma. Epilepsy Res. 2011;96(1–2):24–8.
416. Shalev O, Silverberg R. Dexamethasone for acute radiation encephalopathy. J Lancet. 1978;2(8089):574–5.
417. Shoji M, Ninomiya I, Makino I, et al. Valproic acid, a histone deacetylase inhibitor, enhances radiosensitivity in esophageal squamous cell carcinoma. Int J Oncol. 2012;40(6):2140–6.
418. Zivkovic SA, Abdel-Hamid H. Neurologic manifestations of transplant complications. Neurol Clin. 2010;28(1):235–51.
419. Senzolo M, Ferronato C, Burra P. Neurologic complications after solid organ transplantation. Transpl Int. 2009;22(3):269–78.
420. Cappadona R, De Giorgi A, Di Simone E, et al. Infodemiology of solid organ transplantation: relationship to the Global Observatory on Donation and Transplantation data. Eur Rev Med Pharmacol Sci. 2020;24(24):12630–7.
421. Wszolek ZK, Steg RE. Seizures after orthotopic liver transplantation. Seizure. 1997;6(1):31–9.
422. Saner FH, Sotiropoulos GC, Gu Y, et al. Severe neurological events following liver transplantation. Arch Med Res. 2007;38(1):75–9.
423. Vernon HJ, Sperati CJ, King JD, et al. A detailed analysis of methylmalonic acid kinetics during hemodialysis and after combined liver/kidney transplantation in a patient with mut (0) methylmalonic acidemia. J Inherit Metab Dis. 2014;37(6):899–907.
424. Haughey D, Narsipur SS. Posterior reversible encephalopathy syndrome after renal transplant: a simple solution for a complicated patient. Case Rep Nephrol Dial. 2015;5(1):20–5.
425. Moris D, Vernadakis S, Lionaki S, et al. An uncommon cause of acutely altered mental status in a renal transplant recipient. Ups J Med Sci. 2014;119(1):50–4.
426. Ocal R, Sezer T, Kibaroglu S, et al. Epilepsy after heart transplant: a single center experience. Exp Clin Transplant. 2016; https://doi.org/10.6002/ect.2016.0047.
427. Zhang XH, Xu LP, Liu DH, et al. Epileptic seizures in patients following allogeneic hematopoietic stem cell transplantation: a retrospective analysis of incidence, risk factors, and survival rates. Clin Transpl. 2013;27(1):80–9.

428. Maheshwari A, Torbenson MS, Thuluvath PJ. Sirolimus monotherapy versus sirolimus in combination with steroids and/or MMF for immunosuppression after liver transplantation. Dig Dis Sci. 2006;51(10):1677–84.
429. Saner F, Gu Y, Minouchehr S, et al. Neurological complications after cadaveric and living donor liver transplantation. J Neurol. 2006;253(5):612–7.
430. Klawitter J, Gottschalk S, Hainz C, et al. Immunosuppressant neurotoxicity in rat brain models: oxidative stress and cellular metabolism. Chem Res Toxicol. 2010;23(3):608–19.
431. Katsarou AM, Moshe SL, Galanopoulou AS. Interneuronopathies and their role in early life epilepsies and neurodevelopmental disorders. Epilepsia Open. 2017;2(3):284–306.
432. Pittock SJ, Rabinstein AA, Edwards BS, et al. OKT3 neurotoxicity presenting as akinetic mutism. Transplantation. 2003;75(7):1058–60.
433. Kunnathu Puthanveedu ND, Lum J. Central nervous system infections after solid organ transplantation. Curr Opin Infect Dis. 2021;34(3):207–16.
434. van Veen KE, Brouwer MC, van der Ende A, et al. Bacterial meningitis in solid organ transplant recipients: a population-based prospective study. Transpl Infect Dis. 2016;18(5):674–80.
435. Charlier C, Perrodeau E, Leclercq A, et al. Clinical features and prognostic factors of listeriosis: the MONALISA national prospective cohort study. Lancet Infect Dis. 2017;17(5):510–9.
436. Hun M, Xie M, She Z, et al. Management and clinical outcome of posterior reversible encephalopathy syndrome in pediatric oncologic/hematologic diseases: a PRES subgroup analysis with a large sample size. Front Pediatr. 2021;9:678890.
437. Bartynski WS, Tan HP, Boardman JF, et al. Posterior reversible encephalopathy syndrome after solid organ transplantation. AJNR Am J Neuroradiol. 2008;29(5):924–30.
438. Song T, Rao Z, Tan Q, et al. Calcineurin inhibitors associated posterior reversible encephalopathy syndrome in solid organ transplantation: report of 2 cases and literature review. Medicine (Baltimore). 2016;95(14):e3173.
439. Vizzini G, Asaro M, Miraglia R, et al. Changing picture of central nervous system complications in liver transplant recipients. Liver Transpl. 2011;17(11):1279–85.
440. Cheng CY, Wang HY, Liou WS, et al. Hazards of stroke in renal transplant recipients and patients with end-stage renal disease. Transplant Proc. 2019;51(5):1402–5.
441. Liou L, Mostofsky E, Lehman L, et al. Racial disparities in post-transplant stroke and mortality following stroke in adult cardiac transplant recipients in the United States. PLoS One. 2023;18(2):e0268275.
442. Yang M, Qamer SZ, Hill AP, et al. Postoperative myocardial injury and outcomes in liver and kidney transplant patients. Cardiovasc Revasc Med. 2022;41:154–8.
443. Tanaka T, Ihara M. Post-stroke epilepsy. Neurochem Int. 2017;107:219–28.
444. Chabolla DR, Wszolek ZK. Pharmacologic management of seizures in organ transplant. Neurology. 2006;67(12 Suppl 4):S34–8.
445. Scheffner D, Konig S, Rauterberg-Ruland I, et al. Fatal liver failure in 16 children with valproate therapy. Epilepsia. 1988;29(5):530–42.
446. Patsalos PN. Clinical pharmacokinetics of levetiracetam. Clin Pharmacokinet. 2004;43(11):707–24.
447. Meehan AL, Yang X, McAdams BD, et al. A new mechanism for antiepileptic drug action: vesicular entry may mediate the effects of levetiracetam. J Neurophysiol. 2011;106(3):1227–39.
448. Brodie MJ, Perucca E, Ryvlin P, et al. Comparison of levetiracetam and controlled-release carbamazepine in newly diagnosed epilepsy. Neurology. 2007;68(6):402–8.
449. Glass GA, Stankiewicz J, Mithoefer A, et al. Levetiracetam for seizures after liver transplantation. Neurology. 2005;64(6):1084–5.
450. Nicolas JM, Collart P, Gerin B, et al. In vitro evaluation of potential drug interactions with levetiracetam, a new antiepileptic agent. Drug Metab Dispos. 1999;27(2):250–4.
451. Franzoni E, Sarajlija J, Garone C, et al. No kinetic interaction between levetiracetam and cyclosporine: a case report. J Child Neurol. 2007;22(4):440–2.

452. Lin CH, Chen CL, Lin TK, et al. Levetiracetam in the treatment of epileptic seizures after liver transplantation. Medicine (Baltimore). 2015;94(38):e1350.
453. Kilic B, Gungor S, Arslan M, et al. Seizures in pediatric patients with liver transplant and efficacy of Levetiracetam. J Child Neurol. 2017;32(8):740–5.
454. Shepard PW, St Louis EK. Seizure treatment in transplant patients. Curr Treat Options Neurol. 2012;14(4):332–47.
455. Urbanowicz T, Pawlowska M, Buczkowski P, et al. Seizures after heart transplantation–two cases of non-immunosuppressant drug interactions in young patients. Ann Transplant. 2014;19:417–20.
456. Masetti R, Cordelli DM, Zama D, et al. PRES in children undergoing hematopoietic stem cell or solid organ transplantation. Pediatrics. 2015;135(5):890–901.
457. Peyrl A, Weichert N, Kuhl JS, et al. Levetiracetam as a possible cause of secondary graft failure after allogenic hematopoietic stem cell transplantation. Eur J Paediatr Neurol. 2015;19(1):75–7.
458. Ouyang J, Peng S, Wu G, Liu R. Association between neurodegenerative diseases and an increased risk of epilepsy based on single nucleotide polymorphisms: a Mendelian randomization study. Mol Neurobiol. 2024;61:5950.
459. Bronisch FW, Rauch HJ. Pathogenesis of epileptic seizures in multiple sclerosis. Dtsch Z Nervenheilkd. 1947;158:322–43.
460. Hamlin PG. Convulsive states and multiple sclerosis: report of a case. Ann Intern Med. 1955;42:201–5.
461. Rafalowska J, Warecka K. Epidemic seizures in the course of multiple sclerosis. Neurol Neurochir Psychiatr Pol. 1962;12:317–23.
462. Boudin G, Masson S, Vacheron-Baglin F, Désignolle L. Apropos of 2 anatomo-clinical cases of multiple sclerosis having presented epileptic attacks. Rev Neurol (Paris). 1965;113:267–8.
463. van Klink N, Tousseyn S, Schijns O, van Eijsden P, Vos P, Hilkman D, et al. Successful epilepsy surgery in two cases with multiple sclerosis. Epileptic Disord. 2023;25:890–4.
464. Ciolac D, Gonzalez-Escamilla G, Winter Y, Fleischer V, Grothe M, Groppa S. Brain network correlates of epilepsy occurrence in multiple sclerosis and neuroinflammation. Neural Regen Res. 2023;18:1717–8.
465. Drulovic J, Pekmezovic T, Tamas O, Adamec I, Aleksic D, Andabaka M, et al. The impact of the comorbid seizure/epilepsy on the health related quality of life in people with multiple sclerosis: an international multicentric study. Front Immunol. 2023;14:1284031.
466. Nurre ER, Shah A, Hansen CJ, Dowling C, Thakolwiboon S, Mao-Draayer Y, et al. Multiple sclerosis and seizures: a retrospective observational study in a multiple sclerosis autoimmunity center of excellence. Seizure. 2024;115:44–9.
467. Sanchez M, Marone A, Silva WH, Marrodan M, Correale J. Clinical characteristics, course and prognosis of Multiple Sclerosis patients with epilepsy. A case control study: MS and epilepsy. Mult Scler Relat Disord. 2024;83:105422.
468. Ghezzi A, Montanini R, Basso PF, Zaffaroni M, Massimo E, Cazzullo CL. Epilepsy in multiple sclerosis. Eur Neurol. 1990;30:218–23.
469. Zuo H, Peng L, Li W, Wang Y, Du X, Zou X, et al. Assessment of bidirectional relationships between multiple sclerosis and epilepsy: a two-sample Mendelian randomization study. Mult Scler Relat Disord. 2024;81:105148.
470. Sokic DV, Stojsavljevic N, Drulovic J, Dujmovic I, Mesaros S, Ercegovac M, et al. Seizures in multiple sclerosis. Epilepsia. 2001;42:72–9.
471. Striano P, Orefice G, Brescia Morra V, Boccella P, Sarappa C, Lanzillo R, et al. Epileptic seizures in multiple sclerosis: clinical and EEG correlations. Neurol Sci. 2003;24:322–8.
472. Gurtubay IG, Gila L, Morales G, Gállego-Culleré J, Ayuso MT, Manubens JM. Multiple sclerosis and epileptic seizures. Rev Neurol. 2000;30:827–32.
473. Zhang D, Chen S, Xu S, Wu J, Zhuang Y, Cao W, et al. The clinical correlation between Alzheimer's disease and epilepsy. Front Neurol. 2022;13:922535.

474. Naville F. Epileptiform crises with palilal auras; pick or Alzheimer's disease, or traumatic brain contusion? Rev Med Suisse Romande. 1946;66:50–6.
475. Dascalov D. EEG findings in Alzheimer's disease. Electroencephalogr Clin Neurophysiol. 1969;27:447.
476. Giménez-Roldan S, Peraita P, López Agreda JM, Abad JM, Esteban A. Myoclonus and photic-induced seizures in Alzheimer's disease. Eur Neurol. 1971;5:215–24.
477. Paul LA, Scheibel AB. Structural substrates of epilepsy. Adv Neurol. 1986;44:775–86.
478. Mendez MF, Catanzaro P, Doss RC, ARguello R, Frey WH 2nd. Seizures in Alzheimer's disease: clinicopathologic study. J Geriatr Psychiatry Neurol. 1994;7:230–3.
479. Paudel YN, Angelopoulou E, Jones NC, O'Brien TJ, Kwan P, Piperi C, et al. Tau related pathways as a connecting link between epilepsy and Alzheimer's disease. ACS Chem Neurosci. 2019;10:4199–212.
480. Hautecloque-Raysz G, Sellal F, Bousiges O, Phillipi N, Blanc F, Cretin B. Epileptic prodromal Alzheimer's disease treated with Antiseizure medications: medium-term outcome of seizures and cognition. J Alzheimers Dis. 2023;94:1057–74.
481. Tombini M, Boscarino M, Di Lazzaro V. Tackling seizures in patients with Alzheimer's disease. Expert Rev Neurother. 2023;23:1131–45.
482. Xu Y, Lavrencic L, Radford K, Booth A, Yoshimura S, Anstey KJ, et al. Systematic review of coexistent epileptic seizures and Alzheimer's disease: incidence and prevalence. J Am Geriatr Soc. 2021;69:2011–20.
483. Haoudy S, Jonveaux T, Puisieux S, Epstein J, Hopes L, Maillard L, et al. Epilepsy in early onset Alzheimer's disease. J Alzheimers Dis. 2022;85:615–26.
484. Mendez M, Lim G. Seizures in elderly patients with dementia: epidemiology and management. Drugs Aging. 2003;20:791–803.
485. Lozsadi DA, Larner AJ. Prevalence and causes of seizures at the time of diagnosis of probable Alzheimer's disease. Dement Geriatr Cogn Disord. 2006;22:121–4.
486. Cheng C-H, Liu C-J, Ou S-M, Yeh C-M, Chen T-J, Lin Y-Y, et al. Incidence and risk of seizures in Alzheimer's disease: a nationwide population-based cohort study. Epilepsy Res. 2015;115:63–6.
487. Hommet C, Hureaux R, Barré J, Constans T, Berrut G. Epileptic seizures in clinically diagnosed Alzheimer's disease: report from a geriatric medicine population. Aging Clin Exp Res. 2007;19:430–1.
488. Bosco F, Guarnieri L, Rania V, Palma E, Citraro R, Corasaniti MT, et al. Antiseizure medications in Alzheimer's disease from preclinical to clinical evidence. Int J Mol Sci. 2023;24
489. Hwang K, Vaknalli RN, Addo-Osafo K, Vicente M, Vossel K. Tauopathy and epilepsy comorbidities and underlying mechanisms. Front Aging Neurosci. 2022;14:903973.
490. Martin SP, Leeman-Markowski BA. Proposed mechanisms of tau: relationships to traumatic brain injury, Alzheimer's disease, and epilepsy. Front Neurol. 2023;14:1287545.
491. Zawar I, Kapur J. Does Alzheimer's disease with mesial temporal lobe epilepsy represent a distinct disease subtype? Alzheimers Dement. 2023;19:2697–706.
492. Alves SS, de Oliveira JAC, Lazarini-Lopes W, Servilha-Menezes G, Grigório-de-Sant'Ana M, Del Vecchio F, et al. Audiogenic seizures in the Streptozotocin-induced rat Alzheimer's disease model. J Alzheimers Dis. 2023;94:1179–96.
493. Rizzello E, Pimpinella D, Pignataro A, Titta G, Merenda E, Saviana M, et al. Lamotrigine rescues neuronal alterations and prevents seizure-induced memory decline in an Alzheimer's disease mouse model. Neurobiol Dis. 2023;181:106106.
494. Cretin B, Philippi N, Bousiges O, Dibitonto L, Sellal F, Martin-Hunyadi C, et al. Do we know how to diagnose epilepsy early in Alzheimer's disease? Rev Neurol (Paris). 2017;173:374–80.
495. Horváth A, Szűcs A, Hidasi Z, Csukly G, Barcs G, Kamondi A. Prevalence, semiology, and risk factors of epilepsy in Alzheimer's disease: an ambulatory EEG study. J Alzheimers Dis. 2018;63:1045–54.

496. Samudra N, Ranasinghe K, Kirsch H, Rankin K, Miller B. Etiology and clinical significance of network Hyperexcitability in Alzheimer's disease: unanswered questions and next steps. J Alzheimers Dis. 2023;92:13–27.
497. Yang F, Chen L, Yu Y, Xu T, Chen L, Yang W, et al. Alzheimer's disease and epilepsy: an increasingly recognized comorbidity. Front Aging Neurosci. 2022;14:940515.
498. Lee HC, Kim B-K, Kang K, Lee W-W, Yoo I, Kim YS, et al. Aphasic status epilepticus associated with Alzheimer's disease: clinical and electrographic characteristics. Epilepsy Res. 2023;13:55–8.
499. Romanelli MF, Morris JC, Ashkin K, Coben LA. Advanced Alzheimer's disease is a risk factor for late-onset seizures. Arch Neurol. 1990;47:847–50.
500. Cumbo E, Ligori LD. Levetiracetam, lamotrigine, and phenobarbital in patients with epileptic seizures and Alzheimer's disease. Epilepsy Behav. 2010;17:461–6.
501. Musaeus CS, Nilsson C, Cooper C, Kramberger MG, Verdelho A, Stefanova E, et al. Pharmacological medical treatment of epilepsy in patients with dementia: a systematic review. Curr Alzheimer Res. 2021;18:689–94.
502. Sen A, Akinola M, Tai XY, Symmonds M, Davis Jones G, Mura S, et al. An Investigation of Levetiracetam in Alzheimer's Disease (ILiAD): a double-blind, placebo-controlled, randomised crossover proof of concept study. Trials. 2021;22:508.
503. Giorgi FS, Guida M, Vergallo A, Bonuccelli U, Zaccara G. Treatment of epilepsy in patients with Alzheimer's disease. Expert Rev Neurother. 2017;17:309–18.

Chapter 5
Diagnosis and Treatment of Epilepsy Syndromes

Yin Yan, Yi Wang, Fei Xiao, Xuefeng Wang, Haiqing Zhang, Yue Hu, Rong Luo, Li Jiang, Ye Wu, Xuewu Liu, Xin Tian, Xiangqing Wang, and Tingsong Li

Y. Yan
Epilepsy rehabilitation Center, Beibei Hospital of Chongqing Medical University, Chongqing, China

Y. Wang (✉)
Department of Neurology, Children's Hospital of Fudan University, National Children's Medical Center, Shanghai, China
e-mail: yiwang@shmu.edu.cn

F. Xiao · X. Wang · X. Tian
Department of Neurology, The First Affiliated Hospital of Chongqing Medical University, Chongqing, China

H. Zhang
Department of Neurology, Affiliated Hospital of Zunyi Medical University, Zunyi, Guizhou, China

Y. Hu
Department of Neurology, Children's Hospital of Chongqing Medical University, Chongqing, China

R. Luo
Department of Pediatrics, West China Second University Hospital, Sichuan University, Chengdu, China

L. Jiang
Department of Neurology, Children's Hospital of Chongqing Medical University, National Clinical Research Center for Child Health and Disorders, Chongqing, China

Y. Wu (✉)
Department of Pediatrics, Peking University First Hospital, Beijing, China
e-mail: dryewu@263.net

X. Liu
Department of Neurology, Shandong Provincial Hospital Affiliated to Shandong First Medical University, Jinan, Shandong, China

X. Wang
Department of Neurology, The First Medical Center of Chinese PLA General Hospital, Beijing, China

T. Li
Department of Rehabilitation, Children's Hospital of Chongqing Medical University, National Clinical Research Center for Child Health and Disorders, Chongqing, China

X. Wang, L. Zhou (eds.), *Pharmacological Treatment of Epileptic Seizures*,
https://doi.org/10.1007/978-981-96-8520-2_5

5.1 International League Against Epilepsy (ILAE) Classification and Definition of Epilepsy Syndromes

Epilepsy, seizures, and epileptic syndromes are the main subjects of epileptology. According to the International League Against Epilepsy, epilepsy syndromes refer to a group of epilepsies with characteristic clinical and electroencephalographic manifestations and typical etiologies (structural, genetic, metabolic, immune, or infectious). These features of epileptic syndromes can occur simultaneously, are often age-dependent (e.g., age at onset or age at resolution), and are often associated with specific coexisting conditions. The diagnosis of epilepsy syndromes may be highly important for determining patient prognosis and selecting treatment options [1, 2].

5.1.1 Historical Evolution

The name "epilepsy syndrome" was first described by Tissot [3] in 1770, who considered it to have a unique electroclinical phenotype. In 1841, Dr. West [4] described the clinical presentation of his son during a spasm. In 1950, Lennox and Davis [5] discovered the characteristic EEG pattern of Lennox–Gastaut syndrome (LGS) and subsequently published the first paper on electroclinical manifestations [6]. In 1952, Gibbs and Gibbs [7] reported the characteristic EEG of hypsarrhythmia.

In 1981, the International League Against Epilepsy (ILAE) published the *Proposal for Revised Clinical and Electroencephalographic Classification of Epileptic Seizures*, which indicated that the classification of epileptic syndromes should be the next area addressed [8]. In 1983, a workshop organized at Centre Saint Paul, Marseille, involving 30 international epilepsy specialists from 13 countries, including members of the ILAE Classification and Terminology Committee, agreed for the first time on the definition of epilepsy syndromes, documenting the known etiology and evolution, clinical and EEG features, and diagnostic criteria for each syndrome. The proceedings, known as the *Blue Guide*, were published in 1984 [9]. In 1985, the *Proposal for Classification of Epilepsies and Epileptic Syndromes*, published by ILAE, defined an epileptic syndrome as "a type of epilepsy with a combination of specific symptoms and signs that may be clinical (e.g., medical history, seizure types, seizure and recurrence patterns, neurological and psychological manifestations) or ancillary (e.g., medical history, seizure types, seizure and recurrence patterns, neurological and psychological manifestations (e.g., Electroencephalogram, X-ray, CT and MRI))" [10]. In 1989, the revised classification report published by ILAE provided a similar definition of epileptic syndromes and noted that some epileptic syndromes may evolve from one type to another, such as infantile spasms (ISs) syndrome to Lennox–Gastaut syndrome [11]. Although the ILAE recommendations published in both 1985 and 1989 included many recognized syndromes, their definitions have never been formally accepted by the general public. In 2017, the ILAE Commission for Classification and Terminology published position papers on the *Classification of the Epilepsies* and the *Operational Classification of Seizure Types*. The revised epilepsy classification framework adopts a multilevel classification approach. The third level is epilepsy syndrome, which is defined as "a group of specific epileptic phenomena, including seizure type, electroencephalogram and imaging findings, which tend to occur at the same time." It is important to note that these syndromes are often age-dependent (e.g., age at onset and age at resolution), are precipitating factors, exhibit circadian variation, and are sometimes prognostic; additionally, they may be associated with unique coexisting conditions, such as intellectual and psychiatric disorders [2]. The publication of the position paper was followed by the establishment of the ILAE Task Force on Nosology and Definitions, which is responsible for providing definitions and classifications of epilepsy syndromes. In 2022, ILAE published an online report on the classification and definition of epilepsy syndromes in the journal *Epilepsia*, with a total of six articles: Introduction to the Epilepsy Syndrome Papers; Methodology for Classification and Definition of Epilepsy Syndromes with List of Syndromes: Report of the ILAE Task Force on Nosology and Definitions; ILAE Classification and Definition of Epilepsy Syndromes with Onset in Neonates and Infants: Position statement by the ILAE Task Force on Nosology and Definitions; ILAE Classification and Definition of Epilepsy Syndromes with Onset in Childhood: Position Paper by the ILAE Task Force on Nosology and Definitions; ILAE Classification and Definition of Epilepsy Syndromes with Onset at A Variable Age: Position Statement by the ILAE Task Force on Nosology and Definitions; and ILAE Definition of the Idiopathic Generalized Epilepsy Syndromes: Position statement by the ILAE Task Force on Nosology and Definitions [1]. The main contents, classifications, and terminology of 2017 and 2022 were consistent.

5.1.2 Classification Framework and Definition

In 2022, ILAE described an epilepsy syndrome as a set of features comprising a cluster of typical clinical and EEG features that tend to occur simultaneously and are often age-dependent; these features include age at onset and at remission, seizure triggers, circadian variation, prognosis, and unique comorbidities such as intellectual disability (ID) and psychiatric disorders. Syndromes may have etiological, prognostic, and therapeutic implications [1].

Framework for the Classification of Epilepsy Syndromes

In 2022, ILAE published a two-dimensional classification of epilepsy syndromes (Table 5.1). First, four groups were established according to the age of onset: epilepsy syndromes with neonatal and infantile onset (0–2 years of age), epilepsy syndromes with childhood onset (2–16 years of age), epilepsy syndromes that occur at

Table 5.1 Classification of epilepsy syndromes published by ILAE 2022

Classification	Focal	Generalized	Focal and/or generalized	Syndromes with DEE or with progressive neurological deterioration
Epilepsy syndromes with onset in neonates and infants	SeLNE SeLFNIE SeLIE	MEI	GEFS+	EIDEE EIMFS IESS DS Etiology-Specific Syndromes KCNQ2-DEE · PD-DEE · P5PD-DEE · CKDL5-DEE · PCDH19 clustering Epilepsy · GLUT1DS · SWS · GS-HH
Epilepsy Syndromes with onset in childhood	SeLECTS SeLEAS COVE POLE	EEM EMA		EMAtS LGS DEE-SWAS and EE-SWAS FIRES HHE
Epilepsy syndromes with onset at a variable age	MTLE-HS FMTLE SHE FFEV EAF		EwRIS	RS PME
Idiopathic generalized epilepsies		CAE JAE JME GTCA		

Green: *SeLFEs* self-limited focal epilepsies, red: *GGE* genetic generalized epilepsy, *SLFNE* self-limited familial neonatal epilepsy, *SeLFNIE* self-limited familial neonatal–infantile epilepsy, *SeLIE* self-limited (familial) infantile epilepsy, *MEI* myoclonic epilepsy in infancy, GEFS+ genetic epilepsy with febrile seizures plus, *EIDEE* early infantile developmental and epileptic encephalopathy, *EIMFS* epilepsy of infancy with migrating focal seizures, *IESS* infantile epileptic spasms syndrome, *DS* Dravet syndrome, *KCNQ2-DEE KCNQ2* developmental and epileptic encephalopathy, *PD-DEE* pyridoxine-dependent (ALDH7A1) developmental and epileptic encephalopathy, *P5PD-DEE* pyridox(am)ine 5′-phosphate oxidase (PNPO) developmental and epileptic encephalopathy, *CKDL5-DEE* cyclin-dependent kinase-like 5-related developmental and epileptic encephalopathy, *PCDH19 clustering epilepsy* protocadherin 19 clustering epilepsy, *Glut1-DS* glucose transporter type 1 deficiency syndrome, *SWS* Sturge–Weber syndrome, *GS-HH* gelastic seizure with hypothalamic hamartoma, *SeLECTS* self-limited epilepsy with centrotemporal spikes, *SeLEAS* self-limited epilepsy with autonomic seizures, *COVE* childhood occipital visual epilepsy, *POLE* photosensitive occipital lobe epilepsy, *EEM* epilepsy with eyelid myoclonia, *EMA* epilepsy with myoclonic absences, *EMAS* epilepsy with myoclonic–atonic seizures, *LGS* Lennox–Gastaut syndrome, *DEE-SWAS* DEE with spike-and-wave activation in sleep, *EE-SWAS* EE with spike-and-wave activation in sleep, *FIRES* febrile infection-related epilepsy syndrome, *HHE* hemiconvulsion–hemiplegia–epilepsy, *MTLE-HS* mesial temporal lobe epilepsy with hippocampal sclerosis, *FMTLE* familial mesial temporal lobe epilepsy, *SHE* sleep-related hypermotor epilepsy, *FFEVF* familial focal epilepsy with variable foci, *EAF* epilepsy with auditory features, *EwRIS* epilepsy with reading-induced seizures, *RS* Rasmussen syndrome, *PME* progressive myoclonic epilepsy, *CAE* childhood absence epilepsy, *JAE* juvenile absence epilepsy, *JME* juvenile myoclonic epilepsy, *GTCA* generalized tonic–clonic seizures alone

all ages (children and adults), and idiopathic generalized epilepsies (IGEs). IGEs are considered a special group that first appeared in the *Proposal for Revised Classification of Epilepsies and Epileptic Syndromes* in 1989. They are defined on the basis of age-related onset, special clinical and EEG manifestations, and presumed genetic etiology. The term "idiopathic" refers to the absence of a known or suspected cause other than a possible genetic predisposition [1]. The 2017 *Classification of the Epilepsies* defined six etiological categories—genetic, structural, metabolic, immunological, infectious, and unknown—and replaced older terms such as "idiopathic," "cryptogenic," and "symptomatic"; however, IGEs were retained [2]. At present, IGEs are not considered a syndrome but rather separate syndromes caused by childhood absence epilepsy (CAE), juvenile absence epilepsy (JAE), juvenile myoclonic epilepsy (JME), and epilepsy with generalized tonic–clonic seizures alone (GTCA). IGEs usually have a good prognosis, do not develop into epileptiform encephalopathy, and have similar EEG characteristics [2]. In 2022, ILAE adopted IGEs as a separate group of syndromes [1]. This was followed by further subdivision of the epilepsy syndrome according to the origin of the seizures into focal epilepsy, generalized epilepsy, focal and/or generalized epilepsy, and syndromes with developmental and epileptic encephalopathy (DEE) or progressive neurological deterioration, establishing a separate category for the latter [1]. The term "DEE" was introduced in the 2017 Classification of the Epilepsies to denote epilepsy associated with developmental disorders that may be caused by an underlying disease etiology, superimposed epileptic activity, or both [2]. The 2022 ILAE framework recommended merging epilepsy syndromes with DEE and epilepsy syndromes with progressive neurological deterioration to include syndromes associated with cognitive impairment with or without other neurological deterioration, recognizing that such impairment may result from an underlying etiology, an overlapping epileptic activity, or both [1].

In addition, epilepsy syndromes can be divided into self-limiting epilepsy syndromes, epilepsy syndromes with DEE or with progressive neurological deterioration, and other epilepsy syndromes. The terms "severe" (severe infantile myoclonic epilepsy), "malignant" (malignant infantile migratory focal seizures), and "benign" (benign neonatal seizures) have been changed. Terms such as "severe" and "malignant" have been abandoned. The term "benign" was replaced by "self-limited," and the term "partial" was replaced by "focal." A new class of epilepsy syndromes, such as self-limited focal epilepsies, which refer to a group of age-dependent disorders, has been proposed. Patients with self-limiting epilepsy syndromes can have a good long-term prognosis and avoid prolonged use of antiseizure medications (ASMs) and unnecessary tests or treatments. There are also etiology-specific epilepsy syndromes, which have relatively consistent and unique clinical phenotypes, electrophysiological characteristics, neuroimaging findings, treatment, and prognosis; these include electroclinical syndromes with specific genetic or structural etiologies. Most epilepsy syndromes with specific etiologies are rare diseases, and most of those occurring in neonates and infants are related to DEE. Following the development of molecular and genetic testing, the number of epilepsy syndromes with specific etiologies will increase. The diagnosis of epilepsy syndromes with specific etiologies conveys the possibility of new precise treatments and improvements in long-term prognosis [1, 2].

It is important to classify epilepsy according to the syndrome and etiology. The diagnosis of epileptic syndromes provides an important basis for etiological screening, treatment selection, and prognosis determination. Syndrome differentiation according to age groups highlights the characteristics of different syndromes, suggesting the possibility of optimizing clinical treatment [1, 2].

Criteria for Defining Epilepsy Syndromes

According to the 2022 ILAE published report, each syndrome was defined using a clinical template that included "Overview, epidemiology, clinical features (including age of onset, sex, significant prodromal history, cognitive, developmental, and neurological examination at presentation), natural history (including evolution from one syndrome to another, overall response to ASMs and other therapies, likelihood of remission, and risk of specific comorbidities), seizure type, electroencephalogram, neuroimaging, and sequelae." Biological findings, other laboratory studies, and differential diagnosis can be used to assess these parameters The use of this template requires that the core diagnostic criteria for each syndrome be subdivided into the following: ① mandatory: the criteria that must be present in the diagnosis of the syndrome; ② exclusionary: the criteria that must be absent in the diagnosis of the syndrome; and ③ alerts: the vast majority of patients with epilepsy syndrome do not meet the criteria, but the warning alone cannot rule out the syndrome; this should prompt clinicians to reconsider the diagnosis and further examine the patient to rule out other diseases. The appeal template is applicable to both resource-limited and well-resourced areas [1].

5.2 Epilepsy Syndromes with Onset in Neonates and Infants

In May 2022, a report by the ILAE Task Force on Nosology and Definitions proposed the classification and definition of epileptic syndromes in newborns and infants. The age of onset ranged from birth to 2 years (for both premature and full-term infants). Syndromes are divided into self-limiting epilepsy syndromes (epilepsies that may spontaneously remit), developmental and epileptic encephalopathy, and etiology-specific epilepsy syndromes. The incidence of epilepsy in this age group is greater than that in other age groups, with a greater risk of associated cognitive impairment and behavioral comorbidities, a greater mortality rate, and a less effective response to conventional antiseizure medications [1, 2, 12, 13].

5.2.1 Self-Limiting Epileptic Syndrome

5.2.1.1 Self-Limited Familial Neonatal Epilepsy

Overview

Self-limited familial neonatal epilepsy (SLFNE) is a rare autosomal dominant inherited neonatal idiopathic epilepsy that can be divided into self-limited neonatal epilepsy and self-limited familial neonatal epilepsy according to family history [14–16]. The first seizure usually occurs 2–7 days after birth and usually presents as focal tonic, clonic or focal secondary bilateral tonic, or clonic with an uncertain lateralized onset. Seizures occur at intervals of hours or days. The patient's neuropsychological development and electroencephalogram (EEG) results are normal.

History and Epidemiology
SLFNEs were previously called benign neonatal seizures or convulsions and were first reported by Rett [17] and Teubel in 1964. In 2017, ILAE used the terms "self-limiting" and "drug-responsive" to replace "benign" [2]. The incidence of SLFNE is estimated to be 5.3 per 100,000 live births [18].

Etiology
SLFNE is an autosomal dominant ion channelopathy with incomplete penetrance. Pathogenic mutations are found in up to 90% of SLFNE families [16]. Some mutations in *KCNQ2* (located on chromosome 20q13.3), *KCNQ3* (8q24), and *SCN2A* (2q24.3) are related to SLFNE, among which *KCNQ2* is the most common pathogenic gene, while *KCNQ3* and *SCN2A* are expressed at markedly lower levels [16, 18, 19]. The *KCNQ2* and *KCNQ3* genes encode the voltage-gated potassium channel subunits Kv7.2 and Kv7.3.7, respectively. *KCNQ2* mutations causing SLFNE include missense mutations, gene deletions, and frameshift mutations, which cause haploid dose insufficiency and thus reduce potassium channel currents.

Clinical Manifestations
Patients experience seizure onset 2–7 days after birth, usually on day 2 or 3. They generally exhibit spontaneous remission within 6 months, mostly within 6 weeks, and are relieved within several weeks if antiseizure medications are used. In preterm infants, onset occurs at the corresponding corrected gestational age. The incidence ratio is similar for both males and females. There are no significant abnormalities during pregnancy or in the perinatal period [14–16].

Seizures: Patients first experience a focal tonic seizure, which may involve the head, face, and limbs, followed by autonomic nervous symptoms (such as apnea, violet, heart rate changes, etc.), motor symptoms (such as bilateral, local tonic or clonic, or myoclonus, first affecting one side and then the other), and automatic symptoms (such as sucking, chewing, etc.). Focal motor seizures may evolve into bilateral tonic or clonic seizures as the predominant seizure type, with frequent lateral changes occurring during each seizure, which may be clustered with normal interictal periods [15, 16, 20].

Development: Growth and development are usually normal, and head circumference and nervous system physical examination results are normal.

Auxiliary Examination
1. Cranial imaging: No significant abnormalities or epileptogenic focus
2. EEG: A normal background or mild nonspecific abnormalities. The interictal period is mostly normal, or focal abnormalities are common in the central, temporal central, or frontotemporal areas. Typical ictal EEG signals show bilateral

asynchronous low-voltage activity that progresses into spike-and-sharp-wave rhythms [21–23].

3. Genetic testing: The most common abnormality is *KCNQ2* gene mutation, and other abnormalities include *KCNQ3* and *SCN2A* mutations.

Diagnosis

In 2022, the International League Against Epilepsy proposed diagnostic criteria for SLFNE [12], emphasizing its division into three parts:

Mandatory condition: Seizures presented as focal tonic seizures involving the head, face, and limbs. Focal clonic or tonic seizures may alternate from seizure to seizure and may progress to bilateral tonic or clonic seizures.

If the following conditions exist, other diseases should be considered: (1) a clinical history suggesting intrauterine seizures; (2) a slow interictal EEG background; (3) a significant neurological examination; (4) lack of relevant mutations in pathogenic genes, most commonly *KCNQ2* or *KCNQ3*, or lack of family history suggesting Alzheimer's disease (AD) inheritance with incomplete penetrance; (5) long-term mild developmental delay; and (6) persistent seizures after 6 months of age, such as drug-resistant epilepsy.

Diagnosis should be excluded if the patient has any of the following conditions: (1) clinical seizures present with spasm, myoclonus, generalized tonic seizures or generalized tonic–clonic seizures (GTCSs); (2) EEG: persistent focal slowing or moderate-to-severe background slowing (non-postictal) on interictal EEG, burst suppression pattern, hypsarrhythmia, and lack of EEG data associated with clinical seizures during the ictal period; (3) onset after the first month of age; (4) encephalopathy manifestations; (5) neuroimaging suggesting an epileptogenic focus; (6) other causes of seizures, including intracranial infection, ischemia or hemorrhage, hypoxic-ischemic brain injury, or significant metabolic abnormalities; and (7) moderate-to-severe neurodevelopmental disability.

Differential Diagnosis

Acutely provoked seizures induced by hypoxic-ischemic encephalopathy, metabolic diseases, electrolyte imbalances, and cerebrovascular diseases are more common than self-limited neonatal epilepsy. Provoked seizures occur earlier, usually on the first day of life, and have a longer course. Self-limited neonatal epilepsy can be excluded if the patient has manifestations of encephalopathy.

Focal structural abnormalities can also manifest as typical focal clonic seizures.

Benign neonatal sleep myoclonus: The neurological examination and EEG results of a child with benign neonatal sleep myoclonus are normal. Myoclonic seizures are found only in sleep at variable seizure sites, with or without a rhythm, lasting for several seconds, and sometimes even up to 30–60 min, which may lead to misdiagnosis of status epilepticus. Symptoms gradually disappear with age.

Self-limited familial infantile epilepsy: Children develop normally and have cluster seizures, with the first seizure occurring at 4–8 months of age. The most common pathogenic gene is *PRRT2*.

Self-limited familial neonatal–infantile epilepsy: This disease shows onset in the neonatal stage or in infancy. The most common pathogenic gene is *SCN2A*.

Treatment
SLFNE can be resolved spontaneously or with antiseizure medications. Often, it is not directly diagnosed when the first seizure occurs. First-line drugs such as phenobarbital, phenytoin (PHT), and levetiracetam are usually selected for treatment. When a child has frequent seizures, combination drugs are chosen, but their efficacy is poor [22, 24]. Phenobarbital is often ineffective in treating neonatal hereditary epilepsy and has more side effects than new antiseizure medications, such as phenobarbital and phenytoin [23, 25, 26].

Clinical studies have shown that sodium channel blockers, such as carbamazepine (CBZ) or oxcarbazepine (OXC), could be more effective at controlling SLFNE, with faster onset and greater safety [22, 27]. Previous studies have demonstrated that the potassium channel blocker retigabine has a significant effect on epilepsy caused by *KCNQ2*/*KCNQ3* mutations [27, 28]. However, the study of this treatment in clinical trials was halted due to severe adverse reactions. Currently, analogues of retigabine are being studied [29].

Prognosis
Most SLFNE patients achieve remission within 6 months and usually experience normal development. A few may have learning difficulties or mild motor disorders, and a few may have recurrent seizures after infancy, including febrile seizures (FSs) or afebrile seizures. Additionally, a few patients present with self-limited epilepsy with centrotemporal spikes [15, 16, 30].

5.2.1.2 Self-Limited Familial Neonatal–Infantile Epilepsy

Overview
Self-limited familial neonatal–infantile epilepsy (SeLFNIE) is an autosomal dominant epilepsy syndrome characterized by neonatal or infantile onset in different family members [31]. The most common cause is a pathogenic mutation in the *SCN2A* gene [32, 33]. New disease-causing gene variants have been detected in patients without a family history. From 1 day to 23 months of age, nearly half of the children experience neonatal onset [34]. The condition mainly manifests as focal clonus/focal rigidity or secondary generalized attack, revealing the characteristics of cluster onset. Developmental milestones are generally normal [17].

Historical Evolution and Epidemiological Investigation
SeLFNIE, previously known as benign familial neonatal–infantile epilepsy (BFNIS) [2], is the first reported phenotype for SCN2A-related diseases [32, 33]. In 2017, ILAE replaced the term "benign" with "self-limited" and "drug-responsive" [15]. Currently, there is lack of comprehensive epidemiological data on self-limited familial neonatal–infantile epilepsy.

Etiology

SeLFNIE is associated with pathogenic genes such as *SCN2A*, *KCNQ2*, and *PRRT2*. The *SCN2A* gene, reported by Heron et al. in 2002 as the causative gene for SeLFNIE, is located on chromosome 2q24.3 [32]. This gene encodes the α2 subunit of the voltage-gated sodium ion channel (Nav1.2). Most *SCN2A* mutations in SeLFNIE patients are missense mutations, which are generally less harmful [35]. Functional analysis of *SCN2A* variants indicated that gating changes leading to gain-of-function effects explain why many patients respond to sodium channel blockers [36]. Mouse model studies have demonstrated that the expression of Nav1.2 in key hippocampal and cortical neurons diminishes over time; Nav1.2 is eventually replaced by Nav1.6, which rescues channel function. This replacement contributes to the transient and self-limited nature of SeLFNIE during early infancy.

KCNQ2 is the primary pathogenic gene involved in self-limiting (familial) neonatal epilepsy. Research has indicated that self-limited convulsive seizures associated with *KCNQ2* can persist beyond the neonatal period in some families [31, 37, 38]. *PRRT2* gene mutations are infrequently observed in families with SeLFNIE [38].

Clinical Manifestations

Course of the Disease

The disease course ranges from 1 day to 23 months [33]. The ratio of males to females is similar. No special circumstances exist during the perinatal period. Compared with others of the same age, the child has normal growth and development and a normal head circumference and nervous system physical examination. No other clinical manifestations, such as motor disorders, are present.

Seizures

Seizures typically begin with deviated focal tonic movements, followed by tonic and clonic movements. Episodes can sometimes include apnea and binocular gaze, lasting from 20 s to 4 min, with febrile convulsions being rare. The frequency of seizures varies. Some children have infrequent episodes that do not need treatment, while others experience cluster seizures multiple times per day.

Auxiliary Inspection

Cranial Imaging

No significant abnormalities or pathological lesions are observed.

Electroencephalogram

Patients with a normal background activity and an interictal period may exhibit focal or multifocal spikes, with some presenting a completely normal EEG. During frequent seizures, focal discharges, posterior head dominant, or diffuse slow waves are visible [39].

Diagnosis

In 2022, the International Anti-epileptic Alliance proposed three diagnostic criteria [12]:

Preconditions

These include: (1) focal tonic seizures with head and eye deviation, followed by tonic–clonic seizures that may progress to bilateral involvement; (2) onset age: 1 day to 23 months post-birth; and (3) no lesions on magnetic resonance imaging (MRI) of the head.

Notes

Conditions suggesting alternative diagnoses include (1) continuous attack (sequential seizures); (2) a mild, slow background in the interval; (3) history of intracranial infection, ischemia or hemorrhagic attention, ischemia, hypoxic cerebral injury, or significant metabolic disorders; 4) notable neurological deficits; (4) lack of relevant pathogenic genes (typically *SCN2A*); and (5) long-term mild developmental delay, ongoing seizures, or drug-resistant epilepsy after 2 years of age.

The following conditions should be excluded: (1) clinical seizures are spasmic and myoclonic; (2) EEG: persistent focal slowing or moderate-to-severe background slowing (non-seizure), suppression of waveform and high arrhythmia; (3) lack of EEG data related to clinical seizures during the seizure; (4) encephalopathy; (5) neuroimaging suggests epileptogenic lesions; and (6) moderate-to-severe neurodevelopmental disorders.

In medically underserved areas, even if there are no head MRI or EEG results, a diagnosis of SeLFNIE can be made if it is present in a child's family as long as the diagnostic criteria and other conditions are met and all exclusion conditions and precautions are not met. However, the patient should be closely monitored for SeLFNIE features.

Differential Diagnosis

Distinguishing between self-limited (familial) neonatal epilepsy and self-limited (familial) infantile epilepsy can be challenging; a detailed family history of epilepsy is critical for differentiation.

Symptomatic epilepsy in newborns or infants may result from hypoxic-ischemic encephalopathy, infections, stroke, or metabolic diseases.

Structural etiologies such as brain malformations should be considered in infants with persistent focal convulsions.

Treatment

SeLFNIE may resolve spontaneously or require medical treatment. For SeLFNIE related to *SCN2A* mutations, antiepileptic drugs, especially sodium channel blockers such as phenytoin, oxcarbazepine, and carbamazepine, are effective [34, 38, 39]. Sodium channel blockers are particularly useful for treating seizures under 3 months of age. However, these agents might be less effective or even worsen seizures in patients whose symptoms begin after 3 months of age. The early stage of the disease may be resistant to standard antiepileptic drugs, such as phenobarbital, topiramate (TPM), levetiracetam, and valproate. Phenobarbital and phenytoin sodium are effective for treating SeLFNIE due to *KCNQ2* mutations [40]. Considering their adverse effects in newborns, the use of sodium ion channel blockers (carbamazepine or oxcarbazepine) is recommended.

Prognosis
Some children's symptoms may resolve spontaneously. While some children experience only a few attacks and do not require treatment, others may have several cluster attacks daily. Seizures typically cease between 12 and 24 months of age and do not recur. They are usually well-controlled with antiepileptic drugs. Development is usually normal [38].

5.2.1.3 Self-Limiting Familial Infantile Epilepsy

Overview
Self-limited familial infantile epilepsy (SeLIE) is a syndrome of infancy onset that mostly occurs at 3–20 months [41]. Infants with a family history and normal development often experience frequent cluster seizures, which occur 8–10 times every 1–3 days [41]. The attack type is mostly focal with conscious damage, often combined with hemilateral clonus and head and eye deviation, and can also be combined with facial or limb automatisms. In patients with a family history, *PRRT2* pathogenic variants can be detected in more than 80% of patients [42, 43], and other related genes include *SCN8A*, *KCNQ2*, *KCNQ3*, and *SCN2A* [32].

Historical Evolution and Epidemiological Investigation
In 1963, Fukuyama reported a group of patients under 2 years of age with epilepsy characterized by focal convulsions, an unknown etiology, and favorable outcomes [44]. Vigevano et al. further described epilepsy patients with a family history and good prognosis, with autosomal dominant genetic characteristics, and proposed benign infantile familial convulsions [45]. Subsequently, studies investigating several different populations identified this new epilepsy syndrome [46–51]. In 2001, the Working Group of the International Alliance (International League Against Epilepsy, ILAE) formally included this syndrome [52]. In 2010, ILAE classified benign familial infantile epilepsy as an electroclinical syndrome and recommended the application of the term "self-limiting" instead of "benign" [53]. According to the new definition and concept of the 2017 ILAE classification, the term "benign" was replaced by "self-limiting" or "drug-responsive" [2].

SeLIE is relatively common, accounting for 7–9% of all epilepsy cases before 2 years of age [2], with an estimated incidence of 14.2 per 100,000 live births [54].

Etiology
PRRT2 is the most common causal gene in this syndrome [18, 54, 55]. In patients with a family history, it is autosomal dominant with high penetrance. Causative genes can be identified in approximately 80% of patients [54].

Clinical Manifestations

The age of onset is 3–20 months, and the highest incidence age is 6 months. Patients typically have no special perinatal history and exhibit normal head circumference and neurological examination results.

Patients with Pathogenic Variants of *PRRT2*

Seizures in these patients are mainly focal with consciousness disorders, and they originate in the temporal, central, parietal, and occipital regions, with or without secondary generalized seizures [56]. Seizures are mostly cluster seizures. Among them, motor cessation, decreased consciousness, and automatism are relatively rare [57], and patients rarely develop status epilepticus. Approximately 30% of the paroxysmal dyskinesias caused by *PRRT2* lead to SeLIE. Another group of patients with a 16p11.2 microdeletion (including the *PRRT2* gene) may also be associated with developmental delay, mental retardation, and/or autism [58–61].

Patients with the Pathogenic *SCN8A* Variant

Epilepsy often occurs before 1 year of age (the mean age of onset is 6 months). Seizure types may include focal seizures, focal generalization to bilateral tonic–clonic seizures, and bilateral tonic–clonic seizures. Patients may also experience paroxysmal dyskinesia, triggered by stretching, initiating actions, or emotional stimulation, often occurring during adolescence [62].

Patients with the *KCNQ2* Pathogenic Variant

Among some members of the SeLIE family, there is increased peripheral excitability of the nerve, manifested as myotonia [63].

Patients with the *KCNQ3* Pathogenic Variant

Children with normal development develop transient, recurrent, focal, and secondary systemic seizures within 1 year of age, and these seizures disappear after 1–2 years of age. These seizures are usually short, lasting for approximately 2 min, and have cluster onset characteristics. For infants, seizures are normal, and, despite these seizures, psychomotor development is also usually normal [64].

Auxiliary Examination

The EEG background is normal, and focal slow waves can be observed after the attack [41]. Interictal EEG signals are usually normal, and midline areas also exhibit specific activity patterns [64–66]. Focal discharges can be monitored during seizure EEG signals; these discharges usually start in the temporal region or posterior head and may spread to the bilateral hemispheres [41]. In the same patient, epileptic seizures can arise from various brain regions or both hemispheres; however, the EEG pattern remains consistent for each individual seizure.

If the patient's clinical and EEG features are highly typical, if they have a corresponding family history, and/or if a *PRRT2* pathogenic variant is present, cranial imaging is not necessarily needed; if a focal lesion associated with the episode is found, the syndrome needs to be revisited.

Diagnosis
The International Anti-epilepsy Alliance has proposed diagnostic criteria for this disease, which include three parts: ① Necessary criteria: behavioral cessation, impaired consciousness, automatism, head/eye deviation, and focal tonic features (often from one side to the contralateral side and progressing to bilateral tonic or clonic seizures). The attack is usually brief (<3 min). For long-range or focal (hemi) clonic seizures (>10 min), the interphase EEG background is mildly slower, with late onset (18–36 months of age) ② Exclusionary criteria: Special seizure types (epileptic spasms (ESs), myoclonus, combined epilepsy, tonic seizure); persistent focal slow waves or moderate or above moderate background slowing after onset; high degree of arrhythmia; age of onset <1 month or >36 months; moderate-to-significant regression in neurocognitive development; and the presence of brain MR lesions that could explain the onset, neurocognitive developmental regression associated with myoclonic epilepsy, ataxia, or spasticity. ③ Alerts: Mild developmental delay; significant neurological examination abnormalities (except for incidental findings); lack of evidence of pathogenic variants (*PRRT 2*, *SCN2A*, *KCNQ2*, *KCNQ3*) or family history (autosomal dominant inheritance with incomplete penetrance); and symptoms persisting into older age [12].

At diagnosis, seizure EEG is not essential, and brain MRI is performed to exclude lesions [67].

In areas with limited medical resources, SeLIE can be diagnosed without EEG or brain MRI, provided that infants with a family history meet all necessary clinical criteria, excluding other conditions. However, the evolution of the medical history of the affected family members should be consistent with SeLIE, and the child should be closely followed up to determine whether the evolution of the disease course is consistent with SeLIE [12].

Differential Diagnosis
Self-Limited Familial Neonatal Epilepsy

It is necessary to distinguish between self-limited familial neonatal epilepsy and self-limited familial neonatal–infantile epilepsy syndrome, which typically presents earlier in family members.

Infant Convulsions

Infant convulsions are caused by acute illness, such as cerebral hemorrhage, heat stroke infection, or hypoglycemia.

Epilepsy Caused by Structural Etiology

Epilepsy can occur due to cortical dysplasia or brain damage.

Baby ant Focal Epilepsy

Patients with a single focal seizure can be observed via synchronous EEG monitoring, often accompanied by developmental delays.

Dravet Syndrome (DS)

Dravet syndrome patients can also present with focal clonus or lateral clonic seizures, but these seizures are often long-term attacks and mostly heat-sensitive, and most of them are drug-refractory.

Metabolic Diseases

In addition to focal convulsions, such patients often present with progressive epileptic encephalopathy and/or other organ insufficiency, sometimes accompanied by biochemical abnormalities or enzymatic abnormalities.

Treatment

PRRT2-Induced SeLIE

For 33 *PRRT2* gene-related epilepsy patients, sodium channel blockers (carbamazepine, oxcarbazepine, etc.) were the most effective antiseizure medications (ASMs) [66]. However, there is lack of special drugs available for preventing paroxysmal dyskinesia.

KCNQ2-Related SeLIE

A systematic review of 40 patients (approximately 30%) with 133 self-limited familial neonatal seizures has been recently conducted [66]. *KCNQ2*-related seizures are usually controlled by conventional ASM therapy, with phenobarbital and sodium channel blockers (CBZ, OXC, lamotrigine (LTG), and PHT) being the most common [22].

SCN8A Association of SeLIE Therapy

Studies have shown that people with focal seizure phenotypes (*SCN8A*-DEE, *SCN8A* mild-onset developmental and epileptic encephalopathy (mild/MODEE), and *SCN8A*-SeLIE) respond well to sodium channel blockers (e.g., phenytoin, sodium valproate, carbamazepine, lacosamide (LSM), lamotrigine, rufinamide, and oxcarbazepine). Other categories of ASMs may also be useful [68–70]. The effectiveness of sodium channel blockers is consistent with pathogenic gain-of-function variants in SCN8A [71–73].

KCNQ3 Correlation with SeLIE Treatment

SeLIE seizures can be usually completely controlled by the antiepileptic drugs phenobarbital, carbamazepine, or sodium valproate. If adequately treated, few recurrences occur; seizure recurrence is usually caused by a low starting dose of ASM [74].

Prognosis

This disease has a good prognosis. Although it often occurs in the initial stage, it usually resolves within 1 year of onset. During the onset of epilepsy, untreated patients can have independent or transient cluster seizures [64]. In a few cases, patients may continue to experience epilepsy into old age.

5.2.1.4 Genetic Epilepsy with Febrile Seizures Plus

Overview

Genetic epilepsy with febrile seizures plus (GEFS+) is a familial syndrome that usually has an autosomal dominant mode of inheritance or complex inheritance patterns [1, 12]. The most common types of phenotypes are febrile seizures (FSs) and febrile seizures plus (FS+) [2], when seizures with fever persist beyond the age of 6 years or when they are associated with afebrile tonic–clonic seizures [12]. However, other seizure types can also occur in family members, with the most common being genetic generalized epilepsy, focal epilepsy without FSs, developmental and epileptic encephalopathy, such as Dravet syndrome (DS), and epilepsy with myoclonic–atonic epilepsy (MAE) [2].

History and Epidemiology

GEFS+ was previously known as generalized epilepsy with febrile seizures plus. In 1997, Professors Scheffer and Berkovic [2] first reported GEFS+, which was defined as a familial epilepsy syndrome with marked phenotypic heterogeneity [13]. Later studies revealed that some patients with GEFS+ also had focal epilepsy. Therefore, this disease was renamed genetic epilepsy with febrile seizures plus.

GEFS+ is relatively common in patients with epilepsy syndromes, but epidemiological data are lacking.

Etiology

Although most GEFS+ patients exhibit complex inheritance patterns, up to one-third of cases are clearly caused by single-gene abnormalities and are usually autosomal dominant [2]; among these cases, the most commonly mutated genes are *SCN1A*, *SCN1B*, *SCN2A*, *SCN9A*, *GABRG2*, and *STX1B* [2], and the proportions of *SCN1A*, *GABRG2*, and *SCN1B* variation are 19%, 9%, and 8%, respectively [2].

Clinical Manifestations

GEFS+ is genetically heterogeneous and shows diverse clinical manifestations. FS is the most common symptom in patients with GEFS+, followed by FS+ [14]. Neurological examination and cognitive function are often normal in children with FS/FS+. In addition to presenting with FS/FS+, some patients also have other generalized seizures, such as absence, myoclonic, and atonic seizures. Furthermore, GEFS+ can also coincide with focal seizures, such as frontal lobe epilepsy and temporal lobe epilepsy. MAE and DS are the most severe symptoms in GEFS+ patients (details are reported in the corresponding sections). If children present with long-range focal clonic seizures (hemiclonic) with fever before 15 months of age, especially when the disease recurs, they should be alerted for DS.

FS

FS often presents with tonic–clonic seizures associated with fever (38 °C), typically accompanied by bilateral involvement; most patients spontaneously resolve in a short time, and a few cases may persist for more than 30 min [15–17]. In GEFS+

patients, onset may occur earlier than 6 months of age or still recur at more than 6 years of age, unlike in typical FSs [1, 13].

FS+

Nine percent of patients with FS progress to FS+ [18], which refers to febrile seizures that recur and/or progress to afebrile seizures after the age of 6 years, and the most common of which are typical febrile seizures that persist after 6 years. The age at which afebrile seizures appear is often variable.

Auxiliary Examination

The EEG background is normal, and focal generalized spinous slow waves are occasionally observed on interictal EEG. Ictal EEG is often consistent with the seizure type. When diagnosing GEFS+, brain MRI is required to rule out epileptogenic focus.

Diagnosis

GEFS+ refers to familial epilepsy syndrome in which at least two family members have phenotypes that fit within the GEFS+ spectrum and at least one of them is diagnosed with FS+. If the family members do not have FS+ phenotypes, at least three family members are required to have other classic GEFS+ phenotypes (e.g., febrile seizures or MAE) [2].

Differential Diagnosis

Familial Febrile Seizures

If all members of the family present only with FS, familial febrile seizures should be diagnosed instead of GEFS+ [2].

Infant Seizures Caused by Other Etiologies

Examples include ischemia, infection, and hypoglycemia.

Structural Etiology

In the diagnosis of GEFS+, structural etiology, such as cortical dysplasia or brain injury, needs to be excluded.

Treatment

GEFS+ includes a variety of phenotypes, on the basis of which appropriate drugs are selected. Among these, the most common phenotypes are FS and FS+. Approximately one-third of GEFS+ cases are related to pathogenic variants in *SCN1A*, *SCN1B*, *GABRG2*, and other genes, and medications that can increase seizures should be avoided during treatment. In summary, treatment of GEFS+ should involve a combination of phenotypic and pathogenic gene information. Specific treatments for patients with MAE or DS according to the GEFS+ criteria are described in the relevant sections.

Patients with FS and FS+

Patients with FS+ respond well to antiseizure medications, and patients with FS or FS+ generally do not need long-term drug therapy. However, for some patients with FS or FS+, it is difficult to prevent seizures with intermittent medication during fever.

Treatment of Febrile Convulsive Status Epilepticus

Acute-phase febrile convulsive status epilepticus should be treated according to the general treatment guidelines for status epilepticus. Benzodiazepines (BZDs) administered via the vein, buccal mucosa, or rectum can terminate most febrile convulsive status epilepticus. Midazolam administered through the buccal mucosa may be more effective than intrarectal diazepam [19].

GEFS+ Caused by *SCN1A* Pathogenic Variants

For these patients, especially those with DS, it is necessary to avoid sodium channel blockers, such as carbamazepine, lamotrigine, and oxcarbazepine, which may aggravate seizures through blocking intermediate (inhibitory) neuronal sodium channels. In such patients, it is necessary to be vigilant for sudden unexpected death in epilepsy (SUDEP). Prolonged seizure activity may lead to lasting brain damage, and attention needs to be paid to treating convulsive status epilepticus.

Prognosis
Not all FS+ patients require prophylaxis, and antiseizure medications are usually effective. If patients present only with FS+, the disease is usually self-limiting before adolescence [13]. Patients with different phenotypes of GEFS+ receive different treatments and have different prognoses.

5.2.1.5 Myoclonic Epilepsy of Infancy (MEI)

Overview
MEI, a rare neurological disorder that can occur during infancy, is characterized by myoclonic jerks as the primary manifestation of epilepsy onset [12]. Approximately one-third of patients exhibit reflexive myoclonic seizures triggered by stimuli such as noise, touch, or startle [75]. In the majority of cases, epileptic episodes demonstrate a self-limiting nature [12].

Historical Evolution and Epidemiological Investigations
MEI was previously termed "benign myoclonic epilepsy in infants (BMEI)." Dravet and Bureau first described this disease in 1981 [76]. In 1989, ILAE categorized BMEI under age-related idiopathic generalized epilepsy syndromes [11]. In the 2022 ILAE classification of epilepsy syndromes, MEI was categorized as an infantile-onset generalized epilepsy syndrome. MEI is a rare condition that affects <0.8% of epileptic children treated at epilepsy centers and 1.1% of all epilepsy patients with onset before 36 months of age in population cohorts [12]. It is more common in boys than in girls. This syndrome is characterized by brief generalized myoclonic seizures occurring within the first 2 years of life in developmentally

healthy children. Pre-seizure developmental trajectories are typically normal. However, mild cognitive, behavioral, or motor impairments can accompany onset, and neurological examination usually yields normal findings.

Etiology

The genetic basis of this condition remains unclear. Stephane et al. [75] reported no significant correlation between MEI and prenatal, perinatal, or postnatal factors. Approximately 10% of patients have a family history of epilepsy or febrile seizures [75].

Clinical Presentation

MEI manifests between the ages of 4 months and 3 years, with a peak incidence occurring between 6 and 18 months [12]. Neurodevelopmental assessments conducted before or during the onset of the disease typically reveal normal findings, or mild developmental anomalies may be observed.

Myoclonic Seizures

Myoclonus is a pivotal diagnostic criterion, and myoclonic seizures in MEI typically involve the head and upper arms and occur during both wakefulness and sleep. These seizures are characterized by their brief duration, occurring as solitary events or in clusters, with variability in frequency and intensity among individuals. Clinical manifestations commonly include jerking movements of the head, while bending or extension of the body is relatively less frequent. During myoclonic jerks, the upper limbs often rapidly abduct and elevate, while the eyes may exhibit upward movement. Transient vocalizations may arise from diaphragmatic contractions and can sometimes accompany myoclonic movements of the limbs. In a minority of cases, patients may experience falls, primarily due to involvement of the lower limbs.

Apart from clustered presentations, which may involve mild alterations in consciousness, awareness during seizures is typically preserved.

Myoclonus occurs spontaneously during wakefulness and is often self-limiting, although its frequency may increase during drowsiness and slow-wave sleep. Some patients exhibit a propensity for clustered myoclonic events during the first hour of awakening or when asleep. Roberto H et al. [77] reported several brief and isolated myoclonic events occurring in 38 patients during the wakefulness period and the first 2 stages of sleep, several times a day, lasting between 3 and 7 s. Only 7.8% of patients experienced myoclonic events exclusively in states of drowsiness. A total of 21% of the patients displayed extensive myoclonus, primarily involving the lower limbs, resulting in sudden drop attacks. A total of 28.9% of the seizures occurred in clusters, while 31.5% presented with reflexive myoclonus.

Other Seizure Types

One-fifth of patients often experience infrequent and brief simple febrile seizures preceding myoclonic seizures, and another one-fifth of patients may exhibit infrequent generalized tonic–clonic seizures (GTCSs) in early adolescence. Unclassified afebrile seizures may precede myoclonic seizures or emerge during the disease course [78].

Triggering Factors

Approximately one-third of patients exhibit reflexive myoclonic seizures triggered by stimuli such as noise, touch, or startle [75, 79, 80].

Ancillary Investigations

The awake-state electroencephalogram (EEG) background activity of MEI patients is typically normal. The interictal EEG pattern manifests as generalized spike-and-wave complexes, occasionally evolving into generalized polyspike-and-wave discharges, which are particularly evident during early sleep stages [77]. Flash stimulation does not elicit spike-and-wave discharges in the absence of concurrent myoclonic jerks; however, photosensitivity bursts may be observed in some patients after the cessation of myoclonic seizures. During myoclonic seizure episodes, EEG activity reveals transient generalized spike-and-wave complexes, polyspikes, and discharges at approximately 3 Hz [12]. Myoclonus can be activated during drowsiness and sleep, triggered by sudden noises, tactile stimuli, or startles, and occasionally by intermittent photic stimulation [81]. Synchronized electromyographic recording aids in diagnosis. Laboratory investigations are typically within normal limits, and neuroimaging studies reveal no epileptogenic lesions [11, 75–77, 79, 81].

Diagnosis

ILAE has proposed diagnostic criteria, emphasizing three components: (1) Essential criteria: The presence of myoclonic seizures with a normal EEG background. (2) Additional noteworthy points: At onset, seizures may present as afebrile generalized tonic–clonic seizures or generalized clonic seizures; interictal EEG lacks generalized spike-and-wave discharges during sleep and demonstrates a low-frequency photoparoxysmal response (indicative of ceroid lipofuscinosis type 2 (CLN2) disease). The diagnostic criteria include concurrent language developmental delay, moderate-to-severe intellectual disability (ID), and prominent neurological examination abnormalities. These features may not necessarily signify MEI. (3) Exclusion criteria: Patients with onset of myoclonic seizures at ≤6 months or >3 years of age are excluded. The exclusion criteria include absence seizures, atonic seizures, tonic–clonic seizures, focal sensory impairment seizures, focal clonic (hemifacial clonic) seizures, myoclonic–atonic seizures, and tonic seizures. Seizure EEG may record myoclonic events without EEG changes, or interictal EEG may display high-amplitude dysrhythmia or generalized slow spike-and-wave activity (<2.5 Hz). Exclusion is required in the presence of significant neuroimaging abnormalities, malformation, or other congenital anomalies (suggesting chromosomal disorders) or neurocognitive regression. In patients with low cerebrospinal fluid (CSF) glucose or pathogenic SLC2A1 variants (those with glucose transporter type 1 deficiency syndrome (Glut1-DS)), exclusion is necessary [12].

Differential Diagnosis

Infantile Spasms Syndrome

This syndrome is characterized by epileptic spasms rather than myoclonic seizures. Epileptic spasms tend to occur shortly after awakening, unlike the myoclonic jerks observed in infantile myoclonic epilepsy, which can occur during both wakefulness and sleep. The duration of epileptic spasms exceeds 1 s. Interictal EEG signals in this syndrome are often abnormal and show high-amplitude dysrhythmia or multifocal discharges. Seizure EEG monitoring can also distinguish between epileptic spasms and myoclonic seizures.

Dravet Syndrome

Dravet syndrome is characterized by prolonged seizures triggered by fever and status epilepticus. Myoclonic seizures typically appear later in the course of the syndrome.

Lennox–Gastaut Syndrome

This syndrome is characterized by prominent atonic seizures, tonic seizures, and atypical absence seizures and is not observed in patients with infantile myoclonic epilepsy.

Myoclonic–Atonic Seizures

Epilepsy is characterized by myoclonic–atonic seizures, atypical absence seizures, generalized tonic–clonic seizures, and nonconvulsive status epilepticus (NSE). These occur during preschool and school-age years. These seizure types are not observed in infantile myoclonic epilepsy.

Early Infantile Developmental and Epileptic Encephalopathy (EIDEE)

Apart from myoclonic seizures, multiple seizure types are present, with significant developmental delay and severe EEG abnormalities.

Various Neurological Metabolic Disorders

Various neurological metabolic disorders include small molecule, mitochondrial, and storage disorders, which may lead to the early postnatal onset of myoclonic seizures. These conditions are often associated with progressive neurological dysfunction and dysfunction of other organ systems.

Glucose Transporter Type 1 Deficiency Syndrome (Glut1-DS)

This syndrome is characterized by mild-to-moderate microcephaly; epilepsy involving seizure types other than myoclonic seizures; low cerebrospinal fluid (CSF) glucose levels; low CSF-to-blood glucose ratio; and pathogenic variants in the *SLC2A1* gene (if feasible, genetic testing can be performed).

Progressive Myoclonic Epilepsy (PME)

This disease is characterized by significant language or motor regression and is often accompanied by seizure types other than myoclonic seizures, MRI findings frequently revealing brain atrophy, and the occurrence of a photoparoxysmal response to low-frequency photic stimulation (indicative of a possible CLN2 disease).

Nonepileptic Seizures

1. The distinction of infantile benign myoclonus lies in the absence of ictal electroencephalogram (EEG) changes during myoclonic locking.
2. Startle seizures present pathological startle reactions without any abnormalities in the EEG.
3. Sleep-related myoclonus constitutes a normal sleep-related event that most commonly occurs during light sleep stages.
4. Tremor episodes involve repetitive, rapid tremulous movements typically induced by excitement; however, there is no correlation with EEG findings.

Treatment
There are currently no evidence-based treatment guidelines specific to MEI. Standard broad-spectrum antiepileptic drugs (such as levetiracetam, clobazam (CLB), and valproate) are utilized to manage seizures [77].

Prognosis
Myoclonic seizures in MEI patients often resolve spontaneously within 6 months to 5 years of onset, and most patients can discontinue antiepileptic medications [75]. Approximately 10% of patients may develop other seizure types in the future, with adolescent myoclonic epilepsy being the most common [75, 77]. The majority of patients have favorable neurodevelopmental outcomes, although some individuals might experience intellectual disabilities, learning difficulties, or attention issues [12, 76].

5.2.2 Developmental and Epileptic Encephalopathy

5.2.2.1 Early Infantile Developmental and Epileptic Encephalopathy

Overview
Early infantile developmental and epileptic encephalopathy (EIDEE) is characterized by an early onset and frequent seizures occurring within the first 3 months of life and often demonstrates drug resistance. Abnormalities, including posture, tone, or motor abnormalities, are noted on neurological examination. Electroencephalography (EEG) reveals burst suppression, slow-wave activity, and abundant multifocal discharges, and, as the disease progresses, this can lead to severe developmental delay [12, 82, 83].

Historical Evolution and Epidemiological Investigations
EIDEE is a rare disorder with an estimated incidence of 10 per 100,000 live births [13]. In the 2022 update of the ILAE classification, the previously designated Ohtahara syndrome and early myoclonic encephalopathy (EME) were reclassified under EIDEE. This is due to substantial overlap in their electroclinical features and similar underlying etiologies.

Etiology
EIDEE has several potential underlying causes, including genetic, metabolic, and structural factors [18, 82]. The most common causes include brain malformations and congenital metabolic disorders, such as hemispheric dysplasia, agenesis of the corpus callosum, developmental brain anomalies, focal cortical dysplasia (FCD), nonketotic hyperglycinemia, organic acidemia, Menkes disease, and molybdenum cofactor deficiency [18, 84, 85].

Clinical Presentation
Onset occurs within the first 3 months of birth. Neurological examination at onset might reveal hypotonia or spasticity, often accompanied by asymmetric movements [12]. Developmental delay can occur at seizure onset or rapidly follow. The diagnosis of EIDEE requires the presence of tonic or myoclonic seizures. Other seizure types include focal clonic seizures and epileptic spasms. Sequential seizures may be observed [12].

EIDEE encompasses one or more of the following seizure types: tonic seizures, myoclonic seizures, epileptic spasms, and sequential seizures involving tonic, clonic, and/or autonomic and autonomic symptomatology. However, there is no single predominant seizure type. Tonic seizures are frequent and can occur singly or in clusters of 10–20 per day. The distinction between clusters of tonic seizures and spasms includes the following: (1) Tonic seizures are typically unrelated to the sleep cycle, whereas spasms usually occur during wakefulness and (2) tonic seizures have a longer duration than spasms (tonic seizures last longer than 3 s, while spasms last less). Tonic seizures in the neonatal period can be focal or asymmetric.

Focal or multifocal myoclonus may be the predominant seizure type. The frequency of myoclonus can vary from isolated to nearly continuous. Myoclonus may be erratic or symmetrical, manifesting as large-amplitude bilateral movements. Erratic myoclonus is characterized by asynchronous, asymmetrical, and random movements that can involve the face, limbs, eyebrows, lips, or fingers. It can occur during wakefulness and sleep. This type of erratic myoclonus is more commonly associated with metabolic etiologies.

Some patients might experience epileptic spasms, which typically appear after the first month of life and often cluster during wakefulness.

Sequential seizures are characterized by the occurrence of different seizure manifestations in succession during a single seizure episode. For example, a sequence may start with focal tonic seizures, followed by focal clonic seizures and then epileptic spasms, without a single predominant symptom. In addition to the abovementioned seizure types, focal motor seizures might also be present.

Diagnostic Workup
Electroencephalogram (EEG)

The characteristic EEG background pattern of EIDEE is burst suppression, which may occur not only during sleep but also during all sleep–wake periods. While myoclonic seizures may not always exhibit a distinctive EEG seizure pattern, focal, clonic, or tonic seizures often manifest with evident epileptic patterns. In later stages of the disease, EEG signals can evolve to show high-amplitude disorganization or multifocal spikes and sharp waves.

1. *Interictal period*: The background can appear abnormal and is characterized by burst suppression and multifocal spike/spike-and-slow-wave complexes with or without slow waves or intermittent and/or diffuse slow waves. In some patients, the background may normalize early in the course of the disease but deteriorate rapidly with increasing seizure frequency. Burst suppression includes high-voltage mixed spikes and sharp-slow wave bursts (150–300 spikes) lasting for 1–5 s, followed by a marked suppression phase lasting for 3–10 s (<5 μV), although the duration may be affected by medication. Burst suppression can be recorded during both wakefulness and sleep and is unresponsive to stimulation. Typically, bilateral abnormalities are observed, but they can also be asymmetrical, asynchronous, or even unilateral. Focal low-voltage activity may also be observed. In some children, an abnormal EEG background may be evident before the onset of seizures and burst suppression becomes apparent only after the onset of seizures. Burst suppression may disappear with age, but abnormal EEG patterns persist. In infants evolving to infantile epileptic spasms syndrome (IESS), high-amplitude disorganization may appear as they grow older. If the cause is treatable (metabolic or surgically correctable structural lesion), the EEG may improve or even normalize.
2. *Ictal period*: The seizure pattern depends on the seizure type. In the neonatal period, seizures often exhibit focal or asymmetric patterns. With the onset of tonic seizures, burst suppression can decrease with the appearance of low-voltage, high-frequency fast activity. Myoclonus may be related to spike-and-wave or sharp-wave complexes. Erratic or fragmented myoclonus may not cause the occurrence of EEG changes during the ictal period. Focal seizures correlate with focal ictal recruitment rhythms. The ictal pattern of sequential seizures changes with evolving clinical presentation. Epileptic spasms may be accompanied by generalized or focal high-amplitude sharp or slow waves, followed by low-voltage fast rhythm and voltage attenuation. Additionally, ictal EEG discharges may or may not correlate with clinical seizures.

Imaging

Structural brain abnormalities are significant and common causes of EIDEE; thus, all affected children should undergo brain imaging to assess structural abnormalities. If drug-resistant epilepsy or evident focal symptoms are present, further imaging should be considered to exclude surgically treatable lesions. For certain genetic etiologies, initial imaging may be normal or demonstrate reduced brain volume or abnormal white matter myelination. Progressive brain atrophy may become evident as the disease progresses.

Genetics

The following investigations are recommended: ① chromosomal microarray analysis (CMA) and karyotype (especially in infants with dysmorphic features or associated extracranial anomalies, e.g., ring chromosome 14) and ② next-generation sequencing (NGS) techniques: epilepsy gene panel, whole exome sequencing (WES), or whole genome sequencing (preferred for infants without obvious dysmorphic features).

Epileptic seizure types and electroencephalograms (EEGs) combined with phenotypic features can predict genotypes:

1. Pathogenic variations in *KCNQ2*-DEE are associated with sequential seizures (primarily involving tonic components but also related to spasms and tonic, myoclonic, tonic–clonic, or autonomic seizures) (see subsequent section). These variations can also be observed in patients with tonic seizures with only burst suppression or multifocal EEG abnormalities. There may be affected individuals in the family with self-limited familial infantile epilepsy.
2. Patients with pathogenic variations in *SCN2A*-DEE may manifest sequential seizures predominantly characterized by tonic seizures and autonomic features.
3. *SCN8A*-DEE pathogenic variations are associated with focal epileptic seizures.
4. Pathogenic variations in *STXBP1*-DEE are related to asymmetric tonic or sequential seizures (tonic, autonomic, spasms, and tonic–clonic seizures).
5. Other chronic diseases, such as cyclin-dependent kinase-like 5-related developmental and epileptic encephalopathy (*CDKL5*-DEE), are linked to tonic seizures; sequential seizures often recur with the "hyperkinetic–tonic–clonic" phenotype. Pathogenic variations in *KCNT1*-DEE may present as focal tonic seizures with autonomic symptoms; *UBA5*-DEE pathogenic variations primarily manifest as myoclonic seizures.

Recommended Metabolic Investigations

These include the following:

1. Urinary organic acids and amino acids (including S-sulfo homocysteine) and urinary α-amino isocaproic semialdehyde
2. Plasma amino acids, lactate, uric acid, copper/ceruloplasmin, blood ammonia, acylcarnitine profile, and very long-chain fatty acids
3. Cerebrospinal fluid glucose, lactate, pyruvate, amino acids, and neurotransmitters

Diagnosis

The International League Against Epilepsy has proposed diagnostic criteria for EIDEE: ① Essential criteria: Onset of tonic and/or myoclonic seizures within the first 3 months of life (adjusted based on prematurity) with burst suppression or multifocal discharges on interictal EEG. Developmental abnormalities are present either before or shortly after the onset of seizures, with subsequent neurodevelopmental abnormalities, including intellectual disability. ② Cautionary criteria: Patients with normal disease onset are less likely to have EIDEE.

Differential Diagnosis

Seizures related to ischemic-hypoxic encephalopathy, infections, acute reversible metabolic disturbances, and stroke or intracranial hemorrhage can manifest as myoclonic, focal clonic, or focal tonic seizures. There may be pronounced encephalopathy and burst suppression patterns on EEG. Symptomatic seizures are more common than EIDEE-related seizures, and relevant investigations should be carried out to exclude acute etiologies. However, certain genetic causes of EIDEE, including molybdenum cofactor deficiency and sulfite oxidase deficiency, can display imaging features similar to those of hypoxic-ischemic brain injury.

Treatment

Initial treatment involves the use of standard antiepileptic drugs to manage seizures, although EIDEE is often drug-resistant. As our understanding of the genetic basis of EIDEE has increased, there has been growing interest in more targeted therapies, leading to a more optimistic outlook [86]. Sodium channel-blocking antiepileptic drugs may be effective in treating EIDEE caused by pathogenic variations in the *KCNQ2*, *SCN2A*, or *SCN8A* genes. Drugs such as carbamazepine, oxcarbazepine, lacosamide, or phenytoin could be considered. For certain metabolic disorders and vitamin-dependent epilepsies, treatment with specific vitamins may be beneficial [87]. A ketogenic diet (KD) has been shown to have efficacy for some patients with EIDEE [88]. Additionally, surgical interventions, such as hemispherectomy or more individualized focal cortical dysplasia resections [89–91], might be effective in select patients. Importantly, treatment approaches should be personalized based on the specific genetic and metabolic factors contributing to EIDEE in each patient.

Prognosis

The overall prognosis for patients with EIDEE is poor, and patients often exhibit severe developmental delay, motor impairments, and shortened life expectancy [92]. Approximately 50% of affected infants do not survive infancy. Many patients with EIDEE may progress to a high-amplitude slowing of the background rhythm on their EEG, which might be asymmetric if there is hemispheric or unilateral focal cortical dysplasia. Other patients might develop multifocal or focal spikes on EEG.

EIDEE represents earliest-onset age-dependent encephalopathy, which also includes infantile epileptic spasms syndrome with suppression bursts (IESS) and Lennox–Gastaut syndrome [93]. These three diseases share common features including (1) specific onset age, (2) profound intellectual disability, (3) EEG readings revealing abundant epileptiform abnormalities, (4) frequent and drug-resistant seizures, and (5) potential progression from one syndrome to another depending on the patient's age.

As a result, when infants or young children with EIDEE reach several months of age, they might develop IESS and subsequently develop Lennox–Gastaut syndrome during childhood. This progression is often associated with specific seizure types and prognoses corresponding to each stage.

5.2.2.2 Infantile Epileptic Spasms Syndrome

Overview

Infantile epileptic spasms syndrome (IESS) is a common refractory developmental and epileptic encephalopathy characterized by epileptic spasm (ES) onset between 1 and 24 months of age (with a peak between 3 and 12 months), hypsarrhythmia on EEG, and developmental stagnation or regression. The pathogenesis of the disease is unclear, the etiology is complex, and the disease is usually drug-refractory with a poor prognosis.

Historical Evolution and Epidemiological Investigation

William James West [94] first described his son's spasms in 1841, which became known as West syndrome (WS), with epileptic spasms, hypsarrhythmia on EEG, and developmental stagnation or regression as the typical clinical features. With a better understanding of the disorder, its terminology has been adapted and made more accurate. The term "infantile spasms (ISs)" was first adopted based on clinical features. The term "epileptic spasms (ESs)" was adopted because this disorder may develop outside of infancy. Both of these terms have been incorporated into the definition of infantile spasticity syndromes. ILAE defined the term "IESS" in 2022 to include West syndrome and children who presented with epileptic spasms but did not meet all the criteria for the diagnosis of West syndrome [12], emphasizing the importance of early diagnosis and treatment of IESS.

Epidemiological studies have shown the prevalence of IESS to be approximately 2–5/10,000. Studies in Sweden, Finland, and Denmark have shown that the prevalence is higher in areas of higher geographic latitude [12, 18, 95]. A population-based cohort study showed that IESS accounted for 10% of patients with epilepsy whose onset age was within 36 months; both sexes were affected, with a higher prevalence in males [18].

Etiology

In 2015, the National Infantile Spasms Consortium (NISC) classified the etiology of IESS into eight categories: hereditary, genetic structural, congenital structural, acquired structural, metabolic, immune, infectious, and an unknown etiology. These categories update the spectrum of etiological components of IESS, define them in detail, and are more clinically applicable [96]. In 2022, ILAE categorized IESS into developmental and epileptic encephalopathy syndromes, where developmental encephalopathy (DE) in patients with IESS may be due to the underlying etiology of the disease, to epileptic activity, or to both [97].

The etiologies of IESS can be clarified in 70–80% of cases by cranial imaging (cranial CT, magnetic resonance imaging (MRI), etc.), metabolic tests (blood ammonia, blood lactate, blood pyruvate, blood homocysteine, folic acid, copper cyanine, urinary organic acids, etc.), and genetic testing (chromosomal karyotyping, array comparative genomic hybridization (aCGH), epilepsy gene panel, etc.) [98].

Following the development and application of genetic techniques, an increasing number of genes and chromosomal copy number variants have been shown to be associated with IESS, and most of them are highly phenotypically heterogeneous and can cause disease by affecting transcription factors, neuronal migration, signaling, and altered synaptic development and function. *ARX* and *CDKL5* were the earliest genes identified in patients and are most directly associated with IESS. Other common genes, including *STXBP1*, *KCNQ2*, *GRIN2B*, *GRIN2A*, *MAGI2*, *SPTAN*, *FOXG1*, and *NSD1* [98, 99], and additional candidate genes associated with IESS have been reported [24]. Trisomy 21, 7q11.23 deletion, 12p tetrasomy, 1p36 deletion, 15q11-q13 duplication, 2q23 deletion, and 17p13 deletion are chromosomal abnormalities closely associated with IESS [99].

Structural etiologies can be categorized as congenital, acquired, or hereditary. Common structural brain abnormalities causing IESS include anencephaly, focal cortical dysplasia, polymicrogyria, effusive anencephaly, and hemimegalencephaly. Ischemic-hypoxic encephalopathy and hypoglycemic brain injury are the most commonly acquired structural causes [98]. Neurocutaneous syndromes are common genetic structural causes, with tuberous sclerosis complex (TSC) caused by mutations in the *TSC1* or *TSC2* gene being the most common. A total of 85.2% of patients with TSC present with seizures, and 37.8% have epileptic spasms [100]. In addition, 80% of IESS patients with anencephaly exhibit *PAFAH1B1/LIS1* or *DCX* gene variants.

Approximately 3–22% of patients with IESS have metabolic etiologies. There are more than 30 metabolic etiologies associated with IESS, commonly including phenylketonuria (PKU), pyridoxine (PN)-dependent epilepsy (PDE), and organic aciduria [98, 99]. Congenital infections involving the central nervous system, including rubella and cytomegalovirus infections, can lead to IESS. The immune response is a rare etiology of IESS [96, 101], and there are now clinical and animal models that show multiple neuroinflammatory pathways that are associated with IESS [102–104]. A number of genes that play important roles in various inflammatory cascades and signaling pathways are associated with IESS.

Clinical Presentation

The age of onset of IESS ranges from 1 to 24 months, with a peak at 3–12 months. The typical clinical features of IESS include epileptic spasms, hypsarrhythmia on EEG, and developmental stagnation or regression. However, not all patients present with the complete triad of symptoms, especially in the first few weeks of the disease course. Epileptic spasms are transient contractions (flexion, extension, or mixed) of the neck, trunk, and upper and lower extremities that occur in strings or in isolation, ranging from a few to more than a hundred per string, and are evident just after sleep or upon awakening. Extension spasms are characterized by sudden extension of the trunk or head and neck tilt, with or without extension or adduction of the limbs. Flexion spasms are characterized by flexion of the trunk, limbs, head, and neck, resulting in a typical "nodding and hugging" seizure. The mixed type is characterized by flexion of the head and neck, trunk muscles, and upper limbs and extension of the lower limbs. Some patients have spasms characterized by gaze, eye spasms, shoulder twisting, yawning, jaw movements, and pouting, which are sometimes mild and difficult to detect [105]. IESS can evolve from Ohtahara syndrome, and some cases may gradually transform to Lennox–Gastaut syndrome (LGS).

Auxiliary Examination

Electroencephalogram (EEG)

Interictal EEG signals from IESS patients are commonly hypsarrhythmia, with the highest detection rate in the nonrandom eye movement (NREM) phase. Some patients may have multifocal epileptiform discharges without typical hypsarrhythmia. Fixed consistent focal epileptiform discharges or focal fast-wave rhythmic activity suggest underlying structural abnormalities. Hypsarrhythmia may be absent in the early stage of the disease or in older patients. The new 2022 ILAE definition of IESS suggests that patients with IESS who do not have hypsarrhythmia should also be treated by standard means.

Ictal EEGs of epileptic spasms show widespread high-amplitude sharp or slow waves compounded by low-amplitude fast-wave activity and may also show transient voltage decay. Hypsarrhythmia usually diminishes or ceases during a series of epileptic spasms. Synchronized electromyography (EMG) is helpful for detecting epileptic spasms, myoclonic seizures, and tonic seizures.

Neuroimaging

ILAE strongly recommends neuroimaging in children with IESS to clarify the etiology, and approximately two-thirds of patients with IESS have abnormalities on cranial MRI. When myelin formation is completed after 2 years of age, neuroimaging should be repeated in patients with refractory epileptic spasms who are suspected of having a focal structural lesion or whose etiology is unknown. For patients with subtle focal cortical dysplasia, optimized imaging and analysis may be required for further clarification. When MRI is negative, other methods, such as ^{18}F-fludeoxyglucose positron emission tomography (FDG-PET) or arterial spin labeling, may be used to detect focal structural abnormalities, and early referral for epilepsy surgery evaluation is recommended.

Genetics

Genetic testing should be performed in patients whose clinical examination and MRI results do not reveal an etiology or those with genetically related structural abnormalities. A genetic etiology can be identified in up to 41% of cases. In addition, a range of chromosomal abnormalities and copy number variants have been associated with IESS, so chromosomal microarray analysis and routine karyotyping should also be considered.

Metabolic and Other Laboratory Tests

Metabolic etiologies are rare but important causes of IESS. In the absence of a clinically known etiology, pyridoxine-dependent epilepsy should be considered and treated with a pyridoxine test [12].

Diagnosis

IESS is often diagnosed on the basis of clinical symptoms of spasms. After the clinician confirms the clinical features of IESS, an electroencephalogram (EEG) is first performed, which should include a complete sleep–wake cycle and a set of seizure events. Hypsarrhythmia is a characteristic of IESS.

To clarify the structural etiology, neuroimaging tests, such as cranial MRI, could be performed. In some cases, diffuse structural brain abnormalities with no lateral features are observed on cranial MRI. These parameters can be further evaluated by positron emission tomography.

To assess the metabolic etiologies of IESS, a series of metabolic tests, such as those for pyridoxine, urinary organic acid, serum lactate and amino acid, biotinidase, lactate, amino acid, and folate levels, should be performed.

Genetic testing should include an epilepsy gene panel, and whole exome or whole genome sequencing should be considered if no clear etiologies are found after a thorough gene panel and metabolic evaluation.

Differential Diagnosis

First, IESS should be differentiated from other epileptic disorders. Early infantile developmental and epileptic encephalopathy (EIDEE) begins within 3 months of age, and, in addition to spasms, other forms of seizures (including tonic, myoclonic, and sequential) can occur.

Myoclonic epilepsy of infancy (MEI) presents as myoclonic seizures rather than epileptic spasms. EEG and EMG can distinguish between myoclonic seizures and epileptic spasms. MEI has a normal EEG background with widespread spike and slow waves.

In addition, IESS should be differentiated from nonepileptic disorders. Benign myoclonus during sleep is characterized by twitching, which is normal. Interictal and ictal EEGs of benign myoclonus patients in infancy are both normal. Benign infantile nodding mostly starts at 3–6 months of age and is a self-limiting disorder characterized by a normal EEG. In addition, IESS should be differentiated from other nonepileptic disorders, such as gastroesophageal reflux and benign tremors, in infancy [12].

Treatment

First-Line Treatment

IESS is a severe epileptic syndrome that is refractory to most ASMs and has a poor prognosis. Currently, adrenocorticotropic hormone (ACTH), corticosteroids, and vigabatrin (VGB) are considered to be the most effective agents [105].

1. *Hormonal therapy*: Hormones are the first-line drugs for the treatment of IESS. ACTH, methylprednisolone, and prednisone are used clinically. The dosage and duration of ACTH therapy for IESS vary widely in different regions. At present, intravenous infusion or intramuscular injection at a dose of 1–2 U/(kg·day) is recommended, and treatment should be continued for 2 weeks, followed by sequential treatment with prednisone or prednisolone orally, gradually

decreasing the dosage until discontinuation. The total course of the treatment is 3–6 months. A high dose of 2–4 mg/(kg·day) of oral prednisone or prednisolone is also recommended for patients after ACTH therapy.

A retrospective study showed that 47.3% of patients responded well after 2 weeks of ACTH therapy and that 55% were seizure-free at the 6-month follow-up; thus, the short-term therapeutic effect of ACTH has significant predictive value for long-term prognosis [103]. A meta-analysis of randomized controlled trials (RCTs) showed that for patients with new-onset IESS, hormone monotherapy was more efficacious than VGB monotherapy was (odds ratio (OR) = 0.37, 95% confidence interval (95% CI = 0.20–0.67). Moreover, there was no significant difference in efficacy between the combination of hormone and VGB or hormone monotherapy for IESS (OR = 0.75, 95% CI = 0.09–6.45) [106].

2. *Vigabatrin*: Vigabatrin (VGB) is a gamma-aminobutyric acid (GABA) transaminase inhibitor that can increase the concentration of the inhibitory neurotransmitter GABA in the brain to control spasms. The recommended therapeutic dose in foreign countries is 50–150 mg/(kg·day), and it is considered that the efficacy of a high dose (100–150 mg/(kg·day)) is more favorable. However, most of the experiences in China show that a dose of 50–100 mg/(kg·day) may be optimally effective. Therefore, the effective dosage range may vary among different races [107].

VGB is the first choice for patients with IESS combined with TSC, for which the overall response rate is 67% [108]. Administration of the drug before the patient becomes symptomatic may reduce the risk of IESS. However, VGB can cause retinopathy and visual field defects [109] and vigabatrin-associated brain abnormalities on magnetic resonance imaging (VABAM) [110]. Mammalian target of rapamycin (mTOR) inhibitors such as rapamycin, everolimus, and sirolimus have potential value in the treatment of patients with IECSS combined with TSC.

Second-Line Therapy

For patients who do not respond to first-line therapy, second-line treatments, including pyridoxine, a ketogenic diet, and traditional ASMs, should be used.

Pyridoxine is first recommended for screening for pyridoxine-dependent epilepsy. It has also been used in combination with ACTH as an add-on therapy, but the results show no significant advantage. A ketogenic diet is widely used to treat patients with various refractory epilepsies, and it can reduce the frequency and duration of seizures and improve EEG abnormalities in patients who do not respond to first-line treatment [111]. In addition, some ASMs, such as topiramate, sodium valproate, zonisamide, levetiracetam, and lamotrigine, can also be used to treat IESS.

Third-Line Treatment

Cannabidiol (CBD) is a nonpsychoactive derivative of cannabis that has been shown to have good anticonvulsant efficacy as well as anxiolytic, antidepressant, neuroprotective, anti-inflammatory, and immunomodulatory effects. Cannabidiol

(Epidiolex®) passed the US Food and Drug Administration (FDA) approval in 2018, and studies related to the application of CBD in the treatment of IESS were launched. The efficacy of CBD in IESS patients for whom first-line treatment has failed is currently controversial, and additional clinical evidence is still needed to support its effectiveness. Preliminary clinical studies have shown that flunarizine does not significantly control seizures but may improve cognition in patients with IESS. Insulin-like growth factor, perampanel, and sulthiame may be effective in treating IESS [112]. A combination regimen of magnesium sulfate and ACTH was used in patients with IESS who did not respond to first-line treatment; the results showed that the seizure-free rate was 48.5% and that the remission rate of hypsarrhythmia on EEG was 72.1% [113]. However, the efficacy of these medications needs to be further verified. In addition, patients with poor drug efficacy may undergo preoperative evaluation and surgical interventions such as lesionectomy and vagus nerve stimulation (VNS).

Prognosis

The overall prognosis of IESS is poor, with a mean annual mortality rate of approximately 15.3/1000 [114]. The frequency or severity of spasms caused by IESS decreases with age, with only a minority of patients having spasms by the age of 5 years; however, these spasms are often accompanied by severe global developmental delay. Spasms cannot be controlled in 33–56% of patients after standardized treatment, and, even if medication is effective, some patients may still experience relapses; moreover, there is no medication available to prevent relapses of IESS, except for surgical resection of lesions in appropriate patients [115]. In addition, the possibilities of mental development and movement disorders associated with IESS are not optimistic. The underlying etiologies and the duration of the interval between the onset of spasms and the initial treatment are closely related to the prognosis. Early diagnosis and treatment can significantly improve neurological development.

5.2.2.3 Epilepsy in Infancy with Migrating Focal Seizures

Overview

Epilepsy of infancy with migrating focal seizures (EIMFS) was previously known as migrating partial seizures of infancy (MPSI), malignant migrating partial seizures of infancy (MMPSI), or migrating focal seizures of infancy (MFSI). EIMFS is a rare epilepsy syndrome that usually occurs within 6 months of birth and manifests as frequent, migrating, and various types of focal seizures that are almost continuous and originate independently from multiple brain regions of both hemispheres. A typical ictal EEG signal is epileptic abnormal discharge that successively occurs in multiple independent regions of both hemispheres. The efficacy of antiseizure medications is often poor, resulting in severe psychomotor delay or even regression.

Historical Evolution and Epidemiological Investigation

EIMFS is an early epileptic encephalopathy in infants that was first described in 1995 by Coppola et al. [116] and was reported as an electroclinical syndrome of

EIMFS by ILAE in 2010. The condition was grouped as developmental or epileptic encephalopathy according to the new ILAE classification in 2022.

EIMFS is a rare disease with equal prevalence in both boys and girls. Its prevalence was estimated to range from 0 to 0.11/100,000 children in the United Kingdom [117].

Etiology

EIMFS was previously believed to be an epileptic syndrome of an unknown etiology. *KCNT1* encodes a sodium-activated potassium channel and was reported to be the main pathogenic gene, accounting for approximately 50% of EIMFS etiologies. *KCNT1* encodes the sodium-activated potassium channel protein KNa1.1. It mediates the outward rectifying K^+ current associated with slow hyperpolarization after a depolarization potential. All pathogenic *KCNT1* gene mutations are missense mutations with gain of function, which lead to activation of sodium-gated potassium channels and hyperpolarization of inhibitory intermediate neurons, leading to an imbalance between excitatory and inhibitory neurons and subsequent seizures. With the development of genetic technology, more pathogenic genes, such as *SCN1A*, *SCN2A*, *SCN8A*, *TBC1D24*, *SLC25A22*, and *SLC12A5*, have been found to be associated with EIMFS. Burgess et al. conducted genetic testing on 135 patients with EIMFS and found that pathogenic mutations existed in 69% of them. The most common genes involved were *KCNT1* and *SCN2A*, accounting for 27% and 7%, respectively. Other genes included *GABRA1*, *GABRB1*, *ATP1A3*, *CDKL5*, *PIGA*, *ITPA*, *AIMP1*, *KARS*, and *WWOX* [118]. The etiologies of EIMFS are heterogeneous, and many of them are still unclear.

Clinical Manifestations

Epileptic seizures usually start within 6 months of birth and are characterized by focal motor seizures followed by significant cognitive and motor developmental regression.

Seizures

The natural course of seizures in this syndrome can be divided into three stages: (1) The first stage lasts for 1 week to several months after birth, with an average onset age of 3 months. At this stage, seizures are usually sporadic, and their frequency is approximately once a week. Most of these seizures are focal motor seizures that involve one or more limbs; half of the patients experience focal motor seizures secondary to generalized seizures, and a few may progress to persistent status epilepticus. Spontaneous symptoms such as apnea, flushing, or cyanosis are common in the early stages of attacks; these symptoms can be misinterpreted as nonepileptic attacks and may be difficult to diagnose in a timely manner. (2) The second stage is also defined as a “stormy period.” At 3 weeks to 10 months of age, a variety of seizures can occur on a daily basis, but focal motor seizures are still the prevalent ones. Clinical manifestations include head and eye deflection, staring, eyelid clonic convulsions, and clonic or tonic convulsions of unilateral or bilateral limbs; these conditions often progress to secondary generalized tonic–clonic seizures. Bilateral limbs could be alternately involved. Manifestation of autonomic attacks such as apnea, facial flushing and/or cyanosis, masticatory movements, swallowing, sweating, and salivation is significant. Different severities, durations, and different varieties of attacks can be expected for the same patient. (3) The age at which stage 3 starts can vary widely, from 1 year to more than 5 years of age. Seizures are gradually reduced and relatively stable at this stage. Certain disease states, such as infection or fever, are prone to induce cluster seizures or episodic status epilepticus.

Developmental Disorders

Most of the children develop normally before the onset of epileptic seizures, and significant regression of cognition and motor functions occur after cluster epileptic seizures. If the frequency of attack is reduced and seizures are alleviated, psychomotor development can be restored to a certain extent. However, only those with fully controlled seizures are likely to gain the ability to hold objects, recognize their surroundings, and walk. Burgess et al. studied 135 children with EIMFS and reported that 127 of them had severe to extremely severe psychomotor developmental delay [118].

Other Features

These include microcephaly, dyskinesia, and dystonia. Burgess et al. reported that 40/135 (30%) patients had spasticity or spastic tetraplegia. Of the 135 children, 82 (61%) had hypotonia, 16 (12%) had scoliosis, and 36 (27%) had dyskinesia, including choreoathetosis and dystonia. Of 124 patients, 61 (49%) had microcephaly [118].

Auxiliary Examination

Patients with EIMFS have no specific neuroimaging changes, and cranial CT or magnetic resonance imaging (MRI) results are usually normal. Burgess et al. analyzed the cranial MRI data of 133 patients with EIMFS and showed that 55/133 (41%) patients were normal, 54/133 (41%) had brain atrophy, 17/133 (13%) had a high T2 signal in the white matter, and 14/133 (11%) had delayed myelination [118].

The EEG may be normal at disease onset, with an abnormal manifestation of diffuse slowing of background activity, but epileptic discharges usually occur within 1 month of the first seizure. In the first stage, slow waves of the EEG background are characterized by asymmetric migration, often transferring from one hemisphere to the other. Sleep–wake cycles can still be identified in this stage, but spindles are significantly reduced and bilateral asymmetry is observed. Interictal multifocal abnormal discharges were activated during sleep, and the typical manifestations of interictal EEG signals disappeared with an increasing number of seizures.

Ictal focal abnormal discharge has typical migratory characteristics and can manifest as rhythmic electrical activity that starts in one cortical area and gradually spreads to other areas. Different focal seizures may occur independently or simultaneously in different brain regions for different periods of time, and the onset area may shift from one region to other regions of the ipsilateral or contralateral hemisphere, resulting in a complex multifocal seizure state. Electroclinical events usually last for 1–4 min. If attacks are very frequent, the onset zone can move from one brain region to other regions or from one hemisphere to the other. Successive episodes may overlap; that is, one episode has not yet ended before another episode has begun. This leads to continuous, migrating epileptic discharges and the development of status epilepticus.

The abnormal paroxysmal discharges recorded by video EEG are closely related to clinical manifestations. Occipital discharge can cause eye clonus and head deviation. Contralateral limb clonus can be caused by discharge in the Rolandic region. Temporal discharges can cause chewing, swallowing, staring, and salivating. Frontal area discharges can cause hypertonia of the contralateral limbs.

Diagnosis

ILAE's proposed diagnostic criteria are as follows: ① Mandatory criteria: <12 months of age, focal/multifocal tonic or clonic seizures, and motor arrest or obvious autonomic features. Seizures shift from one hemisphere or lobe to another or other brain regions. The seizure frequency quickly increases in the first few weeks and months, and seizures usually progress to status epilepticus. Developmental plateauing or regression can be caused by frequent seizures. ② Warning criteria that require attention: Onset age of 6–12 months, severe developmental delay before seizure onset, significant abnormalities on neurological examination before seizure onset, burst suppression or hypsarrhythmia pattern of interictal EEG, and ictal EEG of single focal persistent abnormal discharges. The exclusion criteria for patients are as follows: myoclonic seizures and neuroimaging abnormalities with obvious structural lesions.

Differential Diagnosis

Self-Limited Familial Neonatal Epilepsy (SLFNE), Self-Limited Familial Infantile Epilepsy (SeLIE), and Self-Limited Familial Neonatal–Infantile Epilepsy (SeLFNIE)

The main distinguishing points between these other conditions and EIMFS are the absence of a migrating pattern within the same seizure upon ictal EEG and normal development.

Other Focal Early-Onset Epilepsies Due to Structural Etiologies

These seizures can be distinguished by the presence of stereotypical seizures, usually with a single constant seizure pattern without a migrating pattern on the EEG.

Other Early Infantile Developmental and Epileptic Encephalopathies

Patients may have multifocal and/or generalized seizures with severe neurodevelopmental delay but not exhibit the typical migrating pattern on EEG.

Dravet Syndrome

This syndrome manifests as prolonged focal clonic (hemiclonic) seizures that may alternate from side to side at different times. However, they do not show migrating patterns within the same seizure.

Treatment

Treatment of EIMFS is challenging, especially since seizures of EIMFS are highly resistant to ASMs, and there are currently no specific treatment regimens available.

Treatment of Epileptic Seizures

1. *Levetiracetam*: Cilio et al. [119] reported that intravenous infusion of levetiracetam at a loading dose of 60 mg/kg followed by 30 mg/kg levetiracetam twice daily rapidly terminated refractory status epilepticus (RSE) in two patients with EIMFS and effectively prevented the recurrence of status epilepticus. The treatment was safe and well-tolerated. Djuric et al. [120] reported that two patients with EIMFS were treated with a combination of levetiracetam, sodium bromide, and stiripentol, which showed significant efficacy. Multiple therapies can effectively reduce the frequency and severity of seizures in EIMFS patients but have no significant impact on psychomotor development [120].
2. *Rufinamide*: Vendrame et al. [121] conducted a retrospective analysis regarding the efficacy of rufinamide treatment in five EIMFS patients aged 25–41 months with a median age of 30 months. The age of epilepsy onset ranged from 15 days to 3.5 months with a median age of 1.5 months; four patients were treated with additional therapy; and one patient was treated with monotherapy. The dosage of rufinamide ranged from 5 to 75 mg/kg*day. The number of seizures of two patients was reduced by more than 50%, and the treatment was well-tolerated. Side effects of vomiting and loss of appetite were reported [121].
3. *Stiripentol*: Merdariu et al. [122] reported on an EIMFS patient aged 2 months who showed poor response to oxcarbazepine treatment, topiramate treatment, and a ketogenic diet. Seizures were temporarily relieved after treatment with levetiracetam and clonazepam (CZP) and were later controlled following treatment with additional stiripentol. At the final follow-up at 20 months of age, the patient had remained seizure-free for 12 months under the combined therapy of levetiracetam, clonazepam, and stiripentol. As seizures were controlled, psychomotor development improved. At 20 months of age, the patient could crawl, stand, grab, and interchange objects and exhibited good social behavior.
4. *Cannabidiol*: Saade and Joshi reported on an EIMFS patient who experienced onset on the first day after birth. The patient exhibited poor response to phenobarbital and levetiracetam treatments, and frequent seizures presented as status epilepticus. At 4 months of age, the child underwent ketogenic diet therapy (KDT), which was effective, and she subsequently received cannabidiol treatment. The dosage was increased from 10 mg/kg*day to 25 mg/

kg*day without causing obvious adverse effects. The patient was followed for 6 months after taking cannabidiol, and the frequency of seizures decreased from 10–20 times a day to 5 times a week with polytherapy comprising levetiracetam, clonazepam, and cannabidiol. EEG readings showed extensive slow waves with abnormal discharges in the right occipital region, but no clinical seizures were observed. After treatment with cannabidiol, psychomotor development improved and her head circumference increased normally. Therefore, cannabidiol supplementation may be beneficial for controlling seizures and improving psychomotor development in children with EIMFS [123]. In a study of 27 patients with *KCNT1* gene variants, Borlot et al. reported that 7 of them were treated with cannabidiol, 71% of whom experienced significant improvement (a >50% reduction) or partial improvement (a 25–50% reduction) in seizures [124].

5. *Potassium bromide*: Caraballo et al. retrospectively analyzed the efficacy of potassium bromide supplementation in six children with EIMFS who received 30–80 mg/kg*day. Four patients responded well; one was seizure-free but still had severe cognitive impairment. Two responders, currently 4 and 6 years of age, had monthly seizures with axial hypotonia and severe language impairment. The final responder had weekly seizures and displayed moderate psychomotor developmental delay. Except for one child who was seizure-free, the focal seizures of the other three responders did not progress to generalized seizures, no longer showed status epilepticus, and did not require hospitalization. Two patients did not respond well to potassium bromide therapy. Three patients experienced adverse effects, including vomiting in one patient, lethargy in one patient, and an acne-like facial rash in the third, but these reactions were relieved with reduced dosage. Patients with EIMFS should be treated with potassium bromide as early as possible to control seizures, prevent status epilepticus, and avoid progressive cognitive dysfunction [125].
6. *Quinidine*: The *KCNT1* gene encodes the sodium-activated potassium channel subunit and plays an important role in regulating neuronal excitability. Quinidine has been used as an antimalarial and antiarrhythmic drug in clinical practice. Having been shown to be a partial antagonist of the KCNT1 channel in experimental studies, it may be used as a targeted therapy for children with a *KCNT1* gain-of-function variant. Borlot et al. [124] studied 27 patients with *KCNT1* gene variants and reported that 11 of them received quinidine therapy, 45% of whom had a significantly reduced (a >50% reduction) or partially reduced (a 25–50% reduction) number of attacks. Patil et al. [126] reported the clinical characteristics of two patients with EIMFS caused by *KCNT1* gene variation who did not respond to ASMs or a ketogenic diet. One patient experienced a 30% reduction in the number of seizures when treated with a dosage of 20 mg/kg*day quinidine and an 80% reduction when the dosage was increased to 36 mg/kg*day. Another patient experienced a

30% reduction in seizure number when treated with a dosage of 20 mg/kg*day quinidine [126]. Barcia et al. [127] reported that two patients with *KCNT1* gene variants received additional quinidine treatment, but neither of them showed clinical seizure or EEG abnormality improvement.

7. *Dietary treatment*: Borlot et al. [124] studied 27 patients with *KCNT1* gene variants and reported that 14 of them received dietary therapy, including 12 patients placed on a ketogenic diet and 2 who received treatment with a low-glycemic-index diet. Fifty-seven percent of the patients achieved significant improvement (a >50% reduction in the number of seizures) or partial improvement (25–50% reduction in the number of seizures). In patients for whom enteral nutrition is not feasible, parenteral nutrition could be considered. Armeno et al. [128] reported three patients with EIMFS who received treatment with a parenteral ketogenic diet due to intestinal nutrient absorption disorders. The ketogenic ratio of the diet was <1.5:1 due to a limited fat intake through the parenteral pathway, and the patients showed good response to a parenteral low ketogenic ratio diet.
8. *Antisense oligonucleotides*: Burbano L et al. [129] injected KCNT1 antisense oligonucleotides into the lateral ventricles of mice harboring the *KCNT1* p.P924L pathogenic mutation. The frequency of seizures was significantly reduced in the treated group compared with the control group, abnormal behaviors improved, and the overall survival period was prolonged. Antisense oligonucleotide therapy showed good efficacy and tolerance for controlling seizures and prolonging lifespan. Therefore, gene silencing based on antisense oligonucleotides is a promising treatment for *KCNT1* mutation-associated epilepsy [129]

Prognosis

The long-term prognosis of patients with EIMFS is poor. All of these patients may exhibit severe psychomotor delay or even regression, quadriplegia with axial hypotonia, pyramidal bundle signs, extrapyramidal signs, and athetosis. Patients often die within the first year of disease. Burgess et al. [118] reported that 45/135 (33%) patients died at a median age of 2 years and 7 months (34 days to 12 years), and the causes of death included persistent seizures, status epilepticus, and complications such as pneumonia and heart and/or respiratory failure [118].

Kuchenbuch et al. [130] followed 17 patients with EIMFS caused by *KCNT1* gene variants and reported that only 1 patient was seizure-free over the long term, while the rest were affected by neurological sequelae and active epilepsies. Symptoms, in addition to those of the nervous system that may be associated with *KCNT1* gene variation, include arteriovenous fistula, dilated cardiomyopathy, and precocious puberty. Eight (47%) patients died between 2 months and 19.5 years of age, four in the acute stage, four in the chronic stage, and three of the eight patients were suspected to have experienced sudden unexpected death in epilepsy.

5.2.2.4 Dravet Syndrome

Overview

Dravet syndrome was classified in 1989 as an epilepsy or epileptic syndrome that could not be definitively categorized as either focal or generalized. ILAE (2022) classifies this disease as developmental or epileptic encephalopathy. Typically, this disease manifests between 1 and 20 months after birth and primarily presents as drug-resistant seizures characterized by unilateral focal or focal-to-bilateral tonic–clonic seizures. Cognitive and behavioral impairments become apparent after the age of 1 year. Eighty percent of cases are associated with abnormalities in the sodium channel gene *SCN1A* [12, 131–138].

Historical Evolution and Epidemiological Investigations

Previously known as severe myoclonic epilepsy of infancy, Dravet syndrome was first reported in 1945 by Tolone [131] as myoclonic epilepsy of an unknown cause. In 1951, this disease was further described as myoclonic encephalopathy. Subsequent discoveries revealed that myoclonic components were not always present and that clinical manifestations were not entirely consistent. Consequently, in 1989, the syndrome was renamed Dravet syndrome. In 2005, Dravet summarized the clinical features and diagnostic methods used to identify this syndrome, and, in 2010, patients with Dravet syndrome were found to have mutations in the *SCN1A* gene. In 2011, attention was given to cognitive impairments in patients. Subsequently, Dravet outlined the core symptoms of this syndrome, elevating its prevention and treatment to a new level [139].

Many pediatric epilepsy patients exhibit similarities to those with Dravet syndrome but lack myoclonic features. These patients have distinct electroencephalogram characteristics from those of patients with myoclonic epilepsy but share similar clinical processes and prognoses. Therefore, they are also included within the spectrum of Dravet syndrome, referred to by Dravet as borderline Dravet syndrome [137].

This condition is rare, with an estimated incidence of 6.5/100,000 according to ILAE. Epidemiological studies by Hurst suggest an incidence of 1/40,000, with a male predominance (2:1 ratio). Some patients have a family history of epilepsy or febrile seizures.

Etiology

There are no reported associations between birth trauma or perinatal injuries and this condition. Among the 42 patients included in the study by Dravet [137, 139], only 3 had neonatal asphyxia. The majority of patients show no abnormalities upon CT or MRI scanning, with occasional instances of diffuse brain atrophy observed in imaging studies. Pathological studies have revealed minor abnormalities in the cortices and cerebella of some patients as well as spinal cord malformations. There have been no reports of other abnormalities, and muscle and skin biopsies have shown negative results [12].

Approximately 15–25% of patients have a family history of epilepsy or febrile seizures, suggesting a genetic basis for this disease. Studies on monozygotic twins have shown similar clinical features, electroencephalogram patterns, and prognoses, although the genetic factors and inheritance patterns remain unclear. Recent research has indicated that approximately 80% of patients have *SCN1A* mutations, while 10% have mutations in other genes. Therefore, the cause of this condition appears most likely to be genetic in nature [12, 139].

Clinical Manifestations

Seizures

Onset occurs within the first year of birth. Prior to the onset of seizures, most children exhibit normal development. Seizures typically begin with generalized or unilateral myoclonic jerks, followed by reflex myoclonic jerks and focal seizures. Affected children experience impediments in psychomotor development and other neurological dysfunctions [12, 137, 139–141].

Generalized or unilateral myoclonic jerks are the most common seizure types. The duration of seizures varies, ranging from short to prolonged. In many cases, the initial seizure occurs with fever, and these febrile seizures often recur after 6–8 weeks or may be delayed, sometimes progressing to status epilepticus. Subsequent seizures manifest as afebrile myoclonic jerks, with unusual characteristics and electroencephalogram patterns differing from those of generalized tonic–clonic seizures. Careful analysis requires video electroencephalography [12, 137, 139–141].

Myoclonic jerks followed by generalized tonic–clonic or tonic seizures are also common. Seizures may originate locally, often starting on one side of the limbs or head before becoming generalized. Reflex myoclonic jerks are frequent and occur several times a day. Initially, tonic seizures with or without clonic components are more evident in the face or head, and bilateral involvement may lead to impaired consciousness. If the seizure duration is short, vegetative symptoms may not be present [12, 140, 142].

Short-duration atypical absence seizures are not uncommon. In a study by Genton et al. [142], 6 out of 24 patients exhibited atypical absences. Abnormal spikes and waves were present on electroencephalography, and clinical monitoring revealed that these wandering myoclonic jerks could persist for several hours.

Tonic–clonic seizures predominantly occur during sleep and often in clusters, becoming more pronounced in the later stages of the disease and in adulthood. Genton et al. [142] reported that in adulthood, generalized tonic–clonic seizures (GTCSs) are the sole type of seizure observed in nearly all patients. Some of these seizure events may have atypical features, such as bilateral or asymmetrical tonic postures.

Status epilepticus is quite common before the age of 5 and often affects patient prognosis. De Liso et al. [143] reported on seven patients who died from intractable status epilepticus; the average age was 6.9 years (1.3–23.4 years). All patients had a history of status epilepticus. Fatal status epilepticus is often triggered by fever, which can persist anywhere from 80 min to 9 h. Four patients died during the occurrence of status epilepticus or within a few hours, while three died 13–60 days later.

Other manifestations include psychomotor seizures with loss of tone or torsion, autonomic symptoms, or automatisms. Occasionally, generalized seizures may also occur [143].

Developmental Impairment

Developmental delay becomes evident in the second year following the onset of seizures. Subsequently, progressive neurological dysfunction, such as ataxia and corticospinal tract signs, occurs. A study by Battaglia et al. [140] involving 34 Italian patients revealed that 16 patients exhibited mild developmental delays within 2–3 years of birth, particularly in visual motor skills, progressing to global developmental impairment. Twelve patients experienced early-onset global developmental delays of greater severity. Two patients showed essentially normal neurodevelopment but had behavioral and language issues. Another study by Olivieri et al. involving 20 adolescent patients revealed that all patients had behavioral and intellectual impairments; these included 6 mild cases, 7 moderate cases, and 7 severe cases. Visual function, especially visual motor skills, was most highly impaired in mildly intellectually disabled patients, while language skills were relatively preserved.

Other Injuries

A recent study by Perulli et al. [144] has investigated heart rate variability in 56 DS patients and showed that it was significantly lower in these patients than in the control group. A recent history of status epilepticus has been identified as the only significant predictive factor.

Auxiliary Examinations

In the early stages of the disease, electroencephalograms may not reveal apparent abnormalities. As the disease progresses, diffuse spikes and waves or polyspikes and waves gradually appear. Single or multiple burst activities may occur and are typically more pronounced in one hemisphere. Intermittent photic stimulation and drowsiness can induce burst-like electroencephalographic activity. In addition to generalized discharges, localized spikes and waves and sharp waves are common and often multifocal. Burst activity disappears in awake-state electroencephalograms, while sleep-state electroencephalograms show prominent burst activity. The laboratory test results for these patients are usually normal. CT and MRI scans, besides occasionally showing mild diffuse atrophy or enlargement of the cerebellar medullary pontine cistern, are mostly normal [12, 140, 141].

Diagnosis

ILAE proposed diagnostic criteria emphasizing three components:

Essential: Onset between 1 and 20 months after birth, focal seizures or secondary generalized tonic–clonic seizures, often drug-resistant. Physical examination may reveal signs of cognitive dysfunction and neurological disorders.

Cautionary: Lack of sensitivity to febrile seizure induction and a normal background on electroencephalogram after 2 years of age; absence of interictal discharges; developmental impairment during seizures; absence of pathogenic *SCN1A* mutations or other pathogenic variants; and good efficacy of sodium channel drugs, including carbamazepine, oxcarbazepine, and phenytoin, which may indicate a condition other than Dravet syndrome.

Patients were excluded if they had epileptic spasms, early-onset infantile *SCN1A*-DEE, or localized lesions suggested by head MRI [12].

Although more than 80% of Dravet syndrome patients have *SCN1A* gene mutations, the diagnosis still relies primarily on typical clinical presentations. It is crucial not to rely solely on gene mutations to confirm Dravet syndrome, as similar genetic changes can be found in patients with non-Dravet syndrome diseases. The absence of gene mutations also does not rule out Dravet syndrome, and treatment should not be delayed [12, 139].

Differential Diagnosis

Febrile Seizures

Initial seizures often accompany febrile convulsions and require differentiation from febrile seizures. The differentiation points include:

1. Onset occurs at a younger age, typically within the first year of birth; febrile seizures often occur between 18 and 22 months of age.
2. Seizures are mainly characterized by myoclonic jerks, often unilateral, as opposed to the generalized tonic–clonic seizures observed in febrile convulsions.
3. Longer and more frequent seizure episodes
4. The presence of other seizure types, especially reflex myoclonic jerks, and photoparoxysmal responses according to electroencephalograms, supporting the diagnosis.
5. Consideration of atypical variants even in the absence of myoclonic jerks [12, 139]

Lennox–Gastaut Syndrome (LGS)

Differentiation from LGS involves the following points: LGS typically manifests after the first year of birth and involves drop attacks, atypical absence seizures, axial tonic seizures, and characteristic abnormalities on electroencephalograms.

Myoclonic Astatic Epilepsy (MAE) or Doose Syndrome

Onset is later than that seen in Dravet syndrome, with the main presentation being myoclonic astatic seizures. There is minimal occurrence of focal seizures and localized electroencephalogram abnormalities. Although children may experience myoclonic nonconvulsive status epilepticus, recurrent convulsive status epilepticus is rare [12, 139].

Treatment

Treatment of Seizures

1. *Initial treatment*: Broad-spectrum antiseizure medications (ASMs), such as valproic acid (VPA) and clobazam (CLB), are commonly used for initial treatment. However, these methods are often insufficient for controlling seizures.
2. *Adjunctive therapies*: (1) Stiripentol (Diacomit®): Stiripentol, a unique antiseizure medication with multiple potential mechanisms, including enhancing central γ-aminobutyric acid transmission, has been approved for the treatment of seizures in Dravet syndrome patients. It is often used in combination with clobazam and valproic acid for refractory generalized tonic–clonic seizures. Stiripentol has shown efficacy in reducing seizure frequency, although common adverse events include drowsiness, decreased appetite, weight loss, ataxia, and tremor [145]. (2) Cannabidiol (CBD): High-purity, plant-derived cannabidiol, known as Epidiolex, has demonstrated efficacy in reducing seizure frequency in Dravet syndrome patients. It is administered orally, and studies have indicated a significant reduction in seizure frequency compared to that in a placebo group, although this change was lower than that observed with clobazam treatment. The onset of action for cannabidiol was observed during the titration period, with a significant difference in symptoms appearing on days 12–13 [146, 147].
3. *Fenfluramine*: Fenfluramine, a derivative of amphetamines that affects serotonin neurotransmitter levels, has been studied for its efficacy in treating Dravet syndrome. Research has suggested that fenfluramine can significantly reduce seizure frequency with good tolerability, providing valuable evidence for clinical practice [148].
4. *Other options*: Topiramate, levetiracetam, bromides, and a ketogenic diet can be considered adjunctive treatments. Some patients may respond to phenobarbital and ethosuximide, while carbamazepine, oxcarbazepine, phenytoin, and lamotrigine might exacerbate seizures. However, the role of vigabatrin is uncertain. The primary goal of treatment is to circumvent prolonged, widespread, or unilateral seizures triggered by infections or fever, and surgical intervention is not recommended [12].

Treatment of Status Epilepticus

For status epilepticus in patients with Dravet syndrome, benzodiazepines (BZDs) are the preferred initial treatment. If BZDs are ineffective, other options, such as midazolam, phenobarbital, or phenytoin, may be considered. Kikuchi et al. reported that BZDs had an efficacy rate of 61.8%, with subsequent use of midazolam, phenobarbital, or phenytoin having varying efficacy rates [149].

Prognosis

Dravet syndrome generally has a poor prognosis, with most children experiencing persistent seizures. Fever is a triggering factor that may lead to status epilepticus. Almost all patients suffer from cognitive impairment, but it typically does not worsen after the age of 4. Behavioral disturbances, such as psychiatric symptoms, may occur. Additionally, 14% of patients may die during seizures, often due to infection or accidents. A study by Genton et al. on the long-term prognosis of Dravet syndrome in adulthood revealed that of 24 patients, 5 (20.8%) died at an average age of 24.8 years. One patient died from status epilepticus, three from sudden unexpected death in epilepsy (SUDEP), and one from an unknown cause. Seizures tended to become less frequent and more severe in adulthood, with only 3 out of 24 adult patients being able to live independently [142].

5.2.3 Epileptic Syndromes with Specific Etiology

5.2.3.1 *KCNQ2*-Related Disorders

Overview

KCNQ2-related disorders are a spectrum of diseases of varying severity caused by mutations in the *KCNQ2* gene. The most common phenotypes include a mild form of self-limited familial neonatal epilepsy (SLFNE) and a severe form of developmental and epileptic encephalopathy (*KCNQ2*-DEE) with neonatal onset [150]. Some *KCNQ2* gene variants can also manifest as neurodevelopmental delays, non-epileptic myoclonic neonatal encephalopathy, developmental delays, etc.

SLFNE usually occurs within 2–8 days of birth, presenting with focal tonic seizures, and often resolves itself at 4–5 months of age. Indices of neurodevelopment, physical examination of the nervous system, and intermittent electrophysiological examinations are generally normal. Most patients have a family history of neonatal epilepsy. Approximately 15–30% of patients have recurrent epilepsy in childhood or early adulthood, and some patients progress to refractory epilepsy and encephalopathy.

The clinical manifestations of *KCNQ2*-DEE are serious, and intractable epilepsy occurs in the first week after birth. The seizures are mainly tonic, often accompanied by cyanosis or apnea, and some patients have myoclonic and infantile spasms. Interictal electroencephalograms often show burst suppression or multifocal epileptiform discharges. Early brain MRI reveals abnormal T2 hyperintensity in the basal ganglia and thalamus, while later brain MRI may reveal white matter lesions or brain atrophy. Seizures are relieved between the age of 9 months and 4 years, but most patients still have moderate-to-severe developmental delays and cognitive impairment.

Historical Evolution and Epidemiological Investigation

Rett and Teubel first reported familial neonatal epilepsy syndrome in 1964; seizures occurred across three generations during the neonatal period, disappeared after 6–8 weeks in girls, and persisted throughout adolescence in boys. Neonatal seizures were not associated with perinatal complications. In 1968, Bjerre and Corelius described five generations of a family with neonatal convulsions and normal motor and intellectual development, naming this disease benign familial neonatal convulsion syndrome. In 1998, it was first reported that an autosomal dominant variant of the *KCNQ2* gene can cause benign familial neonatal epilepsy (BFNE), which manifests as seizures 3–7 days after birth and gradually progresses to frequent spontaneous remission at 4–6 months of age without affecting psychomotor development outcomes [151, 152]. In 2004, several researchers reported that several *KCNQ2* gene variants could also lead to neonatal epileptic encephalopathy syndrome [153]. These patients presented with early-onset refractory epilepsy. In contrast to patients with SLFNE, these patients had abnormal EEG backgrounds during intermittent periods and moderate-to-severe neurodevelopmental delays remained even though epilepsy was gradually alleviated. However, the role of epileptic seizures in the process of neurodevelopmental delay, stagnation, and regression, known as *KCNQ2*-related developmental and epileptic encephalopathy, is unclear [154].

KCNQ2-related diseases are rare. However, mutation of this gene remains one of the most common causes of hereditary epilepsy [155]. In neonatal epilepsy, an autosomal dominant inherited heterozygous variant of *KCNQ2* is the most common cause [55]. To date, more than 200 families with self-limited familial neonatal epilepsy and more than 200 cases of developmental and epileptic encephalopathy have been reported. A recent prospective national epidemiological cohort study in Scotland evaluating monogenic epilepsy, which is common in early childhood, has estimated that *KCNQ2* is the most common causative gene in infants under 6 months of age, with an incidence of approximately 5.9 per 100,000 [55].

Etiology and Pathophysiology

The *KCNQ2* gene is located on chromosome 20. This gene encodes the Kv7.2 subunit, which, together with the Kv7.3 subunit encoded by the *KCNQ3* gene in vivo, forms a heterotetramer (Kv7.2/Kv7.3) that is a voltage-gated potassium ion channel that plays an important role in the generation of M-type currents regulated by muscarinic acid in neurons [55]. The 7.2/Kv7.3 channel is widely expressed throughout the central nervous system and plays an important role in controlling the excitability of neural networks, especially in the immature brain; here, the gamma-aminobutyric acid (GABA) energy system is not yet the main inhibitory system but has depolarization and excitability effects [156]. The Kv7.2/Kv7.3 channel is rapidly replaced by the GABA receptor in the first few months of life, so this *KCNQ2* gene variant causes epilepsy in the neonatal period but leads to spontaneous remission in early infancy.

KCNQ2-related SLFNE is mainly caused by truncating mutations (nonsense, shear, and frameshift), exon deletion, heterozygous missense mutations, and other loss-of-function variants [152]. In cells with heterozygous mutations, wild-type and mutant subunits are coexpressed, resulting in a 20–30% decrease in M current density.

KCNQ2-DEE is generally caused by missense mutations or in-frame deletion/insertion mutations, and some scholars speculate that this phenomenon is related to the dominant negative effect caused by gene variants [157]. In contrast to SLFNE patients, *KCNQ2*-DEE patients exhibit more serious potassium current dysfunction, and the M current amplitude decreases by 50% [157]. *KCNQ2*-DEE-related gene mutations are mostly distributed in four high-risk regions—the S4 voltage sensor, the pore channel, the near end of the C-terminal region, and the B-helix near the C-terminal—all of which are key ion channel regions [157].

Clinical Presentation

Seizures

SLFNE always initiates at 2–8 days after birth and presents with focal tonic seizures, often accompanied by apnea, vocalization, and autonomic nervous system manifestations; cluster seizures are also common. Seizures generally resolve spontaneously in the first month of life or at 6–12 months of age. Approximately 15–30% of children develop recurrent seizures after infancy [157], including simple febrile convulsions (13%), childhood convulsions (10%), and adolescent or adult seizures (14%).

KCNQ2-DEE often presents with intractable epilepsy in the first week after birth; most of the seizures are tonic and accompanied by cyanosis or apnea. Some patients have frequent myoclonus and infantile spasms and a poor response to drugs. The frequency of attacks decreases with age, but they may still recur.

Other Nervous System Manifestations

Patients with SLFNE exhibit normal development, while *KCNQ2*-DEE is associated with moderate-to-severe developmental delay, mostly including hypotonia of trunk muscles and/or spastic quadriplegia. Motor development is significantly delayed, language development is impaired, and patients cannot speak or speak only single words or short sentences. Some patients are unable to sit alone, lack the ability to make eye contact, and lack interest in their surroundings. Other clinical features of *KCNQ2*-DEE include dystonia, spasticity, hypotonia, cortical visual impairment, abnormal eye movement, and feeding intolerance [158, 159].

Laboratory Findings

In patients with SLFNE, EEG signals during the intermittent period are mostly normal, while some patients exhibit spikes and sharp waves in the central temporal region [160]. Intermittent EEG data from patients with *KCNQ2*-DEE always show significant discharge, which often indicates burst suppression in the neonatal period, after which the disease disappears and evolves to diffuse slow background EEG signals and multifocal epileptic discharge. In a Korean study of 13 patients with *KCNQ2*-related diseases, 7 exhibited burst suppression and 6 exhibited a slow background and multifocal epileptic discharge [161]. Early brain MRI of *KCNQ2*-DEE indicated abnormal signals in the basal ganglia and thalamus, which may spontaneously disappear after 3 years of age.

Diagnosis
Based on the clinical manifestations, associated laboratory findings, and family history, a clinical diagnosis is obtained. With the detection of pathogenic heterozygous mutations in the *KCNQ2* gene, a diagnosis can be confirmed. Among mutations, 90% of *KCNQ2* gene mutations are point mutations and 10% are copy number variations [162].

Differential Diagnosis
Self-Limited Familial Neonatal Epilepsy Caused by *KCNQ3* Mutations

Clinical manifestations are similar and cannot be distinguished, and molecular detection is needed.

Self-Limited Familial Infantile Epilepsy and Self-Limited Familial Neonatal–Infantile Epilepsy Caused by Mutations in *PRRT2*, *SCN2A*, *SCN8A*, and Other Genes

The former patients develop epilepsy at more than 6 months of age, while the latter can develop epilepsy from the newborn stage to infancy; the age of onset varies within the same family.

Treatment
To date, there is a lack of clinical practice guidelines for the treatment of *KCNQ2*-related diseases, and the treatment mainly involves symptomatic support.

Antiseizure Therapy

SLFNE generally responds well to traditional antiepileptic drugs, and 30% of patients improve without medication.

The epilepsy caused by *KCNQ2*-DEE is mostly drug-resistant (insensitive to either single or combination drugs). Sodium channel blockers, such as oxcarbazepine, phenytoin, carbamazepine, lamotrigine, topiramate, and zonisamide, are more likely to achieve seizure control [161–163]. In a study of children with *KCNQ2*-DEE, 53% were seizure-free after carbamazepine treatment and 33% responded to phenytoin [163]. Oxcarbazepine is also effective and well-tolerated in patients with neonatal epilepsy caused by *KCNQ2* mutations (SLFNE or DEE).

In a retrospective study of 23 patients with *KCNQ2*-DEE, 11 were treated with the selective potassium channel opening agent ezogabine, and it was found that ezogabine may be effective and well-tolerated for the impaired type of *KCNQ2*-DEE, especially in patients treated within 6 months of onset [159]. However, use of the drug was discontinued in 2017 due to risks such as retinal pigmentation and skin discoloration.

Pyridoxine may be effective against *KCNQ2*-DEE.

Individualized Treatment

Children with intellectual disabilities or developmental delays should be treated individually.

Other Treatments

For patients with *KCNQ2* gene mutations and their families, genetic counseling and prenatal diagnosis education should be provided.

Prognosis
The epilepsy in SLFNE patients usually relapses after infancy without residual neurodevelopmental abnormalities. The epilepsy in *KCNQ2*-DEE patients improves between 9 months and 4 years of age, but most patients have moderate-to-severe developmental delays and cognitive impairment.

5.2.3.2 Pyridoxine-Dependent (ALDH7A1) Developmental and Epileptic Encephalopathy (PD-DEE)

Overview
Pyridoxine-dependent developmental and epileptic encephalopathy (PD-DEE), also known as PDE-ALDH7A1, was categorized as an epilepsy syndrome of undetermined localization or generalization in 1989. However, in the 2022 reclassification, ILAE placed this disease within the spectrum of developmental and etiology-specific epileptic encephalopathies. PD-DEE patients typically present with seizures within the first few weeks to months of life; these seizures are characterized by various seizure types, including focal seizures, spasms, myoclonic seizures, tonic–clonic seizures, and status epilepticus [164]. Conventional antiepileptic drugs often fail to control seizures, and up to 75% of patients may experience cognitive and behavioral disturbances [165, 166]. This rare autosomal recessive genetic disorder is primarily caused by mutations in the *ALDH7A1* gene, located on the long arm of chromosome 5.

Historical Evolution and Epidemiological Investigations
In 1953 and 1954, the role of vitamin B6 in epilepsy was recognized through observations of seizures in infants with vitamin B6 deficiency [167, 168]. In 1954, hereditary epilepsy caused by pyridoxine was first described [169]. In 2006, Mills et al. confirmed that mutations in the aldehyde dehydrogenase 7 family member A1 (*ALDH7A1*) gene are responsible for PD-DEE [170]. To date, more than 200 cases have been reported. The prevalence of PD-DEE ranges from 1:65,000 to 1:273,000 newborns, with some reports showing its incidence is as rare as 1:783,000 newborns [165, 171, 172].

Etiology

Pyridoxine-dependent epilepsy is a congenital metabolic disorder with an autosomal recessive inheritance pattern. The *ALDH7A1* gene is located at chromosomal region 5q32.2, and more than 165 pathogenic mutations in *ALDH7A1* have been reported [165]. A mutation in the *ALDH7A1* gene leads to a loss of α-aminoadipic semialdehyde (α-AASA) dehydrogenase expression during lysine decomposition, after which harmful metabolites, such as piperidine acid, α-AASA, and Δ1-piperidine-6- carboxylate (Δ1-P6C), accumulate in the body, leading to the inactivation of pyridoxal 5′-phosphate (PLP) [173]. PLP is an active form of vitamin B6 that maintains the normal activities and orderly work of cells in the central nervous system through transamination, decarboxylation, and regulation of gene expression. The transamination and decarboxylation of neurotransmitters (γ-aminobutyric acid (GABA), dopamine, and serotonin) require the participation of PLP. A decrease in the activity of PLP-dependent glutamate decarboxylase leads to an increase in glutamate abundance and a decrease in GABA abundance. An imbalance between excitatory (glutamate) and inhibitory (GABA) neurotransmitter levels may lead to PD-DEE encephalopathy and seizures [165].

Clinical Presentation

PD-DEE patients typically experience seizures within hours to days of birth. Approximately 25% of PD-DEE patients may have seizures starting in the first 3 years of life [174]. It is difficult for antiepileptic drugs to completely stop epileptic seizures. Most patients exhibit intellectual and developmental abnormalities.

Seizures

PD-DEE patients present with a wide range of seizure types, including multifocal myoclonic seizures, focal seizures, spasms, tonic–clonic seizures, and status epilepticus [174]. Infants with PD-DEE may also have febrile seizures, status epilepticus, or focal seizures before the onset of recognizable epilepsy. The presence of various seizure types makes PD-DEE a consideration in any infant with drug-resistant seizures.

The typical clinical manifestation of PDE-DEE is that the newborn undergoes seizures within hours to days of birth. Baxter [175] noted that fetuses may experience epileptic seizures in the second or third trimester of pregnancy, which are characterized by abnormal intrauterine activity. PDE-DEE conveys many forms of clinical seizures, including generalized tonic–clonic seizures, myoclonic seizures, atonic seizures, spastic seizures, etc., and often conveys status epilepticus and frequent seizures; patients may also have electrical seizures. Before a seizure, newborns may experience encephalopathy manifestations, such as irritability, crying, abnormal breathing, and vomiting; simultaneously, a low Apgar score and abnormal umbilical cord blood gas can be observed, which may lead to misdiagnosis of neonatal hypoxic-ischemic encephalopathy [176]. Similar manifestations of encephalopathy can also be observed in infants, possibly because the growth and development of patients and/or the progression of infectious diseases are associated with a greater demand for vitamin B6.

Atypical clinical manifestations of PDE-DEE include seizures that occur late, most of which begin after birth, at 1 year of age, or even in adolescence. In the initial stage of the disease, antiepileptic drugs can control the seizure, and, as the disease progresses, intractable epilepsy presents. Treatment with pyridoxine has no obvious effect on the disease course in the initial stage of the disease, but, after several months of pyridoxine treatment, the seizures can be controlled; when the treatment is stopped, its effects can persist long term and the patient becomes seizure-free (interval $\leq$5 months) [177].

Developmental Impairment

Patients with PDE-DEE often have severe intellectual impairment, particularly those who require multiple antiepileptic drugs for seizure control [177]. Even when seizures are controlled, many patients still exhibit varying degrees of cognitive impairment [178]. The duration of an epileptic seizure is related to the prognosis of the affected child's cognitive function. The earlier the seizure occurs, the more delayed the cognitive development of the child. Therefore, it is impossible to diagnose and treat children with pyridoxine as soon as possible, as this will increase the risk of developmental delays [179, 180]. In the late-onset population, a better cognitive prognosis can be observed, which may be due to the comprehensive effects of many factors. Among these factors, the most obvious is that the patient does not experience brain damage caused by epileptic seizures during the neonatal period [180].

Auxiliary Examinations

Studies by Mills et al. [181] and Schmitt et al. [182] have indicated that PDE-DEE does not exhibit characteristic electroencephalogram abnormalities. Nabbout et al. [183] reported that neonates may exhibit sustained high-voltage, rhythmic delta slow waves before receiving pyridoxine treatment, suggesting the possibility of pyridoxine-dependent epilepsy. Prior to pyridoxine treatment, EEG readings may show burst suppression or focal/multifocal spikes and waves in a slow-wave background. After pyridoxine treatment, abnormal EEG signals are suppressed and patients may return to a normal background within hours or days [174]. To date, there are no distinct MRI characteristic features of PDE-DEE. MRI findings, including thinning of the corpus callosum, hydrocephalus, ventricular enlargement, and cortical dysplasia, among others, occur in more than half of PDE-DEE patients [184, 185]. Most PD-DEE cases are associated with biallelic mutations in the *ALDH7A1* gene, while a few have been linked to biallelic mutations in pyridoxal 5′-phosphate-binding protein (PLPBP) [186]. Elevated levels of α-aminoadipic semialdehyde (α-AASA) and pipecolic acid (PA) in urine, plasma, and cerebrospinal fluid can serve as diagnostic biomarkers [173].

Diagnosis

According to the diagnostic criteria proposed by the International League Against Epilepsy in 2022 [12], the diagnosis includes three steps: ① Mandatory: Multiple seizure types, including focal/multifocal seizures, epileptic spasms, generalized tonic seizures, and generalized clonic seizures; resistance to antiepileptic drugs (usually progressing to status epilepticus); and a rapid response to pyridoxine treatment. During the interictal periods of seizures, patients exhibit a slowing of background brain activity and may have focal or multifocal abnormal discharges or burst suppression on EEG. Laboratory evidence supporting the diagnosis includes an increase in pipecolic acid (PA) and/or α-aminoadipic semialdehyde (α-AASA) levels in urine, plasma, and/or cerebrospinal fluid or the identification of pathogenic variants in the *ALDH7A1* gene. Lifelong use of pyridoxine can sustainably and significantly reduce or eliminate seizures. ② Alerts: Onset of seizures after 3 years of age, representing rare, late-onset, pyridoxine-dependent epilepsy and normal neurodevelopment. ③ Exclusions: None. MRI and ictal EEG are not required for diagnosis, but MRI is strongly recommended for excluding other causes. In resource-limited areas where laboratory evidence cannot be obtained and the patient meets all essential and exclusionary clinical criteria and whose seizures stop with pyridoxine supplementation, recur upon discontinuation, and cease once again upon reinitiation, a diagnosis of pyridoxine-dependent epilepsy syndrome may be made.

Differential Diagnosis

Hypoxic-Ischemic Encephalopathy

Fifty-five percent of children with *PDE-ALDH7A1* experience fetal distress and have a low Apgar score and seizures; therefore, PDE needs to be differentiated from hypoxic-ischemic encephalopathy. Key differentiating factors include drug resistance to common antiepileptic medications, preterm birth, severe or persistent EEG abnormalities, and the presence of alterations in AASA and PA levels, along with pathogenic gene mutations.

Vitamin B6-Responsive Infantile Spasms

This disease begins in infancy and mainly manifests as spasms. During the interictal periods of seizures, EEG signals show marked hypsarrhythmia. A distinguishing factor is that in most cases, vitamin B6 supplementation can control spasms; however, vitamin B6 loses effectiveness when the disease progresses to focal epilepsy or Lennox–Gastaut syndrome. Moreover, the vitamin B6 treatment scheme depends on changes in the patient's clinical condition and does not necessarily require lifelong medication.

Pyridox(am)ine 5′-Phosphate Oxidase (PNPO) Deficiency

This autosomal recessive inherited disease is caused by *PNPO* gene mutations and mainly presents as neonatal epileptic encephalopathy refractory to treatment with pyridoxamine or pyridoxine. Diagnosis requires *PNPO* gene testing. The distinguishing factor is the presence of alterations in AASA and PA levels in this condition with confirmed pathogenic mutations in *ALDH7A1*; the seizures can be controlled with pyridoxine supplementation.

Treatment

Pyridoxine

PDE-ALDH7A1 requires lifelong pyridoxine supplementation. After summarizing the observational studies and expert opinions, the current recommendations of the International PDE Association regarding the recommended dose of pyridoxine treatment are as follows [173]: for neonates, 100 mg/day; for infants, 30 mg/kg/day (maximum dose of 300 mg/day); and for adults, 200–500 mg/day (maximum dose of 500 mg/day). During acute illness, such as gastroenteritis or febrile respiratory infections, daily doses of pyridoxine can be doubled for the first 3 days to prevent seizures and/or worsening encephalopathy. In most patients, once the pyridoxine dosage has effectively controlled seizures, all other antiepileptic drugs can be discontinued. The pyridoxine dosage should not exceed 500 mg/day, as the neurotoxicity of pyridoxine can lead to reversible sensory neuropathy [187].

Folate

If pyridoxine does not completely control seizures, supplementation with folate can be considered, with a recommended dosage of 3–5 mg/kg/day. However, the mechanism of folate treatment is not yet clear.

Arginine

Arginine and lysine compete for transport via cationic amino acid transporter 1 in the blood–brain barrier (BBB) and mitochondrial ornithine carriers in the mitochondrial membrane; thus, by increasing arginine content, excess lysine can be eliminated through the blood–brain barrier and cerebrospinal fluid lysine concentration can be reduced [188]. Studies have shown that supplementing arginine alongside pyridoxine can improve motor and language function in patients [189]. The management consensus of the International PDE Association suggests an initial arginine dosage of 200 mg/day [173].

Lysine-Restricted Diet

Research has suggested that limiting dietary lysine intake may lower lysine-derived substrate levels and help improve brain function [188]. According to the management consensus of the International PDE Association, only 10 out of 27 patients achieved neurological development outcomes related to lysine-restricted diets [173]. Therefore, restricting dietary lysine intake can be considered only an adjunctive therapy for patients.

Prognosis

Seventy-five percent of patients experience varying degrees of cognitive and behavioral impairments, with most of these patients achieving complete seizure control [165, 166]. The younger the age of seizure onset is, the greater the likelihood of cognitive developmental delay, and delayed diagnosis and pyridoxine treatment increase the risk of intellectual disabilities [179, 180]. In the late-onset population, the cognitive prognosis is better than that in the early-onset population, which is a result of the comprehensive actions of many factors [180]. The prognoses of PDE-DEE patients are related to many factors, including the age of seizure onset, the duration of treatment with pyridoxine, and the presence of complications.

5.2.3.3 Pyridox(am)ine 5′-Phosphate Deficiency (PNPO) Developmental and Epileptic Encephalopathy

Overview

Pyridox(am)ine 5′-phosphate oxidase (PNPO) developmental and epileptic encephalopathy (P5PD-DEE) was first proposed by Kuo and Wang [190] in 2002. Beginning in 2022, patients were classified as having developmental and epileptic encephalopathy or etiology-specific epileptic encephalopathy according to the new ILAE classification. P5PD-DEE usually presents as severe epileptic encephalopathy in newborns or young infants, and conventional antiepileptic drugs are ineffective; therefore, the treatment of P5PD-DEE depends on lifelong pyridoxal 5′-phosphate (PLP) treatment [191]. This disease is a rare autosomal recessive genetic disease, and its pathogenesis is due to PNPO deficiency caused by a mutation in the *PNPO* gene on chromosome 17.

Historical Evolution and Epidemiological Investigation

In 2002, Kuo and Wang [190] first discovered PNPO deficiency. By 2005, research by Mills et al. suggested that PNPO deficiency is caused by mutations in the *PNPO* gene, with clear characteristics of autosomal recessive inheritance [191]. This condition is relatively rare, and 90 cases have been reported across 32 studies. However, the exact incidence rate of P5PD-DEE is still unknown.

Etiology

P5PD-DEE is a rare autosomal recessive genetic disorder caused by pathogenic mutations in the *PNPO* gene. The *PNPO* gene encodes pyridox(am)ine 5′-phosphate oxidase (PNPO) and is located on chromosome 17. This gene consists of 7 exons and has a length of approximately 7500 base pairs. PNPO catalyzes the conversion of pyridoxine (PN) to pyridoxal 5′-phosphate (PLP), and a deficiency in PNPO expression leads to reduced PLP production. PLP serves as a cofactor for numerous enzymes and participates in more than 140 enzymatic reactions in the human body [192]. These reactions include the metabolism of amino acids, glycogen phosphorylation, and the synthesis of nucleic acids, hemoglobin, sphingolipids, phospholipids, and neurotransmitters (serotonin, dopamine, norepinephrine, γ-aminobutyric acid), among others [193, 194]. PLP promotes the decarboxylation of glutamate via glutamate decarboxylase, increasing the production of the inhibitory neurotransmitter γ-aminobutyric acid. Abnormalities in γ-aminobutyric acid synthesis often lead to seizures in infants.

Clinical Presentation

The primary clinical manifestation of P5PD-DEE is seizures, which occur during the neonatal period and early infancy, with more than half of the patients presenting with seizures within 24 h of birth. Seizures are refractory to conventional antiepileptic drugs and are accompanied by neonatal distress, irritability, vomiting, metabolic acidosis, and low Apgar scores [195]. P5PD-DEE patients present with various forms of seizures, 80% of which are characterized by focal/multifocal clonic seizures and generalized tonic–clonic seizures. Some patients may experience absence seizures and spasms [196, 197], often accompanied by frequent seizures and status epilepticus; these patients are typically unresponsive to antiepileptic drugs or pyridoxine treatment.

P5PD-DEE may also exhibit non-neurological manifestations, including premature birth and fetal distress, as well as less common features, such as anemia, abnormal fetal movements, intrauterine growth restriction, and amniotic fluid abnormalities. Rarely, patients may exhibit pigmentary retinopathy [82], abdominal distension [191], constipation [198], and feeding intolerance [197]. Despite treatment with PLP, more than half of P5PD-DEE patients continue to experience developmental delays or intellectual disabilities.

Auxiliary Examinations

The electroencephalogram (EEG) characteristics of patients with P5PD-DEE are variable. In more than half of patients, the interictal periods exhibit burst suppression. A few of EEG readings show multifocal sharp waves, spikes, and intermittent spikes. In some cases, the EEG may show no abnormal discharges. To date, there are still no distinctive MRI features specific to P5PD-DEE. However, more than half of P5PD-DEE patients have MRI abnormalities [195]. Common MRI changes include diffuse atrophy, ischemic changes, brain softening, delayed myelination, diffuse or focal edema, and, in rare cases, intracranial venous sinus thrombosis, subdural hemorrhage, or abnormal periventricular white matter signals. P5PD-DEE is associated with pathogenic *PNPO* gene mutations. According to laboratory tests, most patients exhibit elevated organic acid levels in urine, low PLP levels in cerebrospinal fluid, and elevated glycine and threonine levels.

Diagnosis

According to the diagnostic criteria proposed by ILAE in 2022 [12], the diagnosis includes three steps: ① Mandatory: Multiple seizure types, including focal/multifocal seizures, spasms seizures, generalized tonic seizures, and generalized clonic seizures, with resistance to antiepileptic drugs (typically leading to status epilepticus) but responsive to pyridoxal 5′-phosphate (PLP) treatment. Interictal EEG signals show a slowing background with focal or multifocal discharges or a burst suppression pattern. The diagnostic evidence obtained from laboratory tests includes reduced PLP levels in cerebrospinal fluid or identification of pathogenic variants of the *PNPO* gene. Lifelong PLP supplementation significantly reduces or stops seizures. ② Alerts: Onset of symptoms after age 3, with normal neurodevelopment. ③ Exclusions: None. MRI and ictal EEG are not necessary for diagnosis but are strongly recommended for ruling out other causes. In resource-limited regions where laboratory evidence cannot be obtained, if the patient meets all the essential and exclusionary clinical criteria, has seizures that stop with PLP supplementation, recur upon discontinuation, and stop again upon reinitiation, they may be diagnosed with pyridox(am)ine 5′-phosphate deficiency (PNPO) syndrome [12].

Differential Diagnosis

1. *Hypoxic-ischemic encephalopathy*: P5PD-DEE patients often have a history of fetal distress, low Apgar scores, and clinical seizures, making it necessary to differentiate them from those with hypoxic-ischemic encephalopathy. P5PD-DEE is characterized by drug-resistant seizures, a history of premature birth, severe or persistent EEG abnormalities, and pathogenic gene mutations.
2. *Ohtahara syndrome*: Typically, this syndrome begins within the first 3 months of life and is characterized by a burst suppression pattern upon EEG and drug-resistant seizures. The key distinguishing factor is that P5PD-DEE, as confirmed by *PNPO* gene testing, is refractory to commonly used antiepileptic drugs but can be controlled with PLP treatment.
3. *Pyridoxine-dependent (ALDH7A1) developmental and epileptic encephalopathy*: Caused by pathogenic mutations in the *ALDH7A1* gene and confirmed by *ALDH7A1* gene testing, this disease is an autosomal recessive genetic disorder. Clinical presentation often occurs during the neonatal period in patients with drug-resistant seizures; these patients require pyridoxine treatment. A distinguishing feature of this disease is that P5PD-DEE patients may exhibit reduced PLP levels in cerebrospinal fluid, and seizures can be controlled with PLP treatment.

Treatment

Patients with P5PD-DEE require lifelong supplementation with PLP or PN.

PLP

To date, there has been no unified consensus on the optimal long-term treatment dosage for PLP. Determination of the treatment dosage primarily depends on the patient's response to PLP therapy and is typically in the range of 30–60 mg/kg/day; the treatment is divided into three to four rounds of oral administration [199]. Individual dosing should be based on the minimum effective dose of PLP. There is currently no specified safe dosage for PLP, but the potential side effects may include hepatotoxicity. It has been reported that patients taking 50 mg/kg/day PLP show elevated transaminase levels, and those taking 50–100 mg/kg/day PLP show indications of cirrhosis [200]. The occurrence of side effects may be due to excessive PLP dosage or the formation of toxic degradation products during PLP tablet dissolution. Therefore, PLP tablets should be taken directly or immediately after dissolution, and liver function should be regularly monitored when PLP is used for treatment.

PN

For P5PD-DEE patients who respond to PN therapy and have controlled seizures, there is no need to switch to PLP treatment. The PN treatment dosage can be determined according to expert opinions published by the International PDE

Association for treating PDE-ALDH7A1: for newborns, 100 mg/day pyridoxine; for infants, 30 mg/kg/day pyridoxine (maximum dose of 300 mg/day); and for adults, 200–500 mg/day pyridoxine (maximum dose of 500 mg/day). The pyridoxine dosage should not exceed 500 mg/day, as its neurotoxicity may lead to reversible sensory neuropathy [187].

Prognosis

The prognosis for P5PD-DEE varies widely, with approximately half of patients experiencing intellectual and motor developmental delays at 18–24 months of age. Premature infants have a higher incidence of adverse outcomes, but patients who receive early or preventative PLP treatment tend to have a better prognosis [201]. In a minority of patients, seizures may continue despite treatment with pyridoxine and PLP. This could be due to delayed diagnosis and effective treatment. Therefore, early diagnosis and treatment of this condition can lead to better outcomes. Without timely treatment, most patients may die between 2 and 24 weeks after birth, and survivors may have severe neurological sequelae [170]. In addition, different genotypes are important factors affecting patient prognosis [170].

5.2.3.4 CDKL5 Developmental and Epileptic Encephalopathy

Overview

CDKL5 deficiency disorder (CDD), also known as developmental and epileptic encephalopathy, is an X-linked dominantly inherited neurodevelopmental disorder. It is an important cause of very-early-onset epilepsy (median age 6 weeks) with significant hypotonia. It is characterized by onset within the first few months of life and clusters of combined spasmodic and tonic seizures, although multiple seizure types may occur. Seizures usually have multiple phases and typically present as sequential hyperkinetic–tonic–convulsive seizures. Severe-to-very-severe global developmental delays are present in almost all cases [202]. In 2022, the new ILAE classification of epilepsy syndromes categorized this disease as developmental or epileptic encephalopathy [12].

Historical Evolution and Epidemiological Investigations

In 1985, Hanefeld first described early-onset epilepsy in Rett syndrome (RTT) patients prior to the diagnosis of intellectual disability [203], and, in 2003, Kalscheuer et al. localized the gene encoding a serine threonine kinase (STK9) on the X chromosome (Xp22.3), suggesting that mutations in this gene are involved in the pathogenesis of X-linked infantile spasms syndrome (ISSX) [204]. Two female patients with infantile spasms and severe mental developmental delays were analyzed. In 2004 and 2005, the occurrence of CDKL5 mutations was confirmed in patients previously diagnosed with Rett syndrome, which suggested an atypical form of the disease. In 2022, the new ILAE classification of epileptic syndromes classified this disease as developmental or epileptic encephalopathy. The prevalence of CDKL5 mutations is estimated to be approximately 1/40,000 to 1/60,000 live births. Ninety percent of patients with CDKL5 deficiency are girls.

Etiology
The causative gene for developmental and epileptic encephalopathy is *CDKL5*, which is located at Xp22. This gene encodes a protein belonging to the serine–threonine kinase family that is widely distributed in all tissues of the human body, with the highest expression in the brain (cerebral cortex, hippocampus, cerebellum, thalamus, and brainstem), testis, and thymus. CDKL5 expression is lowest during the prenatal period and highest in the later stages of rapid postnatal neurological development (especially in the cortex and hippocampus) [205]. The CDKL5 protein plays an important role in neuronal formation and maturation, participating in proliferation, neuronal migration, neurite formation and neurite growth, and synaptic development and function during brain maturation [206]. CDKL5 is involved in the phosphorylation of MeCP2 products. Its mutation underlies the pathophysiology of Rett syndrome. This finding suggests that the two proteins share a common metabolic pathway, thus partially explaining the clinical presentation with similarities to Rett syndrome [207].

Clinical Manifestations
The causative gene for CDD is located on the X chromosome and affects girls more dramatically than boys, with X chromosome inactivation being one of the most important determinants of symptom severity in girls [208]. Approximately 8–16% of girls with early-onset epilepsy carry the *CDKL5* gene mutation, while the clinical symptoms are more pronounced in boys with CDD [202]. The main clinical symptoms of these patients are as follows:

Seizures

Seizures are usually the first symptom of CDD [209]. The median age at which seizures occur is 6 weeks, with 90% of them starting within 3 months of birth. Initial seizure types vary, but tonic, convulsive, generalized tonic–clonic, or focal seizures are common. As the disease progresses, other seizure types may appear. Most patients will have epileptic spasticity and/or tonic seizures. Hyperkinetic–tonic–convulsive sequential seizures are the typical seizure type and are observed in most but not all cases. The first phase of this type of seizure begins with hypermobility accompanied by rocking, kicking, and vocalization and lasts for 10–60 s. This is followed by a tonic phase involving extension of the limbs or straightening of the upper limbs and flexion of the lower limbs, lasting for 20–45 s. This is followed by a series of extensor spasms lasting for 1–15 min. Similarly, multitemporal episodes include clusters of tonic and spastic episodes, but the order in which the types of episodes occur may be different. Autonomic symptoms include flushing, dilated pupils, and irregular breathing. Myoclonic, clonic, catatonic, and atonic seizures may occur as the disease progresses. Typical CDKL5-DEE-associated epilepsy is divided into three consecutive stages [210]: ① Stage 1: Early-onset epilepsy with brief tonic seizures, often accompanied by flushing. Interictal EEG is normal, and the tonic seizure phase shows generalized voltage reduction followed by rapid activity in the frontal or central regions. There is no burst inhibition pattern in this phase. ② Stage 2: Epileptic encephalopathy with tonic seizures and infantile spasms.

Interictal EEG is markedly abnormal, showing bilateral slow waves or widespread spikes, slow waves or polyspikes, and slow waves. There is rarely a burst inhibition pattern in this stage. ③ Stage 3: Late multifocal and myoclonic epilepsy with tonic seizures, myoclonic seizures, absence seizures, or multifocal seizures. The interictal phase is characterized by diffuse high-amplitude δ slow waves with pseudo-periodic bursts of spikes, polyspikes, and spike complex waves in the central, temporal, or temporo-occipital regions.

Developmental Disorders

Developmental disorders are present at the onset of epilepsy and become more pronounced as the disease progresses [211]. However, definite developmental regression is rare. In almost all cases, there is severe-to-very-severe global developmental regression. Neurological examination suggests diffuse hypotonia with a normal head circumference at onset. Cortical vision is impaired, often accompanied by a lack of eye contact and poor pursuit vision. Minor physical deformities, such as deep eye sockets, wide forehead, protruding lips, deep manubrium, and bulging finger/toe bones with tapered fingers, are present.

Diagnosis

Epileptic seizures, including tonic seizures, epileptic spasms, generalized tonic–clonic seizures, and/or focal hyperkinetic–tonic–spasmodic sequential seizures, are characteristic phenotypes, but not all patients present with these types of seizures. Genetic testing suggests a pathogenic mutation in the *CDKL5* gene.

Differential Diagnosis

Rett Syndrome

Rett syndrome (RTT) [212] is an X-linked dominant genetic disorder in which a mutation in the *MECP2* gene causes severe intellectual impairment. Patients exhibit normal growth and development in the early years of life, followed by slow development. They show slow brain and head growth, intellectual impairment, seizures, breathing disorders, rigid hand movements, and gastrointestinal problems.

Infantile Epileptic Spasm Syndrome

This is characterized by epileptic spasms rather than myoclonic seizures. The onset of epileptic spasm occurs early after awakening, and it has a duration of >1 s. Most patients with IESS have abnormal inter-episodic EEG signals, accompanied by high arrhythmia or multifocal discharge. Early monitoring during seizures can also distinguish epileptic spasms from myoclonic seizures.

Treatments

Choice of Antiseizure Medications (ASMs) [55]

CDD usually does not respond well to standard ASMs, and the improvement is usually short-term. Multidrug combination therapy, the most commonly used regimen of ASMs for CDD, can include clobazam, valproic acid, topiramate, levetiracetam, and vigabatrin, but the treatment effect of ASMs is limited.

Other Nonpharmacological Treatments

Other nonpharmacological treatments may include a ketogenic diet and vagus nerve stimulation. A ketogenic diet may provide short-term benefits in controlling seizures that may not be sustained in the long term. Some patients respond to VNS therapy [213].

Recent Advances in Gene Therapy for *CDKL5* Expression Deficiency [214–216]

1. *ZTALMY oral suspension*: ZTALMY oral suspension, the first FDA-approved drug specifically for the treatment of CDD, is a neuroactive steroid that acts as a positive allosteric regulator of GABAA receptors.
2. *Enzyme replacement therapy*: Enzyme replacement therapy involves regular injections of the CDKL5 protein to compensate for the protein deficiency caused by gene mutations.
3. *Exogenous gene introduction*: The purpose of this therapy is to introduce the exogenous *CDKL5* gene into the body through a viral vector to express normal protein. Another treatment option is to activate the *CDKL5* gene on the silenced X chromosome in female patients. Treatment that targets nonsense mutations forces cells to ignore this abnormal termination signal, allowing them to produce full-length functional proteins.

Prognosis

CDD often results in drug-resistant epilepsy, and most patients have severe intellectual disabilities [216]. Most patients have seizures on a daily basis, although less than half experience episodic periods of up to 2 months or more without seizures. Less than a quarter of patients are able to walk and speak independently. Movement disorders such as dance athetosis, asthenia, dystonia, and Parkinson's disease can affect a small number of patients. Men are more severely affected by this disease than women.

5.2.3.5 *PCDH19* Clustering Epilepsy

Overview

PCDH19 gene-associated epilepsy, also known as *PCDH19* clustering epilepsy, is a rare genetic disorder. Its clinical manifestations include a wide spectrum and overlap with those of a variety of diseases; the core symptoms are heat sensitivity and cluster seizures, accompanied by varying degrees of intellectual disability [217]. This disease has a special X-linked inheritance mode; that is, heterozygous women who carry the gene mutation develop the disease, while semizygous men who carry the mutation do not [218, 219]. However, it has been reported that men with chimeric mutations in the *PCDH19* gene can develop this disease, and its clinical phenotype is epilepsy accompanied by different degrees of intellectual disability.

Historical Evolution and Epidemiological Investigation

Mutations in the *PCDH19* gene were first clinically described in 1971 in a female-limited family with epilepsy and mental developmental delays [220]. It has subsequently been reported that men with chimeric *PCDH19* gene mutations may also be affected. There have also been a few cases in which intellectual delays are not associated. In 2008, systematic sequencing of X chromosome exons from seven large families diagnosed with epilepsy and mental retardation limited to females (EFMR) revealed that *PCDH19* gene mutations were the cause of this disease, which was subsequently classified as PCDH19-related epilepsy [221]. The 2022 ILAE Task Force on Classification and Definition of Disease classified epilepsy with *PCDH19* clustering epilepsy as DEE or a syndrome of progressive neurological impairment (etiological-specific epileptic encephalopathy) that is associated with a specific etiology and clearly defines its distinct phenotype [12]. A recent population-based study has shown that PCDH19 is the most common form of single-gene epilepsy among young children, with an incidence of 1/20600 female births, although definitive epidemiological survey data are lacking in China.

Etiology

The cadherin 19-encoding gene (*PCDH19*) is localized to Xq22.1. PCDH19 is expressed in multiple tissues but is mainly expressed in the peripheral regions of the nervous system. The *PCDH19* gene encodes a transmembrane adhesion molecule of the cadherin family, which is a member of the protocadherin delta 2 subfamily and is a single transmembrane protein involved in neuronal connection and signal transduction. The main pathogenic mechanisms of *PCDH19* mutation include the following [222–224]: (1) affecting the early stage of neuronal formation via its involvement in the proliferation of neuronal progenitor cells and the regulation of cell motility; (2) PCDH19 mutations may alter the correct position of the mitotic spindle, resulting in asymmetric cell division, which leads to accelerated neural differentiation; and (3) the interaction between the cytoplasmic domain of PCDH19 and the α-subunit of the GABAA receptor may alter the excitation–inhibition balance in patients with epilepsy, and PCDH19 is involved in regulating channel gating and blood–brain barrier (BBB) dysfunction. *PCDH19* gene-related epilepsy is inherited in a specific X-linked manner; heterozygous females carrying the *PCDH19* mutation are affected, while hemizygous males are not.

Clinical Manifestations

1. The clinical phenotype of *PCDH19* gene-related epilepsy is heterogeneous, and identical twins may have different phenotypes. The core phenotypes include early-onset seizures, heat-sensitive seizures, and cluster seizures. The age of onset ranges from 1 to 70 months, and the peak age of onset is 10–12 months.
2. Most children with *PCDH19* gene-related epilepsy have two or more types of seizures, mainly including general tonic, clonic, or tonic–clonic seizures; focal seizures; and focal seizures accompanied by generalization. Other rare seizure types include atypical absence, atonic, and myoclonic seizures. Epileptic seizures are characterized by heat sensitivity; that is, fever easily induces epileptic seizures, and fever seizures are significantly aggravated. Clusters of seizures are an important seizure characteristic; these are several to dozens of attacks over a

few consecutive days, with each attack lasting 1–5 min. A few seizures can also have a longer duration of attack or even status epilepticus. In most patients, seizures are difficult to control in infancy and childhood, but the frequency of the seizures gradually decreases with age, and some patients can be completely seizure-free in adolescence and adulthood.

3. *PCDH19* gene-related epilepsy has a wide spectrum of manifestations that can overlap with those of other epilepsy types and clinical phenotypes of neurological diseases. The main presentations include the following [221, 225–227]: ① *PCDH19* gene mutation can lead to a Dravet syndrome (DS) phenotype. The phenotype of DS caused by the *PCDH19* gene mutation overlaps with that of DS caused by the *SCN1A* gene mutation, which includes an early onset (before 1 year of age), heat sensitivity at onset, multiple attack types, poor efficacy of antiseizure drugs, normal development before onset, and developmental delay, cognitive impairment, and behavioral abnormalities after onset. However, there are also differences between the two groups of patients. Children with *PCDH19* mutation-associated DS have shorter seizure durations; the characteristics of cluster seizures are more prominent; myoclonic seizures, epileptic status, and light sensitivity are rare; and the long-term prognosis is mostly better than that of children with *SCN1A* mutation-positive DS. ② *PCDH19* is associated with focal epilepsy. Focal epilepsy accompanied by emotional symptoms (screaming in fear during seizures etc.) is a major feature of *PCDH19* gene-associated epilepsy. EEG during focal attacks shows that the frontotemporal region of the brain is the main area involved [205]. Although most patients with *PCDH19* gene-related epilepsy have normal cranial imaging, focal cortical dysplasia is observed in a small number of patients. Patients with focal epilepsy with heat sensitivity and cluster seizures should be excluded for *PCDH19* gene mutations.
4. The developmental trajectories of children with *PCDH19*-gene-related epilepsy can be divided into several patterns: normal, delayed, or initially normal with subsequent regression or delay. Intelligence ranges from normal to severe intellectual disability, and most patients are diagnosed with low or borderline intellectual disability [217]. It can be accompanied by attention disorders, hyperactivity, anxiety, autism, obsessive–compulsive disorder, impulsivity, irritability, aggressive behavior, and other mental behavioral disorders. Patients with *PCDH19* gene-related epilepsy may have an ASD phenotype.
5. Electroencephalogram (EEG) signals may have generalized or focal discharge, and the interval between episodes may be normal. Magnetic resonance imaging (MRI) of the head shows no abnormalities in most patients, and a few patients are diagnosed with or suspected of having focal cortical dysplasia.

Diagnosis

The main seizure varieties include early-onset, heat-sensitive, and cluster seizures; focal seizures; and seizures accompanied by emotional symptoms. Molecular tests for pathogenic mutations in PCDH19 are used to confirm the diagnosis.

Differential Diagnosis

Generalized Epilepsy with Febrile Seizures Plus

This is a familial epilepsy syndrome diagnosed on the basis of the characteristics of the whole family, and its onset occurs at 3 months of age. At 6 years of age, multiple phenotypes can be observed, such as FS or FS+. Most patients with these forms of epilepsy develop normally, and there is no developmental regression after febrile convulsions.

Dravet Syndrome (DS)

Dravet syndrome (DS) [225] is characterized by obvious thermal sensitivity before 1 year of age and a convulsive state. After 1 year of age, many types of seizures can occur. In children with *PCDH19* mutation-associated DS, the seizure duration is shorter (generally <5 min); the characteristics of cluster seizures are more prominent; however, myoclonic seizures, epileptic status, and light sensitivity are rare; and the long-term prognosis is mostly better than that of children with *SCN1A* mutation-associated DS.

Treatment

PCDH19-related epilepsy usually has poor response to antiseizure drugs, and it is difficult to achieve complete control of seizures. The main purpose of treatment is to reduce both the frequency of seizures and the occurrence of status epilepticus, so multidrug combination therapy or ketogenic diet therapy is needed [228].

Antiseizure Medications (ASMs)

There are currently no antiseizure medications that explicitly prevent recurrent seizures, and treatment depends on the type and severity of the seizure and the associated neurological characteristics. A combination of ASMs is commonly used to control different types of seizures. Commonly used first-line drugs are bromide, clobazam, valproic acid, and levetiracetam.

Ketogenic Diet (KD) and Vagus Nerve Stimulation (VNS)

A ketogenic diet (KD) and vagus nerve stimulation (VNS) can be used to treat refractory epilepsy and status epilepticus. A ketogenic diet has been associated with a positive response in 50% of patients.

Corticosteroids

Corticosteroids can be used for treatment during acute attacks, and the effect is significant. Hormone therapy can significantly improve patient symptoms in the acute phase and help cluster attacks disappear quickly in all patients, but this effect is only temporary. In addition, mutations in the *PCDH19* gene have been shown to cause allopregnanolone (AP) deficiency in female patients [229, 230]. AP is a neurosteroid hormone and the most effective regulator of the γ-aminobutyric acid (GABA) receptor. It can be used as a forward allosteric regulator of the GABAA inhibitory neurotransmitter receptor, a type A receptor of GABA [218]. This leads to prolonged hyperpolarization of neurons and inhibits excessive firing of neurons during seizures.

Prognosis

In addition to early-onset and refractory disease, cluster seizures can occur. In most patients, these seizures are difficult to control in infancy and childhood, but the frequency of seizures gradually decreases with age, and some patients can be completely seizure-free in adolescence and adulthood. *PCDH19* gene-related epilepsy is associated with varying degrees of cognitive and sensory impairment as well as mental and behavioral problems. Associations with depression, autism, obsessive–compulsive disorder, and aggressive behavior, among other disorders, have been observed in patients with *PCDH19* gene-related epilepsy, and other neurological abnormalities may also occur, including sleep disturbances, episodic apnea, movement disorders, hypotonia, speech delays, sensory integration problems, and autonomic disorders. The overall prognosis is poor.

5.2.3.6 Glucose Transporter Type 1 Deficiency Syndrome (Glut1-DS)

Overview

Glucose transporter type 1 deficiency syndrome (Glut1-DS) is a group of diseases characterized by a continuous phenotypic spectrum due to a defect in the *SLC2A1* gene encoding glucose transporter type 1 (Glut1), which causes dysfunction in the transport of glucose into brain tissue through the blood–brain barrier. The classic phenotypes are paroxysmal motion-induced dyskinesia and epilepsy (formerly known as DYT18), paroxysmal chorea with spasticity (formerly known as DYT9), atypical childhood absence epilepsy, myoclonic unstable epilepsy, and paroxysmal nonepileptic manifestations, including intermittent ataxia, chorea, dystonia, and alternating hemiplegia. Seizure, paroxysmal dyskinesia, and psychomotor developmental delay are the three major clinical manifestations of Glut1-DS, and early initiation of a ketogenic diet can significantly improve the prognosis of this disease.

Historical Evolution and Epidemiological Investigation

Glut1-DS was first described in 1991 by de Vivo, and cases have since been reported worldwide. The exact incidence and prevalence of Glut1-DS, a rare nervous system disease, are lacking. The incidence/prevalence in Queensland, Australia, is approximately 1:90,000 [231], while a recent Nordic study has estimated that the incidence/prevalence was approximately 1:83,000 [232]. Due to the difficulty in diagnosing this disease, the true incidence/prevalence rate is likely greater.

Etiology and Pathophysiology

Sugars are the primary energy source for the brain. Glucose transporter type 1 (Glut1), encoded by the *SLC2A1* gene, is a major carrier that facilitates the passage of glucose through the blood–brain barrier into the brain. The metabolic rate of brain sugar is very low in the fetal period; it rises rapidly after birth, reaches a peak at approximately 3 years of age, and gradually decreases after 10 years of age until it reaches the metabolic level of early adulthood. Therefore, the clinical symptoms of Glut1-DS are most common in infants and young children. Both human and animal data show that the safe range of glucose content that reaches the brain through the blood–brain barrier to meet the needs of brain metabolism and brain function is very narrow. A 25–35% decrease in Glut1 transport function causes mild phenotypes such as paroxysmal dyskinesia [233], while a significant decrease causes more severe clinical phenotypes [234].

Clinical Manifestations

In Glut1-DS, 90% of patients present with the typical syndrome and 10% with atypical phenotypes. Neonatal seizures, paroxysmal dyskinesia, and psychomotor developmental delay are the main clinical manifestations of typical Glut1-DS. The atypical phenotype is relatively mild and usually lacks seizures, while movement disorders, such as intermittent ataxia, chorea, dystonia, and alternating hemiplegia, are more common.

Seizures

Approximately 90% of Glut1-DS patients have epilepsy, which usually starts in infancy (most often within 2 years of age, especially at 1–6 months of age). The phenotypes of seizures vary and include generalized tonicity/clonus, focal, myoclonus, atypical absence, atonic, and unclassifiable types [235]. Generalized tonic–clonic seizures and absence seizures are most common, and more than two-thirds of patients can have more than two types of seizures. The frequency, severity, and types of seizures are not associated with the severity of the disease.

Dyskinesia

Complex movement disorders characterized by ataxia, dystonia, and chorea may occur in any combination and may be paroxysmal or persistent, with their severity fluctuating depending on environmental factors such as fasting or infectious stress [235–238]. A summary of movement disorders in 57 Glut1-DS patients revealed that the most common was gait disorder (89%), including ataxia with or without spasms; other manifestations included motor limb dystonia (86%), mild chorea (75%), cerebellar activity tremor (70%), nonepileptic events (28%), apraxia (21%), and myoclonus (16%) [238].

In early infancy, distinctive paroxysmal oculo-cephalic movement, characterized by involuntary, transient, repetitive multidirectional nystagmus, often conjugated, and often accompanied by head movements in the same direction, is the second most common initial symptom of Glut1-DS. It is also known as an abnormal gaze saccade, is sometimes accompanied by apnea and cyanosis, and is usually resolved by age 6. In some infants, apnea and paroxysmal eye–head movements may precede epilepsy [239].

Atypical Glut1-DS patients present with paroxysmal motion-induced dyskinesia and late-onset epilepsy, and the neurological examination and head circumference of the child are normal during intermittent seizures [240–242]. It has been reported that heterozygous mutations in *SLC2A1* can also lead to chronic progressive spastic paraplegia and paroxysmal chorea and that movement disorders can be induced by prolonged exercise, anxiety, or emotional problems, which gradually decrease or stop with age [243].

Cognitive and Language Impairments

Generally, varying degrees of cognitive impairment are present, ranging from mild learning disabilities to severe intellectual disability. All patients have varying degrees of dysarthria, including decreased comprehension and expression. However, patients with Glut1-DS are often well-adapted to groups and school settings and interact well with others, and autism spectrum disorder symptoms are not obvious.

Microcephalus

Patients are born with a normal head circumference and gradually develop varying degrees of microcephaly as the disease progresses. Microcephaly can appear in infancy to varying degrees and may correspond to the severity of the disease.

Laboratory Findings

Electrophysiological Tests

The intermittent EEG signal is generally normal but can also indicate epileptic discharge and slow background activity.

Neuroimaging Results

Brain MRI is usually normal. Some patients may exhibit nonspecific abnormalities, such as ventricular widening and a lag in myelin development.

Cerebrospinal Fluid Findings

A low CSF glucose concentration combined with a normal blood glucose level are an important piece of evidence for the diagnosis of Glut1-DS. Lumbar puncture examination should be performed after 4–6 h of fasting, preferably before breakfast, and a synchronous blood glucose test should be performed before lumbar puncture. To date, the CSF glucose concentrations of all patients are <3.3 mmol/L (60 mg/dL, normal range: 16.2–52 mg/dL), and 90% of patients have a CSF glucose concentration <2.2 mmol/L (40 mg/dL) [234, 244, 245]. The glucose concentration in the cerebrospinal fluid of patients with atypical Glut1-DS (41–52 mg/dL) is greater than that in typical patients [27]. In terms of diagnostic value, an absolute decrease in CSF glucose content is better than a decrease in the CSF glucose/glycemic index, and this finding is consistent with the severity of clinical symptoms.

In addition, the level of lactic acid in cerebrospinal fluid is generally reduced or at the low normal limit, which is also helpful for disease diagnosis.

Erythrocyte Glucose Uptake Assay

In addition to being expressed throughout the central nervous system, Glut1 is also highly expressed on erythrocyte cell membranes, so the ability of Glut1 to take up glucose in the brain can be indirectly assessed by the red blood cell 3-*O*-methyl-D-glucose (3-OMG) uptake test. It is generally believed that a finding falling within 35–74% of normal control values is helpful for diagnosis.

Genetic Tests

Patients can be diagnosed according to the presence of pathogenic variations in the *SLC2A1* gene. Most patients inherit autosomal dominant patterns, among whom 90% of patients represent sporadic cases and 10% have a family history. A few patients are autosomal recessive or have HELLP (hemolysis, elevated liver enzymes, and low platelets) syndrome; 84% have point mutations, and 13% have deletions or duplications. The type of mutation may be related to the severity of the clinical phenotype. Heterozygous missense mutations usually cause mild-to-moderate clinical manifestations, while shear, nonsense, insertion, and deletion mutations occur only in moderate-to-severe patients, and complete exon deletion leads to severe clinical manifestations. Some patients with heterozygous mutations may have parents who are mild or asymptomatic carriers.

Diagnosis

Based on the clinical manifestations of the proband, combined with a normal blood glucose level and low cerebrospinal fluid glucose concentration (<3.3 mmol/L or 60 mg/dL), the possibility of this disease should be considered. Heterozygous (or rare biallelic) pathogenic variants in *SLC2A1* can lead to a definite diagnosis. Glut1-DS is highly suspected when a patient has characteristic clinical manifestations and cerebrospinal fluid hypoglycemia but lacks a pathogenic variation of *SLC2A1* or when the patient does not have characteristic clinical manifestations but has cerebrospinal fluid hypoglycemia and pathogenic variation of *SLC2A1* and needs to start ketogenic diet therapy. If the ketogenic diet is effective or there is a family history of Glut1-DS, the diagnosis of Glut1-DS is more warranted. If the patient has the characteristic clinical manifestations of Glut1-DS and a pathogenic *SLC2A1* mutation but the glucose level in the cerebrospinal fluid is normal or if the patient does not have characteristic clinical manifestations, and a low glucose level in the cerebrospinal fluid or a pathogenic variant of *SLC2A1* is found, the patient should be diagnosed with possible Glut1-DS and a ketogenic diet should be considered.

Differential Diagnosis

Other conditions that can cause chronic or intermittent hypoglycemia, such as familial hyperinsulinemia, should be ruled out. It is also necessary to exclude other diseases that can cause early-onset epilepsy and acquired microcephaly, such as early Rett syndrome, Angelman syndrome, and infantile neuronal ceroid lipofuscinosis (NCL). Opsoclonus–myoclonus syndrome should be excluded. It should be distinguished from other causes of dystonia.

Treatment

Ketogenic Diet

A ketogenic diet therapy (KDT) is the most effective treatment for Glut1-DS; this treatment can significantly improve seizures and gait abnormalities and is well-tolerated. The earlier the treatment is started, the better the effect [214]. Therefore,

KDT should be given as early as possible after a clear diagnosis, maintained at least until adolescence, and can also be used for a long time until adulthood. However, whether lifelong KDT is necessary is still uncertain.

In general, the classic ketogenic diet usually provides a greater level of ketosis and is preferred for younger children, especially infants and toddlers. Children, adolescents, and adults with poor compliance should be treated with modified Atkins dietary therapy.

Patients following a ketogenic diet may lack sufficient L-carnitine intake, and dietary supplementation is needed. Proper hydration and avoidance of carbonic anhydrase inhibitors should be considered. Foods containing carbohydrates, intravenous fluids, and medications that interrupt ketosis should be avoided. Blood ketone concentrations should be monitored regularly, with a target β-hydroxybutyrate concentration of 3–5 mmol/L.

Antiseizure Medications

Antiseizure medications are generally ineffective or only mildly effective. The responses of a small number of patients with similar idiopathic generalized epilepsy to conventional antiepileptic drugs and generalized tonic–clonic seizures at a late age of onset may be predictors of the effectiveness of antiepileptic drugs. Barbiturates and valproic acid can cause impaired Glut1 transport and should be avoided. Acetazolamide, topiramate, and zonisamide inhibit carbonic liver enzymes, can cause metabolic acidosis, and should also be avoided as much as possible.

Other Treatments

Triheptanoin is a specially designed and synthesized triglyceride compound consisting of three seven-carbon (C7) fatty acids that is designed to provide medium-length, odd-chain fatty acids to patients. A preliminary study of the effects of triheptanoin as a dietary supplement in Glut1-DS patients showed that it increased the cerebral metabolic rate, reduced the number of seizures, and improved neuropsychological performance. Another study showed that triheptanoin significantly improved paroxysmal dyskinesia in ketogenic diet-intolerant Glut1-DS patients [246, 247].

Studies of AAV9 (adeno-associated virus serotype 9)-mediated gene therapy in mouse models revealed that early Glut1 protein supplementation may effectively treat Glut1-DS [247]. These results demonstrate the therapeutic effect of restoring Glut1 protein expression early in life and represent an important step toward modifying disease therapy for Glut1-DS patients.

Prevention and Early Detection

For newborns, infants, and other family members at risk of disease, early detection is necessary for early diagnosis and early treatment. For probands, there is a 50% chance that their offspring will develop the disease and prenatal diagnosis should be made.

Prognosis

Glut1-DS symptoms mainly manifest as seizures and cognitive impairment from infancy to early childhood and movement disorders in adolescence and adulthood. Early initiation of KDT has a significant effect on improving prognosis.

5.2.3.7 Sturge–Weber Syndrome (SWS)

Overview

Sturge–Weber syndrome (SWS) is a neurocutaneous syndrome characterized by facial and leptomeningeal hemangiomas, epilepsy, neurological dysfunction, and glaucoma. In 1860, Schirmer first named this syndrome Sturge–Weber syndrome [248]. The main skin manifestation of SWS is port-wine stain (PWS), which usually affects one side of the face along the trigeminal nerve branch, along with microvascular malformations of the ipsilateral parenchyma of the brain and the eye. The ophthalmic trigeminal skin group (V1) is most commonly involved; PWS is less common in the V2 and V3 areas, and facial hemangioma strongly suggests SWS, with a risk of 15–50%.

Epidemiology

The incidence of SWS is unclear and is estimated to be approximately 1/20,000 live-born infants [249]. In a recent study of the Olmsted County population, the incidence of SWS has been reported to be 0.19 per 100,000 persons/year, with Caucasians (85%) and women (69%) having a higher incidence [250] than other races and men, respectively.

Etiology

SWS is associated with somatic mutations during embryonic development, and the earlier the mutation occurs, the more widespread the clinical phenotype. Among these somatic mutations, chimeric mutations in G-α subunit q (GNAQ) and in the proteins associated with the phosphoinositide 3-kinase (PI3K) pathway and their interactions are considered the most important mutation types [251, 252]. GNAQ chimeric mutations are critical because the G-αq subunit is the signaling mediator between the G protein receptor (e.g., endothelin) and its downstream effectors [252]. Alterations in these pathways, leading to the dysregulation of vascular development during embryogenesis, underlie the pathogenesis of SWS. A recent study has shown that *GNA11* and *GNAQ* are highly homologous genes encoding different G-α subunits of the G-αq subfamily. Mutations in the *GNA11*-encoding gene can also cause SWS, but, compared with those of classic *GNAQ*-SWS, *GNA11*-SWS conveys different neurological symptoms and skin changes, mainly manifested as capillary malformation. This presents as pink and spotted skin at birth, which gradually fades with age and evolves into purple, and less severe nervous system symptoms than classic *GNAQ*-SWS [253].

Clinical Manifestations

The clinical manifestations of SWS patients include the classical triad of PWSs distributed along the trigeminal nerve, neurological dysfunction (seizures, developmental delay, and motor impairment), and glaucoma. The traditional classification method divides SWS into three types according to the Roach scale of facial hemangiomatosis: type I, with both facial and leptomeningeal hemangiomas, possibly with glaucoma ("classic" or "complete" SWS); type II, isolated facial hemangioma (without central nervous system involvement), with or without glaucoma; and type III, isolated leptomeningeal cerebral hemangioma, usually without glaucoma [254]. Currently, the correlation between SWS symptoms and the risk of brain and eye involvement can be more accurately stratified based on the scope and location of facial capillary malformations [255].

Skin Changes

PWSs are the most common cutaneous skin alterations in SWS patients. Typically, they are red in childhood, become darker and more purple with age, and accompany hypertrophy of the surrounding soft tissue, with approximately 8–20% of facial capillary malformations associated with SWS [256]. The distribution of facial PWSs follows the distribution of the trigeminal sensory innervation branch (ophthalmic (V1), maxillary (V2), and mandibular (V3)), with children having involvement of the first branch (V1) having the highest risk of SWS [257]. Moreover, the site and degree of deformity of PWSs are associated with SWS risk in children, and children with bilateral anterior head and unilateral facial capillary malformations have the highest risk of SWS [255].

Neurological Symptoms

The most common neurological symptom observed in SWS patients is infantile seizures, which affect 75–100% of patients and are usually accompanied by focal motor seizures that can range from being partly secondary to generalized. Other common episodes include febrile convulsion, status epilepticus, and stroke-like episodes [258]. Status epilepticus is usually related to stroke-like episodes and can be observed in 30–50% of pediatric patients [258]. Of patients with unilateral brain involvement, 75% had combined epilepsy and 90% with bilateral brain involvement had combined epilepsy [259]. Approximately 75% of patients develop epilepsy before 1 year of age, 85% before 2 years of age, and 90–95% before 5 years of age [260].

The second most common neurological symptoms in SWS patients are intellectual delays and behavioral problems, which are closely associated with the early onset of refractory epilepsy. Approximately 50% of SWS patients experience different degrees of cognitive decline. The degree of cognitive decline is associated with the number of affected brain lobes, and bilateral brain involvement may lead to severe intellectual disability and language impairment [261]. Early seizures and active seizures are associated with intellectual and language disorders.

The incidence of hemiplegic or stroke-like attacks is 31–46% in SWS patients [262]. SWS-affected children usually exhibit varying degrees of motor dysfunction on the side of the body contralateral to the affected hemisphere, which is more severe in patients with early-onset epilepsy. Usually, onset occurs within 6 months of birth and is exacerbated by repeated stroke-like episodes in infancy and childhood. Approximately 50% of SWS patients have residual permanent motor dysfunction, and approximately 30% develop transient stroke-like motor dysfunction [199].

Headache in SWS patients can be characterized by migraine, which is observed in approximately 20–30% of patients and is significantly more common in these patients than in healthy children. The median age of onset of the illness is 8 years [263], and this condition can sometimes occur together with epilepsy.

Patients with SWS are at a higher risk of having an autism spectrum disorder. A 13-year UK study showed that 24% of SWS patients were diagnosed with autism spectrum disorder and 45% had social dysfunction [264]. Patients with SWS may also experience other social behavioral problems, including severe behavioral difficulties and sleep difficulties.

Ocular Symptoms

Up to 50% of SWS patients develop varying degrees of ocular lesions, the most common of which are glaucoma and choroidal angioma [265]. Glaucoma can occur on either the ipsilateral or the contralateral side to the PWS. Glaucoma occurs in 30–70% of SWS patients [266] at any age, with three significant peaks (<1 year (40%), 5–9 years (23%), and >20 years (20%) [267]). Glaucoma may be the result of increased superior scleral venous pressure and an abnormal anatomy of the anterior chamber (leading to reduced eye drainage). In SWS patients, open-angle glaucoma is the most common type of glaucoma, and symptoms include vision loss, conjunctiva, eye pain, and eye protrusion; if not treated in a timely manner, this can cause ischemic damage to the optic nerve, thus threatening vision [268]. Therefore, annual eye assessment and intraocular pressure measurement are recommended to prevent optic nerve atrophy and blindness.

Other Symptoms

Other systemic symptoms of SWS include growth hormone deficiency, hypothalamic–pituitary axis damage, central hypothyroidism, oral vasculopathy, giant malformation, renal hypertension, etc.

Auxiliary Inspection

Enhancing cranial MRI, which can detect leptomeningeal enhancement, abnormal venous drainage, cortical atrophy, leptomeningeal myeloma, and calcification, is the main means of diagnosing brain involvement in SWS patients. Susceptibility-weighted imaging (SWI), which is an MRI technique, and contrast-enhanced fluid attenuated inversion recovery (FLAIR) sequences provide optimal sensitivity [253] for detecting leptomeningeal vascular abnormalities in SWS patients.

Positron emission tomography (PET) or perfusion imaging with single-photon emission computed tomography (SPECT) can be used to monitor disease progression in SWS patients, and PET can detect subtle changes in the extent and asymmetry of glucose activity/levels in the brain that are sensitive markers of cognitive decline and seizure activity in SWS [269].

Electroencephalography (EEG) is helpful for detecting cortical lesions and epilepsy in patients with SWS, subclinical epileptic activity, which is more common than epileptic discharges, and is associated with rhythm and voltage asymmetry.

Diagnosis

The diagnosis of SWS relies on typical clinical features, ophthalmological examination, and imaging examination. Cranial MRI is the gold standard for diagnosing SWS and for evaluating the brain features in SWS patients: hemangioma, brain atrophy, and possible cortical malformations or injuries. Enhanced T1- and susceptibility-weighted images facilitate visualization of leptomeningeal hemangioma, dilated choroid plexus, and venous abnormalities (abnormal cortical veins, dilated trans-dark and subependymal veins) [270]. Compared with MRI, CT is more favorable for revealing special imaging features of SWS, such as subcortical calcification ("trolley track" appearance) and scalp bone hyperplasia, which can be used to exclude emergency intracranial hemorrhage and three-dimensional (3D) angiography.

EEG is an important diagnostic tool for SWS, with standard EEG revealing voltage decay, slow background activity, and seizure discharge [270] in the affected hemisphere; moreover, EEG is important in the differential diagnosis of seizures, migraine, and stroke-like seizures.

Differential Diagnosis

Neonatal Nevus (Salmon Patches)

The characteristic distribution locations of neonatal nevus are the bilateral upper eyelid, eyebrow, neck, and scalp. PWSs are usually located on one side of the face but also appear on the medial forehead; however, they are sometimes difficult to distinguish from the rash distribution, and close follow-up or related examinations such as cranial MRI are needed.

Arteriovenous Malformations (AVMs)

Arteriovenous malformations usually present as warmer and more unevenly colored areas, with archipelagic borders and mostly punctate and patchy calcifications along with recurrent bleeding. Mucinous magnetic resonance angiography (MRA), computed tomography angiography (CTA), and digital subtraction angiography (DSA) can help in differential diagnosis.

Macrocerebral Capillary Malformation Syndrome (MCAP)

This syndrome can manifest as facial (medial forehead) or trunk network capillary malformation, partial overgrowth, or giant malformation and is often accompanied by other overgrowth symptoms, such as toe deformation, without leptomeningeal hemangioma or glaucoma. Gene testing is helpful for differential diagnosis.

Nodous Sclerosis

Nodous sclerosis is a typical triad that includes sebaceous adenoma, seizures, and intellectual delays. Cranial MRI shows characteristic nodular calcification in bilateral lateral paraventricular and subependymal areas or within the cortex.

Treatment

The treatment strategy for SWS relies mainly on symptomatic treatment. As SWS is a multisystem disease, the management of pediatric patients requires the support of a multidisciplinary team, which includes pediatricians, neurologists, neurosurgeons, radiologists, ophthalmologists, dermatologists, geneticists, psychologists, and physiotherapists.

Treatment of PWSs

Laser therapy is the standard treatment for PWSs, and pulsed dye laser (PDL) therapy is currently the recommended first-line therapy and gold standard. It is safer for pediatric patients and early treatment, especially before the age of 1, and is associated with a better prognosis [271]. Laser treatment is recommended every 6 weeks, and shortening the treatment cycle does not increase efficacy. If conventional laser therapy is ineffective, medication, photodynamic therapy (intravenous photosensitizer administration), surgery, or corrective masking should be administered [272].

Treatment of Neurological Symptoms

The preferred treatment for seizures is medication; oxcarbazepine is the most commonly used antiepileptic drug [273], and other antiepileptic drugs include levetiracetam, carbamazepine, and topiramate. Oxcarbazepine and carbamazepine are the most effective agents for treating SWS patients with complicated epilepsy, followed by levetiracetam and topiramate [273]. Low-dose aspirin (35 mg/kg/day) can be used as an additional therapy alongside antiepileptic drugs, significantly reducing the frequency and severity of headaches, seizures, and stroke-like episodes in patients with SWS [274]. Some specialists recommend low-dose aspirin for all patients under 3 years or young patients with three or more lobes involved [266]. However, there is a lack of reports on the effects of long-term aspirin use on cognitive function and quality of life in SWS patients.

Migraine patients are usually treated with triptan drugs, and the preventive use of flunarizine can reduce the severity, frequency, and duration of headaches [275]. Sleep deprivation has been found to be the main cause of headaches in SWS patients [276], so adequate and regular sleep and exercise may help prevent headaches.

Surgery should be considered in patients with drug-refractory epilepsy and unilateral brain injury [277]. Surgical treatment is usually not preferred for SWS patients with bilateral cerebral involvement because of the increased risk of neurological and cognitive dysfunction. Hemispherectomy is performed only in patients with bilateral involvement and severely disabling epilepsy in the unilateral brain.

Presymptomatic Treatment

As SWS is a persistent progressive disease, early intervention is very important. Infants receiving presymptomatic treatment with low-dose aspirin and antiepileptic drugs have lower seizure scores and older age of seizure onset [278]. However, it has also been shown that there is no significant difference in frequency of seizures among SWS patients receiving valproate or carbamazepine for prophylactic treatment [279]. More prospective studies are therefore needed to clarify the optimal presymptomatic treatment options.

Prognosis

The natural history of SWS is extensively heterogeneous, with the age of onset being a crucial factor [280]. Early seizures are associated with learning disability, intellectual disability, stroke-like seizures, hemiparesis, visual field defects, and a necessity for brain surgery. The extent of cutaneous capillary malformations is related to the possibility of epilepsy and necessity of glaucoma surgery, while bilateral cerebral involvement is associated with learning disability and intellectual disability.

5.2.3.8 Gelastic Epilepsy with Hypothalamic Hamartoma

Overview

Hypothalamic hamartoma (HH) is a congenital benign tumor originating from the hypothalamus with an incidence of approximately 1/100,000–50,000 people [281]. The typical clinical symptoms include seizures, central precocious puberty, cognitive impairment, and behavioral problems. Gelastic seizure (GS), also known as laughter epilepsy (gelastic epilepsy), is the main manifestation of epilepsy and is the most common form of seizure in hypothalamic hamartoma patients. As the disease progresses, other focal or comprehensive seizure types may gradually appear. Hypothalamic hamartoma is the most common cause of gelastic seizures.

Historical Evolution and Epidemiology

In 1873, Trousseau first described the phenomenon of gelastic seizures [282]. In 1957, Daly and Mulder [283] first described two patients with epileptic seizures (gelastic seizure) as the seizure type [259]. In 1971, Gascon and Lombroso defined the first clinical features of gelastic seizures (GSs) as "stereotyped, repetitive, with other clinical features corresponding to seizures and interictal EEG abnormalities" [284]. ILAE officially defined GS in 2001 as a type of focal seizure and a rare type of seizure [52], accounting for <1% of all patients with epilepsy [285].

Etiology
The most common disease leading to epilepsy is hypothalamic hamartoma, followed by temporal and frontal lobe lesions [286]. In recent years, parietal and cerebellar lesions have also been reported to cause this type of epilepsy [287, 288], but a few (8%) of these lesions are cryptic [288]. According to cerebral MRI results, hypothalamic hamartomas can be divided into "intrahypothalamic type" (mainly manifested as epilepsy) and "parahypothalamic type" (mainly manifested as precocious puberty) [289].

Clinical Manifestations
GSs mainly manifest as rigid, repetitive, or unrelated to the environment; involuntary laughing; sudden stopping for 5 s to 1 min; frequent attacks; and can occur when the individual is awake or asleep and can be accompanied by many other types of seizures, including focal or secondary full tonic seizures. The diagnosis of epilepsy is based on the following conditions: (1) recurrent and stereotyped laughter, (2) no external inducement, (3) the presence of other types of epileptic seizures, and (4) seizures or interictal EEG discharge. Most seizures occur in infancy and can also occur during childhood or adolescence. In early infancy, laughter epilepsy usually results in daily attacks, less so in disorders of consciousness; as the duration of the disease increases, the onset of seizures often progresses in combination with disorders of consciousness [290]. Seizures typically carry significant drug resistance [291].

5.2.4 *Auxiliary Inspection*

EEG
Due to the deep location of hypothalamic hamartoma lesions and the complex connections within hamartomas, scalp EEG has a limited role in monitoring epileptic activity. In the early stages of the disease, when only gelastic seizures occur, the results of scalp EEG during the interictal period may be normal or mildly abnormal. As the disease progresses, the type of epileptic seizure that occurs gradually evolves and focal/multifocal epileptiform discharges or diffuse episodic abnormal discharges can usually be observed in one or both frontal and temporal lobes during the intervals between seizures [292].

CT Examination
Hypothalamic hamartoma is equally dense on CT and is a space-occupying lesion located behind the pituitary stalk, intermedullary cistern, anterior pontine cistern, and suprasellar cistern. There is no enhancement after injection of the contrast agent.

MRI
MRI is the gold standard for diagnosing hypothalamic hamartomas. Hypothalamic hamartomas have characteristic MRI features and are characterized by small

circular or oval masses with clear edges in the suprasellar cistern and hypothalamic region; these masses are closely related to gray nodules and papillary bodies, with diameters mostly ranging from 10 to 30 mm. The lesions show equal signals on T1-weighted imaging (T1WI) and equal or slightly greater signals on T2-weighted imaging (T2WI). Given that hypothalamic hamartomas do not exhibit blood–brain barrier disruption, lesions are not enhanced after injection of contrast agents [293]. Positron emission tomography (PET) and single-photon emission computed tomography (SPECT) can reveal high metabolic and perfusion rates in the hypothalamic region during epileptic seizures.

Diagnosis

In 1971, Gascon and Lombroso stated that diencephalic lesions are an important cause of GSs and proposed the diagnostic criteria for GSs: ① recurrent GS episodes in the presence or absence of external stimulation, ② the presence of other seizure types, ③ epileptic discharge during episodic or inter-seizure EEG, and ④ GS with or without disturbance of consciousness [284].

Differential Diagnosis

Other Epilepsy/Epilepsy Syndromes Leading to Laughter

Laughter onset itself has no lateral or localization significance. In addition to hypothalamic hamartomas, seizures can also be observed at other locations, such as the frontal lobe, temporal lobe, parietal lobe, or insular cortex; these lesions need to be identified via EEG, cranial MRI, or PET findings.

Other Sellar Tumors

Other sellar tumors, such as low-grade gliomas and suprasellar germ cell tumors, are difficult to identify via T1WI and T2WI, but the two lesions are enhanced, and the tumors are progressive and enlarged, allowing them to be differentiated from hypothalamic hamartomas.

Pallister–Hall Syndrome

Hypothalamic hamartomas are one of the main symptoms of Pallister–Hall syndrome. This syndrome is an autosomal dominant disease caused by a *GLI3* gene mutation on chromosome 7p14. In addition to hypothalamic hamartomas, it is often accompanied by other developmental malformations, such as epiglottis, anal atresia, polydactyly (toe deformity), and a good response to antiepileptic drug treatment.

Treatment

Early diagnosis and appropriate treatment options are needed to improve cognitive and behavioral abnormalities in patients with giggling attacks accompanied by hypothalamic hamartoma [294].

Antiseizure Medication Therapy

Approximately 95% of patients do not respond to antiepileptic drug therapy [295]. There is no optimal antiepileptic drug strategy for laughter seizures caused by hypothalamic hamartomas, but, because of the nature of the focal seizures, carbamazepine and lamotrigine may be preferred [291]. However, gelastic seizures accompanied by hypothalamic hamartomas are mostly drug-resistant, and, as the condition progresses, cognitive function, learning ability, and behavioral abnormalities gradually decrease. Therefore, the main treatment goal for patients is to delay their progression to convulsive attacks rather than to control the gelastic seizures themselves because simple gelastic seizures do not directly affect cognitive function [291].

Surgical Treatment of Hypothalamic Hamartoma

Surgery is the most effective treatment for hypothalamic hamartoma with dementia onset [296]. The surgical methods mainly include: (1) Lesion resection: Surgical resection can achieve direct tumor resection, and endoscopic-assisted lesion resection is mainly used for tumors in which the lesion body is located in the third ventricle. Lesion resection is effective in refractory epilepsy, precocious puberty, and cognitive behavior disorders but can also cause serious complications. (2) Vagal nerve stimulation: This is mainly used in patients with hypothalamic hamartoma with refractory epilepsy that are found to be unsuitable for surgery. (3) Stereotactic radiotherapy: For smaller hypothalamic hamartomas, gamma knife therapy alone has good efficacy and safety, but, after surgery, it has a lag effect; long-term follow-up is needed to evaluate its efficacy [297]. For larger hamartomas, gamma knife therapy combined with other surgical methods is used. (4) Patients may undergo stereotactic radiofrequency thermocoagulation. Kuzniecky et al. [298] first reported the use of stereotactic radiofrequency damage in hypothalamic hamartomas, which has been widely used in clinical practice. Compared with traditional lesion resection, stereotactic radiofrequency damage is safer and more effective. It is more suitable for small- to medium-sized hypothalamic hamartomas [299], but it can also treat larger hamartomas and multiple damaged targets through multiple needle channels.

Assessment of the Endocrine System

In addition to epilepsy, many patients with hypothalamic hamartomas have subtle, subclinical, or undiagnosed endocrine dysfunction (mainly disorders of growth and puberty), and comprehensive dynamic assessment and follow-up of pituitary function is necessary even in the absence of obvious clinical features.

Prognosis

Patients with epilepsy caused by hypothalamic hamartoma exhibit varying degrees of cognitive impairment, especially of speech memory and executive dysfunction. Frequent seizures and an excessive dose of antiepileptic drugs may lead to cognitive impairment. For patients who have already developed cognitive impairment, early surgical evaluation is necessary to improve the prognosis [300].

5.3 Childhood-Onset Epilepsy Syndromes

The onset of epileptic syndromes is often age-related. The new classification of epilepsy syndromes by ILAE includes epilepsy syndromes with onset in the neonatal period and infancy, epilepsy syndromes with onset in childhood (2–12 years), and epilepsy syndromes with variable ages of onset. According to ILAE, childhood-onset epilepsy syndromes can be roughly divided into three categories: self-limited focal epilepsies, epilepsy syndromes with a genetic basis, and developmental and/or epileptic encephalopathies [301].

5.3.1 Self-Limited Focal Epilepsy Syndrome in Children

Although this type of epilepsy syndrome, previously known as benign epilepsy syndrome, has a good overall prognosis, some patients have severe seizures before their condition is significantly relieved and some seizures show drug resistance. Therefore, in the new classification of epilepsy syndromes, ILAE refers to it as self-limited focal epilepsy syndrome, especially regarding epilepsy syndromes that have been effectively identified at this age [301].

5.3.1.1 Self-Limited Epilepsy with Centrotemporal Spikes (SeLECTS)

Overview

Self-limiting epilepsy with centrotemporal spikes is an epilepsy syndrome proposed in the new classification of epilepsy syndromes by ILAE. It was previously called benign epilepsy of childhood with centrotemporal spikes (BECTS), epilepsy of childhood with centrotemporal spikes, or benign Rolandic epilepsy. It is a common clinical epilepsy syndrome. The characteristic electroencephalogram (EEG) signals include biphasic spikes and waves or spikes and slow waves with high amplitude in the temporal regions, which are easily induced by sleep. The overall prognosis is good, and EEG signals gradually return to normal with the cessation of seizures [301].

Historical Evolution

In 1966, Blom and Brorson [302] first noticed the existence of this syndrome, and, in 1972, Beaussart [303] analyzed the clinical characteristics of 221 patients, thus deepening our understanding of this syndrome. In 1975, Lerman and Kivity [304] studied the long-term efficacy of 100 patients with SeLECTS and found that all patients had recovered before adulthood and that their clinical manifestations and EEG results disappeared, suggesting that SeLECTS had a good prognosis. In 1975, Heijbel et al. [305] noted that the occurrence of this syndrome may be related to genetic factors, which promoted people's understanding of this syndrome; recently, Lu et al. [306] have reported that patients with this syndrome may have status epilepticus during slow-wave sleep, which may affect the prognosis. Ji et al. [307] reported that high-frequency oscillatory waves of the scalp could better predict the recurrence of epilepsy than sharp waves, which enriched the research in this field.

Epidemiology
Sidenvall et al. [308] conducted a survey of 500,000 children aged 0–16 years in northern Sweden and found that 155 had epilepsy, for a prevalence rate of 42/10000; among these children, the incidence of benign childhood epilepsy with centrotemporal spikes was 17.4%. Alshahawy et al. [309] conducted a questionnaire survey on 9545 students and found that 25 had epilepsy with centrotemporal spikes, suggesting a prevalence of 26/10,000. Ramírez et al. [310] investigated 60,000 children under 11 years of age and found that 136 of them had epilepsy, 29% of whom had SeLECTS. Heijbel et al. [311] conducted an epidemiological survey of 52,252 children under the age of 15 and reported that the prevalence of SeLECTS was 21/100,000, accounting for 16% of epilepsy patients. These studies showed that the prevalence of SeLECTS ranged from 2.6 to 4.2%, and the prevalence ranged from 17.4% to 29% in people with epilepsy.

Causes of the Disease
Patients with SeLECTS have a good prognosis, and there are few positive findings on imaging and electrophysiology, suggesting that this disease is not caused by structural damage. The current view tends to be that its incidence is due to genetic factors, but the genetic pattern involved is very complex. In 1975, Heijbel et al. [305] performed a genetic study on probands, including 19 patients, 36 biological parents, and 34 biological siblings, and reported that 15% (5/34) of these siblings had seizures and Rolandic discharges and that 19% (6/32) had only Rolandic discharges. Among adult parents, 11% had seizures in childhood but did not experience seizures in adulthood, demonstrating an age-dependent autosomal dominant inheritance. Degen and Degen [312] studied the families of 43 patients and found that 22 (51.16%) of them had at least 1 sibling with epileptic activity recorded on EEG; 26 (37.68%) of the 69 siblings had epileptiform discharges, with the largest number of epileptic discharges occurring upon awakening during hyperventilation and during slow-wave sleep. Neng et al. [313] performed whole exome sequencing on three patients in a family and found that the *CHRNA4* c.1007G>A mutation in the gene is associated with the incidence of SeLECTS. Ma et al. [314] screened for novel genetic variants in 292 SeLECTS patients and family members and found that 5 patients had *RYR2* mutations and that at least 3 web-based prediction tools indicated that the missense mutations were destructive.

Clinical Presentation
Age of Onset

Stephani [315] noted that SeLECTS is age-related and that the age of onset ranged from 3 to 13 years (the peak occurred at 9–10 years), with recovery before the age of 15–16 years. Bouma et al. [316] studied 2561 patients involved in 32 studies and found that the age of onset ranged from 3 months to 14 years and that the age of the last seizure ranged from 3 to 18 years. The 19 patients included in a study reported by Lima et al. [317] had an average age of 10.95 years. These studies suggest that the onset age of SeLECTS may range from 3 months to 14 years.

1.1.4.2 *Sex:* Sidenvall et al. [308] reported that the male-to-female ratio of patients was 1:1.1; 38% of the 19 patients included in the report by Lima et al. [317] were male, and Dalla Bernardina et al. [318] reported that 14 of the 20 patients included in their study were female, suggesting that there are slightly more women among SeLECTS patients.

Duration of the Attack

Most patients have seizures only during sleep. If seizures occur during sleep, focal motor seizures occur within 1–2 h of falling asleep or 1–2 h before waking up. In all 10–20% of children have seizures while awake; other types of seizures should be considered if they occur only during the day [301].

Frequency of Seizures

The frequency of BECTS varies greatly, but the overall number of episodes is not large. Ambrosetto et al. [319] studied the seizure frequency of 72 patients and reported that 11 of them (15%) had only 1 seizure, 40 patients (56%) had 2–6 seizures, and 21 patients (29%) had more than 6 seizures.

Presentation at the Time of Attack

Dysarthria, sialorrhea, language disorders, and focal epilepsy manifest as unilateral myoclonus or tonic–clonic seizures at the mouth corner. Bilateral tonic–clonic seizures tend to occur at night [301].

1. *Focal myoclonus*: Self-limited seizures with centrotemporal spikes typically present with orofacial focal myoclonus. Due to the involvement of the muscles on one side of the face, tongue, lips, and throat, patients present with mouth-to-side tilt, clonic or tonic–clonic tics in the mouth, and ipsilateral face. The seizures may rapidly extend to the upper limbs (face–arm seizures) but less often to the lower limbs; sometimes the seizures only convey sensory symptoms, and approximately 4.3% of patients have complex partial seizures [301].
2. *Salivation and speech stops*: Roulet et al. [320] reported that SeLECTS patients can present with drooling, tongue movement disorders, and drooling at one side of the mouth. Boulloche et al. [321] reported a case involving a 5.4-year-old patient with recurrent oropharyngeal spasm, salivation and speech cessation, and synchronous EEG-recorded bilateral central temporal lobe spike discharges, suggesting that the patient had SeLECTS.
3. *Status epilepticus*: The prognosis of SeLECTS is good, and the seizures are mostly mild; however, status epilepticus may also occur. Colamaria et al. [322] reported status epilepticus in four patients with SeLECTS, characterized by speech cessation, salivation, and epileptiform discharges on EEG, which were relieved by treatment with diazepam and valproic acid. Electrical status epilepticus is a special type of status epilepticus in children with epilepsy that can affect their neurodevelopment and cognitive integrity; it is mainly characterized by

persistent epileptiform discharges on EEGs. It is one of the most common manifestations of self-limiting epilepsy in patients with centrotemporal spikes. Ucar et al. [323] followed 126 patients with self-limited epilepsy with centrotemporal spikes and found that 33 of them had electrical status epilepticus, including 13 females and 20 males.

4. *Others*: Steinruecke et al. [324] investigated 114 patients who had self-limited epilepsy with centrotemporal spikes identified in 10 epilepsy centers in England and reported that 26 of them (23%) had poor academic performance and 15 (13%) had a neurodevelopmental disorder (6 with autism spectrum disorder and 6 with attention-deficit/hyperactivity disorder (ADHD)). Hosseinpour et al. [325] found that self-limiting epilepsy patients with centrotemporal spikes may be accompanied by exercise-induced myotrophic disorder.

Electroencephalographic Findings

Recurrent spikes or spikes and slow waves in the central temporal region are the most obvious EEG changes in patients with self-limited epilepsy with centrotemporal spikes. Beydoun et al. [326] studied the EEG characteristics of 41 children and reported that 14.6% of them had extensive spike discharges on EEG and that 9.8% had multiple independent sharp wave lesions. This epileptic discharge was not fixed but could move from one side to the opposite side; from the central temporal region to the ipsilateral occipital region; and the spike-and-slow-wave frequency increased significantly after the patients had fallen asleep. In some patients, this epileptiform discharge occurs only during sleep.

Tekgul et al. [327] studied the change rule of sharp waves in the EEG signals of 127 children with self-limiting epilepsy and centrotemporal spikes and evaluated the sharp wave velocity, morphology, and position. The results showed that there was no significant difference in the sharp wave composition between patients who relapsed and those who did not after drug withdrawal. There was no difference across the antiseizure medications used in the rate of peak clearance. Günay et al. [328] calculated the spike indices on EEG signals for 136 patients and reported that the median spike indices on the first and last EEG signals were 39% (7.6–89%) and 0 (0–112%), respectively. Sex, age of seizure onset, and psychiatric disorders did not significantly affect the spike index.

Diagnosis

The diagnosis of this disease mainly depends on a detailed history and characteristic electroencephalogram changes. In general, the diagnosis and prognosis can be confirmed only when typical clinical symptoms and specific EEG signals are available. According to ILAE, the main clinical manifestations of self-limiting epilepsy patients with centrotemporal spikes are paroxysmal dysarthria, salivation, language disorder, unilateral myoclonus or tonic–clonic seizures in the mouth, and focal seizures at night that can be followed by bilateral tonic–clonic seizures. There are high-amplitude biphasic spikes in the middle temporal region on EEG [301]. The diagnosis can be ruled out in the presence of waking generalized tonic–clonic seizures, atypical absence, seizures with gustatory hallucinations, fear, or autonomic features [301]. Neurological and neuroimaging findings are usually normal, and psychomotor development is normal. When the above conditions are met, the diagnosis of self-limiting epilepsy with centrotemporal spikes is generally not difficult.

Treatment

Patients with self-limiting epilepsy with centrotemporal spikes have a good prognosis, and the frequency of seizures is low. Most patients do not need treatment, but some with a greater number of seizures need treatment. Treatment for self-limiting epilepsy with centrotemporal spikes can be divided into two categories: drug treatment and nondrug treatment.

Precautions in Drug Therapy

1. Indications for drug therapy: Because the prognosis of self-limiting epilepsy patients with centrotemporal spikes is good, most patients do not require long-term antiseizure therapy. Antiseizure medications should be considered only when the patient has frequent seizures accompanied by other atypical clinical and EEG manifestations.
2. Most children respond well to monotherapy, and high-dose or combination therapy is not necessary. Liu et al. [329] summarized the treatment of 1817 patients and reported that 62.9% of them received monotherapy and that only 10.6% needed multidrug combination therapy.

Selection of Antiseizure Medications

Valproic acid, carbamazepine (oxcarbazepine), levetiracetam, and alprazolam are the most widely used drugs for the treatment of self-limiting epilepsy with centrotemporal spikes; however, there is considerable controversy surrounding their use. Valproic acid is the most commonly used antiseizure drug in clinical practice, and it is also the first choice for treatment. However, Cheng et al. [330] compared the efficacy of valproic acid, levetiracetam, and oxcarbazepine in patients with self-limiting epilepsy with centrotemporal spikes and reported no significant difference in seizure frequency across the three drugs. Ahadi et al. [331] conducted experiments on 92 patients treated with levetiracetam and carbamazepine and found that there was no significant difference in the reduction in seizure frequency between the two groups. Gerstl [332] conducted a systematic review of drug treatment for self-limiting epilepsy with centrotemporal spikes, including 19 studies involving 308 patients, and found that children treated with levetiracetam and clobazam had higher success rates than those treated with carbamazepine (oxcarbazepine) or topiramate. Many scholars believe that levetiracetam and clobazam may be more reasonable first-line drugs for treatment, but some scholars advocate for oxcarbazepine as the first choice [333].

Nonpharmacological Treatments

Jin et al. [334] performed transcranial magnetic stimulation (TMS) on four patients, during which their seizures were stopped for 3 months. Three patients showed a significant decrease in SWI after repetitive transcranial magnetic stimulation (rTMS) compared to baseline, and the attention deficits found at baseline in two patients returned to the normal range after rTMS, which may also be effective in surgical treatment of patients with drug-resistant epilepsy [335].

Prognosis
The overall prognosis of patients with self-limiting epilepsy with centrotemporal spikes is good, and most seizures stop during adolescence. De Romanis et al. [336] conducted a 16-year clinical and EEG follow-up of 150 patients aged 3–12 years with self-limited epilepsy with centrotemporal spikes and reported that the frequency of seizures decreased with age and that no seizures occurred after 14 years of age or 8 years after the final cessation of drug treatment. Therefore, long-term drug treatment is not necessary. Ucar et al. [323] studied the remission of status epilepticus in 33 patients with self-limiting epilepsy with centrotemporal spikes and reported that 42.4% of them experienced remission of status epilepticus, with a median remission time of 10.5 months and an average age at remission of 9.8 ± 2.0 years. The mean duration of response was 8.8 months.

5.3.1.2 Self-Limited Epilepsy with Autonomic Seizures (SeLEAS)

Overview
In 2022, ILAE defined early-onset benign childhood occipital epilepsy, or Panayiotopoulos syndrome, as self-limited epilepsy with autonomic seizures. It is one of the most common benign local epilepsies and has a childhood onset. The onset of the disease is age-dependent and related to genetic factors, and the prognosis is good. The peak age of onset is 4–6 years, and the frequency of attacks is low. Prominent symptoms are autonomic symptoms, such as abnormal behavior, vomiting, sweating, deviation of the head and eyes, and disturbance of consciousness [301]. Secondary seizures can often occur, and interictal EEG signals often include a burst of spikes in the occipital region as well as multifocal spikes.

Historical Evolution
The understanding of self-limited epilepsy with autonomic seizures has gradually improved. In the 1940s, several scholars noticed spike discharge in the occipital lobe and proposed a variety of theories to explain this phenomenon; however, Panayiotopoulos et al. made the greatest contribution to this area of research [337–339]. ILAE directly equates self-limited epilepsy with autonomic seizures with Panayiotopoulos syndrome in its new classification of epilepsy syndromes. In 1970, Panayiotopoulos et al. [337] first noted sharp waves in the occipital lobe and suggested that these waves were related to epilepsy. In 1980, Panayiotopoulos noted that patients with a previous diagnosis of basilar migraine might have a type of seizure associated with photosensitivity [338]. In 1988, in a study of 900 patients with epilepsy, 24 patients, who were all prepubertal children, presented with episodic vomiting. This episodic vomiting was significantly associated with occipital spikes but not centrotemporal spikes. During long-term follow-up, the patients' seizures were completely relieved, which suggested that this might be a new type of epileptic

seizure from a clinical point of view [339]. In 1989, Panayiotopoulos [340] summarized the clinical trial of nocturnal seizures, tonic deviation of the eye, and vomiting; these may occur with symptoms involving the head and limbs and eventually end with generalized tonic–clonic seizures. The age of onset is 3–5 years, and interictal EEG shows occipital sharp waves or spikes and slow complex waves. It is a novel, idiopathic, age-related, benign epilepsy syndrome. He subsequently followed 418 patients for up to 15 years and summarized the clinical manifestations that have been used to date [340]. In 2001, ILAE accepted the observations of Panayiotopoulos et al. and referred to this syndrome as Panayiotopoulos syndrome, which became widely accepted as benign childhood occipital lobe epilepsy [337].

Epidemiology

Weir et al. [341] investigated children under 16 years of age and reported that the prevalence of self-limited epilepsy with autonomic seizures was 0.8/100,000 people. Self-limited epilepsy with autonomic seizures occurs in approximately 6% of children who have one or more seizures before the age of 13 years. Panayiotopoulos [340] investigated 418 children with onset before the age of 13 and reported that 18 patients had clinical and EEG manifestations of early-onset childhood benign occipital lobe epilepsy, accounting for 20% of all benign, age-related idiopathic epilepsies. Covanis A et al. [342] investigated children who had more than one febrile seizure between the ages of 3 and 6 years and reported that 13% of them had self-limited epilepsy with autonomic seizures. Yoshinaga et al. [343] investigated 1794 children aged 1–14 years with first focal seizures and found that 93 (5.2%) had self-limited epilepsy with autonomic seizures. Ramos-Lizana et al. [344] conducted a prospective follow-up of 827 patients with epilepsy and found that 27 of them (3.3%) had self-limited epilepsy with autonomic seizures. Self-limited epilepsy with autonomic seizures occur in approximately 8/10000 people in the general population, with an incidence of approximately 3–4% in patients with epilepsy and 6–20% in patients with benign childhood epilepsy syndromes.

Causes of the Disease

The etiology of self-limited epilepsy with autonomic seizures is unclear, and genetic and developmental factors must be considered due to the marked age differences of the patients. Kivity et al. [345] performed whole exome sequencing on 26 patients with epilepsy and found 16 with *SCN1A* missense mutations—4 patients with self-limited epilepsy with autonomic seizures and 3 patients with self-limited epilepsy with autonomic seizures with *SCN1A* mutations were reviewed in the literature. Livingston et al. [346] reported two families with novel *SCN1A* mutations, one of whom had Panayiotopoulos syndrome, suggesting that the occurrence of self-limited epilepsy with autonomic seizures may be related to certain gene mutations. Rudolf et al. [347] performed whole exome sequencing on 57 children with benign self-limited epilepsy, including self-limited epilepsy with autonomic seizures, and found that 20 patients had gene mutations, among which *GRIN2B* and *CAMK2A* gene mutations may be related to the disease. These findings support that self-limited epilepsy with autonomic seizures may be associated with a genetic predisposition.

Clinical Presentation

Age of Onset

Durá-Travé et al. [348] analyzed 37 patients with self-limited epilepsy with autonomic seizures and reported that the peak age of onset was 5.4 years. The cases reported by Panayiotopoulos [340] all had onset before the age of 13 years, usually 3–6 years, and the peak age of onset was 4–5 years [349]. After the age of 12, seizures no longer occurred, and EEG signals returned to normal. Yoshinaga et al. [343] analyzed 93 patients and reported that the age of onset ranged from 1.1 to 8.6 years, indicating that most patients with self-limited epilepsy with autonomic seizures had onset before the age of 13 years, most of the onset ages ranged from 1 to 8 years, and the peak age of onset was 4–5 years.

Sex

Both men and women can be affected. Durá-Travé T et al. [348] analyzed 37 patients and reported that the female:male ratio was 2.1. The cases reported by Panayiotopoulos [340] also revealed a female majority.

Duration of the Attack

In patients with self-limited epilepsy with autonomic seizures, these seizures occur predominantly at night. Caraballo et al. [350] conducted a study on 192 patients and reported that 187 of them had attacks only at night; two-thirds of the cases reported by Covanis [342] occurred only at night; and Panayiotopoulos [340] reported on 18 patients, of whom 11 had attacks only at night, 5 had both daytime and nighttime attacks, and 2 had only daytime attacks. Durá-Travé et al. [348] conducted a study on 37 patients and reported that 36% of them had attacks at night and that those with daytime onset had a poor prognosis.

Seizure Frequency

Patients with self-limiting epilepsy with autonomic seizures have very few seizures. Of the 192 patients reported by Caraballo et al. [350], 84 (44.2%) had only 1 seizure, 79 (41.2%) had 2–5 seizures, and 29 (14.6%) had frequent seizures.

Duration of Seizures

The duration of seizures in patients with self-limited epilepsy with autonomic seizures is long, and most of the children have seizures lasting for 5–10 min. Kawakami et al. [351] investigated the attack times of 18 patients and reported that only 3 had an attack time of more than 15 min. However, observing when an attack begins at night and accurately calculating its duration are sometimes difficult. In addition, some children have seizures that can last for several hours.

Clinical Presentation

Self-limited epilepsy with autonomic seizures is mainly characterized by autonomic seizures Panayiotopoulos [338] summarized the clinical manifestations of this disease and proposed a clinical trial of nocturnal seizures, tonic ocular deviation, and vomiting, which may involve the head and limbs and eventually end with generalized tonic–clonic seizures. According to ILAE, patients mainly present with focal autonomic seizures, with or without impaired consciousness, often with episodic dry vomiting or vomiting, and may also have pallor, flushing, abdominal pain, pupils, or cardiopulmonary changes [301].

1. *Initial symptoms*: In 2004, Panayiotopoulos [349] summarized the clinical characteristics of more than 800 patients worldwide and reported that most patients with epileptic seizures had paroxysmal vomiting as the first symptom and that most patients were fully awake before other symptoms appeared. Lada et al. [352] analyzed 43 of 90 patients with Panayiotopoulos syndrome and reported that paroxysmal vomiting was often the first symptom and that 86% of patients eventually developed vomiting. Autonomic symptoms may be the sole feature of seizures [338]. Yoshinaga et al. [343] investigated the recurrence rates of 93 patients after the first seizure, and the results showed that the cumulative recurrence probabilities at 6, 12, 24, and 36 months after the first seizure were 57.6%, 45.6%, 35.1%, and 11.7%, respectively.
2. *Paroxysmal ocular deviation*: Paroxysmal ocular deviation is the main manifestation of self-limited epilepsy with autonomic seizures. Of the 18 patients included in the study by Panayiotopoulos [340], 16 had paroxysmal ocular deviation, often secondary to unilateral or generalized convulsions; these patients mainly had clonic or tonic–clonic seizures, occasionally accompanied by tonic seizures or paroxysmal weakness and pallor. Generally, there is no change in consciousness at the beginning of an attack, but, as the attack progresses, there may be disturbance of consciousness or loss of consciousness and some children experience no change in consciousness. In the 43 patients reported by Lada et al. [352], the involuntary manifestations were mainly lateral deviation of the eyeball and some patients had visual abnormalities. All seizures were accompanied by disturbance of consciousness, and half of the seizures ended with unilateral or generalized convulsions.
3. *Status epilepticus*: Although self-limited epilepsy with autonomic seizures is a benign childhood epilepsy syndrome, status epilepticus is common. More than half of the 43 patients reported by Lada et al. [352] had episodes of status epilepticus lasting for more than 30 min. More than half of the more than 800 patients in the world investigated by Panayiotopoulos [349] had seizures lasting for more than 30 min, which constitute epileptic autonomic status epilepticus; these findings indicate that autonomic status epilepticus is very common in individuals with self-limited epilepsy with autonomic seizures and needs to be considered. Verrotti et al. [353] summarized the characteristics of status epilepticus in 37 patients and reported that the average age at first onset of convulsive status epilepticus was 6.5 years, one-third of patients needed to be admitted to the intensive care unit (ICU), and sharp wave activity in the occipital lobe was detected via interictal EEG in 31 patients (83.7%). However, the overall prognosis of the patients was good, all patients were seizure-free at the last follow-up, and the

authors speculate that the presence of status epilepticus did not affect the prognosis of the patients.

4. *Paroxysmal cardiac arrest*: Yamamoto et al. [354] reported on a 10-year-old boy who vomited while sleeping and had abdominal pain on waking up, and his condition deteriorated rapidly when he arrived at the emergency room with loss of breathing and cardiac arrest. After awakening, the patient was diagnosed with self-limited epilepsy with autonomic seizures, while brain MRI showed no abnormalities. EEG revealed repeated multifocal epileptiform activity in the bilateral occipital lobes during sleep. Mujawar et al. [355] described a 3.5-year-old boy with self-limited epilepsy with autonomic seizures who had paroxysmal cardiac arrest after the onset of status epilepticus and who required cardiopulmonary resuscitation to be revived. Mujawar reviewed the literature regarding four other cases of cardiac arrest in patients with self-limited epilepsy with autonomic seizures, and he noted that all four patients recovered spontaneously from cardiac arrest without resuscitation.
5. *Others*: Other autonomic abnormalities, such as pallor or diaphoresis, restlessness, and episodic syncope, may also be observed in self-limited epilepsy syndromes with autonomic seizures [338]. Some patients only feel uncomfortable or nauseated or cough without vomiting. Some become quiet rather than irritable, can experience urinary and fecal incontinence and pupil dilation, and have visual hallucinations, throat twitching, and automatism. Brabec et al. [356] reported a case of a 13-month-old boy diagnosed with self-limited epilepsy with autonomic seizures who presented with genital priapism during seizures. The authors suggested that the epileptic focus of the child might be in the left temporal region.

Yalçin et al. [357] summarized the autonomic symptoms of 43 patients with self-limited epilepsy with autonomic seizures. The results showed that the most common symptoms were nausea (54.8%), vomiting (50.0%), pallor (50.0%), head–eye deviation (45.2%), generalized seizures (35.7%), paroxysmal syncope (33.3%), and stomachache (26.2%). A total of 38.9% of the patients had visual symptoms such as amaurosis, a colored light flicker, a strong light flicker, hallucinations, and blurred vision. Autonomic status epilepticus occurred in 21.4% of the patients.

Electroencephalogram

EEG examination is highly important for diagnosing this disease. According to ILAE, the most prominent manifestations of this disease are high-amplitude, focal, or multifocal epileptiform discharges in the occipital lobe on EEG during sleepiness and sleep [301].

Epileptiform Discharge

Epileptiform discharge on electroencephalogram is the most important basis for the diagnosis of self-limited epilepsy with autonomic seizures. Caraballo et al. [358] studied nine patients with typical clinical manifestations and reported that diffuse spike discharges were observed during the interictal period in both awake and sleeping interictal EEG (100%). Three children had focal spikes during sleep, including one with spikes in the occipital region and one with spikes in the frontal region. The other patient showed spikes in the temporo-occipital region. During the course of the disease, no specific electroclinical pattern was observed.

Sleep EEG

Tata et al. [359] studied the sleep EEG signals of 24 patients with self-limited epilepsy with autonomic seizures and found that the interictal spike activity increased significantly during nonrapid eye movement sleep and could spread to the central and central temporal regions.

Interictal EEG

Variability and multifocal epileptiform discharges may be the main features of interictal EEG signals in patients. Yoshinaga et al. [343] studied the interictal electroencephalogram (EEG) signals of 93 patients and found that there was great variation. A total of 79.5% of the patients experienced changes in the location and peak value of epileptiform discharges over time. Only 16.1% of patients had abnormal EEG backgrounds without obvious epileptiform discharge, and 5.4% of patients had normal EEG data at all times. Specchio et al. [360] analyzed the interictal EEG signals of 20 patients and found that they mainly exhibited sharp waves with variable positions and that these sharp waves often changed with time. Oguni [361] summarized the characteristics of interictal EEG signals in patients with self-limiting epilepsy with autonomic seizures and reported that the interictal EEG signals of patients were characterized by multifocal EEG signals and that the main location was related to age (2–5 years in the occipital lobe, 4–7 years in the occipital and frontal pole, and 6–10 years in the central parietotemporal region). With aging, the signals can evolve into a multifocal EEG that disappears by 12–16 years of age, and, in rare cases, the EEG does not have epileptic discharges. The authors suggest that the interictal EEG lesions may differ in location and appearance pattern, which may be specifically related to the age at the time of EEG recording. This age-dependent EEG pattern may be specific for the diagnosis of self-limiting epilepsy with autonomic seizures.

Ictal EEG

Ictal EEG abnormalities are also variable and typically start in the anterior or posterior regions and propagate to other regions as small sharp waves mixed with rhythmic θ waves [360]. Yoshinaga et al. [343] reported that five patients had unfixed epileptiform discharge sites on EEG during the ictal period; these sites often spread from the posterior or anterior head to other places. Iannetti et al. [362] recorded nocturnal seizures in an 8-year-old girl whose EEG showed diffuse episodic discharges with almost no epileptiform discharges during the interictal period.

To perform electroencephalogram monitoring, Brabec et al. [356] conducted video EEG monitoring of a 4-year-old boy and found that the interictal EEG showed multifocal sharp waves in the central temporal region and the left posterior region and that the ictal EEG showed fast rhythms in the left posterior region, which gradually formed bilateral high-amplitude sharp waves or mixed waves of fast and slow rhythms. Clinical symptoms began to appear 2 min after the onset of the EEG, and these symptoms were mild and difficult to characterize as seizures without ictal EEG recordings.

Diagnosis

It is easy to make a diagnosis based on disease onset before the age of 13 years, typical clinical manifestations, and the EEG characteristics of triad syndrome. The most important basis for the diagnosis of this disease is abnormal EEG data, but these abnormalities are not specific; therefore, these patients need to be differentiated from other patients with occipital lobe EEG abnormalities. Ivanov [363] summarized the clinical manifestations of self-limited epilepsy with autonomic seizures into eight characteristics, namely, infrequent seizures (up to five), seizure duration >5 min, paroxysmal vomiting, paroxysmal ocular deviation, paroxysmal autonomic manifestations, paroxysmal behavior disorder, gradually deepening disturbance of consciousness during seizures, and convulsions. A total of 34 patients were selected for the study, and self-limited epilepsy with autonomic seizures was found to be distinguishable from other similar disorders when 5 of these features were present. For example, age of onset <1 year or >15 years, obvious cognitive decline with persistent electrical discharge during sleep, and structural changes on brain MRI can exclude the possibility of this syndrome [301].

Treatment

Because most patients have only one seizure, treatment is not necessary. When the patient has a first seizure and is subsequently observed for a period of time, if a seizure occurs again, the use of antiseizure medications can be considered. Moreover, current antiseizure drugs only control seizures and have little effect on the development of epilepsy, and patients with this disease have very few seizures. If the children or their parents are unwilling to use drugs, they can also be temporarily treated without drugs. Antiseizure medications are necessary for patients with frequent seizures. Carbamazepine, valproate sodium, and levetiracetam can effectively control seizures. Mellish et al. [364] conducted a survey of 132 doctors. Most doctors preferred carbamazepine and levetiracetam for treatment, but it has also been reported that carbamazepine can cause aggravation of seizures and deterioration of EEG signals in patients [365].

Prognosis

This disease is an age-dependent benign epilepsy of childhood. The overall prognosis is good, and most patients are seizure-free before the age of 13 years. Even patients with frequent status epilepticus have a good prognosis, and this condition has almost no effect on patient development. Only a small percentage of people who have a cardiac arrest episode have serious consequences.

5.3.1.3 Childhood Occipital Visual Epilepsy (COVE)

Overview

Occipital visual epilepsy, formerly known as late-onset childhood occipital epilepsy (Gastaut type), is a rare age-dependent childhood epilepsy syndrome. The etiology is unclear and may be related to genetics. The main clinical manifestations are paroxysmal visual symptoms, eyeball deviation, headache after attack, and disturbance of consciousness and convulsions in severe cases. The attacks are usually more frequent, with more waking episodes that last from a few seconds to 3 min. Interictal EEG shows occipital discharge and is sensitive to open or closed eyes. Some patients have only occasional occipital spikes or occipital spikes during sleep, and a few patients have normal EEGs at all times. Ictal EEG shows transient inhibition in the occipital region, followed by sudden occipital discharge with a fast rhythm or fast spike [301].

Historical Evolution

In 1982, Gastaut [366] proposed the concept of "benign epilepsy with occipital spikes" for the first time and summarized that it could be characterized by seizures dominated by visual symptoms and EEG signals with eye-closure-induced high-amplitude spikes during interictal periods, mainly located in the occipital lobe; it was speculated that this was a new type of epilepsy. In 1984, Deonna et al. [367] studied the characteristics of benign occipital lobe epilepsy described by Gastaut et al. and its relationship with childhood migraine in 195 patients with idiopathic epilepsy and concluded that this "new" type of epileptic syndrome could be well-distinguished from other similar epileptic seizure entities. In 1989, Nalin et al. [368] studied 13 epileptic patients with visual symptoms and found that their symptoms were completely consistent with the clinical and EEG manifestations of occipital lobe epilepsy as reported by Gastaut, which confirmed the existence of occipital visual epilepsy in children. In 1998, Andermann and Zifkin [369] studied the relationship between occipital lobe epilepsy, migraine, and Panayiotopoulos syndrome and posited that they were essentially a different and unique epilepsy syndrome. In 2005, Tedrus and Fonseca [370] studied 63 patients aged 2–14 years with seizures and occipital epileptic activity on EEG and proposed that these cases could be divided into early-onset occipital epilepsy, late-onset occipital epilepsy (Gastaut type), and Rolandic epilepsy syndrome. Subsequently, Caraballo et al. [371] noted that patients with this syndrome may present with absence seizures. In 2019, Akca Kalem et al. [372] explained that early- and late-onset occipital lobe epilepsies are completely different diseases from the perspective of neuropsychology, which deepened the general understanding of this kind of occipital lobe epilepsy in children. In 2022, ILAE named late-onset occipital epilepsy (Gastaut type) "children with occipital visual epilepsy," which led to this syndrome becoming more widely recognized [301].

Epidemiology
Ermolenko et al. [373] conducted a study on 1036 children aged 1–18 years with epilepsy and reported 106 cases of idiopathic focal epilepsy; among these cases, 12.3% were diagnosed with Gastaut syndrome. Gaggero et al. [374] studied 80 children diagnosed with a specific syndrome and reported that 2.8% of them had occipital visual epilepsy. A total of 52 epileptic patients with visual symptoms were investigated, and the incidence of late-onset pediatric occipital epilepsy with the Gastaut variant was 23.1%. Fortini et al. [375] investigated 7705 patients with self-limiting childhood epilepsy aged 2–14 years and found that 356 of them had self-limiting pediatric occipital lobe epilepsy (Gastaut type).

Causes of the Disease
The etiology of occipital visual epilepsy syndrome in children is unclear. Clinically, this association tends to be hereditary, but the specific mechanism of heredity is unclear. Grosso et al. [376] studied two Gastaut epilepsy syndrome patients with a family history of the disease and reported that two generations of the patients' families had epilepsy and could be considered autosomal dominant inherited. Gastaut [366] reported that 36% of the patients had a family history of epilepsy, suggesting that the occurrence of this syndrome is related to genetics; however, Taylor et al. [377] studied twins and families to explore the genetic characteristics of Panayiotopoulos syndrome and Gastaut syndrome. Among the 16 probands, 7 were twins and 9 had a family history of epilepsy. One study revealed that in relatives with epilepsy, there was a mixture of focal and generalized epilepsy, and focal epilepsy was dominant. The authors suggest that Gastaut syndrome may be a multifactorial disorder with low concordance in monozygotic twins, suggesting that unconventional genetic influences or environmental factors play a major role.

Clinical Presentation
Caraballo et al. [378] conducted a study on 33 patients with Gastaut syndrome and reported that visual symptoms and paroxysmal ocular deviation were the most common symptoms; approximately 50% of the patients had migraine-like symptoms, and most of the patients had spike discharges in the occipital region when their eyes were closed, which disappeared or decreased when their eyes were open. Among the 12 children reported on by Caraballo et al. [379], 75.0% had visual hallucinations, 50% had blindness or blurred vision, 50% had headaches, 58.3% had secondary generalized tonic–clonic seizures, and all patients had occipital spikes that could be induced by eye closing and opening.

Age of Onset

Nalin et al. [368] reported that the age of onset ranged from 6 to 14 years. Caraballo et al. [378] reported on three patients, two females and one male, with onset ages of 7.5, 8, and 10 years, respectively. Caraballo et al. [378] studied 33 patients and reported that the peak age of the disease was 8.5 years. Caraballo et al. [379] reported on 12 patients with a median age of onset of 10.3 years. Therefore, the age of onset of Gastaut syndrome is approximately 6–14 years, and the peak age at disease onset is 8–10 years.

Sex

Nine girls and three boys were included in a study by Caraballo et al. [379]. Two of the three patients included in the study reported by Caraballo et al. [371] were girls, indicating that Gastaut syndrome is more common in girls than in boys.

Time of Onset

Most of the patients had seizures during the day while awake, and a small number of patients had seizures during sleep or upon waking at night. Among the 33 patients reported on by Caraballo et al. [379], all had seizures while awake and 11 had seizures during sleep.

Visual Seizures

Gastaut [366] reported the presence of Gastaut syndrome through the visual symptoms of the patients in 1982. He found that amaurosis, visual hallucinations, and complex hallucinations were the main manifestations of these patients. Due to the particularity of this clinical manifestation, he speculated that this was a new epilepsy syndrome. Verrotti et al. [380] analyzed 129 patients and reported that 62% of them had visual hallucinations as the major symptom and 38.8% had visual hallucinations as the only manifestation. In 10 children investigated by Nalin et al. [368], the first symptom was also visual (hallucinations and amaurosis). Most of the visual symptoms were simple visual hallucinations, which presented as flashes of light, red dots, black and white stripes, or colored patterns, while 10% of the patients had complex visual hallucinations, which were perceived as human heads or shadows. Blindness is another common visual symptom following visual hallucinations, and it can also be the only symptom on onset. Blindness occurs suddenly and is usually brief, lasting for 5–15 s and rarely lasting for 1–2 min. In rare cases, blindness can last for 15–20 min or more.

Paroxysmal Head–Eye Deviation

In addition to paroxysmal visual symptoms, paroxysmal head–eye deviation was another common symptom in 33 patients according to Caraballo et al. [379]. One of the three patients investigated by Caraballo et al. [371] was also found to have paroxysmal head and eye deviation. Seven children described by Shu et al. [381] also exhibited head–eye deviation.

Other Seizure Types

In addition to paroxysmal visual symptoms, patients can also experience other types of seizures. Two of the three patients described by Caraballo et al. [371] had absence seizures following occipital seizures, two of the seven patients described by Shu et al. [381] had unilateral seizures, and one had secondary generalized tonic–clonic seizures. Caraballo et al. [379] reported that more than half of the 12 patients had secondary generalized tonic–clonic seizures.

Headache

Paroxysmal headache is another common symptom of this syndrome. Approximately 50% of patients have paroxysmal headache, most of which appear immediately after the end of visual hallucinations or 5–10 min after the headache. The headache is diffuse, and mild-to-moderate headaches occur. A few children may experience severe throbbing headache similar to migraine, which needs to be differentiated from a migraine attack.

Electroencephalographic Features

The characteristic EEG of Gastaut syndrome is that the occipital region epileptiform discharges can be induced by opening or closing the eyes. Gastaut [366] summarized the EEG manifestations of this syndrome as follows: high-amplitude spikes or spikes and slow waves occur when the eyes are closed under normal background activity; these spikes can occur regularly and repeatedly in one or both occipital posterior temporal regions and can be synchronous or asynchronous or symmetric or asymmetric. Nalin et al. [368] reported that 6 of 10 patients had EEG abnormalities (sharp wave, slow wave, or spike and wave) that disappeared after opening their eyes. Caraballo et al. [379] analyzed the EEG signals of 12 patients and reported that the ictal EEG signals exhibited irregular spikes in the bilateral occipital lobes when visual symptoms occurred. The interictal EEG showed occipital spikes sensitive to eye closing and eye opening in all patients, extra-occipital spikes in four patients, and generalized spikes in two patients.

Diagnosis

The age of onset was 3–6 years, and the main manifestations were paroxysmal visual symptoms, eyeball deviation, and headache. EEG signals showed epileptic discharges in the occipital region when the eyes were closed. Gastaut syndrome patients usually have short-lived seizures. According to ILAE, patients diagnosed with Gastaut syndrome should be cautious when seizures last for more than 15 min and when tonic–clonic seizures occur during wakefulness. Patients are excluded if they are <1 or >20 years of age, have dystonia, have structural lesions on MRI of the head, or have occipital lobe calcifications of the brain [301].

Differential Diagnosis

Migraine

Patients present with significant visual symptoms at the time of attack and often have headaches after attack, which is very similar to a migraine attack. Some patients may have both migraine and Gastaut syndrome, constituting a special migraine–epilepsy syndrome, which increases the difficulty of identification. The headache caused by this disease is very mild and mostly consists of dull pain after the seizure. The location of the headache is uncertain, and the disease is rarely accompanied by nausea or vomiting; moreover, the disease does not affect daily activities after the attack, which is different from severe headache, obvious nausea, and vomiting and impacts daily life during a migraine attack. Moreover, the duration of Gastaut syndrome headache is much shorter than that of a migraine headache. It usually lasts for several minutes or tens of minutes, significantly differing from that of migraine headache, which usually lasts for several hours. Although paroxysmal spikes may occur on the EEGs of migraine patients, most of them are not affected by the opening or closing of the eyes, unlike in Gastaut syndrome, which is induced when the eyes are closed and disappears when the eyes are open.

Panayiotopoulos Syndrome

Children with Gastaut syndrome tend to be older, have episodic visual hallucinations as a prominent manifestation, and have epileptiform discharge on EEG that is affected by opening and closing their eyes. This is different from Panayiotopoulos syndrome, which is characterized by episodic autonomic dysfunction, obvious vomiting, and less effect of opening and closing the eyes on EEG epileptiform discharge.

Treatment

The need for treatment of occipital visual epilepsy in children is still being debated. Verrotti et al. [380] reported that 103 of 129 patients did not receive treatment. Although this syndrome has a good overall prognosis and is considered a benign occipital lobe epilepsy in children, most children have frequent seizures and therefore need treatment. If not treated medically, secondary generalized tonic–clonic seizures can occur. Because of the favorable prognosis, no prospective drug treatment has been reported for Gastaut syndrome and administration of valproic acid or carbamazepine has been advocated [380]. In 129 patients described by Verrotti et al. [380], the main treatment drugs were sodium valproate, carbamazepine, levetiracetam, and topiramate. Seventy-six percent of patients responded to a single agent, and 24% required multiple agents. Panayiotopoulos [382] summarized the treatments of nine patients and reported that carbamazepine was effective and advocated for its use in the treatment of Gastaut syndrome. However, Skrijelj and Mulić [383] used carbamazepine to treat symptomatic occipital lobe epilepsy and reported that the patient's seizures were aggravated and required attention. Verrotti et al. [384] treated 12 patients with levetiracetam; 11 patients (91.6%) subsequently had no seizures, and 10 patients (83.3%) had complete normalization of EEG abnormalities.

Prognosis

When Gastaut [366] first proposed the existence of this syndrome, he noted that despite susceptibility to epilepsy, the overall prognosis was good, with 60% of the patients experiencing seizure remission after 2–4 years of onset. Nalin et al. [368] reported that 9 out of 10 patients had paroxysmal visual symptoms that disappeared after antiseizure medication treatment and that more than half of the patients had no intellectual or behavioral abnormalities. Seizures were relieved in 81.8% of 12 patients described by Caraballo et al. [379], half of whom stopped medication after puberty, and their EEGs also returned to normal. Although the overall prognosis of this syndrome is good, antiseizure therapy is effective. However, the prognoses of patients with other diseases or epilepsy syndromes is worse than that of children with simple Gastaut syndrome with occipital lobe epilepsy. Verrotti et al. [380]

categorized 129 cases of occipital lobe epilepsy in children with Gastaut syndrome into simple and combined with other syndromes for comparison and reported that the prognoses of patients with other syndromes was worse than that of children with simple Gastaut syndrome with occipital lobe epilepsy. Two children had unilateral seizures, and only one had secondary generalized tonic–clonic seizures. In all patients, seizures occurred while awake and two patients also had seizures while sleeping. EEG signals showed that occipital spikes were discharged when the eyes were closed and disappeared when the eyes were open in five patients. Despite treatment with antiseizure drugs, two of the seven patients described by Shu et al. [381] developed hemiconvulsion, and one had secondary generalized tonic–clonic seizures. These patients also exhibited learning difficulties and behavioral disorders after seizures.

5.3.1.4 Idiopathic Photosensitive Occipital Lobe Epilepsy (POLE)

Overview

Photosensitive epilepsy is a common reflex seizure seen in clinical practice and is characterized by paroxysmal epileptiform discharges and visual seizures on an EEG under intermittent light stimulation. Clinically, it can be categorized into hereditary generalized epilepsy (HGE), symptomatic generalized epilepsy, and idiopathic photosensitive occipital lobe epilepsy, and its occurrence may be related to genetic factors [301].

Historical Evolution

In 1965, Charlton [385] first noted the existence of this syndrome. In 1966, von Hedenström and Schorsch [386] described the relationship between this syndrome and light stimulation. In 1967, Hishikawa et al. [387] referred to seizures caused by visual or intermittent flash stimulation as photosensitive epilepsy. In 1973, Dimov et al. [388] replicated this type of seizure in animals, deepening the understanding of this photosensitive epilepsy. In 1980, Bruni et al. [389] reported that valproic acid could reduce photosensitivity in these patients. In 1987, Mayr et al. [390] studied 32 epileptic patients whose EEG signals revealed a photoconvulsive response when flashing light appeared, but they did not experience seizures due to exposure to light or absence of light when watching TV, which enriched the related research. In 2013, Taylor et al. [391] studied the genetic characteristics of this syndrome and reported that its occurrence is related to genetic factors.

Epidemiology

Shiraishi et al. [392] conducted a study on light stimulation in 2817 patients with epilepsy and reported that 37 of them (1.7%) had classic photosensitive seizures, which accounted for 2.0% of symptomatic generalized epilepsy patients and 5.6% of idiopathic generalized epilepsy patients. Xue et al. [393] investigated 22 cases of photosensitive generalized epilepsy and found that 12 cases were idiopathic photosensitive occipital lobe epilepsy.

Causes of the Disease

The occurrence of idiopathic photosensitive occipital lobe epilepsy is related to genetic factors. Keren [394] studied 16 children and adolescents with this syndrome and found the occurrence of seizures in 2 groups of siblings and 7 first- or second-degree relatives of the patients, all of whom presented with occipital lobe seizures, suggesting that genetic factors were involved in its occurrence. Sadleir et al. [395] performed whole exome sequencing on eight patients with photosensitive epilepsy and reported that *RORB* gene mutations were related to idiopathic photosensitive occipital lobe epilepsy. Li et al. [396] studied 585 patients with generalized genetic epilepsy and described a p.S632W mutation in a patient with idiopathic photosensitive occipital lobe epilepsy. A study by ILAE also confirmed that 30% of patients had a family history of this disease [385], which supports the hypothesis that idiopathic photosensitive occipital lobe epilepsy is related to genetic factors.

Clinical Presentation

Age of Onset

Guerrini et al. [397] studied 10 patients with idiopathic photosensitive occipital lobe epilepsy aged 8–30 years, whose age of onset ranged from 5 to 17 years, with an average age of 11 years, and identified 29 patients diagnosed with POLE at an average age of 20.1 ± 7.6 years. Cerrahoğlu Şirin et al. [398] studied 29 patients with photosensitive occipital lobe epilepsy, with an average onset age of 20.1 ± 7.6 years. Shiraishi et al. [392] studied the clinical manifestations of 37 patients with idiopathic photosensitive occipital lobe epilepsy and reported that the average age of onset was 17 years, most were 15 years of age, and the number of patients decreased significantly after 20 years of age. According to ILAE, although this syndrome is more common in children, adults can also have idiopathic photosensitive occipital lobe epilepsy [301]. Koutroumanidis et al. [399] studied 30 patients with adult photosensitive epilepsy and found that 15 of them had specific photosensitive occipital lobe epilepsy.

Sex

In a study by Guerrini et al. [397], eight patients were female and two were male. Yazar et al. [400] studied 44 patients with photosensitive seizures, 17 of whom had idiopathic photosensitive occipital lobe epilepsy; more patients were female than male. Similarly, ILAE has reported that more patients with this disease are female than male [301].

Predisposing Factors

The main precipitating factor is light. Flickering sunlight and television may be the most common precipitating factors, and a small number of patients are affected by opening or closing their eyes during sleep [301]. Guerrini et al. [397] reported that all 10 patients in his study had seizures induced by light, and the inducing factors were mainly television and computer lights.

Seizures of Epilepsy

1. *Visual occipital seizures*: Light-induced visual seizures are the core symptoms of this syndrome. These visual symptoms include flashes of light, colored macules, visual hallucinations, or visual blurring/loss, usually of short duration and generally <3 min [401]. Most patients subsequently develop a slow headache, epigastric discomfort, and vomiting with a delayed response [397]. Such light-induced occipital seizures are often accompanied by frequent secondary generalized seizures [301].
2. *Evolution of seizure types*: Bonini et al. [402] described the evolution of seizure types in a patient: the proband developed idiopathic photosensitive occipital lobe epilepsy in childhood, which evolved into absence and generalized tonic–clonic seizures in early adolescence. Guerrini et al. [401] reported that two patients developed Rolandic seizures at the age of 4 and 5 years and developed photosensitive occipital lobe seizures in adolescence.
3. *Other seizure types*: In some patients, focal visual occipital seizures, myoclonus, absence, and generalized tonic–clonic seizures are also observed, with variable frequency. Varotto et al. [403] studied the connectivity of EEG signals in patients with photosensitive epilepsy and found tit to be abnormal. Even though the occipital cortex is the receiving area of stimulation, the anterior cortex is also involved in the hypersynchronization of epileptiform discharges in patients with photosensitive epilepsy, so a variety of seizure types could occur.

EEG Findings

EEG background activity is usually normal, and spikes, sharp waves, or spikes and slow waves can be induced in the occipital region by eye closure or intermittent light stimulation. Ricci et al. [404] studied the EEG signals of five patients with idiopathic photosensitive occipital lobe epilepsy and reported that the EEG signals of two patients exhibited occipital epileptiform discharges during interictal EEG, while the other exhibited bilateral spontaneous and evoked sharp waves followed by generalized epileptiform discharges. Ictal EEG signals in three patients showed focal lateralized θ activity, with a fast recruitment rhythm in one patient and an anterior occipital fast rhythm in another.

Diagnosis

Optic-sensory occipital epilepsy induced by eye closure or intermittent light stimulation is the most prominent manifestation of idiopathic light-sensitive occipital epilepsy. Combined with interictal light stimulation, epileptiform discharges can be induced on occipital EEG. Owing to the combination of the young onset age and short onset time, this disease is not difficult to diagnose. ILAE proposed in its new classification of epilepsy syndromes that if the seizure lasts for more than 3 min, attention should be given to whether it is another type of photosensitive epilepsy. Patients with myoclonus, cognitive impairment, or structural damage on brain MRI can be excluded [301].

Treatment

Most patients with idiopathic photosensitive occipital lobe epilepsy experience self-limiting seizures that are fewer in number and shorter in duration. However, existing antiseizure medications can only control seizures, so it is not necessary to treat patients who experience few and mild seizures if they can effectively avoid light stimulation. Guerrini et al. [401] described two patients: one had only a few visual seizures and did not have seizures again for 4 years and the other had seizures that stopped after using valproic acid and carbamazepine.

Valproic acid is the most commonly used drug for the treatment of idiopathic photosensitive occipital lobe epilepsy. Koutroumanidis et al. [399] treated 15 patients with photosensitive occipital lobe epilepsy with valproic acid and reported that the patients responded well to it. Carbamazepine may be an alternative agent when valproic acid is unavailable.

Prognosis

Idiopathic photosensitive occipital lobe epilepsy is associated with a good prognosis. Politi-Elishkevich et al. [405] observed 16 patients with idiopathic photosensitive occipital lobe epilepsy and reported that 8 of them achieved complete control of seizures after monotherapy, 5 patients needed a second drug, and 3 had no drug treatment.

5.3.2 *Inherited Generalized Epilepsy Syndrome in Children*

5.3.2.1 Eyelid Myoclonic Epilepsy (EMA) (Jeavons Syndrome)

Overview

Eyelid myoclonic epilepsy (EMA) is a type of hereditary generalized epilepsy (HGE) characterized by eyelid myoclonus, eye closure sensitivity, and photosensitivity and is also known as Jeavons syndrome. The new classification of epilepsy syndromes in 2022 by ILAE classifies it as a childhood-onset epilepsy syndrome [301].

Historical Evolution

In 1977, Jeavons [406] first noted this kind of eyelid myoclonic seizure in his study of six types of myoclonic epilepsies in children. The following year, Ichikawa et al. [407] reported a case of eyelid myoclonic seizures caused by eye closure and subsequent authors reported the existence of similar cases [408]. It was also noted that such cases may be accompanied by absence seizures [409]. Its etiology is related to heredity. In 1992, Veggiotti P et al. [410] reported that eyelid myoclonus induced by eye closure can occur in patients with status epilepticus. In 1999, Baykan-Kurt et al. [411] reported that eye closure could induce sharp waves and spikes and slow waves on EEG. Yalçin et al. [412] emphasized that this epilepsy syndrome is not the same as juvenile myoclonus and proposed two clinical differentiation points, which promoted the diagnosis of this eyelid myoclonus. Striano et al. [413] reported that levetiracetam is effective in treating this epilepsy syndrome and that it can also be used to treat eyelid myoclonic seizures with or without absence. Initially, ILAE did not recognize this epilepsy syndrome; until 2001, ILAE included it in the new classification of epilepsy syndromes. In 2022, ILAE again confirmed the presence of Jeavons syndrome [301].

Epidemiological Investigations
Because Jeavons syndrome has not long been recognized by ILAE, there are few epidemiological studies on eyelid myoclonus. Zawar et al. [414] studied 249 patients with photosensitive epilepsy and found that 70 of them (28.1%) had eyelid myoclonic seizures. Asadi-Pooya et al. [415] studied 601 patients with idiopathic epilepsy and found that 12 of them (5.6%) had eyelid myoclonus. Kotov [416] studied 26 children with absence seizures and found that 14 had eyelid myoclonic seizures. Wang et al. [417] found 50 cases of eyelid myoclonic epilepsy among 4230 epileptic patients, suggesting that the incidence of eyelid myoclonic epilepsy in epileptic patients is approximately 1–53%.

Causes of the Disease
Eyelid myoclonic seizures are mainly related to genetic factors. Nilo et al. [418] reported that 13 of 40 patients (32.5%) had a positive family history of epilepsy. Parfyonov et al. [419] described a 2-year-old female patient with eyelid myoclonus whose gene sequencing results suggested that an *ATP1A3* gene mutation was the cause of this disease, suggesting that *ATP1A3* gene mutation should be considered in patients with early-onset epilepsy with eyelid myoclonus. Mutations in the *SYNGAP1*, *GLUT1*, *KLAA*, *SLC6A1*, *PLCB1*, *STAG2*, *NEXMIF*, *RORB*, and *CHD2* genes are also associated with eyelid myoclonus [420–425].

Clinical Presentation
Sex

Eyelid myoclonic epilepsy is common in women. Nilo et al. [418] studied 40 patients with eyelid myoclonus—31 females and 9 males—with a female-to-male ratio of 3.44, indicating that this syndrome is more common in female patients. Zawar et al. [414] described 70 patients, 62 (88.6%) of whom were female. Kelsey M Smith et al. [426] reported that 80% of 30 patients with eyelid myoclonic seizures were female, supporting the view that eyelid myoclonic seizures are more common in women.

Emanuele Cerulli Irelli [427] studied 267 patients and found that in female patients, multivariate logistic regression analysis showed that age of seizure onset, eyelid myoclonus, status epilepticus, psychiatric comorbidities, and menstrual seizures were important predictors of drug resistance. In male patients, a history of febrile seizures was the only predictor of drug resistance.

Age

Eyelid myoclonic epilepsy is more common in childhood. The average onset age of 30 patients described by Smith et al. [426] was 7.3 years, and the average onset age of 50 patients with eyelid myoclonic epilepsy studied by Wang et al. [417] was 8 years. Zawar et al. [414] reported that the average age of onset in 70 patients was 7 years, and, in most cases, the age of onset of eyelid myoclonic epilepsy was 3–12 years [427].

Sensitivity to Light

Among 40 cases of eyelid myoclonic epilepsy reported by Nilo et al. [418], 34 were sensitive to intermittent flash stimulation. The most common precipitating factor is conscious or involuntary or reflexive eye closure, and most episodes are triggered immediately after eyelid closure in the presence of continuous light; eyelid closure cannot be induced in total darkness. Intermittent flash stimulation can also cause seizures when the eyes are open or closed. Photosensitivity decreases with age, and eyelid closure may be a lifelong trigger; however, in some patients, ocular spasms occur only in response to bright light.

Seizures of Epilepsy

There are two types of eyelid myoclonic epilepsies, that is, those with absence seizures and those without. There are two main manifestations of ocular muscle spasms with absence seizures: ① Initially, the most evident manifestation is blepharospasm, which can occur with or without subsequent absence seizures and ② mildly altered consciousness (absence). Attacks start abruptly and end rapidly, lasting for approximately 3–5 s.

Blepharospasm mainly occurred in the second of EEG epileptiform discharge and manifested as rhythmic, 4–6-Hz blepharospasm with different amplitudes. Even in the same patient, the duration, strength, amplitude, and number of ocular myoclonus episodes are variable and there are more than three repeated episodes of blepharospasm per attack, except for an occasional lone ocular myoclonus. Typically, eyelid myoclonus is accompanied by tonic contraction; the eye is half open and half closed, and the eyeballs often jump up and down or stare upward, with eyebrow jitter and head swing. This can also manifest as eyeball or head-to-one-side deviation. Ocular muscle spasms accompanied by hand twitching can occur in some patients. Rarely is the tonicity of the eyelid partially open and partially closed, and deviation of the head and eye may be more pronounced than in clonus, which is quite different from random or rhythmic eyelid closure or beating in individuals with absence seizures in other epilepsy syndromes.

The second feature of the syndrome is disturbance of consciousness (absence). With the gradual alleviation of eyelid myoclonus, disturbance of consciousness follows. This disturbance of consciousness is usually mild, with respiratory arrest, delay, and rhythm disturbance observed on video EEG, and no automata have been reported.

Another rare symptom is a euphoric feeling that occurs during absence episodes, which may be associated with self-induction in some patients.

Abortive blepharospasm manifests as palpebral tremor that resembles a twitch or rapid eye flutter. Rapid flutter is difficult to identify in the absence of video EEG monitoring. The episodes are brief, usually <1 s, and rarely 1–3 s. These two types may coexist with other seizure types or may be the only seizure type. Ictal EEG shows multiple spikes, but the spikes on EEG usually appear before the eyelid closure artifact disappears, indicating that the clonic phenomenon of blepharospasm is an ictal phenomenon.

Status Epilepticus

Inagaki et al. [428] reported that an infant boy with myoclonic epilepsy had eyelid myoclonic seizures when his eyes were closed; these authors considered this to be a case of eyelid myoclonic status epilepticus. Both drug withdrawal and inappropriate treatment can cause persistent blepharospasm in the absence of infection. This status epilepticus is more likely to occur during wakefulness [429].

Relationship with Other Epilepsy Syndromes

Moutaouakil et al. [430] described a patient with infantile benign myoclonic epilepsy who had onset at the age of 3 and whose condition disappeared after treatment. The treatment was stopped at the age of 5, eyelid myoclonic epilepsy developed at the age of 10, and the authors concluded that patients with infantile benign myoclonic epilepsy were likely to need long-term monitoring.

Others

Among the 40 patients described by Nilo et al. [418], 11 had generalized tonic–clonic seizures, 14 had intellectual delays, and 18 had psychiatric symptoms. Ballarà Petitbò et al. [431] analyzed 17 patients and reported that 76.4% of them had neuropsychiatric comorbidities, 75% had neurocognitive manifestations, and 66.6% had cognitive impairment, mainly manifested as difficulties in executive function, language comprehension, and motor skills.

Ancillary Tests

Ocular muscle spasms with absence are part of generalized epilepsy. EEG, especially video EEG, is the most important tool for diagnosing this blepharospasm. On EEG, there are generalized 3–6-Hz (mostly above 4 Hz) high-amplitude spikes or spikes and slow waves lasting for 1–5 s (usually 3 s, rarely more than 5 s), appearing within 0.5–2 s of closing the eyes in a brightly lit room, most prominently within 1–2 s of the onset of seizures, and often persisting. Most patients have varying degrees of clinical seizures at this time. In most cases, epileptiform discharges on EEG precede ocular myoclonus, and, in a few cases, they precede clinical onset. Flash stimulation induces epileptiform discharges in untreated young patients but not in medicated older patients. Even in fully controlled patients, normal EEG signals are rare and hyperventilation can increase epileptic discharges on EEG. There may be an increase in generalized spikes and slow waves during sleep as well as an occasional decrease, a shorter duration of epileptic discharges, a lack of identifiable clinical manifestations, and an increase in EEG and clinical seizures upon awakening [432].

Differential Diagnosis

Eyelid myoclonic seizures are easily misdiagnosed. Of the 70 patients included in the study by Zawar et al. [414], 54 (77.1%) were initially diagnosed with another type of epilepsy and 40 (57.1%) were initially diagnosed with hereditary generalized epilepsy or juvenile myoclonic epilepsy.

Symptomatic or Cryptogenic Ocular Myoclonus with Absence

Ocular myoclonus with absence is usually the main seizure type of ocular myoclonus with absence syndrome. However, ocular myoclonus with absence can also occur in symptomatic or cryptogenic ocular muscle spasms and needs to be differentiated. The following points help distinguish between the two. ① Ocular spasticity with or without symptoms of photosensitive seizures or cryptogenic epilepsy often manifests as impairment of mental developmental, neurological signs, or diffuse abnormal background EEG activity that is rarely observed in patients with primary ocular spasticity with absence. ② Focal EEG abnormalities are common in patients with symptomatic or cryptogenic blepharospasm with absence. If they are significant and of prolonged duration, they often indicate structural damage. ③ Symptomatic or cryptogenic eyelid myoclonus with absence is usually short and stereotyped; occasionally, myoclonus of the limb or body may occur alone, and other seizure types with different durations may occur, such as atypical absence, tonic, atonic, or focal seizures. Eye-closing activation is less common than primary ocular myoclonus with absence.

Primary Generalized Epilepsy with Absence

Primary generalized epilepsy with absence may also present with eyelid myoclonus. Childhood absence seizures, juvenile absence seizures, myoclonic absence (MA) seizures, single myoclonic absence seizures, and other generalized epilepsies with typical absence seizures that cannot be classified may be associated with myoclonus similar to eyelid myoclonic epilepsy; however, these patients are rarely photosensitive and can be used for identification.

Self-Induced Eye Closure or Ocular Myoclonus in Photosensitive Epilepsy

Eyelid myoclonus with absence is usually triggered by eye closure in the presence of light and often exacerbated by intermittent flash stimulation. EEG discharges precede or coincide with ocular muscle spasms, which can be induced by simple eye closure without the need for intermittent light stimulation. Self-induced photosensitive epilepsy requires intermittent photostimulation for induction and confirmation. Eye opening and closing are paroxysmal events that often occur in conjunction with spikes, especially in the first half of a second in patients without EEG abnormalities. In patients subjected to intermittent flash stimulation, generalized epileptic discharges appear before the eyes are closed when ordered, suggesting that some paroxysmal events are caused by the eyes closing and light stimulation.

Passive Eye Closure and Eyelid Flutter in Occipital Lobe Epilepsy

Passive eye closing or blinking is an episodic event in primary or symptomatic occipital lobe epilepsy. Early signs may be helpful in differentiating this syndrome from other focal seizures, and it usually appears after visual hallucinations as a stage of impairment of consciousness, indicating subsequent generalized tonic–clonic seizures. However, it may also occur alone and can be confirmed by video EEG only in occipital photosensitive individuals.

Myoclonic Seizures in Adolescents

Eyelid myoclonus with absences (EMA) and juvenile myoclonus epilepsy (JME) are two separate epilepsy syndromes. Both of these conditions are idiopathic generalized epilepsies. Absence, light sensitivity, and eyelid myoclonus are the main features of eyelid myoclonus epilepsy. Juvenile myoclonic epilepsy has three types of generalized seizures: typical absence, myoclonic convulsion, and generalized tonic–clonic seizures. Myoclonic jerks occur almost exclusively upon awakening and mainly involve the upper limbs, rarely affecting the lower limbs or the whole body. Severe episodes may be accompanied by falls. Generalized myoclonic convulsions are rare in eyelid myoclonic epilepsy, and, when they do occur, they are usually mild and often confined to the upper limbs.

Eyelid Clonus in the Normal Population

Eyelid-related symptoms of eyelid myoclonic epilepsy can be observed in the normal population, and spontaneous eye closure can increase significantly when the eye muscles are relaxed, with some people reaching 3–5 times/second. This closure of the eyes is similar to that in self-induced photosensitive epilepsy; it begins or ends when speaking and exacerbates when talking about sensitive things. Slow and persistent eye closure is rare and mainly occurs when talking about sadness, anger, or frustration. This spontaneous eye closure is not accompanied by epileptic discharges on EEG, and the absence of eye opening or closing is the main distinguishing point.

Treatment

Antiseizure Medications

Long-term use of antiseizure drugs is necessary. Valproate plus ethosuximide may be the most effective regiment. Clonazepam is also effective in treating myoclonus, and small doses of lamotrigine plus valproate also improve eyelid myoclonus without drug interactions.

An international group led by Smith et al. [433] reached a consensus after extensive discussion: there was a strong consensus on valproic acid as a first-line treatment, levetiracetam or lamotrigine was the preferred alternative for women of reproductive age, and ethosuximide and clobazam were effective. Participants also agreed that sodium channel-blocking drugs other than lamotrigine should be avoided because they may worsen seizure control and that carbamazepine, oxcarbazepine, cannabidiol, valproic acid, and phenytoin have the potential to worsen this condition [434, 435].

Ketogenic Diet

Paibool et al. [436] administered a ketogenic diet to six patients with eyelid myoclonic epilepsy, and the results showed that the seizure frequency was reduced by more than 50% in all patients, suggesting that a ketogenic diet may be helpful for these patients. Ballarà Petitbò et al. [431] also suggested that a ketogenic diet is effective in eyelid myoclonic epilepsy.

Others

Electrical stimulation of the thalamus in a patient with drug-refractory absence eyelid myoclonus was found to reduce absence seizures from an average of 60–10 or fewer per day, suggesting a potential treatment for drug-resistant eyelid myoclonus [437].

Prognosis
The prognosis of eyelid myoclonic epilepsy is poor, seizures usually persist into adulthood, and, in the case of medical treatment, <50% of patients achieve remission with medication [418]. However, Nilo et al. [438] have recently reported that 20 of their 40 patients experienced seizure remission for more than 1 year and that those who received effective treatment were seizure-free after an average of 13.85 ± 13.43 years (range: 1–44). Intellectual delay and early onset (≤ 5 years of age) were the strongest predictors of poor seizure control.

5.3.3 *Epileptic Syndromes with Myoclonic Absence Seizures*

Overview
Myoclonic absence epilepsy (EMA) is a type of childhood epilepsy characterized by myoclonic absence (MA) seizures. ILAE considers it a rare childhood epilepsy syndrome and classifies it as a class of childhood-onset epilepsy syndromes [439].

Historical Evolution
In 1969, Tassinari et al. [440] first noted the existence of this epilepsy with myoclonic absence and reported the characteristics of their cases, but this topic has not attracted widespread attention. It was not until 1987 that Fois et al. [441] again noted the existence of this syndrome. He found that such patients had absence seizures on EEG, as well as clonic jerks of the upper limbs, and some had other types of seizures. Additionally, Mikol et al. [442] described patients with myoclonic absence in their investigation of 197 adults with epilepsy. In 1988, Bourgeois [443] proposed that patients with both absence seizures and myoclonus should be treated with ethosuximide combined with valproic acid, and they found that the combined use of drugs was much better than single-drug treatment. In 1990, Salas Puig et al. [444] summarized the characteristics of this syndrome and found that it was mainly observed in children and was more common in males. When there was epileptiform

discharge on EEG, myoclonus of the upper limbs at 3 Hz could be observed on electromyography, there was an obvious relationship between the two, and valproic acid plus ethosuximide had a good effect. He speculated that this type of seizure may be an excessive type of idiopathic epilepsy and symptomatic epilepsy, which attracted widespread attention and was subsequently recognized as a rare epilepsy syndrome by ILAE [445]. Subsequently, Bureau and Tassinari [446] summarized its clinical features and concluded that myoclonic absence epilepsy is characterized by absence accompanied by rhythmic myoclonus, usually associated with progressive tonic contractions. Ictal EEG shows bilateral, synchronous, and symmetrical sharp waves. In 2022, ILAE reaffirmed the existence of this syndrome, and people began to widely accept its existence.

Epidemiology
No population-based epidemiological findings related to EMA have been reported. In a study by Roberto Horacio Caraballo [439], 39 patients were diagnosed with epilepsy syndromes, 6 of whom (15%) had consistent EMA manifestations.

Causes of the Disease
EMA is relatively rare, and its etiology is mainly related to genetic factors.

Genetic Factors

Tang et al. [447] analyzed the clinical characteristics of 101 EMA patients and found that 12 of them had pathogenic mutations in genes, including *SYNGAP1* ($n = 3$), *KIAA2022* ($n = 2$), and *SLC6A1* ($n = 2$). Pathogenic genetic variants in *KCNA2*, *SCN2A*, *STX1B*, *KCNB1*, and *MECP2* were also found ($n = 1$ each). Moreover, the authors also found that *ASH1L* and *CHD4* were related to EMA. The authors therefore speculate that EMA is genetically heterogeneous. Hiraide et al. [448] described a patient with myoclonic absence with mild intellectual disability and language impairment. The video EEG showed characteristic diffuse synchronous 3-Hz sharp waves accompanied by upper limb myoclonus. Whole exome sequencing revealed a mutation in the *SETD1B* gene, and this patient had had a similar attack in the past. Therefore, the authors suggested that the occurrence of EMA may be related to genetic factors. Ogawa et al. [449] reported that a patient with EMA had a 2q13 microstatus deletion, suggesting that EMA may be related to genetic mutations. d Frydson et al. [450] described a 7-year-old boy with paroxysmal rhythmic myoclonus accompanied by disturbance of consciousness. The ictal EEG pattern included bilateral synchronous and symmetrical 3-Hz sharp waves. Genetic testing revealed pathogenic variants in the *FOXP1* gene and variants of unknown significance in the *MBD5* gene.

Developmental and Metabolic Disorders

In the 14 patients described by Elia et al. [451], 1 had neuronal heterotopia and another had metabolic disorders, indicating that developmental disorders and metabolic abnormalities are also common causes of EMA syndrome.

Others

Elia et al. [451] reported that 7 out of 14 EMA patients had chromosomal abnormalities; moreover, abnormal expression of the K^+ channel subfamily and the *GABRB3* gene were possible causes of chromosomal abnormalities; 5 patients were cryptogenic.

Pathogenesis

The pathogenesis of EMA has not been fully elucidated. Ikeda et al. [452] performed SPECT studies on one patient of each sex and reported that the cerebral blood flow in the pericortical, thalamic, caudate, and precuneus regions increased in male patients, while the cerebral blood flow in the middle frontal gyrus and bilateral orbitofrontal cortex decreased. Female patients have increased cerebral blood flow in the thalamus, putamen, and globus pallidus. The authors hypothesize that the changes in pericortical blood perfusion caused by oscillations in the corticothalamic network may cause seizures in EMA patients and that changes in cerebral blood flow may be the key to the pathophysiological mechanism of EMA.

Clinical Presentation

The most obvious clinical manifestation of EMA is absence seizures accompanied by 3-Hz myoclonus. Ictal EEG data reveal bilateral synchronous and symmetrical 3-Hz sharp waves, which is similar to the EEG findings in childhood absence epilepsy.

Age of Onset

Tang et al. [447] described 101 patients with EMA; the median age of onset was 34 months (6–72 months) and 70% of them were male. Zanzmera et al. [453] described 12 patients with EMA from India whose mean age of onset was 3.5 years. Elia et al. [451] described seven cases of EMA caused by chromosomal disorders. The average age of onset was 2.9 years (range: 4 months to 6.5 years). Bureau and Tassinari [446] reported that the age of onset of the patient was 7 years. Cherian et al. [454] reported that the age of onset in two siblings was 3.5 years. According to these findings, the age of EMA onset may be between 0.5 and 7 years. Ikeda et al. [455] reported that the age of EMA onset in six patients ranged from 18 to 92 months. Verrotti et al. [456] studied six children with early-onset cryptogenic myoclonic absence seizures whose ages of seizure onset ranged from 6 to 27.8 months. Recently, ILAE has summarized the clinical characteristics of EMA and suggested that the peak age of onset be approximately 7 years, ranging from 1 to 12 years.

Sex

Tang et al. [447] reported that 70% of 101 EMA patients were male. Four of the six patients studied by Verrotti et al. [456] were female and two were male. Zanzmera et al. [453] described 12 cases of EMA, including 50% males and 50% females. Among the patients described by Bureau and Tassinari [446], more were male than female. ILAE supports the idea that there are more men than women with this disease [301].

Durations of Seizures

In the two EMA patients described by Myers and Scheffer [457], the durations of seizures ranged from 10 to 60 s. The duration of seizures in the studies by Zanzmera et al. [453] was 4–20 s.

Types of Seizures

1. *Myoclonic absence seizures*: Myoclonic absence seizures are the main seizure type. They were present in 100% of the cases reported by Zanzmera et al. [453], and most patients first presented with absence seizures, which are characterized by sudden loss of consciousness, followed by 3-Hz myoclonus, mostly located in the head or limbs, accompanied by disturbance of consciousness. This myoclonus is generalized, symmetrical, and rhythmic and can occur many times per day [450, 451].
2. *Myoclonic status epilepticus*: Myoclonic absence status epilepticus occurs in 20% of the patients according to Emma G [458]. Of the 10 patients described by Zanzmera et al. [453] 1 died due to convulsive status epilepticus.
3. *Other seizure types*: Bureau and Tassinari [446] reported that 45% of cases were accompanied by generalized tonic–clonic seizures and that the prognosis of patients with generalized tonic–clonic seizures was worse once they occurred. Generalized tonic–clonic seizures also occurred in 42% of the cases described by Zanzmera et al. [453]. Myers and Scheffer [457] described two children who presented with myoclonus absence at the ages of 3 and 8 years, characterized by bilateral 3-Hz myoclonus superimposed on tonic abduction of the upper limbs, complex gestural automatism during seizures, and extensive 3-Hz spikes on ictal EEG. The authors speculate that this is the first report of complex automatism in patients with myoclonic absence seizures.

ILAE has summarized the characteristics of seizures in EMA: Seizures often have sudden onset, falls are rare, and myoclonic convulsions are usually bilateral symmetric but can be unilateral or asymmetric. Perioral myoclonus and rhythmic jerks of the head and legs may also occur, and, occasionally, autonomic symptoms such as changes in breathing, urinary incontinence, or complex automaticity of gestures may occur. Myoclonic absence is the only type of seizure, and status epilepticus is rare. Generalized tonic–clonic, clonic, atonic, or typical absence seizures may also occur. Multiple seizure types may indicate a more unfavorable prognosis [301].

EEG

An EEG shows rhythmic, bilateral, synchronous, and symmetrical 3-Hz sharp waves, which have an obvious relationship with 3-Hz myoclonus and are mostly superimposed on gradually increasing tonic muscle contractions. Background activity on interictal EEG is normal, and spikes and sharp waves could be independently detected in bilateral temporal and frontal regions [454]. Frydson et al. [450] reported that the ictal EEG of a patient showed bilateral 3-Hz, synchronous and symmetric sharp waves.

Others

Tang et al. [447] analyzed 101 patients with EMA and reported that 62% of them had intellectual disability, 24% had autistic symptoms, and 37% had attention-deficit/hyperactivity symptoms. The authors speculated that EMA was related to severe neurodevelopmental disorders. EMA is genetically heterogeneous.

Diagnosis

ILAE considers myoclonic absence seizures to be a necessary condition for the diagnosis of EMA. Absence seizures accompanied by rhythmic, 3-Hz myoclonus of the upper limbs, often accompanied by tonic abduction of the upper limbs, and epileptiform discharges with myoclonic locks on EEG are the main bases for diagnosis [301]. Iyer [459] emphasized that proximal convulsions of the upper limbs are very important in the diagnosis of EMA.

Differential Diagnosis

Idiopathic Absence Seizures

Idiopathic absence seizures are mainly characterized by paroxysmal, transient loss of consciousness but rarely obvious myoclonus. EMA myoclonus is the prominent manifestation of idiopathic absence seizures.

Idiopathic Generalized Seizures

Myoclonus and absence seizures may occur in this type of epilepsy, but it is rare for both to occur at the same time. Combined with the occurrence of 3-Hz myoclonus during absence seizures, the epileptiform discharges on EEG have an obvious relationship with the myoclonus of the patient, and the latter can be distinguished from the former.

Treatment

Medical Treatment

1. *Ethosuximide combined with valproic acid*: Bourgeois [443] proposed the combination of ethosuximide and valproate for the treatment of EMA in 1988, and Salas Puig et al. [444] also found that ethosuximide plus valproate was the most effective regimen.
2. *Valproate plus topiramate*: Cherian et al. [454] administered carbamazepine in combination with phenobarbital in two siblings with EMA, and the frequency of seizures increased from 5 to 100 times/day; valproic acid was used to reduce the frequency of seizures, suggesting that it is an important drug for the treatment of EMA. They also tried adding lamotrigine as a supplement to valproic acid, and the patients' seizures did not improve; however, when topiramate was added, the seizures improved significantly, suggesting that topiramate plus valproic acid is also a beneficial option.
3. *Valproic acid combined with phenobarbital*: In more than 30% of patients, seizures are drug-resistant and special methods are required to treat them. Ito et al. [460] described a 10-year-old boy who began to have drug-resistant

myoclonic absence seizures and occasional generalized tonic–clonic seizures at the age of 7. He was successively treated with sodium valproate, levetiracetam, ethosuximide, clobazam, zonisamide, topiramate, clonazepam, and lamotrigine but had no significant effect. Phenobarbital was added to valproic acid and clobazam at 8 years of age, after which the concentration gradually increased to 1.2 mg/kg/day (blood concentration 8.6 μg/mL). Within 1 month, the seizures stopped completely, 2 years of follow-up were seizure-free, and his EEG was normal, suggesting that small doses of phenobarbital may be of secondary benefit.

4. *Rufinamide combined with levetiracetam*: Häusler et al. [461] described three patients with drug-resistant EMA, two of whom were treated with levetiracetam combined with rufinamide, during which the seizures stopped. The authors speculate that the combination of rufinamide and levetiracetam is useful for treating drug-resistant EMA.

Surgical Treatment

Emma G Carter et al. [458] reported that two patients who failed to respond to drug therapy underwent callosotomy. The results showed that one patient was seizure-free for 8 months after surgery and that the other had a more than 50% reduction in the number of seizures within 5 months, indicating that surgical treatment is also a beneficial option for drug-resistant EMA.

Prognosis

The overall picture of tEMA is not pessimistic. Zanzmera et al. [453] followed the 12 patients he described for an average of 23.9 months and reported that 9 of them experienced seizure remission, 4 experienced no seizures for at least 1 year, 2 experienced more than 90% seizure reduction, and 3 experienced more than a 50% reduction in seizure frequency.

The progression of EMA is variable. Responses occur in approximately 40% of patients. In the remaining patients, myoclonic symptoms persist or epilepsy may develop with the progression of other generalized seizure types. If myoclonic absence seizures are the only seizure type and are controlled medically, the prognosis improves.

5.3.4 Developmental and Epileptic Encephalopathy

Overview

Developmental and epileptic encephalopathy (DEE) was first described by ILAE in 2017, and it is distinguished from developmental encephalopathy (DE) and epileptic encephalopathy (EE). Developmental encephalopathy primarily implicates growth and development without frequent epileptic activity, while EE is characterized by frequent seizure-like discharges, leading to severe developmental, cognitive, and behavioral abnormalities. Children usually exhibit normal development at

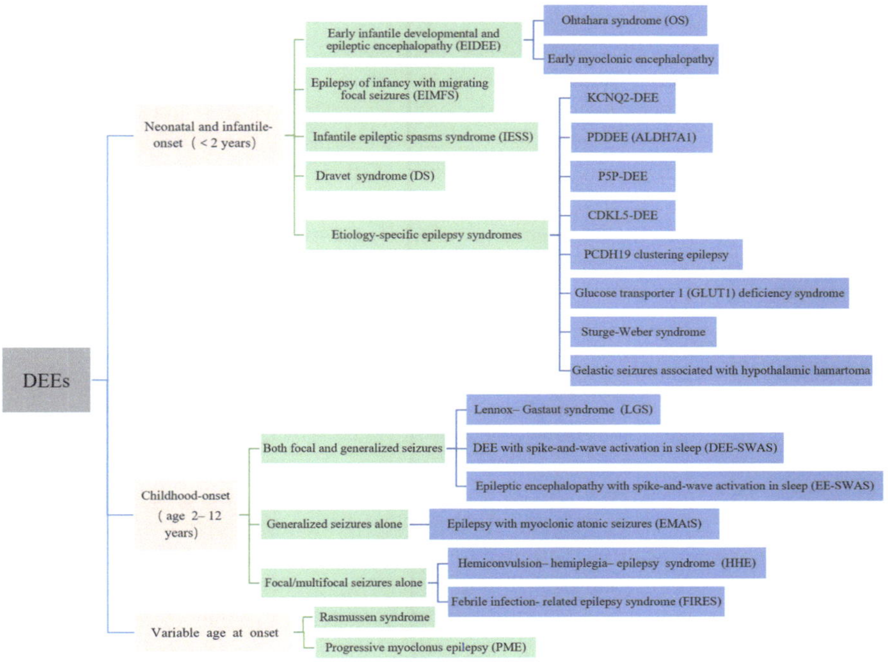

Fig. 5.1 Classification of DEEs. DEE developmental and epileptic encephalopathy, PDDEE (ALDH7A1) pyridoxine-dependent developmental and epileptic encephalopathy (ALDH7A1 pathogenic variant), P5P-DEE pyridoxamine 5′-phosphate oxidase deficiency-developmental and epileptic encephalopathy, CDKL5-DEE cyclin-dependent kinase-like 5-related DEE

the time of seizures and later develop developmental delay. In DEE patients, developmental delays occur prior to the onset of seizures, with the exacerbation of brain dysfunction due to etiology and frequent seizure-like discharges. Even if seizure control is achieved, the neurological manifestations of the brain disorder cannot be fully restored, and they may worsen with age. DEE can affect patients at any age, and developmental and epileptic factors interact synergistically [301]. Potential underlying pathologies include epigenetic and genetic factors, which may contribute to the developmental disturbances observed in DEEs [462–464].

Classification

DEEs are primarily classified based on age of onset and can generally be divided into three categories: neonatal and infantile-onset DEEs (onset before 2 years of age), childhood-onset DEEs (onset between 2 and 12 years of age), and DEEs with onset at various age stages (Fig. 5.1).

Neonatal and infantile-onset (before 2 years of age) DEEs include early infantile developmental and epileptic encephalopathy (EIDEE), epilepsy of infancy with migrating focal seizures (EIMFS), infantile epileptic spasms syndrome (IESS), Dravet syndrome (DS), and epilepsy syndromes with specific etiologies. EIDEE encompasses previously classified Ohtahara syndrome and early myoclonic encephalopathy of infancy. The electroclinical features of these two syndromes overlap, and they share similar underlying causes. Therefore, categorizing EIDEE into Ohtahara encephalopathy and early myoclonic encephalopathy does not provide additional valuable information for clinical decisions or prognostic assessments. Etiology-specific epilepsy syndromes are caused by specific genetic, structural, metabolic, immunological, or infectious factors and are associated with consistent clinical electrophysiological characteristics, treatment approaches, and prognoses. Most etiology-specific syndromes with neonatal or infantile onset are considered DEEs [301].

Genetic Etiology

In 1995, the first gene associated with epilepsy, *CHRNA4*, was discovered, marking the advent of the era of channelopathy-related epilepsy genes. Numerous genes related to benign familial epilepsy, such as *SCN1A*, *SCN1B*, *KCNQ2*, *KCNQ3*, and *GABRG2*, were subsequently found. The genes associated with DEEs are primarily aristaless-related homeobox (ARX) genes. While the discovery of epilepsy genes slowed at the turn of the century, candidate gene studies and research on rare recombination abnormalities have continued to unveil some common epilepsy genes, such as *CDKL5*, whose function is related to Rett syndrome. The emergence of whole genome and next-generation sequencing (NGS) technologies has facilitated simultaneous testing of numerous samples, resulting in the discovery of a multitude of new genes and variants, such as the *STXBP1* gene, which was identified through whole genome duplication and deletion analysis in patients with severe epilepsy. Subsequently, the discovery of epilepsy genes benefitted from a new era of large-scale parallel sequencing. The discovery of epilepsy genes has now progressed into the postgenomic era, comprising the ongoing discovery of new genes and increased understanding of phenotype characterization.

Genetic panels are the most cost-effective method for detecting DEE, with diagnostic rates ranging from 15% to 48% (possibly as low as 0.8%), but they may miss detection of unknown pathogenic genes. Whole exome sequencing (WES) has a diagnostic rate of 25–44%, covering the entire coding sequence. Trio exome sequencing can identify novel de novo mutations, allowing for reanalysis and potential detection of copy number variations (CNVs). Multiple variants of uncertain significance (VUSs) must be interpreted, and carriers or nonparental relationships can be identified. However, deep intronic mutations, structural rearrangements, or large deletions/duplications cannot be detected [463]. WES is recommended as a first-line test for patients with developmental delay and intellectual disability. However, genetic testing has limitations, as genetic etiology does not explain all cases. Furthermore, functional studies are needed to verify the gene–phenotype correlations of many newly discovered gene mutations to guide clinical management strategies [464].

DEE has a complex etiology, and more than 400 genes are associated with it. Among patients with infantile-onset DEE, more than 50% have genetic causes, often involving single-gene disorders (30–40%) [465, 466]. These gene mutations affect ion channel function, synaptic function, transport protein function, transcription process dysregulation, DNA repair process impairment, chromosomal reshaping, energy metabolism, mitochondrial dysfunction, and impaired neuronal differentiation and migration [467]. Ion channel-related genes account for approximately 25% of DEE-related genes, with sodium, potassium, and calcium ion channel genes being the most common [468]. Sodium channel genes include *SCN1A*, *SCN2A*, *SCN3A*, *SCN8A*, and *SCN1B*, and mutations in the *SCN1A* and *SCN1B* genes can cause Dravet syndrome [469]. Potassium channel-related genes such as *KCNA*, *KCNB*, *KCNQ*, and *KCNT* are commonly associated with DEE. The *CACNA1H* gene encodes the T-type calcium ion channel Cav3.2 and is closely related to DEE, and pathogenic mutations enhance calcium channel function, leading to seizures and functional impairments. Dysfunctional genes encoding SNAP and SNARE proteins can lead to disease through vesicular transport abnormalities, synaptic vesicle deformities, and interrupted neurotransmitter transmission, such as *STXBP1*-associated epileptic encephalopathy [470]. Some early-onset DEEs result from functional abnormalities in enzymes, such as *ALDH7A1*-related epilepsy. De novo mutations in *CACNA1E* have been identified in individuals with DEE [471, 472]. There is a correlation between DEE and neurodevelopmental disorders, exemplified by *NBEA*, *FBXO11*, and *SMARCC2* [473–475], especially *NBEA*, a candidate gene for neurodevelopmental disorders and autism [476]. The results of a large-scale diagnostic study involving more than 25,000 individuals indicate that 50 genetic genes, including *SCN1A*, *KCNQ2*, *SCN2A*, and *PRRT2*, are associated with epilepsy [477].

Autosomal recessive inheritance, X-linked inheritance, and mosaic variations can also contribute to disease [118, 467]. Autosomal recessive epilepsy is associated with congenital metabolic disorders and cortical malformations [478]. Genes involved in the biosynthesis and reshaping of glycosylphosphatidylinositol-anchored proteins (GPI-APs), such as PIGB, can lead to autosomal recessive epilepsy [479]. Autosomal recessive early infantile epileptic encephalopathy (EIEE) accounts for 50% of the cases in a cohort of 72 EIEE patients from Saudi Arabia with a consanguineous family history [310]. CNVs, including DEE, cause 5–10% of childhood epilepsies [480–482]. Therefore, when clinical manifestations include dysmorphisms, intellectual disabilities, and other neurological and psychiatric manifestations, chromosomal microarray analysis (CMA) is recommended as a first-line genetic test [483]. Exome or whole genome sequencing methods can currently be used to detect single nucleotide variations and CNVs [484]. DNA methylation and histone modifications may be involved in the occurrence of DEE [485–487]. Research has identified differentially methylated regions in two individuals with epilepsy and unexplained intellectual disabilities [488].

With an increasing number of epilepsy patients undergoing genetic testing, many new epilepsy genes and novel phenotypes, mechanisms, and variants associated with known epilepsy genes have been discovered. To date, the number of genes associated with developmental and epileptic encephalopathies (DEEs) in children exceeds 40%. International collaborations have facilitated the discovery of more relatively common genes that cause DEEs, such as *SCN3A*.

The second category with an increasing number of epilepsy-related genes is primarily associated with synaptic abnormalities, such as *AP2M1*, *SNAP25*, and *UNC13B*. Recently, novel variants in *SCN1A* have been shown to lead to a severe early-onset phenotype that is distinct from Dravet syndrome. This phenotype is characterized by seizures occurring significantly earlier than the typical 5–6 months of age and results in unique developmental features. The application of traditional and innovative methods, such as international data sharing (Epi4K and Epi25 collaborations), large-scale sequencing (Deciphering Developmental Disorders (DDD) project), and computational analysis driven by Human Phenotype Ontology (HPO), has also facilitated the discovery of new epilepsy genes. For instance, the Epi25 collaboration project aims to sequence the exomes or genomes of 25,000 epilepsy patients, making it the largest project dedicated to epilepsy gene discovery to date and providing unprecedented opportunities for global clinical trials. In addition to genotyping, new methods such as phenotype similarity analysis have also contributed to the discovery of new genes. In terms of genetic mechanisms, novel disease mechanisms, including pathogenic intronic variants and repeat expansions, as well as innovative integration of genetic data with polygenic risk scoring, have been instrumental in advancing the field.

In addition to the discovery of new genes and phenotypes, novel methods for providing and interpreting data crucial for accessing variant databases, aggregating, functional testing, and interpreting data have grown exponentially in recent years. Accessible open resources combine genetic, phenotypic, and functional data to aid variant interpretation. For example, large-scale collaborations within the National Institutes of Health (NIH)-funded consortia, such as the Center Without Walls (CWOW), have led to the extensive characterization of variations in numerous epilepsy genes. Additional testing of variants of uncertain significance, such as parental testing of candidate variants and reanalysis of exome or genome sequencing, has also contributed to the determination of disease causation.

Other Factors

Other etiologies associated with DEEs include structural causes (such as tuberous sclerosis complex (TSC), hypothalamic hamartoma, and hemimegalencephaly), metabolic disorders (such as pyridoxine or biotinidase deficiency and Glut1 deficiency), and immune-related diseases (such as Rasmussen syndrome) [489–491].

Pathophysiological Mechanisms

DEE has various genetic causes and molecular pathways, including ion channels and proteins necessary for synaptic, regulatory, and developmental functions [491, 492]. At this time, disease occurrence and progression can be predicted based on certain known mutations, such as in *SCN8A* encephalopathy or *CDKL5*-DEE. Although genetic testing can predict the prognosis of DEE, it is not the sole factor influencing the clinical course [493].

Pathological processes leading to comprehensive cognitive impairment may originate from hyperexcitable epileptic cortices and include (1) focal abnormalities, such as focal cortical dysplasia; (2) generalized abnormalities, such as genetic etiologies; and (3) functional changes in subcortical regions that regulate cortical input/output, such as the thalamus and brainstem [494]. Despite the diverse etiologies of DEE, its generation is associated with network involvement [495]. Various functional and structural neuroimaging studies have attempted to elucidate brain characteristics and cortico-subcortical networks in DEE patients at the network level. In patients with Lennox–Gastaut syndrome (LGS) or West syndrome (WS), the (prefrontal) cortex–thalamus–brainstem loop is activated during epileptic discharges [496–501]. Temporoparietal networks, including continuous spikes and waves during slow-wave sleep (CSWS), are affected in patients with idiopathic focal epilepsy [497, 501–503]. The temporoparietal network plays a critical role in specific cognitive functions and is closely connected to thalamic structures [503]. Neuroimaging studies indicate that epilepsy waves interfere with the activity of the default mode network (DMN), which contributes to creating a favorable neural metabolic environment and improving cognitive function [504]. The DMN is associated with epilepsy activity in LGS, CSWS, and self-limited focal epilepsy patients [497–499]. Hence, cognitive impairments in DEEs might be due to pathological processes (the process causing epilepsy waves), disrupting the resting-state activity of the DMN. However, these studies only partially explain this phenomenon, as the activity of the DMN is also affected in patients without cognitive impairments, such as those with genetic generalized epilepsy [492]. Despite evident developmental abnormalities and cognitive deficits, the DMN is not involved in Dravet syndrome or West syndrome [496, 501]. Furthermore, other networks in DEEs are disrupted, affecting cognition [504–506]. Normal cognition requires the stable synaptic plasticity of nonrapid eye movement (NREM) sleep, which is disrupted by frequent epileptic discharges during sleep [507–509]. Sleep-related cognitive impairments may be associated with epileptic networks involving the thalamocortical and hippocampal cortical memory encoding systems [510]. High-frequency spike-and-wave discharges observed during NREM sleep in patients with CSWS interfere with the plasticity function of sleep, particularly the homeostatic slow-wave process [509, 511].

The pathophysiology of DEEs in adulthood is complex and involves the interaction of multiple factors, including neurodegenerative changes caused by genetic variations, chronic recurrent seizures, and the impact of antiseizure medications on brain neuropathology [512].

Epidemiology and Natural History

The overall incidence of DEE is estimated to be approximately 0.27–0.54 per 1000 newborns, with a mortality rate of 17–50%. Even among survivors, the vast majority of affected children have severe neurological sequelae [462]. DEE patients can have comorbidities, including movement disorders, cerebral palsy, behavioral disorders, autism spectrum disorders, psychiatric disorders, sleep disorders, gait disturbances, speech impairments, respiratory issues, and gastrointestinal diseases [513–515]. For newborn-onset DEE, the mortality rate can exceed 50% by the age of 2 [118, 516]. A Danish study revealed that more than 40% of caregivers in DEE families suffer from depression, anxiety, or posttraumatic stress disorder [517]. Most patients require daily care and lifelong support [118, 518].

Different gene mutations exhibit phenotypic heterogeneity. For instance, mutations in *KCNQ2* and *SCN2A* can lead to benign familial neonatal epilepsy (BFNE), early infantile epileptic encephalopathy (EIEE), late-onset epilepsy, developmental delay/intellectual disabilities, movement disorders, autism, and brain malformations [40]. Different developmental functions may vary during different windows of brain maturation. For instance, children with Dravet syndrome initially exhibit normal development in the first few years but gradually experience cognitive impairment or regression. Newborn-onset DEE is often caused by mutations in *SCN2A*, *KCNQ2*, and *STXBP1*. Seizure activity may improve during infancy, but severe developmental impacts persist [155, 464, 519].

Some DEE patients survive into adulthood and exhibit clinical feature characteristics different from those in childhood. Stamberger et al. [520] followed the natural history of 30 STXBP1-DEE patients from early infancy to adulthood. The median age of survival was 24 years (range: 18–58 years), and some patients survived up to 60 years. All patients had a history of seizures, but 38% of them had a prolonged period (up to 16 years) without seizures during childhood or adolescence, followed by seizure recurrence. Similar patterns have been observed in adult patients with *KCNQ2*-DEE or *SCN1A*-DEE [521, 522]. Eighty-seven percent of adult *STXBP1*-DEE individuals and some *SCN1A*-DEE adults experience tremors, gait disturbances, and motor delays [520, 522]. All adult *STXBP1*-DEE individuals exhibit intellectual disability, with 27% experiencing loss of previously acquired skills [520]. There is no correlation between seizures and cognition, similar to findings in patients with *CDKL5*-DEE, *SCN2A*/*SCN8A*-DEE, or TSC [464].

DEE is more common than several other severe inherited childhood diseases [55, 516], such as cystic fibrosis (1:3650) and spinal muscular atrophy (SMA) (1:7000) [523, 524]. However, DEE exhibits significant genetic heterogeneity [154]. Each individual genetic cause of DEE is rare and fits the criteria for "orphan" diseases [525, 526]. For example, the incidence of *SCN1A*-related epilepsy is 1/12,200, and the most common phenotype, Dravet syndrome (*SCN1A*-DEE), has an incidence of 1/15,500. The incidence of *KCNQ2*-related epilepsy is 1/17,000, and that of *SLC2A1*-related epilepsy is 1/24,300 [55]. Orphan disease drug research requires special development pathways and incentives, such as orphan product funding programs in the United States, Europe, Japan, Canada, and Australia [527]. High-quality global natural history studies (NHSs) are recognized as crucial for the development of new therapies for rare diseases and subsequent regulatory approval [523, 524, 528, 529].

Based on the underlying pathophysiology, each genetic DEE typically has a specific genotype–phenotype spectrum. The development of novel targeted therapies for specific genetic DEE phenotypes is essential for improving patient prognosis. Clinical trials rely on a deep understanding of phenotype–genotype correlations and disease progression over time to select appropriate patients for testing. Understanding the natural history of the disease helps in assessing its clinical relevance and identifying biomarkers.

Diagnostic Strategy

Medical history should include risk factors and seizure history. Electroencephalography (EEG) helps in determining electroclinical syndromes and distinguishing DEEs. Different epilepsy syndromes have relatively specific patterns of discharge, such as burst suppression EEG patterns in Ohtahara syndrome patients, highly disorganized EEG patterns in West syndrome patients, slow spike–wave complexes in LGS patients, and nonconvulsive status epilepticus patterns in patients with myoclonic-metastatic epilepsy [477]. For patients with tuberous sclerosis complex (TSC), long-term EEG monitoring is recommended to detect subtle or subclinical seizures. Neuroimaging, especially brain MRI, can reveal the presence of structural abnormalities such as cortical dysplasia or hypoxic injury. Other investigations include metabolic and immunological evaluations. Metabolic disorders such as biotinidase and vitamin B6 deficiency can be diagnosed through early detection and treatment, leading to improved outcomes [530]. Comprehensive genetic testing is recommended for patients with clinical features of DEE [531–533].

Treatment

Pharmacological Treatment

Most patients with DEEs are resistant to antiseizure medications (ASMs); therefore, combination therapy with two or more ASM agents is recommended. A comprehensive evaluation should be conducted, taking into account the etiology, prognosis, efficacy of various treatment options, treatment risks, costs, and treatment preferences of the family to weigh the pros and cons and assess the risk–benefit ratio to determine the ideal treatment approach. However, despite the development of any new treatments, ASMs remain the first-line treatment for epileptic encephalopathies. In clinical practice, in addition to considering surgical evaluation or other potentially effective nonpharmacological treatment options, it is still important to continue the use of different ASMs, especially newer ones. Many currently available ASMs are administered with the aim to restore the excitatory/inhibitory balance in the brain through the use of drugs that modulate voltage-gated ion channels, synaptic neurotransmission, and excitatory glutamatergic pathways, to enhance GABA-mediated inhibition, and to mediate multiple mechanisms [534].

Precision Treatment

Epilepsy is a highly heterogeneous disease in terms of clinical presentation and etiology. Rapid progress in genetic research has significantly changed diagnostic and treatment strategies for epilepsy, forming the cornerstone of precision medicine for epilepsy treatment. Precision treatment includes substitution therapy, modulation of signaling pathways, and potential treatments based on ion channel/receptor-mediated mechanisms (Table 5.2) [535]. For example, clinical trials of drugs for the treatment of Dravet syndrome have shown that oxcarbazepine is an effective drug for treating *SCN2A* gain-of-function variants, while sodium channel blockers are more suitable for treating *KCNQ2* loss-of-function variants. Furthermore, genetic diagnosis has prompted the repurposing of drugs not traditionally used for antiepileptic purposes. For example, in 2020, fenfluramine was approved by the FDA and the European Medicines Agency for the treatment of Dravet syndrome. Precision treatment drugs newly discovered for DEE include everolimus, sirolimus, and NBI 921352. New antiseizure medicines include stiripentol, cannabidiol, soticlestat, ganaxolone, and radiprodil. Newly repurposed drugs include anabasine, quinidine, ezogabine/retigabine, XEN101, memantine, and high-dose phenytoin. Repurposed antiseizure drugs include fenfluramine, flunarizine, and clorazepate. A systematic approach to drug identification may accelerate the development of precision therapy. Numerous reports on targeted treatments for individual variants have already

Table 5.2 Targets for the precise treatment of epilepsy [535–541]

Treatment pathway	Gene	Related diseases	Therapy
Supplementation or restriction of substrates	*SLC2A1*	Glut1 deficiency syndrome	Ketogenic diet
	SLC6A8	Cerebral creatine deficiency syndrome 1	Creatine combined with L-arginine and L-glycine
	GAMT	Cerebral creatine deficiency syndrome 2	Creatine
	AGAT	Creatine deficiency syndrome 3	Creatine
	SLC35A2	Glycosylation disorder	Galactose
	ALDH7A1	Pyridoxine-dependent epilepsy (PDE)	Pyridoxine
	PNPO	Pyridoxamine 5′-phosphate oxidase deficiency	Pyridoxal 5′-phosphate(P5P)
	PIG-Q, A, N, P, S	Ohtahara syndrome, early myoclonic encephalopathy, Infantile spasms syndrome (including WEST syndrome), EIMFS	Pyridoxine or P5P
	FOLR	Folinic acid-responsive seizures	Folinic acid
	MOCS	Molybdenum cofactor deficiency	c-PMP
	TPP1	Neuronal ceroid lipofuscinosis type 2	Cerliponase alfa
	TRPM6	Hypomagnesemia 1	Magnesium sulfate
Modifications of signaling pathways	*DEPDC5* *NPRL2, NPRL3* *TSC1, TSC2*	FFEVF, FTLE, West syndrome FFEVF Tuberous sclerosis complex	Rapamycin and rapamycin derivatives

(continued)

Table 5.2 (continued)

Treatment pathway	Gene	Related diseases	Therapy
Changing channel functions	*Sodium channels*		
	SCN1A	Dravet syndrome, GEFS+, EIMFS	Avoid sodium channel blockers
		DEE6	Sodium channel blockers
	SCN2A	BFNIE, GEFS+, infantile spasms syndrome (including WEST syndrome) EIMFS, Ohtahara syndrome, DEE11, onset within 3 months	Gain of function: Na channel blockers
		Seizures associated with autism spectrum disorder; onset after 3 months	Loss of function: Avoid sodium channel blockers
	SCN8A	DEE13, familial myoclonic epilepsy	Loss of function: Avoid sodium channel blockers
		BFNIE, EIMFS	Gain of function: Sodium channel blockers
	Potassium channels		
	KCNT1, *KCNT2*	ADSHE, EIMFS, DEE14	Quinidine
	KCNQ2, *KCNQ3*	BFNE, Ohtahara syndrome, neonatal epileptic encephalopathy, EIMFS, DEE7, EOEE	Sodium channel blockers, retigabine, VPA
	KCNA1	Episodic ataxia type 1	CBZ, phenytoin, sulthiame
		EE	Sodium channel blockers
	KCNB1	DEE26	Ketogenic diet
	KCNA2	DEE32, ESES	Aminopyridine; sodium channel blockers
	KCNJ10	SeSAME syndrome	CBZ, VPA, LTG, TPM
	Calcium channels		
	CACNA1A	West syndrome, DEE, idiopathic generalized epilepsy	ETX/LTG
	NMDA receptor		
	GRIN2A	Atypical SELECTS, CSWS, infantile spasms syndrome (including WEST syndrome), DEE, Landau–Kleffner syndrome	Memantine
	GRIN2B	Infantile spasms syndrome (including WEST syndrome), DEE, LGS	Memantine
	GRIN2D	DEE	Ketamine, memantine
	nAcH-R		
	CHRNA2, *CHRNA4*, *CHRNAB2*	Nocturnal frontal lobe epilepsy (NFLE)	Nicotine
	cAMP		
	HCN1	GEFS+; DEE	LTG/gabapentin, ketamine/propofol

(continued)

Table 5.2 (continued)

Treatment pathway	Gene	Related diseases	Therapy
Other potential therapies	*SCN1A*		STP (+VPA+CLB)/CBD/FFA
	PCDH19	Infantile spasms syndrome (including WEST syndrome), DEE, Dravet syndrome	LEV/CLB
	CDKL5	Epileptic spasms syndrome, DEE 2	Ganaxolone
	STXBP1	Ohtahara syndrome，epileptic spasms syndrome, NSID，DEE4	LEV
	SLC6A1	Epilepsy with myoclonic atonic seizure (EMAS)	VPA+LTG
	PRRT2	BFIE, ICCA, PKD	Sodium blockers，CBZ

STP stiripentol, *CBD* cannabidiol, *FFA* fenfluramine, *LEV* levetiracetam, *CLB* clobazam, *VPA* valproic acid, *CBZ* carbamazepine, *TPM* topiramate, *ETX* ethosuximide, *LTG* lamotrigine, *ESES* electrical status epilepticus during sleep, *BFNE* benign familial neonatal epilepsy, *BFNIE* benign familial neonatal–infantile epilepsy, *EIMFS* early infantile migrating focal seizures, *ADSHE* autosomal dominant sleep-related hypermotor epilepsy, *BFIE* benign familial infantile epilepsy, *EOEE* early-onset epileptic encephalopathy, *SeSAME* seizure, sensorineural deafness, ataxia, mental retardation, and electrolyte imbalance, *ICCA* infantile convulsions with paroxysmal choreoathetosis, *PKD* paroxysmal kinesigenic dyskinesia, *GEFS+* genetic epilepsy with febrile seizures plus, *NSID* non-syndromic intellectual disability, *FFEVF* familial focal epilepsy with variable foci, *FTLE* familial mesial temporal lobe epilepsy, *CSWS* continuous spikes and waves during slow-wave sleep, *SeLECTS* self-limited epilepsy with centrotemporal spikes

been published. Over the past 25 years, more than 15 new compounds have been used in the treatment of epilepsy, but the prevalence of refractory epilepsy has not fundamentally changed. The control of seizures toward targeted epileptic etiology will inevitably lead to transformation. Currently, there are multiple compounds in the clinical development stage [542], including (1) those with novel mechanisms similar to those of marketed ASMs, such as ganaxolone (a GABA receptor modulator), allopregnanolone (a $GABA_A$ receptor modulator (SAGE-547), selurampanel (BGG492) (an alpha-amino-3-hydroxy-5-methyl-4-isoxazolepropionic acid (AMPA) and kainate receptor competitive antagonist), ICA-105665 (a selective opener of neuronal Kv7 potassium channels), and YKP3089 (cenobamate) (a selective blocker of sodium channels in the inactivated state that enhances presynaptic GABA release); (2) those with novel mechanisms: beprodone (a melatonin receptor 3 agonist) and huperzine A (an acetylcholinesterase (AChE) receptor inhibitor); (3) repurposed drugs originally used for other diseases, such as everolimus (a selective inhibitor of the TOR pathway), fenfluramine (a serotonin reuptake inhibitor), naluzotan (nonazapirone, a partial agonist of 5-HT1_A), pitolisant (a histamine H3 receptor antagonist), quinidine (a partial antagonist of KCNT1), valnoctamide (a $GABA_A$ receptor agonist), and verapamil (a P-glycoprotein inhibitor); and (4) those with unknown mechanisms: JNJ-26489112 (multiple mechanisms, unknown).

In addition to conventional drug treatments, gene therapy is gradually becoming more commonly used. For instance, adeno-associated virus vectors and gene editing through antisense oligonucleotides (ASOs) have been applied for precision treatment in conditions such as spinal muscular atrophy (SMA), Duchenne muscular dystrophy, and familial amyloid polyneuropathy. ASOs are synthetic single-stranded oligonucleotides with lengths ranging from 8 to 50 nucleotides that can bind to messenger RNA (mRNA) through various mechanisms to modify protein expression. Well-designed ASOs can induce targeted degradation, translational arrest, inhibition of RNA-binding proteins, splicing modulation, and protein expression upregulation/downregulation [465]. Preclinical and clinical studies related to ASOs have been conducted in the field of epilepsy treatment. Due to the limited penetration and stability of drugs in the central nervous system and the lack of suitable delivery vehicles, many gene therapy approaches require intrathecal administration, which presents a challenge for developing safe gene therapy approaches.

To date, high- or medium-throughput preclinical models have been developed to facilitate the rapid transition from biological mechanisms to precision treatment. These models include heterologously expressed proteins or genetic materials that promote protein function, patient-derived induced pluripotent stem cells (iPSCs), zebrafish models, and others. Throughout the development of epilepsy genetics and treatment, efforts have been made to explore the genetic mechanisms involved in epilepsy, leading to the discovery of a series of precise new targets and clinical trials. In the future, from the initiation of genetic discoveries to the implementation of innovative therapies, the coordinated and systematic approach of precision epilepsy medicine, combined with the collaborative efforts of multidisciplinary teams and international coordination, could lead epilepsy treatment into a new era.

5.3.5 Epilepsy with Myoclonic–Atonic Seizures (EMASs)

Overview

Epilepsy with myoclonic–atonic seizures (EMAS) is also known as Doose syndrome. It was first described in 1970 by Hermann Doose in Germany, who described this type of seizure as not fully defined and called it a separate epilepsy syndrome [543]. In 2017, the International League Against Epilepsy classified this disease as a childhood-onset epilepsy syndrome. This is also called myoclonic–atonic seizures. Epidemiological surveys show that its prevalence is approximately 1/10000, accounting for approximately 1–2% of childhood-origin epilepsy cases, and the onset of this disease usually occurs between 2 and 6 years of age. Ninety-four percent of the patients presented within the first 5 years of life. It is more common in boys than in girls, but the incidence in males and females is equal during the first year of life. In contrast to general DEE, although its seizure frequency is high and its seizure forms are diverse, its overall prognosis is better than that of other developmental and epileptic encephalopathies and it responds well to antiseizure medications and ketogenic diet treatment.

Historical Evolution

In 1945, TOLONE S [131] noted this type of seizure in the study of myoclonic epilepsy. In 1970, Doose et al. [543] described the characteristics of this epilepsy syndrome in detail through the clinical manifestations of 51 patients. General development is normal, multiple types of seizures are common after 2 years of age, especially clonic seizures, and cognitive impairment may occur in the later stages of the disease. In 1975, Degen et al. [544] described the efficacy of nitrazepam in the treatment of children with myoclonic–atonic seizures. They found that nitrazepam was more effective in treating this type of seizure than other types of myoclonic seizures and that the EEG changes were consistent with the treatment response of the children to the drug. In the same year, Skarpa and Erak [545] described the electrophysiological characteristics of Doose syndrome. In 1989, the International League Against Epilepsy classified it as symptomatic epilepsy in the classification of epilepsy syndromes and the associated seizures were classified as generalized seizures. Diagnostic criteria were proposed. Recently, Caraballo et al. [546] have described the efficacy of cannabidiol in the treatment of Doose syndrome and reported that it reduced seizures by more than 50% in 57.7% of patients. In 2010, Kelley and Kossoff [547] summarized the research progress on Doose syndrome in the past 40 years and proposed that corticosteroids, sodium valproate, levetiracetam, and zonisamide may be effective in its treatment of, but the most effective treatment seems to be a ketogenic diet. Nickels et al. [548] proposed a diagnostic method for Doose syndrome through a survey of 76 participants. Electroencephalography and MRI (essential), amino acid, organic acid, fatty acid/acylcarnitine profile, microarray, genomic, lactate/pyruvate, cerebrospinal fluid, and serum glucose/lactate (strong) tests are encouraged to help confirm the diagnosis.

Causes of Myoclonic–Atonic Epilepsy

Genetic Factors

Genetic factors play an important role in the etiology of Doose syndrome. A high percentage of patients have immediate family members and even distant relatives who experience similar seizures and EEG abnormalities. The most common EEG manifestations in such a family are light sensitivity and abnormal theta background rhythm. The pattern of inheritance is complex polygenic, so there can be many different phenotypes in the same family. Tang et al. [447] studied the genetic factors of 101 patients and reported that 14% of them had gene mutations, including 3 with *SYNGAP1* gene abnormalities, 2 with *KIAA2022* gene abnormalities, and 2 with *SLC6A1* gene abnormalities. One patient each had *KCNA2*, *SCN2A*, *STX1B*, *KCNB1*, and *MECP2* gene abnormalities. In addition to these existing reports, the authors also found that the *ASH1L* and *CHD4* genes may have a pathogenic role. Hinokuma et al. [549] collected blood samples from 29 patients with Doose syndrome for whole exome sequencing and found 4 new variants: missense variants of *SLC6A1* and *HNRNPU* as well as a microdeletion of 2q24.2 involving *SCN1A* and a microdeletion of Xp22.31 involving *STS*. The authors suggest that these gene mutations may underlie the genetic susceptibility of the patient and that *HNRNPU* and *STS* may be candidate pathogenic genes for this disease.

Structural Damage

Structural brain damage is another common cause of Doose syndrome. Denervaud et al. [550] conducted neuroimaging studies on 14 patients and found obvious structural differences between the brain structures of the patients and those of the healthy control group. Some patients with trigeminal hemangioma were also reported to have Doose syndrome [547].

Clinical Manifestations of Myoclonic–Atonic Seizures

Belcastro et al. [551] studied 18 patients with Doose syndrome and reported that in addition to myoclonic–atonic seizures, they also had myoclonic seizures, absence, and nonconvulsive status epilepticus, 7 patients had epileptic encephalopathy, and some patients had generalized tonic–clonic seizures [75].

Multiple Seizure Forms

1. *Myoclonic–atonic seizures*: These are the only seizure form necessary for the diagnosis of this syndrome. They often occur in the first year after onset and are characterized by transient myoclonus in the proximal muscles (in the trunk or axial direction). These seizures are often accompanied by mild vocalis and followed by transient atonic seizures, which may include a slight nod or sudden fall, but most patients recover quickly. A mild startle may be perceived only subjectively by the child or may be sustained only as a slight sound.
2. *Generalized tonic–clonic seizures*: These seizures are most commonly observed in patients with other seizure forms of Doose syndrome. Nickels et al. [548] conducted a long-term follow-up study of 166 patients with Doose syndrome and reported that 60% of them had generalized tonic–clonic seizures, which were similar to tonic–clonic seizures in generalized clonic seizures or generalized clonic seizures similar to large myoclonic seizures.
3. *Seizures of absence*: These are seen in 50–80% of patients, accompanied by full-lead asymmetric spike-and-wave complexes (SWCs) at 2–3 Hz.
4. *Seizures of tonicity*: Although used as an exclusion criterion, a small number of patients develop tonic episodes later in the course of the disease, suggesting a poor long-term prognosis.
5. *Nonconvulsive status epilepticus*: This disease is common and may occur in almost all types of patients.

Cognitive Impairment

The overall prognosis of patients with Doose syndrome is good, and seizures eventually stop for most of them, but they may still experience cognitive dysfunction. Nickels et al. [548] studied 166 children with Doose syndrome and reported that 2% of them had developmental delay at disease onset and 49% had overall developmental delay during the course of the disease.

Epileptic Encephalopathy

The course of EMAS often has clinical manifestations similar to those of acute epileptic encephalopathy, with sudden clinical and EEG deterioration. In addition to the increase in the number of seizures, patients have decreased cognition, vigilance, and social activities; lethargy; decreased oral motor function; increased drooling; dysarthria; ataxia; and so on. Most patients eventually develop nonconvulsive status epilepticus. It usually occurs 2–60 months after the onset of seizures. A quarter of EMAS patients have hyperactivity and behavioral problems, and half have developmental delay.

Electroencephalogram

Nickels et al. [548] reported that 28% of patients had a normal EEG, 20% had a slowed background, and 69% had epileptiform discharges or seizures at the onset of epilepsy. Subsequent EEG revealed slowing in 62% and epileptiform discharges or seizures in 90% of patients.

Background activity was usually normal at onset, and an age-appropriate posterior head dominant rhythm was observed. EMAS is characterized by a single θ rhythm (4–6 Hz) in the bilateral parietal region. With increasing seizure frequency, there may be generalized, higher-amplitude background slowing, spikes and waves, and spikes and slow waves, which mainly manifest as generalized sharp waves (3–6 Hz), and absence of electromyographic activity in the deltoid, neck, and sternocleidomastoid muscles as revealed by an electromyography test. EEG abnormalities disappear within 4 years of onset in all patients. EMAS should be excluded if patients have persistent focal discharge and high arrhythmia on EEG, LGS should be excluded if patients have generalized paroxysmal fast activity and generalized slow spikes and waves <2.5 Hz during sleep, and CLN2 disease should be excluded if patients have a low-frequency photoparoxysmal response.

Diagnosis of Myoclonic–Atonic Seizures

Each epilepsy syndrome has its own unique etiology, pathogenesis, clinical manifestations, and treatment methods. According to the 2022 ILAE diagnostic criteria for myoclonic–atonic epilepsy syndrome, (1) seizures are preceded by normal development and cognition; (2) seizures occur from 6 months to 6 years of age (peak: 2–4 years); (3) myoclonic–atonic seizures are the core manifestations; (4) generalized spike firing at 2–3 Hz is present, but there is no sustained focal spike firing; and (5) other myoclonic epilepsy syndromes are excluded [552]. Thus, generalized myoclonic–atonic seizures, EEG signals with generalized 3–6-Hz sharp waves or spikes and slow waves, and normal pre-seizure development are the main features of Doose syndrome. Tonic seizures occurring within 12 months of life, age of onset <6 months or >8 years of age, or the presence of a specific etiological lesion on imaging are not considered for the diagnosis of the syndrome. Care should be taken to rule out other disorders if a child has moderate-to-severe developmental delay or focal neurological abnormalities on neurological examination before seizures. In resource-limited settings, EMAS can be diagnosed without EEG or MRI support only if a clinician witnessing a myoclonic–atonic seizure (either by direct observation of the patient or by means of video provided by the family) meets all mandatory and exclusionary clinical criteria.

Identification of Myoclonic–Atonic Seizures

EMAS should be distinguished from LGS, MEI, and DS with "petit mal" characteristics. In the early recognition of these syndromes, they are not distinguished. The types of epilepsies that are most difficult to distinguish from Doose syndrome are benign myoclonic epilepsy, severe myoclonic epilepsy, and LGS.

LGS

The two syndromes are not distinguishable in the early stage and are often considered two manifestations of a syndrome. Later, general understanding of the two syndromes gradually became clearer.

It is difficult to distinguish EMAS from cryptogenic LGS. The main seizure types of LGS include tonic, atypical absence, and atonic seizures. The main seizure forms of EMAS are myoclonic–atonic, atonic, and myoclonic-flexor seizures (MASs), among which tonic seizures are the characteristic seizures of LGS, but they are the basis for the exclusion of EMAS. On EEG, the background activity is usually abnormal in LGS but normal in EMAS, especially in the early stage. The generalized spike-wave discharges (GSWD) frequency of LGS is usually <2.5 Hz, while that of EMAS is 3–6 Hz. Paroxysmal fast activity and fast spikes are characteristic EEG changes in LGS but not in EMAS. Most LGS patients have abnormal premorbid development, while EMAS patients have normal premorbid development. The prognosis of LGS is poor, while that of EMAS is relatively good.

Myoclonic Epilepsy of Infancy (MEI)

Myoclonic epilepsy of infancy is an age-related idiopathic generalized epilepsy and is a rare self-limited epilepsy syndrome. The patient is healthy and develops normally before the age of 3 years. The main manifestations of seizures are myoclonic seizures involving the upper body, which occur multiple times per day. Ictal EEG shows extensive spikes or slow-wave discharges. Interictal electroencephalograms are usually normal, with few atonic seizures that can be distinguished from Doose syndrome [75].

Severe Myoclonic Epilepsy

This disease is also known as Dravet syndrome. The younger age of onset, usually characterized by generalized tonic–clonic seizures, resistance to antiseizure drugs, and marked intellectual impairment, can be distinguished from Doose syndrome.

Treatment

The prognosis of EMAS varies greatly. Early seizure control and no persistent EEG abnormalities are good prognostic factors. Early diagnosis and timely treatment are necessary.

Antiseizure Medications

Doose syndrome is responsive to a variety of broad-spectrum antiseizure drugs, among which valproic acid, lamotrigine, levetiracetam, and benzodiazepine have good therapeutic effects, although lamotrigine may aggravate myoclonic seizures. It is not recommended for the early treatment of EMAS in children with myoclonic seizures. Although there is not much evidence for clobazam in EMAS, the Chinese expert consensus in 2022 listed clobazam as an additive treatment for EMAS. Felbamate, rufinamide, ethosuximide, and acetazolamide are also therapeutic options, while cannabidiol is not recommended for the treatment of EMAS.

1. *Valproic acid*: Nickels et al. [548] analyzed drug therapy in 166 patients and reported a valproic acid response rate of 31%. Nickels et al. [553] studied 76 patients and reported that valproic acid, topiramate, zonisamide, levetiracetam, benzodiazepines, and a ketogenic diet were effective; however, valproic acid was recommended as a first-line drug.
2. *Levetiracetam*: Nickels et al. [548] reported that levetiracetam was 19% effective in the treatment of Doose syndrome.
3. *Others*: Carbamazepine, oxcarbazepine, vigabatrin, and phenytoin can aggravate the myoclonus–atonic seizures of EMAS and should be avoided in clinical practice.

Corticosteroids

Corticosteroids are the main treatment for EMAS. Adrenocorticotropic hormone and high-dose glucocorticoids are effective in treating children with refractory nonconvulsive status epilepticus. The main problems are recurrence and side effects of glucocorticoids after drug withdrawal. It can be used for nonconvulsive status epilepticus or after the failure of rational use of one to two antiseizure medications.

Ketogenic Diet Treatment

Stenger et al. [554] conducted a ketogenic diet study on 50 patients who failed to respond to an average of 4.3 antiseizure medications. The results showed that 54% of the patients had seizures that disappeared after 6 months of ketogenic diet treatment and that 86% had seizures that were reduced by more than 70% after 2 months of ketogenic diet treatment. Among them, 44% of patients significantly benefited from early KD treatment. The authors concluded that early ketogenic diet treatment for resistant EMAS can lead to long-term remission and better cognitive outcomes, suggesting that a ketogenic diet is a more effective treatment for EMAS. Wiemer-Kruel et al. [555] fed 30 patients (24 boys) modified ketogenic diets at 4 centers and found that 25 of the 30 patients (83%) had a ≥50% reduction in seizures and that 14 of them (47%) experienced seizure cessation. Nickels et al. [548] administered a ketogenic diet with 79% efficacy and suggested that this diet may be the most effective in treating Doose syndrome; however, long-term ketogenic diet treatment can induce liver damage, hepatic steatosis, and gallstone formation, and liver enzymes need to be monitored to prevent these side effects from causing irreversible damage to patients [555]. Therefore, ketogenic therapy can be considered early in patients with poor seizure control after treatment with one to two reasonable antiseizure drugs.

A ketogenic diet, a low glycemic index diet, and a modified Atkins diet are recommended.

Prognosis

The prognosis of myoclonic–atonic epilepsy varies widely, ranging from normal cognition to severe cognitive impairment and from seizure-free to experiencing seizures that are difficult to control. Approximately two-thirds of patients achieve remission within 3 years of onset, and antiseizure drugs can be withdrawn or discontinued. The other third of patients may have persistent seizures, cognitive impairment, aggression, or hyperactivity. It is difficult to predict patient prognosis by clinical and EEG changes in the early stage of the disease. The factors associated with poor prognosis included generalized tonic–clonic seizures before the age of 2 years, myoclonic state, absence or convulsive status, tonic seizures, abnormal background activity on EEG, obvious θ rhythm, and absence of alpha background rhythm.

5.3.6 Lennox–Gastaut Syndrome (LGS)

Overview

Lennox–Gastaut syndrome (LGS) is a childhood-onset epileptic encephalopathy. In 2022, the new classification of epilepsy syndromes by the International League Against Epilepsy classified it as childhood-onset epilepsy syndrome, which is part of developmental or epileptic encephalopathy. The characteristic seizure types of this epileptic syndrome include axial tonic, atypical absence, and atonia. The characteristic electroencephalogram (EEG) changes include slow spikes and slow waves <3 Hz and are often accompanied by intellectual delay or regression. Moreover, seizures are often difficult to control, and the prognosis is poor because of the characteristics of LGS as an epileptic encephalopathy. The peak age of the disease is 3–5 years, and there are more boys affected than girls, accounting for approximately 5–10% of childhood epilepsy cases [478–480].

Historical Evolution

In 1950, Lennox and Davis [5] first noted the difference between slow and fast spikes and slow waves. In 1966, Gastaut et al. [6] noticed this kind of pediatric epileptic encephalopathy with diffuse slow spikes and slow waves, which he called Lennox syndrome. Because the occurrence of slow spikes and slow waves is similar to that of typical absence seizures or generalized tonic–clonic seizures, it is called a variant of generalized tonic–clonic seizures. Subsequently, Bernard et al. [556] summarized the clinical features and evolution of this kind of epileptic encephalopathy and proposed diagnostic methods. In 1968, Gastaut et al. [557] again studied the characteristics of epilepsy in children with diffuse slow spikes and waves (or small variations). Because these children had other brain injuries in addition to seizures, he considered this a special encephalopathy and named this Lennox epileptic encephalopathy in children. In the same year, Niedermeyer [558] proposed Lennox–Gastaut syndrome for the first time and emphasized that it was a severe childhood epilepsy. In 1972, Tassinari et al. [559] reported that five patients with Lennox–Gastaut syndrome developed tonic status epilepticus after using diazoxide for treatment, indicating that the treatment of this disease was different from that of other diseases; these findings attracted special attention to the treatment of this disease and promoted the understanding of this syndrome. Moreover, its electrophysiological characteristics have also been noted [486]. In 1974, Speciali JG et al. [560] summarized the clinical characteristics of status epilepticus in Lennox–Gastaut syndrome patients, helping to foster a deeper understanding of this syndrome.

Epidemiological Data

Poke et al. [85] investigated the epidemiology of developmental encephalopathy and epileptic encephalopathy as well as intellectual disability and epilepsy in children and reported that the cumulative incidence of Lennox–Gastaut syndrome in children was 13.2/100000. A survey conducted by Strzelczyk et al. [561] in Germany showed that the prevalence of LGS was 6.5–39.2/100,000. Asadi-Pooya [562] conducted a survey of 3737 outpatients with epilepsy and found that 300 of them had LGS, suggesting a prevalence of 8%.

Etiology

Lennox–Gastaut syndrome can be divided into three categories: idiopathic, cryptogenic, and symptomatic. Those with no obvious cause and no history of central nervous system abnormalities are considered cryptogenic. Epidemiological investigations have shown that such patients account for approximately 20–30% of the total number of patients. Although the reason for this difference is unclear, the prognosis of patients with cryptogenic Lennox–Gastaut syndrome is better than that of those with symptomatic Lennox–Gastaut syndrome. Idiopathic Lennox–Gastaut syndrome is mostly related to genetic factors, and 3–27% of patients with typical Lennox–Gastaut syndrome have a family history. Pathogenic variants in many genes can cause LGS. These include *CDKL5*, *FASTKD2*, *CACNA1A*, and *TANC2* gene mutations; chromosomal abnormalities; and copy number variations [491–494].

Lennox–Gastaut syndrome can also be classified as symptomatic. The etiology of LGS can be identified in 60–75% of cases, and it can include various brain injuries before, during, and after delivery. The most common causes are malformation of brain development, hypoxic-ischemic brain damage, encephalitis, meningitis, and tuberous sclerosis complex. Among the six causes of ILAE epilepsy, the most common is structural etiology. Malformations of cortical development are common causes of LGS. Focal cortical dysplasia can lead to typical or incomplete LGS. Almost all children with LGS have abnormal brain MRI and PET findings. In approximately one-third of children with LGS with normal MRI results, FDG-PET usually reveals focal or multifocal hypometabolism, which is often consistent with malformations of cortical development and white matter abnormalities and common global hypometabolism. When the etiology is not clear upon imaging or genetic examination, metabolic examination should be performed.

Clinical Manifestations

Age of Onset

There are different opinions on the age of onset of LGS. The new classification of the International League Against Epilepsy in 2022 emphasized that the age of onset should be under 18 years, and Asadi-Pooya and Farazdaghi [563] analyzed this in 3737 patients with epilepsy. They found that LGS patients had onset at the age of 21 years. LGS can be ruled out by an age of onset older than 18 years, which is a limitation of the new classification system. Asadi-Pooya [562] investigated the ages of 300 LGS patients and reported that the age of onset was 3.3 ± 4.1 years. In 10 patients (3%), the disease onset age was 14 years or older. Although the majority of patients present with the disease before the age of 8 years, some have disease onset in late childhood or adolescence. Moreover, the age of onset is significantly related to clinical manifestations, and tonic–clonic seizures are more common in patients older than 8 years. These findings support that the first seizure in Lennox–Gastaut syndrome occurs mostly at 1–8 years of age and that the peak occurs at 3–5 years of age. Patients with symptomatic Lennox–Gastaut syndrome with typical onset before the age of 3 years have poor seizure control and mental development. Occasional seizures and abnormal EEGs may also occur in young people aged 10–20 years [496].

Seizures of Epilepsy

Jose Luis et al. [564] investigated 331 LGS patients and reported that the most common seizure type was axial tonic (89%), followed by atypical absence (84%) and atonic seizures (69%).

1. *Seizures of tonicity*: Tonic seizures are tonic contractions of muscles without clonic phenomena. These can be divided into three types: axial, axial limb band, and generalized. It is the most common (80–100%) and the most characteristic type of seizure. It mainly occurs in slow-wave sleep and can occur in clusters, and the intensity of the attacks varies. Axial tonic seizures often involve the face, neck, trunk, paraspinal muscles, respiratory muscles, and abdominal muscles. They may also involve the proximal muscles of the upper limbs, called axial–proximal tonic seizures, and the distal limbs. The extent of motor involvement in tonic episodes also varies considerably. Mild episodes are limited to a slight upward gaze of the eyeball and are associated with transient disturbances in breathing. Such episodes are most common during sleep and are difficult to detect without video EEG recording. Tonic seizures may be confined to the cervical flexors, facial muscles, and masticatory muscles (body axial seizures); may affect the muscles of the proximal limbs, causing elevation and abduction of the arms (axial limb girdle); or may involve rigidity of the muscles of the distal limbs (generalized tonic seizures). In such episodes, flexion of the lower limbs and extension of the upper limbs represent the hypertonic type, often resulting in

sudden falls. Tonic episodes lasting for more than 20 s may be accompanied by a rapid fibrillation component (tonic-fibrillation episodes), with altered consciousness occurring after the onset of EEG discharges and recovering after the end of the discharges. After the tonic phase, automatism related to posture and ambulation may occur, especially in late-onset Lennox–Gastaut syndrome. Damage to the respiratory tract is also common and may lead to apnea. Facial flushing, tachycardia, and dilated pupils have also been reported.

2. *Atypical absence seizures*: In approximately two-thirds of children with LGS, the seizures gradually develop and abate with blurred consciousness. During seizures, changes in muscle tone and myoclonic seizures may be prominent. Postural loss of muscle tone in the trunk and head, facial or neck rigidity, eyelid or perioral myoclonus, and irregular head or limb jerks and nodding are often observed. Atypical absence seizures are a component of generalized seizures and differ from typical absence seizures in terms of clinical manifestations, electroencephalogram characteristics, and etiology. Absence seizures are characterized by sudden onset and sudden cessation of consciousness, while atypical absence seizures may have a longer duration of loss of consciousness and incomplete loss of alertness. Some patients can even answer simple questions during seizures and partially recall the details of seizures afterward. The accompanying tone changes may be more pronounced, and the onset and recovery of seizures are somewhat slower than those of typical absence seizures, often accompanied by tonic, clonic, and autonomic dysfunction. Ictal EEG signals are usually diffuse, asymmetric, and have irregular 2–2.5-Hz spikes and slow waves rather than the typical absence of 3-Hz spikes and slow waves, sometimes accompanied by fast waves and spikes.
3. *Atonic seizures*: These seizures occur in approximately half of children with LGS, and attacks tend to be frequent and involve the whole body or only the head. Generalized loss of postural tone can lead to "lightning" cataplexy, with mild and brief episodes of atonic seizures involving just nodding or bending the knee.
4. *Myoclonic seizures*: Myoclonic seizures occur in 11–28% of children with LGS. It usually occurs bilaterally and symmetrically, and the axial flexors and abductors of the upper limbs are easily affected.
5. *Status epilepticus*: The prevalence of status epilepticus in Lennox–Gastaut syndrome patients ranges from 54% to 97%. Tonic seizures and mental disorders are the most common manifestations of Lennox–Gastaut syndrome. Patients are often not diagnosed with epilepsy, which can be attributed to the side effects of drugs or other paroxysmal diseases. Nonconvulsive status epilepticus (NSE) is found in half of LGS children. NSE can occur in all types of epilepsies; it usually lasts for a long time and is recurrent and refractory. For example, absence status epilepticus is a mild (occasionally severe) state of clouded consciousness that lasts for days or weeks. Mixed tonic–absence status epilepticus is probably the most common type and is characterized by repeated and uninterrupted alternating episodes of brief tonic seizures and atypical absence seizures.

6. *Epileptic falls*: Many seizure forms of LGS can lead to epileptic falls (fall attacks), such as atonic, tonic, myoclonic–atonic, or myoclonic. Cataplexy often leads to repeated trauma and is a dangerous form of epileptic seizure. A reduction in the frequency of epileptic falls is of great clinical significance [497].

Cognitive Behavioral Disorders

Cognitive impairment does not always occur at disease onset but becomes increasingly obvious with increasing age. Thirty-four percent of patients have normal intellectual development at the age of 4 years, but 78–96% of the patients eventually experience cognitive impairment. The severity of intellectual disability is associated with onset before the age of 3 years, frequent seizures, recurrent status epilepticus, and symptomatic Lennox–Gastaut syndrome. Approximately 20–60% of children with LGS have cognitive and behavioral abnormalities before epileptic seizures, especially symptomatic LGS children, who often have obvious psychomotor deficits before the onset of disease that manifest as global developmental delay, decreased learning ability, and behavioral problems and worsen with age. Behavioral problems include irritability, hyperactivity, and psychosis, and it is sometimes difficult to distinguish them from seizures in LGS.

EEG Characteristics

Extensive <2.5-Hz slow spikes and waves or generalized paroxysmal fast activity during sleep are essential EEG changes. If there is a low-frequency photoparoxysmal response in an EEG, which often indicates CLN2 disease rather than LGS, attention should be given to excluding this disease. If the EEG shows persistent focal discharge without a generalized spike-and-wave pattern, LGS could be excluded.

1. *Background activity abnormalities*: Background activity abnormalities are observed in almost all patients, with or without slow GSWD at the beginning of the disease, manifested as a slow patchy alpha rhythm, diffuse slow-wave increase, and disorganized EEG rhythm. Focal slow waves are more common in symptomatic LGS.
2. *Paroxysmal electroencephalographic abnormalities*: Patients with <2.5 Hz-slow GSWD have bilateral, synchronous, and symmetrical characteristics, with high amplitudes in the anterior head region; additionally, GSWD can occur asymmetrically and unilaterally. The approximately 10-Hz paroxysmal rhythm during slow-wave sleep is a characteristic manifestation of LGS. The clinical manifestations accompanied by paroxysmal fast activity may not be obvious, or transient tonic seizures (mainly in facial muscles) may occur; these seizures often require video EEG monitoring. At this time, the rhythm of paroxysmal fast activity is usually faster than 10 Hz. Interictal spikes, multifocal spikes or sharp-and-slow complex waves are mainly observed in the frontal and temporal lobes in 75% of patients. Multiple, independent spike foci may occur during development from West syndrome to LGS. EEG findings vary from person to person and change

over time. Low EEG activity with or without paroxysmal fast activity is also common.

3. *Ictal EEG*: An extremely fast rhythm with amplitude changes is a common ictal feature of LGS. Low EEG activity with or without paroxysmal fast activity is also a common ictal EEG change in LGS. The clinical seizure types and ictal EEG patterns observed are mostly consistent. Tonic seizures often have a characteristic paroxysmal fast rhythm, while atypical absence seizures often have a slow GSWD (<2.5 Hz), which can be observed both in the clinical quiescent phase (interictal phase) and in clinical seizures of varying severity. Atonic seizures are associated with generalized polyspikes, slow GSWD, and accelerated fast rhythm, which could occur alone or in combination. Myoclonic seizures are characterized by generalized polyspikes with or without slow waves and fast rhythms. An EEG of massive myoclonus, atonic seizures, and myoclonic–atonic seizures may reveal a mixture of slow and multiple spikes. In the late stage of seizures, generalized slow waves or slow GSWD may appear instead of low EEG.

Diagnosis

According to the 2022 ILAE diagnostic criteria for epilepsy syndromes, the diagnosis of LGS must include the characteristic seizure forms and EEG changes in LGS and the triad of cognitive impairment [565].

Approximately 20% of patients have basically normal memory and cognition, so the existence of cognitive impairment is not considered a necessary criterion in the literature. However, these patients have lags in cognitive information processing and other aspects, and more detailed or accurate clinical evaluations and judgments are needed.

Multiple forms of epileptic seizures depend on the presence of at least one of the following seizure types in addition to tonic seizures: atypical absence, atonia, myoclonic, generalized tonic–clonic, nonconvulsive status epilepticus, epileptic spasms, etc. The most characteristic seizures of LGS are tonic seizures, atypical absence seizures, and atonic seizures.

ILAE's 2022 diagnostic criteria for LGS require tonic seizures to be indispensable, but some scholars also speculate that atypical absence seizures are indispensable, indicating the characteristics and importance of these two types of seizures in LGS [565].

Treatment

Treatment should not only control seizures but also address cognitive and behavioral disorders.

Basic Principles of Treatment

1. *Treatment goals*: Because LGS is a very severe type of epileptic encephalopathy in children, seizures are often not successfully controlled. Existing treatments for epilepsy are extremely limited in terms of seizure control and

improvement of cognitive behavior. Therefore, minimizing the number of seizures and improving the quality of life are often the main goals of treatment.
2. *Control triggers*: Controlling the triggers of seizures is part of the rational management of LGS. Recurrent fever, vomiting, diarrhea, and medication changes may precipitate seizures or lead to status epilepticus. Excessive excitation or lack of adequate external stimulation can also lead to increased seizures. Regular diet and sleep, medication, and a stable environment are important for reducing the number of daily seizures.
3. *Treatment during rehabilitation*: Most LGS patients have severe cognitive and behavioral disorders and movement disorders and need corresponding rehabilitation training and management. It is necessary to pay attention to the educational, behavioral, and psychological needs of children, and multidisciplinary means are needed to support children and their families.
4. Considering the efficacy and safety of LGS treatments as a whole, reducing rather than increasing ASM use with increasing seizure frequency is a better choice. Drug effects are often temporary, often lasting weeks to 4 months, and side effects of sedatives can lead to a vicious cycle. For example, sedation may increase tonic episodes during sleep. Phenytoin, carbamazepine, oxcarbazepine, gabapentin, lacosamide, and phenobarbital may aggravate some seizure types associated with LGS and should be used with caution.
5. LGS is resistant to ASMs, and it is often necessary to use a reasonable combination of drugs. ASMs should be combined according to the main seizure type, and it is generally not recommended to use more than three kinds of ASMs in combination. ASM treatment can temporarily reduce seizures but cannot completely control them. Tonic seizures during sleep are the most difficult to control. Patients with atypical absence seizures, myoclonic seizures, and atonic seizures respond relatively well to drugs.

Antiseizure Medications

It is difficult to control seizures in Lennox–Gastaut syndrome patients using antiseizure medications. Although multiple drug combinations are generally used, monotherapy is still advocated for in the early stage because of the sedative and neurotoxic effects of antiseizure medications, and the side effects of these drugs must be maintained at the minimum extent possible.

Frank M C Besag et al. [566] summarized the results of randomized double-blind placebo trials for the treatment of Lennox–Gastaut syndrome and found evidence to support the use of lamotrigine, cannabidiol, felbamate, fenfluramine, rufinamide, and topiramate as adjunctive treatments for seizures, with clobazam being the most effective. Valproic acid is still considered the drug of choice, despite a lack of support from randomized, double-blind trials. Riva et al. [567] summarized the current status of drug treatment for LGS in Italy and found that although lamotrigine, rufinamide, topiramate, cannabidiol, and clobazam are popular treatment options, valproic acid remains the main treatment option for patients with

LGS. Devi et al. [568] used a network meta-analysis to study six drugs for the treatment of LGS and found that clobazam, cannabidiol, and rufinamide were the most effective and safest.

1. *Valproate*: Valproic acid is the first-line treatment for LGS. Its effect on cryptogenic Lennox–Gastaut syndrome is better than that on symptomatic Lennox–Gastaut syndrome, mainly for myoclonic seizures, atypical absence seizures, and akinesia seizures. There is an increased risk of severe hepatotoxicity in children under 2 years of age, especially in those receiving combination therapy. Attention should be given to the risk of polycystic ovaries in adolescent women.
2. *Clobazam*: In 1982, Pechadre et al. [569] first reported the use of clobazam for the treatment of Lennox–Gastaut syndrome. Subsequently, Ng et al. [570] described a clinical trial of clobazam in the treatment of 305 patients with LGS. They found that clobazam could significantly reduce the seizure rate in LGS patients, which verified its clinical efficacy in treating LGS.
3. *Cannabidiol (CBD)*: Cannabidiol use for LGS-related seizures in children older than 2 years of age was initiated in 2018. Espinosa-Jovel et al. [571] studied the efficacy of cannabidiol in the treatment of refractory epilepsy and reported that its rate was 67.8% and that the drug retention rate was 78.2%. It is especially suitable for treating falling attacks and other seizure types. When combined with other ASMs, attention should be given to drug interactions. The main adverse reactions are diarrhea and somnolence, and there is also a risk of aggravating seizures.
4. *Lamotrigine*: In 1992, Timmings and Richens [572] studied the clinical efficacy of lamotrigine as an adjuvant in the treatment of Lennox–Gastaut syndrome and reported that it could reduce the frequency of seizures by more than 50% in 81% of patients. It is effective in treating various seizure conditions, such as cataplexy and absence seizures, but can aggravate myoclonic seizures in LGS patients. Rash is the main side effect of lamotrigine, which can also cause severe Sjogren's syndrome and even be life-threatening. Lamotrigine and sodium valproate have beneficial pharmacokinetic effects, and the combined use of lamotrigine and sodium valproate should be reduced.
5. *Felbamate*: As an earlier drug approved by the FDA (1993) for the treatment of LGS, felbamate can reduce fall attacks, absence attacks, and other forms of seizures. Because of its fatal adverse effects (liver damage), this drug should be used with caution and should not be used for more than 2 months if there is no clear effect.
6. *Rufinamide*: This drug was approved by the FDA in 2008 for the treatment of LGS in children older than 4 years or in adults. Treatment of atonic and tonic–clonic epilepsies with this drug has the outstanding feature of not worsening other types of seizures.
7. *Vigabatrin*: Similar to its use for West syndrome, vigabatrin may be effective in treating LGS due to cortical dysplasia, but there is a greater risk of irreversible visual field defects.

Nonpharmacological Treatment

In many cases, drug therapy needs to be rationally combined with surgery, a ketogenic diet, and vagus nerve stimulation, including the choice of timing, age, and condition. A ketogenic diet and vagus nerve stimulation have limited effects on seizure control in LGS patients. It is more helpful for improving children's cognitive behavior, attention and arousal, activity level, and socialization. For some genetic causes of LGS, the efficacy of a ketogenic diet will be more prominent. In patients with definite local lesions, focal lesion resection can be performed. Corpus callosotomy is an effective surgical method for neurosurgical treatment of epileptic encephalopathy complicated with severe atonic seizures and cataplexy [506] and is also suitable for refractory tonic seizures and occasionally for GTCSs. Those with fewer seizures after surgery also have improved behavior and alertness. However, other seizure types do not improve. Recurrence can occur up to 2 years after surgery and may lead to more severe focal seizures [507, 508, 510].

Prognosis

Traditionally, the prognosis of LGS is poor; 5% of LGS patients die, 80–90% continue to have seizures in adulthood, and 85–92% develop severe cognitive and behavioral disorders that eventually require specialized institutional care. However, Kim et al. [573] studied the long-term prognosis of 68 LGS patients aged 18–35 years. During an average follow-up of 19.3 years, 16 patients (23.5%) stopped experiencing seizures, 26 (38.2%) of whom only received AED treatment. Six of these patients were seizure-free. Nineteen patients were treated with a ketogenic diet, 5 of whom were seizure-free during treatment. However, the cognitive function of the patients was significantly impaired; 94.7% of the patients had moderate-to-severe intellectual delay, only 39.7% of had the complete ability to perform independent daily living, and 25.4% could not walk even with support. The factors suggesting a poor prognosis are as follows: early onset, frequent refractory seizures, recurrent status epilepticus, fixed slow background activity on EEG, focal or multifocal EEG abnormalities, symptomatic etiology, history of West syndrome, etc. The factors suggesting a better prognosis include normal premorbid development, normal EEG background activity, rapid GSWD, normal brain imaging, and hyperventilation-induced generalized spike–slow complex.

5.3.7 Developmental and Epileptic Encephalopathy with Spike Activation During Sleep

Overview

In 2022, the new classification of epilepsy syndromes by the International League Against Epilepsy included Landau–Kleffner syndrome (LKS), epileptic encephalopathy with continuous spikes and waves during slow-wave sleep (EE-CSWS), and atypical benign partial epilepsy (ABPE) (also known as pseudo-Lennox syndrome), which are classified as "developmental and epileptic encephalopathy with childhood onset and epileptic encephalopathy" or "developmental/epileptic encephalopathy with spike-and-wave activation in sleep (D/EE-SWAS)." These diseases are defined as a series of regressions in cognitive, language, behavioral, and motor function associated with characteristic spike-and-slow-wave activity during sleep (non-REM 1.5–2-Hz spike–slow complex) [53]. Usually, spikes and slow waves are nearly continuous and can exceed 85% of the entire nonrapid eye movement (NREM) duration; that is, spike–wave indices (SWIs) >85%. This EEG pattern is also known as electrical status epilepticus during sleep (ESES) [574, 575]. Patients usually exhibit regression of the above functions within weeks of the onset of SWAS. EE-SWAS refers to patients with previous normal neurological development, while DEE-SWAS refers to patients with previous neurodevelopmental disorders. After the occurrence and persistence of SWAS, patients show significant regression of the above functions. Since LKS is characterized by language regression and acquired auditory agnosia, it is reserved as a special subclass of DEE-SWAS, while CSWS and ABPE are not mentioned [53].

Historical Evolution and Epidemiological Investigations
Patry et al. [574] first described "subclinical electrical status epileptiform during sleep in children" in 1971 and proposed that this condition is characterized by spike-and-slow-wave activity accounting for more than 85% of NREM sleep time. In 1985, epilepsy with continuous spikes and waves during slow-wave sleep (CSWS) was defined by ILAE as a syndrome related to various types of seizures (focal or generalized but without tonic seizures) occurring during sleep and atypical absence seizures occurring during waking, with persistent diffuse spikes and slow-wave patterns occurring during NREM sleep after the onset of seizures [10]. In the 1989 classification, CSWS was placed in the group of "epilepsy syndromes with both generalized and partial seizures" of the "classification of epilepsy and epileptic syndromes" [11]. In 2001, ILAE classified these diseases into the "epileptic encephalopathy" group when they were grouped into epilepsy syndromes [576]. In the 2010 ILAE classification of epilepsy syndromes by age, CSWS was classified into the "childhood-onset epilepsy syndromes" group and renamed EE-CSWS [53]. EE-CSWS was considered an acquired, age-related childhood disorder characterized by (1) focal and/or generalized seizures; (2) ESES in EEG; and (3) cognitive or behavioral disorders [574, 577–580].

The atypical variant of benign epilepsy with centrotemporal spikes (BECTs) was first reported by Aicardi and Chevrie [581] in 1982. The characteristics of BECTs include the following: (1) onset age of 2–7 years and clinical characteristics consistent with those of the early stage; (2) gradual appearance of negative myoclonus, atypical absence, and oropharyngeal dyskinesia (average 18 months after onset); (3) typical bilateral epileptic discharges in the Rolandic areas, as revealed by EEG, and activation of spikes and slow waves during sleep; and (4) probable occurrence of cognitive dysfunction [581–583].

LKS was first reported by Landau and Kleffner [584] in 1957. Its main clinical features include (1) acquired aphasia in childhood and rare seizures and (2) EEG signals showing epileptic discharges mainly in the temporal region during waking and ESES during sleep [577, 585–587]. In the 1989 classification, LKS and CSWS were classified into the "epilepsy syndromes with generalized and partial seizures" group in the "classification of epilepsy and epilepsy syndromes" [11] and into the "epileptic encephalopathy" group in 2001 [52]. In 2006, the ILAE Working Group stated that there was insufficient evidence for a difference in pathogenesis between LKS and CSWS to indicate that the two syndromes are separate [588]. In the 2010 ILAE classification of epilepsy syndromes by age, LKS and CSWS were grouped together into the "childhood-onset epilepsy syndromes" group [53]. LKS and epilepsy with CSWS are now recognized to include all epilepsy disorders characterized by cognitive or behavioral disorders in childhood and significant activation of epileptic waves during interictal sleep. This spectrum of disorders also includes ABPE.

In 2022, the new ILAE classification includes LKS, EE-CSWS, and ABPE under the DEE-SWAS group of "developmental and epileptic encephalopathy with onset in childhood" [301].

DEE-SWAS is a rare disease, and there is no sex difference in its incidence. Studies have shown that it accounts for 0.5–0.6% of all epilepsy types in tertiary pediatric epilepsy centers [589–591].

Causes of the Disease

Researchers have reported that structural brain damage is a risk factor for DEE-SWAS. Kersbergen et al. [592] reported that of 14 patients with thalamic hemorrhage in the neonatal period, 3 were diagnosed with ESES in childhood (SWI > 85%), 2 had SWI between 50 and 85%, and 2 had significant activation of epileptic waves during sleep. Second, unilateral, or bilateral polymicrogyria is also associated with ESES [593, 594]. Van Hirtum-Das et al. [595] reported that among 67 children with ESES, approximately half had imaging abnormalities, including cortical dysplasia, stroke, diffuse brain atrophy, white matter changes, abnormal or delayed myelination, nodules, and Chiari malformation type II; however, structural brain damage was uncommon in LKS [595]. In addition, ESES has been reported in four patients with congenital Zika virus syndrome [596]. Neuronal antibody-related autoimmune diseases can also lead to ESES [597, 598].

Up to 50% of patients with DEE-SWAS have a family history of seizures [599], suggesting a genetic basis for the syndrome. Among them, the most important pathogenic gene is *GRIN2A* [600]. Lesca et al. [601] reported that approximately 20% of LKS, EE-CSWS, and ABPE incidences were caused by de novo mutations to *GRIN2A*. Pathogenic variants in GRIN2A are associated with the severity of the DEE-SWAS phenotype [601–603]; DEE-SWAS caused by this gene variation can present with specific language disorders, mainly dysarthrias and coordination disorders; some patients may have lifelong impaired speech intelligibility [604]. Second, researchers have reported that *SCN2A*, *SLC9A6*, *ATN 1*, *SRPX2*, *KCNQ2*, *OPA3*,

KCNA2, *CNKSR2*, *SLC6A1*, and *KCNB1* gene variants are also related to the pathogenesis of DEE-SWAS [34, 605–610]. In addition, *ATP13A4*, *CDH9*, *CDH13*, *CNTNAP2*, *CTNNA3*, *DIAPH3*, *MDGA2*, *SHANK3*, and other genes that are associated with autism spectrum disorders and copy number variations of cell adhesion proteins are also associated with DEE-SWAS [615].

Clinical Presentation

Epileptic seizures usually occur between 2 months and 12 years of age, and the peak age is 4–5 years [616, 617]. Spike and slow-wave activation occurs on EEG during sleep 1–2 years after epileptic seizures and is accompanied by cognitive and/or behavioral regression. The SWAS pattern on EEG may disappear with the cessation of seizures or gradually disappear after the cessation of seizures. Sleep structure also gradually returns to normal, but focal epileptic discharges may persist during waking and/or sleeping periods [618–620]. With the disappearance of the SWAS pattern, cognitive and/or behavioral disorders can improve, and some patients still experience long-term severe functional impairment [577, 621, 622].

Seizures in Epilepsy

There are many different types of seizures, depending on the cause, and some patients do not experience clinical seizures. In the early stage of the disease, most of the seizures are motor seizures of focal origin with or without impaired consciousness, which can be followed by bilateral tonic–clonic seizures. Subsequently, the seizures worsen, and a variety of seizure forms can occur, including focal seizures with or without impaired consciousness, typical or atypical absence seizures, atonic seizures, and focal motor seizures with negative myoclonus.

In 2006, a study classified the seizures of 90 patients with ESES according to their clinical and EEG characteristics. Among them, 34 patients (38%) had complex partial seizures, 3 (3.3%) had benign Rolandic seizures, 11 (12%) had generalized or nonconvulsive seizures, and 23 (26%) had mixed seizure types. Six patients had no clinical seizures and 13 had unclear seizure types. The average duration of seizures before the first discovery of ESES was 36 months (1 day to 13 years), and the frequency of seizures ranged from several times per day to two times per year when ESES was identified [595].

Fernández et al. [623] categorized EE-CSWS into three stages in 2012. The first stage occurs before the appearance of CSWS (mostly at the age of 4–5 years) and is usually characterized by occasional nighttime interfocal motor seizures. In addition, there are often unilateral limb-clonic status, absence seizures, atonic seizures, complex partial seizures, and generalized tonic–clonic seizures. In the second stage, the average age at which the seizures occur is 6.8 years and the seizures are more frequent and complex and include typical or atypical absence, status absence, atonic seizures, clonic seizures, and generalized tonic–clonic seizures. In the third stage, after a few months to 2–7 years, the seizures decrease or even stop.

Regression of Function

1. *Regression of language function*: LKS is characterized by acquired aphasia. The onset of the disease is subacute, usually at 3–12 years (with a peak age of 5–7 years). Before disease onset, the patient has developed normally and acquired age-appropriate language ability but lost acquired language function after disease onset. Auditory agnosia is a typical manifestation of this syndrome and is characterized by normal hearing, loss of ability to understand the language of others or oneself, and inability to execute commands issued by language. In severe cases, there is no response to calling one's name, and, at the same time, there is a loss of understanding of nonverbal sounds (such as dog barking and doorbells) [624–626]. Subsequently, impaired oral expression may occur, manifesting as paraphasia, phonological errors, sentence shortening, dysphonia, etc., and eventually mutism [626–629]. Some patients may have reading and writing dysfunction [626, 629–631]. The above symptoms may fluctuate over days to months and may worsen and resettle several times during the course of the disease [626, 632]. If language skills improve, receptive skills usually improve earlier than expressive skills [629, 633].

   A study of 29 follow-up LKS patients showed that auditory agnosia was present in all. The median age of aphasia onset was 5 years (2–9 years). Among the 29 patients, 16 (55.1%) had insidious symptoms, 10 (34.4%) had subacute onset, and 3 (10.3%) had acute aphasia. Twenty-four patients (82.8%) had severe aphasia, 5 (17.2%) had moderate aphasia, and 7 had fluctuations in symptoms. Among the 29 patients, 15 (51.7%) had normal nonverbal cognitive function and 14 (48.3%) had moderate impairment [634].
2. *Other neuropsychological and higher-functioning disorders*: After the occurrence of ESES, patients usually exhibit more serious functional disorders, including intellectual disability, language function degradation, spatial and temporal disorientation, and behavioral disorders (attention deficit, hyperactivity, aggression, and difficulty getting along with one another), and very few may develop mental disorders [586]. A follow-up study of 29 LKS patients showed that 15 patients had attention-deficit/hyperactivity disorders (51.7%), 4 had aggression (13.7%), 4 had memory dysfunction (13.7%), and 2 had spatial and temporal disorientation (6.8%). No mental disorders or autism were found [634].
3. *Motor dysfunction*: ESES patients can also have motor dysfunctions, such as dyskinesia, dystonia, ataxia, unilateral limb movement disorder, and negative myoclonus [616].

Ancillary Tests

The EEG characteristics in the early stage of the disease are related to the type of seizure. After the occurrence of SWAS, a normal sleep structure during sleep is absent and even difficult to distinguish. Significant diffuse 1.5–2-Hz spikes and slow-wave activation are observed during NREM and sleep II, usually with a susceptibility-weighted imaging (SWI) of at least 50%, which could be persistent, fragmented, or periodic. Spike and slow-wave activation are reduced or even disappear during REM sleep.

The background of the waking period may be focal or diffuse slowing, and focal, multifocal, unilateral, or asymmetric bilateral epileptic discharges may occur, but they are not persistent. Some patients have normal EEG signals during the waking period [635].

Therefore, SWI and epileptic discharges should be carefully described during the waking period, during each sleep cycle, and throughout the night via 24-h video EEG. SWI refers to the percentage of epileptic discharge activity during sleep as measured by the spike index [577]. The numerical criteria for assessing SWI in ESES differ and include 85%, 90%, 50%, 60%, and 25%. Several researchers have used grading scales to quantify SWI. Mikati et al. [636] used grades 0–4, including "no SW, 0-25%, 25-50%, and 75-100%." Beaumanoir et al. [637] used "no SW, <50%, 50-85% and 85 percent." Second, the presence of structural lesions can be further screened by improving head imaging.

Diagnosis

DEE-SWAS is diagnosed if the patient meets the clinical characteristics, has an EEG pattern, and has a series of cognitive, language, behavioral, and motor function regressions related to SWAS.

Differential Diagnosis

Lennox–Gastaut Syndrome (LGS)

The EEG of LGS patients shows significant slow spikes and slow complex waves in the waking and sleeping periods and diffuse fast activity bursts in the sleeping period, and the patients often have tonic seizures.

Structural Focal Epilepsy

In some cases of structural focal epilepsy, a large number of focal epileptic discharges may be activated during sleep, but patients do not exhibit cognitive impairment or behavioral problems related to the EEG pattern of SWAS.

Self-Limited Focal Epilepsies (SeLFEs)

SeLFEs can present with significant epileptic wave activation during sleep, but this disorder is not associated with cognitive impairment or behavioral problems associated with the SWAS EEG pattern.

Treatment

The aim of treatment is to control seizures and improve neuropsychological dysfunction abnormal EEG patterns.

Antiseizure Medications (ASMs)

A retrospective study of 88 patients with ESES revealed that avoiding multidrug combination therapy as much as possible was associated with improvement in ESES [638]. Although phenytoin sodium, carbamazepine, and phenobarbital can reduce seizures, they are contraindicated for ESES because they may aggravate epileptic discharges on EEG and lead to deterioration of neuropsychological dysfunction [639]. Carbamazepine is associated with the occurrence of CSWS and the persistence of EEG patterns [638, 640, 641]. Valproic acid, ethosuximide, benzodiazepines, clobazam, and levetiracetam were found to be beneficial [642–647]. Aeby et al. reported that after levetiracetam treatment of 12 children with ESES, the amplitude and range of epileptic discharges on EEG improved in 7 patients but only 25% of those patients showed a reduction in SWI [644]. Second, acetazolamide and sulthiame are also safe and effective for EE-CSWS and LKS [638, 639], and sulthiame is also effective for patients with benign partial epilepsy (APBE) developing into ESES [640–652].

De Negri et al. [653] studied 16 patients with CSWS or LKS who were given a high dose of diazepam (1 mg/kg) via the rectum, and the EEGs of all the patients were significantly improved. Subsequently, 14 patients showed significant improvement after a short course of diazepam (0.5–0.75 mg/kg/d) for 3–4 weeks. Five patients experienced recurrence and were again treated with diazepam. Ten patients underwent neuropsychological testing after 6 months of treatment; 7 patients experienced improvement or even disappearance of dysfunction, 1 had no significant improvement, and 2 had deterioration.

Glucocorticoid and Adrenocorticotropic Hormone

At present, hormone therapy is considered to be the first choice for treatment of this disease. Marescaux et al. [639] administered glucocorticoids to three patients with LKS, which improved the severity of language dysfunction and led to a normal EEG. Therefore, they suggested that high-dose glucocorticoids be given immediately after diagnosis and that maintenance doses be given for several months to several years. Subsequently, it has been reported that the use of prednisone (2–5 mg/kg/day), methylprednisolone (20 mg/kg/day for 3 days), and adrenocorticotropic hormone (ACTH, 80 IU/day, given for 3 months with a taper period) can improve abnormal EEG and dysfunction [654–657]. The earlier the use of glucocorticoids is, the shorter the course of treatment and the better the curative effect. A retrospective study reported that eight children with LKS and two children with ESES were treated with oral prednisone (1 mg/kg for at least 6 months) and were followed up for a mean duration of 4 years, with significant improvements in language, cognition, and behavior in all seven children [658].

Intravenous Gamma Globulin

The treatment efficacy of intravenous immunoglobulin (IVIG) is uncertain. Some case reports have suggested that IVIG may benefit some patients with ESES [633, 659]. Mikati et al. [636] administered IVIG (2 g/kg, 4 days) to five patients with newly diagnosed LKS, and two cases of language disorders and EEG abnormalities were relieved. Arts et al. [660] administered IVIG 400 mg/kg/day to six ESES patients (three with LKS and three with EE-CSWS) for 5 consecutive days, after which 400 mg/kg IVIG was given every 3 weeks beginning at the fourth week until the twenty-fifth week. One patient completed the treatment, and only one patient (the EE-CSWS patient) responded; however, the condition deteriorated immediately after stopping treatment and improved again after restarting treatment. In two patients (one with LKS and one with EE-CSWS), the treatment was ineffective. The other three patients stopped treatment after 8–12 weeks because of ineffective treatment and changed to prednisone treatment. Among them, one patient (LKS) had a good response and almost completely recovered, and the other two patients (one with LKS and one with EE-CSWS) experienced improvements in condition and EEG signals after a follow-up period of 12 months. Moreover, this study retrospectively analyzed 12 patients with LKS and EE-CSWS previously diagnosed and treated. Five patients were treated with IVIG, of which one experienced improvement in their condition 3 months after treatment, one had improved language function and electroencephalogram results that returned to normal, one had improved language function and electroencephalogram results 1 year after treatment, one had some improvement in electroencephalogram results, and one had aggravated clinical symptoms [660].

Surgical Treatment

At present, the main surgical treatment for this disease worldwide is multiple subpial transection (MST). Morrell et al. performed MST on 14 patients with refractory LKS. After a follow-up period of 13–78 months, six patients' language function recovered to that of the same age level without seizures and EEGs were normal; five patients' language dysfunction improved without seizures (three patients had normal EEG signals), and three patients' EEG abnormalities persisted without significant remission [625]. Grote et al. [661] conducted a longer follow-up of 14 LKS patients (including 10 cases reported by Morrell et al.) and included another 8 LKS patients whose age of onset was mostly approximately 4 years, while the average age of receiving MST was 7.4 years (5.1–13.1 years). The follow-up time ranged from 6 to 6.3 years. Thirteen patients completed the Peabody test, 7 significantly improved in score compared with the preoperative period, 5 exhibited no significant change compared with preoperative scores, and 1 exhibited more severe disease. Fourteen patients completed the Expressive One-Word Picture Vocabulary Test–Revised (EOWPVT/R) test, of which 8 exhibited significant improvement in score, 5 exhibited no significant change, 1 exhibited more severe disease, and only 4 exhibited significant improvement in the 2 tests.

A British study of five patients with ESES who underwent MST showed that behavioral problems and seizure frequency improved in all patients after surgery and that language function improved but not to the level of children of the same age [662]. However, Blount et al. [663] performed an MST on four LKS patients, and only one achieved improved language function after the MST.

In addition, vagus nerve stimulation (VNS) has been reported to be effective [664]. A retrospective study of six LKS patients treated with VNS showed that approximately 50% of patients experienced improvements in seizure frequency and quality of life at 6 months after surgery [665]. Very few patients with associated temporal lobe lesions can be considered for early preoperative evaluation of epilepsy, and surgical resection can be considered [666].

Other Treatments

Bergqvist et al. used a ketogenic diet to treat three patients with drug-refractory LKS who had durable improvements in speech disorders, behavioral problems, and seizures [667]. A ketogenic diet can theoretically improve ESES through the GABA pathway and inhibit inflammation. Overall, in 38 patients who had previously undergone ketogenic diet treatment, 53% of the EEGs improved and 41% of the seizures decreased by >50%. Cognitive impairment improved by 45%, and only 9% had a normal EEG [668]. In addition, sign language may help patients with language dysfunction communicate and may even facilitate recovery from language dysfunction [669].

Prognosis

Patients usually stop having seizures in the adolescent stage. Sánchez Fernández et al. reported that some patients can stop having seizures at the age of 6–9 years [670] and that the average duration of epilepsy is 12 years (4–15 years). On average, SWAS persists until 11 years of age and eventually resolves [577], whereas focal epileptic discharges can persist for some time after SWAS has resolved [671]. Clinical seizures may stop at the same time as the SWAS disappears or before or after its disappearance [671]. After the disappearance of SWAS, cognitive function and behavioral disorders improve, but some patients may experience moderate-to-severe cognitive impairment. Approximately 70% of 117 patients with ESES can recover to the baseline level of cognitive impairment, and patients without structural lesions have a better prognosis [672, 673].

Studies have shown that an increased frequency of interictal epileptic discharges, bilateral spikes and waves in the prefrontal region, and frequent generalized epileptic discharges during wakefulness and sleep indicate a poor prognosis [674]. Saltik et al. showed that the recovery of cognitive function in patients with nonstructural lesion-related epilepsy with ESES after the disappearance of SWAS was dependent on the duration and severity of SWAS [675]. Early recognition and effective treatment to reduce seizures and alleviate SWAS are essential for improving long-term outcomes [673]. In addition, ABPE has a good prognosis, while children whose disease develops into LKS or EE-CSWS have a poor prognosis of language, cognitive, and behavioral dysfunction [582], and the prognosis of LKS is generally better than that of EE-CSWS [595].

5.3.8 Febrile Infection-Related Epilepsy Syndrome (FIRES)

Overview

Febrile infection-related epilepsy syndrome (FIRES) is a subtype of childhood-onset epilepsy syndrome according to the new classification of the International League Against Epilepsy [301], especially in healthy children. Multiple severe types of seizures occur within 24 h to 2 weeks of nonspecific fever and often progress to refractory status epilepticus (RSE) within 2 weeks, with or without febrile symptoms at the onset of status epilepticus (SE) [676]. It is a kind of epileptic encephalopathy that is not rare in clinical practice. It is easy for patients to develop drug-resistant epilepsy, which can lead to cognitive impairment [677]. Its pathogenesis is still unclear, but there is increasing evidence that acute, non-antibody-mediated neuroinflammation can be caused by a variety of factors [678]. At present, specific biomarkers for diagnosis are lacking, and diagnosis mainly relies on clinical manifestations and the exclusion of other diseases [679].

Definitions of New-Onset Refractory Status Epilepsy (NORSE) and FIRES
NORSE is a clinical manifestation rather than a specific diagnosis. New-onset refractory status epilepticus is defined in patients without active epilepsy or other preexisting associated neurological conditions, and patients with a definite acute or active structural, toxic, or metabolic cause are excluded. Several points should be noted: (1) Patients diagnosed with viral encephalitis and autoimmune encephalitis are not excluded from NORSE diagnosis. (2) NORSE can include patients with a history of long-term brain injury as well as those who are "seizure-free" (seizure-free for at least 10 years and withdrawal of antiseizure medications >5 years). Diagnosis requires exclusion of patients with active epilepsy. (3) Cryptogenic NORSE or NORSE of an unknown etiology refers to NORSE whose etiology cannot be determined after adequate investigation (which may take several weeks). (4) NORSE does not include refractory SE with fully preserved consciousness (e.g., epilepsia partialis continua (EPC)) [676].

FIRES is one of the subcategories of NORSE and is the most predominant diagnosis in children with NORSE. FIRES patients have prodromal febrile infection before NORSE. Fever usually occurs between 24 h and 2 weeks before status epilepticus (SE), and body temperature can return to normal or remain febrile when SE occurs. It should be noted that (1) patients of all ages can be diagnosed, not just children; however, most patients are between 2 and 17 years of age and the median age is 8 years, and (2) the definition of more than 24 h excludes most children with febrile seizure status [676].

Historical Evolution
It has been more than half a century since the discovery of FIRES, and the evolution of its nomenclature reflects the continuing understanding of the disease by researchers. The disease was first described in 1961 by Lyon et al. [680] as acute encephalopathy of an unknown origin. In 1986, Awaya [681] described this category of disease as chronic-onset, similar to the acute onset of encephalitis. In 2001, Sakuma et al. [682] named this disease acute encephalitis with recurrent refractory focal epilepsy (AERRPS), proposed diagnostic criteria for the disease, and evaluated the efficacy of different treatment regimens. In 2006, Mikaeloff et al. [683] retrospectively analyzed the clinical characteristics of 14 patients with intractable epilepsy of the lateral fissure, which started with SE caused by unexplained fever and was accompanied by severe cognitive impairment; these authors named this disease devastating epileptic encephalopathy in school-aged children (DESC) for the first time. In 2009, van Baalen et al. [684] named this phenomenon "school-age febrile infection-responsive epileptic encephalopathy (FIRES)." In 2010, van Baalen et al.

[685] retrospectively analyzed the medical histories of 22 patients with this disease and found no evidence of encephalitis; these authors considered this to indicate that this was another infection-related pathogenesis, so they named this disease febrile infection-related epilepsy syndrome (FIRES). In 2018, a multidisciplinary group of experts from eight different countries developed a consensus definition of FIRES, classifying it as a subtype of new-onset refractory status epilepticus (NORSE). This classification has been approved by the Intensive Care EEG Monitoring Research Consortium [676]. In 2022, the International League Against Epilepsy classified FIRES as developmental and/or epileptic encephalopathy in childhood-onset epilepsy syndrome, which has led to a deeper understanding of the disease [301].

Epidemiological Survey

FIRES is very rare in clinical practice. In Germany, the incidence of FIRES is 1/1000,000 and the prevalence is 1/1000,000 [686]. Because FIRES is a diagnosis of exclusion, it may be missed, such as when patients are misdiagnosed with encephalitis or other diseases due to characteristics that are very similar to those of FIRES, so the true incidence and prevalence of this disease may be greater than reported [677].

Pathogenesis

The pathogenesis of FIRES is still unclear, and, recently, many scholars have proposed two possible pathogenetic mechanisms [677].

Neuroinflammation

In recent years, many studies have shown that the levels of inflammation-related factors in the serum or cerebrospinal fluid of FIRES patients are increased, and some anti-inflammatory treatments are effective, indicating that this disease may be related to neuroinflammation [687]. Kothur et al. [688] reported that, compared with those in patients with epilepsy or noninflammatory neurological diseases, the levels of Th1-associated cytokines/chemokines (including tumor necrosis factor-α (TNF-α), C–X–C motif chemokine ligand (CXCL)9, CXCL10, and CXCL11), interleukin (IL)-6, C–C motif ligand (CCL)2, CCL19, and CXCL1 were significantly elevated in the cerebrospinal fluid of FIRES patients, indicating that elevated cytokine/chemokine levels are significantly associated with the underlying etiology. They argue that despite clear signs of neuroinflammation, it is not clear whether this inflammation is primary and causal or secondary and reactive. Clarkson et al. [689] examined the levels of IL-1β and IL-1RA in the serum and CSF of FIRES patients and in those of healthy controls and reported that they were significantly greater in the former than in the latter group. These authors suggested that FIRES was associated with reduced expression of intracellular IL-1RA isoforms and functional defects in IL-1RA inhibitory activity, possibly related to neuroinflammation. Muccioli et al. [690] reported that cranial MRI of a 40-year-old patient with FIRES showed abnormalities mainly on the right side, with a claviform nucleus sign, which they speculated may represent FIRES related to cytokine-mediated neuroinflammation. Lin and Hsu [691] suggested that FIRES is associated with excessive activation of the inflammasome/IL-1 axis in microglia. A study by Sakuma et al. [692]

revealed significant upregulation of proinflammatory cytokine and chemokine levels in the CSF of FIRES patients.

Mechanisms of Immunity

Recent studies have also found specific antibodies in the serum and CSF of some FIRES patients, and some studies have shown that some FIRES patients have a good response to immunomodulation-related treatment, indicating that immune-mediated mechanisms may play a role in the occurrence and development of FIRES, but this view is still controversial [677]. Caputo et al. [693] first reported that GABAAR antibodies were found in the CSF and serum of FIRES patients and that these patients responded to high-dose intravenous steroid treatment; they suggested that autoimmune responses may play an important role in the pathogenesis of FIRES. Basso et al. [694] reported that a 5-year-old child with FIRES had a strong response after immunohistochemical detection of neuronal antibodies in the striatum, indicating the presence of antibodies against an uncharacterized neuronal target. The condition of the patients treated with plasma exchange was significantly improved, and the antibody titer was also significantly decreased. These authors suggested that immunological mechanisms may be involved in FIRES. Kurimoto et al. [695] successfully treated a patient with FIRES with anti-inflammatory and immunosuppressive therapy and suggested that autoimmune mechanisms may play a role in the development of FIRES. A study by Hsieh et al. [696] revealed that impaired TLR3, TLR4, TLR7/8, and TLR9 expression may exist in FIRES patients, which may be related to weakened phagocytic function and a decrease in T-regulatory cells, indicating that impaired immunity may be involved in FIRES. However, van Baalen et al. [686] found no antibodies associated with autoimmune encephalitis in the cerebrospinal fluid or serum of 12 FIRES patients and that treatment with steroids, immunoglobulin, or plasma exchange had no significant effect. Alparslan et al. [697] described the first case in Turkey in which IVIG was used to successfully treat a previously healthy 8-year-old boy with FIRES, but no autoimmune-related antibodies were found in the cerebrospinal fluid.

Clinical Presentation

Age and Sex at Disease Onset

FIRES is most common in school-aged children (average age of 8 years), generally ranging from 2 to 17 years, and can occur at different ages but rarely occur in children under 2 years or in adults [696]. Both males and females can be affected, but, generally, males are more affected than females [677, 698].

Howell et al. [699] followed seven FIRES patients, whose mean age was 10.8 years (6.7–14 years), and all patients were male. Among the 29 patients studied by Lee and Chi [700], the median age was 8.9 years (range: 1.2–17.8) and 12 were males and 17 were females. The median age of the 77 FIRES patients included in the multicenter study by Kramer et al. [698] was 8 years (range: 2–17 years), for a 4:3 male-to-female ratio. Lam et al. [701] followed 25 FIRES patients—11 females and 14 males—with ages of onset ranging from 1.6 to 17.2 years (mean 9.6 ± 4.4 years). According to a retrospective study conducted by Caraballo et al.

[702], the average and median ages of 12 FIRES patients were 8.5 and 10 years, respectively (range: 2–13.5 years) and included 8 males and 4 females; thus, the peak age of FIRES was 2–17 years, and more males were included.

Clinical Features

Patients usually develop normally before disease onset and have no family history. Agarwal et al. [703] proposed that FIRES can be categorized into three phases: the febrile infectious phase, followed by acute seizures or SE with poor response to drugs, and, ultimately, a chronic phase, including refractory seizures, cognitive decline, and behavioral problems; however, the boundaries between the phases are not distinct: (1) The prodromic phase is often characterized by infection with fever and may be accompanied by respiratory or gastrointestinal symptoms, but the fever is not always high. There are no specific neurological symptoms at this stage, but symptoms such as headache can occur. Among the 29 FIRES patients studied by Lee et al. [700], 21 (72%) had upper respiratory tract infections. Kramer et al. [698] analyzed the clinical characteristics of 77 FIRES patients and found that most of them had upper respiratory tract infections, followed by gastrointestinal infections. Fever preceded seizures with a median duration of 4 days (range: 1–14 days). Caraballo et al. [702] conducted a retrospective study of 12 FIRES patients, 9 of whom had fever-related upper respiratory tract infections and 3 of whom clinically presented with fever, headache, lethargy, and delirious encephalitis-like features for 2–10 days prior to seizures. (2) In the acute phase, seizures occurred within 24 h to 2 weeks of prodromal fever, and the body temperature was normal or still febrile at the time of seizures. The initial seizure may be transient or manifest as status epilepticus, and the frequency of seizures increases rapidly within a few days. These seizures usually manifest as binocular strabismus on one side with or without mouth or facial twitching and can be accompanied by unilateral limb twitching or progress to bilateral tonic–clonic seizures. Patients progress to SE within several days, usually referred to as super-refractory SE with encephalopathy symptoms such as disturbance of consciousness. Rivas-Coppola et al. [704] reviewed the clinical features of seven children with FIRES and found that the antecedent infection in these patients was mainly upper respiratory tract or gastrointestinal tract infection and that all patients presented with complex partial seizures <24 h after onset. In 71.42% of the patients, seizures were rapidly aggravated and progressed to SE. Byler and Grageda [705] reported that seizures in children with FIRES could be characterized by lip smacking, right or left gaze, facial twitching, and progression to generalized rigidity or clonic movements. This phase usually lasts for weeks to months, depending on the severity of the patient's condition and appropriate and timely treatment. (3) Chronic phase: After a few weeks or months, status epilepticus gradually improved, first changing to frequent electroclinical seizures or electrical seizures, and gradually evolving into chronic recurrent seizures. The frequency of seizures is usually daily to weekly, and the seizures are usually focal [679]. Most patients are not seizure-free at all between the acute and chronic phases, and some patients receiving early and reasonably aggressive treatment may be seizure-free after the acute phase (usually 1–2 months), after which the chronic phase of seizures returns.

A small number of patients who undergo reasonably aggressive treatment during the acute phase can achieve long-term freedom from attacks. Chronic-phase seizures are usually drug-refractory. In the chronic stage of FIRES, in addition to seizures, most patients have advanced cortical dysfunction, such as cognitive decline, communication disorders, or emotional disorders. Rachfalska et al. [706] reported that FIRES patients can present with extrapyramidal symptoms such as dystonia in the chronic stage.

Ancillary Tests

Electroencephalogram (EEG)

In acute-phase EEG, generalized or multifocal slow waves are abnormal. EEG typically has the following three features: (1) repeated paroxysmal 15–18-Hz beta signals superimposed on 1–3-Hz delta signals, often observed in the frontal and central regions; (2) a gradual increase in seizure burden; continuous VEEG monitoring shows a gradual increase in seizure burden within 1 week of onset, which is gradually characterized by frequent multifocal electrical or electroclinical seizures; and (3) an episodic EEG pattern: the typical seizure pattern is a focal low- to medium-amplitude fast rhythm (>10 Hz) that begins and evolves into rhythmic spikes or spike–slow complexes, with electrical activity usually moving from one hemisphere to the opposite hemisphere (Fig. 5.2) [306]. EEG in the chronic phase usually shows a slow background rhythm and multifocal slow waves, spikes, and spikes during the interictal phase.

Farias-Moeller et al. [707] studied the EEG signals of seven children with FIRES in neurological intensive care and analyzed two sets of EEG signals from each patient (i.e., 12 h at the beginning of recording and 12 h before the induction of burst-suppressed coma). They found the following:

1. The EEG background of all patients contained a prominent extreme delta brush (EDB), which consisted of paroxysmal β–δ complex waves with 15–18-Hz β-activity superimposed on 1–3-Hz δ in the frontal and central regions and was recurrent in all patients.
2. The onset of refractory status epilepticus was preceded by a progressive increase in seizures.
3. During the course of the disease, there was a characteristic EEG seizure pattern that evolved from focal activity of small-to-moderate amplitude >10 Hz to rhythmic spikes and sharp and slow complexes. Ictal activity can shift from one hemisphere to the contralateral side. During the first 12 h of recording, most seizures were from the frontal, central, or temporal regions in either hemisphere. In the second EEG recording, seizures were also present in the occipital and parietal regions. Fast activity is usually still present and is superimposed on spikes and sharp–slow complex waves. These authors suggested that these EEG features of FIRES could help in the early diagnosis of this disease. A study of the EEG signals of 12 FIRES patients by Caraballo et al. [702] showed that interictal EEG recordings revealed diffuse δ–θ background slowing in all the patients. Initial ictal EEG recordings revealed temporal seizures in four children (33%), fronto-

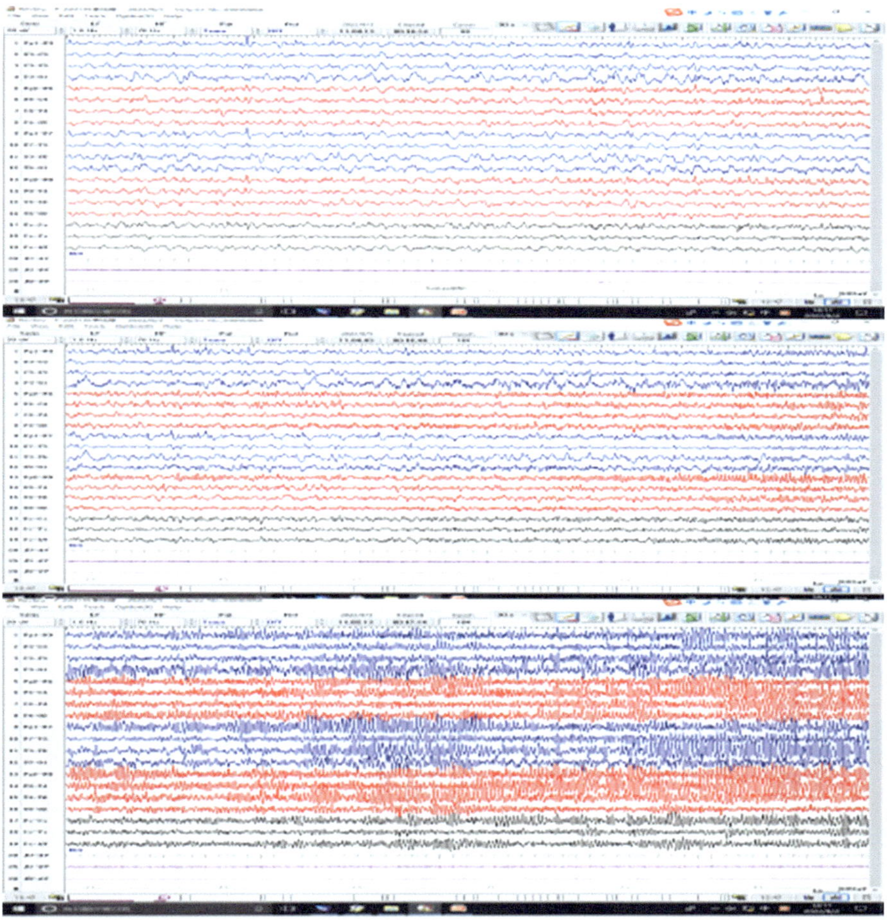

Fig. 5.2 EEG in the acute phase of a child with FIRES: fast rhythm firing in the left parietal, occipital, and middle and posterior temporal regions and fast-wave firing in the right frontal pole, frontal, and anterior temporal regions → dominant fast-wave firing in the left posterior head and bilateral anterior head → fast rhythm firing in bilateral hemispheres. FIRES, febrile infection-related epilepsy syndrome

temporal seizures in four children (33%), and frontofrontal seizures in two children (16.5%), all of whom rapidly progressed to multifocal and independent seizures, unilateral or bilateral, spreading to three different lobes in the same hemisphere and to the contralateral hemisphere in nine patients. Several other studies have reported similar findings [698, 703–705].

Imaging Studies

In the acute phase, MRI is negative in approximately two-thirds of patients and T2WI hyperintensity in the bilateral temporal lobe, insular lobe, or basal ganglia can be observed in approximately one-third of patients. In 2019, Culleton et al. [708] summarized the MRI characteristics of FIRES patients published in the literature and reported that among 129 patients in the acute stage, 61.2% had normal MRI findings, 25.5% had abnormal signals in the temporal lobe, 6.9% had abnormal signals in the basal ganglia, 5.4% had abnormal signals in the insular lobe, and 4.6% had cortical swelling in other brain lobes. Leptomeningeal enhancement was 4.6%, thalamic abnormal signals were 1.5%, and brain stem abnormal signals were 1.5%. In the chronic phase, in 97 patients, MRI showed extensive brain atrophy (49.4%), medial temporal lobe sclerosis (24.7%), a normal brain (18.5%), white matter abnormalities (11.3%), basal ganglia/thalamus changes (5.3%), insular or periinsular abnormalities (3.1%), and gliosis (2.1%). In recent years, it has been reported that FIRES patients have symmetrical T2WI, T2/FLAIR hyperintensity with limited diffusion (DWI hyperintensity) in the bilateral claustrum in the acute phase; this phenomenon is called the claustrum sign (Fig. 5.3). Approximately half of patient lesions can extend to the insular lobe or the medial temporal lobe [682]. The claustrum sign, which usually appears several days (average, 10 days) after status epilepticus and resolves in most patients within a few weeks, is considered to be a relatively characteristic MRI finding in FIRES patients, but it has also been reported in other inflammation-related acute encephalopathies (e.g., COVID-19).

Byler et al. [705] reported cranial imaging features of a 5-year-old child with FIRES who showed bilateral hippocampal atrophy only on day 37 of illness.

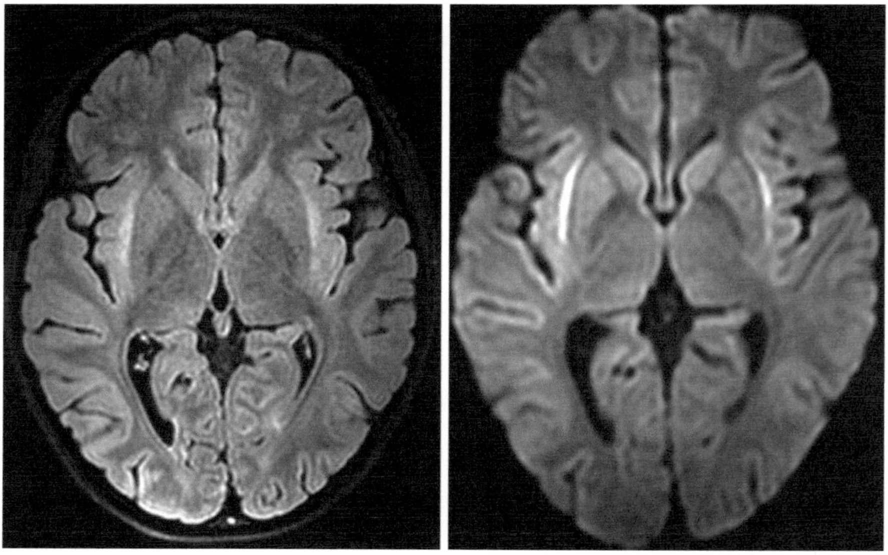

Fig. 5.3 Claustrum signs on MRI in the acute phase in a child with FIRES: T2/FLAIR sequence on the left and DWI sequence on the right. A high signal intensity in the claustrum was observed symmetrically. FIRES, febrile infection-related epilepsy syndrome; T2/FLAIR, T2/fluid attenuated inversion recovery; DWI, diffusion-weighted imaging

Agarwal et al. [703] also described a 5-year-old child with FIRES whose head MRI was initially normal and whose condition gradually progressed to hippocampal edema; ultimately, hippocampal atrophy was found at 7 months after onset. Similar findings have been reported in two other studies [698, 702]. Tan [709] described a case of FIRES in which the patient had extensive subcortical infarcts on cranial MRI, mainly in the temporo-occipital lobe. Nozaki et al. [710] reported that a head MRI of a 7-year-old patient with FIRES revealed a reversible splenial lesion of the corpus callosum.

Blood and CSF Examination

In the acute phase, the number of nucleated cells in the CSF was usually normal or slightly increased, the CSF biochemistry was usually normal, and a few patients had slightly increased protein levels. In addition, inflammatory cytokines/chemokine levels in the blood are mainly related to the innate immune system. The cytokines include IL-12p70, IL-6, TNF-α, CXCL8, MIP-1α, and CCL2 in the serum and IL-6, CXCL8, MIP-1α, and CCL2 in the CSF. However, the elevation of these cytokines/chemokine levels was not specific to FIRES. It can also be observed in patients with other causes of NORSE or non-de novo status epilepticus [683]. Tests performed to exclude other causes, including blood lactic acid, blood NH3, electrolytes, blood glucose, and other metabolic indicators; blood/CSF antibodies related to autoimmune encephalitis; and infection-related etiological tests, are all negative.

Diagnosis

A FIRES diagnosis first requires the coincidence of NORSE, which is a case of de novo status epilepticus in a previously healthy patient, and the presence of a prodromal febrile infection between 24 h and 2 weeks before NORSE onset. In addition, it is important to diagnose FIRES to rule out other causes of status epilepticus, including infectious encephalitis (e.g., viral encephalitis), autoimmune encephalitis, genetic metabolic encephalopathy, and toxic encephalopathy caused by toxins.

According to the *Classification and Definition of Epilepsy Syndromes* published by ILAE in 2022, clinical diagnosis is made according to the following necessary, cautionary, and exclusion criteria [301]. The necessary criteria for diagnosis are as follows: (1) a history of nonspecific febrile infection within 2 weeks of seizure onset; (2) focal or multifocal seizures, often progressing to bilateral tonic–clonic seizures; (3) progression to super-refractory SE within 2 weeks of onset; and (4) an electroencephalogram reading revealing background slow waves, multifocal epileptic discharges, frequent focal electrical seizures, or electroclinical seizures. When the following warning signs are present, the diagnosis should be cautious and other diseases should be considered: (1) the origin site of the focal seizures should be fixed; (2) the patient should be under 2 years of age; (3) the patient should have intellectual delay before the onset of the disease; (4) the patient should have an abnormal nervous system examination before onset; and (5) the long-term prognosis should be good: there should be no drug-resistant epilepsy, learning difficulties/intellectual disability, or brain atrophy. The presence of the following features rules out the diagnosis of FIRES: (1) a previous history of epilepsy; (2) age <1 year or

>30 years; (3) presence of definite epileptogenic structural lesions on brain MRI at the onset of epilepsy; and (4) clear evidence of other causes: CNS infection, autoimmune encephalitis, metabolic or genetic etiology, or toxic encephalopathy. At the time of diagnosis, the following auxiliary tests are usually required to screen for causes [711, 712]: (1) head imaging: plain MRI scan + enhanced; if necessary, head CT, MRA, and magnetic resonance venography (MRV) are performed. The exclusion criteria for individuals are as follows: (2) whole blood and serum samples: routine blood test, blood biochemistry, C-reactive protein (CRP), autoimmune encephalitis and SLE autoantibodies, cytokine/chemokine detection, and pathogen detection; and (3) CSF samples: routine, biochemical, lactic acid, neopterin, cytokine/chemokine, and pathogen detection. (4) Toxin testing and genetic testing are performed when necessary.

Differential Diagnosis

Other Epilepsy Syndromes

PCDH19-related cluster epilepsy: This disease mainly occurs in children under 3 years of age and manifests as a cluster of seizures caused by fever, but RSE is rare [713].

Encephalitis

1. *Limbic encephalitis*: Patients with this disease have a subacute onset and late onset of seizures and may have memory impairment. MRI signal changes are more obvious than those in other patients and can also affect the temporal lobe, but the imaging manifestations and clinical course are different, and the CSF antibody test is positive [708].
2. *Acute disseminated encephalomyelitis (ADEM)*: Seizures are not a prominent clinical feature; MRI imaging predominantly reveals white matter involvement, and, in some cases, the basal ganglia may also be involved [708].

Treatment

At present, there is still a lack of high-quality clinical research evidence for the treatment of FIRES, and the research results are mostly based on small sample case series or case reports [677, 687, 688]. In 2022, experts from the International NORSE Consensus Group published a consensus document on the treatment process of NORSE (including FIRES) and reached a consensus on the treatment of the disease [694, 695]. However, this consensus does not distinguish FIRES alone but rather is an overall consensus on the diagnosis and treatment of NORSE, which includes FIRES. In 2021, the FIRES Working Group, composed of 21 experts, made recommendations for the evaluation and treatment of FIRES [714]. The following is a treatment for FIRES that combines the above documents and is proposed based on our own experience.

Key Points in Acute FIRES Treatment

1. Patients are tested within 48–72 h of the onset of SE.

   1. Antiseizure medications and anesthetics are used to terminate SE according to the treatment process. However, SE is usually ultra-refractory and has a poor response to the above drugs.
   2. Anti-infective therapy against potential pathogens
   3. Respiratory and circulatory support
   4. Complete all etiological examinations as soon as possible.

2. Within 1 week:

   1. Initiation of first-line immunotherapy: *A. Immunotherapy*: Despite limited evidence, some scholars have chosen to treat FIRES patients with immunomodulatory therapy in recent years [677]. These include first-line therapies (e.g., steroids, intravenous immunoglobulin (IVIG), and plasma exchange) and second-line therapies (e.g., tacrolimus, rituximab, cyclophosphamide, and anacana) [687]. Caraballo et al. [702] analyzed the clinical characteristics and treatment of 12 FIRES patients at the Garrahan Hospital in Buenos Aires between 1997 and 2012 and reported that 2 patients treated with IVIG and 1 treated with steroids had a better prognosis than the other patients. Horino et al. [715] treated six FIRES patients with intrathecal dexamethasone and ultimately found improvements in symptoms and EEG characteristics as well as cytokines and chemokines in CSF. Coban et al. [716] reported successful control of seizures with immunoglobulin combined with plasma exchange in a 4-year-old patient with FIRES. However, Howell et al. [699] followed seven FIRES patients long term (5–17 years) and reported that none of the four patients who received immunotherapy, including IVIG, corticosteroids, plasma exchange, and rituximab, were responsive. *B. Anti-inflammatory treatment*: Interleukin-1 (IL-1α and Il-1β) are central mediators of immunity and are considered to be the main cytokines involved in local and systemic inflammation. IL-1 has become a key factor in the pathogenesis of autoinflammatory diseases, and blocking this pathway has become a key goal of treatment [717]. Anakinra (ANA) is a recombinant IL-1β receptor antagonist and the first anti-IL-1 drug used in clinical practice. Recent studies have shown that ANA can effectively improve the symptoms of FIRES patients. Kenney-Jung et al. [718] first reported successful treatment of super-refractory status epilepticus (SRSE) secondary to FIRES with ANA in children, suggesting a potential pathogenic role of neuroinflammation in FIRES. Several studies have shown that ANA can improve the prognosis of FIRES patients [719–721].
   2. Initiation of a ketogenic diet
   3. Initiation of second-line immunomodulatory therapy: If first-line therapy does not lead to a response and evidence of autoimmune encephalitis is lacking, the interleukin-1 receptor antagonist ANA or the IL-6 antagonist tocilizumab should be administered as soon as possible.

3. After 1 week, the patients are advised to (1) continue ANA (daily) or tocilizumab (repeated after 2 weeks and then once a month) for at least 3 months; (2) continue a ketogenic diet; (3) adjust their oral antiseizure medications and reduce their intravenous anesthetics as much as possible; and (4) receive supportive care.
4. Key points of treatment in the chronic phase of FIRES:

    1. Controlling seizures: Seizures are the most prominent manifestation of FIRES, so controlling them becomes an important measure for FIRES treatment. However, seizures in FIRES patients are usually insensitive to high-dose antiseizure medications (ASMs) and require the use of anesthetics [420]. High doses of barbiturates induce burst suppression on EEG signals and may be the only effective anti-status epilepticus agent used in the acute phase [719, 722]. Howell et al. [699] followed seven patients diagnosed with FIRES for 5–17 years, and each patient received a variety of ASMs (such as phenobarbital, benzodiazepines, carbamazepine, gabapentin, lamotrigine, and levetiracetam). However, only burst suppression induced by barbiturates could effectively control the onset of status epilepticus. Some studies have also investigated the use of anesthetics such as midazolam, pentobarbital, sodium thiopental, propofol, ketamine, lidocaine, and a combination of lidocaine and magnesium for the treatment of patients with status epilepticus [694, 715–717, 723]. Cannabidiol has been proposed as a possible effective drug for the treatment of epilepsy in recent years, and some scholars have noted that it can be used to treat FIRES. Gofshteyn et al. [724] analyzed the clinical characteristics of seven children from five centers who were treated with cannabidiol during the acute or chronic phase of FIRES. The seizure frequency and duration improved in six of the seven patients. These authors suggested that cannabidiol could be an effective treatment for FIRES. A similar conclusion was reached in a study by Duda and Reinert [725].
    2. Ketogenic diet (KD): A KD is a high-fat, low-carbohydrate, protein-sufficient diet. It can alter brain energy metabolism from the processing of glucose to that of ketone bodies and has multiple antiepileptic, antiseizure, neuroprotective, antioxidant, and anti-inflammatory effects; thus, it may be an effective measure for alleviating this disease [726, 727]. Although a KD is commonly used in the chronic phase of drug-resistant epilepsy, recent studies have shown its efficacy in patients with SE [728].

FIRES patients exhibit a good response to KD, and early diagnosis of FIRES can rapidly lead to the initiation of KD treatment and improve patient prognosis [729]. Peng et al. [730] conducted a retrospective analysis of patients who met the diagnostic criteria of FIRES, were diagnosed with super-refractory status epilepticus (SRSE), and received KD treatment at the Department of Pediatrics, Xiangya Hospital, Central South University, from 2015 to 2018. After the initiation of KD, all patients developed ketosis and SE disappeared within an average of 5 days. Seizures were reduced in number and duration, the background in the EEG recordings was restored, and sleep architecture was normalized. Therefore, the authors suggest that a KD may be a safe and effective therapy for FIRES with SRSE and that early initiation of KD yields a good prognosis. Kessi et al. [731] conducted a systematic review of the PubMed and Embase literature on FIRES up to May 2019 and reported that KD use in the acute phase was positively associated with the outcome of FIRES. Obara and Ono [732] reported that a KD is also applicable to adult patients with chronic FIRES. Koh et al. [714], in order to propose a treatment plan to improve the outcome of FIRES, in a workshop held in conjunction with the annual meeting of the American Epilepsy Society between 2017 and 2019, suggested that KDs be given early once a patient is suspected of having FIRES. Li et al. [733] described a 3-year-old FIRES patient with SE who was admitted to the pediatric intensive care unit for 55 days. Despite treatment with multiple ASM agents in addition to intravenous anesthetics, the patient remained in SRSE, EEG continued to show generalized epileptic activity, and KD treatment started on day 14 after onset. The patient's neurological function recovered completely after KD treatment, and the symptoms were completely controlled during the remainder of the hospital stay. Singh et al. [734] described two FIRES patients who underwent KD during the acute phase of the disease, and both ultimately had good outcomes, suggesting that early KD treatment may optimize seizure control and cognitive outcomes after FIRES.

Prognosis

FIRES has an uncertain, usually very poor prognosis [677]. Lee and Chi [700] conducted a retrospective analysis of the follow-up of 29 FIRES patients from December 2000 to May 2016. They found that 87% of these patients still had seizures or converted to refractory epilepsy, 26% had normal cognitive function, and 26% had learning disabilities and mild-to-moderate intellectual delay. Forty-eight percent of patients had severe intellectual delay or developed into a vegetative state. Mortality was 10% in the acute phase and 13% in the chronic phase. Howell et al. [699] followed seven patients with FIRES for 5–17 years; four patients eventually developed moderate-to-severe intellectual delay, and two patients developed mild intellectual delay. Lam et al. [701] analyzed the outcomes of 25 FIRES patients; ultimately, 61% of the patients had cognitive deficits, the duration and amount of anesthetic use were associated with poor long-term outcomes, the in-hospital mortality was 16%, and the incidence of significant functional decline at discharge was 100%. Patil et al. [735] conducted a retrospective analysis of 15 children with FIRES in southern India between January 2007 and January 2012 and reported that 3 children eventually died in the acute phase, 7 children had refractory epilepsy with encephalopathy, 8 had SRSE, and 3 children died in the acute phase. The authors suggested that the duration and severity of seizures in the acute phase are directly related to short- and long-term clinical outcomes. Boor and colleagues [685] conducted a retrospective study of 22 FIRES patients and found that 2 of them eventually died, 8 remained consciousness-impaired, 8 developed refractory epilepsy, 2 developed behavioral disorders, and 2 eventually recovered. Kramer et al. [698] analyzed 77 FIRES patients from 8 centers and reported that 9 (11.7%) died in the acute phase and only 12 (18%) of 68 survivors maintained normal cognitive levels; however, most of those patients had learning disabilities. At follow-up, 63 (93%) patients had refractory epilepsy. The longer the duration of BSC and the younger the age at onset of FIRES, the worse the cognitive level of the patients at follow-up. Kramer et al. [698] conducted a retrospective multicenter study of children enrolled in eight studies published between November 2001 and July 2010 to explore the association between BSC and FIRES outcomes and suggested that the prognosis of FIRES was poor and that the duration of BSC therapy was correlated with patient cognitive outcomes.

Future Research Directions
As a newly recognized inflammation-related encephalopathy, FIRES still has many problems to be resolved. Its pathogenesis needs to be clarified to identify and explore new therapeutic targets and the mechanism of inflammatory susceptibility factors in patients; prospective studies are needed to determine the best algorithm for acute-phase care and to explore more specific biomarkers for differential diagnosis, condition judgment, and efficacy evaluation in patients with FIRES.

5.3.9 Hemiconvulsion–Hemiplegia–Epilepsy (HHE) Syndrome

Overview
Hemiconvulsion–hemiplegia–epilepsy syndrome is a rare paroxysmal disorder characterized by the sudden onset of prolonged unilateral clonic seizures followed by persistent hemilateral hemiplegia in healthy children during a febrile illness. This progression progresses to focal epilepsy. The syndrome was first described by Gastaut et al. [736]. The age of onset was generally 5 months to 4 years, and the peak age was <2 years. In contrast to other common epilepsy syndromes, the onset of this syndrome conveys acute fever and there are characteristic brain imaging changes.

Historical Evolution
HHE was first reported by Gastaut et al. in 1957 [736]. In 1958, Vigouroux et al. [737] reported the EEG characteristics of HHE syndrome. In 1960, Gastaut et al. [738] named this syndrome HHE syndrome. Hemiconvulsions, hemiplegia, and seizures are the main clinical manifestations. The clinical features of five HHE syndrome patients were summarized. In 1979, Mori [739] described the pathological characteristics of HHE syndrome and explored the possible underlying mechanism involved. In 1988, Kataoka et al. [740] summarized the neuroimaging characteristics of 22 patients with HHE syndrome and described the syndrome in detail.

Epidemiology
Since HHE is a relatively rare disease, its prevalence has not been reported in relevant databases and most of the available data are from surveys of patients visiting hospitals. Assadeck et al. [741] studied 882 patients with epilepsy aged <20 years who came to the hospital and found 22 patients with HHE syndrome, suggesting a hospital incidence of 2.5%. There were 14 males and 8 females. Kataoka et al. [740]

conducted a 5-year follow-up study of 25 patients with hemiplegia after seizures and reported that 22 of them developed HHE. Goetz et al. [742] investigated 289 patients aged <18 years infected with influenza virus, 37 of whom had neurological symptoms; ultimately, 1 patient was diagnosed with HHE.

Causes of the Disease

The etiology and pathogenesis of HHE are still unclear. Previous studies have shown that the etiology of HHE may be diverse. Infection, genetic mutations, prolonged seizures, high fever, inflammation, and blood–brain barrier damage can all contribute to HHE syndrome. It is generally speculated that the etiology of HHE is related to infection resulting from persistent seizures after fever, followed by hemiplegia and chronic seizures in some patients. Vestergaard and Uldall [743] reported that a 2-year-old girl with adreno-reproductive system disease developed HHE syndrome after coinfection with a bacterial infection, suggesting that its etiology is related to infection. Anuar et al. [744] reported that among 11 patients with nervous system damage after COVID-19 infection, 1 had HHE. Gong et al. [745] reported that a patient developed ultra-refractory focal status epilepticus after COVID-19 infection. Neurological examination revealed right hemiplegia, and brain MRI showed edema in the left cerebral hemisphere, which was consistent with the diagnosis of HHE syndrome. Despite the high prevalence of fever, the cause of infection is often not known, suggesting that there are other factors involved in the development of HHE.

In addition to infection, cerebral thrombosis or cerebral hypoxia can also cause HHE progression. In 2022, Kumar et al. [746] reported the occurrence of HHE syndrome due to perinatal hypoxic-ischemic injury and suggested that the change in blood–brain barrier function after cerebral ischemia may be an important factor in the formation of HHE and a possible cause of this syndrome. Joshi et al. [747] described the case of a 33-month-old girl with unilateral cerebral edema in the right hemisphere, left hemiplegia and aphasia, and complex partial seizures in the left upper limb, which developed status epilepticus. Progressive atrophy of the right cerebral hemisphere was found during the 3-month follow-up. The authors speculated that cerebral hypoxia might induce HHE formation.

Predisposing Factors

Itamura et al. [748] described three patients with HHE syndrome after virus infection. They performed surgical treatment on these three patients, and postoperative pathological examination showed that the patients had focal cortical developmental infertility, which may have contributed to the development of HHE. Miteff et al. [749] reported that a patient with HHE had a microdeletion at chromosome 16p13.11, suggesting that this microdeletion may be a potential pathogenic factor for HHE. Myers et al. [750] presented findings regarding a 4-year-old girl with inherited cobalamin C deficiency who presented with dramatic manifestations of hemiconvulsion–hemiplegia–epilepsy that was resistant to most drugs and required craniectomy to relieve intracranial hypertension. The authors suggest that disturbance of cobalamin metabolism may be a contributing factor to hemiconvulsion, hemiplegia, epilepsy, and febrile seizures in general.

Possible Mechanisms

Auvin et al. [751] summarized his experience in the diagnosis and treatment of HHE syndrome for more than 20 years and proposed that the occurrence of HHE syndrome may be related to (1) inflammation caused by febrile seizures leading to necrosis of nerve cells; (2) long-term inflammation caused by neuronal damage affecting the permeability of the blood–brain barrier; (3) the presence of several predisposing factors that can lead to long-term seizures, such as genetic factors or focal epileptogenic foci, with some cases being related to genetic factors (the *CACNA1A* gene).

Clinical Presentation

According to the 2022 diagnostic criteria for ILAE, HHE onset generally occurs at <4 years of age and the acute phase is characterized by fever, followed by homonymous and permanent hemiplegia. Patients in this phase enter the chronic phase after a period of seizure-free time, and 85% of HHE patients usually have unilateral focal motor or focal to bilateral tonic–clonic seizures within 3 years of initial status epilepticus and more than 1–2 years later [92].

General Characteristics

Assadeck et al. [741] analyzed 22 patients with HHE syndrome and reported that the male-to-female ratio was 1.75, the average age was 3.76 (1–20) years, and 81.8% of the patients were younger than 6 years at the time of visit.

Fever

Fever is the most common symptom of infection, but a survey by Assadeck et al. [741] revealed that only 31.8% of the patients had febrile seizures, suggesting that fever is common but not a prerequisite for diagnosis.

Seizures

The mean age at seizure onset is 2.94 years (1–8 years). Hemiseizures often occur suddenly and include unilateral clonic seizures. Without appropriate treatment, symptoms may persist for hours or days, but if they persist for very long, they may spread to the other side of the body or alternate sides. Eye and head deflection may be the first signs of a seizure. After the acute phase, the seizures are controlled, and after a seizure-free period, generally within 3 years—mostly within 1–2 years—approximately 80% of the patients have seizures again, resulting in chronic focal epilepsy, mostly manifesting as complex partial seizures of temporal lobe origin and becoming drug-refractory epilepsy.

Hemiplegia

Homonymous hemiplegia after a seizure is observed in all patients; the face is often involved, it lasts more than 7 days, and it is mostly persistent. The mean age of onset of hemiplegia is 1.9 years (9 months to 5 years), and the mean interval between seizure onset and onset of hemiplegia is 9 months (1 month to 4 years)

[741]. Permanent focal dyskinesia is a prerequisite for diagnosis, and aphasia can occur with involvement of the dominant hemisphere [92].

Others

van Toorn et al. [752] described eight patients from South Africa and reported that most of the children had cognitive dysfunction.

Imaging Studies
Albakaye et al. [753] performed brain MRI on 35 patients with HHE syndrome, and the results showed that all the patients had abnormal results. Kataoka et al. [740] described the head CT manifestations of 22 patients with HHE syndrome and reported that 13 of them had obvious cerebral hemisphere atrophy, 1 had moderate or mild cerebral atrophy, and 4 had focal atrophy or ventricular malformation, suggesting that the imaging changes associated with HHE syndrome were mainly unilateral signal abnormalities involving the whole hemisphere. In some cases, the mass had an effect on the contralateral side. Early on, DWI showed limited diffusion of cytotoxicity and low density on the apparent diffusion coefficient (ADC). Cytotoxic edema was reduced, and the apparent diffusion coefficient (ADC) was pseudonormalized from day 8 to day 15; however, gliosis caused T2 hyperintensity, the brain volume began to decrease, and the brain showed atrophic changes after 1 month of hemiplegia. MRS revealed a decrease in the N-acetylaspartate (NAA) concentration and a slight increase in the lactate concentration. MRI performed immediately after febrile status epilepticus can reveal diffuse signal changes with T2 hyperintensity and limited diffusion in subcortical regions of the affected hemisphere, often accompanied by severe edema [92]. Atrophy of the involved cerebral hemisphere is a necessary criterion for the diagnosis of HHE.

Electroencephalogram (EEG)
Electroencephalogram (EEG) in the acute phase is used only to confirm clinical seizure status and does not reveal specific changes in the underlying cause or progression. In the acute phase of HHE, ictal EEG reveals bilateral high-amplitude, rhythmic 2–3-Hz slow waves; mixed spikes; sharp waves; spike and slow complex waves; and paroxysmal fast rhythms of 10–12 Hz on the affected side. In the posterior part of the affected hemisphere, the amplitude is greater and the spikes and waves are more prominent. After a period of attacks, the spikes and slow waves on the affected side are gradually replaced by delta waves with high amplitude. Background activity is slowed in the affected hemisphere. Focal or multifocal epileptiform discharges in the involved hemisphere in the chronic phase are essential for diagnosis [92].

Diagnosis
The International League Against Epilepsy proposed diagnostic criteria for HHE syndrome in 2021. It is suggested that individuals in the acute phase of HHE syndrome have fever and hemiclonic status epilepticus, followed by permanent hemiplegia, and that patients in the chronic phase have unilateral focal motor or focal to

bilateral tonic–clonic seizures; moreover, there should be special EEG and neuroimaging changes in HHE patients [92].

Differential Diagnosis

Patients were excluded from diagnose with HHE according to the International League Against Epilepsy if they are aged ≥6 years, have significant intellectual disability prior to the seizure, have a structural cause of focal status epilepticus, or have Todd's palsy. Rasmussen encephalitis should be considered if unilateral focal motor seizures progressively worsen over months to years and progress to hemiplegia in the later stages [92].

Treatment

Etiological Treatment

Although the etiology of HHE has not been fully elucidated and treatment is limited, some scholars are exploring etiological treatment methods. Shimakawa et al. [754] reported that a normally developing 1-year-old girl developed HHE syndrome after rotavirus infection and was treated with sodium valproate, clonazepam, zonisamide, phenytoin, phenobarbital, topiramate, and lamotrigine for seizures. At the age of 7, ACTH treatment was administered, and on the tenth day, the seizures stopped.

Symptom Treatment

Because the etiology of most HHE patients is unclear, treatment is symptomatic and can be divided into acute and chronic stages.

1. *Treatment in the acute phase*: In the acute phase, the main goal is to control epilepsy and status epilepticus. Anti-status epilepticus drugs such as diazepam can be used, and complications can be managed (see treatment of status epilepticus for details). A ketogenic diet may be effective in patients with refractory status epilepticus [754].
2. *Treatment in the chronic phase*: In the chronic phase, seizures should be controlled as much as possible, the disability rate should be reduced, and the motor function of patients should be improved as much as possible. Some scholars have proposed that the prevention of febrile seizures seems to be an effective way to prevent HHE syndrome [753].
3. *Control of seizures*: According to the type of seizure, antiseizure medications such as oxcarbazepine and lacosamide can be used; however, most patients have drug-resistant seizures and the control of epilepsy is not ideal. Reduction of disability: There is no effective treatment for hemiplegia, and rehabilitation training can help improve function.
4. *Surgical treatment*: HHE syndrome is not effective, especially in patients with elevated intracranial pressure, and surgical treatment may reduce mortality.

Prognosis

Patient prognosis mainly depends on the cause and timely effective treatment in the acute phase. In 80% of patients with acute seizures, focal seizures of focal temporal, lateral temporal, or multifocal origin occur within 1–5 years. Most patients also present with secondary GTCSs, and epileptiform status epilepticus is frequently present. These types of seizures are usually resistant to antiseizure medications. Moreover, some patients may have learning difficulties and even severe cognitive impairment and some patients may die. Jayakody and Joshi [755] described the case of a 3-year-old girl with HHE who died due to malignant cerebral edema and herniation, indicating that the overall prognosis of HHE syndrome is poor.

5.4 Epilepsy Syndromes with Onset at a Variable Age

5.4.1 Generalized Epilepsy Syndromes (See Sect. 5.3)

5.4.1.1 Sleep-Related Hypermotor Epilepsy (SHE)

Overview

Sleep-related hypermotor epilepsy (SHE) is a subtype of epilepsy syndrome that occurs at different ages according to the new International League Against Epilepsy (ILAE) classification. It is characterized by a series of motor seizures that occur during sleep. This type of epileptic seizure often occurs suddenly, usually lasting no more than 2 min, and mainly manifests as stereotyped hyperactivity or asymmetric tension disorder/tonic motor patterns. This type of epilepsy syndrome, especially that associated with brain structural abnormalities or specific genes (such as *KCNT1*), may lead to drug resistance. SHE includes and replaces certain previous epilepsy syndromes, such as hypnogenic nocturnal paroxysmal dystonia epilepsy and autosomal dominant nocturnal frontal lobe epilepsy (ADNFLE) [92, 756].

Historical Evolution

Nocturnal frontal lobe epilepsy (NFLE) was first described in 1981. Patients with this disease develop a special movement disorder during sleep characterized by vigorous limb movement or rigidity muscle tone disorders. Whether it is a phenomenon of epilepsy or a new motor disorder is highly controversial according to different authors [756, 757]. In 1990, Tinuper et al. [758] reported on three patients, demonstrating that this type of seizure is an epileptic seizure originating from the frontal lobe. In 1994, Scheffer et al. [759] noted that this type of nocturnal seizure was easily misdiagnosed as episodic sleep disorder. In 1995, Scheffer et al. [760] summarized the clinical manifestations of this syndrome and proposed that this autosomal dominant nocturnal frontal lobe epilepsy is an independent disease, which has attracted widespread attention. In the same year, Phillips et al. [761] discovered that this autosomal dominant nocturnal frontal lobe epilepsy had a pathogenic genetic linkage on chromosome 20, confirming that it was a disease with a genetic basis. In 1997, Berkovic [762] noted that this patient had a genetic mutation, which may be a new syndrome. On August 30, 2014, a consensus development conference was held in Bologna, which identified it as a new epilepsy syndrome and proposed changing its name to SHE [756, 763].

Epidemiological Investigation

Menghi et al. [764] reported that the lowest incidence rate of SHE in patients was 1.8/100000, accounting for approximately 10% of drug-resistant surgical cases. Vignatelli et al. [765] reported the prevalence of SHE in two northeastern regions of Italy, with rates of 1.8/100000 and 1.9/100000. Therefore, it can be determined that the incidence rate of SHE is approximately 1.8–1.9/100000.

The Etiology of SHE

SHE is a newly identified epilepsy syndrome by ILAE and includes various previously distinct diseases with different etiologies. Overall, most SHE patients do not have a clear family history or other confirmed causes. In some drug-resistant SHE patients, the etiology may involve surgically treatable lesions, especially type II focal cortical dysplasia. The most common syndrome is ADNFLE, and the etiology of this syndrome is related to genetics.

Clinical Manifestations

Age

The incidence rate of SHE is 1.8/100000 people [766], which falls under the category of rare diseases. Although seizures can occur at any age, they are more common between the ages of 14 and 20 years, and cases described by Vignatelli et al. [765] mostly occurred during adolescence (median age 11–13 years).

Sex

Both males and females are affected, but males are affected to a greater extent. Licchetta et al. [767] described 103 SHE patients, including 61 males and 42 females. Out of the 100 patients described by Provini et al. [768], 70% were male.

Frequency of Seizures

The frequency of seizures may be very high, as they can occur every night or almost every night and may occur multiple times every night, sometimes with a quasiperiodic pattern.

Onset Time

SHE occurs mainly during non-REM sleep and rarely during REM sleep. There may also be occasional seizures while awake during the patient's lifetime.

Seizure Manifestation

There may be sudden awakening or obvious premonstration before epileptic seizures. In addition, transient (no more than 2 min), stereotypical, and sudden awakenings, more complex dystonia–dyskinesia, and long-term "sleepwalking" behavior can be observed, mainly manifested as follows [768].

1. *Paroxysmal arousals*: Paroxysmal arousals are among the most common manifestations of SHE and can manifest as short (no more than 2 min), stereotypic, or sudden arousals. These are characterized by the patient suddenly staring or sitting up from bed with their eyes open during sleep, in strange postures, with expressions of fear or surprise on their face, sometimes screaming, and returning to sleep after an attack. Patients may complain of poor sleep and fatigue during the day.
2. *Nocturnal paroxysmal dystonia*: Nocturnal paroxysmal dystonia is characterized by a long duration (20 s to 2 min); often large and sharp movements; generalized dystonia, such as performance, such as head swing; trunk flexion; and limb dancing-athetoid movements accompanied by vocalization. These patients often exhibit a variety of vocal movements, such as drones, screams, roars or unprovoked laughter, and attacks that cannot be heard. There is a tendency toward periodic cluster attacks at night.
3. *Paroxysmal nocturnal wandering*: Paroxysmal nocturnal wandering is less common, lasting for up to 1–3 min, characterized by stereotyped episodic walking during sleep, generally more intense, with screaming and dystonic movements.
4. *"Hyperkinesia"*: Explosive movements, such as rapid jumping, swinging back and forth, and behavioral automatism, such as repeatedly tapping items etc., are the main manifestations. Manifestations can also include involuntary movements (sudden jumping from the bed, turning quickly in place, or bicycle-like motion). The amplitude is large and abundant, which is called hypermotor automatism. Repeated, stereotypically unilateral myoclonus may also occur, extending to the upper arms, shoulders, neck, and upper trunk, and may be conscious and recalled later.
5. *Others*: In the highly stereotypical "hyperactive state," in addition to intense hyperactive movements, such as complex body movements, limb kicks, and body swings, it is usually accompanied by autonomic signs, emotional facial expressions, sudden fear, and purposeless crying.

Auxiliary Examination

Interictal EEGs may reveal continuous generalized sharp waves, spikes, and slow waves; however, since epilepsy in most patients originates from the deep frontal lobe, scalp EEGs may be negative. Among the 100 patients included in the study reported by Provini et al. [768], 44% had normal EEGs during the ictal period and 51% had normal EEGs during the interictal period. Intracranial recordings made in SHE-resistant patients clearly indicate that interictal discharges may originate not only from the frontal lobe but also from different additional regions, including the insula, temporal cortex, and parietal cortex, and then spread to the frontal cortex to cause hypermotor seizures. This could indicate critical involvement of cortical–subcortical networks or an inherent release phenomenon of innate fixed motor patterns.

Diagnosis

In 2022, the International League Against Epilepsy proposed the diagnostic criterion for SHE, which states that transient focal motor seizures, characterized by hyperactivity or asymmetric tonic/dystonia, mainly occur during sleep as the core symptom of the diagnosis, and those that occur mainly during wakefulness or only during the day, can exclude the diagnosis of SHE. The diagnosis of SHE does not require cranial MRI or EEG to provide a diagnostic basis. The diagnosis of SHE is not considered if the patient has obvious intellectual delay [92].

Differential Diagnosis

Abnormal Nonrapid Eye Movement Sleep

SHE may be misdiagnosed as abnormal sleep. SHE episodes are usually short-lived (<2 min), sudden onset/offset, with stereotypic motor features from episode to episode, can occur during the night and cluster throughout the night (from sleep onset to early morning), and consciousness is usually retained during episodes. A longer duration of NREM sleep disorder (>10 min) occurs less frequently, usually once a night, and is more common 1–2 h after the patient has fallen asleep. The patient is delirious at the time of the event and does not have any memory afterward.

Psychogenic Nonepileptic Seizures (PNESs)

Patients with SHE may be misdiagnosed with PNESs because they may remain conscious in bilateral movements during seizures and because their initial EEG may not show a clear initial pattern. SHE may be distinguished from PNESs in terms of stereotyped hyperactive features, transient nature, and clustering of episodes during nocturnal sleep, whereas the events of PNESs are less stereotyped and occur during wakefulness.

Rapid Eye Movement Behavior Disorder

Rapid eye movement sleep disorder usually occurs after the age of 50 years. Hypermobility is not stereotyped but corresponds to vivid dreams.

Focal Seizures Occurring Mainly During Sleep

These seizures do not have the characteristic hyperactivity or asymmetric tonic/dystonic features observed in SHE.

Treatment

Antiseizure Medications (ASMs)

Carbamazepine (CBZ) inhibits the nicotinic receptor $\alpha 4\beta 2$ and $\alpha 2\beta 4$ subunits associated with SHE, thereby inhibiting glutamatergic excitability of the thalamocortical system and hippocampus, and enhancing GABAergic activity, thereby altering neuronal excitability. Low-dose CBZ (200–1000 mg/kg) is effective in some SHE patients but not in one-third of patients [768]. Oxcarbazepine (OXC) and topiramate (TPM) have been shown to be effective in both familial and sporadic ADSHE in uncontrolled trials [769, 770]. Raju et al. [771] reported that OXC was effective at treating eight patients who were not treated with CBZ or other ASMs, and Provini et al. [768] also reported that CBZ could stop seizures in 20% of patients and significantly relieve seizures in another 48%.

Other Drug Treatments

Most epilepsy cases are caused by mutations in the *KCNT1* gene, which encodes the sodium-activated potassium channel and induces epilepsy that is resistant to commonly used ASMs. Milligan et al. [772] suggested that quinidine, a partial antagonist of *KCNT1* channels, could treat *ADSHE* due to *KCNT1* mutations. Quinidine has been approved by the US Food and Drug Administration for the treatment of epilepsy caused by *KCNT1* mutations. The efficacy of quinidine, an emerging ASM, needs to be verified by clinical studies with large sample sizes. Lacosamide (LCM), which acts on slowly inactivated sodium channels, is a potentially effective adjuvant therapy for refractory SHE. Samarasekera et al. [773] used lacosamide (300–600 mg/kg) to treat eight patients with refractory SHE, and the frequency of seizures was reduced by more than 50% in five patients and 25% in one patient.

Surgery

Gibbs et al. [774] conducted a 2-year follow-up of 127 patients with SHE who underwent surgery; 104 (82%) achieved Engel grade I outcomes, and 86 (68%) achieved Engel grade Ia outcomes. The location of the lobule in the seizure onset zone (SOZ) had no significant effect on postoperative outcomes. Surgical treatment is effective in some severely drug-resistant SHE patients with FCD. Although there are few studies on surgical outcomes in patients with known genetic mutations, genetic etiology is not contraindicated during preoperative evaluation.

Prognosis

The overall prognosis of SHE is poor. Menghi et al. [764] reported that the cumulative probability of achieving terminal remission 10 years after the disease onset is 20.4%.

5.4.2 Familial Focal Epilepsy with Variable Foci (FFEVF)

Overview

Familial focal epilepsy with variable foci (FFEVF) is a subtype of age-onset epilepsy syndrome according to the new ILAE classification [92]. It is an autosomal dominant familial focal epilepsy syndrome with incomplete penetrance. According to previous reports of familial focal epilepsy, seizures in family members originate from the same cortical area, but, in familial focal epilepsy of variable origin, focal epilepsy in different family members originates from different cortical areas. One study reported that seizures in patients may originate from the frontal lobe, temporal lobe, parietal lobe, or occipital lobe and that the clinical manifestations may also differ. However, there are focal epileptiform discharges of different origins on EEG [92, 775, 776].

Historical Evolution

In 1997, Hayman et al. [775] conducted a study on two pairs of patients from two different families and found that although the clinical features of each patient in each family were almost the same, their EEGs showed that their seizures originated from different brain regions, one from the left frontal pole and the other from the right parasagittal and middle frontal regions. The authors attributed this to autosomal dominant nocturnal frontal lobe epilepsy. In 1998, Scheffer et al. [776] published the first paper on familial focal epilepsy of variable origin. They described an Australian family of 10 members with 4 generations of focal seizures, but their epileptic foci originated from the frontal, temporal, occipital, and central parietal regions. It was proposed that this special type of seizure is characterized by similar focal seizures in different family members but different electroclinical features between affected patients and family members. In 1999, Xiong et al. [777] reported that the pathogenic gene underlying this special type of familial epilepsy may be located at the chromosomal region 22q11-q12, which promoted the progress of research on this variable-origin familial focal epilepsy. In 2001, ILAE first included it as a new epilepsy syndrome in the new classification of epilepsy syndromes [778].

Epidemiology

No investigations of FFEVF syndrome have been reported in the population. Wang et al. [779] conducted a survey of 5300 patients and reported that 1 family met the diagnostic criteria for FFEVF syndrome. Picard et al. [780] investigated 19 families with autosomal dominant focal epilepsy and found 4 FFEVF families.

Etiology

Familial focal seizures of a variable origin are an autosomal dominant disorder. The initial linkage analysis suggested that the pathogenic gene was located on chromosome 2q, but its logarithm of odds (LOD) was only 2.74 [776]. Subsequent analysis of a five-generation Australian family of patients suggested that the pathogenic gene may be located at chromosome 22q12 that was considered to be a separate locus of the disease [778]. In recent years, research has focused on *DEPDC5* gene mutations. In 2013, Dibbens et al. [781] detected *DEPDC5* mutations in FFEVF families and subsequently found mutations in five patients in six other published large FFEVF families. Further studies of FFEVF families revealed that approximately 12% (10/82) of the patients had *DEPDC5* mutations, thus establishing that they are a common cause of FFEVF. Functional studies suggest that *DEPDC5* may play a role in neuronal signaling. In 2022, Samanta [782] and Gu et al. [783] again demonstrated the pathogenicity of *DEPDC5*. The new classification of ILAE also mentions that *TSC1*, *TSC2*, *NPRL2*, *NPRL3*, and other genes may also be related to FFEVF [92, 784, 785]. Structural damage mainly occurs in FCD (usually type II FCD).

Main Clinical Manifestations

Age of Onset and Sex

The age of onset is usually between 10 and 20 years (peak: 12–13.5 years), but there is considerable variation even within the same family. Scheffer et al. [776] described 10 patients in 4 generations of an Australian family; 2 patients had disease onset at the age of 60 years, and the average age of disease onset in the remaining 8 was 10 years (9 months to 43 years). Among the five patients included in the study by Klein et al. [778], the average age at seizure onset was 13 years (range: 0.75–43 years) and there was no difference between the sexes [92].

Clinical Features

The clinical manifestations are diverse. Since the frontal and temporal lobes are the most frequently affected regions, focal seizures with or without damage are the main manifestations, while symptoms are related to the focal cortical area of origin but are constant in the same patient [92]. Each patient has a focal seizure, such as focal cognitive, sensory, autonomic, or motor seizures, with psychiatric symptoms and oropharyngeal hallucinations when originating in the temporal lobe, and 60–86% of patients have secondary generalized tonic–clonic seizures, the severity of which varies greatly among individuals. There were 10 patients in 4 generations of an Australian family, all of whom had focal seizures—4 of whom presented with olfactory hallucinations or psychiatric symptoms of unconscious impairment. Six patients had focal seizures with disturbance of consciousness, and the other two family members had no clinical seizures but had epileptic discharges on EEG, with an average seizure duration of 13 years [778]. Scheffer et al. [776] reported seven patients, among whom five had seizures originating from the temporal lobe and two had frontal lobe epilepsy. Seizure frequency varies widely among individuals. One patient had lifelong refractory seizures, but his father had 16 seizures while asleep during a 28-year course, and his cousin had his first seizure at the age of 43. In the FFEVF family, patients had a variety of seizure types (febrile seizures, infantile spasms, focal seizures, or focal secondary generalized tonic–clonic seizures) caused by the *NPRL2* gene mutation reported by Zhang et al. [784]. Electroencephalography (EEG) revealed frequent discharges in the left frontal and central regions. Fabio A et al. [786] described a family with epilepsy caused by FFEVF due to *DEPDC5* mutation; two of these patients died suddenly and were diagnosed with unexplained sudden death after autopsy.

Development is usually normal during both birth and the neonatal period. Early development, intelligence, and cognition are usually normal, and mild intellectual disability and abnormalities, including autism spectrum disorders and behavioral disorders, have also been reported [92]. Neuroimaging studies may be normal or reveal focal cortical dysplasia.

Auxiliary Examination

An EEG shows normal background activity in most patients. However, 60–75% of patients have epileptiform discharges on EEG, mainly originating from the frontal lobe, temporal lobe, and central parietal lobe or occipital lobe; however, the origin of the EEG signal may be different for each affected individual in the same family. Epileptiform discharges can be exacerbated by sleep deprivation and sleep. There was no significant relationship between the epileptiform discharges on EEG and the clinical manifestations. Some patients still had significant epileptiform discharges on EEG for many years after the cessation of seizures, and 16–18% of their family members without seizures also had epileptiform discharges on EEG, suggesting that they may be carriers of the focal variant familial focal epilepsy gene. One of the important clinical features of this disease is the detection of epileptic discharges in family members without clinical seizures via routine EEG, which can be considered a genetic marker [92].

Diagnosis

FFEVF is a rare epilepsy syndrome characterized by focal seizures of different origins in different family members. Its clinical manifestations are consistent with the localization of EEG. In patients with generalized seizures but without focal seizures, EEG also suggests focal seizures. However, the patient's performance is fixed. The presence of epileptiform discharges on EEG in family members without clinical seizures may be a prominent feature of this disease. Interictal EEG abnormalities are more likely to be observed in sleep recordings [92, 776, 778].

Differential Diagnosis

FFEVF is easily confused with other monogenic hereditary epilepsies, especially autosomal nocturnal frontal lobe epilepsy and familial temporal lobe epilepsy, which require differential diagnosis.

FFEVF differs from other familial focal epilepsies. First, it is very rare, and, second, it has a very high penetrance, which may be related to the roles of genes and environmental occurrences. The absence of nocturnal clusters and transient motor seizures is the main distinguishing point from autosomal dominant nocturnal frontal lobe epilepsy. Epileptiform discharges may be found in patients with different origins of EEG signals and in patients without clinical seizures. A history of traumatic injury, febrile seizures, and hippocampal sclerosis are the key points in the differential diagnosis of familial mesial temporal lobe epilepsy. The affected patients have different origins according to EEG. The absence of obvious auditory hallucinations can be differentiated from lateral temporal lobe epilepsy with auditory hallucinations.

Treatment

FFEVF is a benign epilepsy, and 85–96% of cases respond well to traditional ASMs. It can be treated according to the general principles of epilepsy medication, and the broad-spectrum ASM agent valproic acid (VPA) may be the most effective. Some patients with *NPRL2* mutations respond well to vitamin B6 and TPM; however, 30% of patients still exhibit drug resistance. Epilepsy surgery can effectively relieve seizures in epilepsy patients, and death has also been reported [786].

5.4.3 Epilepsy with Auditory Features (EAF)

Overview

Epilepsy with auditory features (EAF) is a focal epilepsy syndrome that appears in adolescence/adulthood without any medical history and is characterized by focal onset with auditory symptoms and/or acquired aphasia. Patients rarely have focal to bilateral tonic–clonic seizures. Some patients have seizures induced by specific sounds. The syndrome was previously referred to as autosomal dominant lateral temporal lobe epilepsy and autosomal dominant partial epilepsy with auditory features. EAF may be a familial focal epilepsy syndrome, and familial EAF may be inherited in an autosomal dominant manner.

Historical Evolution and Epidemiological Investigation

Auditory symptoms are closely related to epilepsy, and the earliest description can be traced back to 1883 [787]. Auditory hallucinations can be simple (monotonous sounds, such as buzzing in tinnitus) or complex (hearing sounds or music); in these cases, auditory hallucinations can be defined as hallucinations. In 1995, on the basis of the first description of the genetic basis of SHE, Ottman et al. [788] published a study in which they found a linkage site on chromosome 10q related to focal epilepsy in 11 members of a large family showing autosomal dominant inheritance with high penetrance. Of the 11 members affected, 55% reported auditory symptoms. The first observation was confirmed in 1999 by Poza et al. [789], who described 19 individuals from Basque families with similar focal epilepsy, even in the case associated with chromosome 10q. However, these patients also exhibited other sensory symptoms, such as visual hallucinations, than did those in previous studies. Thus, a new term, "autosomal dominant lateral temporal lobe epilepsy (ADLTE)," was proposed for its anatomical origin rather than for medial temporal lobe epilepsy. Subsequently, Winawer et al. [790] further described the clinical condition of a family. The authors introduced an alternative name, autosomal dominant partial epilepsy with auditory features (ADPEAF), to emphasize the high prevalence of sudden auditory symptoms. In 2022, the ILAE Working Group proposed the term "EAF" to include ADLTE and ADPEAF and defined the genetic form as familial EAF (FEAF) through a position paper on the definition of epilepsy syndromes and new nomenclature [92].

Etiology

Most of these cases involve autosomal recessive inheritance. In 2002, Kalachikov et al. [791] discovered *LGI1*, the first pathogenic gene involved in ADLTE, on chromosome 10q24, which was a decisive turning point in the identification of ADLTE/ADPEAF. In particular, five different pathogenic *LGI1* variants were identified, three of which were frameshift variants, one was a missense variant, and the last was a splice site variant. *LGI1* mutations are also associated with temporal lobe epilepsy with aphasia seizures, suggesting that other manifestations should be considered in the phenotypic spectrum of temporal lobe epilepsy with auditory features. In 2015, pathogenic variants in a second gene, *RELN*, were identified in seven families, and other related genes, including *DEPDC5*, *MICAL-1*, *CNTNAP2*, and *SCN1A*, were subsequently identified [792].

Main Clinical Manifestations

Age of Onset and Sex

The prevalence of this syndrome is unknown. The age of seizure onset is usually between 10 and 30 years. No sex difference has been reported. The medical, birth, and neonatal histories are generally normal. A neurological examination is normal. Early developmental milestones and intelligence/cognition are usually normal.

Clinical Features

Focal sensory (auditory) and/or cognitive (acquired aphasia) seizures are obligatory symptoms of this syndrome. Auditory symptoms typically include simple unformed sounds (such as buzzing or ringing), less common auditory distortions (such as volume changes), or complex sounds (such as specific songs or sounds). Acute acquired aphasia is the inability to understand spoken language in the absence of a disturbance of consciousness. Other focal onset symptoms can also be present, including changes in vision (face/object deformation) and vertigo. Focal impaired consciousness and focal to bilateral tonic–clonic seizures (usually from sleep) may also occur. Some patients have reflex seizures that are triggered by sounds, such as a ringing telephone.

Auxiliary Examination

Interictal EEG is normal in most patients. If abnormalities are found, they are characterized by focal, often temporary, epileptiform discharges. EEGs may be activated by hyperventilation, sleep deprivation, and sleep. Neuroimaging is usually normal, but the cause of structural damage can rarely be identified.

Diagnosis and Differential Diagnosis

Diagnosis

The clinical diagnosis of EAF is based on the presence of the above clinical features, normal brain imaging (magnetic resonance imaging (MRI) or CT), and a family history of autosomal dominant inheritance. If other findings are inconclusive, molecular genetic testing is needed to confirm the diagnosis by identifying heterozygous pathogenic (or likely pathogenic) variants in LGI1, MICAL1, or RELN [793].

Differential Diagnosis

1. *FFEVF*: Although individuals in a family with FFEVF may present with seizures consistent with those of EAF, to diagnose FEAF, all affected individuals in the family must present with seizures consistent with those of EAF.
2. *Psychiatric disorders*: Auditory hallucinations can be easily distinguished from EAF hallucinations because mental auditory hallucinations are non-episodic and more complex in terms of presentation.
3. *Tinnitus*: This symptom is so common that it may appear coincidentally within the patient's family. The difference between tinnitus and focal sensory auditory episodes is that the duration of tinnitus in patients with peripheral auditory system disorders is usually longer.

Treatment

EAF is considered to be a focal epilepsy syndrome sensitive to ASMs, and CBZ monotherapy may be effective [764]. In drug-resistant patients, surgical treatment can be used. Another consideration is that discontinuation often leads to clinical relapse and does not always lead to retreatment. These issues should be emphasized when discussing treatment options with patients.

5.4.4 Epilepsy with Reading-Induced Seizures (EwRIS)

Overview

Epilepsy with reading-induced seizures (EwRIS) is a rare epilepsy syndrome characterized by reflexive myoclonic seizures triggered by language-related activities, especially reading, affecting orofacial muscles [92]. If reading continues, seizures may worsen with generalized tonic–clonic seizures. This special syndrome was once classified into the category of reflex epilepsy, but people later noted that the patient may have a family history of this disease; therefore, it was classified as idiopathic generalized epilepsy. In 2022, the new classification of epilepsy syndromes by the International League Against Epilepsy placed it into the category of generalized and focal seizures with multiple etiologies [92]. Most patients respond to drug treatment, and seizures can be reduced by avoiding precipitating factors. The overall prognosis of this syndrome is good.

Historical Evolution

Sequence-induced seizures were first discovered and described as epileptic syndrome by Bickford et al. [794] In 1981, Lorizio and Franciosi [795] reported the long-term follow-up results of two cases of reading epilepsy, which were considered to be reflex seizures. In 1989, the International League Against Epilepsy classified primary reading epilepsy into the category of partial idiopathic (age-dependent onset) epilepsy syndrome. In 1995, Radhakrishnan et al. [796] summarized the clinical characteristics of 20 patients, who attracted widespread attention. In 1998, Koutroumanidis et al. [797] summarized the clinical manifestations of 17 patients with variant reading epilepsy. In the same year, Wolf et al. [798] reported that these patients had a good response to VPA treatment, but the use of CBZ could aggravate these seizures, which enriched the related research. The latest classification of the International League Against Epilepsy in 2022 classified it as generalized or focal epilepsy syndrome with multiple etiologies [92].

Epidemiological Investigation

Because the prevalence of this type of epilepsy syndrome is very low, no epidemiological data are available.

Causes

The etiology is unclear, and a small number of patients have a family history, which is speculated to be related to genetic factors. Puteikis et al. [799] described 101 patients, of whom 30.8% had a family history of epilepsy, and Radhakrishnan et al. [796] described 20 patients with a family history of epilepsy, suggesting that genetic factors play an important role in the pathogenesis of epilepsy. However, the details are not clear.

Triggers and Possible Mechanisms

Reading is the main cause of epileptic seizures. The reading methods for inducing seizures include reading aloud and silent reading, which can be performed on the same patient. Reading can include paper books or materials, TV and computer screens, mobile phones, tablets, etc. It often appears when patients are staying up late, when they are reading complex materials, when they are reading small fonts, and when they are tired. It is often sporadic [92], but it is not the only precipitating factor. Radhakrishnan et al. [796] reported that 9 out of 20 patients had precipitating factors involving verbal or nonverbal high-level cognitive processes in addition to reading. The pathogenesis is unclear, and it may be that the cortical areas related to reading are sensitive and produce a highly excitatory state, which makes it easier for the cortex to respond to reading stimuli. Puteikis et al. [799] suggested that reading-induced seizures are an abnormal response to external or proprioceptive input to the cortical network supporting reading upregulation [92].

Clinical Manifestations

Age

Puteikis et al. [799] studied the clinical manifestations of 101 patients and reported that the average age of onset was 18.3 ± 7.9 years. Radhakrishnan et al. [796] reported on 20 patients whose onset age ranged from 10 to 46 years (median age 17.5 years). The onset ages of 17 patients studied by Koutroumanidis et al. [797] was 11–22 years (median age 15 years). Therefore, the range of onset age of patients with reading epilepsy is wide, and both childhood- and adulthood-onset may occur; however, the incidence in adults is much greater than that in children.

Sex

Although it can occur in both sexes, the syndrome of reading epilepsy is more common in males. Among the 100 patients identified by Puteikis et al. [799], 67 (66.3%) were male and 34 (33.7%) were female.

Seizures

1. *Seizures*: The main manifestation of epileptic seizures is low-amplitude myoclonus affecting the face, pharynx, and masseter muscles [92]. Puteikis et al. [799] reported 68 cases (67.3%) of orofacial reflex myoclonus in 101 patients and that these patients had no obvious disturbance of consciousness during seizures. However, some patients described a "light bulb turning on/off," a feeling of interrupted thinking, being stuck in the current sentence and not being able to move on, or not knowing where to read and thus having to start again. These phenomena may be related to the severity of motor symptoms. The accompanying stuttering can be explained by perioral spasms or tonic activity that prevents articulation, and it is also possible that it is related to transient cognitive dysfunction. In a small number of patients, orofacial myoclonus can extend to the upper limbs. Continuing reading can lead to secondary generalized tonic–clonic seizures (GTCSs). Some patients also had juvenile myoclonic epilepsy, manifested as episodic myoclonus in the

morning, showing overlap between reading epilepsy and juvenile myoclonic epilepsy. This overlap suggests that cortical hyperexcitability is more widespread in these patients than in those with pure reading- or language-induced seizures.

2. *Other manifestations*: In 101 patients described by Puteikis et al. [799], in addition to orofacial reflex myoclonus; visual, sensory, or cognitive symptoms; non-orofacial myoclonic seizures; and absence seizures were observed.

Others

The medical, birth, and neonatal histories are generally normal. Here, development and cognition are normal. A neurological examination is normal.

Auxiliary Examination

EEG background activity is normal. There may be no interictal epileptiform discharges. During myoclonic seizures, EEG may reveal transient epileptiform discharges, which can manifest as focal or generalized epileptiform discharges or slow activity. Local EEG abnormalities occur more frequently in the left (dominant hemisphere) midline, left frontotemporal region, and other regions and can also be manifested on the right (nondominant side) or even both sides. The myoclonus of the mandible appears 30–35 ms after the epileptiform discharges on EEG, and focal discharges in the temporoparietal region also appear, suggesting that these regions play important roles in language output and reading epilepsy. Radhakrishnan et al. [796] performed EEG examinations on 20 patients, and the results showed that 12 of them (60%) had abnormal interictal EEG signals, 75% had generalized symmetric ictal EEG signals, and only 2 had focal (temporoparietal) discharge.

Neuroimaging studies are normal. If the clinical presentation is atypical, imaging should be considered to rule out a structural cause. PET hypometabolism appears bilaterally in the occipito-temporal cortex, with a left predominance, or only in the left temporo-occipital cortex. It may also appear in frontal/orbitofrontal locations, suggesting that reading epilepsy may involve a wider network.

Diagnosis

The necessary criterion for the diagnosis of reading epilepsy is reflex myoclonic seizures affecting the orofacial muscles triggered by reading/language-related tasks [92]. The patient has a normal developmental status, and interictal neurological examination and imaging abnormalities are generally not present. According to the International League Against Epilepsy, clinicians should be cautious when diagnosing reading epilepsy when the patient has myoclonic convulsions affecting the upper limbs and when the age of onset is more than 20 years. If all seizure types, except generalized tonic–clonic seizures are present and the EEG background slows down, the diagnosis of reading epilepsy can be excluded [92].

Differential Diagnosis

1. *Nonepileptic stuttering*: Nonepileptic stuttering is characterized by involuntary repetition and prolongation of sounds, syllables, words, or phrases as well as

involuntary silence and pauses during which the person is unable to produce a sound.

2. *Juvenile myoclonic epilepsy (JME)*: In reading epilepsy, myoclonus is all or almost all (i.e., 80–90%) related to reading or language and is limited to the jaw. In JME, myoclonus occurs spontaneously, affects the upper limbs, is more common in the morning, and elicits photosensitive paroxysmal responses on EEG.

Treatment

Although the overall prognosis of primary reading epilepsy is good and spontaneous remission may occur within 3 years of onset, most patients still require antiepileptic drugs to control seizures. Radhakrishnan et al. [796] followed up with 20 patients and reported that only 3 achieved remission without medication. Other patients require antiepileptic drugs to control their seizures.

The most commonly used clinical drug is VPA, and most patients respond well to this treatment. Only a small number of patients need to use other ASM agents; levetiracetam (LEV) and clonazepam (CZP) are optional drugs [796, 798, 800]. It has been reported that CBZ may aggravate reading seizures, so caution should be exercised when prescribing CBZ.

Prognosis

Patients with reading epilepsy have a good prognosis, and it has been confirmed that there is no trend toward deterioration of the syndrome during long-term follow-up [798].

5.4.5 Progressive Myoclonic Epilepsy

Overview

Traditionally, an epileptic syndrome is defined as a unique phenomenon with a specific etiology, pathogenesis, clinical and EEG features, and treatments that differ from those of other disorders. ILAE refers to a group of epilepsies with typical clinical and electroencephalographic features and specific etiological findings (structural, genetic, metabolic, immune, and infectious), the diagnosis of which is often prognostic and therapeutic, as epileptic syndromes [92, 801–803]. Progressive myoclonic epilepsy (PME) is an epileptic syndrome classified by ILAE as developmental or epilepsy-associated encephalopathy (DAE). In DAEs, a specific disorder causes developmental and functional brain dysfunction as well as epilepsy-induced brain damage [92, 801–803].

PMEs are a group of genetically heterogeneous disorders that commonly present with myoclonic and generalized tonic–clonic seizures as well as neurological deterioration, such as dementia and ataxia. They can develop at any age but typically appear during late childhood or adolescence. Genetic defects that characterize the majority of patients have been identified. These include Unverricht–Lundborg disease (ULD), Lafora disease (LD), various forms of neuronal ceroid lipofuscinoses, myoclonic epilepsy with ragged red fibers (MERRF), and sialidosis types I and II [92, 803].

Classification of Progressive Myoclonic Epilepsy
The ILAE Working Group's methodology identifies PME as primarily consisting of ULD, Lafora disease, neuronal ceroid lipofuscinosis (NCL), mitochondrial disorders (MERRF, polymerase gamma (POLG)-related disorders, MELAS (mitochondrial encephalomyopathy, lactic acidosis, and stroke-like episodes)), and sialidosis. Additionally, less common causes include Niemann–Pick disease type C, dentate erythropoietic glaucomatous atrophy, and juvenile Huntington's disease. The following diseases and conditions are mentioned: action myoclonus–renal failure syndrome, juvenile neuroaxonal dystrophy, pantothenic acid kinase-associated neurodegeneration, neuroserine protease inhibitor inclusion body disease, leukoencephalopathy with leukoencephalomalacia, early-onset Alzheimer's disease, pathogenic variants of GOSR2, myoclonic epilepsy in Down's syndrome, GM2 gangliosiderosis, tetrahydrobiopterin deficiency, noninfantile neuronal disease, Goshen disease, and celiac disease. Most of these conditions are associated with inherited metabolic disorders and require genetic testing for diagnosis and determination of their cause [92, 801–803].

Clinical Characteristics of Different Types of PMEs
Unverricht–Lundborg Disease (ULD)

Unverricht–Lundborg disease (ULD) is also known as epilepsy with progressive myoclonic or Baltic myoclonic epilepsy due to its initial case reports from Europe, particularly the Baltic region, and North Africa [301].

ULD is a neurodegenerative disorder that is autosomal recessive and typically presents with stimulus-sensitive myoclonic and tonic–clonic seizures between the ages of 6 and 16. Several years after the onset of seizures, patients may experience ataxia, intentional tremors, and dysarthria. Over time, mood instability, depression, and mild intellectual decline may also occur [803].

Historical Evolution

In 1949, Van Bogaert [804] described the existence of ULD and named it myoclonic epilepsy. In 1950, Caron and Michel [805] noted its familial features, followed by Wohlfart and Hook [806], who summarized its clinical features, drawing significant attention from their peers. In 1955, Kelly and Laurence [807] explored the use of mephenesin (methylphenidate) to treat ULD. In 1967, Anraku [808] described the pathological changes associated with ULD. Later, Iatsuk and Samoĭlov [809] analyzed 40 patients with Kozhevnikov syndrome, 24 with Sokolianskiĭ–Kliuchikov syndrome, 6 with cerebellar myoclonic ataxia, and 10 with ULD, proposing differential diagnostic criteria. In 2022, the International League Against Epilepsy Working Group classified epileptic syndromes as developmental and epileptic encephalopathies of different ages of onset, providing authoritative annotations and advancing their normative application [92]. In 2023, Acharya and Acharya [801] summarized the clinical features of familial adult myoclonic epilepsy (FAME) and proposed a method for differentiating it from ULD to improve diagnosis and management.

Epidemiology

In 2014, Franceschetti et al. [810] collected data on 204 patients with myoclonic epilepsy at 25 Italian epilepsy centers, 77 of whom were diagnosed with ULD, 37 with Lafora disease, 31 with PME due to rare genetic factors (mainly neuronal ceroid lipofuscinoses), and 2 with celiac disease. Despite extensive investigations, no clear cause was found in 57 patients. In 2022, Sipilä et al. [811] published a Finnish population-based epidemiological survey of ULD, which identified 135 patients (54% female) with EPM1, 105 of whom were alive (prevalence 1.91/100,000 people). The age-standardized (European Standard Population 2013) incidence was 1.53/100,000 people. The mean age at disease onset was 9.4 ± 2.3 years (7.0–14.6 years, no sex difference). The median age at death among the 34 patients was 53.9 years, with no difference between the sexes. Lower respiratory tract infections were the immediate causes of death. The risk of death decreased with increasing age of onset, suggesting that ULD, although rare in Finland, is still more prevalent and severe than elsewhere worldwide.

Clinical Manifestations

In a report by Muccioli et al. [812], the main clinical manifestations of a patient with genetically confirmed ULD were myoclonus, generalized tonic–clonic seizures, intellectual disability, ataxia, and dysarthria. The patient's myoclonus and gait disorders significantly improved with alcohol consumption. Tandon et al. [813] investigated three patients with ULD. The main manifestations were noise- or touch-induced myoclonus, ataxia, and cognitive decline. Seizures with myoclonus, ataxia due to impaired potassium metabolism, cognitive dysfunction, and autosomal recessive inheritance are the most prominent clinical manifestations of ULD.

1. *Epileptic seizures*: Van Bogaert [814] summarized the characteristics of epileptic seizures in ULD patients. Myoclonus is the most common type of epileptic seizure in ULD and is triggered by tactile or light stimulation. It is usually more pronounced upon waking up and can be exacerbated by phenytoin administration. Hypponen et al. [815] summarized the characteristics of epileptic myoclonic seizures in ULD patients. The myoclonus is aggravated by activity and disappears at rest. It is usually regular and of short duration. In addition to myoclonic seizures, patients may also experience absence seizures and generalized tonic–clonic seizures. In the study by Bosak et al. [816] comprising 16 patients, myoclonus was identified as the primary manifestation of ULD. Similarly, Lasek-Bal et al. [817] reported that 11 of their ULD patients mainly presented with generalized tonic–clonic seizures and myoclonus, which resulted in 91% of these patients being unable to move independently.
2. *Cognitive dysfunction*: Äikiä et al. [818] assessed the intelligence, verbal memory, executive function, and psychomotor functioning of 68 patients with genetically verified ULD. Compared with 46 healthy volunteers, 49% of these patients

had verbal IQs below the average range and their performance was worse than that of the control group in immediate and delayed story recall, suggesting that there were impairments in executive function and psychomotor speed.

3. *Comorbidities in ULD*: Tandon and Pradhan [813] reported 3 patients with ULD, all of whom exhibited autistic features. Sipilä and Kälviäinen [802] conducted a study on comorbidities in 135 ULD patients with a mean follow-up of 31.4 years. This study revealed that 107 patients (79%) developed at least 1 comorbidity and 53 patients (39%) exhibited ≥3 comorbidities. This study also revealed that the most prevalent comorbidities among the patients were trauma; psychiatric and behavioral disorders; and endocrine, nutritional, and metabolic disorders. Additionally, depression was observed in 13% of the patients, indicating the need for specific attention to their needs.

Ancillary Examinations

1. *Electroencephalographic manifestations*: In a study conducted by Gargouri-Berrechid et al. [819], 47 electroencephalogram (EEG) signals were analyzed across 17 patients. The results showed that 30 EEGs (64%) were normal, 17 (36%) had slowed background activity, and 11 (23%) were abnormal. Epileptiform abnormalities were found in 22 EEGs (47%). Myoclonus was recorded in 13 EEGs (28%), and all of them improved after appropriate antiseizure medication treatment.
2. *Genetic testing*: Hosny et al. [820] retrospectively analyzed the genetic sequences of 20 patients with a diagnosis of ULD from 13 unrelated families and confirmed the occurrence of *EPM1* repeat amplification in 14 patients from 8 families (frequency 70%).

Diagnosis

ILAE's diagnosis of ULD emphasizes the presence of generalized myoclonic seizures and diffuse epileptiform discharges on EEG as well as cognitive dysfunction and motor deficits in the early stages of life, which stabilize in adulthood. Genetic testing has shown that 90% of patients have EPM1 abnormalities [92]. Silvennoinen et al. [821] proposed that the diagnosis of EPM1-ULD can be confirmed by identifying the causative mutation in the cysteine protease inhibitor cysteine protease inhibitor B (*CSTB*) gene.

Lafora Disease (LD)

Lafora disease (LD), also known as Lafora microsomia, is a rare form of PME. It is caused by mutations in the *EPM2A* and *EPM2B* (*NHLRC1*) genes and is more prevalent in Southern Europe, Central Asia, South Asia, and North Africa. LD typically begins in adolescence, with onset occurring between the ages of 6 and 19 years (peak: 14–16 years). Before onset, patient neurological function is typically normal and a few patients have a history of febrile or nonfebrile convulsions. In the early stages of the disease, symptoms may include headache, decreased academic performance, depression, and apathy [822, 823]. As the disease progresses, patients may experience rapidly progressing dementia with refractory or super-refractory status epilepticus, myoclonus, cerebellar ataxia, or dysarthria. Death usually occurs years after the first symptoms, and the most common causes of death are status epilepticus and respiratory failure [824].

Historical Evolution, Etiology, and Epidemiology

First reported in 1911 by Lafora and Glueck [825], the global prevalence of this disease is close to 4/1000,000, and it is more common in the Mediterranean, North Africa, the Middle East, and regions where consanguineous marriages are practiced. Currently, more than 100 pathogenic mutations involving 2 genes, *EPM2A* (6q24) and *EPM2B/NHLRC1* (6p22.3), have been identified in association with more than 90% of LD patients [823, 826]. Turnbull et al. preliminarily demonstrated that mutations of a third gene, *PRDM8* (4q21.21), are associated with a new type of early-onset LD [827].

Lafora disease is a rare condition, and, as such, investigations of its incidence, natural regression, and prognostic factors have been limited. To date, single-center cohort studies have been virtually impossible due to the rarity of this disease. In 2021, Pondrelli et al. [828] conducted a meta-analysis of 73 papers that included 298 patients with Lafora disease. Their study revealed that the mean age of onset was 13.4 years (SD 3.7) and that only 9.1% of the patients were aged 18 years or older. Their study also revealed that the 5-year survival rate of the 272 patients was 93% (95% CI = 89–96), the 10-year survival rate was 62% (95% CI = 54–69), and the 15-year survival rate was 57% (95% CI = 49–65). The median survival time was 11 years. Additionally, 45% (95% CI = 36–55) of the 110 patients experienced loss of self-care ability at 5 years and 75% (95% CI = 66–84) experienced this loss at 10 years. The negative prognostic factors included Asian origin and onset age <18 years, while mutant gene type and onset symptoms were not associated with survival.

Clinical Presentation

1. *Seizures*: Seizures are important clinical manifestations of LD. Half of the patients experience onset with focal seizures, so they are mostly diagnosed with epilepsy in the early stage; they develop epilepsy progressively over a few months, accompanied by the appearance of myoclonus and generalized tonic–clonic seizures. Seizures can be triggered or exacerbated by noise, fright, agitation, unexpected tactile stimuli, or some kind of sustained activity and even develop into a series of myoclonus with secondary generalized convulsions accompanied by loss of consciousness [823].

    1. Generalized tonic–clonic seizures are common clinical manifestations and are often the first symptom in patients with Lafora disease, accounting for 35.7% and 50% of patients with two gene mutations in *EPM2A* and *EPM2B*, respectively.
    2. Following generalized tonic–clonic seizures, visual seizures are often the next symptom and occur in approximately 18% of cases. These seizures are characterized by transient blindness and simple or complex visual hallucinations.

3. Myoclonus is a common clinical manifestation in LD patients, although it is not often the first symptom. It is more prevalent in patients with *EPM2A* mutations than in those with *EPM2B* mutations (14.3% vs. 6.3%). Myoclonus is most frequently observed in a quiet state and can be triggered by mood swings, physical activity, and light stimuli. As the disease progresses, myoclonus remains asymmetric and segmental but may persist.
4. Additionally, secondary bilateral tonic–clonic seizures are often the first symptom in LD patients.

2. *Cognitive dysfunction*: As the disease progresses, patients develop impaired speech, altered muscle tone, cerebellar ataxia, and cognitive dysfunction. Before the onset of myoclonus and epileptic seizures, some patients may exhibit irritability, eccentricity, and progressive cognitive decline. Nomani et al. [829] reported a case of delayed diagnosis in a 17-year-old girl who presented with intractable epileptic seizures and progressive cognitive impairment. She was later confirmed to have Lafora disease through a skin biopsy. Skin biopsy is recommended for definitive diagnosis in individuals with intractable myoclonus and rapidly progressive cognitive impairment. d'Orsi et al. [830] studied the characteristics of the late stage of Lafora disease and reported that neurological symptoms further deteriorated. All five patients were bedridden and had severe psychocognitive deficits (Montreal Cognitive Assessment (MoCA) <10). The main difference between Lafora disease and ULD is early cognitive decline and rapid progression of PME.
3. *Visual impairment and retinal changes*: LD patients often present with visual impairment in its early stages. Heitkotter et al. [831] reported that retinal thickness was reduced in two patients with a history of seizures but remained normal in one asymptomatic patient. Orsini et al. [832] used full-field electroretinogram to evaluate the function of retinal cones and rod cells in Italian LD patients. This study revealed linear correlations between disease stage and the degree of cone and rod cell dysfunction and between the type of mutation and dysfunction of cone and rod cells.
4. *Progression and comorbidities of Lafora disease*: Gómez-Abad [833] showed that patients with *NHLRC1* mutations had a slightly longer disease course than did those with *EPM2A* mutations. Franceschetti et al. [834] noted that the clinical phenotypic variability associated with *NHLRC 1* mutations is large and includes patients with mild or severe outcomes. Baykan [835] described a Turkish family with LD carrying a pure *D146N* mutation that progressed slowly (three out of four subjects were followed for more than 10 years). Ferlazzo et al. [836] described the clinical, neurophysiological, and genetic characteristics of a series of Italian patients with LD to determine the differential features of those with slow progression. Twenty-three patients with LD were included (17 females and 6 males). The mean age at onset was 14.5 ± 3.9 years, and the mean age at follow-up was 13.2 ± 8.0 years. There were 18 *NHLRC1* mutations and 5 *EPM2A* mutations. Six of the 23 patients had mild disease, with a delayed onset, lower

neurological dysfunction scores at 4 years after onset, and milder myoclonic seizures. Patients with mild LD had *NHLRC1* mutations and 5 out of the 6 patients carried pure or compound heterozygous *D146N* mutations, which are not typically found in LD patients. According to d'Orsi et al. [830], patients with LD may experience malnutrition, dysphagia, aspiration pneumonia, acute respiratory failure with tracheotomy, sepsis, and decubitus ulcers in the late stages of the disease. Therefore, a multidisciplinary medical and nursing team, including epileptologists/neurologists, gastroenterologists, infectious disease physicians, surgeons, ENTs, and anesthesiologists, should be involved in the prevention and treatment of multiple complications. Oksel et al. [837] described the case of a 6-year-old boy with third-degree atrioventricular block and dementia who was eventually diagnosed with LD.

Ancillary Examinations

Routine laboratory tests for blood analysis, biochemical analysis, and cerebrospinal fluid analysis often yield normal results.

1. *EEG*: At onset, the EEG background appears normal, and low-frequency, light-stimulation- induced spiking slow-wave and polyspike discharges may be present during the interictal period. In contrast to juvenile myoclonus epilepsy (JME), generalized epileptiform discharges are not activated during sleep. However, focal epileptiform discharge activation in the posterior head may be present [92]. Patients with Lafora disease may present with irregular myoclonus without correlation with EEG signals, which distinguishes it from JME. As the disease progresses, there is a noticeable increase in irregular spiking in the occipital lobe on the EEG, both in a generalized and focal manner. Additionally, there is an increase in interictal discharge during sleep. This form of EEG evolution is suggestive of the diagnosis of LD. In the late stage of the disease, there is further slowing of background activity, disappearance of the sleep physiological cycle, and visible full-conductance 4–6-Hz high-amplitude irregular spikes and polyspikes. Flash stimulation can induce spike bursts and myoclonic seizures.
2. *Genetic testing*: LD is a genetic disorder caused by mutations in the *EPM2A* and *NHLRC1* genes, which encode the laforin and malin proteins, respectively. Both laforin and malin act on glycogen to maintain its solubility in the central nervous system. Mutations in these genes result in abnormal storage of insoluble glycogen in the brain, leading to the formation of Lafora vesicles. A study of 250 families with LD revealed that 42% of cases were caused by *EPM2A* mutations, while 58% were caused by *EPM2B* mutations. Pathogenic variants include missense mutations, nonsense mutations, splice site mutations, and small intragenic deletions and insertion mutations that result in loss of function [838]. Riva et al. [839] demonstrated that patients with *NHLRC1* mutations tend to have a milder clinical course, with later onset and slower progression, than patients with *EPM2A* mutations.
3. *Imaging*: Cranial MRI findings appear to be mostly normal, while MRS may indicate a significant decrease in the *N*-acetylaspartate/creatine ratio in the fron-

tal cortex, basal ganglia, and cerebellar hemispheres [840]. ^{18}-Ffludeoxyglucose positron emission tomography (FDG-PET) may reveal widespread regional reduction in glucose metabolism [841].

4. *Pathological manifestations*: Pathologic manifestations are characterized by the presence of intracellular inclusion bodies (Lafora vesicles) that stain positive for PAS. These inclusion bodies are found in various organs, including the kidneys, heart, liver, muscles, skin, and central nervous system.

Diagnosis

ILAE emphasizes early and rapidly progressive cognitive, visual, and motor decline in the diagnosis of LD. Most deaths occur within 10 years of onset, and focal seizures with visual symptoms are often an early feature. Laforin (*EPM2A*) causative gene variants account for 70% of the cases, malin (*EPM2B*) causative gene variants account for 27% of the cases, and 3% are not found to have a causative gene. Lafora vesicles are observed in sweat gland cells or other tissues. The main difference between LD and ULD is the early cognitive decline and rapid progression of PME.

Clinical Features of Other Types of PMEs

1. *Sialidosis*: Sialidosis is a rare autosomal recessive lysosomal storage disease. It was first described by Cantz et al. [842] in 1977 and was later named "cherry erythema-myoclonus syndrome" by Lowden and O'Brien [843] in 1979. Type I is a less severe, late-onset form of the disease, also known as "cherry erythema-myoclonus syndrome." It has an incidence of approximately 1/200,000 people. Patients typically present with myoclonus, visual impairment, and ataxia between the ages of 20 and 30. Sialidosis is a disease that progresses slowly and does not cause developmental regression or malformations. A definitive diagnosis of sialidosis is made when mutations in the *NEU1* gene are detected through genetic testing or when laboratory tests reveal neuraminidase deficiency. Type II has an earlier onset and more severe clinical presentation, with a prevalence of 1/250,000–2,000,000. The condition is characterized by malformations such as barrel chest, spinal deformities, and skeletal abnormalities as well as cognitive impairment. The age of onset can range from infancy to teenage years. Clinical features include myoclonus, rough facial features, clouding of the cornea, hepatomegaly, and cherry erythema of the retina [844].

   EEG signals of these patients indicate low-amplitude fast activity. Massive myoclonus is associated with strings of positive spikes at 10–20 Hz that appeared prior to EMG. Cranial MRI is normal in the early stages, with progressive atrophy of the cerebellum, pons, and cerebral cortex as the disease progresses. According to Lai et al. [845], 17 Taiwanese patients were diagnosed with sialidosis type I and cherry erythema on the fundus was detected in only 3 patients, while myoclonus, ataxia, and epilepsy all appeared within 5 years. Sialidosis type I commonly causes progressive visual loss through retinopathy and optic neuropathy. The authors [845] also reported that 94.1% of patients had abnormalities in visual evoked potentials (VEPs), which suggests that VEPs are an early diagnostic tool for visual impairment in this disorder.

2. *NCL*: NCL is a neurogenetic disorder associated with lysosomal storage. Clinical manifestations include myoclonus, visual impairment, developmental regression, dementia, and ataxia. EEG findings reveal slowed background activity in 95% of the patients and widespread epileptiform discharges in 80% of the patients. Additionally, somatosensory-evoked potentials are present in approximately one-quarter of patients. Cranial MRI demonstrates cerebral cortex and cerebellar atrophy. Nerve conduction tests confirm neuroaxonal degeneration in approximately 30% of patients. Skin or lymphocyte biopsy can reveal autofluorescent lipofuscin deposits within neuronal or glial cell lysosomes, including osmiophilic granules, curvilinear bodies, fingerprint bodies, rectilinear bodies, and mixed deposits in the brain, interosseous plexus, muscle, and skin.

   Based on the age of onset, NCL includes infantile, late infantile, adolescent, and adult types. The infantile type often starts at 1 year of age with intellectual and motor development regression, followed by myoclonic seizures and other forms of seizures. Blindness due to retinal atrophy and continuous deterioration of the disease occur, with the majority of children dying before the age of 10 years [846]. The late infantile type most often starts at 3 years of age and features refractory epilepsy, myoclonus, hypotonia and ataxia, and progressive intellectual and motor regression. Most patients die in adolescence due to aspiration pneumonia, and a few survive until 40 years of age. The adolescent type starts with visual impairment at 4–10 years of age. Most often, blindness at 10–20 years of age, milder myoclonus, tonic–clonic seizures, behavioral and psychosomatic problems, progressive dementia, extrapyramidal symptoms, and death at approximately 8 years after disease onset may occur. Adults have dementia, ataxia, and extrapyramidal symptoms as the first symptoms, and myoclonus develops at approximately 30 years of age, with normal vision. The new NCL classification system considers both the genotype and the age of disease onset, and there are 14 subtypes of NCL that can correspond to different clinical phenotypes.

3. *Neurological Gaucher's disease*: Neurologic Gaucher's disease, also known as Gaucher's disease, is a lysosomal storage disorder. Type I patients may present with multisystemic symptoms involving the liver, spleen, and bone marrow but not typically involving the nervous system. Types II and III, on the other hand, involve neurological symptoms, with varying ages of onset and rates of progression but no absolute boundaries. Type III can result in severe neurological damage, such as abnormal horizontal gaze, generalized seizures, convulsive seizures, progressive dementia, and ataxia and is classified as a PME phenotype. Gaucher's disease is caused by a mutation in the *GD1* gene, which encodes a lysosomal glucocerebrosidase [847]. Its pathology involves extensive deposition of macrophages that phagocytose lysosomal glucocerebrosides.

4. *Niemann–Pick disease*: Niemann–Pick disease is classified into three types: type A is characterized by acute neurological symptoms in the early stages, with large amounts of sphingomyelin deposits in the viscera and brain; type B is predominantly characterized by chronic visceral involvement; and type C is characterized by chronic neurological impairment and chronic visceral sphingomyelin deposits [848]. The incidence rate of type C Niemann–Pick disease is approximately 1/1,500,000–1/1,200,000 in Western European countries and 1/15,000–1/12,000 in China [848]. The clinical features of this disease include vertical supranuclear gaze palsy, dysarthria, dysphagia, cerebellar ataxia, seizures, progressive dementia, and dystonia, with retinal cherry erythema. Myoclonus is rare, and a small number of people die from persistent epileptic states. Type C Niemann–Pick syndrome is an autosomal recessive disorder caused by mutations in either the *NPC1* gene, which is located at 18q11.2 (found in 95% of families), or the *NPC2* gene, which is located at 14q24.3. This disease is characterized by the excessive deposition of cholesterol and sphingolipids in lysosomes. Its pathology is characterized by the presence of numerous foam cells containing lipids, known as "Niemann–Pick cells," found in mononuclear macrophages throughout the body and nervous system.
5. *Action myoclonus–renal failure syndrome*: Andermann et al. [849] first described this condition in 1986, with clinical features including progressively worsening myoclonus, ataxia, dysarthria, and renal failure. There is significant gene–phenotype heterogeneity, and only neurologic or renal impairment may manifest in patients carrying the same mutation in one family line. Seizures are relatively infrequent and easily controlled during the course of the disease. Most patients present with proteinuria and glomerulosclerosis before puberty or at the time of neurological onset. Death can occur due to renal failure or neurogenic respiratory failure. It is autosomal recessive and caused by mutations in the *SCARB2* gene. This gene is localized at 4q21.1. This gene encodes a lysosomal membrane type 2 protein, a member of the CD36 scavenger receptor protein family involved in the translocation of β-glycosylphosphatidylinositol enzymes from the endoplasmic reticulum to the lysosome [850].
6. *North Sea progressive myoclonic epilepsy*: North Sea progressive myoclonic epilepsy is a disease first described by Corbett et al. [851] in 2010. Its name is derived from the location of the index patient's family near the north coast. The clinical features of this disease include ataxia, loss of reflexes, and elevated serum creatine kinase levels at approximately 2 years of age. Myoclonic and epileptic seizures typically occur at approximately 6 years of age, with scoliosis developing during adolescence. Patients are unable to walk independently between the ages of 10 and 20 years, although some cognitive function may be preserved until the late stages of the disease. The gene responsible for these findings is *GOSR2*, which encodes the Golgi SNAP receptor complex 2. This complex is responsible for mediating Golgi vesicle transport. All the described patients had a missense mutation at position c.430G>T in the

GOSR2 gene. This mutation results in the inability of the GOSR2 protein to localize to the *cis*-Golgi.
7. *MERRF*: MERRF is a mitochondrial syndrome associated with point mutations in mitochondrial DNA [852]. The four "classic" features of MERRF include myoclonus, generalized epilepsy, cerebellar ataxia, and fragmented red fibers in muscle biopsies [853]. The onset of this disease usually occurs in childhood and early adulthood, but adult onset is not uncommon. Other common presentations include hearing loss, short stature, optic atrophy, and cardiomyopathy with Wolff–Parkinson–White syndrome [854].

Treatment of Progressive Myoclonic Seizures
Treatment for PME focuses on controlling seizures and myoclonus as well as providing palliative, supportive, and rehabilitative care. While the initial response to treatment may be relatively favorable, seizures may become more frequent and progressive neurological decline may occur.

Etiological Treatment

Currently, treatment options are available only for infantile CLN2-related late-onset neuronal wax-like lipofuscinosis. It is important to note that these treatments are specific to the disease and are not applicable to other conditions. Cerliponase alfa (Brineura®) contains the active ingredient cerliponase alfa, which is a recombinant form of human tripeptidyl peptidase 1 (TPP1). This treatment is specifically designed for patients with CLN2-related PME and is administered through intracerebroventricular infusion every other week at a dosage of 300 mg. The FDA approved its use in 2017 for children aged ≥3 years in the United States and for patients of all ages in the EU. Clinical trials are currently underway to determine the long-term efficacy of this therapy. It is important to note that this is one of the most expensive therapies approved by the FDA, costing approximately $702,000 per year.

In addition, enzyme replacement and substrate reduction therapies have been used to treat Gaucher's disease type 1 [855] but are ineffective at treating the neurological damage caused by Gaucher's disease type 2 [856, 857]. Splenectomy is indicated for patients with giant spleen due to hypersplenism who are older than 5 years of age and is recommended for patients with type I and some type III Gaucher's disease to prevent splenic rupture and to improve symptoms of hemorrhage and infection. Although supplementation with coenzyme Q10 and carnitine has been proposed for MERRF patients, there is no evidence from clinical studies that these treatments can alter the course of the disease or help control epilepsy [858]. Research on mitochondria-targeted gene therapy is ongoing [859]. Research on the accelerated degradation and reduced synthesis of Lafora vesicles through antisense oligonucleotides, RNA interference, genome engineering, small molecule therapies, and virus-mediated gene replacement is ongoing [823]. Gene therapy for ULD is under investigation [860]. There is no specific treatment for sialidosis.

Antiseizure Medications (ASMs)

Although seizures in PMEs, such as generalized tonic–clonic seizures, usually respond to ASMs, myoclonic seizures are often difficult to control. The efficacy of ASMs for treating seizures in PME patients appears to be syndrome-independent, i.e., medications effective at controlling myoclonic seizures in patients with LD may also be effective at controlling seizures in patients with ULD. However, some ASMs may exacerbate MERRF [861].

1. *Sodium valproate*: Sodium valproate is usually the drug of choice and the first line of treatment for myoclonic seizures in children and adults because it is a broad-spectrum ASM, with a recommended average daily dose of 250–1500 mg. However, it is contraindicated for patients with myoclonus associated with mitochondrial disease [861].
2. *Benzodiazepines (BDZs)*: Benzodiazepines (BDZs), mainly clonazepam (CZP) and clobazam (CLB), are used to treat myoclonic seizures in children and adults by binding to the gamma subunit of the GABAA receptor and enhancing GABAergic inhibition CZP is the only FDA-approved single-agent treatment for myoclonic seizures. The average doses of CZP and CLB are 3–6 mg/day and 10 mg/day, respectively. In adults with PME, drugs such as clonazepam and phenobarbital are more effective than phenytoin sodium and carbamazepine [862].
3. *Perampanel*: Assenza et al. [863] reported the effectiveness of perampanel in the treatment of epileptic myoclonus and seizures in 11 patients with epilepsy, 5 with ULD, 3 with LD, 2 with sialidosis, and 1 with an undetermined type of PME. Myoclonus and associated disability improved in 9 of the 11 patients (2 LD patients did not improve), and action myoclonus improved significantly in more than half of the 104 patients with myoclonus who were treated with perampanel and analyzed in the systematic evaluation. Compared with other more severe myoclonus, ULD appears to have the best clinical response to perampanel, with a significant reduction in the number of active seizures in all patients. The authors concluded that perampanel had beneficial effects on the treatment of myoclonus, disability, and seizures and that it was well-tolerated in patients with PME. Saito et al. [864] described the case of a 49-year-old male with severe bronchial asthma attack, resulting in cardiopulmonary arrest due to the development of Lance–Adams syndrome (LAS) with significant myoclonus, which was highly responsive to treatment with perampanel, and they concluded that perampanel should be considered for the treatment of extremely refractory myoclonus due to LAS.

   Oi et al. [865] described a 32-year-old female patient who had been experiencing myoclonic and generalized tonic–clonic seizures since the age of 9 and was diagnosed with ULD by genetic analysis. Despite multiple antiepileptic medications used to control her seizures, her cortical myoclonus remained intractable and severely affected her daily life activities. On admission, she presented with mild cognitive dysfunction, dysarthria, severe postural and motor myoclonus of the extremities, severe motor coordination disorder, inability to stand and walk independently, and severe phobias. The administration of perampanel at an initial dose of 1 mg/day, which was increased to 2 mg/day after 16 days, resulted in a significant improvement in myoclonus and a reduction in phobias within 30 days of initiation. In addition, the abnormal release of short-latency somatosensory-evoked potentials induced by median nerve stimulation was substantially reduced, suggesting a decrease in abnormal cortical hyperexcitability primarily in the primary sensorimotor cortex. Perampanel was found to be an effective drug for the treatment of refractory cortical myoclonus, even at small doses.

4. *Brivaracetam*: Ben-Menachem et al. [866] treated 94 patients with ULD at 100 mg/day and reported seizure-free rates of 22.2% and 15.8% at 6 and 12 months, respectively. The authors concluded that brivaracetam was well-tolerated as a long-term adjunctive therapy for patients with ULD, with improvement in focal seizure frequency over time.
5. Several novel ASM agents, including levetiracetam (LEV), topiramate, zonisamide, and clobazam [867–871], have been shown to be effective in some studies. LEV has been recommended as a first-line therapy for myoclonic seizures at a dose of 1000–3000 mg per day, and a retrospective and observational study of 789 patients in China showed that among 6 antimyoclonic seizure drugs, LEV is a drug with good efficacy, safety, tolerability, and the fewest adverse effects.
6. *Drugs with no clear effect or possible exacerbation of PME*: These include Na^+ channel blockers (phenytoin sodium, carbamazepine, oxcarbazepine, lamotrigine), tiagabine, aminocaproic acid, and pregabalin [872]. The mechanism by which these drugs exacerbate myoclonus is unknown.
7. *ASMs that affect MERRF*: These include valproate, carbamazepine, phenytoin sodium, and phenobarbital. Valproic acid causes mitochondrial complex I and complex IV dysfunction, reduces adenosine triphosphate (ATP) production, and causes damage to mitochondrial endosomal tissue and secondary carnitine deficiency. Carbamazepine, phenytoin sodium, and phenobarbital decrease ATP production and the mitochondrial membrane potential and impair Ca^{2+} uptake/release. Therefore, sodium valproate is a contraindicated drug for treating mitochondrial disease.
8. *Combination of medications*: Patients with progressive myoclonic epilepsy are mostly refractory to medications and usually require a combination of medications. Several studies have shown that LEV combined with CZP is a better choice for treating myoclonic seizures in patients with MERRF. The antiepileptic mechanisms of LEV and CZP are different; LEV does not have sedative side effects, CZP is also widely used to treat psychiatric disorders, and CZP can counteract some of the psychoemotional side effects of LEV. Therefore, it is reasonable to combine LEV and CZP to treat myoclonic seizures. We admitted two siblings with sialidosis type I who had good control of myoclonus with a low-dose combination of LEV, clonazepam, topiramate, and perampanel and

who basically recovered to a normal life, and the older brother was able to perform more than 10 consecutive push-ups. Therefore, when monotherapy is ineffective, a combination of drugs is reasonable and may benefit the patient.

Nondrug Treatment

Several studies have applied a ketogenic diet to treat LD because the genes encoding the laforin and malin proteins are involved in glycogen metabolism and a ketogenic diet may slow the progression of LD by decreasing the synthesis of glycogen and excessive glucose accumulation [873].

Research regarding treatments such as vagus nerve stimulation (VNS) [874, 875], deep brain stimulation (DBS) [876], and transcranial magnetic stimulation (TMS) has made some progress but has not had a significant impact on epileptic control. The mechanism of action of VNS has not been clearly defined but may involve the inhibition of excitability in the limbic system, thalamus, and thalamocortical cortex; increased activity in the locus coeruleus and raphe nucleus; and modulation of the downstream release of norepinephrine and serotonin, both of which have been shown to have antiepileptic effects. Attention should also be given to seizure triggers, such as sleep deprivation and stress. Intractable myoclonic seizures occur more frequently and/or are more severe when the patient is under physical or emotional stress, which can create a vicious cycle.

5.5 Idiopathic Generalized Epilepsy Syndrome

Idiopathic generalized epilepsy (IGE) syndrome refers to a broad group of epilepsies characterized by generalized seizures and generalized spikes and waves (GSWs) on electroencephalography (EEG), which is presumed to be related to genetic causes. It generally has a favorable prognosis for seizure outcomes. According to the proposal of the Task Force on Nosology and Definitions of ILAE, the most common subtypes of IGEs are childhood absence epilepsy (CAE), juvenile absence epilepsy (JAE), juvenile myoclonic epilepsy (JME), and epilepsy with generalized tonic–clonic seizures alone (GTCA).

5.5.1 Childhood Absence Epilepsy (CAE)

Overview

In 1989, ILAE classified CAE into the age-related idiopathic subgroup of generalized epilepsy and epileptic syndromes, also known as "pyknolepsy" [11]. In 2022, the latest ILAE classification named it idiopathic generalized epilepsy syndrome. The onset of CAE occurs between the ages of 2 and 13 years (peak: 4–10 years). Absence seizures are frequent and can be induced by hyperventilation. Epilepsy

EEG signals are characterized by comprehensive 2.5–4-Hz spike-and-wave discharges with a normal background [565]. Patients with CAE usually exhibit normal neural development and no significant abnormalities on neuroimaging.

Historical Evolution and Epidemiological Investigation
Absence seizures were first described by Poupart in 1705 [877], and, approximately a century later, Calmeil first named them “absence” and described the meaning and clinical features in detail in 1824 [878]. Esquirol used the term “petit mal” to describe this form of seizure [879]. Sauer created the Greek term “pyknolepsy” in 1916, after which it was gradually popularized [880]. Pyknolepsy specifically refers to a typical absence epilepsy that starts at 4–12 years of age, is associated with frequent seizures and self-alleviates, and does not affect psychology or cognition. In 1989, ILAE named the syndrome CAE [11, 881] based on its unique seizure type and EEG features, while the term “pyknolepsy” was retained. In 2022, ILAE retained only the term “CAE” in the classification of epileptic syndromes and stopped mentioning the term “pyknolepsy”. The incidence of CAE is approximately 5.8–8.0/year/100,000 children, accounting for approximately 18% of epilepsy cases in school-aged children, and, in the pediatric cohort, the prevalence is estimated to be 0.4–0.7/1000 [565, 882].

Etiology
The brain imaging findings of CAE patients are normal, and there have been no reports of abnormal brain structures. CAE is now believed to be a form of idiopathic epilepsy determined by genetic factors, but the exact way in which it is inherited remains unclear. Among the families of CAE patients, approximately only one-quarter of affected relatives have a CAE phenotype, approximately one-quarter have febrile convulsions, and the other half have other IGE manifestations [883]. At present, the main risk genes associated with CAE are identified as *CACNA1H*, *CACNG3*, *CLCN2*, *GABRA1*, *GABRA6*, *GABRB3*, *GABRG2*, *SCN1A*, *SCN8A*, *NIPA2*, etc. [884–892] and a small number of patients have copy number variations in complex genetic patterns (e.g., 15q11.2, 15q13.3, and 16p13.11 microdeletions). Of absence seizures occurring in patients younger than 4 years of age, 10% are related to glucose transporter type 1 defects and *SLC2A1* gene testing should be performed [565].

Clinical Manifestations
Seizures

CAE presents as frequent typical absence seizures (often dozens per day in untreated patients) and is difficult to identify, with 98% of seizures induced by hyperventilation and a small percentage induced by light stimulation (16%) [893]. GTCSs rarely present during frequent absence seizures to CAE.

Absence Seizures

An absence seizure manifests as sudden, transient, and severe impairment of consciousness. Significant impairment of consciousness is the basic feature of CAE absence seizures, and the most common features are interruption of ongoing activities or staring spells, automatism (face or hand movements), blinking, and mild eyelid or perioral myoclonus [894]. Normal activity can be resumed immediately after the attack, usually lasting for 3–20 s (median duration is 10 s). Urinary incontinence or instability while standing may occur [565].

Generalized Tonic–Clonic Seizures

During frequent seizures of absence, generalized tonic–clonic seizures are rare and generally occur 5–10 years after absence seizures. For example, CAE patients with GTCS should be vigilant about whether they develop other epileptic syndromes, such as JAE, JME, or eyelid myoclonic seizures [1, 882, 895].

Myoclonic Seizures

Except for minor eyelid or perioral myoclonus that accompany absence seizures, children with CAE do not have myoclonic seizures elsewhere. If an upper limb myoclonus of 3 Hz is present with absence, this is an alert for the possibility of myoclonic absence epilepsy (EMA).

Other Impairments

Patients with CAE usually have normal neurodevelopment, but some children with CAE may have learning difficulties and hyperactivity, which are usually mild and easily ignored. Caplan et al. [896] reported that 25% of children with CAE had mild cognitive deficits, 43% had language difficulties, and 61% had language difficulties compared with the normal group.

Laboratory Testing

The background of interictal EEG signals is generally normal. Generalized spikes and waves (GSWs) can be detected in almost all CAE EEGs and occur mainly during sleep, and multispike waves or segmented GSWs can be detected in sleepy or sleeping children with CAE [897, 898]. Approximately one-third of children with CAE have 2.5–4-Hz occipital intermittent rhythmic delta activity (OIRDA), which can be enhanced by hyperventilation [897]. Focal or multifocal spike-and-wave discharge can also be observed in the EEGs of CAE patients during the interictal period, but the area of occurrence is not fixed; most of these discharges occur in the anterior head, and the morphology of these spikes is similar to that of comprehensive spikes and waves. Both focal spike-and-wave and generalized spike-and-wave discharges can be enhanced by hyperventilation [899]. Approximately 21% of CAE patients develop generalized spikes and waves after flash stimulation.

Seizure EEG is characterized by regular 3-Hz (range: 2.5–4 Hz) global spikes and waves in the first second after a seizure and accompanied by absence seizures. Approximately 21% of patients have at least part of their absence onset with GSWs at 2.5 Hz, and 43% have at least part of their absence onset with GSWs at 4 Hz [565]. Compared with those in the JME and JAE cohorts, the number of spikes and disorganized discharges per GSW in the CAE cohort was smaller [897]. Hyperventilation can induce typical generalized spike-and-wave discharges and absence seizures. If an untreated child with CAE does not exhibit generalized spike-and-wave release after hyperventilation for more than 3 min, CAE can be excluded [565].

When the clinical manifestations of CAE patients are typical, the neurological examination results are normal, there are characteristic electroencephalograms, and further neurological imaging examinations are not needed [900].

Diagnosis

ILAE put forward the latest diagnostic criteria [565], emphasizing that they can be divided into three levels:

1. Diagnostic requirements: Typical absence seizures; absence seizure begins with an episodic 3-Hz (range: 2.5–4 Hz) global spike and wave on electroencephalogram.
2. It is necessary to pay attention to the manifestations that are distinguished from other epilepsy complexes: appearance of GTCSs before or during frequent absence seizures; gaze duration >30 s or confusion or fatigue after onset; frequency of seizures in untreated patients <1 per day; persistent epileptoid discharges in unilateral brain region; the fact that 2.5-Hz total spikes and waves are not induced despite untreated and complete hyperventilation for ≥3 min; persistent background slow waves without sedation; age of onset 2–3 years or 11–13 years; mild intellectual delay; and the presence of potential neurological abnormalities and neuroimaging abnormalities that may be associated with seizures.
3. The diagnosis of JAE was excluded if any of the following types of seizures occur: Myoclonic seizures, eyelid myoclonic seizures, myoclonic seizures, tonic seizures, ataxic seizures, atypical seizures, or focal consciousness impairment seizures; EEG, diffuse background slowing; aging; age of onset <2 years or >13 years; moderate-to-very-severe intellectual delay; delayed or regressive cognitive development; and decreased cerebrospinal fluid glucose levels or if *SLC2A1* mutations are associated with epilepsy [565].

Differential Diagnosis

Adolescent Absence Epilepsy

JAE usually develops after 10 years of age, absence seizures are more frequent in patients with CAE than in those with JAE, GTCSs are less frequent, febrile convulsions are more common, and absence persistence is more common in patients with JAE [565, 901].

Eyelid Myoclonic Epilepsy

Eyelid myoclonic epilepsy is characterized by absence seizures accompanied by repetitive and rhythmic rapid eyelid twitching, upward displacement of the eyeball, and slight extension of the head. Eye closure, sunlight, and flash stimulation can induce seizures [565].

Myoclonic Seizures

Myoclonic seizures are a typical feature of this disease, and a 3-Hz myoclonic seizure of the upper limb accompanied by gradual lifting of the arm occurs during an absence seizure [565].

Other Generalized Epilepsies with Atypical Absence

There is usually a longer period of loss of consciousness and a greater frequency of generalized spikes and waves (<2.5 Hz). It usually occurs in the context of developmental and/or epileptic encephalopathy, such as in Lennox–Gastaut syndrome [565].

Focal Impaired Awareness Seizures

These seizures refer to focal nonmotor seizures and are characterized by prolonged unresponsive staring (usually >30 s) and postattack features (including confusion, drowsiness, and headache). An electroencephalogram shows focal epileptiform discharges [565].

Treatment

Ethosuximide, valproic acid, and lamotrigine are usually used as initial monotherapies for CAE, and two double-blind randomized controlled trials have supported ethosuximide as the best initial monotherapy for CAE [902, 903]. Several studies have also recommended valproic acid combined with lamotrigine as a first-line treatment; however, the failure rate of the combined treatment is significantly greater than that of ethosuximide, valproic acid, or lamotrigine alone ($P = 0.012$) and the dose of the combined treatment group is lower than that of the monotherapy group [904]. Perampanel, a novel antiseizure drug, has also been used to treat CAE. However, the therapeutic effects of levetiracetam and topiramate are unclear. Sodium channel blockers such as carbamazepine, oxcarbazepine, sodium pentobarbital, and vigabatrin can aggravate absence seizures and should be avoided.

Ethosuximide

Ethosuximide is the drug of choice for CAE patients with only absence seizures, and the available evidence suggests that it prevents synchronous firing of corticothalamic neurons primarily by blocking the instantaneous low-threshold calcium current generated by T-type calcium channels in thalamic neurons. A class I randomized controlled trial by Glauser et al. [903] also showed a similar failure-free rate in the valproic acid group (53% vs. 58%, $P = 0.35$) that was significantly greater than that in the lamotrigine group; however, attention deficit was more common in the valproic acid group (49% vs. 33%, $P = 0.03$). In a second randomized controlled trial of monotherapy in which another initial monotherapy failed [905], the failure rate of ethosuximide was similar to that of valproic acid (57% vs. 49%) after 12 months of follow-up but significantly greater than that of lamotrigine (36%). The main side effects of ethosuximide include gastrointestinal dysfunction (abdominal discomfort, nausea, vomiting, diarrhea), headache, and drowsiness, and rare side effects include behavioral and psychiatric disorders, blood disorders, and allergic reactions [906].

Sodium Valproate

VPA is the drug of choice for CAE patients with GTCSs because ethosuximide has no control effect on GTCSs. Valproic acid and ethosuximide have been shown to cause similar failure rates in multiple studies [894, 907]. In 5 noncontrolled trials of valproic acid, 82 of 89 patients (92%) who had previously had a lapse seizure did not have one. Davis et al. [908] analyzed noncontrolled trials of valproic acid (either monotherapy or in combination with other antiseizure agents) in children and reported that 90% of patients had a ≥75% reduction in the number of absence seizures. Common adverse reactions associated with this drug include nausea, vomiting, dyspepsia, weight gain, polycystic ovaries, tremors, transient alopecia and blood system abnormalities such as thrombocytopenia and leukopenia, and liver function impairment [909–911]. Therefore, blood cell indices and liver function should be followed regularly during valproic acid treatment.

Lamotrigine

Frank et al. [912] conducted a study on the single-drug treatment of lamotrigine for typical absence seizures in children and adolescents aged 3–15 years; the seizure-free rate was 62% in the lamotrigine group and 21% in the placebo group ($P < 0.02$), revealing a significant difference between the two groups, and no patients dropped out of the study for any safety-related reasons. Coppola et al. [913] introduced lamotrigine monotherapy to 20 typical children with absence, and, after an average follow-up of 10.8 months, seizures in 11 children (55%) were 100% controlled, seizures in 4 children (20%) were significantly reduced by 75%, and seizures in 5 children (25%) were reduced by 50%. Most of the patients tolerated the treatment well. Although adverse reactions occurred in three patients, no one stopped the drug. However, in a randomized double-blind trial regarding CAE [53], lamotrigine (29%) had a significantly lower failure-free rate than ethosuximide (53%) and valproic acid (58%) and only approximately one-third of patients achieved seizure remission. The main disadvantage of lamotrigine is that it can cause Stevens–Johnson syndrome and toxic epidermal necrolysis [914], which are severe and potentially life-threatening rashes. Therefore, lamotrigine must be titrated slowly and strictly according to drug instructions. The adverse reactions that have been identified involve serious adverse effects of lamotrigine on the liver and hematopoietic system, especially in young children; therefore, regular testing of blood ammonia, platelet, and transaminase levels is necessary to detect and prevent these side effects early [915].

Perampanel

Although most CAE patients respond well to pharmacological therapy, a small number of them fail to achieve epilepsy remission under monotherapy. As a new broad-spectrum antiepileptic drug, perampanel has shown good efficacy in the control of absence seizures both as a single agent and as an additive therapy. In a retrospective cohort study of IGE patients receiving perampanel monotherapy or combination therapy, at the last visit (≥12 months), the response rate and remission rate of absence seizures were 90.5% and 81.0%, respectively, and the most common adverse reactions were irritability, dizziness/vertigo, drowsiness, and withdrawal due to adverse events, accounting for 12.4% (52/419) within 12 months [916]. Another study that included perampanel as an additive therapy included 20 CAE patients with incomplete seizure control under other monotherapies [917] and revealed that 15 patients responded to perampanel and were seizure-free, 3 had a <50% reduction in seizure frequency, and 15 without seizures were switched to perampanel monotherapy, of whom 9 patients remained seizure-free with monotherapy. Only 2 out of the 20 patients reported mild, transient side effects such as irritability, headache, and dizziness, but none stopped treatment.

Others

The effectiveness of levetiracetam and topiramate in patients with CAE is unclear. In a randomized controlled trial [918], compared with the placebo, LEV failed to achieve statistical significance for the primary end point. According to Nolan et al. [919], only approximately one-quarter of patients were seizure-free after LEV introduction and 74% (53/72) of patients discontinued LEV due to poor seizure control (59%, 35/72) and/or adverse side effects that were difficult to tolerate (41%, 24/72). In addition, some studies have even shown that LEV may aggravate the onset of absence [920]. Topiramate was introduced in five CAE patients, of whom one patient with CAE achieved no seizures; after drug titration, the seizures of two patients improved, while the seizures of the remaining two patients did not improve significantly [921].

Prognosis

The prognosis of CAE is good. Under strict diagnostic criteria, most children with CAE experience seizure remission and no recurrence after drug withdrawal; <10% of patients with CAE have GTCS, and the average treatment time is approximately 2 years [922]. Notably, factors that predict epilepsy recurrence after ASM discontinuation include a history of GTCS and the use of two or more ASMs [923]. However, some studies have shown that if GTCSs or myoclonic seizures occur during the course of CAE, then the disease may evolve into another type of epilepsy syndrome; it has been found that CAEs can evolve into juvenile absence epilepsy, juvenile myoclonic epilepsy, and eyelid myoclonus with absence epilepsy [895, 924]. Although it is generally believed that the neurodevelopment of CAE patients is usually normal, a growing body of literature indicates that mild neuropsychological disorders are common in children with CAE, and even if the IQ score of CAE patients is within the normal range, intellectual function performance seems to be worse than that of healthy children. In addition, studies have reported that the language skills and learning ability of CAE patients are affected and that executive function is slightly impaired [925].

5.5.2 *Juvenile Absence Epilepsy (JAE)*

Overview
In 1989, ILAE classified JAE into the age-related idiopathic subgroup of generalized epilepsies and syndromes [11]. In 2022, the latest ILAE classification categorized this disease as idiopathic generalized epilepsy [565]. The age of onset of JAE is mostly 8–20 years. Absence seizures are the main seizure type, and some JAE patients may have generalized tonic–clonic or myoclonic seizures. JAE patients usually exhibit normal neurodevelopment and no significant abnormalities on neuroimaging [565, 926]. An EEG is characterized by generalized 3–5.5-Hz spike-and-wave discharge with a normal EEG background [565].

Historical Evolution and Epidemiological Investigation
The first documented reports of absence seizures date back to 1705, when they were referred to as petit mal. In 1824, the meaning and clinical features of absence were formally described [927] until 1989, when ILAE named the syndrome juvenile absence epilepsy based on its age of onset, unique seizure type, and EEG features. Studies have shown that newly diagnosed JAE accounts for 2.4–3.1% of new-onset epilepsy in children and adolescents [565], and the epidemiological investigation of Gesche et al. [928] showed that the prevalence of typical absence (including eyelid myoclonic absence) in adults is 0.8/1000, with no difference in incidence between men and women [924].

Etiology
The brain imaging results of patients with JAE are usually normal [929], and there are no reports of brain structural abnormalities leading to JAE. JAE is a disease determined by genetic factors. Carla et al. [930] reported that 31% of the affected relatives of grade 1 and grade 2 epileptic patients with JAE suffer from CAE, while some relatives also suffer from JME and febrile convulsion, suggesting that these epileptic patients may carry the same pathogenic gene or have a similar genetic background. However, JAE is not inherited based on a single gene and may involve complex inheritance of two or more genes [931–934]. The complex genetic basis of JAE has not been fully elucidated, and rare mutations and susceptibility alleles, mainly for GABAA receptors and voltage-activated calcium channels, have been identified [9, 935]. In addition, a small number of patients, including *GABRG2*, *GABRA1*, *CACNA1A*, *SLC2A1*, and *ADGRV1*, were found to carry single pathogenic gene mutations [565, 935, 936].

Clinical Manifestations
Seizures

A typical absence seizure is the characteristic seizure type of JAE and can usually be triggered by flashing light or hyperventilation [893]. In JAE patients, the impairment of consciousness during a loss seizure is less severe than that in children with absence epilepsy (CAE), and partial consciousness can be retained, but the duration of a seizure is usually longer [929, 937]. Almost all patients have generalized tonic–clonic seizures (GTCSs) [929], and approximately one-fifth of patients have mild myoclonic seizures.

1. *Absence seizures*: These generalized, transient, and consciousness-impaired nonmotor seizures [13] are characterized by sudden impairment of consciousness, loss of facial expression, interruption of activity, and no oral automatism and can last for approximately 5–30 s, followed by an immediate return to normal activity. The frequency of absence seizures is usually not daily [11]. Absence is present in approximately 20% of patients and is truly a generalized nonconvulsive epileptic status [938].
2. *GTCSs*: GTCSs occur in more than 80% of JAE patients [565, 901, 929, 939], usually after absence seizures, but in 14–27% of cases before absence seizures [565]. The presence of a GTCS is a predictor of poor prognosis in JAE patients [926, 940].
3. *Myoclonus*: The occurrence of myoclonic seizures alone can exclude JAE, but 20% of patients can have mild myoclonic seizures during absence seizures [939].

Other Damages

Magnus et al. [941] reported that the risk of JAE requiring special education for patients was significantly greater than that of individuals in the normal age group and that the average IQ point was lower than that of children with non-neurological chronic diseases. Moreover, children with JAE have an increased risk of taking antidepressants, melatonin drugs, and outpatient visits to psychological doctors. In addition, patients with JAE are at risk of difficulty in discontinuing medications after coexisting ADHD treatment. Patients with mental disorders such as learning difficulties and anxiety also require vigilant oversight [565].

Laboratory Testing

The interparoxysmal EEG background of JAE patients is usually normal. In untreated JAE patients, EEG signals are abnormal, often due to absence seizures induced by hyperventilation. It is not easy to distinguish between the onset and interictal EEG signals of JAE, both of which are 3–5.5-Hz comprehensive spike-and-wave arrays. In almost all patients, polyspikes can be recorded in the sleepy or sleep phase of the interparoxysmal period, and some patients may experience fragmentary generalized spike-and-wave release. JAE produces more spikes per spike and wave than does CAE and is similar to juvenile myoclonic epilepsy (JME). Disorganized discharges are approximately eight times more common in JAE than in CAE [565, 898].

Neuroimaging in patients with JAE is usually normal. If the clinical manifestations and EEG results are consistent with the diagnosis of typical JAE, additional neuroimaging is not necessary.

Diagnosis

ILAE put forward the latest diagnostic criteria for JAE [565], emphasizing that they can be divided into three levels: (1) *Diagnostic requirements*: Typical absence seizure; EEG criteria include 3–5.5-Hz spike-and-wave episodic discharge. (2)

Findings that distinguish it from other epilepsy syndromes need to be noted: GTCS occurs before or during frequent absence seizures; gaze duration >30 s or post-episodic confusion or during frequent absence seizures; the frequency of attacks in untreated patients is <1 time per day; persistent unilateral epileptiform discharge of the brain area; failure to elicit 2.5-Hz global spikes and waves with untreated hyperventilation for a full 3 min or more; background slow waves sustained without sedation; age of onset 2–3 or 11–13 years; mild intellectual developmental disability; and underlying neurological abnormalities and neuroimaging abnormalities that may be associated with seizures. (3) *Exclusion of JAE diagnosis*: any of the following seizure forms: predominant myoclonic seizures, predominant eyelid myoclonic seizures, myoclonic absence seizures, tonic seizures, clonic seizures, atypical absence seizures, focal impairment of consciousness seizures; EEG showing persistent unilateral focal epileptiform discharge, diffuse background slowing, and no EEG-related changes recorded at typical gaze episodes; age of onset <8 years or >20 years; moderate-to-severe intellectual disability; delayed or regressive cognitive development; and decreased glucose content in cerebrospinal fluid or pathogenic variants of *SLC2A1*.

Differential Diagnosis

Childhood Absence Epilepsy

According to the latest diagnostic criteria of ILAE 2022, CAE and this disease partially overlap in terms of diagnosis but the age of onset of CAE is usually younger, absence seizures are more frequent, GTCSs are less frequent, and febrile convulsions are more common [565, 901].

JME

In JME, some patients experience loss seizures, but the duration of the loss seizure is shorter than that in JAE and the impairment of consciousness is less severe. In addition, myoclonic seizures are typical symptoms of JME, and no single myoclonic seizure occurs in JAE [565].

Myoclonic Absence Seizures

Myoclonic absence seizures are a typical feature of this disease. A 3-Hz myoclonic absence seizure usually occurs in the upper limb accompanied by gradual lifting of the arm, and perioral myoclonus is frequent [565]. Children may experience cognitive or developmental regression as the disease progresses.

Treatment

At present, there is a lack of high-quality evidence-based medical data to support ASM selection. Valproic acid and lamotrigine alone or in combination are the drugs of choice for the treatment of JAE seizures, and benzodiazepines may be chosen when the above treatments are ineffective. Levetiracetam and perampanel, novel antiepileptic agents, have also been used to treat JAE. Since almost all patients with JAE have GTCSs, ethosuximide alone is not recommended. Sodium channel blockers such as carbamazepine, oxcarbazepine, phenytoin sodium, and aminohexanoic acid can aggravate absence seizures and thus should be avoided.

Sodium Valproate

Valproate is the drug of choice for patients with JAE and is the most effective in the treatment of generalized seizures, including absence, tonic–clonic, and myoclonic seizures. In 5 uncontrolled trials of valproic acid monotherapy, 82 of 89 patients (92%) who had a lapse seizure did not have even 1 subsequent treatment [907]. Berkovic et al. [942] evaluated the value of valproic acid monotherapy in preventing relapse of absence status epilepticus in 18 IGE patients. After a mean follow-up duration of 4 years, the number of attacks decreased from 5.7 to 0.6 per year ($p = 0.0005$) and 14 patients (78%) experienced no recurrence. In 2007, Davis et al. [908] analyzed noncontrolled trials of valproic acid (either monotherapy or in combination with other antiseizure agents) in children; 90% of patients had a ≥75% reduction in the frequency of absence seizures, while 69–94% and 68% had a ≥75% reduction in the frequency of myoclonic or tonic–clonic seizures, respectively. Common adverse reactions associated with sodium valproate include nausea, vomiting, dyspepsia, weight gain, polycystic ovaries, tremors, transient alopecia, and blood system abnormalities such as thrombocytopenia and leukopenia [909–911]. In addition, studies have shown that pregnant women who receive valproic acid treatment have a significantly greater risk of fetal malformation, intellectual disability, and autism spectrum disorders than women who do not and may be dose-related. Valproic acid is two to four times more likely to be effective than other ASMs [943, 944]. Therefore, it is not recommended for the treatment of female patients of reproductive age due to the risk of teratogenesis to the female reproductive system and the fetus, but its effects on the reproductive system of girls have not been systematically studied.

Lamotrigine

Lamotrigine is the first choice for women of childbearing age due to the teratogenicity of sodium valproate to their offspring. Sabrina et al. [945] studied the effect of lamotrigine in the treatment of typical absences, including JAE, and showed that after an average of 19 days of lamotrigine addition therapy, the clinical manifestations of eight patients with refractory (valproic acid combined with ethosuximide or no response alone) typical absence seizures completely disappeared. Of the seven patients who received lamotrigine monotherapy after newly diagnosed classic absence, six had absence seizures disappear after treatment and one stopped taking lamotrigine because of a rash. Gericke et al. [946] showed that among 12 patients with JAE who used lamotrigine monotherapy ($n = 4$) or additive therapy ($n = 8$), 10 had no seizures and 2 had a >50% reduction; among 5 patients with generalized tonic–clonic seizures, 3 had no seizures and 1 had a >50% reduction. With the exception of one parent who reported transient tremors, emotional agitation, and difficulty concentrating after lamotrigine, no other patient reported lamotrigine-related side effects, suggesting that lamotrigine is well-tolerated and effective at preventing both typical absence seizures and GTCSs.

Common adverse effects of lamotrigine include headache, drowsiness, dizziness, irritability, tremor, difficulty falling asleep, diarrhea, and nausea. Lamotrigine can also have serious adverse effects on the liver and hematopoietic system, especially in young children; therefore, regular testing of blood ammonia levels, platelet counts, and transaminase levels is necessary to detect these side effects early [915]. Another relatively rare but serious side effect of lamotrigine that needs to be closely watched clinically is allergic rash, especially Stevens–Jonson syndrome. The rash mainly occurs in pediatric patients and in the first 8 weeks of drug use, when the drug is added too quickly. In such circumstances, the patient must immediately return to the original dose and be treated with valproic acid.

Ethosuximide

Ethosuximide is comparable to valproic acid for the treatment of absence seizures but is not effective at controlling the onset of GTCSs; therefore, it is often not used solely to control seizures in patients with JAE [947–949].

Perampanel

Perampanel is a noncompetitive and selective AMPA receptor antagonist that has shown broad-spectrum anticonvulsant activity in animal models of epilepsy [86]. Vicente et al. [950] studied a multicenter retrospective cohort with typical absence ($n = 47$) and reported that the frequency of absence seizures (days per month) decreased by 48.3% in patients treated with perampanel in combination with 12 months compared with the baseline level before treatment and that 51.1% of patients reached 6 consecutive months of absence at 12 months of treatment. There were almost no withdrawals due to adverse events. A recent retrospective cohort study of IGE patients treated with perampanel alone or in combination with other ASM agents has also revealed that perampanel was effective and well-tolerated in patients with typical absence, with a response rate of 90.5% and a remission rate of 81.0% at the last visit (≥12 months). The most common adverse reactions were irritability, dizziness/vertigo, and drowsiness, and 12.4% (52/419) of the patients discontinued treatment due to adverse events within 12 months [916]. A systematic review [88] showed that although only one RCT provided class I evidence that perampanel was effective in primary generalized tonic–clonic seizures, other weaker evidence also showed that perampanel was effective in absence seizures and myoclonic seizures, and there was no evidence that perampanel worsened seizures. These studies suggest the potential of perampanel as a broad-spectrum antiseizure agent and as a candidate treatment for patients with JAE.

Levetiracetam

Alberto et al. [89] administered levetiracetam antiseizure therapy to 12 patients with typical absence; 12 months after treatment, 10 patients had no seizures and 2 patients had sporadic spike–slow-wave complexes in EEGs after hyperventilation.

In this study, no adverse effects were reported, except for in two patients who reported temporary drowsiness and irritability. However, in another randomized controlled trial [918], compared to the placebo, levetiracetam failed to achieve statistical significance for the primary end point. Nolan et al. [919] also reported that the effectiveness of levetiracetam in controlling absence seizures was unclear; only approximately one-quarter of patients were seizure-free after levetiracetam was used, and the percentage of patients who stopped taking levetiracetam was as high as 74% (53/72) due to poor seizure control (59%, 35/72) and/or adverse side effects that were difficult to tolerate (41%, 24/72). However, in patients who are responsive, levetiracetam can control absence seizures at relatively low doses. It is important to note that levetiracetam may aggravate the onset of absence. Among children using levetiracetam, two had CAE, three had JAE, one had myoclonic apnea, and one had aggravated absence seizures, and the dosage of levetiracetam administered was between 17 and 50 mg/kg/d [920].

Benzodiazepines

The National Institute for Health and Care Excellence (NICE) recommends that clonazepam and clobazam be used as additive therapies when VPA and LTG therapies fail [90]. A clinical study with a small sample of 10 patients showed that the addition of 3–6 mg/day clonazepam could cause 8 patients to reach a seizure-free state and that 1 patient experienced a reduction in absence seizures by more than 75% [91]. Additionally, clonazepam had a good effect on the persistence of seizures [93, 951]. Common side effects of clonazepam include sedation, excitement, excessive movement, ataxia, etc. In severe cases, respiratory depression may occur, which requires clinical attention. However, the side effects of clobazam are relatively mild. In addition, inattention is more common in children.

Prognosis

Although seizures in most patients with JAE can be controlled with ASM, antiseizure treatment is usually lifelong [926]. The late remission rate of epilepsy showed a trend toward gradual remission with increasing age. Martin et al. [952] showed through multifactor analysis that at the end of follow-up, only age was independently correlated with 5-year end-stage epilepsy remission and that the greater the age was, the greater was the remission rate. A study on the prognosis of IGE patients [953] revealed that the duration of follow-up was associated with seizure remission, with a longer duration of follow-up associated with a greater rate of seizure remission. In addition, the onset of GTCSs in JAE patients is considered to be a predictor of poor prognosis [926, 940]. Trinka et al. [929] studied a retrospective cohort of patients with typical absence seizures (n = 163), which included JAE, CAE, and untypable seizures. Patients who had daily seizures at the beginning of the disease and combined GTCSs and myoclonic seizures during the course of the disease had a lower rate of seizure remission, while CAE and JAE syndrome status were not associated with prognosis.

5.5.3 *Juvenile Myoclonic Epilepsy (JME)*

Overview
In 1989, the International League Against Epilepsy (ILAE) classified "juvenile myoclonic epilepsy" and "impulsive petit mal" as synonyms in the age-related idiopathic epilepsy subtype of generalized epilepsy and epileptic syndromes [11]. In 2022, the ILAE classification of epileptic syndromes classified JME as idiopathic generalized epilepsies (IGEs), which are also a subgroup of genetic generalized epilepsies (GGEs) [565]. JME is the most common adolescent and adult-onset IGE, with onset occurring at 10–24 years of age [565]. It is characterized by myoclonic and generalized tonic–clonic seizures in otherwise healthy adolescents or adults, with sleep deprivation and excessive alcohol consumption as common triggers [565, 954]. Up to 90% of patients have photosensitive EEG changes [565, 955].

Historical Evolution and Epidemiological Investigation
JMEs were also previously known as "Janz syndrome" and "impulsive petit mal seizures." In 1867, Herpin [956] first described the clinical features of JME in one patient. In 1957, Janz and Christian [954] reported 47 cases of epilepsy and proposed the name "impulsive minor epileptic seizures." In the same year, Castells and Mendilaharsu [957] characterized it as a specific IGE. The name JME was proposed by Lund et al. [958]. In 1989, ILAE used JME as a synonym for "impulsive minor epileptic seizures," and, to date, JME names that reflect the clinical features of the syndrome have been widely used [11].

Studies have suggested that the prevalence of JME in the population is 1–3/10000 [565], accounting for 25–30% of all IGEs [959]. Additionally, the prevalence of JME in adults is reportedly 1.2/1000 [928]; however, this ratio may be lower than the actual prevalence because some patients do not spontaneously mention myoclonic seizures, resulting in missed diagnoses [960].

Etiology
JME is an epileptic syndrome determined by genetic etiology, and 23–35% of JME patients have a family history of epilepsy [394, 961, 962]. Like JAE, it may be more polygenic, and only a few cases have been found with single pathogenic gene variants of *CACNB4*, *GABRA1*, *GABRD*, and *EFHC1*. In addition, single nucleotide polymorphisms of *BRD2*, *Cx-36*, and *ME2* and microdeletions of 15q13.3, 15q11.2, and 16p13.11 have been found to be associated with JME susceptibility [565, 963].

Clinical Manifestations
Onset of JME

The onset of JME is most common in patients aged 10–24 years, and myoclonus is the characteristic clinical manifestation of JME and usually occurs after awakening, sleep deprivation, or alcohol consumption, alone or in combination with general tonic–clonic seizures and/or absence seizures.

1. *Myoclonus*: Myoclonus is the core symptom of JME. It usually occurs within 1 h of awakening and can be induced by sleep deprivation and flash stimulation. It manifests as electric shock, such as movements of the proximal or distal muscles, mainly in the upper limbs, and can also involve the lower limbs and lead to falls [565]. Focal myoclonus may occur in a small number of patients, but synchronous video EEG often indicates generalized spike-and-wave release [964]. Persistent myoclonus is very rare in patients with JME [965].
2. *Generalized tonic–clonic seizures*: GTCSs occur in more than 90% of JME patients [966]. In most patients, they occur after myoclonus, and myoclonus occurs in succession, gradually increasing in frequency and degree, followed by GTCSs, which manifest as generalized myoclonic–tonic–clonic seizures characteristic of JME [565, 954, 967]. However, in approximately 25% of patients, GTCSs occur before the onset of myoclonus [954].
3. *Absence seizures*: Approximately one-third of patients have typical absence seizures, and although 15% of patients with CAE progress to JME [924], JME absence seizures are different from CAE or JAE because they are short in duration (3–8 s), the impairment of consciousness is usually mild, less frequent, and generally does not occur every day [565], and the severity of absence seizures may be age-related. Absence seizures occurring before the age of 10 may be more severe, and their frequency and severity may decrease with age [968, 969].

Other Damages

Magnus et al. [941] reported that JME patients had a lower average score than did children with non-neurological chronic diseases. Moreover, JME patients had an increased risk of taking sleeping drugs. JME patients generally have good long-term results in terms of psychosocial aspects. According to relevant studies, JME patients have a greater quality of life, and mental illness comorbidity is a factor that is significantly associated with a lower quality of life score [970].

Laboratory Testing

Generalized polyspikes and waves are a typical EEG feature of JME patients. Irregular generalized 3–5.5-Hz spikes and waves or polyspikes and waves are observed during wakefulness and sleep. EEG reveals the simultaneous occurrence of generalized polyspikes and waves during myoclonic seizures, and no diagnosis of JME is supported without their presence.

The EEG signals of patients with JME may show focal abnormal discharges (spikes, spikes and waves, or slow waves), but they do not appear repeatedly in the same location. Fragmented generalized spike-and-wave discharges may appear in all JME patient states, and their morphology is similar to that of generalized spikes and waves. The likelihood of irregular discharge in patients with JME is much greater than that in patients with other idiopathic generalized epilepsy syndromes and is 110 times greater than that in patients with CAE. The presence of at least two generalized spikes or spikes and waves during intermittent light stimulation is called the photosensitivity of JME, and, in a study by Appleton et al., 90% of JME patients had a photosensitive response [565, 898, 955, 971].

Neurological and neuroimaging studies of JME patients are usually normal [968, 972]. If typical clinical manifestations and EEG characteristics are present, neuroimaging is not necessary. JME is a genetically determined epilepsy syndrome, but genetic testing is not required or preferred.

Diagnosis

The diagnostic criteria of ILAE for JME are divided into three levels: ① Essential: myoclonic seizure; 3–5.5-Hz generalized spikes and waves or polyspikes and waves (available from previous data). ② Must pay attention to the identification of other seizure types: generalized tonic–clonic status epilepticus; constant focal symptoms at the beginning of a generalized tonic–clonic seizure (e.g., symptoms are always present in the same part of one side); persistent focal myoclonic seizures; 8–9 or 25–40 years of age; mild intellectual disability; and potential and exclusion of incidental findings of neurological and neuroimaging abnormalities. ③ The diagnosis of JME is excluded if any of the following seizures are present: myoclonic seizures, tonic seizures, atonic seizures, atypical seizures, focal seizures with perceptual impairment, myoclonus occurring mainly or only during sleep, myoclonus associated only with reading, and cortical tremor with myoclonus. EEG detected regular myoclonic events without polyspike or spike-and-wave releases, focal slow waves, persistent unilateral focal epileptoid discharges, and <2.5-Hz generalized polyspikes and waves (except near the end of a high-frequency spike–wave burst), except for a diffuse slow-wave background in the post-seizure period. Patients aged <8 years or >40 years (CAE may occasionally progress to JME; such patients may have absence seizures before 8 years of age but no GTCSs or myoclonic seizures); moderate to severe intellectual delay; progressive cognitive impairment; and progressive myoclonus with fine motor impairment [565].

Differential Diagnosis [565]

Infantile Myoclonic Epilepsy

Myoclonic seizures occur before 3 years of age.

JAE

Absence is the main manifestation, there is no single myoclonic seizure, and only minor myoclonic seizures can occur during absence seizures.

Myoclonic Seizures

Myoclonic seizures are a typical feature of this disease. A 3-Hz myoclonic absence seizure usually occurs in the upper limb accompanied by gradual lifting of the arm and frequent myoclonus around the mouth. Children may develop cognitive impairment or developmental regression as the disease progresses.

Progressive Myoclonic Epilepsy

Patients with progressive cognitive decline and ataxia, drug-resistant epilepsy, a slower EEG background, or photosensitivity to low-frequency (<3 Hz) flash stimuli should be considered.

Familial Adult Myoclonic Epilepsy (FAME)

FAME is associated with significant cortical tremor. This tremor is very common, although there are obvious individual differences in its severity; however, with age, it can affect the limbs, face, and voice. Such tremors are often misdiagnosed as iatrogenic tremors secondary to valproic acid or lamotrigine treatment.

Treatment

The predisposing factors of JME patients are clear, and their control is crucial in daily management. Patients should be guided to develop good living habits, try not to stay up late, develop good sleeping habits, drink less alcohol, and try not to contact flashlights and other objects that can easily induce seizures. In terms of ASM selection, valproic acid is the first-line drug of choice, while in female patients or girls, LEV or lamotrigine may be the first choice due to the potential side effects of VPA [973]. Additionally, sodium channel blockers and vigabatrin are avoided to prevent aggravating myoclonic seizures.

Valproic Acid

Valproic acid (VPA) is a branched-chain fatty acid that is structurally distinct from other ASMs. It has multiple antiseizure mechanisms, including inhibition of GABA-T (GABA-aminotransferase) and increased GAD (glutamate decarboxylase) activity to increase GABA synthesis and increase GABA release into synapses; inhibition of protein kinase C epsilon (PKC-ε) causes synchronous spontaneous Ca^{2+} oscillations in cortical cells [974]. VPA is currently the most effective ASM for controlling JME attacks.

Studies have shown that VPA can effectively inhibit myoclonus, generalized tonic—clonic, and absence seizures in more than 80% of patients [975]. A retrospective analysis by Atakli et al. [976] showed that 85.5% of JME patients achieved remission of seizures for at least 1 year under VPA monotherapy. Calleja et al. [977] followed 22 JME patients for an average of 7.7 years. Except for three patients with refractory epilepsy who needed combined medication to control seizures, the seizure control efficacy of VPA alone exceeded 80%. VPA is the drug of choice for many patients with generalized epilepsy syndrome (which included 119 JME patients; 26%). According to a 2007 nonblind, randomized, controlled trial, the Standard and New Antiepileptic Drugs (SANAD) study included 716 patients and compared the effects of VPA, LTG, and TPM on ASM. It was found that VPA was more effective than LTG and better tolerated than TPM [978]. The adverse reactions to this drug are described in the JAE section.

Lamotrigine (LTG)

LTG is a phenyltriazine derivative. It acts by inhibiting voltage-activated sodium channels and possibly calcium channels, thereby preventing the release of glutamate [979].

A prospective, nonblind randomized controlled trial in adults showed no difference between LTG and VPA in the treatment of JME patients in terms of withdrawal time (December vs. November) or long-term attack remission rate; more than 80% attack remission was achieved at the 4-month follow-up, including 4 patients in the LTG group (5.6%). $n = 41$) rashes developed, including 2 patients with Stevens–Johnson syndrome [980]. A study by Bodenstein-Sachar et al. [981] involving 62 JME patients showed that 35 (56%) were responsive to LTG treatment and 27 (44%) were nonresponsive. LTG showed better efficacy in JME patients without generalized tonic–clonic seizures (GTCSs), and good antiepileptic effects were also observed in patients who switched to LTG due to adverse reactions to VPA. Another open-label study evaluating LTG as an alternative to valproate (63 patients switched from valproate to LTG) showed improvement in 67% of patients, and no worsening of clinical symptoms was reported [982]. However, there have also been cases of myoclonus and GTCS aggravation caused by LTG, which may be related to higher doses, but the specific reasons are still unclear [983, 984]. The main adverse effects of LTG are described in the JAE chapter. Special attention should be given to the frequency of rash occurrence when LTG is combined with VPA, and, in a few cases, the rash may develop into toxic epidermal necrolysis or Stevens–Johnson syndrome [914].

Levetiracetam

LEV, a pyrrolidone derivative, is involved in the regulation of neurotransmitter release by binding to the synaptic vesicular protein (SVA2) during vesicular neurotransmitter exocytosis to achieve antiepileptic effects [985].

Noachtar et al. [986] studied 120 patients with myoclonic seizures (112 JME and 8 JAE) treated with LEV in a double-blind, multicenter, placebo-controlled trial, and the results showed that the frequency of seizures decreased in all seizure types, the absence of seizures was maintained for a long period of time, and myoclonic seizure status was achieved. LEV showed significant efficacy compared with the placebo. A multicenter, prospective study of 32 newly diagnosed JME patients by Alberto et al. [987] showed that LEV monotherapy effectively controlled seizures in 29 patients, reduced seizures by >50% in another 3 patients, and eliminated photosensitivity in 21 of 26 patients at follow-up 1 year later. Nineteen patients were followed for up to 2 years; 17 experienced remission of seizures, 2 experienced a >50% reduction in seizures, and no significant side effects were observed during follow-up. These studies suggest that LEV can be used as a first-line treatment for patients with JME.

Benzodiazepines

Benzodiazepines act mainly through binding to GABAA receptors to enhance the inhibition of GABA activity [988]. The most commonly used benzodiazepine is clonazepam (CZP). Obeid and Panayiotopoulos [989] reported that CZP was very effective at controlling myoclonic seizures in all patients but was less effective in patients with GTCSs. Since GTCSs often occur after myoclonus, the early use of CZP in JME allows the onset of myoclonus to be controlled. However, this approach may inhibit the suspicion of myoclonic–tonic–clonic seizures in patients diagnosed with JME. Therefore, benzodiazepines are commonly used as additional therapies for JME. In addition to some patients who only have myoclonic seizures, benzodiazepines can be used alone, and they also have a good effect on controlling the persistent state of myoclonus [965].

Others

Topiramate and zonisamide have been found to be effective against JME in several small cohort studies, but both are second-line agents and are more commonly used in female patients. In addition, phenobarbital, clobazam, and acetazolamide may be effective against JME. Perampanel also has good antiepileptic effects.

Liu et al. [990] included 3 randomized controlled studies in a meta-analysis involving a total of 83 patients with JME. In terms of efficacy, a greater proportion of subjects in the topiramate group than in the placebo group had a 50% or greater reduction in generalized tonic–clonic seizures, while the proportions of patients in the topiramate and VPA groups were not significantly different, with a 50% or greater reduction in myoclonic seizures and GTCS-free states. A review study analyzing the antiepileptic effect of zonisamide in 15 JME patients (13 patients receiving zonisamide monotherapy and 2 receiving combined valproate) reported remission of GTCSs, myoclonus, and absence seizures in 69%, 62%, and 38% of patients, respectively, with side effects reported in 20% of patients. The main side effects are weight loss, headache, and dizziness during gradual dosage increase [991]. Eugen et al. [916] reported that among 96 patients with JME, 77.9% remained seizure-free for 6–12 months after treatment with perampanel monotherapy or in combination with other agents, and 80.9% of myoclonic seizures were seizure-free during the follow-up period, suggesting that perampanel has a good effect on the treatment of JME. However, 1.4–4.5% of the JME patients in this cohort were found to have an increased attack frequency at different follow-up times. The most common adverse events in this IGE cohort were irritability (9.6%), dizziness/vertigo (9.2%), and drowsiness (6.3%), and 12.4% (52/419) of the patients discontinued due to adverse events within 12 months.

Prognosis

Typically, JME requires ASM therapy for life. JME patients who develop adolescent absence epilepsy from childhood absence epilepsy have seizures that are more difficult to control than those of other JME patients [924]. Meta-analyses have also shown that the following nine variables are independent risk factors for drug-resistant JME: three seizure types (simultaneous myoclonus, absence, and GTCS seizures); comorbidities; catamenial epilepsy; focal discharges; ethnicity (European and Latino descent are at a higher risk); history of childhood absence epilepsy; family history of epilepsy; convulsive status epilepticus; and febrile convulsions. Early withdrawal age, short flare-free maintenance time, and use of more ASM types are risk factors for relapse after JME withdrawal [992]. Studies have shown that reproductive-age JME patients have poor seizure control, which may be related to the restriction of VPA use in these women [993]. A study of long-term follow-up outcomes in JME patients showed that although a majority of patients still had seizures after 20 years of follow-up, almost all patients experienced 5-year remission of seizures or significant remission of myoclonic seizures and the severity of myoclonic seizures was significantly reduced in JME patients by the fourth decade [994].

5.5.4 Epilepsy with Generalized Tonic–Clonic Seizures Alone (GTCA)

Overview
GTCA was previously referred to as "epilepsy with grand mal seizures upon awakening," and it was classified as genetic epilepsy and syndrome in the 1989 classification [11]. The new ILAE 2022 classification will be attributed to idiopathic generalized epilepsies (IGEs), and comprehensive epilepsy with GTCA accounts for approximately one-third of the cases in adolescents with IGEs, usually at an onset time of 10–25 years of age. Insufficient sleep, early awakening, and excessive drinking are common inducing factors. Seizures, which are generalized tonic–clonic seizures alone, usually do not occur frequently. ASMs can effectively control seizures but can easily relapse after drug withdrawal [565, 995].

Historical Evolution and Epidemiological Investigation
The concept of GTCA was proposed when it was first described in 1885 in a group of patients with seizures only in the early morning [996]. In 1953, several scholars named this epileptic syndrome "epilepsy of awakening period." In subsequent research, people found that GTCA occurs at any time of day. The term "epilepsy with grand mal seizures on awakening" is not rigorous. Therefore, in 2017, ILAE used the term "epilepsy with generalized tonic–clonic seizures alone" to describe this syndrome, which is still used today [2, 997]. Epidemiological investigations have shown that the prevalence of GTCA in adults is 0.3/1000 [928].

Etiology
The prevalence of epilepsy in family members of GTCA patients is high [998, 999]. Like those with other IGEs, family members with GTCA usually present with IGEs or GGEs [565], suggesting that this disease is a genetically related disorder. However, there are limited data on GTCA susceptibility genes.

Clinical Manifestations
1. Generalized tonic–clonic seizures are a prerequisite for the diagnosis of GTCA, but other seizure forms do not support this diagnosis. GTCA often occurs after awakening but can also occur during wakefulness and sleep and may be induced by insufficient sleep, sleep deprivation, or alcohol consumption [565, 998, 1000].

2. Patients with GTCA usually do not have mental or intellectual developmental disabilities, but some may suffer from other diseases, including behavioral disorders (including ADHD), psychiatric disorders (such as depression or schizophrenia), and problems with learning difficulties [998, 1000].

Laboratory Testing

Generalized spikes and waves or polyspikes and waves of 3–5.5 Hz are often recorded during the interictal period. One study revealed that these abnormal discharges could be recorded in 100% of patients after sleep deprivation. In some patients (approximately 3%), focal epileptiform discharge is rare [1001], but the location of discharge is usually not determined; otherwise, it often indicates brain structural abnormalities. The paroxysmal EEG is often covered by artifacts, with a generalized fast spike rhythm observed in the tonic phase, followed by simultaneous burst spikes and waves and irregular slow-wave activity in the clonic phase. Neuroimaging findings are usually normal in GTCA patients, and, if the clinical manifestations and EEG results are consistent with the characteristics of GTCA, neuroimaging is not needed [565].

Diagnosis

ILAE proposed the latest diagnostic criteria for GTCA, which emphasize that GTCA diagnosis can be divided into three components: ① Essential: generalized tonic–clonic seizures, generalized spikes and waves (3–5.5 Hz), or polyspikes and waves on EEG. ② Must pay attention to other identifications of epileptic syndrome at the beginning of persistent focal symptoms (such as in the same parts on one side of the onset of symptoms); 5–9 or 26–40 years of age onset; mild intellectual disability; underlying neurological examination abnormalities (other than incidental findings); and potential neuroimaging abnormalities (other than incidental findings). ③ Exclusion criteria: generalized myoclonic tonic–clonic seizure (suggestive of JME); any other type of seizure; EEG prompt focal slow-wave, continuous unilateral focal epileptic discharge, <2.5-Hz overall spikes and waves (unless there is a high-frequency spike at the end of the outbreak of slow waves), in addition to the late onset of diffuse slow-wave background; onset age <5 years or >40 years; moderate to extremely severe intellectual retardation; and progressive cognitive decline [565].

Differential Diagnosis [565]

Juvenile Absence Epilepsy

A history of characteristic absence seizures.

Juvenile Myoclonic Epilepsy

A history of characteristic myoclonic seizures.

Febrile Seizures with Additional Signs

Febrile seizures with additional signs should be considered first in patients with a history of continued febrile seizures from the age of 6 years accompanied by tonic–clonic seizures with or without fever.

Convulsive Syncope

Tonic–clonic seizures can be caused by cerebral hypoxia caused by prolonged syncope but are often preceded by standing for a long time or rapid change in position, and all of these events occur in the awake state.

Treatment

Daily patient management is important for seizure control. In daily life, patients should develop good sleep habits to avoid sleep deprivation/early waking up and excessive alcohol consumption.

In terms of ASM selection, JAE or JME patients with GTCA can be referred to the use of VPA and LTG as first-line drugs. In addition, new antiepileptic drugs have gradually shown efficacy in the treatment of primary tonic–clonic seizures. In a double-blind, randomized, placebo-controlled study of 242 patients with primary stiffness clonus attack, the results showed that lacosamide can be used as an additive therapy to significantly increase attack time and reduce the risk of recurrence. Its side effects are relatively mild and include dizziness, somnolence, and headache [1001]. Another placebo-controlled study of LEV revealed that in 299 patients with poorly controlled generalized tonic–clonic seizures, LEV was administered as an add-on therapy at a dosage of 3000 mg/day in adults and 60 mg/kg/day in children. Among these, 34.2% of the patients achieved a seizure-free state of generalized tonic–clonic seizures and 24.1% achieved a seizure-free state of all seizure types, which was significantly greater than that of the control group. During the study, only 1.3% of the patients could not tolerate the side effects of LEV and stopped taking the drug [1002]. Moreover, perampanel showed promising efficacy in treating primary tonic–clonic seizures as an add-on therapy in a double-blind, multicenter study [1003].

Prognosis

GTCA is a relatively benign epilepsy syndrome. In two recent studies, it has been found that more than 90% of patients could remain seizure-free for a long time with appropriate ASMs and that 62–75% of patients discontinued the drug after being seizure-free and remained seizure-free from 2 years to more than 20 years of follow-up [998, 1000]. However, some studies have shown a high recurrence rate in patients with GTCA, with a recurrence rate of 70% after discontinuation of treatment. In a cohort study of 77 IGE patients, including 43 GTCA patients, the risk factors related to epilepsy recurrence after drug withdrawal included the first seizure at the age of 13 years or older, the beginning of ASM reduction at the age of 16 years or older, the absence of seizures within 36 months of drug withdrawal, and the self-withdrawal of ASM treatment [995]. Martin et al. [952] studied 42 patients with at least 20 years of follow-up; 19 patients were in the follow-up process and tried to stop treatment at least once, but among them, 12 patients (63.2%) experienced epilepsy recurrence. Their study revealed that the remission rate of epilepsy increased with patient age, so it is possible to discontinue ASMs with increasing age and treatment duration.

References

1. Wirrell EC, Nabbout R, Scheffer IE, Alsaadi T, Bogacz A, French JA, et al. Methodology for classification and definition of epilepsy syndromes with list of syndromes: report of the ILAE Task Force on Nosology and Definitions. Epilepsia. 2022;63(6):1333–48.
2. Scheffer IE, Berkovic S, Capovilla G, Connolly MB, French J, Guilhoto L, et al. ILAE classification of the epilepsies: position paper of the ILAE Commission for Classification and Terminology. Epilepsia. 2017;58(4):512–21.
3. Tissot SAD. Traité de l'epilepsie, faisant le tome troisieme du Traité des nerfs & de leurs maladies, 1770.
4. West WJ. On a peculiar form of infantile convulsions. Lancet. 1841;34:724–5.
5. Lennox WG, Davis JP. Clinical correlates of the fast and the slow spike-wave electroencephalogram. Pediatrics. 1950;5(4):626–44.
6. Gastaut H, Roger J, Soulayrol R, Saint-Jean M, Tassinari CA, Regis H, et al. Epileptic encephalopathy of children with diffuse slow spikes and waves (alias "petit mal variant") or Lennox syndrome. Annales de pediatrie. 1966;13(8):489–99.
7. Gibbs FA, Gibbs EL. Atlas of eletroencephalography: Adisson-Wesley. Editora Cambridge-Massesguster; 1952.
8. Proposal for revised clinical and electroencephalographic classification of epileptic seizures. From the Commission on Classification and Terminology of the International League Against Epilepsy. Epilepsia. 1981;22(4):489–501.
9. Roger J, Dravet C, Bureau M, Dreifuss FE, Wolf P. Epileptic syndromes in childhood and adolescence, 1984.
10. Proposal for classification of epilepsies and epileptic syndromes. Commission on Classification and Terminology of the International League Against Epilepsy. Epilepsia. 1985;26(3):268–78.
11. Proposal for revised classification of epilepsies and epileptic syndromes. Commission on Classification and Terminology of the International League Against Epilepsy. Epilepsia. 1989;30(4):389–99.
12. Zuberi SM, Wirrell E, Yozawitz E, Wilmshurst JM, Specchio N, Riney K, et al. ILAE classification and definition of epilepsy syndromes with onset in neonates and infants: position statement by the ILAE Task Force on Nosology and Definitions. Epilepsia. 2022;63(6):1349–97.
13. Fisher RS, Cross JH, French JA, Higurashi N, Hirsch E, Jansen FE, et al. Operational classification of seizure types by the International League Against epilepsy: position paper of the ILAE Commission for Classification and Terminology. Epilepsia. 2017;58(4):522–30.
14. Shevell MI, Sinclair DB, Metrakos K. Benign familial neonatal seizures: clinical and electroencephalographic characteristics. Pediatr Neurol. 1986;2(5):272–5.
15. Ronen GM, Rosales TO, Connolly M, Anderson VE, Leppert M. Seizure characteristics in chromosome 20 benign familial neonatal convulsions. Neurology. 1993;43(7):1355–60.
16. Grinton BE, Heron SE, Pelekanos JT, Zuberi SM, Kivity S, Afawi Z, et al. Familial neonatal seizures in 36 families: clinical and genetic features correlate with outcome. Epilepsia. 2015;56(7):1071–80.
17. Rett ATR. Neugeborenenkra?mpfe im Rahmen einer epileptisch belasteten Familie. Wien Klin Wochenschr. 1964;
18. Symonds JD, Elliott KS, Shetty J, Armstrong M, Brunklaus A, Cutcutache I, et al. Early childhood epilepsies: epidemiology, classification, aetiology, and socio-economic determinants. Brain. 2021;144(9):2879–91.
19. Heron SE, Cox K, Grinton BE, Zuberi SM, Kivity S, Afawi Z, et al. Deletions or duplications in KCNQ2 can cause benign familial neonatal seizures. J Med Genet. 2007;44(12):791–6.
20. Dedek K, Kunath B, Kananura C, Reuner U, Jentsch TJ, Steinlein OK. Myokymia and neonatal epilepsy caused by a mutation in the voltage sensor of the KCNQ2 K+ channel. Proc Natl Acad Sci USA. 2001;98(21):12272–7.

21. Hirsch E, Velez A, Sellal F, Maton B, Grinspan A, Malafosse A, et al. Electroclinical signs of benign neonatal familial convulsions. Ann Neurol. 1993;34(6):835–41.
22. Sands TT, Balestri M, Bellini G, Mulkey SB, Danhaive O, Bakken EH, et al. Rapid and safe response to low-dose carbamazepine in neonatal epilepsy. Epilepsia. 2016;57(12):2019–30.
23. Cornet MC, Morabito V, Lederer D, Glass HC, Ferrao Santos S, Numis AL, et al. Neonatal presentation of genetic epilepsies: early differentiation from acute provoked seizures. Epilepsia. 2021;62(8):1907–20.
24. Peng J, Wang Y, He F, Chen C, Wu LW, Yang LF, et al. Novel West syndrome candidate genes in a Chinese cohort. CNS Neurosci Ther. 2018;24(12):1196–206.
25. Scher MS, Alvin J, Gaus L, Minnigh B, Painter MJ. Uncoupling of EEG-clinical neonatal seizures after antiepileptic drug use. Pediatr Neurol. 2003;28(4):277–80.
26. Pressler RM, Lagae L. Why we urgently need improved seizure and epilepsy therapies for children and neonates. Neuropharmacology. 2020;170:107854.
27. Sharma D, Hussain AM, Sharma SS. Efficacy of Levetiracetam in neonatal seizures: a systematic review. J Matern Fetal Neonatal Med. 2022;35(20):3923–30.
28. Rundfeldt C, Netzer R. The novel anticonvulsant retigabine activates M-currents in Chinese hamster ovary-cells tranfected with human KCNQ2/3 subunits. Neurosci Lett. 2000;282(1–2):73–6.
29. Musella S, Carotenuto L, Iraci N, Baroli G, Ciaglia T, Nappi P, et al. Beyond Retigabine: design, synthesis, and pharmacological characterization of a potent and chemically stable neuronal Kv7 channel activator with anticonvulsant activity. J Med Chem. 2022;65(16):11340–64.
30. Maihara T, Tsuji M, Higuchi Y, Hattori H. Benign familial neonatal convulsions followed by benign epilepsy with centrotemporal spikes in two siblings. Epilepsia. 1999;40(1):110–3.
31. Kaplan RE, Lacey DJ. Benign familial neonatal-infantile seizures. Am J Med Genet. 1983;16(4):595–9.
32. Heron SE, Crossland KM, Andermann E, Phillips HA, Hall AJ, Bleasel A, et al. Sodium-channel defects in benign familial neonatal-infantile seizures. Lancet. 2002;360(9336):851–2.
33. Berkovic SF, Heron SE, Giordano L, Marini C, Guerrini R, Kaplan RE, et al. Benign familial neonatal-infantile seizures: characterization of a new sodium channelopathy. Ann Neurol. 2004;55(4):550–7.
34. Wolff M, Johannesen KM, Hedrich UBS, Masnada S, Rubboli G, Gardella E, et al. Genetic and phenotypic heterogeneity suggest therapeutic implications in SCN2A-related disorders. Brain. 2017;140(5):1316–36.
35. Gardiner M. Molecular genetics of infantile nervous system channelopathies. Early Hum Dev. 2006;82(12):775–9.
36. Liao Y, Deprez L, Maljevic S, Pitsch J, Claes L, Hristova D, et al. Molecular correlates of age-dependent seizures in an inherited neonatal-infantile epilepsy. Brain. 2010;133(Pt 5):1403–14.
37. Zara F, Specchio N, Striano P, Robbiano A, Gennaro E, Paravidino R, et al. Genetic testing in benign familial epilepsies of the first year of life: clinical and diagnostic significance. Epilepsia. 2013;54(3):425–36.
38. Zeng Q, Yang X, Zhang J, Liu A, Yang Z, Liu X, et al. Genetic analysis of benign familial epilepsies in the first year of life in a Chinese cohort. J Hum Genet. 2018;63(1):9–18.
39. Herlenius E, Heron SE, Grinton BE, Keay D, Scheffer IE, Mulley JC, et al. SCN2A mutations and benign familial neonatal-infantile seizures: the phenotypic spectrum. Epilepsia. 2007;48(6):1138–42.
40. Spoto G, Saia MC, Amore G, Gitto E, Loddo G, Mainieri G, et al. Neonatal seizures: An overview of genetic causes and treatment options. Brain Sci. 2021;11(10):1295.
41. Vigevano F. Benign familial infantile seizures. Brain Dev. 2005;27(3):172–7.
42. Heron SE, Grinton BE, Kivity S, Afawi Z, Zuberi SM, Hughes JN, et al. PRRT2 mutations cause benign familial infantile epilepsy and infantile convulsions with choreoathetosis syndrome. Am J Hum Genet. 2012;90(1):152–60.
43. Ono S, Yoshiura K, Kinoshita A, Kikuchi T, Nakane Y, Kato N, et al. Mutations in PRRT2 responsible for paroxysmal kinesigenic dyskinesias also cause benign familial infantile convulsions. J Hum Genet. 2012;57(5):338–41.

44. Fukuyama Y. Borderland of epilepsy with special reference to febrile convulsions and so-called infantile convulsions. Seishin-Igaku (Clin Psychiatry). 1963;5:211–23.
45. Vigevano F, Fusco L, Di Capua M, Ricci S, Sebastianelli R, Lucchini P. Benign infantile familial convulsions. Eur J Pediatr. 1992;151(8):608–12.
46. Lee WL, Low PS, Rajan U. Benign familial infantile epilepsy. J Pediatr. 1993;123(4):588–90.
47. Luovigsson P. Benign infantile familial epilepsy: three families with multiple affected members in three generations. Epilepsia. 1993;34(2):18.
48. Echenne B, Humbertclaude V, Rivier F, Malafosse A, Cheminal R. Benign infantile epilepsy with autosomal dominant inheritance. Brain Dev. 1994;16(2):108–11.
49. Capovilla G, Giordano L, Tiberti S, Valseriati D, Menegati E. Benign partial epilepsy in infancy with complex partial seizures (Watanabe's syndrome): 12 non-Japanese new cases. Brain Dev. 1998;20(2):105–11.
50. Giordano L, Accorsi P, Valseriati D, Tiberti A, Menegati E, Zara F, et al. Benign infantile familial convulsions: natural history of a case and clinical characteristics of a large Italian family. Neuropediatrics. 1999;30(2):99–101.
51. Callenbach PM, de Coo RF, Vein AA, Arts WF, Oosterwijk J, Hageman G, et al. Benign familial infantile convulsions: a clinical study of seven Dutch families. Eur J Paediatr Neurol. 2002;6(5):269–83.
52. Engel J Jr. International League Against E. A proposed diagnostic scheme for people with epileptic seizures and with epilepsy: report of the ILAE Task Force on Classification and Terminology. Epilepsia. 2001;42(6):796–803.
53. Berg AT, Berkovic SF, Brodie MJ, Buchhalter J, Cross JH, van Emde BW, et al. Revised terminology and concepts for organization of seizures and epilepsies: report of the ILAE Commission on Classification and Terminology, 2005-2009. Epilepsia. 2010;51(4):676–85.
54. Ramos-Lizana J, Martinez-Espinosa G, Rodriguez-Lucenilla MI, Aguirre-Rodriguez J, Aguilera-Lopez P. Frequency, semiology and prognosis of benign infantile epilepsy. Rev Neurol. 2018;66(8):254–60.
55. Symonds JD, Zuberi SM, Stewart K, McLellan A, O'Regan M, MacLeod S, et al. Incidence and phenotypes of childhood-onset genetic epilepsies: a prospective population-based national cohort. Brain. 2019;142(8):2303–18.
56. Heron SE, Dibbens LM. Role of PRRT2 in common paroxysmal neurological disorders: a gene with remarkable pleiotropy. J Med Genet. 2013;50(3):133–9.
57. Caraballo RH, Cersosimo RO, Amartino H, Szepetowski P, Fejerman N. Benign familial infantile seizures: further delineation of the syndrome. J Child Neurol. 2002;17(9):696–9.
58. Watanabe K, Yamamoto N, Negoro T, Takaesu E, Aso K, Furune S, et al. Benign complex partial epilepsies in infancy. Pediatr Neurol. 1987;3(4):208–11.
59. Dale RC, Grattan-Smith P, Nicholson M, Peters GB. Microdeletions detected using chromosome microarray in children with suspected genetic movement disorders: a single-centre study. Dev Med Child Neurol. 2012;54(7):618–23.
60. Silveira-Moriyama L, Gardiner AR, Meyer E, King MD, Smith M, Rakshi K, et al. Clinical features of childhood-onset paroxysmal kinesigenic dyskinesia with PRRT2 gene mutations. Dev Med Child Neurol. 2013;55(4):327–34.
61. Weber A, Kohler A, Hahn A, Neubauer B, Muller U. Benign infantile convulsions (IC) and subsequent paroxysmal kinesigenic dyskinesia (PKD) in a patient with 16p11.2 microdeletion syndrome. Neurogenetics. 2013;14(3–4):251–3.
62. Termsarasab P, Yang AC, Reiner J, Mei H, Scott SA, Frucht SJ. Paroxysmal kinesigenic dyskinesia caused by 16p112 microdeletion. Tremor Other Hyperkinet Mov (N Y). 2014;4:274.
63. Gardella E, Becker F, Moller RS, Schubert J, Lemke JR, Larsen LH, et al. Benign infantile seizures and paroxysmal dyskinesia caused by an SCN8A mutation. Ann Neurol. 2016;79(3):428–36.
64. Miceli F, Soldovieri MV, Ambrosino P, Barrese V, Migliore M, Cilio MR, et al. Genotype-phenotype correlations in neonatal epilepsies caused by mutations in the voltage sensor of K(v)7.2 potassium channel subunits. Proc Natl Acad Sci USA. 2013;110(11):4386–91.

65. Bureau M, Cokar O, Maton B, Genton P, Dravet C. Sleep-related, low voltage Rolandic and vertex spikes: an EEG marker of benignity in infancy-onset focal epilepsies. Epileptic Disord. 2002;4(1):15–22.
66. Flesler S, Sakr D, Cersosimo R, Caraballo R. Benign infantile focal epilepsy with midline spikes and waves during sleep: a new epileptic syndrome or a variant of benign focal epilepsy? Epileptic Disord. 2010;12(3):205–11.
67. Capovilla G, Beccaria F, Montagnini A. 'Benign focal epilepsy in infancy with vertex spikes and waves during sleep'. Delineation of the syndrome and recalling as 'benign infantile focal epilepsy with midline spikes and waves during sleep' (BIMSE). Brain Dev. 2006;28(2):85–91.
68. Kong W, Zhang Y, Jiang Y. In response: SCN8A mutations in Chinese children with early onset epilepsy and intellectual disability. Epilepsia. 2015;56(8):1320.
69. Larsen J, Carvill GL, Gardella E, Kluger G, Schmiedel G, Barisic N, et al. The phenotypic spectrum of SCN8A encephalopathy. Neurology. 2015;84(5):480–9.
70. Boerma RS, Braun KP, van den Broek MP, van Berkestijn FM, Swinkels ME, Hagebeuk EO, et al. Remarkable Phenytoin sensitivity in 4 children with SCN8A-related epilepsy: a molecular neuropharmacological approach. Neurotherapeutics. 2016;13(1):192–7.
71. Wagnon JL, Barker BS, Hounshell JA, Haaxma CA, Shealy A, Moss T, et al. Pathogenic mechanism of recurrent mutations of SCN8A in epileptic encephalopathy. Ann Clin Transl Neurol. 2016;3(2):114–23.
72. Wagnon JL, Korn MJ, Parent R, Tarpey TA, Jones JM, Hammer MF, et al. Convulsive seizures and SUDEP in a mouse model of SCN8A epileptic encephalopathy. Hum Mol Genet. 2015;24(2):506–15.
73. Wagnon JL, Meisler MH. Recurrent and non-recurrent mutations of SCN8A in epileptic encephalopathy. Front Neurol. 2015;6:104.
74. Okumura A, Hayakawa F, Kuno K, Watanabe K. Benign partial epilepsy in infancy. Arch Dis Child. 1996;74(1):19–21.
75. Auvin S, Pandit F, De Bellecize J, Badinand N, Isnard H, Motte J, et al. Benign myoclonic epilepsy in infants: electroclinical features and long-term follow-up of 34 patients. Epilepsia. 2006;47(2):387–93.
76. Dravet C, Bureau M. The benign myoclonic epilepsy of infancy (author's transl). Rev Electroencephalogr Neurophysiol Clin. 1981;11(3–4):438–44.
77. Caraballo RH, Flesler S, Pasteris MC, Lopez Avaria MF, Fortini S, Vilte C. Myoclonic epilepsy in infancy: an electroclinical study and long-term follow-up of 38 patients. Epilepsia. 2013;54(9):1605–12.
78. Lin Y, Itomi K, Takada H, Kuboda T, Okumura A, Aso K, et al. Benign myoclonic epilepsy in infants: video-EEG features and long-term follow-up. Neuropediatrics. 1998;29(5):268–71.
79. Ricci S, Cusmai R, Fusco L, Vigevano F. Reflex myoclonic epilepsy in infancy: a new age-dependent idiopathic epileptic syndrome related to startle reaction. Epilepsia. 1995;36(4):342–8.
80. Capovilla G, Beccaria F, Gambardella A, Montagnini A, Avantaggiato P, Seri S. Photosensitive benign myoclonic epilepsy in infancy. Epilepsia. 2007;48(1):96–100.
81. Dravet C, Bureau M, Genton P. Benign myoclonic epilepsy of infancy: electroclinical symptomatology and differential diagnosis from the other types of generalized epilepsy of infancy. Epilepsy Res Suppl. 1992;6:131–5.
82. Olson HE, Kelly M, LaCoursiere CM, Pinsky R, Tambunan D, Shain C, et al. Genetics and genotype-phenotype correlations in early onset epileptic encephalopathy with burst suppression. Ann Neurol. 2017;81(3):419–29.
83. Djukic A, Lado FA, Shinnar S, Moshe SL. Are early myoclonic encephalopathy (EME) and the Ohtahara syndrome (EIEE) independent of each other? Epilepsy Res. 2006;70(Suppl 1):S68–76.
84. Dulac O. Epileptic encephalopathy. Epilepsia. 2001;42 Suppl 3(s3):23–6.
85. Poke G, Stanley J, Scheffer IE, Sadleir LG. Epidemiology of developmental and epileptic encephalopathy and of intellectual disability and epilepsy in children. Neurology. 2023;100(13):e1363–e75.

86. Hanada T, Hashizume Y, Tokuhara N, Takenaka O, Kohmura N, Ogasawara A, et al. Perampanel: a novel, orally active, noncompetitive AMPA-receptor antagonist that reduces seizure activity in rodent models of epilepsy. Epilepsia. 2011;52(7):1331–40.
87. Villanueva V, Montoya J, Castillo A, Mauri-Llerda JA, Giner P, Lopez-Gonzalez FJ, et al. Perampanel in routine clinical use in idiopathic generalized epilepsy: The 12-month GENERAL study. Epilepsia. 2018;59(9):1740–52.
88. Trinka E, Lattanzi S, Carpenter K, Corradetti T, Nucera B, Rinaldi F, et al. Exploring the evidence for broad-spectrum effectiveness of Perampanel: a systematic review of clinical data in generalised seizures. CNS Drugs. 2021;35(8):821–37.
89. Verrotti A, Cerminara C, Domizio S, Mohn A, Franzoni E, Coppola G, et al. Levetiracetam in absence epilepsy. Dev Med Child Neurol. 2008;50(11):850–3.
90. National Institute for Health and Care Excellence: clinical guidelines. Epilepsies: diagnosis and management. National Institute for Health and Care Excellence: clinical guidelines. London: National Institute for Health and Care Excellence (NICE); 2021.
91. Mikkelsen B, Birket-Smith E, Bradt S, Holm P, Bparm LM, et al. Clonazepam in the treatment of epilepsy. A controlled clinical trial in simple absences, bilateral massive epileptic myoclonus, and atonic seizures. Arch Neurol. 1976;33(5):322–5.
92. Riney K, Bogacz A, Somerville E, Hirsch E, Nabbout R, Scheffer IE, et al. International League Against Epilepsy classification and definition of epilepsy syndromes with onset at a variable age: position statement by the ILAE Task Force on Nosology and Definitions. Epilepsia. 2022;63(6):1443–74.
93. Genton P, Ferlazzo E, Thomas P. Absence status epilepsy: delineation of a distinct idiopathic generalized epilepsy syndrome. Epilepsia. 2008;49(4):642–9.
94. West WJ. On a peculiar form of infantile convulsions. Lancet. 1841;35:724–5.
95. Riikonen R. Epidemiological data of West syndrome in Finland. Brain Dev. 2001;23(7):539–41.
96. Wirrell EC, Shellhaas RA, Joshi C, Keator C, Kumar S, Mitchell WG, et al. How should children with West syndrome be efficiently and accurately investigated? Results from the National Infantile Spasms Consortium. Epilepsia. 2015;56(4):617–25.
97. Wirrell E, Tinuper P, Perucca E, Moshe SL. Introduction to the epilepsy syndrome papers. Epilepsia. 2022;63(6):1330–2.
98. Pavone P, Polizzi A, Marino SD, Corsello G, Falsaperla R, Marino S, et al. West syndrome: a comprehensive review. Neurol Sci. 2020;41(12):3547–62.
99. Chopra SS. Infantile spasms and west syndrome - a clinician's perspective. Indian J Pediatr. 2020;87(12):1040–6.
100. Chu-Shore CJ, Major P, Camposano S, Muzykewicz D, Thiele EA. The natural history of epilepsy in tuberous sclerosis complex. Epilepsia. 2010;51(7):1236–41.
101. Surana P, Symonds JD, Srivastava P, Geetha TS, Jain R, Vedant R, et al. Infantile spasms: etiology, lead time and treatment response in a resource limited setting. Epilepsy Behav Rep. 2020;14:100397.
102. Galanopoulou AS, Moshe SL. Neonatal and infantile epilepsy: acquired and genetic models. Cold Spring Harb Perspect Med. 2015;6(1):a022707.
103. Meng Y, Geng G, Ren Y, Zhang H, Gao Z, Liu Y, et al. Long-term outcome of Adrenocorticotropic hormone therapy in children with new-onset infantile spasms. Pediatr Neurol. 2023;143:100–5.
104. Pardo CA, Nabbout R, Galanopoulou AS. Mechanisms of epileptogenesis in pediatric epileptic syndromes: Rasmussen encephalitis, infantile spasms, and febrile infection-related epilepsy syndrome (FIRES). Neurotherapeutics. 2014;11(2):297–310.
105. Paprocka J, Malkiewicz J, Palazzo-Michalska V, Nowacka B, Kuzniak M, Kopyta I. Effectiveness of ACTH in patients with infantile spasms. Brain Sci. 2022;12(2):254.
106. O'Callaghan FJ, Edwards SW, Alber FD, Hancock E, Johnson AL, Kennedy CR, et al. Safety and effectiveness of hormonal treatment versus hormonal treatment with vigabatrin for infantile spasms (ICISS): a randomised, multicentre, open-label trial. Lancet Neurol. 2017;16(1):33–42.

107. O'Callaghan FJK, Edwards SW, Alber FD, Cortina Borja M, Hancock E, Johnson AL, et al. Vigabatrin with hormonal treatment versus hormonal treatment alone (ICISS) for infantile spasms: 18-month outcomes of an open-label, randomised controlled trial. Lancet Child Adolesc Health. 2018;2(10):715–25.
108. Prezioso G, Chiarelli F, Matricardi S. Efficacy and safety of vigabatrin in patients with tuberous sclerosis complex and infantile epileptic spasm syndrome: a systematic review. Expert Rev Neurother. 2023;23(7):661–71.
109. Krueger DA, Northrup H. International Tuberous Sclerosis Complex Consensus G. Tuberous sclerosis complex surveillance and management: recommendations of the 2012 international tuberous sclerosis complex consensus conference. Pediatr Neurol. 2013;49(4):255–65.
110. Hussain SA, Tsao J, Li M, Schwarz MD, Zhou R, Wu JY, et al. Risk of vigabatrin-associated brain abnormalities on MRI in the treatment of infantile spasms is dose-dependent. Epilepsia. 2017;58(4):674–82.
111. Hanifiha M, Shervin Badv R, Mahmoudi M, Tavasoli AR. The efficacy of the Ketogenic diet in improving seizures and EEG findings in patients with refractory infantile spasms. Iran J Child Neurol. 2022;16(4):45–54.
112. Matsuura R, Hamano SI, Ikemoto S, Daida A, Takeda R, Horiguchi A, et al. Adjunctive perampanel therapy for patients with epileptic spasms. Pediatr Int. 2022;64(1):e15364.
113. Wang Q, He W, Wang Y, Liu L, Zhang M, Yang X, et al. Response to magnesium sulfate and adrenocorticotropic hormone combination therapy for infantile spasms with failed first-line treatments. Pediatr Investig. 2023;7(1):29–35.
114. Sillanpaa M, Riikonen R, Saarinen MM, Schmidt D. Long-term mortality of patients with West syndrome. Epilepsia Open. 2016;1(1–2):61–6.
115. Rajaraman RR, Lay J, Alayari A, Anderson K, Sankar R, Hussain SA. Prevention of infantile spasms relapse: Zonisamide and topiramate provide no benefit. Epilepsia. 2016;57(8):1280–7.
116. Coppola G, Plouin P, Chiron C, Robain O, Dulac O. Migrating partial seizures in infancy: a malignant disorder with developmental arrest. Epilepsia. 1995;36(10):1017–24.
117. McTague A, Appleton R, Avula S, Cross JH, King MD, Jacques TS, et al. Migrating partial seizures of infancy: expansion of the electroclinical, radiological and pathological disease spectrum. Brain. 2013;136(Pt 5):1578–91.
118. Burgess R, Wang S, McTague A, Boysen KE, Yang X, Zeng Q, et al. The genetic landscape of epilepsy of infancy with migrating focal seizures. Ann Neurol. 2019;86(6):821–31.
119. Cilio MR, Bianchi R, Balestri M, Onofri A, Giovannini S, Di Capua M, et al. Intravenous levetiracetam terminates refractory status epilepticus in two patients with migrating partial seizures in infancy. Epilepsy Res. 2009;86(1):66–71.
120. Djuric M, Kravljanac R, Kovacevic G, Martic J. The efficacy of bromides, stiripentol and levetiracetam in two patients with malignant migrating partial seizures in infancy. Epileptic Disord. 2011;13(1):22–6.
121. Vendrame M, Poduri A, Loddenkemper T, Kluger G, Coppola G, Kothare SV. Treatment of malignant migrating partial epilepsy of infancy with rufinamide: report of five cases. Epileptic Disord. 2011;13(1):18–21.
122. Merdariu D, Delanoe C, Mahfoufi N, Bellavoine V, Auvin S. Malignant migrating partial seizures of infancy controlled by stiripentol and clonazepam. Brain Dev. 2013;35(2):177–80.
123. Saade D, Joshi C. Pure cannabidiol in the treatment of malignant migrating partial seizures in infancy: a case report. Pediatr Neurol. 2015;52(5):544–7.
124. Borlot F, Abushama A, Morrison-Levy N, Jain P, Puthenveettil Vinayan K, Abukhalid M, et al. KCNT1-related epilepsy: An international multicenter cohort of 27 pediatric cases. Epilepsia. 2020;61(4):679–92.
125. Caraballo R, Pasteris MC, Fortini PS, Portuondo E. Epilepsy of infancy with migrating focal seizures: six patients treated with bromide. Seizure. 2014;23(10):899–902.
126. Patil AA, Vinayan KP, Roy AG. Two south Indian children with KCNT1-related malignant migrating focal seizures of infancy - clinical characteristics and outcome of targeted treatment with quinidine. Ann Indian Acad Neurol. 2019;22(3):311–5.

127. Barcia G, Chemaly N, Kuchenbuch M, Eisermann M, Gobin-Limballe S, Ciorna V, et al. Epilepsy with migrating focal seizures: KCNT1 mutation hotspots and phenotype variability. Neurol Genet. 2019;5(6):e363.
128. Armeno M, Verini A, Araujo MB, Reyes G, Caraballo RH. Ketogenic parenteral nutrition in three paediatric patients with epilepsy with migrating focal seizures. Epileptic Disord. 2019;21(5):443–8.
129. Burbano LE, Li M, Jancovski N, Jafar-Nejad P, Richards K, Sedo A, et al. Antisense oligonucleotide therapy for KCNT1 encephalopathy. JCI Insight. 2022;7(23):e146090.
130. Kuchenbuch M, Barcia G, Chemaly N, Carme E, Roubertie A, Gibaud M, et al. KCNT1 epilepsy with migrating focal seizures shows a temporal sequence with poor outcome, high mortality and SUDEP. Brain. 2019;142(10):2996–3008.
131. Tolone S. On Unverricht's myoclonus-epilepsy. Prog Med (Napoli). 1945;1:150–5.
132. Harriman DG, Millar JH, Stevenson AC. Progressive familial myoclonic epilepsy in three families: its clinical features and pathological basis. Brain. 1955;78(3):325–49.
133. Dravet C, Bureau M, Oguni H, Fukuyama Y, Cokar O. Severe myoclonic epilepsy in infancy: Dravet syndrome. Adv Neurol. 2005;95:71–102.
134. Wolff M, Casse-Perrot C, Dravet C. Severe myoclonic epilepsy of infants (Dravet syndrome): natural history and neuropsychological findings. Epilepsia. 2006;47(Suppl 2):45–8.
135. Depienne C, Trouillard O, Gourfinkel-An I, Saint-Martin C, Bouteiller D, Graber D, et al. Mechanisms for variable expressivity of inherited SCN1A mutations causing Dravet syndrome. J Med Genet. 2010;47(6):404–10.
136. Ragona F, Granata T, Dalla Bernardina B, Offredi F, Darra F, Battaglia D, et al. Cognitive development in Dravet syndrome: a retrospective, multicenter study of 26 patients. Epilepsia. 2011;52(2):386–92.
137. Dravet C. The core Dravet syndrome phenotype. Epilepsia. 2011;52(Suppl 2):3–9.
138. Hurst DL. Epidemiology of severe myoclonic epilepsy of infancy. Epilepsia. 1990;31(4):397–400.
139. Dravet C. Dravet syndrome history. Dev Med Child Neurol. 2011;53(Suppl 2):1–6.
140. Battaglia D, Chieffo D, Lucibello S, Marini C, Sibilia V, Mei D, et al. Multicenter prospective longitudinal study in 34 patients with Dravet syndrome: neuropsychological development in the first six years of life. Brain Dev. 2021;43(3):419–30.
141. Olivieri G, Battaglia D, Chieffo D, Rubbino R, Ranalli D, Contaldo I, et al. Cognitive-behavioral profiles in teenagers with Dravet syndrome. Brain Dev. 2016;38(6):554–62.
142. Genton P, Velizarova R, Dravet C. Dravet syndrome: the long-term outcome. Epilepsia. 2011;52(Suppl 2):44–9.
143. De Liso P, Pironi V, Mastrangelo M, Battaglia D, Craiu D, Trivisano M, et al. Fatal status Epilepticus in Dravet syndrome. Brain Sci. 2020;10(11):889.
144. Perulli M, Battista A, Sivo S, Turrini I, Musto E, Quintiliani M, et al. Heart rate variability alterations in Dravet syndrome: The role of status epilepticus and a possible association with mortality risk. Seizure. 2022;94:129–35.
145. Frampton JE. Stiripentol: a review in Dravet syndrome. Drugs. 2019;79(16):1785–96.
146. Gunning B, Mazurkiewicz-Beldzinska M, Chin RFM, Bhathal H, Nortvedt C, Dunayevich E, et al. Cannabidiol in conjunction with clobazam: analysis of four randomized controlled trials. Acta Neurol Scand. 2021;143(2):154–63.
147. Madan Cohen J, Checketts D, Dunayevich E, Gunning B, Hyslop A, Madhavan D, et al. Time to onset of cannabidiol treatment effects in Dravet syndrome: analysis from two randomized controlled trials. Epilepsia. 2021;62(9):2218–27.
148. Simon K, Sheckley H, Anderson CL, Liu Z, Carney PR. A review of fenfluramine for the treatment of Dravet syndrome patients. Curr Res Pharmacol Drug Discov. 2022;3:100078.
149. Kikuchi K, Hamano SI, Matsuura R, Nonoyama H, Daida A, Hirata Y, et al. The effectiveness of intravenous benzodiazepine for status epilepticus in Dravet syndrome. Brain Dev. 2022;44(5):319–28.

150. Goto A IASMIYCECHS. Characteristics of KCNQ2 variants causing either benign neonatal epilepsy or developmental and epileptic encephalopathy. Epilepsia. 2019;60(9):1870.
151. Singh NA, Charlier C, Stauffer D, DuPont BR, Leach RJ, Melis R, et al. A novel potassium channel gene, KCNQ2, is mutated in an inherited epilepsy of newborns. Nat Genet. 1998;18(1):25–9.
152. Soldovieri MV, Miceli F, Bellini G, Coppola G, Pascotto A, Taglialatela M. Correlating the clinical and genetic features of benign familial neonatal seizures (BFNS) with the functional consequences of underlying mutations. Channels (Austin). 2007;1(4):228–33.
153. Borgatti R, Zucca C, Cavallini A, Ferrario M, Panzeri C, Castaldo P, et al. A novel mutation in KCNQ2 associated with BFNC, drug resistant epilepsy, and mental retardation. Neurology. 2004;63(1):57–65.
154. Symonds JD, McTague A. Epilepsy and developmental disorders: next generation sequencing in the clinic. Eur J Paediatr Neurol. 2020;24:15–23.
155. Shellhaas RA, Wusthoff CJ, Tsuchida TN, Glass HC, Chu CJ, Massey SL, et al. Profile of neonatal epilepsies: characteristics of a prospective US cohort. Neurology. 2017;89(9):893–9.
156. Zhu G, Okada M, Murakami T, Kamata A, Kawata Y, Wada K, et al. Dysfunction of M-channel enhances propagation of neuronal excitability in rat hippocampus monitored by multielectrode dish and microdialysis systems. Neurosci Lett. 2000;294(1):53–7.
157. Orhan G, Bock M, Schepers D, Ilina EI, Reichel SN, Loffler H, et al. Dominant-negative effects of KCNQ2 mutations are associated with epileptic encephalopathy. Ann Neurol. 2014;75(3):382–94.
158. Weckhuysen S, Ivanovic V, Hendrickx R, Van Coster R, Hjalgrim H, Moller RS, et al. Extending the KCNQ2 encephalopathy spectrum: clinical and neuroimaging findings in 17 patients. Neurology. 2013;81(19):1697–703.
159. Millichap JJ, Park KL, Tsuchida T, Ben-Zeev B, Carmant L, Flamini R, et al. KCNQ2 encephalopathy: features, mutational hot spots, and ezogabine treatment of 11 patients. Neurol Genet. 2016;2(5):e96.
160. Ishii A, Miyajima T, Kurahashi H, Wang JW, Yasumoto S, Kaneko S, et al. KCNQ2 abnormality in BECTS: benign childhood epilepsy with centrotemporal spikes following benign neonatal seizures resulting from a mutation of KCNQ2. Epilepsy Res. 2012;102(1–2):122–5.
161. Kim HJ, Yang D, Kim SH, Won D, Kim HD, Lee JS, et al. Clinical characteristics of KCNQ2 encephalopathy. Brain Dev. 2021;43(2):244–50.
162. Stenson PD, Mort M, Ball EV, Chapman M, Evans K, Azevedo L, et al. The Human Gene Mutation Database (HGMD((R))): optimizing its use in a clinical diagnostic or research setting. Hum Genet. 2020;139(10):1197–207.
163. Pisano T, Numis AL, Heavin SB, Weckhuysen S, Angriman M, Suls A, et al. Early and effective treatment of KCNQ2 encephalopathy. Epilepsia. 2015;56(5):685–91.
164. Gospe SM Jr. Pyridoxine-dependent epilepsy - ALDH7A1. In: Adam MP, Feldman J, Mirzaa GM, Pagon RA, Wallace SE, Bean LJH, et al., editors. GeneReviews((R)). Seattle; 1993.
165. Coughlin CR 2nd, Swanson MA, Spector E, Meeks NJL, Kronquist KE, Aslamy M, et al. The genotypic spectrum of ALDH7A1 mutations resulting in pyridoxine dependent epilepsy: a common epileptic encephalopathy. J Inherit Metab Dis. 2019;42(2):353–61.
166. Crowther LM, Mathis D, Poms M, Plecko B. New insights into human lysine degradation pathways with relevance to pyridoxine-dependent epilepsy due to antiquitin deficiency. J Inherit Metab Dis. 2019;42(4):620–8.
167. Snyderman SE, Holt LE Jr, Carretero R, Jacobs K. Pyridoxine deficiency in the human infant. J Clin Nutr. 1953;1(3):200–7.
168. Molony CJ, Parmelee AH. Convulsions in young infants as a result of pyridoxine (vitamin B6) deficiency. JAMA J Am Med Assoc. 1954;154(5):405–6.
169. Hunt AD Jr, Stokes J Jr, Mc CW, Stroud HH. Pyridoxine dependency: report of a case of intractable convulsions in an infant controlled by pyridoxine. Pediatrics. 1954;13(2):140–5.
170. Mills PB, Struys E, Jakobs C, Plecko B, Baxter P, Baumgartner M, et al. Mutations in antiquitin in individuals with pyridoxine-dependent seizures. Nat Med. 2006;12(3):307–9.

171. Ebinger M, Schultze C, Konig S. Demographics and diagnosis of pyridoxine-dependent seizures. J Pediatr. 1999;134(6):795–6.
172. Baxter P. Epidemiology of pyridoxine dependent and pyridoxine responsive seizures in the UK. Arch Dis Child. 1999;81(5):431–3.
173. Coughlin CR 2nd, Tseng LA, Abdenur JE, Ashmore C, Boemer F, Bok LA, et al. Consensus guidelines for the diagnosis and management of pyridoxine-dependent epilepsy due to alpha-aminoadipic semialdehyde dehydrogenase deficiency. J Inherit Metab Dis. 2021;44(1):178–92.
174. Jiao X, Xue J, Gong P, Wu Y, Zhang Y, Jiang Y, et al. Clinical and genetic features in pyridoxine-dependent epilepsy: a Chinese cohort study. Dev Med Child Neurol. 2020;62(3):315–21.
175. Baxter P. Pyridoxine-dependent and pyridoxine-responsive seizures. Dev Med Child Neurol. 2001;43(6):416–20.
176. Srinivasaraghavan R, Parameswaran N, Mathis D, Burer C, Plecko B. Antiquitin deficiency with adolescent onset epilepsy: molecular diagnosis in a mother of affected Offsprings. Neuropediatrics. 2018;49(2):154–7.
177. van Karnebeek CD, Tiebout SA, Niermeijer J, Poll-The BT, Ghani A, Coughlin CR 2nd, et al. Pyridoxine-dependent epilepsy: An expanding clinical spectrum. Pediatr Neurol. 2016;59:6–12.
178. Bok LA, Halbertsma FJ, Houterman S, Wevers RA, Vreeswijk C, Jakobs C, et al. Long-term outcome in pyridoxine-dependent epilepsy. Dev Med Child Neurol. 2012;54(9):849–54.
179. Basura GJ, Hagland SP, Wiltse AM, Gospe SM Jr. Clinical features and the management of pyridoxine-dependent and pyridoxine-responsive seizures: review of 63 North American cases submitted to a patient registry. Eur J Pediatr. 2009;168(6):697–704.
180. de Rooy RLP, Halbertsma FJ, Struijs EA, van Spronsen FJ, Lunsing RJ, Schippers HM, et al. Pyridoxine dependent epilepsy: is late onset a predictor for favorable outcome? Eur J Paediatr Neurol. 2018;22(4):662–6.
181. Mills PB, Footitt EJ, Mills KA, Tuschl K, Aylett S, Varadkar S, et al. Genotypic and phenotypic spectrum of pyridoxine-dependent epilepsy (ALDH7A1 deficiency). Brain. 2010;133(Pt 7):2148–59.
182. Schmitt B, Baumgartner M, Mills PB, Clayton PT, Jakobs C, Keller E, et al. Seizures and paroxysmal events: symptoms pointing to the diagnosis of pyridoxine-dependent epilepsy and pyridoxine phosphate oxidase deficiency. Dev Med Child Neurol. 2010;52(7):e133–42.
183. Nabbout R, Soufflet C, Plouin P, Dulac O. Pyridoxine dependent epilepsy: a suggestive electroclinical pattern. Arch Dis Child Fetal Neonatal Ed. 1999;81(2):F125–9.
184. Friedman SD, Ishak GE, Poliachik SL, Poliakov AV, Otto RK, Shaw DW, et al. Callosal alterations in pyridoxine-dependent epilepsy. Dev Med Child Neurol. 2014;56(11):1106–10.
185. Oesch G, Maga AM, Friedman SD, Poliachik SL, Budech CB, Wright JN, et al. Geometric morphometrics reveal altered corpus callosum shape in pyridoxine-dependent epilepsy. Neurology. 2018;91(1):e78–86.
186. Darin N, Reid E, Prunetti L, Samuelsson L, Husain RA, Wilson M, et al. Mutations in PROSC disrupt cellular pyridoxal phosphate homeostasis and cause vitamin-B(6)-dependent epilepsy. Am J Hum Genet. 2016;99(6):1325–37.
187. Stockler S, Plecko B, Gospe SM Jr, Coulter-Mackie M, Connolly M, van Karnebeek C, et al. Pyridoxine dependent epilepsy and antiquitin deficiency: clinical and molecular characteristics and recommendations for diagnosis, treatment and follow-up. Mol Genet Metab. 2011;104(1–2):48–60.
188. van Karnebeek CD, Jaggumantri S. Current treatment and management of pyridoxine-dependent epilepsy. Curr Treat Options Neurol. 2015;17(2):335.
189. Mercimek-Mahmutoglu S, Cordeiro D, Cruz V, Hyland K, Struys EA, Kyriakopoulou L, et al. Novel therapy for pyridoxine dependent epilepsy due to ALDH7A1 genetic defect: L-arginine supplementation alternative to lysine-restricted diet. Eur J Paediatr Neurol. 2014;18(6):741–6.

190. Kuo MF, Wang HS. Pyridoxal phosphate-responsive epilepsy with resistance to pyridoxine. Pediatr Neurol. 2002;26(2):146–7.
191. Mills PB, Surtees RA, Champion MP, Beesley CE, Dalton N, Scambler PJ, et al. Neonatal epileptic encephalopathy caused by mutations in the PNPO gene encoding pyridox(am)ine 5′-phosphate oxidase. Hum Mol Genet. 2005;14(8):1077–86.
192. Bairoch A. The ENZYME database in 2000. Nucleic Acids Res. 2000;28(1):304–5.
193. Khayat M, Korman SH, Frankel P, Weintraub Z, Hershckowitz S, Sheffer VF, et al. PNPO deficiency: an under diagnosed inborn error of pyridoxine metabolism. Mol Genet Metab. 2008;94(4):431–4.
194. Veeravigrom M, Damrongphol P, Ittiwut R, Ittiwut C, Suphapeetiporn K, Shotelersuk V. Pyridoxal 5′-phosphate-responsive epilepsy with novel mutations in the PNPO gene: a case report. Genet Mol Res. 2015;14(4):14130–5.
195. Mills PB, Camuzeaux SS, Footitt EJ, Mills KA, Gissen P, Fisher L, et al. Epilepsy due to PNPO mutations: genotype, environment and treatment affect presentation and outcome. Brain. 2014;137(Pt 5):1350–60.
196. di Salvo ML, Mastrangelo M, Nogues I, Tolve M, Paiardini A, Carducci C, et al. Pyridoxine-5′-phosphate oxidase (Pnpo) deficiency: clinical and biochemical alterations associated with the C.347g>A (P..Arg116gln) mutation. Mol Genet Metab. 2017;122(1–2):135–42.
197. Xue J, Chang X, Zhang Y, Yang Z. Novel phenotypes of pyridox(am)ine-5′-phosphate oxidase deficiency and high prevalence of c.445_448del mutation in Chinese patients. Metab Brain Dis. 2017;32(4):1081–7.
198. Guerriero RM, Patel AA, Walsh B, Baumer FM, Shah AS, Peters JM, et al. Systemic manifestations in Pyridox(am)ine 5'-phosphate oxidase deficiency. Pediatr Neurol. 2017;76:47–53.
199. Sudarsanam A, Singh H, Wilcken B, Stormon M, Arbuckle S, Schmitt B, et al. Cirrhosis associated with pyridoxal 5′-phosphate treatment of pyridoxamine 5′-phosphate oxidase deficiency. JIMD Rep. 2014;17:67–70.
200. Coman D, Lewindon P, Clayton P, Riney K. PNPO deficiency and Cirrhosis: expanding the clinical phenotype? JIMD Rep. 2016;25:71–5.
201. Levtova A, Camuzeaux S, Laberge AM, Allard P, Brunel-Guitton C, Diadori P, et al. Normal cerebrospinal fluid Pyridoxal 5'-phosphate level in a PNPO-deficient patient with neonatal-onset epileptic encephalopathy. JIMD Rep. 2015;22:67–75.
202. Leonard H, Downs J, Benke TA, Swanson L, Olson H, Demarest S. CDKL5 deficiency disorder: clinical features, diagnosis, and management. Lancet Neurol. 2022;21(6):563–76.
203. Hanefeld F. The clinical pattern of the Rett syndrome. Brain Dev. 1985;7(3):320–5.
204. Kalscheuer VM, Tao J, Donnelly A, Hollway G, Schwinger E, Kubart S, et al. Disruption of the serine/threonine kinase 9 gene causes severe X-linked infantile spasms and mental retardation. Am J Hum Genet. 2003;72(6):1401–11.
205. Liao W, Lee KZ. CDKL5-mediated developmental tuning of neuronal excitability and concomitant regulation of transcriptome. Hum Mol Genet. 2023;32(23):3276–98.
206. Eyers PA. A new consensus for evaluating CDKL5/STK9-dependent signalling mechanisms. EMBO J. 2018;37(24):e100848.
207. Patnaik A, Spiombi E, Frasca A, Landsberger N, Zagrebelsky M, Korte M. Fingolimod modulates dendritic architecture in a BDNF-dependent manner. Int J Mol Sci. 2020;21(9):3079.
208. Jakimiec M, Paprocka J, Smigiel R. CDKL5 deficiency disorder-a complex epileptic encephalopathy. Brain Sci. 2020;10(2):107.
209. Demarest ST, Olson HE, Moss A, Pestana-Knight E, Zhang X, Parikh S, et al. CDKL5 deficiency disorder: relationship between genotype, epilepsy, cortical visual impairment, and development. Epilepsia. 2019;60(8):1733–42.
210. Demarest S, Pestana-Knight EM, Olson HE, Downs J, Marsh ED, Kaufmann WE, et al. Severity assessment in CDKL5 deficiency disorder. Pediatr Neurol. 2019;97:38–42.
211. Aznar-Lain G, Fernandez-Mayoralas DM, Caicoya AG, Rocamora R, Perez-Jurado LA. CDKL5 deficiency disorder without epilepsy. Pediatr Neurol. 2023;144:84–9.
212. Kadam SD, Sullivan BJ, Goyal A, Blue ME, Smith-Hicks C. Rett syndrome and CDKL5 deficiency disorder: from bench to clinic. Int J Mol Sci. 2019;20(20):5098.

213. Lim Z, Wong K, Downs J, Bebbington K, Demarest S, Leonard H. Vagus nerve stimulation for the treatment of refractory epilepsy in the CDKL5 deficiency disorder. Epilepsy Res. 2018;146:36–40.
214. Vossler DG. Ganaxolone: a new treatment for CDKL5 deficiency disorder. Epilepsy Curr. 2022;22(6):348–50.
215. Knight EMP, Amin S, Bahi-Buisson N, Benke TA, Cross JH, Demarest ST, et al. Safety and efficacy of ganaxolone in patients with CDKL5 deficiency disorder: results from the double-blind phase of a randomised, placebo-controlled, phase 3 trial. Lancet Neurol. 2022;21(5):417–27.
216. Olson HE, Demarest S, Pestana-Knight E, Moosa AN, Zhang X, Perez-Perez JR, et al. Epileptic spasms in CDKL5 deficiency disorder: delayed treatment and poor response to first-line therapies. Epilepsia. 2023;64(7):1821–32.
217. Smith L, Singhal N, El Achkar CM, Truglio G, Rosen Sheidley B, Sullivan J, et al. PCDH19-related epilepsy is associated with a broad neurodevelopmental spectrum. Epilepsia. 2018;59(3):679–89.
218. Moncayo JA, Ayala IN, Argudo JM, Aguirre AS, Parwani J, Pachano A, et al. Understanding Protein Protocadherin-19 (PCDH19) syndrome: a literature review of the pathophysiology. Cureus. 2022;14(6):e25808.
219. Depienne C, LeGuern E. PCDH19-related infantile epileptic encephalopathy: an unusual X-linked inheritance disorder. Hum Mutat. 2012;33(4):627–34.
220. Juberg RC, Hellman CD. A new familial form of convulsive disorder and mental retardation limited to females. J Pediatr. 1971;79(5):726–32.
221. Scheffer IE, Turner SJ, Dibbens LM, Bayly MA, Friend K, Hodgson B, et al. Epilepsy and mental retardation limited to females: an under-recognized disorder. Brain. 2008;131(Pt 4):918–27.
222. Lamers D, Landi S, Mezzena R, Baroncelli L, Pillai V, Cruciani F, et al. Perturbation of cortical excitability in a conditional model of PCDH19 disorder. Cells. 2022;11(12):1939.
223. Tsai TY, Sikora M, Xia P, Colak-Champollion T, Knaut H, Heisenberg CP, et al. An adhesion code ensures robust pattern formation during tissue morphogenesis. Science. 2020;370(6512):113–6.
224. Cwetsch AW, Ziogas I, Narducci R, Savardi A, Bolla M, Pinto B, et al. A rat model of a focal mosaic expression of PCDH19 replicates human brain developmental abnormalities and behaviours. Brain Commun. 2022;4(3):fcac091.
225. Rampazzo ACM, Dos Santos RRP, Maluf FA, Simm RF, Marson FAL, Ortega MM, et al. Dravet syndrome and Dravet syndrome-like phenotype: a systematic review of the SCN1A and PCDH19 variants. Neurogenetics. 2021;22(2):105–15.
226. Samanta D. PCDH19-related epilepsy syndrome: a comprehensive clinical review. Pediatr Neurol. 2020;105:3–9.
227. Trivisano M, Specchio N. The role of PCDH19 in refractory status epilepticus. Epilepsy Behav. 2019;101(Pt B):106539.
228. Moncayo JA, Vargas MN, Castillo I, Granda PV, Duque AM, Argudo JM, et al. Adjuvant treatment for Protocadherin 19 (PCDH19) syndrome. Cureus. 2022;14(7):e27154.
229. Trivisano M, Lucchi C, Rustichelli C, Terracciano A, Cusmai R, Ubertini GM, et al. Reduced steroidogenesis in patients with PCDH19-female limited epilepsy. Epilepsia. 2017;58(6):e91–e5.
230. Tan C, Shard C, Ranieri E, Hynes K, Pham DH, Leach D, et al. Mutations of protocadherin 19 in female epilepsy (PCDH19-FE) lead to allopregnanolone deficiency. Hum Mol Genet. 2015;24(18):5250–9.
231. Coman DJ, Sinclair KG, Burke CJ, Appleton DB, Pelekanos JT, O'Neil CM, et al. Seizures, ataxia, developmental delay and the general paediatrician: glucose transporter 1 deficiency syndrome. J Paediatr Child Health. 2006;42(5):263–7.
232. Larsen J, Johannesen KM, Ek J, Tang S, Marini C, Blichfeldt S, et al. The role of SLC2A1 mutations in myoclonic astatic epilepsy and absence epilepsy, and the estimated frequency of GLUT1 deficiency syndrome. Epilepsia. 2015;56(12):e203–8.

233. Rotstein M, Engelstad K, Yang H, Wang D, Levy B, Chung WK, et al. Glut1 deficiency: inheritance pattern determined by haploinsufficiency. Ann Neurol. 2010;68(6):955–8.
234. Yang H, Wang D, Engelstad K, Bagay L, Wei Y, Rotstein M, et al. Glut1 deficiency syndrome and erythrocyte glucose uptake assay. Ann Neurol. 2011;70(6):996–1005.
235. Leen WG, Klepper J, Verbeek MM, Leferink M, Hofste T, van Engelen BG, et al. Glucose transporter-1 deficiency syndrome: the expanding clinical and genetic spectrum of a treatable disorder. Brain. 2010;133(Pt 3):655–70.
236. Alter AS, Engelstad K, Hinton VJ, Montes J, Pearson TS, Akman CI, et al. Long-term clinical course of Glut1 deficiency syndrome. J Child Neurol. 2015;30(2):160–9.
237. Pearson TS, Akman C, Hinton VJ, Engelstad K, De Vivo DC. Phenotypic spectrum of glucose transporter type 1 deficiency syndrome (Glut1 DS). Curr Neurol Neurosci Rep. 2013;13(4):342.
238. Pons R, Collins A, Rotstein M, Engelstad K, De Vivo DC. The spectrum of movement disorders in Glut-1 deficiency. Mov Disord. 2010;25(3):275–81.
239. Pearson TS, Pons R, Engelstad K, Kane SA, Goldberg ME, De Vivo DC. Paroxysmal eye-head movements in Glut1 deficiency syndrome. Neurology. 2017;88(17):1666–73.
240. Urbizu A, Cuenca-Leon E, Raspall-Chaure M, Gratacos M, Conill J, Redecillas S, et al. Paroxysmal exercise-induced dyskinesia, writer's cramp, migraine with aura and absence epilepsy in twin brothers with a novel SLC2A1 missense mutation. J Neurol Sci. 2010;295(1–2):110–3.
241. Zorzi G, Castellotti B, Zibordi F, Gellera C, Nardocci N. Paroxysmal movement disorders in GLUT1 deficiency syndrome. Neurology. 2008;71(2):146–8.
242. Weber YG, Storch A, Wuttke TV, Brockmann K, Kempfle J, Maljevic S, et al. GLUT1 mutations are a cause of paroxysmal exertion-induced dyskinesias and induce hemolytic anemia by a cation leak. J Clin Invest. 2008;118(6):2157–68.
243. Weber YG, Kamm C, Suls A, Kempfle J, Kotschet K, Schule R, et al. Paroxysmal choreoathetosis/spasticity (DYT9) is caused by a GLUT1 defect. Neurology. 2011;77(10):959–64.
244. De Vivo DC, Wang D. Glut1 deficiency: CSF glucose. How low is too low? Rev Neurol (Paris). 2008;164(11):877–80.
245. Leen WG, Wevers RA, Kamsteeg EJ, Scheffer H, Verbeek MM, Willemsen MA. Cerebrospinal fluid analysis in the workup of GLUT1 deficiency syndrome: a systematic review. JAMA Neurol. 2013;70(11):1440–4.
246. Mochel F, Hainque E, Gras D, Adanyeguh IM, Caillet S, Heron B, et al. Triheptanoin dramatically reduces paroxysmal motor disorder in patients with GLUT1 deficiency. J Neurol Neurosurg Psychiatry. 2016;87(5):550–3.
247. Tang M, Gao G, Rueda CB, Yu H, Thibodeaux DN, Awano T, et al. Brain microvasculature defects and Glut1 deficiency syndrome averted by early repletion of the glucose transporter-1 protein. Nat Commun. 2017;8:14152.
248. Ein SR, von Teleangiektasie F. Arch Ophthalmol. 1860;7(1):119–21.
249. Singh AK, Keenaghan M. Sturge-Weber Syndrome. Treasure Island (FL): StatPearls; 2024.
250. Rihani HT, Dalvin LA, Hodge DO, Pulido JS. Incidence of Sturge-Weber syndrome and associated ocular involvement in Olmsted County, Minnesota, United States. Ophthalmic Genet. 2020;41(2):108–24.
251. Bartoli A, El Hassani Y, Jenny B, Momjian S, Korff CM, Seeck M, et al. What to do in failed hemispherotomy? Our clinical series and review of the literature. Neurosurg Rev. 2018;41(1):125–32.
252. Yin R, Gao L, Tan W, Guo W, Zhao T, Nelson JS, et al. Activation of PKCalpha and PI3K Kinases in hypertrophic and nodular Port Wine stain lesions. Am J Dermatopathol. 2017;39(10):747–52.
253. Dompmartin A, van der Vleuten CJM, Dekeuleneer V, Duprez T, Revencu N, Desir J, et al. GNA11-mutated Sturge-Weber syndrome has distinct neurological and dermatological features. Eur J Neurol. 2022;29(10):3061–70.
254. Roach ES. Neurocutaneous syndromes. Pediatr Clin N Am. 1992;39(4):591–620.

255. Sanchez-Espino LF, Ivars M, Antonanzas J, Baselga E. Sturge-Weber syndrome: a review of pathophysiology, genetics, clinical features, and current management Approache. Appl Clin Genet. 2023;16:63–81.
256. Tamburrini G, Mohsen Amen M, Di Rocco C. Sturge-Weber syndrome. In: Di Rocco C, Pang D, Rutka JT, editors. Textbook of pediatric neurosurgery. Cham: Springer International Publishing; 2018. p. 1–13.
257. Zallmann M, Leventer RJ, Mackay MT, Ditchfield M, Bekhor PS, Su JC. Screening for Sturge-Weber syndrome: a state-of-the-art review. Pediatr Dermatol. 2018;35(1):30–42.
258. Bianchi F, Auricchio AM, Battaglia DI, Chieffo DRP, Massimi L. Sturge-Weber syndrome: an update on the relevant issues for neurosurgeons. Childs Nerv Syst. 2020;36(10):2553–70.
259. Jagtap S, Srinivas G, Harsha KJ, Radhakrishnan N, Radhakrishnan A. Sturge-Weber syndrome: clinical spectrum, disease course, and outcome of 30 patients. J Child Neurol. 2013;28(6):725–31.
260. Pascual-Castroviejo I, Pascual-Pascual SI, Velazquez-Fragua R, Viano J. Sturge-Weber syndrome: study of 55 patients. Can J Neurol Sci. 2008;35(3):301–7.
261. Day AM, McCulloch CE, Hammill AM, Juhasz C, Lo WD, Pinto AL, et al. Physical and family history variables associated with neurological and cognitive development in Sturge-Weber syndrome. Pediatr Neurol. 2019;96:30–6.
262. Tillmann RP, Ray K, Aylett SE. Transient episodes of hemiparesis in Sturge Weber syndrome - causes, incidence and recovery. Eur J Paediatr Neurol. 2020;25:90–6.
263. Klapper J. Headache in Sturge-Weber syndrome. Headache. 1994;34(9):521–2.
264. Gittins S, Steel D, Brunklaus A, Newsom-Davis I, Hawkins C, Aylett SE. Autism spectrum disorder, social communication difficulties, and developmental comorbidities in Sturge-Weber syndrome. Epilepsy Behav. 2018;88:1–4.
265. Hassanpour K, Nourinia R, Gerami E, Mahmoudi G, Esfandiari H. Ocular manifestations of the Sturge-Weber syndrome. J Ophthalmic Vis Res. 2021;16(3):415–31.
266. Comi AM. Update on Sturge-Weber syndrome: diagnosis, treatment, quantitative measures, and controversies. Lymphat Res Biol. 2007;5(4):257–64.
267. Bodensteiner JB, Roach ES. Sturge-Weber syndrome. Sturge-Weber Foundation Mt. Freedom; 1999.
268. Sullivan TJ, Clarke MP, Morin JD. The ocular manifestations of the Sturge-Weber syndrome. J Pediatr Ophthalmol Strabismus. 1992;29(6):349–56.
269. Hatfield LA, Crone NE, Kossoff EH, Ewen JB, Pyzik PL, Lin DD, et al. Quantitative EEG asymmetry correlates with clinical severity in unilateral Sturge-Weber syndrome. Epilepsia. 2007;48(1):191–5.
270. Kasasbeh AS, Kalaria A, Comi AM, Lo W, Lin DDM. Atypical intracerebral developmental venous anomalies in Sturge-Weber syndrome: a case series and review of literature. Pediatr Neurol. 2020;104:54–61.
271. Sabeti S, Ball KL, Burkhart C, Eichenfield L, Fernandez Faith E, Frieden IJ, et al. Consensus statement for the management and treatment of Port-Wine birthmarks in Sturge-Weber syndrome. JAMA Dermatol. 2021;157(1):98–104.
272. Comi AM. Sturge-Weber syndrome. Handb Clin Neurol. 2015;132:157–68.
273. Kaplan EH, Kossoff EH, Bachur CD, Gholston M, Hahn J, Widlus M, et al. Anticonvulsant efficacy in Sturge-Weber syndrome. Pediatr Neurol. 2016;58:31–6.
274. Lance EI, Sreenivasan AK, Zabel TA, Kossoff EH, Comi AM. Aspirin use in Sturge-Weber syndrome: side effects and clinical outcomes. J Child Neurol. 2013;28(2):213–8.
275. Gallop F, Fosi T, Prabhakar P, Aylett SE. Flunarizine for headache prophylaxis in children with Sturge-Weber syndrome. Pediatr Neurol. 2019;93:27–33.
276. Kossoff EH, Hatfield LA, Ball KL, Comi AM. Comorbidity of epilepsy and headache in patients with Sturge-Weber syndrome. J Child Neurol. 2005;20(8):678–82.
277. Arzimanoglou AA, Andermann F, Aicardi J, Sainte-Rose C, Beaulieu MA, Villemure JG, et al. Sturge-Weber syndrome: indications and results of surgery in 20 patients. Neurology. 2000;55(10):1472–9.

278. Day AM, Hammill AM, Juhasz C, Pinto AL, Roach ES, McCulloch CE, et al. Hypothesis: Presymptomatic treatment of Sturge-Weber syndrome with Aspirin and antiepileptic drugs may delay seizure onset. Pediatr Neurol. 2019;90:8–12.
279. Bar C, Pedespan JM, Boccara O, Garcelon N, Levy R, Grevent D, et al. Early magnetic resonance imaging to detect presymptomatic leptomeningeal angioma in children with suspected Sturge-Weber syndrome. Dev Med Child Neurol. 2020;62(2):227–33.
280. Sujansky E, Conradi S. Sturge-Weber syndrome: age of onset of seizures and glaucoma and the prognosis for affected children. J Child Neurol. 1995;10(1):49–58.
281. Khawaja AM, Pati S, Ng YT. Management of epilepsy due to hypothalamic hamartomas. Pediatr Neurol. 2017;75:29–42.
282. Trousseau A, editor. Clinique médicale de l'Hôtel-Dieu de Paris.
283. Daly DD, Mulder DW. Gelastic epilepsy. Neurology. 1957;7(3):189–92. https://doi.org/10.1212/wnl.7.3.189.
284. Gascon GG, Lombroso CT. Epileptic (gelastic) laughter. Epilepsia. 1971;12(1):63–76.
285. Choi JU, Kim DS. Treatment modalities for intractable epilepsy in hypothalamic hamartoma. Adv Tech Stand Neurosurg. 2012;39:117–30.
286. Kovac S, Deppe M, Mohammadi S, Schiffbauer H, Schwindt W, Moddel G, et al. Gelastic seizures: a case of lateral frontal lobe epilepsy and review of the literature. Epilepsy Behav. 2009;15(2):249–53.
287. Machado RA, Astencio AG. Gelastic seizures involving the left parietal lobe. Epilepsy Behav. 2012;23(1):87–9.
288. Striano S, Meo R, Bilo L, Cirillo S, Nocerino C, Ruosi P, et al. Gelastic epilepsy: symptomatic and cryptogenic cases. Epilepsia. 1999;40(3):294–302.
289. Arita K, Ikawa F, Kurisu K, Sumida M, Harada K, Uozumi T, et al. The relationship between magnetic resonance imaging findings and clinical manifestations of hypothalamic hamartoma. J Neurosurg. 1999;91(2):212–20.
290. Alomari SO, Houshiemy MNE, Bsat S, Moussalem CK, Allouh M, Omeis IA. Hypothalamic hamartomas: a comprehensive review of the literature - part 1: neurobiological features, clinical presentations and advancements in diagnostic tools. Clin Neurol Neurosurg. 2020;197:106076.
291. Helen Cross J, Spoudeas H. Medical management and antiepileptic drugs in hypothalamic hamartoma. Epilepsia. 2017;58(Suppl 2):16–21.
292. Specchio N, Rizzi M, Trivisano M, Fusco L, Rebessi E, Cappelletti S, et al. Acute intralesional recording in hypothalamic hamartoma: description of 4 cases. Acta Neurol Belg. 2015;115(3):233–9.
293. Osborn AG. Osborn's brain: imaging, pathology, and anatomy. Salt Lake City; 2013.
294. Ng YT, Rekate HL, Prenger EC, Wang NC, Chung SS, Feiz-Erfan I, et al. Endoscopic resection of hypothalamic hamartomas for refractory symptomatic epilepsy. Neurology. 2008;70(17):1543–8.
295. Kerrigan JF, Ng YT, Chung S, Rekate HL. The hypothalamic hamartoma: a model of subcortical epileptogenesis and encephalopathy. Semin Pediatr Neurol. 2005;12(2):119–31.
296. Shirozu H, Masuda H, Kameyama S. Long-term seizure outcomes in patients with hypothalamic hamartoma treated by stereotactic radiofrequency thermocoagulation. Epilepsia. 2021;62(11):2697–706.
297. Regis J, Scavarda D, Tamura M, Nagayi M, Villeneuve N, Bartolomei F, et al. Epilepsy related to hypothalamic hamartomas: surgical management with special reference to gamma knife surgery. Childs Nerv Syst. 2006;22(8):881–95.
298. Kuzniecky R, Guthrie B, Mountz J, Bebin M, Faught E, Gilliam F, et al. Intrinsic epileptogenesis of hypothalamic hamartomas in gelastic epilepsy. Ann Neurol. 1997;42(1):60–7.
299. Kuzniecky RI, Guthrie BL. Stereotactic surgical approach to hypothalamic hamartomas. Epileptic Disord. 2003;5(4):275–80.
300. Wagner K, Wethe JV, Schulze-Bonhage A, Trippel M, Rekate H, Prigatano GP, et al. Cognition in epilepsy patients with hypothalamic hamartomas. Epilepsia. 2017;58(Suppl 2):85–93.

301. Specchio N, Wirrell EC, Scheffer IE, Nabbout R, Riney K, Samia P, et al. International League Against Epilepsy classification and definition of epilepsy syndromes with onset in childhood: position paper by the ILAE Task Force on Nosology and Definitions. Epilepsia. 2022;63(6):1398–442.
302. Blom S, Brorson LO. Central spikes or sharp waves (Rolandic spikes) in children's EEG and their clinical significance. Acta Paediatr Scand. 1966;55(4):385–93.
303. Beaussart M. Benign epilepsy of children with Rolandic (centro-temporal) paroxysmal foci. A clinical entity. Study of 221 cases. Epilepsia. 1972;13(6):795–811.
304. Lerman P, Kivity S. Benign focal epilepsy of childhood. A follow-up study of 100 recovered patients. Arch Neurol. 1975;32(4):261–4.
305. Heijbel J, Blom S, Rasmuson M. Benign epilepsy of childhood with centrotemporal EEG foci: a genetic study. Epilepsia. 1975;16(2):285–93.
306. Lu G, Cheng Y, Wang Y, Hu J, Zhang F, Li W, et al. The prevalence and risk factors of electrical status epilepticus during slow-wave sleep in self-limited epilepsy with Centrotemporal spikes. Clin EEG Neurosci. 2024;55(2):265–71.
307. Ji Y, Zhang J, Lu H, Yang H, Zhang X, Liu H, et al. Correlation between scalp high-frequency oscillations and prognosis in patients with benign epilepsy of childhood with centrotemporal spikes. CNS Neurosci Ther. 2023;29(10):3053–61.
308. Sidenvall R, Forsgren L, Heijbel J. Prevalence and characteristics of epilepsy in children in northern Sweden. Seizure. 1996;5(2):139–46.
309. Alshahawy AK, Darwish AH, Elsaid Shalaby S, Mawlana W. Prevalence of idiopathic epilepsy among school children in Gharbia Governorate, Egypt. Brain Dev. 2018;40(4):278–86.
310. Onsurbe Ramírez I, Hernández Rodríguez M, Aparicio Meix JM, Carrascosa RC. Incidence of epilepsy and epileptic syndromes in children in the province of Albacete. An Esp Pediatr. 1999;51(2):154–8.
311. Heijbel J, Blom S, Bergfors PG. Benign epilepsy of children with centrotemporal EEG foci. A study of incidence rate in outpatient care. Epilepsia. 1975;16(5):657–64.
312. Degen R, Degen HE. Some genetic aspects of rolandic epilepsy: waking and sleep EEGs in siblings. Epilepsia. 1990;31(6):795–801.
313. Neng X, Xiao M, Yuanlu C, Qinyan L, Li S, Zhanyi S. Novel variant in CHRNA4 with benign childhood epilepsy with centrotemporal spikes and contribution to precise medicine. Mol Genet Genomic Med. 2020;8(7):e1264.
314. Ma MG, Liu XR, Wu Y, Wang J, Li BM, Shi YW, et al. RYR2 mutations are associated with benign epilepsy of childhood with Centrotemporal spikes with or without arrhythmia. Front Neurosci. 2021;15:629610.
315. Stephani U. Typical semiology of benign childhood epilepsy with centrotemporal spikes (BCECTS). Epileptic Disord. 2000;2(Suppl 1):S3–4.
316. Bouma PA, Bovenkerk AC, Westendorp RG, Brouwer OF. The course of benign partial epilepsy of childhood with centrotemporal spikes: a meta-analysis. Neurology. 1997;48(2):430–7.
317. Lima EM, Rzezak P, Guimaraes CA, Montenegro MA, Guerreiro MM, Valente KD. The executive profile of children with Benign Epilepsy of childhood with Centrotemporal Spikes and Temporal Lobe Epilepsy. Epilepsy Behav. 2017;72:173–7.
318. Dalla Bernardina B, Bureau M, Dravet C, Dulac O, Tassinari CA, Roger J. Affective symptoms during attacks of epilepsy in children (author's transl). Rev Electroencephalogr Neurophysiol Clin. 1980;10(1):8–18.
319. Ambrosetto G, Giovanardi Rossi P, Tassinari CA. Predictive factors of seizure frequency and duration of antiepileptic treatment in rolandic epilepsy: a retrospective study. Brain Dev. 1987;9(3):300–4.
320. Roulet E, Deonna T, Despland PA. Prolonged intermittent drooling and oromotor dyspraxia in benign childhood epilepsy with centrotemporal spikes. Epilepsia. 1989;30(5):564–8.
321. Boulloche J, Husson A, Le Luyer B, Le Roux P. Dysphagia, speech disorders and centrotemporal spikes-waves. Arch Fr Pediatr. 1990;47(2):115–7.

322. Colamaria V, Sgro V, Caraballo R, Simeone M, Zullini E, Fontana E, et al. Status epilepticus in benign rolandic epilepsy manifesting as anterior operculum syndrome. Epilepsia. 1991;32(3):329–34.
323. Ucar HK, Arhan E, Aydin K, Hirfanoglu T, Serdaroglu A. Electrical status epilepticus during sleep (ESES) in benign childhood epilepsy with Centrotemporal spikes (BCECTS): insights into predictive factors, and clinical and EEG outcomes. Eur Rev Med Pharmacol Sci. 2022;26(6):1885–96.
324. Steinruecke M, Gillespie C, Ahmed N, Bandyopadhyay S, Duklas D, Ghahfarokhi MH, et al. Care and three-year outcomes of children with Benign Epilepsy with Centro-Temporal Spikes in England. Epilepsy Behav. 2023;148:109465.
325. Hosseinpour S, Tavasoli AR, Rohani M, Emamikhah M. Rolandic epilepsy with paroxysmal exercise-induced dystonia and writer's cramp: a case report. Neurol Sci. 2023;44(1):381–4.
326. Beydoun A, Garofalo EA, Drury I. Generalized spike-waves, multiple loci, and clinical course in children with EEG features of benign epilepsy of childhood with centrotemporal spikes. Epilepsia. 1992;33(6):1091–6.
327. Tekgul H, Kanmaz S, Serin HM, Yilmaz S. Spike wave characteristics and temporal spike evolution on serial EEG in childhood epilepsy with centrotemporal spikes. Seizure. 2021;87:75–80.
328. Günay Ç, Sarikaya Uzan G, Özsoy Ö, Hiz Kurul S, Yiş U. The fate of spikes in self-limited epilepsy with centrotemporal spikes: are clinical and baseline EEG features effective? Epilepsy Res. 2023;193:107165.
329. Liu MJ, Su XJ, Md XS, Wu GF, Zhang YQ, Gao L, et al. Clinical features of benign epilepsy of childhood with centrotemporal spikes in chinese children. Medicine (Baltimore). 2017;96(4):e5623.
330. Cheng W, Yang Y, Chen Y, Shan S, Li C, Fang L, et al. Anti-seizure medication treatment of benign childhood epilepsy with centrotemporal spikes: a systematic review and meta-analysis. Front Pharmacol. 2022;13:821639.
331. Ahadi P, Nasiri J, Ghazavi MR, Mosavian T, Mansouri V. A comparative study on the efficacy of Levetiracetam and Carbamazepine in the treatment of Rolandic seizures in children: An open-label randomized controlled trial. J Res Pharm Pract. 2020;9(2):68–72.
332. Gerstl L, Willimsky E, Rémi C, Noachtar S, Borggräfe I, Tacke M. A systematic review of seizure-freedom rates in patients with benign epilepsy of childhood with Centrotemporal spikes receiving antiepileptic drugs. Clin Neuropharmacol. 2021;44(2):39–46.
333. Gu W, Chen J, Tian W, Tao W, Chen J, Zhang G, et al. Outcome analysis of children with rolandic discharges on EEG: a real-world study. Seizure. 2020;82:105–8.
334. Jin G, Chen J, Du J, He L, Qi L, Wu D, et al. Repetitive transcranial magnetic stimulation to treat benign epilepsy with centrotemporal spikes. Brain Stimul. 2022;15(3):601–4.
335. Wang S, Zhang H, Liu C, Liu Q, Ji T, Wang W, et al. Surgical treatment of children with drug-resistant epilepsy involving the Rolandic area. Epileptic Disord. 2021;23(2):376–84.
336. De Romanis F, Feliciani M, Ruggieri S. Rolandic paroxysmal epilepsy: a long term study in 150 children. Ital J Neurol Sci. 1986;7(1):77–80.
337. Panayiotopoulos CP, Jeavons PM, Harding GF. Occipital spikes during photic stimulation and their relation to visual evoked responses in photosensitive epilepsy. Electroencephalogr Clin Neurophysiol. 1970;29(3):327.
338. Panayiotopoulos CP. Benign nocturnal childhood occipital epilepsy: a new syndrome with nocturnal seizures, tonic deviation of the eyes, and vomiting. J Child Neurol. 1989;4(1):43–9.
339. Panayiotopoulos CP. Vomiting as an ictal manifestation of epileptic seizures and syndromes. J Neurol Neurosurg Psychiatry. 1988;51(11):1448–51.
340. Panayiotopoulos CP. Benign childhood epilepsy with occipital paroxysms: a 15-year prospective study. Ann Neurol. 1989;26(1):51–6.
341. Weir E, Gibbs J, Appleton R. Panayiotopoulos syndrome and benign partial epilepsy with centro-temporal spikes: a comparative incidence study. Seizure. 2018;57:66–9.
342. Covanis A. Panayiotopoulos syndrome: a benign childhood autonomic epilepsy frequently imitating encephalitis, syncope, migraine, sleep disorder, or gastroenteritis. Pediatrics. 2006;118(4):e1237–43.

343. Yoshinaga H, Koutroumanidis M, Kobayashi K, Shirasawa A, Kikumoto K, Inoue T, et al. EEG dipole characteristics in Panayiotopoulos syndrome. Epilepsia. 2006;47(4):781–7.
344. Ramos-Lizana J, Martinez-Espinosa G, Jimenez-Iniesta E, Aguirre-Rodriguez J. Frequency, semiology and prognosis of Panayiotopoulos syndrome. Rev Neurol. 2019;68(9):369–74.
345. Kivity S, Oliver KL, Afawi Z, Damiano JA, Arsov T, Bahlo M, et al. SCN1A clinical spectrum includes the self-limited focal epilepsies of childhood. Epilepsy Res. 2017;131:9–14.
346. Livingston JH, Cross JH, McLellan A, Birch R, Zuberi SM. A novel inherited mutation in the voltage sensor region of SCN1A is associated with Panayiotopoulos syndrome in siblings and generalized epilepsy with febrile seizures plus. J Child Neurol. 2009;24(4):503–8.
347. Rudolf G, de Bellescize J, de Saint MA, Arzimanoglou A, Valenti Hirsch MP, Labalme A, et al. Exome sequencing in 57 patients with self-limited focal epilepsies of childhood with typical or atypical presentations suggests novel candidate genes. Eur J Paediatr Neurol. 2020;27:104–10.
348. Durá-Tráve T, Yoldi-Petri ME, Gallinas-Victoriano F. Panayiotopoulos syndrome: epidemiological and clinical characteristics and outcome. Eur J Neurol. 2008;15(4):336–41.
349. Panayiotopoulos CP. Autonomic seizures and autonomic status epilepticus peculiar to childhood: diagnosis and management. Epilepsy Behav. 2004;5(3):286–95.
350. Caraballo R, Cersosimo R, Fejerman N. Panayiotopoulos syndrome: a prospective study of 192 patients. Epilepsia. 2007;48(6):1054–61.
351. Kawakami S, Kubota M, Terashima H, Nagata C, Ishiguro A. Differentiating early clinical features of Panayiotopoulos syndrome from acute encephalopathy. Brain Dev. 2022;44(6):386–90.
352. Lada C, Skiadas K, Theodorou V, Loli N, Covanis A. A study of 43 patients with panayiotopoulos syndrome, a common and benign childhood seizure susceptibility. Epilepsia. 2003;44(1):81–8.
353. Verrotti A, Sebastiani M, Giordano L, Striano P, Belcastro V, Franzoni E, et al. Panayiotopoulos syndrome with convulsive status epilepticus at the onset: a long-term study. Seizure. 2014;23(9):728–31.
354. Yamamoto H, Naito H, Osako T, Tsukahara K, Yamada T, Yumoto T, et al. Ictal cardiorespiratory arrest associated with status epilepticus in Panayiotopoulos syndrome. Acta Med Okayama. 2018;72(3):297–300.
355. Mujawar QM, Sen S, Ali MD, Balakrishnan P, Patil S. Panayiotopoulos syndrome presenting with status epilepticus and cardiorespiratory arrest: a case report. Pediatr Emerg Care. 2011;27(8):754–7.
356. Brabec J, Chaudhary S, Ng YT. Ictal priapism as an autonomic manifestation of Panayiotopoulos syndrome. J Child Neurol. 2013;28(12):1686–8.
357. Yalçin AD, Ertasoglu TH. Panayiotopoulos syndrome with a special emphasis of ictal semiologic features. Epilepsy Res. 2017;131:37–43.
358. Caraballo RH, Pasteris MC, Portuondo E, Fortini PS. Panayiotopoulos syndrome and diffuse paroxysms as the first EEG manifestation at clinical onset: a study of nine patients. Epileptic Disord. 2015;17(2):143–9.
359. Tata G, Guveli BT, Dortcan N, Cokar O, Kurucu H, Demirbilek V, et al. Panayiotopoulos syndrome and symptomatic occipital lobe epilepsy of childhood: a clinical and EEG study. Epileptic Disord. 2014;16(2):197–202.
360. Specchio N, Trivisano M, Claps D, Battaglia D, Fusco L, Vigevano F. Documentation of autonomic seizures and autonomic status epilepticus with ictal EEG in Panayiotopoulos syndrome. Epilepsy Behav. 2010;19(3):383–93.
361. Oguni H. A reappraisal of interictal EEG characteristics in self-limited epilepsy with autonomic seizures, formerly known as Panayiotopoulos syndrome or early-onset benign occipital epilepsy. Eur J Paediatr Neurol. 2023;47:18–24.
362. Iannetti P, Spalice A, Rocchi V, Verrotti A. Diffuse onset of ictal electroencephalography in a typical case of Panayiotopoulos syndrome and review of the literature. J Child Neurol. 2009;24(4):472–6.

363. Ivanov IS. Proposal for panayiotopoulos syndrome criteria. Folia Med (Plovdiv). 2006;48(3–4):50–5.
364. Mellish LC, Dunkley C, Ferrie CD, Pal DK. Antiepileptic drug treatment of rolandic epilepsy and Panayiotopoulos syndrome: clinical practice survey and clinical trial feasibility. Arch Dis Child. 2015;100(1):62–7.
365. Kikumoto K, Yoshinaga H, Oka M, Ito M, Endoh F, Akiyama T, et al. EEG and seizure exacerbation induced by carbamazepine in Panayiotopoulos syndrome. Epileptic Disord. 2006;8(1):53–6.
366. Gastaut H. Benign spike-wave occipital epilepsy in children. Rev Electroencephalogr Neurophysiol Clin. 1982;12(3):179–201.
367. Deonna T, Ziegler AL, Despland PA. Paroxysmal visual disturbances of epileptic origin and occipital epilepsy in children. Neuropediatrics. 1984;15(3):131–5.
368. Nalin A, Ruggerini C, Ferrari E, Galli V, Ferrari P, Finelli T. Clinical aspects, differential diagnosis and evolution of visual epileptic seizures in children. Neurophysiol Clin. 1989;19(1):25–36.
369. Andermann F, Zifkin B. The benign occipital epilepsies of childhood: an overview of the idiopathic syndromes and of the relationship to migraine. Epilepsia. 1998;39(Suppl 4):S9–23.
370. Tedrus GM, Fonseca LC. Idiopathic childhood occipital epilepsies: clinical and electroencephalographic features in 63 children. Arq Neuropsiquiatr. 2005;63(1):61–7.
371. Caraballo RH, Cersósimo RO, Fejerman N. Late-onset, "Gastaut type", childhood occipital epilepsy:: an unusual evolution. Epileptic Disord. 2005;7(4):341–6.
372. Akca Kalem S, Elmali AD, Demirbilek V, Oktem O, Yapici Z, Saltik S, et al. Panayiotopoulos syndrome and Gastaut syndrome are distinct entities in terms of neuropsychological findings. Epilepsy Behav. 2019;99:106447.
373. Ermolenko NA, Ermakov A, Buchneva IA, Voronkova KV, Zakharova EI. Idiopathic focal epilepsies of infancy and childhood. Zh Nevrol Psikhiatr Im S S Korsakova. 2011;111(11 Pt 1):17–24.
374. Gaggero R, Pistorio A, Pignatelli S, Rossi A, Mancardi MM, Baglietto MG, et al. Early classification of childhood focal idiopathic epilepsies: is it possible at the first seizure? Eur J Paediatr Neurol. 2014;18(3):376–80.
375. Fortini S, Espeche A, Galicchio S, Cersósimo R, Chacon S, Gallo A, et al. More than one self-limited epilepsy of childhood in the same patient: a multicenter study. Epilepsy Res. 2021;177:106768.
376. Grosso S, Vivarelli R, Gobbi G, Di Bartolo R, Berardi R, Balestri P. Late-onset childhood occipital epilepsy (Gastaut type): a family study. Eur J Paediatr Neurol. 2008;12(5):421–6.
377. Taylor I, Berkovic SF, Kivity S, Scheffer IE. Benign occipital epilepsies of childhood: clinical features and genetics. Brain. 2008;131(Pt 9):2287–94.
378. Caraballo RH, Cersósimo RO, Fejerman N. Childhood occipital epilepsy of Gastaut: a study of 33 patients. Epilepsia. 2008;49(2):288–97.
379. Caraballo RH, Fontana E, Darra F, Bongiorni L, Fiorini E, Cersosimo R, et al. Childhood absence epilepsy and electroencephalographic focal abnormalities with or without clinical manifestations. Seizure. 2008;17(7):617–24.
380. Verrotti A, Laino D, Rinaldi VE, Suppiej A, Giordano L, Toldo I, et al. Clinical dissection of childhood occipital epilepsy of Gastaut and prognostic implication. Eur J Neurol. 2016;23(2):241–6.
381. Shu XM, Zhang GP, Yang BZ, Li J. The characterization of childhood occipital epilepsy of Gastaut: a study of seven patients. Cell Biochem Biophys. 2013;67(3):991–5.
382. Panayiotopoulos CP. Elementary visual hallucinations, blindness, and headache in idiopathic occipital epilepsy: differentiation from migraine. J Neurol Neurosurg Psychiatry. 1999;66(4):536–40.
383. Skrijelj FE, Mulić M. Aggravation of symptomatic occipital epilepsy of childhood by carbamazepine. Vojnosanit Pregl. 2014;71(4):404–7.

384. Verrotti A, Parisi P, Loiacono G, Mohn A, Grosso S, Balestri P, et al. Levetiracetam monotherapy for childhood occipital epilepsy of gastaut. Acta Neurol Scand. 2009;120(5):342–6.
385. Charlton MH. Borderlands of petit mal. Am J Psychiatry. 1965;122(6):669–72.
386. von Hedenström I, Schorsch G. Photosensitivity during EEG in epileptics and in oligophrenics with rare attacks. Arch Psychiatr Nervenkr (1970). 1966;208(2):147–61.
387. Hishikawa Y, Yamamoto J, Furuya E, Yamada Y, Miyazaki K. Photosensitive epilepsy: relationships between the visual evoked responses and the epileptiform discharges induced by intermittent photic stimulation. Electroencephalogr Clin Neurophysiol. 1967;23(4):320–34.
388. Dimov S, Lanoir J. Chronic epileptogenic foci in the photosensitive baboon. Papio papio Electroencephalogr Clin Neurophysiol. 1973;34(4):353–67.
389. Bruni J, Wilder BJ, Bauman AW, Willmore LJ. Clinical efficacy and long-term effects of valproic acid therapy on spike-and-wave discharges. Neurology. 1980;30(1):42–6.
390. Mayr N, Wimberger D, Pichler H, Mamoli B, Zeitlhofer J, Spiel G. Influence of television on photosensitive epileptics. Eur Neurol. 1987;27(4):201–8.
391. Taylor I, Berkovic SF, Scheffer IE. Genetics of epilepsy syndromes in families with photosensitivity. Neurology. 2013;80(14):1322–9.
392. Shiraishi H, Fujiwara T, Inoue Y, Yagi K. Photosensitivity in relation to epileptic syndromes: asurvey from an epilepsy center in Japan. Epilepsia. 2001;42(3):393–7.
393. Xue J, Gong P, Yang H, Liu X, Jiang Y, Zhang Y, et al. Genetic (idiopathic) epilepsy with photosensitive seizures includes features of both focal and generalized seizures. Sci Rep. 2018;8(1):6254.
394. Dhanuka AK, Jain BK, Daljit S, Maheshwari D. Juvenile myoclonic epilepsy: a clinical and sleep EEG study. Seizure. 2001;10(5):374–8.
395. Sadleir LG, de Valles-Ibanez G, King C, Coleman M, Mossman S, Paterson S, et al. Inherited RORB pathogenic variants: overlap of photosensitive genetic generalized and occipital lobe epilepsy. Epilepsia. 2020;61(4):e23–e9.
396. Li M, Maljevic S, Phillips AM, Petrovski S, Hildebrand MS, Burgess R, et al. Gain-of-function HCN2 variants in genetic epilepsy. Hum Mutat. 2018;39(2):202–9.
397. Guerrini R, Dravet C, Genton P, Bureau M, Bonanni P, Ferrari AR, et al. Idiopathic photosensitive occipital lobe epilepsy. Epilepsia. 1995;36(9):883–91.
398. Cerrahoğlu Şirin T, Yılmaz T, Elmalı AD, Bebek N, Demirbilek V, Baykan B. Photosensitive occipital lobe epilepsy: delineation of an under-recognized reflex epilepsy syndrome according to the new ILAE criteria and long-term follow-up. Epileptic Disord. 2023;25(2):187–99.
399. Koutroumanidis M, Tsirka V, Panayiotopoulos C. Adult-onset photosensitivity: clinical significance and epilepsy syndromes including idiopathic (possibly genetic) photosensitive occipital epilepsy. Epileptic Disord. 2015;17(3):275–86.
400. Yazar HO, Gul G, Yazar T, Eren F, Kuscu DY, Kirbas D. Electroclinical and prognostic characteristics of epilepsy patients with photosensitivity. Ideggyogy Sz. 2018;71(1–02):43–8.
401. Guerrini R, Bonanni P, Parmeggiani L, Belmonte A. Adolescent onset of idiopathic photosensitive occipital epilepsy after remission of benign rolandic epilepsy. Epilepsia. 1997;38(7):777–81.
402. Bonini F, Egeo G, Fattouch J, Fanella M, Morano A, Giallonardo AT, et al. Natural evolution from idiopathic photosensitive occipital lobe epilepsy to idiopathic generalized epilepsy in an untreated young patient. Brain Dev. 2014;36(4):346–50.
403. Varotto G, Visani E, Canafoglia L, Franceschetti S, Avanzini G, Panzica F. Enhanced frontocentral EEG connectivity in photosensitive generalized epilepsies: a partial directed coherence study. Epilepsia. 2012;53(2):359–67.
404. Ricci S, Vigevano F. Occipital seizures provoked by intermittent light stimulation: ictal and interictal findings. J Clin Neurophysiol. 1993;10(2):197–209.
405. Politi-Elishkevich K, Kivity S, Shuper A, Levine H, Goldberg-Stern H. Idiopathic photosensitive occipital epilepsy: clinical and electroencephalographic (EEG) features. J Child Neurol. 2014;29(3):307–11.

406. Jeavons PM. Nosological problems of myoclonic epilepsies in childhood and adolescence. Dev Med Child Neurol. 1977;19(1):3–8.
407. Ichikawa T, Ohtaka T, Fukuzawa H, Yano K, Yamada R. A case presenting myoclonic seizures of eyelids induced by closing the eyes (author's transl). Seishin Shinkeigaku Zasshi. 1978;80(3):89–103.
408. De Marco P, Miottello P. Eye closure epilepsy, report of an uncomplicated case. Clin Electroencephalogr. 1981;12(2):66–8.
409. DeMarco P. Eyelid myoclonia with absences (EMA) in two monovular twins. Clin Electroencephalogr. 1989;20(3):193–5.
410. Veggiotti P, Viri M, Lanzi G. Electrical status epilepticus on eye closure: a case report. Neurophysiol Clin. 1992;22(4):281–6.
411. Baykan-Kurt B, Gokyigit A, Parman Y, Kinay D, Gurses C. Eye closure related spike and wave discharges: clinical and syndromic associations. Clin Electroencephalogr. 1999;30(3):106–10.
412. Destina Yalçin A, Forta H, Kiliç E. Overlap cases of eyelid myoclonia with absences and juvenile myoclonic epilepsy. Seizure. 2006;15(6):359–65.
413. Striano P, Sofia V, Capovilla G, Rubboli G, Di Bonaventura C, Coppola A, et al. A pilot trial of levetiracetam in eyelid myoclonia with absences (Jeavons syndrome). Epilepsia. 2008;49(3):425–30.
414. Zawar I, Toribio MGG, Xu X, Alnakhli RS, Benech D, Valappil AMN, et al. Epilepsy with Eyelid myoclonias - a diagnosis concealed in other genetic generalized epilepsies with photoparoxysmal response. Epilepsy Res. 2022;181:106886.
415. Asadi-Pooya AA, Homayoun M. Idiopathic (genetic) generalized epilepsies with absences: clinical and electrographic characteristics and seizure outcome. Neurol Sci. 2020;41(12):3677–82.
416. Kotov AS. Pathomorphosis of idiopathic generalized epilepsies. Zh Nevrol Psikhiatr Im S S Korsakova. 2019;119(9):7–11.
417. Wang XL, Bao JX, Liang S, Tie M, Deng YC, Zhao G, et al. Jeavons syndrome in China. Epilepsy Behav. 2014;32:64–71.
418. Nilo A, Crespel A, Genton P, Macorig G, Gigli GL, Gelisse P. Epilepsy with eyelid myoclonias (Jeavons syndrome): An electro-clinical study of 40 patients from childhood to adulthood. Seizure. 2021;87:30–8.
419. Parfyonov M, Ivaniuk A, Parikh S, Pestana-Knight E. Epilepsy with eyelid myoclonia in the setting of de novo pathogenic variant in ATP1A3. Epileptic Disord. 2023;25(4):545–8.
420. Smith KM, Wirrell EC, Andrade DM, Choi H, Trenité DK, Knupp KG, et al. A comprehensive narrative review of epilepsy with eyelid myoclonia. Epilepsy Res. 2023;193:107147.
421. Spurgeon AL, Keaveney SF, Ng YT. Refractory Jeavons syndrome from birth symptomatic to PLCB1 mutation. Child Neurol Open. 2023;10:2329048X231183524.
422. Gokce-Samar Z, de Bellescize J, Arzimanoglou A, Putoux A, Chatron N, Lesca G, et al. STAG2 microduplication in a patient with eyelid myoclonia and absences and a review of EMA-related reported genes. Eur J Med Genet. 2022;65(12):104636.
423. Samanta D, Willis E. KIAA2022-related disorders can cause Jeavons (eyelid myoclonia with absence) syndrome. Acta Neurol Belg. 2020;120(1):205–7.
424. Madaan P, Jauhari P, Chakrabarty B, Gulati S. Jeavons syndrome in a family with GLUT1-deficiency syndrome. Seizure. 2019;71:158–60.
425. Mori T, Sakamoto M, Tayama T, Goji A, Toda Y, Fujita A, et al. A case of epilepsy with myoclonic atonic seizures caused by SLC6A1 gene mutation due to balanced chromosomal translocation. Brain Dev. 2023;45(7):395–400.
426. Smith KM, Youssef PE, Wirrell EC, Nickels KC, Payne ET, Britton JW, et al. Jeavons syndrome: clinical features and response to treatment. Pediatr Neurol. 2018;86:46–51.
427. Cerulli Irelli E, Cocchi E, Ramantani G, Morano A, Riva A, Caraballo RH, et al. Sex-based electroclinical differences and prognostic factors in epilepsy with eyelid myoclonia. Epilepsia. 2023;64(6):e105–e11.

428. Inagaki M, Suzuki N, Koeda T, Kamuro K, Ohtani K. Myoclonic astatic epilepsy presenting eyelid myoclonic seizures induced by closing of eyes. Jpn J Psychiatry Neurol. 1991;45(2):455–7.
429. Oguz Akarsu E, Tekturk P, Yapici Z, Tepgec F, Uyguner ZO, Baykan B. Eyelid myoclonic status epilepticus: a rare phenotype in spinal muscular atrophy with progressive myoclonic epilepsy associated with ASAH1 gene mutation. Seizure. 2016;42:49–51.
430. Moutaouakil F, El Otmani H, Fadel H, El Moutawakkil B, Slassi I. Benign myoclonic epilepsy of infancy evolving to Jeavons syndrome. Pediatr Neurol. 2010;43(3):213–6.
431. Ballarà Petitbò M, González Alguacil E, Gutiérrez Delicado E, Ortiz Cabrera NV, Duat Rodríguez A, Garcia Peñas JJ, et al. Neuropsychiatric comorbidities and cognition in epilepsy with eyelid myoclonia: a retrospective pediatric case series. Epileptic Disord. 2023;25(5):758–68.
432. Zawar I, Pestana Knight EM. An overview of the electroencephalographic (EEG) features of epilepsy with eyelid Myoclonia (Jeavons syndrome). Neurodiagn J. 2020;60(2):113–27.
433. Smith KM, Wirrell EC, Andrade DM, Choi H, Trenité DK, Jones H, et al. Management of epilepsy with eyelid myoclonia: results of an international expert consensus panel. Epilepsia. 2023;64(9):2342–50.
434. Menon R, Baheti NN, Cherian A, Iyer RS. Oxcarbazepine induced worsening of seizures in Jeavons syndrome: lessons learnt from an interesting presentation. Neurol India. 2011;59(1):70–2.
435. Zawar I, Franic L, Kotagal P, Knight EP. Exacerbation of eyelid myoclonia in patients with epilepsy and eyelid myoclonia receiving cannabidiol. Epileptic Disord. 2021;23(6):906–10.
436. Paibool W, Schimpf S, Nordli DR Jr, Phitsanuwong C. Modified Atkins diet in children with epilepsy with eyelid myoclonia (Jeavons syndrome). Epilepsy Behav. 2023;145:109347.
437. Kokkinos V, Urban A, Sisterson ND, Li N, Corson D, Richardson RM. Responsive neurostimulation of the Thalamus improves seizure control in idiopathic generalized epilepsy: a case report. Neurosurgery. 2020;87(5):E578–E83.
438. Nilo A, Crespel A, Genton P, Macorig G, Gigli GL, Gélisse P. Prognostic factors in epilepsy with eyelid myoclonia (Jeavons syndrome). Rev Neurol (Paris). 2023;179(10):1081–5.
439. Caraballo RH, Darra F, Fontana E, Garcia R, Monese E, Dalla Bernardina B. Absence seizures in the first 3 years of life: an electroclinical study of 46 cases. Epilepsia. 2011;52(2):393–400. https://doi.org/10.1111/j.1528-1167.2010.02926.x.
440. Tassinari CA, Lyagoubi S, Santos V, Gambarelli G, Roger J, Dravet C, et al. Study on spike and wave discharges in man. II. Clinical and electroencephalographic aspects of myoclonic absences. Rev Neurol (Paris). 1969;121(3):379–83.
441. Fois A, Malandrini F, Mostardini R. Clinical experiences of petit mal. Brain Dev. 1987;9(1):54–9.
442. Mikol F, Monge-Strauss MF. The timing of crisis and day-night distribution of paroxysmal EEG activities: a study on 197 epileptic patients. Rev Neurol (Paris). 1987;143(5):451–6.
443. Bourgeois BF. Combination of valproate and ethosuximide: antiepileptic and neurotoxic interaction. J Pharmacol Exp Ther. 1988;247(3):1128–32.
444. Salas Puig J, Acebes A, González C, Tuñón A, Guisasola LM, Lahoz CH. Epilepsy with myoclonic absences. Neurologia. 1990;5(7):242–5.
445. Nordli DR Jr. Idiopathic generalized epilepsies recognized by the International League Against Epilepsy. Epilepsia. 2005;46(Suppl 9):48–56.
446. Bureau M, Tassinari CA. Epilepsy with myoclonic absences. Brain Dev. 2005;27(3):178–84.
447. Tang S, Addis L, Smith A, Topp SD, Pendziwiat M, Mei D, et al. Phenotypic and genetic spectrum of epilepsy with myoclonic atonic seizures. Epilepsia. 2020;61(5):995–1007.
448. Hiraide T, Hattori A, Ieda D, Hori I, Saitoh S, Nakashima M, et al. De novo variants in SETD1B cause intellectual disability, autism spectrum disorder, and epilepsy with myoclonic absences. Epilepsia Open. 2019;4(3):476–81.

449. Ogawa K, Tanigawa J, Mukai M, Tominaga K, Kagitani-Shimono K, Nabatame S, et al. Epilepsy with myoclonic absence presenting with unilateral jerks: a case of 2q13 microdeletion syndrome. Seizure. 2023;106:77–9.
450. Frydson I, Avula S, Ahmad SF. A case of a seven-year-old boy with epilepsy with myoclonic absence: importance of seizure semiology, genetic etiology, and electroencephalogram correlation for timely intervention. Child Neurol Open. 2022;9:2329048X221131738.
451. Elia M, Guerrini R, Musumeci SA, Bonanni P, Gambardella A, Aguglia U. Myoclonic absence-like seizures and chromosome abnormality syndromes. Epilepsia. 1998;39(6):660–3.
452. Ikeda H, Imai K, Ikeda H, Matsuda K, Takahashi Y, Inoue Y. Ictal single photon emission computed tomographic study of myoclonic absence seizures. Brain Dev. 2018;40(2):126–9.
453. Zanzmera P, Menon RN, Karkare K, Soni H, Jagtap S, Radhakrishnan A. Epilepsy with myoclonic absences: Electroclinical characteristics in a distinctive pediatric epilepsy phenotype. Epilepsy Behav. 2016;64(Pt A):242–7.
454. Cherian A, Jabeen SA, Kandadai RM, Iype T, Moturi P, Reddy M, et al. Epilepsy with myoclonic absences in siblings. Brain Dev. 2014;36(10):892–8.
455. Ikeda H, Fujiwara T, Shigematsu H, Imai K, Kubota H, Kubota Y, et al. Symptoms and clinical course of epilepsy with myoclonic absences. No To Hattatsu. 2011;43(1):14–8.
456. Verrotti A, Greco R, Chiarelli F, Domizio S, Sabatino G, Morgese G. Epilepsy with myoclonic absences with early onset: a follow-up study. J Child Neurol. 1999;14(11):746–9.
457. Myers KA, Scheffer IE. Myoclonic absence seizures with complex gestural automatisms. Eur J Paediatr Neurol. 2018;22(3):532–5.
458. Carter EG, Armour EA, Pagano LM, Reddy SB. Epilepsy with myoclonic absences: a case series highlighting clinical heterogeneity and surgical management. Epileptic Disord. 2022;24(3):541–47.
459. Iyer RS. Proximal upper limb jerking: important clinical sign to diagnose epilepsy with myoclonic absences. Pediatr Neurol. 2017;71:88–9.
460. Ito S, Nagumo K, Nishikawa A, Oguni H, Nagata S. Low-dose phenobarbital for epilepsy with myoclonic absences: a case report. Brain Dev. 2021;43(5):666–8.
461. Häusler M, Kluger G, Nikanorova M. Epilepsy with myoclonic absences - favourable response to add-on rufinamide treatment in 3 cases. Neuropediatrics. 2011;42(1):28–9.
462. Scheffer IE, French J, Hirsch E, Jain S, Mathern GW, Moshe SL, et al. Classification of the epilepsies: new concepts for discussion and debate-special report of the ILAE Classification Task Force of the Commission for Classification and Terminology. Epilepsia Open. 2016;1(1–2):37–44.
463. Raga S, Specchio N, Rheims S, Wilmshurst JM. Developmental and epileptic encephalopathies: recognition and approaches to care. Epileptic Disord. 2021;23(1):40–52.
464. Specchio N, Curatolo P. Developmental and epileptic encephalopathies: what we do and do not know. Brain. 2021;144(1):32–43.
465. Myers KA, Scheffer IE. Precision medicine approaches for infantile-onset developmental and epileptic encephalopathies. Annu Rev Pharmacol Toxicol. 2022;62:641–62.
466. Hebbar M, Mefford HC. Recent advances in epilepsy genomics and genetic testing. F1000Res. 2020;9:F1000 Faculty Rev-185 [pii].
467. McTague A, Howell KB, Cross JH, Kurian MA, Scheffer IE. The genetic landscape of the epileptic encephalopathies of infancy and childhood. Lancet Neurol. 2016;15(3):304–16.
468. Oyrer J, Maljevic S, Scheffer IE, Berkovic SF, Petrou S, Reid CA. Ion channels in genetic epilepsy: from genes and mechanisms to disease-targeted therapies. Pharmacol Rev. 2018;70(1):142–73.
469. Byrne S, Enright N, Delanty N. Precision therapy in the genetic epilepsies of childhood. Dev Med Child Neurol. 2021;63(11):1276–82.
470. Nashabat M, Al Qahtani XS, Almakdob S, Altwaijri W, Ba-Armah DM, Hundallah K, et al. The landscape of early infantile epileptic encephalopathy in a consanguineous population. Seizure. 2019;69:154–72.

471. Heyne HO, Singh T, Stamberger H, Abou Jamra R, Caglayan H, Craiu D, et al. De novo variants in neurodevelopmental disorders with epilepsy. Nat Genet. 2018;50(7):1048–53.
472. Helbig KL, Lauerer RJ, Bahr JC, Souza IA, Myers CT, Uysal B, et al. De Novo pathogenic variants in CACNA1E cause developmental and epileptic encephalopathy with contractures, macrocephaly, and Dyskinesias. Am J Hum Genet. 2018;103(5):666–78.
473. Mulhern MS, Stumpel C, Stong N, Brunner HG, Bier L, Lippa N, et al. NBEA: developmental disease gene with early generalized epilepsy phenotypes. Ann Neurol. 2018;84(5):788–95.
474. Gregor A, Sadleir LG, Asadollahi R, Azzarello-Burri S, Battaglia A, Ousager LB, et al. De Novo variants in the F-Box protein FBXO11 in 20 individuals with a variable neurodevelopmental disorder. Am J Hum Genet. 2018;103(2):305–16.
475. Machol K, Rousseau J, Ehresmann S, Garcia T, Nguyen TTM, Spillmann RC, et al. Expanding the Spectrum of BAF-related disorders: De Novo variants in SMARCC2 cause a syndrome with intellectual disability and developmental delay. Am J Hum Genet. 2019;104(1):164–78.
476. Castermans D, Wilquet V, Parthoens E, Huysmans C, Steyaert J, Swinnen L, et al. The neurobeachin gene is disrupted by a translocation in a patient with idiopathic autism. J Med Genet. 2003;40(5):352–6.
477. Knowles JK, Helbig I, Metcalf CS, Lubbers LS, Isom LL, Demarest S, et al. Precision medicine for genetic epilepsy on the horizon: recent advances, present challenges, and suggestions for continued progress. Epilepsia. 2022;63(10):2461–75.
478. Calhoun JD, Carvill GL. Unravelling the genetic architecture of autosomal recessive epilepsy in the genomic era. J Neurogenet. 2018;32(4):295–312.
479. Murakami Y, Nguyen TTM, Baratang N, Raju PK, Knaus A, Ellard S, et al. Mutations in PIGB cause an inherited GPI biosynthesis defect with an axonal neuropathy and metabolic abnormality in severe cases. Am J Hum Genet. 2019;105(2):384–94.
480. Epilepsy Phenome/Genome Project Epi KC. Copy number variant analysis from exome data in 349 patients with epileptic encephalopathy. Ann Neurol. 2015;78(2):323–8.
481. Mefford HC, Yendle SC, Hsu C, Cook J, Geraghty E, McMahon JM, et al. Rare copy number variants are an important cause of epileptic encephalopathies. Ann Neurol. 2011;70(6):974–85.
482. Olson H, Shen Y, Avallone J, Sheidley BR, Pinsky R, Bergin AM, et al. Copy number variation plays an important role in clinical epilepsy. Ann Neurol. 2014;75(6):943–58.
483. Orsini A, Zara F, Striano P. Recent advances in epilepsy genetics. Neurosci Lett. 2018;667:4–9.
484. Pfundt R, Del Rosario M, Vissers L, Kwint MP, Janssen IM, de Leeuw N, et al. Detection of clinically relevant copy-number variants by exome sequencing in a large cohort of genetic disorders. Genet Med. 2017;19(6):667–75.
485. Schuster J, Laan L, Klar J, Jin Z, Huss M, Korol S, et al. Transcriptomes of Dravet syndrome iPSC derived GABAergic cells reveal dysregulated pathways for chromatin remodeling and neurodevelopment. Neurobiol Dis. 2019;132:104583.
486. LaCroix AJ, Stabley D, Sahraoui R, Adam MP, Mehaffey M, Kernan K, et al. GGC repeat expansion and Exon 1 methylation of XYLT1 is a common pathogenic variant in Baratela-Scott syndrome. Am J Hum Genet. 2019;104(1):35–44.
487. Barbosa M, Joshi RS, Garg P, Martin-Trujillo A, Patel N, Jadhav B, et al. Identification of rare de novo epigenetic variations in congenital disorders. Nat Commun. 2018;9(1):2064.
488. Aref-Eshghi E, Bend EG, Colaiacovo S, Caudle M, Chakrabarti R, Napier M, et al. Diagnostic utility of genome-wide DNA methylation testing in genetically unsolved individuals with suspected hereditary conditions. Am J Hum Genet. 2019;104(4):685–700.
489. Chang YT, Hong SY, Lin WD, Lin CH, Lin SS, Tsai FJ, et al. Genetic testing in children with developmental and epileptic encephalopathies: a review of advances in epilepsy genomics. Children (Basel). 2023;10(3):556.
490. Scheffer IE, Liao J. Deciphering the concepts behind "Epileptic encephalopathy" and "Developmental and epileptic encephalopathy". Eur J Paediatr Neurol. 2020;24:11–4.
491. Trivisano M, Specchio N. What are the epileptic encephalopathies? Curr Opin Neurol. 2020;33(2):179–84.

492. Myers KA, Johnstone DL, Dyment DA. Epilepsy genetics: current knowledge, applications, and future directions. Clin Genet. 2019;95(1):95–111.
493. von Deimling M, Helbig I, Marsh ED. Epileptic encephalopathies-clinical syndromes and pathophysiological concepts. Curr Neurol Neurosci Rep. 2017;17(2):10.
494. Lado FA, Rubboli G, Capovilla G, Avanzini G, Moshe SL. Pathophysiology of epileptic encephalopathies. Epilepsia. 2013;54 Suppl 8(0 8):6–13.
495. Siniatchkin M, Capovilla G. Functional neuroimaging in epileptic encephalopathies. Epilepsia. 2013;54(Suppl 8):27–33.
496. Siniatchkin M, van Baalen A, Jacobs J, Moeller F, Moehring J, Boor R, et al. Different neuronal networks are associated with spikes and slow activity in hypsarrhythmia. Epilepsia. 2007;48(12):2312–21.
497. Siniatchkin M, Groening K, Moehring J, Moeller F, Boor R, Brodbeck V, et al. Neuronal networks in children with continuous spikes and waves during slow sleep. Brain. 2010;133(9):2798–813.
498. Siniatchkin M, Coropceanu D, Moeller F, Boor R, Stephani U. EEG-fMRI reveals activation of brainstem and thalamus in patients with Lennox-Gastaut syndrome. Epilepsia. 2011;52(4):766–74.
499. Moeller F, Moehring J, Ick I, Steinmann E, Wolff S, Jansen O, et al. EEG-fMRI in atypical benign partial epilepsy. Epilepsia. 2013;54(8):e103–8.
500. Warren AEL, Harvey AS, Vogrin SJ, Bailey C, Davidson A, Jackson GD, et al. The epileptic network of Lennox-Gastaut syndrome: cortically driven and reproducible across age. Neurology. 2019;93(3):e215–e26.
501. Moehring J, von Spiczak S, Moeller F, Helbig I, Wolff S, Jansen O, et al. Variability of EEG-fMRI findings in patients with SCN1A-positive Dravet syndrome. Epilepsia. 2013;54(5):918–26.
502. Siniatchkin M, Van Bogaert P. Pathophysiology of encephalopathy related to continuous spike and waves during sleep: the contribution of neuroimaging. Epileptic Disord. 2019;21(S1):48–53.
503. Halász P, Kelemen A, Rosdy B, Rásonyi G, Clemens B, Szűcs A. Perisylvian epileptic network revisited. Seizure. 2019;65:31–41.
504. Raichle ME, Mintun MA. Brain work and brain imaging. Annu Rev Neurosci. 2006;29:449–76.
505. Pizoli CE, Shah MN, Snyder AZ, Shimony JS, Limbrick DD, Raichle ME, et al. Resting-state activity in development and maintenance of normal brain function. Proc Natl Acad Sci USA. 2011;108(28):11638–43.
506. Bettus G, Guedj E, Joyeux F, Confort-Gouny S, Soulier E, Laguitton V, et al. Decreased basal fMRI functional connectivity in epileptogenic networks and contralateral compensatory mechanisms. Hum Brain Mapp. 2009;30(5):1580–91.
507. Halász P, Bódizs R, Ujma PP, Fabó D, Szűcs A. Strong relationship between NREM sleep, epilepsy and plastic functions - a conceptual review on the neurophysiology background. Epilepsy Res. 2019;150:95–105.
508. Halász P, Szűcs A. Sleep and epilepsy link by plasticity. Front Neurol. 2020;11:911.
509. Bölsterli BK, Schmitt B, Bast T, Critelli H, Heinzle J, Jenni OG, et al. Impaired slow wave sleep downscaling in encephalopathy with status epilepticus during sleep (ESES). Clin Neurophysiol. 2011;122(9):1779–87.
510. Halász P. How sleep activates epileptic networks? Epilepsy Res Treat. 2013;2013:425697.
511. Bölsterli BK, Gardella E, Pavlidis E, Wehrle FM, Tassinari CA, Huber R, et al. Remission of encephalopathy with status epilepticus (ESES) during sleep renormalizes regulation of slow wave sleep. Epilepsia. 2017;58(11):1892–901.
512. Gorodetsky C, Fasano A. Developmental and epileptic encephalopathies in adults: An evolving field. Neurology. 2022;99(3):89–91.
513. Nevin SM, Wakefield CE, Schilstra CE, McGill BC, Bye A, Palmer EE. The information needs of parents of children with early-onset epilepsy: a systematic review. Epilepsy Behav. 2020;112:107382.

514. Rodda JM, Scheffer IE, McMahon JM, Berkovic SF, Graham HK. Progressive gait deterioration in adolescents with Dravet syndrome. Arch Neurol. 2012;69(7):873–8.
515. Licheni SH, McMahon JM, Schneider AL, Davey MJ, Scheffer IE. Sleep problems in Dravet syndrome: a modifiable comorbidity. Dev Med Child Neurol. 2018;60(2):192–8.
516. Howell KB, Eggers S, Dalziel K, Riseley J, Mandelstam S, Myers CT, et al. A population-based cost-effectiveness study of early genetic testing in severe epilepsies of infancy. Epilepsia. 2018;59(6):1177–87.
517. Jakobsen AV, Moller RS, Nikanorova M, Elklit A. The impact of severe pediatric epilepsy on experienced stress and psychopathology in parents. Epilepsy Behav. 2020;113:107538.
518. Harini C, Nagarajan E, Bergin AM, Pearl P, Loddenkemper T, Takeoka M, et al. Mortality in infantile spasms: a hospital-based study. Epilepsia. 2020;61(4):702–13.
519. El Kosseifi C, Cornet MC, Cilio MR. Neonatal developmental and epileptic encephalopathies. Semin Pediatr Neurol. 2019;32:100770.
520. Stamberger H, Crosiers D, Balagura G, Bonardi CM, Basu A, Cantalupo G, et al. Natural history study of STXBP1-developmental and epileptic encephalopathy into adulthood. Neurology. 2022;99(3):e221–e33.
521. Boets S, Johannesen KM, Destree A, Manti F, Ramantani G, Lesca G, et al. Adult phenotype of KCNQ2 encephalopathy. J Med Genet. 2022;59(6):528–35.
522. Selvarajah A, Zulfiqar-Ali Q, Marques P, Rong M, Andrade DM. A systematic review of adults with Dravet syndrome. Seizure. 2021;87:39–45.
523. Susannah A, Geoff S, Mark T, Michael E, John O, Joanna D, et al. The Australian cystic fibrosis data registry annual report, 2015. The ACFD registry. Annu Rep. 2017;18:51.
524. Vill K, Kolbel H, Schwartz O, Blaschek A, Olgemoller B, Harms E, et al. One year of newborn screening for SMA - results of a German pilot project. J Neuromuscul Dis. 2019;6(4):503–15.
525. Richter T, Nestler-Parr S, Babela R, Khan ZM, Tesoro T, Molsen E, et al. Rare disease terminology and definitions-a systematic global review: report of the ISPOR Rare Disease Special Interest Group. Value Health. 2015;18(6):906–14.
526. Institute of Medicine Committee on Accelerating Rare Diseases R, Orphan Product D. The National Academies Collection: reports funded by National Institutes of Health. In: Field MJ, Boat TF, editors. Rare diseases and orphan products: accelerating research and development. Washington (DC): National Academies Press (US); 2010.
527. Miller KL, Mueller C, Liu G, Miller Needleman KI, Maynard J. FDA orphan products clinical trial grants: assessment of outcomes and impact on rare disease product development. Orphanet J Rare Dis. 2020;15(1):234.
528. Gavin P. The importance of natural histories for rare diseases. Expert Opin Orphan Drugs. 2015;3(8):855–7.
529. Palmer EE, Howell K, Scheffer IE. Natural history studies and clinical trial readiness for genetic developmental and epileptic encephalopathies. Neurotherapeutics. 2021;18(3):1432–44.
530. Tabarki B, Thabet F. Vitamin-responsive epilepsies: an update. Arch Pediatr. 2013;20(11):1236–41.
531. Steward CA, Roovers J, Suner MM, Gonzalez JM, Uszczynska-Ratajczak B, Pervouchine D, et al. Re-annotation of 191 developmental and epileptic encephalopathy-associated genes unmasks de novo variants in SCN1A. NPJ Genom Med. 2019;4:31.
532. Berg AT, Levy SR, Testa FM. Evolution and course of early life developmental encephalopathic epilepsies: focus on Lennox-Gastaut syndrome. Epilepsia. 2018;59(11):2096–105.
533. Happ HC, Carvill GL. A 2020 view on the genetics of developmental and epileptic encephalopathies. Epilepsy Curr. 2020;20(2):90–6.
534. Moon JU, Cho KO. Current pharmacologic strategies for treatment of intractable epilepsy in children. Int Neurourol J. 2021;25(Suppl 1):S8–18.
535. Beltrán-Corbellini Á, Aledo-Serrano Á, Møller RS, Pérez-Palma E, García-Morales I, Toledano R, et al. Epilepsy genetics and precision medicine in adults: a new landscape for developmental and epileptic encephalopathies. Front Neurol. 2022;13:777115.

536. Nabbout R, Kuchenbuch M. Impact of predictive, preventive and precision medicine strategies in epilepsy. Nat Rev Neurol. 2020;16(12):674–88.
537. Bayat A, Bayat M, Rubboli G, Moller RS. Epilepsy syndromes in the first year of life and usefulness of genetic testing for precision therapy. Genes (Basel). 2021;12(7):1051.
538. Kay HY, Greene DL, Kang S, Kosenko A, Hoshi N. M-current preservation contributes to anticonvulsant effects of valproic acid. J Clin Invest. 2015;125(10):3904–14.
539. de Kovel CGF, Syrbe S, Brilstra EH, Verbeek N, Kerr B, Dubbs H, et al. Neurodevelopmental disorders caused by De Novo variants in KCNB1 genotypes and phenotypes. JAMA Neurol. 2017;74(10):1228–36.
540. Papavasiliou A, Foska K, Ioannou J, Nagel M. Epilepsy, ataxia, sensorineural deafness, tubulopathy syndrome in a European child with KCNJ10 mutations: a case report. SAGE Open Med Case Rep. 2017;5:2050313X17723549.
541. Mir A, Chaudhary M, Alkhaldi H, Alhazmi R, Albaradie R, Housawi Y. Corrigendum to "Epilepsy in patients with EAST syndrome caused by mutation in the KCNJ10". Brain Dev. 2019;41(8):716.
542. Golyala A, Kwan P. Drug development for refractory epilepsy: The past 25 years and beyond. Seizure. 2017;44:147–56.
543. Doose H, Gerken H, Leonhardt R, Volzke E, Volz C. Centrencephalic myoclonic-astatic petit mal. Clin Genet Investig Neuropadiatr. 1970;2(1):59–78.
544. Degen R, Lassker G, Edelmann R. Long term therapy with nitrazepam in children with infantile spasms and myoclonic-astatic fits. Psychiatr Neurol Med Psychol Beih. 1975;20-21:90–3.
545. Skarpa D, Erak P. Significance and possibility of electroencephalographic definition of epileptic drop attacks and atonic absences. Neuropsihijatrija. 1975;23(1–4):135–9.
546. Caraballo RH, Reyes Valenzuela G, Fortini S, Espeche A, Gamboni B, Silva W, et al. Cannabidiol in children with treatment-resistant epilepsy with myoclonic-atonic seizures. Epilepsy Behav. 2023;143:109245.
547. Kelley SA, Kossoff EH. Doose syndrome (myoclonic-astatic epilepsy): 40 years of progress. Dev Med Child Neurol. 2010;52(11):988–93.
548. Nickels K, Thibert R, Rau S, Demarest S, Wirrell E, Kossoff EH, et al. How do we diagnose and treat epilepsy with myoclonic-atonic seizures (Doose syndrome)? Results of the Pediatric Epilepsy Research Consortium survey. Epilepsy Res. 2018;144:14–9.
549. Hinokuma N, Nakashima M, Asai H, Nakamura K, Akaboshi S, Fukuoka M, et al. Clinical and genetic characteristics of patients with Doose syndrome. Epilepsia Open. 2020;5(3):442–50.
550. Denervaud S, Korff C, Fluss J, Kalser J, Roulet-Perez E, Hagmann P, et al. Structural brain abnormalities in epilepsy with myoclonic atonic seizures. Epilepsy Res. 2021;177:106771.
551. Belcastro V, Giordano L, Pruna D, Peruzzi C, Casellato S, Barca S, et al. Follow-up study of idiopathic generalized epilepsy with associated absence seizure and myoclonic epilepsy of infancy. Epilepsy Res. 2017;136:123–5.
552. Oguni H. Epilepsy with myoclonic-atonic seizures, also known as Doose syndrome: modification of the diagnostic criteria. Eur J Paediatr Neurol. 2022;36:37–50.
553. Nickels K, Kossoff EH, Eschbach K, Joshi C. Epilepsy with myoclonic-atonic seizures (Doose syndrome): clarification of diagnosis and treatment options through a large retrospective multicenter cohort. Epilepsia. 2021;62(1):120–7.
554. Stenger E, Schaeffer M, Cances C, Motte J, Auvin S, Ville D, et al. Efficacy of a ketogenic diet in resistant myoclono-astatic epilepsy: a French multicenter retrospective study. Epilepsy Res. 2017;131:64–9.
555. Wiemer-Kruel A, Haberlandt E, Hartmann H, Wohlrab G, Bast T. Modified Atkins diet is an effective treatment for children with Doose syndrome. Epilepsia. 2017;58(4):657–62.
556. Bernard R, Pinsard N, Dravet C, Gastaut H, Roger J, Soulayrol R, et al. Diagnostic and evolutive aspects of epileptic encephalopathy in children with diffuse slow wave spikes (petit mal variant). Pediatrie. 1966;21(6):712–4.

557. Gastaut H, Tassinari CA, Roger J, Soulayrol R, Saint Jean M, Regis H, et al. Epileptic encephalopathy in children with slow diffuse spike-wares (or petit mal variant) or Lennox syndrome. Recenti Prog Med. 1968;45(2):117–46.
558. Niedermeyer E. The Lennox-Gastaut syndrome: a severe type of childhood epilepsy. Electroencephalogr Clin Neurophysiol. 1968;24(3):283.
559. Tassinari CA, Dravet C, Roger J, Cano JP, Gastaut H. Tonic status epilepticus precipitated by intravenous benzodiazepine in five patients with Lennox-Gastaut syndrome. Epilepsia. 1972;13(3):421–35.
560. Speciali JG, Lison MP. Estados de mal epileptico na síndrome de Lennox-Gastaut. I. Aspectos clinicos [Status epilepticus in the Lennox-Gastaut syndrome. I. Clinical aspects]. Arq Neuropsiquiatr. 1974;32(4):274–83.
561. Strzelczyk A, Schubert-Bast S, Simon A, Wyatt G, Holland R, Rosenow F. Epidemiology, healthcare resource use, and mortality in patients with probable Lennox-Gastaut syndrome: a population-based study on German health insurance data. Epilepsy Behav. 2021;115:107647.
562. Asadi-Pooya AA. The new International League Against Epilepsy (ILAE) definition of Lennox-Gastaut syndrome: practical implications and limitations. J Clin Neurosci. 2023;115:43–6.
563. Asadi-Pooya AA, Farazdaghi M. Age at onset in patients with Lennox-Gastaut syndrome: correlations with clinical manifestations. J Clin Neurosci. 2022;100:138–42.
564. Herranz JL, Casas-Fernández C, Campistol J, Campos-Castelló J, Rufo-Campos M, Torres-Falcón A, et al. Lennox-Gastaut syndrome in Spain: a descriptive retrospective epidemiological study. Rev Neurol. 2010;50(12):711–7.
565. Hirsch E, French J, Scheffer IE, Bogacz A, Alsaadi T, Sperling MR, et al. ILAE definition of the idiopathic generalized epilepsy syndromes: position statement by the ILAE Task Force on Nosology and Definitions. Epilepsia. 2022;63(6):1475–99.
566. Besag FMC, Vasey MJ, Chin RFM. Current and emerging pharmacotherapy for the treatment of Lennox-Gastaut syndrome. Expert Opin Pharmacother. 2023;24(11):1249–68.
567. Riva A, Coppola A, Bonaventura CD, Elia M, Ferlazzo E, Gobbi G, et al. An Italian consensus on the management of Lennox-Gastaut syndrome. Seizure. 2022;101:134–40.
568. Devi N, Madaan P, Ameen R, Sahu JK, Bansal D. Short-term and long-term efficacy and safety of antiseizure medications in Lennox Gastaut syndrome: a network meta-analysis. Seizure. 2022;99:164–75.
569. Pechadre JC, Beudin P, Devoize JL, Gibert J. Anti-epileptic effect of clobazam in Lennox-Gastaut syndrome (author's transl). Encéphale. 1981;7(2):181–90.
570. Ng YT, Conry JA, Drummond R, Stolle J, Weinberg MA, Investigators O-S. Randomized, phase III study results of clobazam in Lennox-Gastaut syndrome. Neurology. 2011;77(15):1473–81.
571. Espinosa-Jovel C, Riveros S, Bolanos-Almeida C, Salazar MR, Inga LC, Guio L. Real-world evidence on the use of cannabidiol for the treatment of drug resistant epilepsy not related to Lennox-Gastaut syndrome, Dravet syndrome or Tuberous Sclerosis Complex. Seizure. 2023;112:72–6.
572. Timmings PL, Richens A. Lamotrigine as an add-on drug in the management of Lennox-Gastaut syndrome. Eur Neurol. 1992;32(6):305–7.
573. Kim HJ, Kim HD, Lee JS, Heo K, Kim DS, Kang HC. Long-term prognosis of patients with Lennox--Gastaut syndrome in recent decades. Epilepsy Res. 2015;110:10–9.
574. Patry G, Lyagoubi S, Tassinari CA. Subclinical "electrical status epilepticus" induced by sleep in children. A clinical and electroencephalographic study of six cases. Arch Neurol. 1971;24(3):242–52.
575. Fernández IS, Chapman KE, Peters JM, Kothare SV, Nordli DR Jr, Jensen FE, et al. The tower of Babel: survey on concepts and terminology in electrical status epilepticus in sleep and continuous spikes and waves during sleep in North America. Epilepsia. 2013;54(4):741–50.
576. Engel J Jr. A proposed diagnostic scheme for people with epileptic seizures and with epilepsy: report of the ILAE Task Force on Classification and Terminology. Epilepsia. 2001;42(6):796–803.

577. Tassinari CA, Rubboli G, Volpi L, Meletti S, d'Orsi G, Franca M, et al. Encephalopathy with electrical status epilepticus during slow sleep or ESES syndrome including the acquired aphasia. Clin Neurophysiol. 2000;111(Suppl 2):S94–S102.
578. Tassinari CA, Cantalupo G, Rios-Pohl L, Giustina ED, Rubboli G. Encephalopathy with status epilepticus during slow sleep: "the Penelope syndrome". Epilepsia. 2009;50(Suppl 7):4–8.
579. Panayiotopoulos CP. The epilepsies: seizures, syndromes and management. Oxfordshire: Bladon Medical Publishing; 2005.
580. Striano P, Capovilla G. Epileptic encephalopathy with continuous spike-and-wave during sleep. In: Panayiotopoulos C, editor. The atlas of epilepsies. London: Springer; 2010. p. 913–8.
581. Aicardi J, Chevrie JJ. Atypical benign partial epilepsy of childhood. Dev Med Child Neurol. 1982;24(3):281–92.
582. Fejerman N, Caraballo R, Tenembaum SN. Atypical evolutions of benign localization-related epilepsies in children: are they predictable? Epilepsia. 2000;41(4):380–90.
583. Tovia E, Goldberg-Stern H, Ben Zeev B, Heyman E, Watemberg N, Fattal-Valevski A, et al. The prevalence of atypical presentations and comorbidities of benign childhood epilepsy with centrotemporal spikes. Epilepsia. 2011;52(8):1483–8.
584. Landau WM, Kleffner FR. Syndrome of acquired aphasia with convulsive disorder in children. Neurology. 1957;7(8):523–30.
585. Gordon N. The Landau-Kleffner syndrome: increased understanding. Brain Dev. 1997;19(5):311–6.
586. Galanopoulou AS, Bojko A, Lado F, Moshé SL. The spectrum of neuropsychiatric abnormalities associated with electrical status epilepticus in sleep. Brain Dev. 2000;22(5):279–95.
587. Nickels K, Wirrell E. Electrical status epilepticus in sleep. Semin Pediatr Neurol. 2008;15(2):50–60.
588. Engel J Jr. Report of the ILAE classification core group. Epilepsia. 2006;47(9):1558–68.
589. Eksioglu YTETM. Clinical presentation and acute treatment of electricalstatus epilepticus in sleep and sleep potentiated spikes. Philadelphia; 2009.
590. Morikawa T, Seino M, Watanabe Y, Watanabe M, Yagi K. Clinical relevance of continuous spike-waves during slow wave sleep. In: Manelis S, Bental E, Loeber JN, Dreifuss FE, editors. Advances in epileptology. New York: Raven Press; 1989. p. 359–3363.
591. Singhal NS, Sullivan JE. Continuous spike-wave during slow wave sleep and related conditions. ISRN Neurol. 2014;2014:619079.
592. Kersbergen KJ, de Vries LS, Leijten FS, Braun KP, Nievelstein RA, Groenendaal F, et al. Neonatal thalamic hemorrhage is strongly associated with electrical status epilepticus in slow wave sleep. Epilepsia. 2013;54(4):733–40.
593. Fohlen M, Dorfmuller G, Ferrand-Sorbets S, Dorison N, Chipaux M, Taussig D. Parasagittal hemispherotomy in hemispheric polymicrogyria with electrical status epilepticus during slow sleep: indications, results and follow-up. Seizure. 2019;71:190–200.
594. Caraballo RH, Cersosimo RO, Fortini PS, Ornella L, Buompadre MC, Vilte C, et al. Congenital hemiparesis, unilateral polymicrogyria and epilepsy with or without status epilepticus during sleep: a study of 66 patients with long-term follow-up. Epileptic Disord. 2013;15(4):417–27.
595. Van Hirtum-Das M, Licht EA, Koh S, Wu JY, Shields WD, Sankar R. Children with ESES: variability in the syndrome. Epilepsy Res. 2006;70(Suppl 1):S248–58.
596. Krueger MB, Magalhaes SC, Pessoa A, Bueno C, Masruha MR, Sobreira-Neto MA. Electrical status epilepticus during sleep in patients with congenital Zika virus syndrome: An unprecedented clinical finding. Seizure. 2020;81:250–3.
597. Nabbout R. Autoimmune and inflammatory epilepsies. Epilepsia. 2012;53(Suppl 4):58–62.
598. Hu LY, Shi XY, Feng C, Wang JW, Yang G, Lammers SH, et al. An 8-year old boy with continuous spikes and waves during slow sleep presenting with positive onconeuronal antibodies. Eur J Paediatr Neurol. 2015;19(2):257–61.
599. Tsai MH, Vears DF, Turner SJ, Smith RL, Berkovic SF, Sadleir LG, et al. Clinical genetic study of the epilepsy-aphasia spectrum. Epilepsia. 2013;54(2):280–7.

600. Lesca G, Moller RS, Rudolf G, Hirsch E, Hjalgrim H, Szepetowski P. Update on the genetics of the epilepsy-aphasia spectrum and role of GRIN2A mutations. Epileptic Disord. 2019;21(S1):41–7.
601. Lesca G, Rudolf G, Bruneau N, Lozovaya N, Labalme A, Boutry-Kryza N, et al. GRIN2A mutations in acquired epileptic aphasia and related childhood focal epilepsies and encephalopathies with speech and language dysfunction. Nat Genet. 2013;45(9):1061–6.
602. Lemke JR, Lal D, Reinthaler EM, Steiner I, Nothnagel M, Alber M, et al. Mutations in GRIN2A cause idiopathic focal epilepsy with rolandic spikes. Nat Genet. 2013;45(9):1067–72.
603. Carvill GL, Regan BM, Yendle SC, O'Roak BJ, Lozovaya N, Bruneau N, et al. GRIN2A mutations cause epilepsy-aphasia spectrum disorders. Nat Genet. 2013;45(9):1073–6.
604. Turner SJ, Mayes AK, Verhoeven A, Mandelstam SA, Morgan AT, Scheffer IE. GRIN2A: an aptly named gene for speech dysfunction. Neurology. 2015;84(6):586–93.
605. Zanni G, Barresi S, Cohen R, Specchio N, Basel-Vanagaite L, Valente EM, et al. A novel mutation in the endosomal Na^+/H^+ exchanger NHE6 (SLC9A6) causes Christianson syndrome with electrical status epilepticus during slow-wave sleep (ESES). Epilepsy Res. 2014;108(4):811–5.
606. Kobayashi K, Hata H, Oka M, Ito M, Yoshinaga H, Kashihara K, et al. Age-related electrical status epilepticus during sleep and epileptic negative myoclonus in DRPLA. Neurology. 2006;66(5):772–3.
607. Coutelier M, Andries S, Ghariani S, Dan B, Duyckaerts C, van Rijckevorsel K, et al. Neuroserpin mutation causes electrical status epilepticus of slow-wave sleep. Neurology. 2008;71(1):64–6.
608. Lee IC, Yang JJ, Li SY. A KCNQ2 E515D mutation associated with benign familial neonatal seizures and continuous spike and waves during slow-wave sleep syndrome in Taiwan. J Formos Med Assoc. 2017;116(9):711–9.
609. Carmi N, Lev D, Leshinsky-Silver E, Anikster Y, Blumkin L, Kivity S, et al. Atypical presentation of Costeff syndrome-severe psychomotor involvement and electrical status epilepticus during slow wave sleep. Eur J Paediatr Neurol. 2015;19(6):733–6.
610. Sachdev M, Gainza-Lein M, Tchapyjnikov D, Jiang YH, Loddenkemper T, Mikati MA. Novel clinical manifestations in patients with KCNA2 mutations. Seizure. 2017;51:74–6.
611. Syrbe S, Hedrich UBS, Riesch E, Djemie T, Muller S, Moller RS, et al. De novo loss- or gain-of-function mutations in KCNA2 cause epileptic encephalopathy. Nat Genet. 2015;47(4):393–9.
612. Masnada S, Hedrich UBS, Gardella E, Schubert J, Kaiwar C, Klee EW, et al. Clinical spectrum and genotype-phenotype associations of KCNA2-related encephalopathies. Brain. 2017;140(9):2337–54.
613. Damiano JA, Burgess R, Kivity S, Lerman-Sagie T, Afawi Z, Scheffer IE, et al. Frequency of CNKSR2 mutation in the X-linked epilepsy-aphasia spectrum. Epilepsia. 2017;58(3):e40–e3.
614. Johannesen KM, Gardella E, Linnankivi T, Courage C, de Saint MA, Lehesjoki AE, et al. Defining the phenotypic spectrum of SLC6A1 mutations. Epilepsia. 2018;59(2):389–402.
615. Lesca G, Rudolf G, Labalme A, Hirsch E, Arzimanoglou A, Genton P, et al. Epileptic encephalopathies of the Landau-Kleffner and continuous spike and waves during slow-wave sleep types: genomic dissection makes the link with autism. Epilepsia. 2012;53(9):1526–38.
616. Dalla Bernardina B, Fontana E, Michelizza B, Colamaria V, Capovilla G, Tassinari CA. Partial epilepsies of childhood, bilateral synchronisation, continuous spike-waves during slow sleep. In: Manelis J, Bental E, Loeber JN, Dreifuss FE, editors. Advances in epileptology: XVII Epilepsy International SymposiumPartial epilepsies of childhood, bilateral synchronization, continuous spike-waves during slow sleep. New York: Raven; 1989. p. 295–302.
617. Bureau M. Outstanding cases of CSWS and LKS: analysis of the data sheets provided by the participants. In: Continuous spikes and waves during slow sleep/electrical status epilepticus during slow sleep, vol. 3. London, UK: John Libbey; 1995. p. 213–6.

618. Caraballo R, Pavlidis E, Nikanorova M, Loddenkemper T. Encephalopathy with continuous spike-waves during slow-wave sleep: evolution and prognosis. Epileptic Disord. 2019;21(S1):15–21.
619. Gardella E, Cantalupo G, Larsson PG, Fontana E, Bernardina BD, Rubboli G, et al. EEG features in encephalopathy related to status epilepticus during slow sleep. Epileptic Disord. 2019;21(S1):22–30.
620. Loddenkemper T, Fernandez IS, Peters JM. Continuous spike and waves during sleep and electrical status epilepticus in sleep. J Clin Neurophysiol. 2011;28(2):154–64.
621. Tassinari CA, Rubboli G. Cognition and paroxysmal EEG activities: from a single spike to electrical status epilepticus during sleep. Epilepsia. 2006;47(Suppl 2):40–3.
622. Roulet Perez E, Davidoff V, Despland PA, Deonna T. Mental and behavioural deterioration of children with epilepsy and CSWS: acquired epileptic frontal syndrome. Dev Med Child Neurol. 1993;35(8):661–74.
623. Fernández IS, Peters JM, Hadjiloizou S, Prabhu SP, Zarowski M, Stannard KM, et al. Clinical staging and electroencephalographic evolution of continuous spikes and waves during sleep. Epilepsia. 2012;53(7):1185–95.
624. Cooper JA, Ferry PC. Acquired auditory verbal agnosia and seizures in childhood. J Speech Hear Disord. 1978;43(2):176–84.
625. Morrell F, Whisler WW, Smith MC, Hoeppner TJ, de Toledo-Morrell L, Pierre-Louis SJ, et al. Landau-Kleffner syndrome. Treatment with subpial intracortical transection. Brain. 1995;118(Pt 6):1529–46.
626. Paquier PF, Van Dongen HR, Loonen CB. The Landau-Kleffner syndrome or 'acquired aphasia with convulsive disorder'. Long-term follow-up of six children and a review of the recent literature. Arch Neurol. 1992;49(4):354–9.
627. Soprano AM, Garcia EF, Caraballo R, Fejerman N. Acquired epileptic aphasia: neuropsychologic follow-up of 12 patients. Pediatr Neurol. 1994;11(3):230–5.
628. Van Dongen HR, Meulstee J, Paquier P, Beaumanoir A, Bureau M, Deonna T, et al. Two contrasting cases of children with acquired epileptic aphasia and continuous spikes and waves during sleep. In: Continuous spikes and waves during slow sleep-electrical status epilepticus during slow sleep: acquired epileptic aphasia and related conditions; 1995. p. 137–41.
629. Deonna T, Peter C, Ziegler AL. Adult follow-up of the acquired aphasia-epilepsy syndrome in childhood. Report of 7 cases. Neuropediatrics. 1989;20(3):132–8.
630. Feekery CJ, Parry-Fielder B, Hopkins IJ. Landau-Kleffner syndrome: six patients including discordant monozygotic twins. Pediatr Neurol. 1993;9(1):49–53.
631. Mantovani JF, Landau WM. Acquired aphasia with convulsive disorder: course and prognosis. Neurology. 1980;30(5):524–9.
632. Rapin I, Mattis S, Rowan AJ, Golden GG. Verbal auditory agnosia in children. Dev Med Child Neurol. 1977;19(2):197–207.
633. Lagae LG, Silberstein J, Gillis PL, Casaer PJ. Successful use of intravenous immunoglobulins in Landau-Kleffner syndrome. Pediatr Neurol. 1998;18(2):165–8.
634. Caraballo RH, Cejas N, Chamorro N, Kaltenmeier MC, Fortini S, Soprano AM. Landau-Kleffner syndrome: a study of 29 patients. Seizure. 2014;23(2):98–104.
635. Scheltens-de BM. Guidelines for EEG in encephalopathy related to ESES/CSWS in children. Epilepsia. 2009;50(Suppl 7):13–7.
636. Mikati MA, Saab R, Fayad MN, Choueiri RN. Efficacy of intravenous immunoglobulin in Landau-Kleffner syndrome. Pediatr Neurol. 2002;26(4):298–300.
637. Beaumanoir A, Bureau M, Mira L. Identification of the syndrome. In: Beaumanoir A, Bureau T, Deonna T, Mira L, Tassinari CA, editors. Continuous spikes and waves during slow sleep. Oxford: John Libbey &Company Ltd; 1995. p. 243–9.
638. Van Lierde A. Therapeutic data. In: Roger J, Bureau M, Dravet C, editors. Epileptic syndromes in infancy, childhood and adolescence. Eastleigh: John Libbey; 1992. p. 225–7.
639. Marescaux C, Hirsch E, Finck S, Maquet P, Schlumberger E, Sellal F, et al. Landau-Kleffner syndrome: a pharmacologic study of five cases. Epilepsia. 1990;31(6):768–77.

640. Snead OC 3rd, Hosey LC. Exacerbation of seizures in children by carbamazepine. N Engl J Med. 1985;313(15):916–21.
641. Lerman P. Seizures induced or aggravated by anticonvulsants. Epilepsia. 1986;27(6):706–10.
642. Inutsuka M, Kobayashi K, Oka M, Hattori J, Ohtsuka Y. Treatment of epilepsy with electrical status epilepticus during slow sleep and its related disorders. Brain Dev. 2006;28(5):281–6.
643. Yasuhara A, Yoshida H, Hatanaka T, Sugimoto T, Kobayashi Y, Dyken E. Epilepsy with continuous spike-waves during slow sleep and its treatment. Epilepsia. 1991;32(1):59–62.
644. Aeby A, Poznanski N, Verheulpen D, Wetzburger C, Van Bogaert P. Levetiracetam efficacy in epileptic syndromes with continuous spikes and waves during slow sleep: experience in 12 cases. Epilepsia. 2005;46(12):1937–42.
645. Larrieu JL, Lagueny A, Ferrer X, Julien J. Epilepsie avec décharges continues au cours du sommeil lent. Guérison sous clobazam [Epilepsy with continuous discharges during slow-wave sleep. Treatment with clobazam]. Rev Electroencephalogr Neurophysiol Clin. 1986;16(4):383–94.
646. Kramer U, Sagi L, Goldberg-Stern H, Zelnik N, Nissenkorn A, Ben-Zeev B. Clinical spectrum and medical treatment of children with electrical status epilepticus in sleep (ESES). Epilepsia. 2009;50(6):1517–24.
647. Wang SB, Weng WC, Fan PC, Lee WT. Levetiracetam in continuous spike waves during slow-wave sleep syndrome. Pediatr Neurol. 2008;39(2):85–90.
648. Fejerman N, Caraballo R, Cersosimo R, Ferraro SM, Galicchio S, Amartino H. Sulthiame add-on therapy in children with focal epilepsies associated with encephalopathy related to electrical status epilepticus during slow sleep (ESES). Epilepsia. 2012;53(7):1156–61.
649. Fine AL, Wirrell EC, Wong-Kisiel LC, Nickels KC. Acetazolamide for electrical status epilepticus in slow-wave sleep. Epilepsia. 2015;56(9):e134–8.
650. Wirrell E, Ho AW, Hamiwka L. Sulthiame therapy for continuous spike and wave in slow-wave sleep. Pediatr Neurol. 2006;35(3):204–8.
651. Gross-Selbeck G. Treatment of "benign" partial epilepsies of childhood, including atypical forms. Neuropediatrics. 1995;26(1):45–50.
652. Wakai S, Ito N, Ueda D, Chiba S. Landau-Kleffner syndrome and sulthiame. Neuropediatrics. 1997;28(2):135–6.
653. De Negri M, Baglietto MG, Battaglia FM, Gaggero R, Pessagno A, Recanati L. Treatment of electrical status epilepticus by short diazepam (DZP) cycles after DZP rectal bolus test. Brain Dev. 1995;17(5):330–3.
654. Hirsch E, Marescaux C, Maquet P, Metz-Lutz MN, Kiesmann M, Salmon E, et al. Landau-Kleffner syndrome: a clinical and EEG study of five cases. Epilepsia. 1990;31(6):756–67.
655. Lerman P, Lerman-Sagie T, Kivity S. Effect of early corticosteroid therapy for Landau-Kleffner syndrome. Dev Med Child Neurol. 1991;33(3):257–60.
656. Tsuru T, Mori M, Mizuguchi M, Momoi MY. Effects of high-dose intravenous corticosteroid therapy in Landau-Kleffner syndrome. Pediatr Neurol. 2000;22(2):145–7.
657. Okuyaz C, Aydin K, Gücüyener K, Serdaroğlu A. Treatment of electrical status epilepticus during slow-wave sleep with high-dose corticosteroid. Pediatr Neurol. 2005;32(1):64–7.
658. Sinclair DB, Snyder TJ. Corticosteroids for the treatment of Landau-kleffner syndrome and continuous spike-wave discharge during sleep. Pediatr Neurol. 2005;32(5):300–6.
659. Fayad MN, Choueiri R, Mikati M. Landau-Kleffner syndrome: consistent response to repeated intravenous gamma-globulin doses: a case report. Epilepsia. 1997;38(4):489–94.
660. Arts WF, Aarsen FK, Scheltens-de Boer M, Catsman-Berrevoets CE. Landau-Kleffner syndrome and CSWS syndrome: treatment with intravenous immunoglobulins. Epilepsia. 2009;50(Suppl 7):55–8.
661. Grote CL, Van Slyke P, Hoeppner JA. Language outcome following multiple subpial transection for Landau-Kleffner syndrome. Brain. 1999;122(Pt 3):561–6.
662. Irwin K, Birch V, Lees J, Polkey C, Alarcon G, Binnie C, et al. Multiple subpial transection in Landau-Kleffner syndrome. Dev Med Child Neurol. 2001;43(4):248–52.

663. Blount JP, Langburt W, Otsubo H, Chitoku S, Ochi A, Weiss S, et al. Multiple subpial transections in the treatment of pediatric epilepsy. J Neurosurg. 2004;100(2 Suppl Pediatrics):118–24.
664. Carosella CM, Greiner HM, Byars AW, Arthur TM, Leach JL, Turner M, et al. Vagus nerve stimulation for electrographic status epilepticus in slow-wave sleep. Pediatr Neurol. 2016;60:66–70.
665. Park YD. The effects of vagus nerve stimulation therapy on patients with intractable seizures and either Landau-Kleffner syndrome or autism. Epilepsy Behav. 2003;4(3):286–90.
666. Cross JH, Neville BG. The surgical treatment of Landau-Kleffner syndrome. Epilepsia. 2009;50(Suppl 7):63–7.
667. Bergqvist AG, Chee CM, Lutchka LM, Brooks-Kayal AR. Treatment of acquired epileptic aphasia with the ketogenic diet. J Child Neurol. 1999;14(11):696–701.
668. Kelley SA, Kossoff EH. How effective is the ketogenic diet for electrical status epilepticus of sleep? Epilepsy Res. 2016;127:339–43.
669. Deonna T, Prelaz-Girod AC, Mayor-Dubois C, Roulet-Perez E. Sign language in Landau-Kleffner syndrome. Epilepsia. 2009;50(Suppl 7):77–82.
670. Sánchez Fernández I, Chapman KE, Peters JM, Harini C, Rotenberg A, Loddenkemper T. Continuous spikes and waves during sleep: electroclinical presentation and suggestions for management. Epilepsy Res Treat. 2013;2013:583531.
671. M. B. 'Continuous spikes and waves during slow sleep' (CSWS): definition of the syndrome. In: Beaumanoir A, Bureau M, Deonna T, Mira L, Tassinari CA, editors. Continuous spikes and waves during slow sleep. Electrical status epilepticus during slow sleep: acquired epileptic Aphasia and related conditions. London, UK: John Libbey; 1995. p. 17–26.
672. Caraballo RH, Veggiotti P, Kaltenmeier MC, Piazza E, Gamboni B, Lopez Avaria MF, et al. Encephalopathy with status epilepticus during sleep or continuous spikes and waves during slow sleep syndrome: a multicenter, long-term follow-up study of 117 patients. Epilepsy Res. 2013;105(1–2):164–73.
673. Liukkonen E, Kantola-Sorsa E, Paetau R, Gaily E, Peltola M, Granström ML. Long-term outcome of 32 children with encephalopathy with status epilepticus during sleep, or ESES syndrome. Epilepsia. 2010;51(10):2023–32.
674. Dalla Bernardina B, Fontana E, Michelizza B, Colamaria V, Capovilla G, Tassinari CA, editors. Partial epilepsies in childhood bilateral synchronization, continuous spike-waves during slow sleep. Advances in epileptology: XVIIth epilepsy international symposium. Raven Press; 1989.
675. Saltik S, Uluduz D, Cokar O, Demirbilek V, Dervent A. A clinical and EEG study on idiopathic partial epilepsies with evolution into ESES spectrum disorders. Epilepsia. 2005;46(4):524–33.
676. Hirsch LJ, Gaspard N, van Baalen A, Nabbout R, Demeret S, Loddenkemper T, et al. Proposed consensus definitions for new-onset refractory status epilepticus (NORSE), febrile infection-related epilepsy syndrome (FIRES), and related conditions. Epilepsia. 2018;59(4):739–44.
677. van Baalen A, Vezzani A, Hausler M, Kluger G. Febrile infection-related epilepsy syndrome: clinical review and hypotheses of epileptogenesis. Neuropediatrics. 2017;48(1):5–18.
678. Payne ET, Koh S, Wirrell EC. Extinguishing febrile infection-related epilepsy syndrome: pipe dream or reality? Semin Neurol. 2020;40(2):263–72.
679. Serino D, Santarone ME, Caputo D, Fusco L. Febrile infection-related epilepsy syndrome (FIRES): prevalence, impact and management strategies. Neuropsychiatr Dis Treat. 2019;15:1897–903.
680. Lyon G, Dodge PR, Adams RD. The acute encephalopathies of obscure origin in infants and children. Brain. 1961;84:680–708.
681. Awaya Y. Epilepsy sequelae of acute encephalitis or encephalopathy (third report). Jpn J Psychiatry Neurol. 1986;40:385–7.
682. Sakuma H, Fukumizu M, Kohyama J. Efficacy of anticonvulsants on acute encephalitis with refractory, repetitive partial seizures (AERRPS). No To Hattatsu. 2001;33(5):385–90.

683. Mikaeloff Y, Jambaque I, Hertz-Pannier L, Zamfirescu A, Adamsbaum C, Plouin P, et al. Devastating epileptic encephalopathy in school-aged children (DESC): a pseudo encephalitis. Epilepsy Res. 2006;69(1):67–79.
684. van Baalen A, Stephani U, Kluger G, Hausler M, Dulac O. FIRES: febrile infection responsive epileptic (FIRE) encephalopathies of school age. Brain Dev. 2009;31(1):91; author reply 2-3.
685. van Baalen A, Hausler M, Boor R, Rohr A, Sperner J, Kurlemann G, et al. Febrile infection-related epilepsy syndrome (FIRES): a nonencephalitic encephalopathy in childhood. Epilepsia. 2010;51(7):1323–8.
686. van Baalen A, Häusler M, Plecko-Startinig B, Strautmanis J, Vlaho S, Gebhardt B, et al. Febrile infection-related epilepsy syndrome without detectable autoantibodies and response to immunotherapy: a case series and discussion of epileptogenesis in FIRES. Neuropediatrics. 2012;43(4):209–16.
687. Gaspard N, Hirsch LJ, Sculier C, Loddenkemper T, van Baalen A, Lancrenon J, et al. New-onset refractory status epilepticus (NORSE) and febrile infection-related epilepsy syndrome (FIRES): state of the art and perspectives. Epilepsia. 2018;59(4):745–52.
688. Kothur K, Bandodkar S, Wienholt L, Chu S, Pope A, Gill D, et al. Etiology is the key determinant of neuroinflammation in epilepsy: elevation of cerebrospinal fluid cytokines and chemokines in febrile infection-related epilepsy syndrome and febrile status epilepticus. Epilepsia. 2019;60(8):1678–88.
689. Clarkson BDS, LaFrance-Corey RG, Kahoud RJ, Farias-Moeller R, Payne ET, Howe CL. Functional deficiency in endogenous interleukin-1 receptor antagonist in patients with febrile infection-related epilepsy syndrome. Ann Neurol. 2019;85(4):526–37.
690. Muccioli L, Pensato U, Di Vito L, Messia M, Nicodemo M, Tinuper P. Teaching NeuroImage: claustrum sign in febrile infection-related epilepsy syndrome. Neurology. 2022;98(10):e1090–e1.
691. Lin WS, Hsu TR. Hypothesis: febrile infection-related epilepsy syndrome is a microglial NLRP3 inflammasome/IL-1 axis-driven autoinflammatory syndrome. Clin Transl Immunol. 2021;10(6):e1299.
692. Sakuma H, Tanuma N, Kuki I, Takahashi Y, Shiomi M, Hayashi M. Intrathecal overproduction of proinflammatory cytokines and chemokines in febrile infection-related refractory status epilepticus. J Neurol Neurosurg Psychiatry. 2015;86(7):820–2.
693. Caputo D, Iorio R, Vigevano F, Fusco L. Febrile infection-related epilepsy syndrome (FIRES) with super-refractory status epilepticus revealing autoimmune encephalitis due to GABA(a)R antibodies. Eur J Paediatr Neurol. 2018;22(1):182–5.
694. Basso M, Gastaldi M, Leonardi V, Izzo G, Olivotto S, Ferrario S, et al. Connections between febrile infection-related epilepsy syndrome and autoimmune encephalitis. A case report of a child with new anti-neuronal antibodies. Front Pediatr. 2022;10:908518.
695. Kurimoto T, Matsuoka T, Ami Y, Kanno K, Fujii T, Fujiwara N, et al. Anti-inflammatory and immune-mediated therapy for a case of febrile infection-related epilepsy syndrome with rapid recurrence. Clin Case Rep. 2022;10(6):e5952.
696. Hsieh MY, Lin JJ, Hsia SH, Huang JL, Yeh KW, Chang KW, et al. Diminished toll-like receptor response in febrile infection-related epilepsy syndrome (FIRES). Biom J. 2020;43(3):293–304.
697. Alparslan C, Kamit-Can F, Anıl AB, Olgaç-Dundar N, Çavuşoğlu D, Göç Z. Febrile infection-related epilepsy syndrome (FIRES) treated with immunomodulation in an 8-year-old boy and review of the literature. Turk J Pediatr. 2017;59(4):463–6.
698. Kramer U, Chi CS, Lin KL, Specchio N, Sahin M, Olson H, et al. Febrile infection-related epilepsy syndrome (FIRES): pathogenesis, treatment, and outcome: a multicenter study on 77 children. Epilepsia. 2011;52(11):1956–65.
699. Howell KB, Katanyuwong K, Mackay MT, Bailey CA, Scheffer IE, Freeman JL, et al. Long-term follow-up of febrile infection-related epilepsy syndrome. Epilepsia. 2012;53(1):101–10.

700. Lee HF, Chi CS. Febrile infection-related epilepsy syndrome (FIRES): therapeutic complications, long-term neurological and neuroimaging follow-up. Seizure. 2018;56:53–9.
701. Lam SK, Lu WY, Weng WC, Fan PC, Lee WT. The short-term and long-term outcome of febrile infection-related epilepsy syndrome in children. Epilepsy Behav. 2019;95:117–23.
702. Caraballo RH, Reyes G, Avaria MF, Buompadre MC, Gonzalez M, Fortini S, et al. Febrile infection-related epilepsy syndrome: a study of 12 patients. Seizure. 2013;22(7):553–9.
703. Agarwal A, Sabat S, Thamburaj K, Kanekar S. Hippocampal changes in febrile infection-related epilepsy syndrome (FIRES). Pol J Radiol. 2015;80:391–4.
704. Rivas-Coppola MS, Shah N, Choudhri AF, Morgan R, Wheless JW. Chronological evolution of magnetic resonance imaging findings in children with febrile infection-related epilepsy syndrome. Pediatr Neurol. 2016;55:22–9.
705. Byler DL, Grageda MR, Halstead ES, Kanekar S. Rapid onset of hippocampal atrophy in febrile-infection related epilepsy syndrome (FIRES). J Child Neurol. 2014;29(4):545–9.
706. Rachfalska N, Pietruszewski J, Paprocka J. Dramatic course of paediatric cryptogenic febrile infection-related epilepsy syndrome with unusual chronic phase presentation-a case report with literature study. Brain Sci. 2021;11(8):1030.
707. Farias-Moeller R, Bartolini L, Staso K, Schreiber JM, Carpenter JL. Early ictal and interictal patterns in FIRES: The sparks before the blaze. Epilepsia. 2017;58(8):1340–8.
708. Culleton S, Talenti G, Kaliakatsos M, Pujar S, D'Arco F. The spectrum of neuroimaging findings in febrile infection-related epilepsy syndrome (FIRES): a literature review. Epilepsia. 2019;60(4):585–92.
709. Tan AP. Febrile Infection-Related Epilepsy Syndrome (FIRES) with multifocal subcortical infarcts, a new imaging phenotype. Neuropediatrics. 2018;49(5):347–52.
710. Nozaki F, Kumada T, Miyajima T, Kusunoki T, Hiejima I, Hayashi A, et al. Reversible splenic lesion in a patient with Febrile Infection-Related Epilepsy Syndrome (FIRES). Neuropediatrics. 2013;44(5):291–4.
711. Wickstrom R, Taraschenko O, Dilena R, Payne ET, Specchio N, Nabbout R, et al. International consensus recommendations for management of New Onset Refractory Status Epilepticus (NORSE) including Febrile Infection-Related Epilepsy Syndrome (FIRES): summary and clinical tools. Epilepsia. 2022;63(11):2827–39.
712. Wickstrom R, Taraschenko O, Dilena R, Payne ET, Specchio N, Nabbout R, et al. International consensus recommendations for management of New Onset Refractory Status Epilepticus (NORSE) incl. Febrile Infection-Related Epilepsy Syndrome (FIRES): statements and supporting evidence. Epilepsia. 2022;63(11):2840–64.
713. Lagae L. Dravet syndrome. Curr Opin Neurol. 2021;34(2):213–8.
714. Koh S, Wirrell E, Vezzani A, Nabbout R, Muscal E, Kaliakatsos M, et al. Proposal to optimize evaluation and treatment of febrile infection-related epilepsy syndrome (FIRES): a report from FIRES workshop. Epilepsia Open. 2021;6(1):62–72.
715. Horino A, Kuki I, Inoue T, Nukui M, Okazaki S, Kawawaki H, et al. Intrathecal dexamethasone therapy for febrile infection-related epilepsy syndrome. Ann Clin Transl Neurol. 2021;8(3):645–55.
716. Coban Y, Akbas Y, Tuncer GO, Koker A, Koker SA. Combined immunoglobulin and plasmapheresis treatment for Febrile Infection-Related Epilepsy Syndrome (FIRES). Transfus Apher Sci. 2022;61(6):103498.
717. Gabay C, Lamacchia C, Palmer G. IL-1 pathways in inflammation and human diseases. Nat Rev Rheumatol. 2010;6(4):232–41.
718. Kenney-Jung DL, Vezzani A, Kahoud RJ, LaFrance-Corey RG, Ho ML, Muskardin TW, et al. Febrile infection-related epilepsy syndrome treated with anakinra. Ann Neurol. 2016;80(6):939–45.
719. Costagliola G, Depietri G, Michev A, Riva A, Foiadelli T, Savasta S, et al. Targeting inflammatory mediators in epilepsy: a systematic review of its molecular basis and clinical applications. Front Neurol. 2022;13:741244.

720. Yamanaka G, Ishida Y, Kanou K, Suzuki S, Watanabe Y, Takamatsu T, et al. Towards a treatment for neuroinflammation in epilepsy: Interleukin-1 receptor antagonist, Anakinra, as a potential treatment in intractable epilepsy. Int J Mol Sci. 2021;22(12):6282.
721. Dilena R, Mauri E, Aronica E, Bernasconi P, Bana C, Cappelletti C, et al. Therapeutic effect of Anakinra in the relapsing chronic phase of febrile infection-related epilepsy syndrome. Epilepsia Open. 2019;4(2):344–50.
722. Sakuma H, Horino A, Kuki I. Neurocritical care and target immunotherapy for febrile infection-related epilepsy syndrome. Biom J. 2020;43(3):205–10.
723. Maniscalco V, Abu-Rumeileh S, Mastrolia MV, Marrani E, Maccora I, Pagnini I, et al. The off-label use of anakinra in pediatric systemic autoinflammatory diseases. Ther Adv Musculoskelet Dis. 2020;12:1759720X20959575.
724. Gofshteyn JS, Wilfong A, Devinsky O, Bluvstein J, Charuta J, Ciliberto MA, et al. Cannabidiol as a potential treatment for Febrile Infection-Related Epilepsy Syndrome (FIRES) in the acute and chronic phases. J Child Neurol. 2017;32(1):35–40.
725. Duda J, Reinert JP. Cannabidiol in refractory status epilepticus: a review of clinical experiences. Seizure. 2022;103:115–9.
726. Martin-McGill KJ, Jackson CF, Bresnahan R, Levy RG, Cooper PN. Ketogenic diets for drug-resistant epilepsy. Cochrane Database Syst Rev. 2018;11(11):CD001903.
727. Li Z, Heber D. Ketogenic Diets. JAMA. 2020;323(4):386.
728. Lin KL, Lin JJ, Wang HS. Application of ketogenic diets for pediatric neurocritical care. Biom J. 2020;43(3):218–25.
729. Nabbout R, Mazzuca M, Hubert P, Peudennier S, Allaire C, Flurin V, et al. Efficacy of ketogenic diet in severe refractory status epilepticus initiating fever induced refractory epileptic encephalopathy in school age children (FIRES). Epilepsia. 2010;51(10):2033–7.
730. Peng P, Peng J, Yin F, Deng X, Chen C, He F, et al. Ketogenic diet as a treatment for super-refractory status epilepticus in febrile infection-related epilepsy syndrome. Front Neurol. 2019;10:423.
731. Kessi M, Liu F, Zhan Y, Tang Y, Wu L, Yang L, et al. Efficacy of different treatment modalities for acute and chronic phases of the febrile infection-related epilepsy syndrome: a systematic review. Seizure. 2020;79:61–8.
732. Obara K, Ono T. Ketogenic diet for a young adult patient with chronic-phase febrile infection-related epilepsy syndrome. Cureus. 2022;14(2):e22099.
733. Li WJ, Xue CL, Zhang Y, Wu LH, Chen DM, Chen F, et al. Ketogenic diet (KD) therapy in the acute phase of febrile infection-related epilepsy syndrome (FIRES): a case report. Transl Pediatr. 2021;10(9):2392–7.
734. Singh RK, Joshi SM, Potter DM, Leber SM, Carlson MD, Shellhaas RA. Cognitive outcomes in febrile infection-related epilepsy syndrome treated with the ketogenic diet. Pediatrics. 2014;134(5):e1431–5.
735. Patil SB, Roy AG, Vinayan KP. Clinical profile and treatment outcome of febrile infection-related epilepsy syndrome in South Indian children. Ann Indian Acad Neurol. 2016;19(2):188–94.
736. Gastaut H, Vigouroux M, Trevisan C, Regis H. Syndrome of hemiconvulsive hemiplegic epilepsy. Rev Neurol (Paris). 1957;97(1):37–52.
737. Vigouroux M. EEG study of hemiconvulsions followed by hemiplegia (the hemiconvulsion-hemiplegia syndrome) & its epileptic sequelae (the hemiconvulsion-hemiplegiaepilepsy syndrome). Rev Neurol (Paris). 1958;99(1):39–53.
738. Gastaut H, Poirier F, Payan H, Salamon G, Toga M, Vigouroux M. H.H.E. syndrome; hemiconvulsions, hemiplegia, epilepsy. Epilepsia. 1960;1:418–47.
739. Mori Y. Anatomopathology and pathogeny of the hemiconvulsion-hemiplegia-epilepsy syndrome. Part II. J Neurosurg Sci. 1979;23(1):1–22.
740. Kataoka K, Okuno T, Mikawa H, Hojo H. Cranial computed tomographic and electroencephalographic abnormalities in children with post-hemiconvulsive hemiplegia. Eur Neurol. 1988;28(5):279–84.

741. Assadeck H, Toudou Daouda M, Mamadou Z, Moussa Konate M, Hassane Djibo F, Douma MD. Hemiconvulsion-hemiplegia-epilepsy syndrome in Niger: a retrospective case series. J Clin Neurosci. 2019;65:121–4.
742. Goetz V, Yang DD, Abid H, Roux CJ, Levy R, Kossorotoff M, et al. Neurological features related to influenza virus in the pediatric population: a 3-year monocentric retrospective study. Eur J Pediatr. 2023;182(6):2615–24.
743. Vestergaard M, Uldall P. Hemiconvulsion-hemiplegia-epilepsy syndrome in a girl with adrenogenital syndrome. Ugeskr Laeger. 2014;176(51):V08140428.
744. Anuar MA, Lee JX, Musa H, Abd Hadi D, Majawit E, Anandakrishnan P, et al. Severe and rare neurological manifestations following COVID-19 infection in children: a Malaysian tertiary centre experience. Brain Dev. 2023;45(10):547–53.
745. Gong P, Karakas C, Morgan B. Child neurology: Hemiconvulsion-Hemiplegia-epilepsy syndrome in the setting of COVID-19 infection and multisystem inflammatory syndrome. Neurology. 2022;99(17):756–60.
746. Kumar P, Nagarajan B, Vyas S, Suthar R, Sankhyan N. Hemiconvulsion Hemiplegia Epilepsy (HHE) syndrome after perinatal hypoxic-ischemic injury. Indian J Pediatr. 2022;89(7):733.
747. Joshi A, Shrestha PS, Dangol S, Shrestha NC, Poudyal P, Shrestha A. Hemiconvulsion-Hemiplegia-Epilepsy syndrome in a girl presented with complex partial seizures. Kathmandu Univ Med J. 2017;15(59):256–60.
748. Itamura S, Okanishi T, Arai Y, Nishimura M, Baba S, Ichikawa N, et al. Three cases of Hemiconvulsion-Hemiplegia-Epilepsy syndrome with focal cortical dysplasia type IIId. Front Neurol. 2019;10:1233.
749. Miteff CI, Smith RL, Bain NL, Subramanian G, Brown JE, Kamien B. 16p13.11 microdeletion in a patient with hemiconvulsion-hemiplegia-epilepsy syndrome: a case report. J Child Neurol. 2015;30(1):83–6.
750. Myers KA, Dudley RWR, Srour M. Hemiconvulsion-Hemiplegia-Epilepsy in a girl with cobalamin C deficiency. Epileptic Disord. 2018;20(6):545–50.
751. Auvin S, Bellavoine V, Merdariu D, Delanoë C, Elmaleh-Bergés M, Gressens P, et al. Hemiconvulsion-hemiplegia-epilepsy syndrome: current understandings. Eur J Paediatr Neurol. 2012;16(5):413–21.
752. van Toorn R, Janse van Rensburg P, Solomons R, Ndondo AP, Schoeman JF. Hemiconvulsion-hemiplegia-epilepsy syndrome in South African children: insights from a retrospective case series. Eur J Paediatr Neurol. 2012;16(2):142–8.
753. Albakaye M, Belaidi H, Lahjouji F, Errguig L, Kuate C, Maiga Y, et al. Clinical aspects, neuroimaging, and electroencephalography of 35 cases of hemiconvulsion-hemiplegia syndrome. Epilepsy Behav. 2018;80:184–90.
754. Shimakawa S, Nomura S, Ogino M, Fukui M, Kashiwagi M, Tanabe T, et al. ACTH therapy on intractable epilepsy in Hemiconvulsion-Hemiplegia-Epilepsy syndrome. Brain Dev. 2015;37(7):733–7.
755. Jayakody H, Joshi C. Fatal outcome in hemiconvulsion-hemiplegia syndrome. J Child Neurol. 2014;29(3):406–11.
756. Tinuper P, Bisulli F. From nocturnal frontal lobe epilepsy to sleep-related Hypermotor epilepsy: a 35-year diagnostic challenge. Seizure. 2017;44:87–92.
757. Lugaresi E, Cirignotta F. Hypnogenic Paroxysmal Dystonia: epileptic seizure or a new syndrome? Sleep. 1981;4(2):129–38.
758. Tinuper P, Cerullo A, Cirignotta F, Cortelli P, Lugaresi E, Montagna P. Nocturnal paroxysmal dystonia with short-lasting attacks: three cases with evidence for an epileptic frontal lobe origin of seizures. Epilepsia. 1990;31(5):549–56.
759. Scheffer IE, Bhatia KP, Lopes-Cendes I, Fish DR, Marsden CD, Andermann F, et al. Autosomal dominant frontal epilepsy misdiagnosed as sleep disorder. Lancet. 1994;343(8896):515–7.
760. Scheffer IE, Bhatia KP, Lopes-Cendes I, Fish DR, Marsden CD, Andermann E, et al. Autosomal dominant nocturnal frontal lobe epilepsy. A distinctive clinical disorder. Brain. 1995;118(Pt 1):61–73.

761. Phillips HA, Scheffer IE, Berkovic SF, Hollway GE, Sutherland GR, Mulley JC. Localization of a gene for autosomal dominant nocturnal frontal lobe epilepsy to chromosome 20q 13.2. Nat Genet. 1995;10(1):117–8.
762. Berkovic SF. Epilepsy genes and the genetics of epilepsy syndromes: the promise of new therapies based on genetic knowledge. Epilepsia. 1997;38(Suppl 9):S32–6.
763. Tinuper P, Bisulli F, Cross JH, Hesdorffer D, Kahane P, Nobili L, et al. Definition and diagnostic criteria of sleep-related hypermotor epilepsy. Neurology. 2016;86(19):1834–42.
764. Menghi V, Bisulli F, Tinuper P, Nobili L. Sleep-related hypermotor epilepsy: prevalence, impact and management strategies. Nat Sci Sleep. 2018;10:317–26.
765. Vignatelli L, Bisulli F, Giovannini G, Licchetta L, Naldi I, Mostacci B, et al. Prevalence of sleep-related Hypermotor epilepsy-formerly named nocturnal frontal lobe epilepsy-in the adult population of the Emilia-Romagna region, Italy. Sleep. 2017;40(2)
766. Vignatelli L, Bisulli F, Giovannini G, Licchetta L, Naldi I, Mostacci B, et al. Prevalence of nocturnal frontal lobe epilepsy in the adult population of Bologna and Modena, Emilia-Romagna region, Italy. Sleep. 2015;38(3):479–85.
767. Licchetta L, Pippucci T, Baldassari S, Minardi R, Provini F, Mostacci B, et al. Sleep-related hypermotor epilepsy (SHE): contribution of known genes in 103 patients. Seizure. 2020;74:60–4.
768. Provini F, Plazzi G, Tinuper P, Vandi S, Lugaresi E, Montagna P. Nocturnal frontal lobe epilepsy. A clinical and polygraphic overview of 100 consecutive cases. Brain. 1999;122(Pt 6):1017–31.
769. Oldani A, Manconi M, Zucconi M, Martinelli C, Ferini-Strambi L. Topiramate treatment for nocturnal frontal lobe epilepsy. Seizure. 2006;15(8):649–52.
770. Romigi A, Marciani MG, Placidi F, Pisani LR, Izzi F, Torelli F, et al. Oxcarbazepine in nocturnal frontal-lobe epilepsy: a further interesting report. Pediatr Neurol. 2008;39(4):298. author reply
771. Raju GP, Sarco DP, Poduri A, Riviello JJ, Bergin AM, Takeoka M. Oxcarbazepine in children with nocturnal frontal-lobe epilepsy. Pediatr Neurol. 2007;37(5):345–9.
772. Milligan CJ, Li M, Gazina EV, Heron SE, Nair U, Trager C, et al. KCNT1 gain of function in 2 epilepsy phenotypes is reversed by quinidine. Ann Neurol. 2014;75(4):581–90.
773. Samarasekera SR, Berkovic SF, Scheffer IE. A case series of lacosamide as adjunctive therapy in refractory sleep-related hypermotor epilepsy (previously nocturnal frontal lobe epilepsy). J Sleep Res. 2018;27(5):e12669.
774. Gibbs SA, Proserpio P, Francione S, Mai R, Cardinale F, Sartori I, et al. Clinical features of sleep-related hypermotor epilepsy in relation to the seizure-onset zone: a review of 135 surgically treated cases. Epilepsia. 2019;60(4):707–17.
775. Hayman M, Scheffer IE, Chinvarun Y, Berlangieri SU, Berkovic SF. Autosomal dominant nocturnal frontal lobe epilepsy: demonstration of focal frontal onset and intrafamilial variation. Neurology. 1997;49(4):969–75.
776. Scheffer IE, Phillips HA, O'Brien CE, Saling MM, Wrennall JA, Wallace RH, et al. Familial partial epilepsy with variable foci: a new partial epilepsy syndrome with suggestion of linkage to chromosome 2. Ann Neurol. 1998;44(6):890–9.
777. Xiong L, Labuda M, Li DS, Hudson TJ, Desbiens R, Patry G, et al. Mapping of a gene determining familial partial epilepsy with variable foci to chromosome 22q11-q12. Am J Hum Genet. 1999;65(6):1698–710.
778. Klein KM, O'Brien TJ, Praveen K, Heron SE, Mulley JC, Foote S, et al. Familial focal epilepsy with variable foci mapped to chromosome 22q12: expansion of the phenotypic spectrum. Epilepsia. 2012;53(8):e151–5.
779. Wang XF, Zhu X, Shen DL, Guan LF, Yan Y. Clinical and epidemiological features of the five kinds of new epileptic syndrome. Zhonghua Yi Xue Za Zhi. 2006;86(47):3319–23.
780. Picard F, Baulac S, Kahane P, Hirsch E, Sebastianelli R, Thomas P, et al. Dominant partial epilepsies. A clinical, electrophysiological and genetic study of 19 European families. Brain. 2000;123(Pt 6):1247–62.

781. Dibbens LM, de Vries B, Donatello S, Heron SE, Hodgson BL, Chintawar S, et al. Mutations in DEPDC5 cause familial focal epilepsy with variable foci. Nat Genet. 2013;45(5):546–51.
782. Samanta D. DEPDC5-related epilepsy: a comprehensive review. Epilepsy Behav. 2022;130:108678.
783. Gu C, Lu X, Ma J, Pu L, Zhi X, Shu J, et al. What is the impact of a novel DEPDC5 variant on an infant with focal epilepsy: a case report. BMC Pediatr. 2022;22(1):459.
784. Zhang J, Shen Y, Yang Z, Yang F, Li Y, Yu B, et al. A splicing variation in NPRL2 causing familial focal epilepsy with variable foci: additional cases and literature review. J Hum Genet. 2022;67(2):79–85.
785. Li Y, Zhao X, Wang S, Xu K, Zhao X, Huang S, et al. A novel loss-of-function mutation in the NPRL3 gene identified in Chinese familial focal epilepsy with variable foci. Front Genet. 2021;12:766354.
786. Nascimento FA, Borlot F, Cossette P, Minassian BA, Andrade DM. Two definite cases of sudden unexpected death in epilepsy in a family with a DEPDC5 mutation. Neurol Genet. 2015;1(4):e28.
787. Ormerod JA. On epilepsy, in its relation to ear-disease. Brain. 1883;6(1):20–43.
788. Ottman R, Risch N, Hauser WA, Pedley TA, Lee JH, Barker-Cummings C, et al. Localization of a gene for partial epilepsy to chromosome 10q. Nat Genet. 1995;10(1):56–60.
789. Poza JJ, Saenz A, Martinez-Gil A, Cheron N, Cobo AM, Urtasun M, et al. Autosomal dominant lateral temporal epilepsy: clinical and genetic study of a large Basque pedigree linked to chromosome 10q. Ann Neurol. 1999;45(2):182–8.
790. Winawer MR, Ottman R, Hauser WA, Pedley TA. Autosomal dominant partial epilepsy with auditory features: defining the phenotype. Neurology. 2000;54(11):2173–6.
791. Kalachikov S, Evgrafov O, Ross B, Winawer M, Barker-Cummings C, Martinelli Boneschi F, et al. Mutations in LGI1 cause autosomal-dominant partial epilepsy with auditory features. Nat Genet. 2002;30(3):335–41.
792. Dazzo E, Fanciulli M, Serioli E, Minervini G, Pulitano P, Binelli S, et al. Heterozygous reelin mutations cause autosomal-dominant lateral temporal epilepsy. Am J Hum Genet. 2015;96(6):992–1000.
793. Michelucci R, Nobile C. Autosomal dominant epilepsy with auditory features. In: Adam MP, Feldman J, Mirzaa GM, Pagon RA, Wallace SE, Bean LJH, et al., editors. GeneReviews(®). Seattle: University of Washington, Seattle. Copyright © 1993–2024, University of Washington, Seattle. GeneReviews is a registered trademark of the University of Washington, Seattle. All rights reserved; 1993.
794. Bickford RG, Whelan JL, Klass DW, Corbin KB. Reading epilepsy: clinical and electroencephalographic studies of a new syndrome. Trans Am Neurol Assoc. 1956;(81st Meeting):100–2.
795. Lorizio A, Franciosi A. Reading epilepsy crises. Riv Patol Nerv Ment. 1981;102(6):269–83.
796. Radhakrishnan K, Silbert PL, Klass DW. Reading epilepsy. An appraisal of 20 patients diagnosed at the Mayo Clinic, Rochester, Minnesota, between 1949 and 1989, and delineation of the epileptic syndrome. Brain. 1995;118(Pt 1):75–89.
797. Koutroumanidis M, Koepp MJ, Richardson MP, Camfield C, Agathonikou A, Ried S, et al. The variants of reading epilepsy. A clinical and video-EEG study of 17 patients with reading-induced seizures. Brain. 1998;121(Pt 8):1409–27.
798. Wolf P, Mayer T, Reker M. Reading epilepsy: report of five new cases and further considerations on the pathophysiology. Seizure. 1998;7(4):271–9.
799. Puteikis K, Mameniskiene R, Wolf P. Reading epilepsy today: a scoping review and meta-analysis of reports of the last three decades. Epilepsy Behav. 2023;145:109346.
800. Gregory JK, Broomall EM. Teaching video neuroimages: reading epilepsy: a seizure in a thousand words (or less). Neurology. 2013;81(13):e100.
801. Acharya JN, Acharya VJ. Neurophysiology of Juvenile and progressive myoclonic epilepsy. J Clin Neurophysiol. 2023;40(2):100–8.

802. Sipilä JOT, Kälviäinen R. Comorbidities in patients with Unverricht-Lundborg disease (EPM1). Acta Neurol Scand. 2022;146(5):690–3.
803. Kälviäinen R, Khyuppenen J, Koskenkorva P, Eriksson K, Vanninen R, Mervaala E. Clinical picture of EPM1-Unverricht-Lundborg disease. Epilepsia. 2008;49(4):549–56.
804. Van Bogaert L. On Unverricht-Lundborg progressive myoclonus epilepsy. Monatsschr Psychiatr Neurol. 1949;118(3–4):170–91.
805. Caron S, Michel P. Unverricht's syndrome (familial and hereditary disease of the nervous system). Laval Med. 1950;15(10):1354–64.
806. Wohlfart G, Hook O. A clinical analysis of myoclonus epilepsy (Unverricht-Lundborg), myoclonic cerebellar dyssynergy (Hunt) and hepatolenticular degeneration (Wilson). Acta Psychiatr Neurol Scand. 1951;26(2):219–45.
807. Kelly RE, Laurence DR. Treatment of progressive myoclonic epilepsy with mephenesin. Br Med J. 1955;1(4911):456–8.
808. Anraku S. Clinical and pathological study on myoclonus epilepsy (Unverricht-Lundborg type). Shinkei Kenkyu No Shimpo. 1967;11(4):717–21.
809. Iatsuk SL, Samoĭlov VI. The differential diagnosis of Kozhevnikov's epilepsy. Zh Nevrol Psikhiatr Im S S Korsakova. 1993;93(1):22–5.
810. Franceschetti S, Michelucci R, Canafoglia L, Striano P, Gambardella A, Magaudda A, et al. Progressive myoclonic epilepsies: definitive and still undetermined causes. Neurology. 2014;82(5):405–11.
811. Sipilä JOT, Hyppönen J, Kytö V, Kälviäinen R. Unverricht-Lundborg disease (EPM1) in Finland: a nationwide population-based study. Neurology. 2020;95(23):e3117–e23.
812. Muccioli L, Farolfi A, Pondrelli F, Matteo E, Ferri L, Licchetta L, et al. FDG-PET findings and alcohol-responsive myoclonus in a patient with Unverricht-Lundborg disease. Epilepsy Behav Rep. 2022;19:100551.
813. Tandon R, Pradhan S. Autistic features in Unverricht-Lundborg disease. Epilepsy Behav Rep. 2019;12:100323.
814. Van Bogaert L. Unverricht-Lundborg progressive epilepsy-myoclonus and the problem of progressive encephalopathies combining epilepsy and myoclonia. Rev Neurol (Paris). 1968;119(1):47–57.
815. Hypponen J, Aikia M, Joensuu T, Julkunen P, Danner N, Koskenkorva P, et al. Refining the phenotype of Unverricht-Lundborg disease (EPM1): a population-wide Finnish study. Neurology. 2015;84(15):1529–36.
816. Bosak M, Sulek A, Lukasik M, Zak A, Slowik A, Lasek-Bal A. Genetic testing and the phenotype of Polish patients with Unverricht-Lundborg disease (EPM1) - a cohort study. Epilepsy Behav. 2020;112:107439.
817. Lasek-Bal A, Lukasik M, Zak A, Sulek A, Bosak M. Unverricht-Lundborg disease: clinical course and seizure management based on the experience of polish centers. Seizure. 2019;69:87–91.
818. Äikiä M, Hyppönen J, Mervaala E, Kälviäinen R. Cognitive functioning in progressive myoclonus epilepsy type 1 (Unverricht-Lundborg disease, EPM1). Epilepsy Behav. 2021;122:108157.
819. Gargouri-Berrechid A, Nasri A, Kacem I, Sidhom Y, Abdelkefi I, Hizem Y, et al. Long-term evolution of EEG in Unverricht-Lundborg disease. Neurophysiol Clin. 2016;46(2):119–24.
820. Hosny H, El Tamawy M, Gouider R, Lesca G, Abdel Naseer M, Kishk N, et al. Clinical and molecular characterization of Unverricht-Lundborg disease among Egyptian patients. Epilepsy Res. 2021;176:106746.
821. Silvennoinen K, Säisänen L, Hyppönen J, Rissanen SM, Karjalainen PA, D'Ambrosio S, et al. Short- and long-interval intracortical inhibition in EPM1 is related to genotype. Epilepsia. 2023;64(1):208–17.
822. Turnbull J, Tiberia E, Striano P, Genton P, Carpenter S, Ackerley CA, et al. Lafora disease. Epileptic Disord. 2016;18(S2):38–62.

823. Nitschke F, Ahonen SJ, Nitschke S, Mitra S, Minassian BA. Lafora disease - from pathogenesis to treatment strategies. Nat Rev Neurol. 2018;14(10):606–17.
824. d'Orsi G, Lalla A, Palumbo O, Di Claudio MT, Valenzano A, Sabetta A, et al. The presenting symptoms of Lafora disease: An electroclinical and genetic study in five Apulian (Southern Italy) families. Seizure. 2020;83:145–53.
825. Lafora GR, Glueck B. Beitrag zur Histopathologie der myoklonischen Epilepsie. Zeitschrift für die gesamte Neurologie und Psychiatrie. 1911;6(1):1–14.
826. Gentry MS, Afawi Z, Armstrong DD, Delgado-Escueta A, Goldberg YP, Grossman TR, et al. The 5th international Lafora epilepsy workshop: basic science elucidating therapeutic options and preparing for therapies in the clinic. Epilepsy Behav. 2020;103(Pt A):106839.
827. Turnbull J, Girard JM, Lohi H, Chan EM, Wang P, Tiberia E, et al. Early-onset Lafora body disease. Brain. 2012;135(Pt 9):2684–98.
828. Pondrelli F, Muccioli L, Licchetta L, Mostacci B, Zenesini C, Tinuper P, et al. Natural history of Lafora disease: a prognostic systematic review and individual participant data meta-analysis. Orphanet J Rare Dis. 2021;16(1):362.
829. Nomani AZ, Rajput HM, Nomani H. Lafora body epilepsy: a challenging diagnosis. J Coll Physicians Surg Pak. 2022;32(8):S133–S5.
830. d'Orsi G, Di Claudio MT, Palumbo O, Carella M. Electro-clinical features and management of the late stage of Lafora disease. Front Neurol. 2022;13:969297.
831. Heitkotter H, Linderman RE, Cava JA, Woertz EN, Mastey RR, Summerfelt P, et al. Retinal alterations in patients with Lafora disease. Am J Ophthalmol Case Rep. 2021;23:101146.
832. Orsini A, Ferrari D, Riva A, Santangelo A, Macri A, Freri E, et al. Ocular phenotype and electroretinogram abnormalities in Lafora disease and correlation with disease stage. J Neurol. 2022;269(7):3597–604.
833. Gómez-Abad C, Gómez-Garre P, Gutiérrez-Delicado E, Saygi S, Michelucci R, Tassinari CA, et al. Lafora disease due to EPM2B mutations: a clinical and genetic study. Neurology. 2005;64(6):982–6.
834. Franceschetti S, Gambardella A, Canafoglia L, Striano P, Lohi H, Gennaro E, et al. Clinical and genetic findings in 26 Italian patients with Lafora disease. Epilepsia. 2006;47(3):640–3.
835. Baykan B, Striano P, Gianotti S, Bebek N, Gennaro E, Gurses C, Zara F. Late-onset and slow-progressing Lafora disease in four siblings with EPM2B mutation. Epilepsia. 2005;46(10):1695–7.
836. Ferlazzo E, Canafoglia L, Michelucci R, Gambardella A, Gennaro E, Pasini E, et al. Mild Lafora disease: clinical, neurophysiologic, and genetic findings. Epilepsia. 2014;55(12):e129–33.
837. Oksel F, Tekgül H, Genç S, Ozyürek R, Akalin T, Tütütüncüoğlu S. A case of Lafora's disease associated with cardiac arrhythmia. J Child Neurol. 1999;14(11):745–6.
838. Singh S, Ganesh S. Lafora progressive myoclonus epilepsy: a meta-analysis of reported mutations in the first decade following the discovery of the EPM2A and NHLRC1 genes. Hum Mutat. 2009;30(5):715–23.
839. Riva A, Orsini A, Scala M, Taramasso V, Canafoglia L, d'Orsi G, et al. Italian cohort of Lafora disease: clinical features, disease evolution, and genotype-phenotype correlations. J Neurol Sci. 2021;424:117409.
840. Villanueva V, Alvarez-Linera J, Gomez-Garre P, Gutierrez J, Serratosa JM. MRI volumetry and proton MR spectroscopy of the brain in Lafora disease. Epilepsia. 2006;47(4):788–92.
841. Muccioli L, Farolfi A, Pondrelli F, d'Orsi G, Michelucci R, Freri E, et al. FDG-PET assessment and metabolic patterns in Lafora disease. Eur J Nucl Med Mol Imaging. 2020;47(6):1576–84.
842. Cantz M, Gehler J, Spranger J. Mucolipidosis I: increased sialic acid content and deficiency of an alpha-N-acetylneuraminidase in cultured fibroblasts. Biochem Biophys Res Commun. 1977;74(2):732–8.
843. Lowden JA, O'Brien JS. Sialidosis: a review of human neuraminidase deficiency. Am J Hum Genet. 1979;31(1):1–18.
844. Winter RM, Swallow DM, Baraitser M, Purkiss P. Sialidosis type 2 (acid neuraminidase deficiency): clinical and biochemical features of a further case. Clin Genet. 1980;18(3):203–10.

845. Lai SC, Chen RS, Wu Chou YH, Chang HC, Kao LY, Huang YZ, et al. A longitudinal study of Taiwanese sialidosis type 1: an insight into the concept of cherry-red spot myoclonus syndrome. Eur J Neurol. 2009;16(8):912–9.
846. Nita DA, Mole SE, Minassian BA. Neuronal ceroid lipofuscinoses. Epileptic Disord. 2016;18(S2):73–88.
847. Girard JM, Turnbull J, Ramachandran N, Minassian BA. Progressive myoclonus epilepsy. Handb Clin Neurol. 2013;113:1731–6.
848. Xiong H, Bao XH, Zhang YH, Xu YN, Qin J, Shi HP, et al. Niemann-Pick disease type C: analysis of 7 patients. World J Pediatr. 2012;8(1):61–6.
849. Andermann E, Andermann F, Carpenter S, Wolfe LS, Nelson R, Patry G, et al. Action myoclonus-renal failure syndrome: a previously unrecognized neurological disorder unmasked by advances in nephrology. Adv Neurol. 1986;43:87–103.
850. Hopfner F, Schormair B, Knauf F, Berthele A, Tölle TR, Baron R, et al. Novel SCARB2 mutation in action myoclonus-renal failure syndrome and evaluation of SCARB2 mutations in isolated AMRF features. BMC Neurol. 2011;11:134.
851. Corbett MA, Schwake M, Bahlo M, Dibbens LM, Lin M, Gandolfo LC, et al. A mutation in the Golgi Qb-SNARE gene GOSR2 causes progressive myoclonus epilepsy with early ataxia. Am J Hum Genet. 2011;88(5):657–63.
852. Finsterer J, Zarrouk-Mahjoub S. Management of epilepsy in MERRF syndrome. Seizure. 2017;50:166–70.
853. Fukuhara N. Clinicopathological features of MERRF. Muscle Nerve Suppl. 1995;3:S90–4.
854. Sparaco M, Bonilla E, DiMauro S, Powers JM. Neuropathology of mitochondrial encephalomyopathies due to mitochondrial DNA defects. J Neuropathol Exp Neurol. 1993;52(1):1–10.
855. Shemesh E, Deroma L, Bembi B, Deegan P, Hollak C, Weinreb NJ, et al. Enzyme replacement and substrate reduction therapy for Gaucher disease. Cochrane Database Syst Rev. 2015;2015(3):CD010324.
856. Tezuka Y, Fukuda M, Watanabe S, Nakano T, Okamoto K, Kuzume K, et al. Histological characterization of visceral changes in a patient with type 2 Gaucher disease treated with enzyme replacement therapy. Blood Cells Mol Dis. 2018;68:194–9.
857. Li M. Enzyme replacement therapy: a review and its role in treating lysosomal storage diseases. Pediatr Ann. 2018;47(5):e191–e7.
858. Rahman S. Mitochondrial disease and epilepsy. Dev Med Child Neurol. 2012;54(5):397–406.
859. Jang YH, Lim KI. Recent advances in mitochondria-targeted gene delivery. Molecules. 2018;23(9):2316.
860. Michelucci R, Pasini E, Riguzzi P, Andermann E, Kalviainen R, Genton P. Myoclonus and seizures in progressive myoclonus epilepsies: pharmacology and therapeutic trials. Epileptic Disord. 2016;18(S2):145–53.
861. Finsterer J. Mitochondrion-toxic drugs given to patients with mitochondrial psychoses. Behav Brain Funct. 2012;8:45.
862. Iivanainen M, Himberg JJ. Valproate and clonazepam in the treatment of severe progressive myoclonus epilepsy. Arch Neurol. 1982;39(4):236–8.
863. Assenza G, Nocerino C, Tombini M, Di Gennaro G, D'Aniello A, Verrotti A, et al. Perampanel improves cortical myoclonus and disability in progressive myoclonic epilepsies: a case series and a systematic review of the literature. Front Neurol. 2021;12:630366.
864. Saito K, Oi K, Inaba A, Kobayashi M, Ikeda A, Wada Y. A case of the successful treatment of severe myoclonus with Lance-Adams syndrome by add-on perampanel showing long term effects. Rinsho Shinkeigaku. 2021;61(1):18–23.
865. Oi Y, Kobayashi K, Hitomi T, Matsumoto R, Ikeda A, Takahashi R. Low-dose perampanel improved cortical myoclonus and basophobia in a patient with Unverricht-Lundborg disease: a case report. Rinsho Shinkeigaku. 2018;58(10):622–5.
866. Ben-Menachem E, Baulac M, Hong SB, Cleveland JM, Reichel C, Schulz AL, et al. Safety, tolerability, and efficacy of brivaracetam as adjunctive therapy in patients with focal sei-

zures, generalized onset seizures, or Unverricht-Lundborg disease: An open-label, long-term follow-up trial. Epilepsy Res. 2021;170:106526.
867. Papacostas S, Kkolou E, Papathanasiou E. Levetiracetam in three cases of progressive myoclonus epilepsy. Pharm World Sci. 2007;29(3):164–6.
868. Roivainen R, Karvonen MK, Puumala T. Seizure control in Unverricht-Lundborg disease: a single-centre study. Epileptic Disord. 2014;16(2):191–5.
869. Aykutlu E, Baykan B, Gurses C, Bebek N, Buyukbabani N, Gokyigit A. Add-on therapy with topiramate in progressive myoclonic epilepsy. Epilepsy Behav. 2005;6(2):260–3.
870. Italiano D, Pezzella M, Coppola A, Magaudda A, Ferlazzo E, Bramanti P, et al. A pilot open-label trial of zonisamide in Unverricht-Lundborg disease. Mov Disord. 2011;26(2):341–3.
871. Ng YT, Collins SD. Clobazam. Neurotherapeutics. 2007;4(1):138–44.
872. Genton P. When antiepileptic drugs aggravate epilepsy. Brain Dev. 2000;22(2):75–80.
873. Cardinali S, Canafoglia L, Bertoli S, Franceschetti S, Lanzi G, Tagliabue A, et al. A pilot study of a ketogenic diet in patients with Lafora body disease. Epilepsy Res. 2006;69(2):129–34.
874. Mikati MA, Tabbara F. Managing Lafora body disease with vagal nerve stimulation. Epileptic Disord. 2017;19(1):82–6.
875. Mostacci B, Bisulli F, Muccioli L, Minardi I, Bandini M, Licchetta L, et al. Super refractory status epilepticus in Lafora disease interrupted by vagus nerve stimulation: a case report. Brain Stimul. 2019;12(6):1605–7.
876. di Giacopo A, Baumann CR, Kurthen M, Capecchi F, Surucu O, Imbach LL. Selective deep brain stimulation in the substantia nigra reduces myoclonus in progressive myoclonic epilepsy: a novel observation and short review of the literature. Epileptic Disord. 2019;21(3):283–8.
877. Poupart F. Histoire de l'Académie Royale des Sciences. DuPont; 1705.
878. Calmeil LF. Faculté de md. De l'épilepsie étudiée sous le rapport de son siège et de son influence sur la production de l'aliénation mentale. Paris: Imp. Didot le Jeune; 1824.
879. Esquirol E. Des maladies mentales, considerées sous les rapports médical, hygiénique et médico-légal. Baillière; 1838.
880. Sauer H. Über gehäufte kleine Anfälle bei Kindern (Pyknolepsie). Eur Neurol. 1916;40:276–300.
881. Brigo F, Trinka E, Lattanzi S, Bragazzi NL, Nardone R, Martini M. A brief history of typical absence seizures - Petit mal revisited. Epilepsy Behav. 2018;80:346–53.
882. Matricardi S, Verrotti A, Chiarelli F, Cerminara C, Curatolo P. Current advances in childhood absence epilepsy. Pediatr Neurol. 2014;50(3):205–12.
883. Marini C, Harkin LA, Wallace RH, Mulley JC, Scheffer IE, Berkovic SF. Childhood absence epilepsy and febrile seizures: a family with a GABA(A) receptor mutation. Brain. 2003;126(Pt 1):230–40.
884. Chen Y, Lu J, Pan H, Zhang Y, Wu H, Xu K, et al. Association between genetic variation of CACNA1H and childhood absence epilepsy. Ann Neurol. 2003;54(2):239–43.
885. Everett KV, Chioza B, Aicardi J, Aschauer H, Brouwer O, Callenbach P, et al. Linkage and association analysis of CACNG3 in childhood absence epilepsy. Eur J Hum Genet. 2007;15(4):463–72.
886. Everett K, Chioza B, Aicardi J, Aschauer H, Brouwer O, Callenbach P, et al. Linkage and mutational analysis of CLCN2 in childhood absence epilepsy. Epilepsy Res. 2007;75(2):145–53.
887. Maljevic S, Krampfl K, Cobilanschi J, Tilgen N, Beyer S, Weber YG, et al. A mutation in the GABA(A) receptor alpha(1)-subunit is associated with absence epilepsy. Ann Neurol. 2006;59(6):983–7.
888. Hernandez CC, Gurba KN, Hu N, Macdonald RL. The GABRA6 mutation, R46W, associated with childhood absence epilepsy, alters 6beta22 and 6beta2 GABA(A) receptor channel gating and expression. J Physiol. 2011;589(Pt 23):5857–78.
889. Gurba KN, Hernandez CC, Hu N, Macdonald RL. GABRB3 mutation, G32R, associated with childhood absence epilepsy alters $\alpha1\beta3\gamma2L$ γ-aminobutyric acid type A (GABAA) receptor expression and channel gating. J Biol Chem. 2012;287(15):12083–97.

890. Kananura C, Haug K, Sander T, Runge U, Gu W, Hallmann K, et al. A splice-site mutation in GABRG2 associated with childhood absence epilepsy and febrile convulsions. Arch Neurol. 2002;59(7):1137–41.
891. Xie H, Su W, Pei J, Zhang Y, Gao K, Li J, et al. De novo SCN1A, SCN8A, and CLCN2 mutations in childhood absence epilepsy. Epilepsy Res. 2019;154:55–61.
892. Jiang Y, Zhang Y, Zhang P, Sang T, Zhang F, Ji T, et al. NIPA2 located in 15q11.2 is mutated in patients with childhood absence epilepsy. Hum Genet. 2012;131(7):1217–24.
893. Hughes JR. Absence seizures: a review of recent reports with new concepts. Epilepsy Behav. 2009;15(4):404–12.
894. Kessler SK, Shinnar S, Cnaan A, Dlugos D, Conry J, Hirtz DG, et al. Pretreatment seizure semiology in childhood absence epilepsy. Neurology. 2017;89(7):673–9.
895. Galli J, Micheletti S, Malerba L, Fazzi E, Giordano L. Childhood absence epilepsy evolving to eyelid Myoclonia with absence epilepsy. Seizure. 2018;61:1–3.
896. Caplan R, Siddarth P, Stahl L, Lanphier E, Vona P, Gurbani S, et al. Childhood absence epilepsy: behavioral, cognitive, and linguistic comorbidities. Epilepsia. 2008;49(11):1838–46.
897. Sadleir LG, Farrell K, Smith S, Connolly MB, Scheffer IE. Electroclinical features of absence seizures in childhood absence epilepsy. Neurology. 2006;67(3):413–8.
898. Sadleir LG, Scheffer IE, Smith S, Carstensen B, Farrell K, Connolly MB. EEG features of absence seizures in idiopathic generalized epilepsy: impact of syndrome, age, and state. Epilepsia. 2009;50(6):1572–8.
899. Koutroumanidis M, Tsiptsios D, Kokkinos V, Kostopoulos GK. Focal and generalized EEG paroxysms in childhood absence epilepsy: topographic associations and distinctive behaviors during the first cycle of non-REM sleep. Epilepsia. 2012;53(5):840–9.
900. Gaillard WD, Chiron C, Cross JH, Harvey AS, Kuzniecky R, Hertz-Pannier L, et al. Guidelines for imaging infants and children with recent-onset epilepsy. Epilepsia. 2009;50(9):2147–53.
901. Asadi-Pooya AA, Farazdaghi M. Childhood vs. juvenile absence epilepsy: how to make a diagnosis. Seizure. 2022;102:125–8.
902. Glauser TA, Cnaan A, Shinnar S, Hirtz DG, Dlugos D, Masur D, et al. Ethosuximide, valproic acid, and lamotrigine in childhood absence epilepsy: initial monotherapy outcomes at 12 months. Epilepsia. 2013;54(1):141–55.
903. Glauser TA, Cnaan A, Shinnar S, Hirtz DG, Dlugos D, Masur D, et al. Ethosuximide, valproic acid, and lamotrigine in childhood absence epilepsy. N Engl J Med. 2010;362(9):790–9.
904. Kim HR, Kim GH, Eun SH, Eun BL, Byeon JH. Therapeutic outcomes and prognostic factors in childhood absence epilepsy. J Clin Neurol. 2016;12(2):160–5.
905. Cnaan A, Shinnar S, Arya R, Adamson PC, Clark PO, Dlugos D, et al. Second monotherapy in childhood absence epilepsy. Neurology. 2017;88(2):182–90.
906. Kessler SK, McGinnis E. A practical guide to treatment of childhood absence epilepsy. Paediatr Drugs. 2019;21(1):15–24.
907. Richens A. Ethosuximide and valproate. In: Duncan JS, Panayiotopoulos CP, editors. Typical absences and related epileptic syndromes. London: ChurchillCommunications Europe; 1995. p. 241–52.
908. Davis R, Peters DH, McTavish D. Valproic acid. A reappraisal of its pharmacological properties and clinical efficacy in epilepsy. Drugs. 1994;47(2):332–72.
909. Epilim. Product monograph. Surrey: Sanofi Winthrop Ltd.; 1995.
910. Chappell KA, Markowitz JS, Jackson CW. Is valproate pharmacotherapy associated with polycystic ovaries? Ann Pharmacother. 1999;33(11):1211–6.
911. Acharya S, Bussel JB. Hematologic toxicity of sodium valproate. J Pediatr Hematol Oncol. 2000;22(1):62–5.
912. Frank LM, Enlow T, Holmes GL, Manasco P, Concannon S, Chen C, et al. Lamictal (lamotrigine) monotherapy for typical absence seizures in children. Epilepsia. 1999;40(7):973–9.

913. Coppola G, Licciardi F, Sciscio N, Russo F, Carotenuto M, Pascotto A. Lamotrigine as first-line drug in childhood absence epilepsy: a clinical and neurophysiological study. Brain Dev. 2004;26(1):26–9.
914. Guberman AH, Besag FM, Brodie MJ, Dooley JM, Duchowny MS, Pellock JM, et al. Lamotrigine-associated rash: risk/benefit considerations in adults and children. Epilepsia. 1999;40(7):985–91.
915. E. DF. Valproate-toxicity. In: Levy RH, Dreifuss FE, Mattson RH, Meldrum BS, Penry JK, editors. Antiepileptic drugs. 3rd ed. New York: Raven; 1989. p. 643–51.
916. Trinka E, Alsaadi T, Goji H, Maehara T, Takahashi S, Jacobs J, et al. Perampanel for the treatment of people with idiopathic generalized epilepsy in clinical practice. Epilepsia. 2023;64(8):2094–107.
917. Operto FF, Orsini A, Sica G, Scuoppo C, Padovano C, Vivenzio V, et al. Perampanel and childhood absence epilepsy: a real life experience. Front Neurol. 2022;13:952900.
918. Fattore C, Boniver C, Capovilla G, Cerminara C, Citterio A, Coppola G, et al. A multicenter, randomized, placebo-controlled trial of levetiracetam in children and adolescents with newly diagnosed absence epilepsy. Epilepsia. 2011;52(4):802–9.
919. Nolan D, Lester SG, Rau SM, Shellhaas RA. Clinical use and efficacy of Levetiracetam for absence epilepsies. J Child Neurol. 2019;34(2):94–8.
920. Auvin S, Chhun S, Berquin P, Ponchel E, Delanoe C, Chiron C. Aggravation of absence seizure related to levetiracetam. Eur J Paediatr Neurol. 2011;15(6):508–11.
921. Cross JH. Topiramate monotherapy for childhood absence seizures: an open label pilot study. Seizure. 2002;11(6):406–10.
922. Grosso S, Galimberti D, Vezzosi P, Farnetani M, Di Bartolo RM, Bazzotti S, et al. Childhood absence epilepsy: evolution and prognostic factors. Epilepsia. 2005;46(11):1796–801.
923. Amianto F, Davico C, Bertino F, Bartolini L, Vittorini R, Vacchetti M, et al. Clinical and instrumental follow-up of childhood absence epilepsy (CAE): exploration of prognostic factors. Children (Basel). 2022;9(10):1452.
924. Wirrell EC, Camfield CS, Camfield PR, Gordon KE, Dooley JM. Long-term prognosis of typical childhood absence epilepsy: remission or progression to juvenile myoclonic epilepsy. Neurology. 1996;47(4):912–8.
925. Verrotti A, Matricardi S, Rinaldi VE, Prezioso G, Coppola G. Neuropsychological impairment in childhood absence epilepsy: review of the literature. J Neurol Sci. 2015;359(1–2):59–66.
926. Tovia E, Goldberg-Stern H, Shahar E, Kramer U. Outcome of children with juvenile absence epilepsy. J Child Neurol. 2006;21(9):766–8.
927. Drury I, Dreifuss FE. Pyknoleptic petit mal. Acta Neurol Scand. 1985;72(4):353–62.
928. Gesche J, Christensen J, Hjalgrim H, Rubboli G, Beier CP. Epidemiology and outcome of idiopathic generalized epilepsy in adults. Eur J Neurol. 2020;27(4):676–84.
929. Trinka E, Baumgartner S, Unterberger I, Unterrainer J, Luef G, Haberlandt E, et al. Long-term prognosis for childhood and juvenile absence epilepsy. J Neurol. 2004;251(10):1235–41.
930. Marini C, Scheffer IE, Crossland KM, Grinton BE, Phillips FL, McMahon JM, et al. Genetic architecture of idiopathic generalized epilepsy: clinical genetic analysis of 55 multiplex families. Epilepsia. 2004;45(5):467–78.
931. Berkovic SF, Howell RA, Hay DA, Hopper JL. Epilepsies in twins: genetics of the major epilepsy syndromes. Ann Neurol. 1998;43(4):435–45.
932. Concordance of clinical forms of epilepsy in families with several affected members. Italian League Against Epilepsy Genetic Collaborative Group. Epilepsia. 1993;34(5):819–26.
933. Beck-Mannagetta G, Janz D. Syndrome-related genetics in generalized epilepsy. Epilepsy Res Suppl. 1991;4:105–11.
934. Janz D, Beck-Mannagetta G, Sander T. Do idiopathic generalized epilepsies share a common susceptibility gene? Neurology. 1992;42(4 Suppl 5):48–55.
935. Yalçın O. Genes and molecular mechanisms involved in the epileptogenesis of idiopathic absence epilepsies. Seizure. 2012;21(2):79–86.

936. Dahawi M, Elmagzoub MS, Baldassari S, Achaz G, Elmugadam FA, et al. Involvement of ADGRV1 gene in familial forms of genetic generalized epilepsy. Front Neurol. 2021;12:738272.
937. Panayiotopoulos CP, Obeid T, Waheed G. Differentiation of typical absence seizures in epileptic syndromes. A video EEG study of 224 seizures in 20 patients. Brain. 1989;112(Pt 4):1039–56.
938. Agathonikou A, Panayiotopoulos CP, Giannakodimos S, Koutroumanidis M. Typical absence status in adults: diagnostic and syndromic considerations. Epilepsia. 1998;39(12):1265–76.
939. Velizarova R, Crespel A, Genton P, Serafini A, Gelisse P. Zonisamide for refractory juvenile absence epilepsy. Epilepsy Res. 2014;108(7):1263–6.
940. Danhofer P, Brazdil M, Oslejskova H, Kuba R. Long-term seizure outcome in patients with juvenile absence epilepsy; a retrospective study in a tertiary referral center. Seizure. 2014;23(6):443–7.
941. Boesen MS, Borresen ML, Christensen SK, Klein-Petersen AW, El Mahdaoui S, Sagar MV, et al. School performance and psychiatric comorbidity in juvenile absence epilepsy and juvenile myoclonic epilepsy: a Danish population-based cohort study. J Neurol. 2022;269(9):4997–5007.
942. Berkovic SF, Andermann F, Guberman A, Hipola D, Bladin PF. Valproate prevents the recurrence of absence status. Neurology. 1989;39(10):1294–7.
943. Meador K. Teratogenicity and Antiseizure medications. Epilepsy Curr. 2020;20(6_suppl):15S-7S.
944. Christensen J, Gronborg TK, Sorensen MJ, Schendel D, Parner ET, Pedersen LH, et al. Prenatal valproate exposure and risk of autism spectrum disorders and childhood autism. JAMA. 2013;309(16):1696–703.
945. Buoni S, Grosso S, Fois A. Lamotrigine in typical absence epilepsy. Brain Dev. 1999;21(5):303–6.
946. Gericke CA, Picard F, de Saint-Martin A, Strumia S, Marescaux C, Hirsch E. Efficacy of lamotrigine in idiopathic generalized epilepsy syndromes: a video-EEG-controlled, open study. Epileptic Disord. 1999;1(3):159–65.
947. Goren MZ, Onat F. Ethosuximide: from bench to bedside. CNS Drug Rev. 2007;13(2):224–39.
948. Callaghan N, O'Hare J, O'Driscoll D, O'Neill B, Daly M. Comparative study of ethosuximide and sodium valproate in the treatment of typical absence seizures (petit mal). Dev Med Child Neurol. 1982;24(6):830–6.
949. Sato S, White BG, Penry JK, Dreifuss FE, Sackellares JC, Kupferberg HJ. Valproic acid versus ethosuximide in the treatment of absence seizures. Neurology. 1982;32(2):157–63.
950. Villanueva V, Montoya J, Castillo A, Mauri-Llerda J, Giner P, López-González FJ, et al. Perampanel in routine clinical use in idiopathic generalized epilepsy: The 12-month GENERAL study. Epilepsia. 2018;59(9):1740–52.
951. Shangguan Y, Liao H, Wang X. Clonazepam in the treatment of status epilepticus. Expert Rev Neurother. 2015;15(7):733–40.
952. Holtkamp M, Janz D, Kirschbaum A, Kowski AB, Vorderwulbecke BJ. Absence epilepsy beyond adolescence: an outcome analysis after 45 years of follow-up. J Neurol Neurosurg Psychiatry. 2018;89(6):603–10.
953. Seneviratne U, Cook M, D'Souza W. The prognosis of idiopathic generalized epilepsy. Epilepsia. 2012;53(12):2079–90.
954. Janz D, Christian W. Impulsiv-Petit mal. Dtsch Z Nervenheilkd. 1957;176(3):346–86.
955. Appleton R, Beirne M, Acomb B. Photosensitivity in juvenile myoclonic epilepsy. Seizure. 2000;9(2):108–11.
956. Herpin T. Des accès incomplets d'épilepsie. Paris: J. B. Baillière et fils; 1867.
957. Castells C, Mendilaharsu C. La epilepsia mioclonica bilateral consciente. Acta Neurol Latinoam. 1958;4:23–48.

958. Lund M, Reintoft H, Simonsen N. En kontrolleret social og psychologisk undersogelse of patienter med juvenil myoklon epilepsi[A controlled social and psychological investigation of patients with juvenile myoclonic epilepsy]. Ugeskr Laeger. 1975;137(41):2415–8.
959. Hauser WA. The prevalence and incidence of convulsive disorders in children. Epilepsia. 1994;35(Suppl 2):S1–6.
960. Syvertsen M, Hellum MK, Hansen G, Edland A, Nakken KO, Selmer KK, et al. Prevalence of juvenile myoclonic epilepsy in people <30 years of age-A population-based study in Norway. Epilepsia. 2017;58(1):105–12.
961. Murthy JM, Rao CM, Meena AK. Clinical observations of juvenile myoclonic epilepsy in 131 patients: a study in South India. Seizure. 1998;7(1):43–7.
962. Jain S, Padma MV, Puri A, Maheshwari MC. Juvenile myoclonic epilepsy: disease expression among Indian families. Acta Neurol Scand. 1998;97(1):1–7.
963. Delgado-Escueta AV, Koeleman BP, Bailey JN, Medina MT, Duron RM. The quest for juvenile myoclonic epilepsy genes. Epilepsy Behav. 2013;28(Suppl 1):S52–7.
964. Usui N, Kotagal P, Matsumoto R, Kellinghaus C, Luders HO. Focal semiologic and electroencephalographic features in patients with juvenile myoclonic epilepsy. Epilepsia. 2005;46(10):1668–76.
965. Larch J, Unterberger I, Bauer G, Reichsoellner J, Kuchukhidze G, Trinka E. Myoclonic status epilepticus in juvenile myoclonic epilepsy. Epileptic Disord. 2009;11(4):309–14.
966. Pietrafusa N, La Neve A, de Palma L, Boero G, Luisi C, Vigevano F, et al. Juvenile myoclonic epilepsy: long-term prognosis and risk factors. Brain Dev. 2021;43(6):688–97.
967. Delgado-Escueta AV, Enrile-Bacsal F. Juvenile myoclonic epilepsy of Janz. Neurology. 1984;34(3):285–94.
968. Panayiotopoulos CP, Obeid T, Tahan AR. Juvenile myoclonic epilepsy: a 5-year prospective study. Epilepsia. 1994;35(2):285–96.
969. Panayiotopoulos CP, Obeid T, Waheed G. Absences in juvenile myoclonic epilepsy: a clinical and video-electroencephalographic study. Ann Neurol. 1989;25(4):391–7.
970. Holtkamp M, Senf P, Kirschbaum A, Janz D. Psychosocial long-term outcome in juvenile myoclonic epilepsy. Epilepsia. 2014;55(11):1732–8.
971. Aliberti V, Grunewald RA, Panayiotopoulos CP, Chroni E. Focal electroencephalographic abnormalities in juvenile myoclonic epilepsy. Epilepsia. 1994;35(2):297–301.
972. Mehndiratta MM, Aggarwal P. Clinical expression and EEG features of patients with juvenile myoclonic epilepsy (JME) from North India. Seizure. 2002;11(7):431–6.
973. (UK) NGA. Effectiveness of antiseizure therapies in the treatment of tonic or atonic seizures/drop attacks: epilepsies in children, young people and adults: evidence review. London: National Institute for Health and Care Excellence (NICE); 2022.
974. Toth M. The epsilon theory: a novel synthesis of the underlying molecular and electrophysiological mechanisms of primary generalized epilepsy and the possible mechanism of action of valproate. Med Hypotheses. 2005;64(2):267–72.
975. Bourgeois B, Beaumanoir A, Blajev B, de la Cruz N, Despland PA, Egli M, et al. Monotherapy with valproate in primary generalized epilepsies. Epilepsia. 1987;28(Suppl 2):S8–11.
976. Atakli D, Sozuer D, Atay T, Baybas S, Arpaci B. Misdiagnosis and treatment in juvenile myoclonic epilepsy. Seizure. 1998;7(1):63–6.
977. Calleja S, Salas-Puig J, Ribacoba R, Lahoz CH. Evolution of juvenile myoclonic epilepsy treated from the outset with sodium valproate. Seizure. 2001;10(6):424–7.
978. Marson AG, Al-Kharusi AM, Alwaidh M, Appleton R, Baker GA, Chadwick DW, et al. The SANAD study of effectiveness of valproate, lamotrigine, or topiramate for generalised and unclassifiable epilepsy: an unblinded randomised controlled trial. Lancet. 2007;369(9566):1016–26.
979. Wang SJ, Huang CC, Hsu KS, Tsai JJ, Gean PW. Inhibition of N-type calcium currents by lamotrigine in rat amygdalar neurones. Neuroreport. 1996;7(18):3037–40.

980. Machado RA, Garcia VF, Astencio AG, Cuartas VB. Efficacy and tolerability of lamotrigine in juvenile myoclonic epilepsy in adults: a prospective, unblinded randomized controlled trial. Seizure. 2013;22(10):846–55.
981. Bodenstein-Sachar H, Gandelman-Marton R, Ben-Zeev B, Chapman J, Blatt I. Outcome of lamotrigine treatment in juvenile myoclonic epilepsy. Acta Neurol Scand. 2011;124(1):22–7.
982. Morris GL, Hammer AE, Kustra RP, Messenheimer JA. Lamotrigine for patients with juvenile myoclonic epilepsy following prior treatment with valproate: results of an open-label study. Epilepsy Behav. 2004;5(4):509–12.
983. Acar B, Dağ E, Turkel Y. Lamotrigine induced seizures in juvenile myoclonic epilepsy. J Exp Clin Med. 2013;30:207–8.
984. Carrazana EJ, Wheeler SD. Exacerbation of juvenile myoclonic epilepsy with lamotrigine. Neurology. 2001;56(10):1424–5.
985. Lynch BA, Lambeng N, Nocka K, Kensel-Hammes P, Bajjalieh SM, Matagne A, et al. The synaptic vesicle protein SV2A is the binding site for the antiepileptic drug levetiracetam. Proc Natl Acad Sci USA. 2004;101(26):9861–6.
986. Noachtar S, Andermann E, Meyvisch P, Andermann F, Gough WB, Schiemann-Delgado J. Levetiracetam for the treatment of idiopathic generalized epilepsy with myoclonic seizures. Neurology. 2008;70(8):607–16.
987. Verrotti A, Cerminara C, Coppola G, Franzoni E, Parisi P, Iannetti P, et al. Levetiracetam in juvenile myoclonic epilepsy: long-term efficacy in newly diagnosed adolescents. Dev Med Child Neurol. 2008;50(1):29–32.
988. Rudolph U, Crestani F, Benke D, Brunig I, Benson JA, Fritschy JM, et al. Benzodiazepine actions mediated by specific gamma-aminobutyric acid(A) receptor subtypes. Nature. 1999;401(6755):796–800.
989. Obeid T, Panayiotopoulos CP. Clonazepam in juvenile myoclonic epilepsy. Epilepsia. 1989;30(5):603–6.
990. Liu J, Tai YJ, Wang LN. Topiramate for juvenile myoclonic epilepsy. Cochrane Database Syst Rev. 2021;11(11):CD010008.
991. Kothare SV, Valencia I, Khurana DS, Hardison H, Melvin JJ, Legido A. Efficacy and tolerability of zonisamide in juvenile myoclonic epilepsy. Epileptic Disord. 2004;6(4):267–70.
992. Stevelink R, Al-Toma D, Jansen FE, Lamberink HJ, Asadi-Pooya AA, Farazdaghi M, et al. Individualised prediction of drug resistance and seizure recurrence after medication withdrawal in people with juvenile myoclonic epilepsy: a systematic review and individual participant data meta-analysis. EClinicalMedicine. 2022;53:101732.
993. Cerulli Irelli E, Morano A, Cocchi E, Casciato S, Fanella M, Albini M, et al. Doing without valproate in women of childbearing potential with idiopathic generalized epilepsy: implications on seizure outcome. Epilepsia. 2020;61(1):107–14.
994. Baykan B, Martinez-Juarez IE, Altindag EA, Camfield CS, Camfield PR. Lifetime prognosis of juvenile myoclonic epilepsy. Epilepsy Behav. 2013;28(Suppl 1):S18–24.
995. Komatsubara T, Kobayashi Y, Hiraiwa A, Magara S, Hojo M, Ono T, et al. Recurrence rates and risk factors for seizure recurrence following antiseizure medication withdrawal in adolescent patients with genetic generalized epilepsy. Epilepsia Open. 2022;7(2):332–43.
996. Gowers WR. Epilepsy and other chronic convulsive diseases: their causes, symptoms, and treatment. London: Churchill; 1885.
997. Janz D. „Aufwach "-Epilepsien. Als Ausdruck einer den „Nacht "oder , „Schlaf "-Epilepsien gegenüberzustellenden Verlaufsform epileptischer Erkrankungen. Arch Psychiatr Nervenkr. 1953;191:73–98.
998. Camfield P, Camfield C. Idiopathic generalized epilepsy with generalized tonic-clonic seizures (IGE-GTC): a population-based cohort with >20 year follow up for medical and social outcome. Epilepsy Behav. 2010;18(1–2):61–3.
999. Gesche J, Antonson S, Dreier JW, Christensen J, Beier CP. Social outcome and psychiatric comorbidity of generalized epilepsies - a case-control study. Epilepsia. 2021;62(5):1158–69.

1000. Caraballo R, Silva S, Beltran L, Calvo A, Caballero R. Childhood-only epilepsy with generalized tonic-clonic seizures: a well-defined epileptic syndrome. Epilepsy Res. 2019;153:28–33.
1001. Vossler DG, Knake S, O'Brien TJ, Watanabe M, Brock M, Steiniger-Brach B, et al. Efficacy and safety of adjunctive lacosamide in the treatment of primary generalised tonic-clonic seizures: a double-blind, randomised, placebo-controlled trial. J Neurol Neurosurg Psychiatry. 2020;91(10):1067–75.
1002. Berkovic SF, Knowlton RC, Leroy RF, Schiemann J, Falter U. Placebo-controlled study of levetiracetam in idiopathic generalized epilepsy. Neurology. 2007;69(18):1751–60.
1003. French JA, Krauss GL, Wechsler RT, Wang XF, DiVentura B, Brandt C, et al. Perampanel for tonic-clonic seizures in idiopathic generalized epilepsy a randomized trial. Neurology. 2015;85(11):950–7.

Chapter 6
Pharmacological Treatment of Status Epilepticus

Xuefeng Wang, Feng Li, Yin Yan, Wei Wang, and Fei Xiao

6.1 Overview of Status Epilepticus

Epileptic status is a common critical condition seen with neurological diseases, and except for cases of accidental death, many of the deaths of patients with epilepsy are caused by epileptic status. Although the understanding of epileptic status has changed over time, the latest understanding of epileptic status is based on the International League against Epilepsy 2015 consensus on epileptic status. According to the International League against Epilepsy provisions, generalized epileptic status means that the disorder of consciousness does not return to normal between two seizures or that a seizure lasts more than 5 minutes (absence seizures last more than 15 minutes). A focal seizure with consciousness impairment lasting more than 10 minutes can also be diagnosed as epileptic status. The duration of focal seizures with unconscious injury is still being investigated [1, 2].

6.1.1 Historical Evolution

The identification of status epilepticus has changed over time. The previous definition of status epilepticus recognized by the World Health Organization was a single seizure lasting more than 30 minutes, and the definition of status epilepticus

X. Wang (✉) · F. Li · W. Wang · F. Xiao
Department of Neurology, The First Affiliated Hospital of Chongqing Medical University, Chongqing, China

Y. Yan
Epilepsy Rehabilitation center, The Affiliated Beibei Hospital of Chongqing Medical University, Chongqing, China

X. Wang, L. Zhou (eds.), *Pharmacological Treatment of Epileptic Seizures*,
https://doi.org/10.1007/978-981-96-8520-2_6

recognized by the International League against Epilepsy in 2015 is a single seizure lasting more than 5–15 minutes; therefore, it is difficult to understand the original source of status epilepticus. The current definition can only be determined based on the results of the database (mainly PubMed).

According to the results collected in the PubMed database, the first paper to mention epileptic status was by Harper et al. [3], who found in their study of 59 children with severe illness that 4 children had epileptic status. Subsequently, Fincham et al. [4] described the serum concentrations of phenytoin sodium in patients with epileptic status. In 1977, Bucking et al. [5] explored a new method of intravenous clonazepam administration for the treatment of epileptic status. They treated 22 patients with epileptic status and achieved very good results, suggesting that an effective method had been found for the treatment of epileptic status. In 1984, A Pilke et al. [6] described 82 patients with epileptic status, and found that tumors, cerebrovascular diseases, and alcoholism could induce epileptic status; for the first time, multiple etiologies of epileptic status were noted. Subsequently, Snodgrass et al. [7] described the electroencephalogram (EEG) manifestations of 147 patients with epileptic status and proposed that EEG plays an important role in the prevention and treatment of epileptic status. A Jagoda et al. [8] later proposed the concept of refractory status epilepticus and discussed its prevention and treatment methods, which promoted progress in the prevention and treatment of status epilepticus. In 2015, the International League Against Epilepsy (ILAE) summarized the causes of status epilepticus and proposed a new perspective on status epilepticus to standardize its prevention and treatment. In 2023, Pilar Bosque Varela [9] et al. described the neuroimaging findings of 206 patients with epileptic status and reported that more than half of the patients with epileptic status had neuroimaging changes and that hyperperfusion was the most common neuroimaging finding. Epilepticus and discussed its prevention and treatment methods, which promoted progress in the prevention and treatment of status epilepticus. In 2015, the ILAE summarized the causes of status epilepticus and proposed a new perspective on status epilepticus to standardize its prevention and treatment. In 2023, Pilar Bosque Varela [9] et al. described the neuroimaging findings of 206 patients with epileptic status and reported that more than half of patients with epileptic status had neuroimaging changes and that hyperperfusion was the most common neuroimaging finding.

6.1.2 Epidemiology

Takafumi Kubota et al. [10] identified 494,790 patients with epilepsy from 53 million electronic medical records in the United States, of whom 19,190 (3.87%) had status epilepticus. Mei Lu et al. [11] conducted a systematic analysis of 69 status epilepticus surveys in the United States and reported that the incidence of status epilepticus in patients of all ages ranged from 10.3 to 41 cases/100,000 cases/year. The incidence of convulsive status epilepticus was 3.5–12.5 cases per 100,000 years and 0–4 years. The peak age of onset was after 60 years, and the mortality rate was 21–31.2%. Bergin et al. [12] investigated 367 patients with seizures lasting more than 10 minutes as epileptic status and reported that the prevalence rate was 22.22–29.25/100,000/year. Vijiala et al. [13] studied 260,855 adults in nonurban areas and found 103 cases of status epilepticus, suggesting that there were 8.6 cases of status epilepticus per 100,000 adults per year, of which 52% were generalized convulsive epileptic status. Thirty-four percent had nonconvulsive status epilepticus with coma.

The incidence of status epilepticus is affected not only by the population but also by the patient's age, etiology, and history of epilepsy. Yi Guo et al. [14] studied 760 newly diagnosed elderly patients with epilepsy and reported that 25% of the patients had one or more epileptic statuses. Alice M Donnan et al. [15] investigated 510 patients with genetic development of epileptic encephalopathy and reported that 47% had convulsive epileptic status and 19% had nonconvulsive epileptic status, suggesting that the incidence of epileptic status in such patients was 67%. Si-Bao Khor et al. [16] investigated 227 patients who died and reported that 4.4% of them died from epileptic status. Yanzi Jin et al. [17] analyzed 216 deaths from 4296 patients with convulsive epilepsy in Northwest China and reported that 22.9% of the patients died from epileptic status.

6.1.3 Causes of Status Epilepticus

Binlu Deng et al. [18] analyzed the etiology of 81 newly diagnosed cases of nonconvulsive epileptic status, and found that the most common causes were central nervous system infection (23.3%), cerebrovascular disease (20%), intracranial tumor (20%), and autoimmune encephalitis (16.4%), and that 36.3% had an unknown etiology. Bo Zhou et al. [19] conducted a study on the etiology of epileptic status in 258 patients, and found that central nervous system infection (33.7%) and inappropriate discontinuation of antiseizure drugs (31.3%) were the most common causes. Other causes were cerebrovascular diseases, cerebral hypoxia, and poisoning.

In 2015, the International League against Epilepsy described more than 150 causes of epileptic status, which can be divided into 17 categories: (1) cerebrovascular diseases, such as cerebral infarction and cerebral hemorrhage; (2) central nervous system infection; (3) neurodegenerative diseases; (4) tumors; (5) cortical developmental disorders; (6) head injury; (7) alcohol poisoning; (8) poisoning; (9) discontinuation of anti-seizure drugs; (10) cerebral hypoxia; (11) metabolic disorders (such as electrolyte imbalance, glucose imbalance, organ failure, acidosis, renal failure, hepatic encephalopathy, radiation encephalopathy, etc.); (12) autoimmune diseases; (13) mitochondrial diseases; (14) chromosomal abnormalities and inheritance; (15) neurocutaneous syndromes; (16) metabolic disorders syndromes (such as porphyria, Wilson's disease, etc.); and (17) others. It has been suggested that epileptic status is a multietiological disease, and all diseases involving central nervous system damage may cause epileptic status.

6.1.4 Possible Pathogenesis of Status Epilepticus

The greatest difference between epilepsy and status epilepticus is that epilepsy generally occurs only once, and then the seizure stops on its own because there is a non-response period to the stimulus after the seizure, during which time extraordinary stimulation is required to induce the next seizure. The greatest characteristic of status epilepticus is that the nonresponse period after the seizure disappears. Therefore, the patient experiences frequent seizures. Another characteristic of the epileptic status is that epileptic status can self-induce, and a previous seizure can become the trigger factor of this seizure. This self-induction enables the seizure to continue, thus leading to an epileptic status. However, the specific underlying mechanism is still under investigation [2].

6.1.5 Classification of Status Epilepticus

In 2015, the International League against Epilepsy divided status epilepticus into two categories: status epilepticus with and without obvious motor symptoms (Figs. 6.1 and 6.2). Epileptic status without obvious motor symptoms is also called nonconvulsive status epileptic [1].

6.1.6 The Main Clinical Manifestations of Status Epilepticus

6.1.6.1 Convulsive Epileptic Status

The International League against Epilepsy divides status epilepticus into two categories: convulsive and nonconvulsive status epilepticus. A seizure resulting in convulsive epilepsy for more than 5 minutes is called convulsive epileptic status. Convulsive seizures are mainly characterized by a sudden loss of consciousness and by continuous activity of clonic seizures after tonic seizures. Continuous contraction of the iliac muscle is called tonic, continuous contraction of the lifting face muscle leads to squinting of both eyes, continuous contraction of the eyeball motor muscle leads to binocular staring, continuous contraction of the masseter muscle leads to tooth clenching, continuous contraction of the throat muscle leads to mouth spitting, and continuous contraction of the vocal cord muscle leads to glottis closing. The tonic contraction of the respiratory muscles forces the air in the lungs through the narrow glottis, and the patient often screams. Tonic contraction of the trunk muscles causes the neck to first bend forward and then stretch strongly. Tonic contraction of the skeletal muscles of the limbs occurs when the hands first rise and turn outward, followed by adduction and rotation. The lower limbs bend first, stretch, and then enter the clonus phase, in which intermittent skeletal muscle

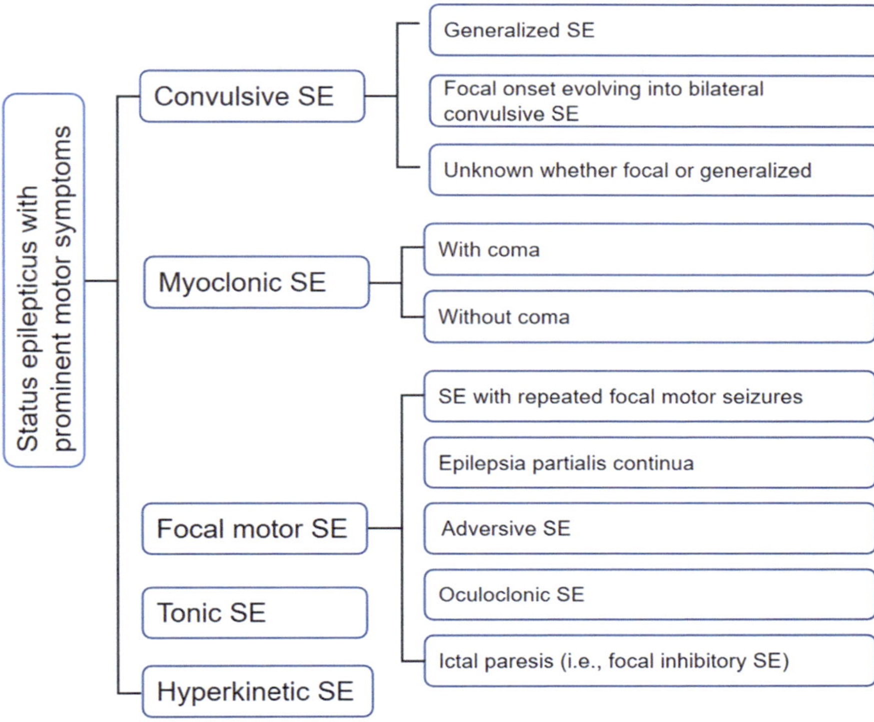

Fig. 6.1 Status epilepticus with prominent motor symptoms [1]

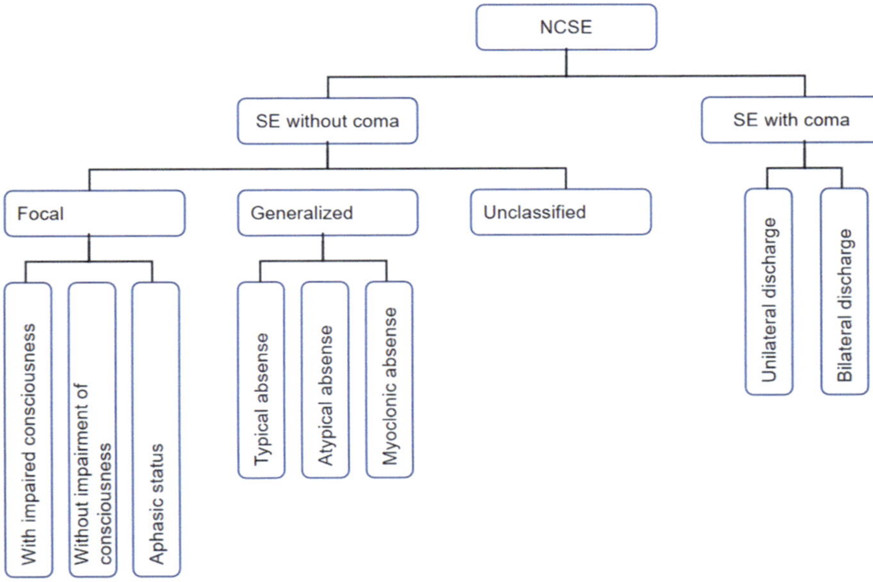

Fig. 6.2 Status epilepticus without prominent motor symptoms [1]

contraction occurs. The literature often refers to the loss of consciousness before the seizure as preeclampsia and the tonic–clonus that appears later as the later eclampsia.

6.1.6.2 Nonconvulsive Status Epilepticus

Nonconvulsive status epilepticus episodes are characterized by psycho-behavioral abnormalities and disturbances in consciousness. Some patients have subtle motor symptoms. Such symptoms include parasympathetic cognitive impairment, subtle facial or limb twitching, head and/or eye disorientation, specific language stasis, sudden behavioral changes, and autonomic disorders. To be diagnosed as nonconvulsive status epilepticus, these manifestations need to last for 10–15 minutes, and since in most cases these manifestations are not specific and the seizures are not obvious, the diagnosis is based on an EEG.

The diagnostic criteria for nonconvulsive epileptic status proposed by the International League against Epilepsy are as follows: (1) the absence of epileptic encephalopathy; and (2) spikes, sharp waves, sharp slow waves, sharp slow waves, and multispinous slow waves >2.5 Hz on EEG. If the EEG only shows epileptic discharge <2.5 Hz or slow waves >0.5 Hz, the EEG and clinical symptoms should improve after the use of antiepileptic drugs or if there were other mild seizures under EEG monitoring. (3) Patients with epileptic encephalopathy: In addition to the significant increase in the above-described EEG discharge frequency, compared with the baseline EEG discharge frequency, the above clinical and EEG manifestations are significantly improved after treatment with antiepileptic seizure drugs [1].

6.1.6.3 Refractory Status Epilepticus

When seizures cannot be controlled with 2–3 antiepileptic status drugs, it is referred to as refractory status epilepticus [2]. Cornwall et al. [20] studied 1200 patients with nonhypoxic refractory status epilepticus and reported that the average duration of this type of epilepsy was 36.3 days, and this accounted for 41.6% and 22.3% of patients with acute symptomatic status epilepticus and unknown etiology, respectively.

6.2 Special Precautions for Status Epilepticus

6.2.1 Epileptic Status in Hypoxic Encephalopathy

6.2.1.1 Historical Evolution

In 1980, Aminoff et al. [21] first reported the existence of an epileptic state in patients with hypoxic encephalopathy. They found that the epileptic state induced by hypoxic encephalopathy mostly manifested as tetanic seizures, the cause of which was sudden cardiac arrest. In 1986, Vincent et al. [22] described the occurrence of myoclonic epileptic status after cardiac arrest induced by lorazepam and proposed the existence of diverse epileptic statuses. Subsequently, Young et al. [23] described myoclonic epileptic status in 11 patients with hypoxic encephalopathy after cardiac arrest and proposed that the cause of death in these patients was hypoxic injury to the brain, and they did not advocate the use of anesthesia to treat such epileptic status. In 1996, Walker et al. [24] described the diagnosis and treatment of epileptic status in the neurological intensive care unit. SP Nordt et al. [25] reported that the sedative and anesthetic midazolam could treat epileptic status patients. Dolinak et al. [26] reported that epileptic status after cardiac arrest can cause neuronal axon damage, which has attracted increased attention due to secondary brain damage in epileptic status. In 2023, Sjoukje Nutma et al. [27] described the clinical characteristics of epileptic myoclonus persistence in EEG rhythmicality and periodic discharge in coma patients after cardiac arrest and noted that such patients had a high mortality rate.

6.2.1.2 Epidemiological Investigation

Dragancea [28] conducted EEG monitoring on 127 patients with cardiac arrest and found that 41 patients (32%) had epileptic status; Stefano et al. [29] studied 11 cohorts with 1092 patients and found that 29–96% of patients had epileptic status. Limotai et al. [30] conducted a systematic review of 78 studies with 16,707 patients and reported that the incidence of nonconvulsive status epilepticus was 6.2–6.3%. Zafar [31] retrospectively analyzed 323 patients with severe neurological conditions and found that 54 (16.7%) had nonconvulsive epileptic status, 22.2% of which were due to hypoxic brain injury. Andal et al. [32] studied 14 patients with nonconvulsive status epilepticus and reported that two of these cases were caused by hypoxic encephalopathy. These studies, despite widely varied subjects and conditions, revealed that epileptic status was very common in post-hypoxic encephalopathy patients, with the highest incidence of epileptic status reaching 96%.

6.2.1.3 Clinical Manifestations

1. Seizure type: Pandian et al. [33] conducted long-term EEG monitoring on 105 patients with severe neurological conditions and found that 45 patients had epileptic status, 19 patients had nonepileptic status, and 7 patients (6.7%) had persistent partial seizures. Young GB et al. [23] reported that 11 adults developed myoclonic epileptic status after cardiac arrest, indicating that epileptic status in hypoxic encephalopathy mainly manifested as (1) convulsive epileptic status; (2) nonconvulsive epileptic status; (3) myoclonic epileptic status; and (4) persistent partial seizures, most of which are refractory status epilepticus [30, 33].

2. Onset time: In the 18 patients included in the study by Hui et al. [34], the average duration of epileptic status onset was 11.7 hours after cardiac arrest, and the average duration was 60.5 hours. As reported by Irina Dragancea et al. [28], the duration of epileptic status in 41 patients was 46 hours on average after cardiac arrest, indicating that the duration of epilepsy in patients with hypoxic encephalopathy could appear as early as 11 hours after the onset of the disease and generally within 2–3 days.

6.2.1.4 Differential Diagnosis

In addition to epileptic status, hypoxic encephalopathy can also cause nonepileptic myoclonus, known as Lance–Adams syndrome, which can coexist with seizures and exhibit abnormal EEG results; therefore, this syndrome is difficult to distinguish from epilepsy and epileptic status. However, this type of myoclonus is not associated with epilepsy, and its impact on the prognosis of patients is different from that of patients with epilepsy and status epilepticus. Different methods are needed to treat this disease, so attention should be given to identification [35].

This syndrome was first reported in 1963, and it has since been found that this complication is not uncommon after hypoxic encephalopathy, which mainly presents as myoclonus in different parts of the body. This kind of myoclonus is mostly induced by, and largely occurs during, exercise, so some literature calls it motor myoclonus. It also easily appears during voluntary activity; therefore, there have also been studies that refer to it as intentional myoclonus, and it can exist for life. At the time of seizure, most patients are subconsciously clear or in a state of drug sedation, unlike those with myoclonic epilepsy, which is usually spontaneous and often carries a loss of consciousness; moreover, myoclonic epilepsy has a shorter duration and does not exist for a lifetime, which is different from Lance–Adams syndrome, which exists for a lifetime. Lance–Adams syndrome is effectively treated by valproic acid, clonazepam, or levetiracetam and can also help distinguish myoclonic from myoclonic epileptic states. Brøchner et al. [36] conducted a follow-up study on myoclonic epileptic state confirmed by EEG and reported that only 2 of 38 patients with myoclonic epileptic state survived for more than one year. Eleven of the 36 patients with nonepileptic myoclonic states survived for more than a year, suggesting a different prognosis.

6.2.1.5 Prognosis

The prognosis of patients with anoxic status epilepticus is very poor, especially for those who present with myoclonic epilepsy. Sixteen of the 18 patients described by Hui et al. [34] died. Kateriine Orav et al. [37] described 64 patients with hypoxic epilepsy, 63 of whom died and only one of whom survived.

6.2.2 Epileptic Status in Autoimmune Encephalopathy

Epileptic patients can have epileptic status, but epileptic status patients do not necessarily have epileptic seizures; epileptic status without epileptic seizures is called acute asymptomatic epileptic status. It is more common in patients with hormone-sensitive encephalopathy, of which autoimmune encephalitis with epileptic status is the most common.

6.2.2.1 Historical Evolution

Although autoimmune encephalitis has existed for a long time, it has not received widespread attention due to a lack of etiological knowledge. In the past 10 years, as a large number of autoimmune antibodies have been identified, status epilepticus in patients with autoimmune encephalopathy has also received widespread attention.

Based on a PubMed database search, Uma Nath et al. [38] first described this type of epileptic status in 2011. This study described a young woman who was hospitalized for severe complex partial epileptic status and required intensive care support and ventilation, which was clinically considered to indicate autoimmune encephalitis. In 2012, Ewa Motta et al. [39] reported that a patient with mental and behavioral abnormalities was clinically diagnosed with multiple sclerosis, followed by a tonic–clonic epileptic status, and a positive serum anti-N-methyl-D-aspartate receptor (NMDAR) antibody test. After immunotherapy, the patient's condition improved, the patient was discharged, and the diagnosis was autoimmune encephalitis. Status epilepticus in patients with AE has attracted increasing attention. In 2013, Lopint-Khoury [40] noted the particularity of this epileptic state, called it the autoimmune epileptic state, and advocated for the use of immunotherapy. In 2016, Chanson et al. [41] noted distinctive delta brushes on the EEGs of patients with NMDA encephalitis, suggesting that it may be electroconvulsive status epilepticus. In 2023, Kachlmeie et al. [42] described a patient who first developed convulsive epileptic status and then developed nonconvulsive epileptic status. After the seizures were controlled, mental and behavioral abnormalities appeared, and the patient was diagnosed with multiple sclerosis, but the NMDA antibody test was positive. The patient was diagnosed with autoimmune encephalitis and multiple sclerosis overlap syndrome.

6.2.2.2 Epidemiological Investigation

Lu Yao et al. [43] investigated 103 patients with AE and found that 18 of them (21.7%) had status epilepticus. Yu Zhang et al. [44] investigated 227 patients with AE and found that 50 patients (22.03%) had epileptic status. Xin-Ping Qu [45] studied 88 patients with AE and found that 27 patients (30.6%) had epileptic status. Two of them had a persistent state of nonconvulsive epilepsy. None of the patients developed refractory status epilepticus. Pandit et al. [46] admitted 15 patients with AE, 4 of whom exhibited epileptic status. Kaaden [47] analyzed 360 patients with autoimmune encephalitis in Germany, 180 of whom had NMDA-type encephalitis, 1/3 of whom had epileptic status. These studies suggest that the prevalence of epileptic status in patients with AE is approximately 20–33%.

6.2.2.3 Clinical Manifestations

Type of Seizure

(1) New refractory status epilepticus (NORSE): New refractory status epilepticus is a special type of epileptic status. Patients do not have epilepsy or other diseases that can cause epileptic status before the disease, and once the onset of the disease occurs, they develop drug-refractory status epilepticus [48]. The International League Against Epilepsy has developed an expert consensus that it represents a unique epileptic status among autoimmune diseases. Murat Alemdar [49] described a 31-year-old woman who developed fever a week prior followed by refractory status epilepticus, and positive NMAD antibodies were detected in her cerebrospinal fluid. Amanda Eisele et al. [50] studied 20 patients with epileptic status who were diagnosed with NORSE and reported that the new epileptic status was refractory. Azevedo et al. [51] analyzed children aged 0–16 years with refractory status epilepticus disorder and reported 15 cases of NORSE. (2) Focal epileptic status: Yoonkyung Lee et al. [52] described focal epileptic status in patients with myelin oligodendrocyte glycoprotein antibody-associated encephalitis. Triplett [53] described a case of anti-GAD antibody-associated encephalitis in which persistent partial epilepsy was the main manifestation. (3) Myoclonic epileptic status: Monnerat et al. [54] described a patient with glutamate decarboxylase antibody (GADA)-associated encephalitis who was admitted to the hospital with focal myoclonic epileptic status in the right facial and lingual pharyngeal region, and the seizures improved after intravenous corticosteroid administration. The authors suggest that patients with encephalitis may develop focal status epilepticus. (4) Nonconvulsive epileptic status: Mitchell et al. [55] analyzed the electroencephalograms of 358 patients with AE and found that 8 patients had nonconvulsive epileptic status. Ugur Cikrikcili [56] described a 63-year-old female patient who was admitted to the hospital with lethargy and psychotic symptoms and was found by EEG to be in a nonconvulsive epileptic state with elevated serum levels of AD-AB antibodies. Uma Nath et al. [38] also described a case of complex partial epileptic status, suggesting that nonconvulsive epileptic status is common in autoimmune encephalitis. Ewa Motta [39] described a case of AE in which the first symptom was complex partial epileptic status, and the patient was admitted to the hospital and their condition improved after receiving intravenous steroids. Pallavi Juneja et al. [57] described a 24-year-old female patient who presented with confusion and myoclonus, whose electroencephalogram indicated a state of continuous epilepsy, and who was positive for GAD65 autoantibodies. (5) Convulsive epileptic status: The most common

type of autoimmune encephalitis is general tonic–clonic epileptic status. Among 28 patients with epileptic status studied by Nils G Margraf et al. [58], 21 patients (75%) suffered from convulsive epileptic status.

Onset Time

(1) Delayed status epilepticus: Ewa Motta [39] et al. described a patient who was diagnosed with multiple sclerosis at the age of 16.5, developed mental abnormalities and limb movement disorders at the age of 20, and developed tonic–clonic epileptic status a few days later. Serum anti-NMDAR antibody was positive, and the patient's condition improved after immunotherapy. (2) The first symptoms of the disease: Many patients with AE also have status epilepticus as the first symptom. This type of status epilepticus is almost always refractory status epilepticus. Stephanie H Chen [59] described a case of autoimmune encephalitis with negative autoantibodies. The patient initially presented with new refractory status epilepticus and later had frequent seizures, which did not respond to four antiepileptic drugs. (3) Early onset of the disease course: Azevedo et al. [51] described 15 patients with autoimmune encephalitis, all of whom had varying degrees of prodromal symptoms before the onset of refractory status epilepticus, and 12 patients had fever 24 hours before the onset of epilepsy. Seungyon Koh et al. [60] described a previously healthy 20-year-old female patient who had epileptic seizures, was diagnosed with AE, and developed status epilepticus while hospitalized.

Duration of Status Epilepticus

Prolonged seizures can cause neuronal damage and brain necrosis, so the International League against Epilepsy divides the new classification of epileptic status into two parts: one for determining the time of epileptic state seizures and the other for determining the time that may cause secondary brain damage, such as tonic–clonic seizures, in patients. The duration of epileptic status was determined to be more than 5 minutes, and the duration of brain damage was determined to be 30 minutes. Margraf et al. [58] studied 21 patients with epileptic status and 7 patients without epileptic status and reported that the median duration of this type of epileptic status was 44 hours.

Prognosis

The course of AE is often self-limiting, and the prognosis is better than that of normal encephalitis. However, the prognosis of patients with epileptic status in AE is poor. In the 28 patients with AE described by Margraf [58], epilepsy persisted, and 6 patients (21%) died. The mortality rate of 15 patients described by Azevedo et al. [51] was 20%. Gugger et al. [61] described 20 patients with newly diagnosed refractory status epilepticus, 7 of whom died. According to these findings, the mortality rate of patients with AE with status epilepticus is approximately 20–35%.

6.2.3 Epileptic Cardiac Arrest

When a heart stops for more than 3 seconds is considered paroxysmal cardiac arrest. Paroxysmal cardiac arrest is an important cause of sudden death. Patients with epilepsy may have sudden cardiac arrest, which may be caused by ASMs, and there are enough studies suggesting that this may be a potential factor for the sudden death of patients with epilepsy [62]. Many scholars have noted that cardiac arrest during epileptic seizures may be a rare manifestation of epileptic seizures. It is an important factor in the death of patients with epilepsy, and it has been noted that cardiac arrest may induce epilepsy and become the cause of recurrent seizures [63]. This complex relationship between cardiac arrest and epilepsy has become an important factor worthy of attention in the prevention and treatment of epilepsy [62].

6.2.3.1 Historical Evolution

Epileptic cardiac arrest was first described by Kowalik et al. [64], who considered it to be a rare but potentially life-threatening phenomenon and proposed treatment methods. Subsequently, Rocamora et al. [65] summarized the clinical and electrophysiological characteristics of epileptic cardiac arrest. In 2006, Ryvlin et al. [66] noted the relationship between cardiac arrest and sudden death in patients with epilepsy and suggested that cardiac arrest may be a potential factor in the sudden death of epilepsy patients with unknown causes, which was subsequently denied by the research of Leung et al. [67]. They suggested that epileptic cardiac arrest has nothing to do with the unexplained sudden death of epilepsy patients and that it is an independent epilepsy phenomenon. With a deeper understanding of epileptic cardiac arrest, Winesett et al. [68] reported that epileptic cardiac arrest was related to temporal lobe seizures and noted the important value of pacemakers in treatment [69]. Bregianni et al. [70] reported that such cardiac arrest may be the only manifestation of focal seizures, which has enriched the research on epileptic cardiac arrest and attracted increased amounts of attention.

6.2.3.2 Epidemiology

Rocamora et al. [65] conducted long-term EEG and electrocardiogram (ECG) monitoring of 1244 patients with epilepsy and found that 11 out of 19 seizures occurred in 5 patients, suggesting that the incidence of seizure cardiac arrest in epileptic patients was 4‰. Casciato et al. [71] analyzed 6494 ECG records from 196 patients with epilepsy and reported that the incidence of cardiac arrest was 2.6%. Tenyi et al.

[72] analyzed 157 patients, 7% of whom experienced recurrent cardiac arrest during secondary general tonic–clonic seizures. Khali et al. [73] reported that the incidence of epileptic cardiac arrest was very low, approximately 0.3–0.4%. The results of a study by Schuele et al. [74] were similar to those of Khali et al. [74]. In a study of 6825 patients with epilepsy, the incidence of cardiac arrest was 0.27%. Ryvlin et al. [66] conducted cardiac monitoring on 20 patients with drug-resistant epilepsy for several months, found that 3 patients experienced paroxysmal cardiac arrest, and speculated that the likelihood of paroxysmal cardiac arrest in patients with epilepsy was 15%. Thus, the incidence of seizure cardiac arrest is likely to be 0.3–2.6%, while the incidence of seizure cardiac arrest in patients with drug-resistant epilepsy and focal epilepsy is more likely to be between 7% and 15%.

6.2.3.3 Etiology

The cause of epileptic cardiac arrest is not clear, but the following factors may be involved: (1) *Epileptic syndrome*: Negishi et al. [75] described a case of a child with SCN8A-related developmental and epileptic encephalopathy accompanied by seizure cardiac arrest during seizures. Since the sudden death rate of such patients exceeded 10%, the author proposed implanting a pacemaker to overcome cardiac arrest during seizures. However, not all patients with epilepsy syndrome experience cardiac arrest during seizures. Shmuely et al. [76] conducted a multicenter observation of 59 patients with Dravet syndrome and found bradycardia or tachycardia during seizures, but no incidence of cardiac arrest. (2) *Structural damage*: patients with epileptic cardiac arrest described by Wali et al. [77] had frequent seizures and repeated syncope; brain magnetic resonance imaging (MRI) revealed abnormalities in the bilateral insula and temporal and right parietal lobes; and pathological reports revealed local cortical dysplasia. LAMC3 gene mutations can cause occipital and multicerebellar gyrus malformations, as well as epileptic seizures. Kasper et al. [78] reported that a patient with multiple cerebellar gyrus malformations experienced cardiac arrest during epileptic seizures and needed pacemaker implantation for treatment. Al-Awwad et al. [79] described a case of right temporal lobe seizure in a traumatic brain injury patient accompanied by cardiac arrest lasting 18 seconds. The patient described by Rossetti et al. [80] also experienced posttraumatic epileptic seizures, which triggered cardiac arrest. (3) *Immune-related seizures*: D'Souza et al. [81] described a 22-year-old woman diagnosed with autoimmune encephalitis with elevated levels of GAD65 antibodies who developed cardiac arrest during seizures. Suski et al. [82] reported a case of seizure cardiac arrest associated with seizures in the left temporal lobe in a previously healthy 15-year-old girl. Focal seizures were present with paroxysmal cardiac arrest, and anti-NMDAR antibodies were detected in both cerebrospinal fluid and serum. (4) *ASMs*: Shmuely et al. [75] described two patients with focal epilepsy who took carbamazepine and phenytoin sodium, and cardiac arrest occurred in each during focal epilepsy. The authors believed that the cardiac arrest of each patient might have been related to the use of sodium channel inhibitors. (5) *Status epilepticus (SE)*: Legriel et al. [83] studied 49 patients with SE who experienced cardiac arrest and reported that 25 patients (51%) experienced cardiac arrest for the first time, and 13 patients (27%) experienced pulseless electrical activity.

6.2.3.4 Possible Mechanisms of Epileptic Cardiac Arrest

Although the mechanism of epileptic cardiac arrest is not clear, there are still some useful explorations. Leung et al. [67] proposed that the function of the central autonomic neural network could be explained by the influence of epilepsy. Leung et al. [84] used intracranial electrodes to study an 18-year-old epileptic patient and found that stimulation of the left cingulate gyrus for more than 3 seconds could induce epileptic cardiac arrest, suggesting that the cingulate gyrus is a part of the central autonomic neural network; this finding supports the hypothesis that epileptic cardiac arrest is related to central autonomic nervous system function. It has been proposed that the occurrence of epileptic cardiac arrest is related to the function of the limbic lobe in both patients [62]. Lagarde et al. [85] studied the brain metabolism of patients with epileptic cardiac arrest and compared them with a healthy control group and an epileptic group without cardiac arrest and found that the metabolism of the right posterior insula in these patients was low.

6.2.3.5 Clinical Manifestations

1. *Time of cardiac arrest*: (1) *Initial symptoms*: Giovannini et al. [86] described the case of a 69-year-old woman. No abnormalities were found in the cardiology examination, but the patient experienced a 9-second cardiac arrest when an EEG showed a seizure in the right frontotemporal lobe. The author suggested that cardiac arrest might have been the first symptom of the patient's seizure. (2) *The only manifestation*: Strzelczyk et al. [87] described a 41-year-old patient with recurrent syncope and head injury. When EEG and ECG combined monitoring revealed epileptiform discharge in the EEG, the ECG showed bradycardia and cardiac arrest. The seizures did not reappear after pacemaker placement, suggesting that epileptic cardiac arrest may be the only manifestation of epileptic seizures. Hagiwara et al. [88] also reported that epileptic cardiac arrest may be the only manifestation of insular epilepsy. (3) *During seizures*: Most epileptic cardiac arrest occurs during a seizure. In the 10 cases described by Khalil et al. [73], the average duration of cardiac arrest was 22 seconds after the onset of seizures, during which the seizures could continue. Nguyen-Michel et al. [89] conducted a study on 9 patients with cardiac arrest among 828 patients with epilepsy and reported that cardiac arrest occurred 32 ± 18 seconds after seizure, with an average duration of 13 ± 7 seconds. Casciato et al. [71] reported that 8 of 1088 patients with epilepsy experienced epileptic cardiac arrest, and the incubation period from the onset of epilepsy to the onset of cardiac arrest was 26.7 seconds.

2. *Duration of cardiac arrest*: Rocamora et al. [65] studied 5 cases of cardiac arrest among 1244 patients with epilepsy and reported that the duration of cardiac arrest ranged from 4–60 seconds. Tenyi et al. [72] studied 157 patients with epileptic cardiac arrest and reported that the duration of cardiac arrest ranged from 3–96 seconds (18 ± 14 seconds). Khalil et al. [73] studied cardiac arrest in 10 patients and reported that the average duration was 15.8 seconds. The duration of cardiac arrest in the 6 patients studied by Kohno et al. [90] was 3.5–20 seconds (12.6 ± 6.2). Therefore, the duration of cardiac arrest in patients with epilepsy is approximately 3–96 seconds.
3. *Relationship with seizure type*: epileptic cardiac arrest is related to seizure type, the most common of which include temporal lobe epilepsy, frontal lobe epilepsy, and focal seizures. (1) *Temporal lobe epilepsy*: Fain et al. [63] described a 33-year-old female patient with recurrent syncope within 3 years. EEG and ECG monitoring revealed temporal lobe epilepsy accompanied by episodic cardiac arrest. Bianco et al. [91] conducted simultaneous brain and ECG monitoring on a patient with recurrent syncope and found that the patient's ECG showed cardiac arrest synchronized with temporal lobe epilepsy on the EEG. After antiseizure treatment, the patient's cardiac arrest disappeared, and the author speculated that the patient's cardiac arrest was related to temporal lobe epilepsy. (2) *Frontal lobe epilepsy*: Zhang et al. [92] described a patient with a 6-year history of frontal lobe seizures who experienced cardiac arrest during frontal lobe seizures, suggesting that epileptic cardiac arrest was related to frontal lobe epilepsy. Mehvari et al. [93] reported that cardiac arrest was recorded by ECG in a patient with left frontal lobe injury during frontal lobe seizure. (3) *Mixed seizures*: Etgen et al. [94] reported that a patient with urination syncope was found to have sinus bradycardia during long-term ECG monitoring and gradually transitioned to a borderline rhythm, followed by sinus pauses of >2.0 seconds (the longest was nearly 10 seconds), and EEG showed focal seizures in the right frontotemporal lobe. Giovannini et al. [86] described the case of a 69-year-old woman who was found to have no abnormalities on cardiology examination upon admission. EEG recorded during a typical seizure revealed a seizure in the right frontotemporal lobe accompanied by progressive bradycardia followed by a 9-second cardiac arrest. They retrospectively analyzed 31 patients with paroxysmal cardiac arrest and found that most of the patients had frontotemporal epilepsy. Serafini et al. [95] described a case of focal seizures originating in the temporal parietal lobe. (4) *Focal seizure:* Casciato et al. [71] monitored 1088 patients with focal epilepsy who underwent preoperative evaluation and found that 8 patients experienced cardiac arrest during seizures, suggesting that focal epilepsy may be the most common type of seizure in patients with cardiac arrest. Wali et al. [77] reported that a patient with focal cortical dysplasia had drug-resistant seizures accompanied by cardiac arrest, suggesting that cardiac arrest may also occur in focal epilepsy. (5) *Others*: Mehvari et al. [93] also reported that a child with a complex partial seizure experienced cardiac arrest during a secondary general tonic–clonic seizure.

4. *Course of epilepsy*: Tényi et al. [72] studied the relationship between paroxysmal cardiac arrest and the course of epilepsy according to the time of occurrence of paroxysmal cardiac arrest and reported that 73% of patients experienced cardiac arrest one year after the onset of epilepsy; only 23% of patients experienced cardiac arrest within one year after the onset of epilepsy, and most of them were young women and people with heart disease.
5. *Relationship with syncope*: Bestawros et al. [96] observed 10 patients with paroxysmal cardiac arrest and found that in 26 of 76 epileptic seizures cardiac arrest occurred, 15 of which resulted in syncope. Moreover, when the duration of cardiac arrest was less than 6 seconds, the patients did not experience syncope. When the duration of cardiac arrest was >6 seconds, syncope occurred in 94% (15/16) of patients. Van Westrhenen et al. [97] studied 29 patients with epilepsy and 38 patients with seizures, 22 of whom had syncope, and the cardiac arrest time ranged from 5–32 seconds (median 20 seconds). Cardiac arrest often occurred 3 seconds before syncope, suggesting that cardiac arrest was the triggering mechanism of syncope. Sowden et al. [98] also reported that syncope occurs in patients with epilepsy after more than 6 seconds of cardiac arrest.
6. Delayed fall seizures, atonic seizures, and simple paroxysmal loss of consciousness may also be important manifestations of epileptic cardiac arrest [71].

6.2.3.6 Diagnosis

Patients with epileptic cardiac arrest should be diagnosed by synchronous EEG-ECG monitoring. Patients with recurrent syncope, delayed falls, atonic seizures, and simple paroxysmal loss of consciousness should be aware of the possibility of epileptic cardiac arrest, and early combined EEG and ECG monitoring is the most important means of diagnosis. Music-induced seizures also require attention for the possibility of epileptic cardiac arrest [99].

6.2.3.7 Differential Diagnosis

Cardiogenic Cardiac Arrest

Cardiogenic paroxysmal cardiac arrest can cause brain ischemia, thereby inducing syncope. If brain stem function is influenced by ischemia, convulsive syncope can occur, and total tonic–clonic seizures can occur, which need to be distinguished from epileptic cardiac arrest. Synchronous monitoring of EEG and ECG signals is the most important means of diagnosis. In patients with heart disease, i.e., initial cardiac arrest and then convulsion, the possibility of cardiogenic cardiac arrest should be considered. In patients with simultaneous seizures, such as limb rigidity, déjà vu, and fall seizures, this is helpful for the diagnosis of epileptic cardiac arrest. The possibility of cardiac arrest should be considered in the presence of organic heart disease.

Sudden, Unexplained Deaths of Epilepsy Patients

Many scholars consider seizure cardiac arrest to be a potential factor of unexplained sudden death in patients with epilepsy, and it was later found that this type of cardiac arrest is different from unexplained sudden death in patients with epilepsy. Severe cardiac arrest is closely related to seizures, and cardiac arrest often occurs after seizures. Even if there is no typical manifestation of seizures, patients with unexplained sudden death of epilepsy often die suddenly in a quiescent state, and in most cases, there is no seizure before death [69]. During the long-term follow-up of these patients, no unexplained sudden deaths from epilepsy were observed, indicating that the prognosis of these patients was relatively good. This is different from the poor prognosis of sudden unexplained death in patients with epilepsy.

6.2.3.8 Treatment

Optimizing the selection of ASMs and placing a pacemaker if necessary are the main treatment methods, and a small number of patients may need surgery for the treatment of epilepsy.

Optimization of ASM Selection

Epileptic cardiac arrest may be one of the causes of sudden death in epileptic patients. Cardiac pacemaker implantation can effectively prevent and treat fatal complications caused by cardiac arrest in epileptic patients. However, Enkiri et al. [100] reported that if drug treatment can effectively and completely control epileptic seizures, cardiac pacemaker implantation is unnecessary. They described a case of a young epileptic patient who, despite the presence of epileptic cardiac arrest, quickly ceased paroxysmal cardiac arrest after effective treatment with oxcarbazepine, suggesting that permanent pacemaker placement was not necessary. Mbizvo et al. [101] conducted a study on two patients with epileptic cardiac arrest, one of whom discontinued ASMs and had a pacemaker implanted, and the other only discontinued ASMs. As a result, the epileptic seizures of both patients worsened, and the epileptic seizures were effectively controlled after the addition of ASMs. It is thus suggested that ASMs may be the main method for treating epileptic cardiac arrest. Strzelczyk et al. [87] described a patient with déjà vu and recurrent syncope who was found to have epileptic cardiac arrest by electrophysiological monitoring. Targeted ASMs were selected for treatment, and no incidence of epileptic cardiac arrest was found after 2 years of follow-up. Kohno et al. [90] optimized ASM use for 6 patients diagnosed with epileptic cardiac arrest. The patients were followed for an average of 19 years, and no seizures or syncope occurred. No pacemaker intervention was found in 4 patients who underwent cardiac pacing. It is believed that adjusting ASMs can control epileptic seizures, and the placement of pacemakers is not necessary.

Implantation of Pacemakers

Optimizing the choice of ASMs can indeed improve seizure cardiac arrest in epilepsy patients, but many patients with cardiac arrest have drug-resistant epilepsy, and adjusting the choice of ASMs may not be effective; at this time, the implantation of pacemakers needs to be considered. Duplyakov et al. [102] studied the treatment of patients with epileptic cardiac arrest and reported that pacemaker implantation seemed to prevent epileptic-related falls and seizure injuries. They reported that patients with drug-resistant epilepsy combined with syncope disappeared after pacemaker implantation, suggesting that if these patients could not completely control their seizures, they would not be able to do so. Thus, implanting a pacemaker is an effective treatment option. Bestawros et al. [96] implanted pacemakers in 8 of the 10 patients with epileptic cardiac arrest who were followed for 72 ± 95 months, and no syncope occurred. Khalil et al. [73] placed pacemakers in 6 out of 10 patients diagnosed with epileptic cardiac arrest, and the seizures completely disappeared in all 6 patients.

Surgical Treatment of Epilepsy

When seizures cannot be completely controlled, the focus of epilepsy is relatively limited, and epilepsy can be clearly positioned; thus, epilepsy surgery may also be an effective treatment method. Russo et al. [103] described a patient with focal epilepsy accompanied by seizure cardiac arrest. Neuroimaging revealed a poorly differentiated tumor in the left temporal neocortex. After anterior temporal lobectomy, the patient was followed for one year without seizures. Ballendine et al. [104] reported that a patient who experienced epileptic cardiac arrest still experienced seizures after pacemaker implantation and subsequently underwent left temporal lobectomy. The incidence of seizures decreased postoperatively, and ASMs were used after the pacemaker was removed, after which the patient's seizures stopped. The author suggests that epilepsy surgery is also an important method for the treatment of epileptic cardiac arrest.

6.2.3.9 Prognosis

The overall prognosis of patients with epileptic cardiac arrest is good. Among the 8 patients studied by Schuele et al. [105], 6 patients were followed for an average of 5 years after receiving pacemaker implantation, and no recurrence of cardiac arrest events was reported in the 10 patients described by Khalil et al. [73].

6.2.4 *Stimulus-Induced Myoclonic Epileptic State with Rhythmic and Periodic Discharge of Electroencephalogram*

Myoclonic epileptic status was first described by TAYLOR FM [106] in 1952; whereas stimulus-induced myoclonic epileptic status was reported much later, and myoclonic epileptic status with rhythmic, periodic, and paroxysmal epileptic discharge on the EEG was reported somewhat later [107].

Patients with stimulus-induced myoclonic epileptic state are particularly sensitive to external stimuli, and any kind of stimulation, including turning over, patting the back, suctioning, and injection, can immediately induce rapid myoclonus in both the upper limbs, shoulders, and trunk, lasting approximately 6–10 minutes. EEG reveals rhythmic, periodic slow-spine or multi-spine-slow complex waves, and synchronous electromyography reveals a positive electromyography burst. EEG-EMG has a significant "electroclinical" lock-in relationship, with an incubation period of approximately 20–50 ms. Unlike traditional epileptic status, this epileptic status has obvious drug resistance, and regardless of which drug is used, it only has a brief effect; once stimulated, the seizure reappears.

The most important feature of this disease is the rhythmic and periodic epileptic discharge on the electroencephalogram. This special EEG phenomenon was discovered by Hirsch et al. [108] in 2004 during the long-term EEG monitoring of patients with severe neurological conditions. They named this previously unrecognized EEG pattern stimulator-induced rhythmic, periodic, or episodic discharge (SIRPID). In 2014, Amanda et al. [109] experimentally confirmed that this particular brain electrical pattern is associated with status epilepticus and traumatic brain injury.

The prognosis of such patients is extremely poor. Ruijter et al. [107] studied 172 patients with epileptic state whose EEG showed rhythmic, periodic, or paroxysmal discharge and reported that the mortality rate was greater than 80% in both the treated group and the untreated group.

6.2.5 *Propofol Infusion Syndrome*

Propofol (2,6-diisopropylphenol) is an intravenous hypnotic drug widely used not only for sedation and anesthesia induction but also for the treatment of refractory status epilepticus. It is favored by medical clinicians because of its rapid onset and quick patient recovery following long-term use. Under normal circumstances, the use of propofol is safe, but long-term, high-dose (>4 mg/kg/h) concentrated use of propofol may lead to a fatal complication known as propofol infusion syndrome [110]. This syndrome can manifest as metabolic acidosis, rhabdomyolysis, and multiorgan failure characterized by arrhythmia and renal failure, which can lead to patient death [111–115].

6.2.5.1 The Historical Evolution of Propofol

Propofol was first used as an anesthetic in 1979 [116]. In 1985, Gepts E et al. [117] described the pharmacokinetic characteristics of a continuous intravenous infusion of propofol in the human body, providing experimental evidence for high-dose, long-term use in the population. In 1989, Raff M [118] conducted a safety trial of a high-dose intravenous infusion of propofol in an animal model of malignant high fever and reported that infusion of propofol at a rate of 12 mg/kg/hr. for 45 minutes did not cause malignant high fever syndrome. It was therefore suggested that the use of propofol was safe. In 1990, propofol was first used for sedation in pediatric patients and achieved good results [119]. Subsequently, it was widely used for sedation, sleep maintenance, and treatment of refractory status epilepticus in intensive care unit patients. In 1995, El European [120] reported that high-dose propofol administration may cause lipid deposition, raising concerns about the safety of propofol. In 1998, Bray [121] described a patient death caused by high-dose infusion of propofol but did not observe the presence of propofol infusion syndrome. In 1999, Hatch DJ [122] and others described the occurrence of infusion syndrome in pediatric patients using propofol. In 2001, Kelly [123] summarized the clinical characteristics of this syndrome and proposed a diagnostic method. Subsequently, Wolf [124] and others discovered that the occurrence of this syndrome may be related to impaired fatty acid oxidation and explored methods for predicting this dangerous syndrome [125]. In 2002, Tep M Kang [126] described propofol infusion syndrome in adult patients and advocated caution when using propofol at doses of >5 mg/kg/h for >48 hours in critically ill patients until further safety data were available [127]. Subsequently, Vasile et al. [128] described the pathological and physiological processes of this patient, deepening people's understanding of this lethal complication.

6.2.5.2 Epidemiological Investigation

Russell J Roberts et al. [129] monitored critically ill adults who received propofol infusion for more than 24 hours at 11 medical centers and found that 11 out of 1017 patients (1.1%) developed propofol infusion syndrome, suggesting that the incidence of propofol infusion syndrome may exceed 1%. Iyer VN et al. [130] studied 41 patients with refractory status epilepticus, 31 (76%) of whom used propofol (propofol group) and 10 (24%) of whom used nonpropofol drugs. Eleven patients (35%) developed non-life-threatening propofol infusion syndrome, three patients died, and none of the nonpropofol group experienced such events. Li et al. [131]

conducted a retrospective study on adult patients who received propofol infusion for ≥48 hours or at a dose ≥60 μg/kg/min for >24 hours in multiple hospitals and reported that the incidence of propofol infusion syndrome was 2.9%, and the associated mortality rate was 36.8%.

6.2.5.3 Pathophysiological Mechanisms

The mechanism of propofol infusion syndrome is not clear, and it is now speculated that its main site of action is the mitochondria, which are related to energy and fatty acid metabolism. Singh et al. [132] reported that propofol infusion syndrome can cause mitochondrial respiratory chain disruption, leading to restricted adenosine triphosphate synthesis and cellular hypoxia. Moreover, excessive lipolysis of adipose tissue produces excess free fatty acids, which cannot be fully utilized during β-oxidation, leading to neuronal degeneration and necrosis. Barajas [5] studied the toxic mechanism of propofol in newborn mice through animal experiments. They found that propofol can cause coenzyme Q (CoQ) substrate oxidation disorders, thereby interfering with CoQ electron transfer. These defects provide new insights into the toxic effects of propofol on the developing heart. Propofol infusion syndrome is also a rare and fatal complication of long-term infusion of propofol in critically ill children. A study conducted by Wolf et al. [124] regarding a child with propofol infusion syndrome revealed a significant increase in plasma concentrations of malonyl carnitine (3.3 μmol/L) and C5 acylcarnitine (8.4 μmol/L) before hemodialysis. After the condition improved, the levels of these indicators returned to normal. This abnormality is consistent with the damage to fatty acid oxidation caused by the entry of long-chain acylcarnitine esters into mitochondria and the failure of the mitochondrial respiratory chain at the 11th complex. Romero et al. [133] also reported that propofol infusion syndrome is associated with mitochondrial long-chain fatty acid oxidation disorder.

6.2.5.4 Risk Factors

Dose and duration of use are risk factors for the induction of propofol infusion syndrome, and a dosage of >4–5 mg/kg/hour and >48 hours of continuous infusion can easily induce the occurrence of propofol infusion syndrome [130]. (1) Drug dosage: Propofol infusion syndrome usually occurs when large doses are used. As reported by Carlos Romero et al. [133], propofol infusion syndrome occurs when a dosage of 7 mg/kg/h is administered; Bray et al. [125] analyzed 18 pediatric patients who received propofol treatment and found that 3 of 9 patients who received propofol infusion at a dosage >4 mg/kg/h and continued for >48 hours had propofol-induced myocardial failure and eventually died. However, propofol infusion syndrome may also occur with the use of conventional doses of propofol. Vincenzo Fodale [110] described a case of propofol infusion syndrome after 1.9–2.6 mg/kg/h propofol was administered; the patient died. Joshua Calvano [134] described a 3-year-old female patient who developed propofol infusion syndrome after being administered very low doses of propofol. We suggest that careful consideration must be given before initiating propofol therapy to avoid infusions of propofol to susceptible individuals. (2) Medication duration: Among the 31 patients described by Vivek N Iyer [130] who used propofol, 3 (10%) experienced cardiopulmonary arrest, 2 of whom died, and 11 (35%) had non-life-threatening propofol infusion syndrome. The authors suggest that using propofol for more than 48 hours is an important cause of this syndrome. (3) In addition to the high-dose and long-term use of propofol, the synchronous administration of steroids, vasopressors, fat emulsions, and low carbohydrates are also important triggering factors.

6.2.5.5 Clinical Manifestations

The propofol infusion syndrome described by Li [131] is mainly characterized by metabolic acidosis (78.9%), cardiac insufficiency (52.6%), hypertriglyceridemia (100%), and rhabdomyolysis (26.3%). Based on case studies and a literature review, Laquay et al. [135] reported that the main clinical manifestations of propofol infusion syndrome are severe metabolic acidosis, rhabdomyolysis, and multiple organ failure, including hyperkalemia, hepatomegaly, renal failure, hyperlipidemia, arrhythmia, and progressive heart failure.

Acidosis

Carlos Romero [132] described a 43-year-old woman who underwent brain surgery for vascular malformations and developed severe lactic acidosis after surgery. During the anesthesia period, she received a propofol infusion at a dosage of 7 mg/kg/hour for more than 8 hours. The author speculates that this acidosis was caused by propofol infusion; Cannon [136] described a 13-year-old girl who was admitted to the hospital after a head injury and received prolonged propofol infusion for sedation. She subsequently developed lactic acidosis and did not respond to treatment. She died 15 hours later. Hanna [137] described two patients who experienced severe metabolic acidosis during the treatment of refractory status epilepticus with propofol. The author speculates that propofol should not be used for prolonged sedation of patients until safety can be guaranteed.

Rhabdomyolysis

Ilya Sabovich [138] described a 16-year-old boy who was admitted to the hospital due to brain injury and received continuous infusion of propofol for sedation and control of intracranial pressure. Three days later, he developed metabolic acidosis and rhabdomyolysis and died 36 hours later of refractory arrhythmia and circulatory failure. Satoshi Karasawa [139] reported that a 22-year-old male patient was admitted to the hospital for Guillain–Barré syndrome. During mechanical ventilation, propofol was administered at a dose of 3.5 mg/kg/hour. On the 13th day, the patient developed severe rhabdomyolysis and compartment syndrome in the lower leg. After symptomatic treatment, the patient gradually recovered.

Mallard [140] confirmed through animal experiments that propofol can cause rhabdomyolysis. The group anesthetized an 8-year-old female dog with propofol for mechanical ventilation, resulting in rhabdomyolysis, myoglobinuria, and methemoglobinemia. The symptoms disappeared after the discontinuation of propofol and the administration of N-acetylcysteine.

Organ Damage

Organ failure is the most common manifestation of propofol infusion syndrome. Satoshi Karasawa [139] reported that a 22-year-old male patient developed hypotension and arrhythmia after mechanical ventilation with propofol. Heterogeneous 18F-FDG uptake was observed in the left ventricle on cardiac 18F-FDG PET, and linear granulocyte myelination was found on myocardial biopsy under electron microscopy, indicating mitochondrial damage to myocardial cells. Bray RJ [121] summarized data from 18 children who received propofol infusions and found 9 patients who received long-term (>48 hours) and high-dose (>4 mg. kg-1. h-1) propofol infusion, 3 of whom died of progressive heart failure.

Barajas MB et al. [141] confirmed the toxic heart effects of propofol through animal experiments. The hearts of newborn mice were exposed to toxic doses of propofol or fat emulsion for 30 minutes. Over time, they found that a toxic dose of propofol induced arrhythmias, decreased ventricular function, and impaired the mitochondrial membrane potential. Subir à González [142] described a patient who developed hepatotoxicity during surgical treatment following administration of conventional-dose propofol.

Multiple organ failure is also common in patients with propofol infusion syndrome. Eriksen [143] described a healthy 20-year-old female patient who was administered propofol at a dose of 1.4–5.1 mg/kg/h for 88 hours after a car accident. Subsequently, she experienced multiple organ failure accompanied by rhabdomyolysis and ultimately died due to multiple organ failure. The patients described by Ilya Sabovich [138] also experienced acute renal failure, refractory myocardial failure, and hyperlipidemia during treatment. Tep M Kang et al. [126] summarized the characteristics of pediatric propofol infusion syndrome and reported that these patients had hyperkalemia, hepatomegaly, lipidemia, and myocardial failure. A 13-year-old girl described by M L Cannon [136] who received a continuous infusion of propofol due to closed head injury died of myocardial failure, metabolic acidosis, and multiple organ failure (involving the kidneys, liver, and heart system) 15 hours after admission.

6.2.5.6 Treatment

Propofol infusion syndrome is a complication of treatment involving the use of propofol, and if its signs are not noticed in a timely manner, its mortality rate is high. There is no remedy for propofol poisoning. The initial treatment includes discontinuing propofol treatment and providing supportive measures; patients with severe injuries can undergo hemodialysis or blood replacement therapy [131].

Stopping or Changing Medication

Stopping or changing medication is the most important treatment for propofol infusion syndrome. Nathalie López [144] described a female patient with refractory status epilepticus. After a continuous intravenous infusion of propofol at a rate of 10 mg/kg/h for 24 hours, her creatine kinase levels were elevated, and metabolic acidosis and lactatemia occurred. After discontinuing treatment with propofol for 24 hours, the patient's condition stabilized; her condition was speculated to have been caused by propofol infusion syndrome. The author suggests that propofol infusion syndrome usually improves gradually after 12 hours of discontinuation; Park [113] described a 59-year-old male patient who developed propofol infusion syndrome after consuming 1.3 mg/kg/hour of propofol. The infusion was stopped, and active support was provided for treatment, leading to a quick recovery. Shimada M [145] described an 82-year-old male who underwent bypass surgery for angina and subsequently developed propofol infusion syndrome. The patient recovered after having the sedatives he was being treated with switched from propofol to midazolam and dexmedetomidine.

Treatment of Metabolic Acidosis

Carlos Romero [133] reported that when severe lactic acidosis occurs due to propofol infusion syndrome, discontinuing propofol treatment and treating acidosis can lead to complete recovery.

Treatment of Circulatory Failure

Christophe Guitton [146] described a case of refractory status epilepticus in a 17-year-old female. After consuming 8.8 mg/kg/h propofol for 58 hours, propofol infusion syndrome, characterized by renal failure, metabolic acidosis, and rhabdomyolysis, developed. A few hours later, cardiac circulatory failure occurred. Despite the possibility of cardiac arrest occurring, the authors still initiated extracorporeal membrane oxygenation therapy, and the patient's circulatory function rapidly improved. The patient was removed from the ventilator after 5 days and left the intensive care unit after 36 days.

Plasma Exchange

Shonola S Da Silva [147] described the case of a child with malignant refractory status epilepticus who developed infusion syndrome while using propofol. After plasma exchange, the patient's abnormal cardiovascular function was restored. The authors suggest that plasma exchange is a safe and effective choice for treating propofol infusion syndrome. Phillip D Levin [148] described a 16-year-old patient with status epilepticus who developed severe lactic acidosis, rhabdomyolysis, and hemodynamic instability after receiving propofol treatment. Propofol infusion syndrome was suspected, and lactate acidosis significantly improved 24 hours after receiving a single therapeutic plasma exchange, with complete recovery occurring within 10 days. Plasma exchange is considered an effective treatment for propofol infusion syndrome.

Drug Therapy

Sun J [149] found through performing animal experiments that dexmedetomidine has a protective effect on myocardial injury caused by propofol infusion syndrome and can thereby reduce pathological damage to the myocardium caused by propofol infusion. The mechanism may be related to the inhibition of iron death caused by the accumulation of reactive oxygen species. The authors suggest that the use of propofol and dexmedetomidine, combined with sedation, may be a potential strategy for preventing and treating propofol infusion-induced cardiac toxicity. The structures of coenzyme Q10 and propofol are similar. Therefore, coenzyme Q may be the main site at which propofol interacts with the mitochondrial respiratory chain in patients with propofol infusion syndrome. To support this hypothesis, Kilicaslan B [150] studied the effects of coenzyme Q10 on survival and organ damage in the propofol infusion syndrome model rabbits and reported that CoQ10 administration can alleviate the toxicity of propofol to the liver, gallbladder, bladder, and spleen.

6.3 Treatment of Status Epilepticus

6.3.1 Treatment for the Cause

There are different causes of epileptic status, and different causes require different treatments. Epileptic status in autoimmune encephalitis, for example, requires the use of hormones to control the primary disease. With acute symptomatic epilepsy, seizures gradually stop as the primary disease improves.

6.3.2 Termination of Seizures in Status Epilepticus Patients

Epileptic seizures can cause neuronal necrosis and secondary brain damage. Although the treatment of epileptic seizures is comprehensive, early termination of epileptic seizures is still the main treatment measure [2].

6.3.2.1 Commonly Used Antiepileptic State Drugs

Currently, there are approximately 14 drugs that can terminate epileptic seizures (Table 6.1), and these drugs can be selected for different therapeutic purposes.

6.3.2.2 Basis for the Selection of Drugs to Terminate Epileptic State Seizures

The basis for the selection of antiepileptic state drugs is mainly the synaptic hypothesis of the epileptic state. According to this hypothesis, the levels of GABA inhibitory neurotransmitters in the presynaptic membrane are mainly reduced in the early stage of epileptic state seizure, so the levels of GABA transmitters need to be supplemented. As the release of presynaptic neurotransmitters is reduced, GABA transmitter receptors in the postsynaptic membrane enter the cytoplasm through exocytosis or endocytosis, thus reducing the number of receptors on the membrane. Due to the decrease in the number of GABA receptors on the postsynaptic membrane and the lack of receptor sites, the levels of glutaminergic neurotransmitters, which do not meet physiological needs, change from intracellular to membrane and subsequently cause a variety of transmitter disorders; thus, epileptic status cannot be terminated by these neurotransmitters [2]. Therefore, the selection of anti-epileptic status drugs needs to be determined according to the following steps (Figs. 6.3 and 6.4):

Table 6.1 Commonly used antiepilepticus status drugs

Commonly used drugs	
1. Lorazepam	8. Ketamine or sodium thiopental
2. Diazepam	9. Fosphenytoin
3. Clonazepam	10. Phenytoin
4. Phenobarbital	11. Lidocaine
5. Valproate	12. Midazolam
6. Propofol	13. Levetiracetam and other new anti-epileptic drugs
7. Pentobarbital	14. Others

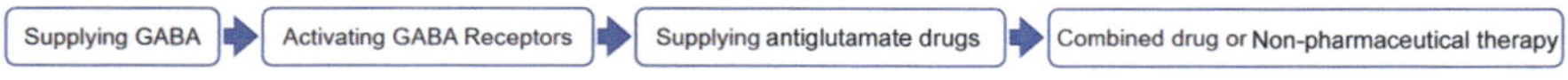

Fig. 6.3 Basis for the selection of drugs to terminate status epilepticus

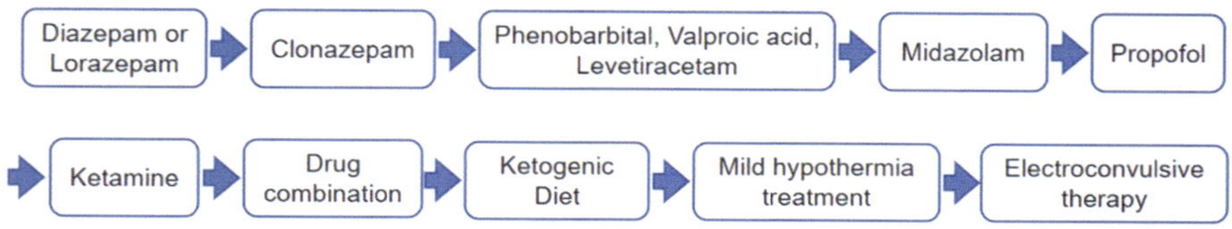

Fig. 6.4 Sequence of drug selection for terminating status epilepticus

6.3.2.3 Clinical Application

Diazepam Injection

Diazepam is a widely used and recognized anti-epileptic state drug, and its efficacy is well-known. In recent years, some countries have recommended the use of lorazepam instead of diazepam, and Mate analysis supports their views. However, considering that lorazepam may not be available in some countries, diazepam is still recommended as the first choice.

1. Indications: It is suitable for the first treatment of epileptic status and for patients who do not meet the criteria for refractory epileptic status, are not resistant to benzodiazepines, and have no contraindications. It is not recommended for epileptic status in patients with hepatic encephalopathy and Lennox–Gastaut syndrome [2].
2. Route of administration: Intravenous administration; prehospital emergencies can also include nonintravenous administration, such as rectal administration, but not intramuscular injection.
3. Dosage: The first dose of 10–20 mg intravenous infusion can be considered when intravenous medication is used for adults with epileptic status. If it is ineffective, intravenous infusion can be repeated 5 minutes later. If effective (seizures stop), intravenous infusion of 80–100 mg with 5% glucose water over 12 hours can be used. If treatment does not work, the drug administration must be stopped, and the patient must be switched to other recommended drugs.
4. Medication precautions: intravenous medication should be used slowly, at a rate of no more than 2 mg/minute, and attention should be given to its impact on respiratory and cardiovascular function; if necessary, respiratory stimulants such as coramine and lobelin should be used to combat respiratory depression.

Clonazepam

Clonazepam is a long-term, highly potent benzodiazepine. It promotes the action of GABA-A by increasing the frequency of chloride channel opening, hyperpolarizing neurons, and reducing firing. As a GABA-A receptor agonist, it can bind to the α and γ subunits of GABA-A, induce conformational changes in GABA-A receptors, promote cell hyperpolarization, and thus play an inhibitory role in the central nervous system [151]. Xiaomeng Zhou et al. [152] conducted a randomized double-blinded experiment on the use of clonazepam in 60 patients with epileptic status and reported that the effective rate of clonazepam was 93.33%, which was better than that of diazepam, which was used as a control. Therefore, Rundfeldt et al. [153] suggested that clonazepam should be the first choice for initial treatment when convulsive status epilepticus persists for more than 5 minutes in infants and children.

1. Indications: The strength of the effect of clonazepam is 10 times greater than that of diazepam. Although many scholars advocate that clonazepam should be the first choice for epileptic status [154], considering the wide drug recognition and the need to accumulate clinical use experience, it is still recommended that clonazepam should be selected only after treatment with diazepam is ineffective [155].
2. Route of administration: intravenous administration.
3. Dosage: Intravenous administration for adult epileptic status can be considered: 1–2 mg intravenous slow infusion, can be repeated once if the drug is ineffective after 10–15 minutes; if still ineffective, the drug should be stopped, and other recommended drugs should be chosen. For patients in which intravenous infusion is effective, 1–2 mg intravenous infusion can be used, which is then maintained every 12 hours, and discontinuation is considered 1–2 days after the seizure stops.

Valproic Acid

1. Indications: These drugs are mainly suitable for benzodiazepine drug-resistant epileptic state patients because they have no significant impact on the patient's consciousness; therefore, they are especially suitable for nonconvulsive epileptic state patients.
2. Route of administration: intravenous administration.
3. Dosage: Adult patients with epileptic status can receive a dose of 20–40 mg/kg/d, and the drug dose needs to be doubled when first used. First, 20–40 mg/kg can be injected intravenously at 3–6 mg/kg/min, then intravenously at the same dose, and then intravenously at 20–40 mg/kg/d the next day for 2–3 consecutive days. Patients in which the treatment is effective can change to oral treatment after the seizure stops and consciousness recovers in order to control long-term seizures in patients with epilepsy. If ineffective, the drug should be discontinued, and other recommended drugs should be chosen.
4. The following precautions should be taken: (1) The first dose of valproic acid used for the treatment of epileptic status needs to be doubled, and it is difficult to achieve the desired effect when a small dose is applied for a long time; and (2) when using valproic acid, it is necessary to pay attention to its special contraindications, such as seizures in mitochondrial encephalomyopathy, etc., and it is not recommended for use in epileptic states caused by hereditary diseases,

epileptic seizures caused by hepatic encephalopathy, and other diseases where its use is obviously not suitable for application [2].

Phenobarbital

1. Indications: It is mainly suitable for epileptic status after treatment diazepam and clonazepam has failed, and may be more effective than other recommended drugs for epileptic status in children and patients with autoimmune diseases.
2. Route of administration: intravenous administration.
3. Dosage: For adult patients with epileptic status, slow intravenous infusion of 10–15 mg/kg (50–100 mg/min) can be administered first, followed by 100–200 mg/time after effective intramuscular infusion twice a day for 1–2 consecutive days. If not effective, the drug should be stopped, and other recommended drugs should be selected.
4. Precautions: (1) Phenobarbital has a significant impact on patient respiratory and cardiovascular function and needs more attention when used in large doses. Once cardiac and pulmonary function inhibition occurs, respiratory stimulants need to be used to combat it. (2) When phenobarbital dosage is excessive, there is often pupil shrinkage, sweating, etc., which requires close observation. (3) Since few large studies have been performed, caution should be exercised in the selection of this drug [2, 156].

Levetiracetam

1. Indications: this drug is mainly suitable for the treatment of epileptic status after the treatment failure of diazepam and clonazepam and the combination of multiple drugs for epileptic status. According to the literature regarding children, it may be effective for electrical status epilepticus during sleep [2, 156, 157].
2. Route of administration: intravenous administration.
3. Dosage: An intravenous infusion of 1000 mg–1500 mg may be considered for adults with epileptic status. The rate of administration is 2–5 mg/kg/min. If the seizure does not stop or the EEG indicates persistent epileptic discharge, the patient should be considered to have refractory epileptic status, and additional dosage should be provided. If ineffective after effective, sustainable infusion of 0.05–2 mg/kg/h, a load capacity of 1500–3000 mg/d, and a maximum dose of 4500 mg, it is necessary to stop the drug and choose other recommended drugs.

   A combination of drugs is mainly used for the treatment of refractory epileptic status and levetiracetam is mainly combined with benzodiazepines. When used in combination with benzodiazepines, the recommended dose of levetiracetam is 2500 mg, which is slowly administered intravenously (>5 minutes). Two methods are used: keeping the original benzodiazepine and then adding levetiracetam or using it in combination with the benzodiazepine [2, 156].

4. Precautions: Although there are a large number of reports in the literature on the use of this drug for the treatment of epileptic status and rich clinical experience has accumulated, large-sample size studies have not been completed, so it is necessary to be careful when choosing this drug.

Yasiry et al. [158] systematically analyzed the relative effectiveness of five drugs for the treatment of epileptic status resistant to benzodiazepines and reported that the efficacy of levetiracetam was 68.5%, that of valproic acid was 75.7%, that of phenobarbital was 73.6%, and that of phenytoin sodium was 50.2%. The authors suggest that valproic acid, levetiracetam, and phenobarbital are all options that can be considered.

Midazolam

1. Indications: Some studies have suggested that the preferred midazolam has better efficacy than diazepam or clonazepam, but it has not been widely recognized by peers, and its influence on respiratory depression and blood pressure is significantly stronger than those of diazepam. This is restricted by the conditions of use, so an expert team still suggests that the use of midazolam for refractory status epilepticus may be more in line with current practice than that of diazepam.
2. Route of administration: intravenous administration.
3. Dosage: Intravenous administration for adult epileptic status can be considered at 0.1–0.2 mg/kg body weight slow intravenous infusion (2–4 mg/min); if ineffective, midazolam can be used again; if still ineffective, it is necessary to stop the drug and choose other recommended drugs. If effective, it can be pumped intravenously at 0.1–0.3 mg/kg/h for 12 hours. Recurrence during maintenance can be repeated once.
4. Precautions: Midazolam significantly inhibits respiration and has an obvious lowering effect on blood pressure. Therefore, it is best to use midazolam under close supervision in the neurological intensive care unit, and mechanical ventilation is required when necessary to maintain respiratory function [2].

Propofol

1. Indications: There is no evidence that the efficacy of the first choice of isopofol is better than that of diazepam or clonazepam, that its influence on respiratory depression and blood pressure is significantly stronger than those of diazepam, and that it is also restricted by the conditions at the time of use. Therefore, the indications for isopofol are mainly refractory epileptic status, and it is used in patients who fail to respond to midazolam or are not suitable for midazolam treatment.
2. Route of administration: intravenous administration.
3. Dosage: Intravenous administration for adult epileptic status can be considered at a slow intravenous injection of 1–2 mg/kg body weight; if ineffective, the

treatment can be repeated once, if the treatment is still ineffective, the drug needs to be stopped, and other recommended drugs can be chosen. If effective, it can be pumped intravenously at 1–4 mg/kg/h for 10–12 hours. If there is recurrence during maintenance, the drug may be reinjected.

4. Precautions: (1) Like midazolam, propofol is best used in the neurological intensive care unit under close supervision, and mechanical ventilation is required when necessary to maintain normal respiratory function; (2) small doses of propofol have been reported to cause epileptic status; therefore, unless a very unique case, generally intravenous application should not be lower than the recommended dose; and (3) large doses and long-term use of propofol, especially when the infusion speed is greater than 100 mcg/kg/min, may cause rhabdomyolysis, which should be noted, and phosphocreatine kinase levels should be checked regularly [157, 159, 160].

Midazolam and propofol are the first-line drugs for the treatment of refractory status epilepticus and are widely accepted. Considering that propofol may aggravate the occurrence of status epilepticus, it is recommended that midazolam be considered after treatment failure [2].

Ketamine

1. Indications: Mainly suitable for the treatment of refractory status epilepticus after failure of treatment with midazolam and propofol, as well as the combination of multiple drugs [161–163]. When studying the efficacy of ketamine, Gaspard et al. [163] reported that the use of ketamine may be effective only after 5–6 other epileptic status drugs have failed. The results of the study by Rosati et al. [164] were similar (5 drugs), and the efficacy rate of ketamine treatment reached 66.7% (6/9), suggesting that ketamine treatment for refractory status epilepticus should generally be used in the late stage and should be used only after 5–6 anti-status epilepticus drugs are found to be ineffective. The animal experiment results of Borris et al. [165] also supported the above conclusion. They found that if ketamine was used 15 min after the onset of epileptic status, the epileptic status could not be controlled in any of the animals (0/4), but if ketamine was used 1 h after the onset of super refractory epileptic status, the epileptic status of all animals could be controlled (4/4). The control rate of status epilepticus was 100%.
2. Route of administration: intravenous administration.
3. Dosage: Adult patients with epileptic status can receive a load dose of 1–3 mg/kg (maximum 4.5 mg/kg), and the maximum speed is 100 mcg/kg/min. Synowiec et al. [166] used ketamine to control refractory status epilepticus by intravenous infusion at an initial dose of 1–2 mg/kg, followed by continuous intravenous infusion at a dose of 0.45–2.1 mg/kg/h. The average duration of use was 9.8 days (4–27). In all patients (11 of 11), status epilepticus was completely controlled, and no side effects occurred.

4. Precautions: (1) Ketamine is an anesthetic and needs to be applied under the guidance of an anesthesiologists. It has an obvious inhibitory effect on respiration. Therefore, it is best to use ketamine under the close supervision of the neurological intensive care unit, and mechanical ventilation is required when necessary to promote normal respiratory function. Due to the obvious respiratory depression effect, the US FDA recommends that the use of ketamine should begin with a small dose and be increased slowly. (2) Because ketamine may have an excitatory effect on the central nervous system, although rare, the US FDA still recommends that it should not be used in people with severe hypertension and allergies to the drug, and it is necessary to perform a head CT scan before treatment to exclude patients with lesions that can cause increased intracranial pressure. (3) Alcohol intoxication causes epileptic state with caution; (4) Symptoms of increased skeletal muscle tone caused by ketamine need to be distinguished from epileptic tonic–clonic seizures [161–163].

Combined Drug Use

1. Potential advantages: Status epilepticus is a heterogeneous disease with multiple etiologies. Not only are there many causes, but the mechanisms are also very complex. The combined application of anti-epileptic status drugs with different mechanisms may be more consistent with the clinical treatment of epileptic state than drugs with a single mechanism [2]. Researchers have also found that the epileptic state is a continuous disease process, and its pathogenesis may not be exactly the same during different occurrences of seizures Wasterlain et al. [167] reported that with repeated seizures and prolonged seizure time, GABA-A receptor activity on the postsynaptic membrane decreased, and the number and activity of NMDA receptors increased, resulting in an increase in the benzodiazepine-resistant epileptic state. The combined application of drugs targeting multiple neurotransmitters may have more obvious advantages. In particular, the combination of some newly listed antiepileptic drugs as additives can improve the prognosis of patients [2].
2. Clinical application: At present, the combined application of anti-epileptic status drugs mainly involves levetiracetam, ketamine, midazolam, phenytoin, barbiturates, steprool, and immunomodulatory drugs, but the most successful drugs are ketamine, midazolam, valproic acid, and levetiracetam. Niquet et al. [168] confirmed through animal experiments that ketamine + midazolam is the best choice when combined drugs are needed, if the treatment has no effect. Ketamine + midazolam + valproic acid can be used in combination.

Ketogenic Diet

This diet is mainly used for patients with ultra refractory epileptic status, and the dosage needs to be determined according to the ingredients of the ketogenic diet.

Mild Hypothermia Treatment

An increasing number of studies supports the inhibitory effect of mild hypothermia on the onset of status epileptic disorder. This effect has attracted the attention of clinicians and has gradually been applied to patients with refractory status epilepticus who have failed drug therapy or who have relapsed after drug withdrawal.

1. Indications: It is mainly used for patients with refractory status epilepticus whose seizures cannot be controlled by the above recommended drug treatment or whose seizures are controlled by the above drug treatment but relapse after withdrawal [169–172].
2. Usage: At the same time as sufficient anti-epileptic status drug treatment, an intravascular hypothermia cooling system or hypothermia therapy instrument is used for low-temperature induction, the body temperature is gradually lowered to the target temperature (31–35 °C), and the temperature is reheated to 36.5 °C after the seizure stops or the EEG bursts are suppressed for 24–48 hours. The rewarming process should not be faster than 0.5–1 °C/day.
3. Onset time: Under normal circumstances, the effect begins 3 to 48 hours after reaching the target body temperature, at which time there is widespread EEG inhibition.
4. Precautions: (1) EEG monitoring should be performed during mild hypothermia induction, treatment and rewarming. After rewarming, the anti-epileptic status drugs can be withdrawn if there is no recurrence, and the seizures can be controlled by oral antiepileptic seizure drugs if necessary. (2) When chills occur during mild hypothermia induction, it is necessary to stop mild hypothermia treatment and simultaneously rewarm the patient; (3) continued use of anti-epileptic status drugs (phenobarbital, midazolam, etc.) for mild hypothermia treatment; and (4) when the temperature is less than 30 °C, ventricular fibrillation, coagulation dysfunction, venous thrombosis and other side effects are more likely to occur [169–171]. In 2009, Cereda et al. [171] described the case of a patient with refractory status epilepticus who suffered from acute intestinal ischemic necrosis due to systemic hypothermia during mild hypothermia treatment and who required surgical resection of the appendix. In 2012, Lin et al. [170] described a case of transient hypokalemia during mild hypothermia. In 2013, Guilliams et al. [169] reported that electrolyte disorders (hypokalemia and hypernatremia) occurred in children during mild hypothermia. Although these adverse reactions return to normal after mild hypothermia treatment, blood gas, coagulation function, electrolytes, and routine blood tests should be monitored every 6 hours during mild hypothermia and rewarming. Weekly ultrasound examinations of the lower extremity veins (if intravascular cooling systems are used) are also necessary [169–172].

Electroconvulsive Therapy

Electroconvulsive therapy for epilepsy was described in the 1930s. In 2001, the American Psychiatric Association listed refractory epilepsy and refractory status epilepticus as indications for electroconvulsive therapy. In 2005, it was first included in the industry specification for the treatment of refractory status epilepticus in the UK guidelines for electroconvulsive therapy. In 2012, Ferlisi et al. [173] once again proposed the use of electroconvulsive therapy as an alternative method for the treatment of epileptic status and promoted the introduction of electroconvulsive therapy for epileptic states into the clinic [173–177].

1. Indications: refractory status epilepticus treated with the above methods after no response.
2. Parameters of electroconvulsive therapy: There are two ways to determine the amount of electroconvulsive therapy given: fixed and titrated doses (gradually increasing doses). Titrated dosing is recommended by the American Psychiatric Association, and because electroconvulsive therapy has the potential to induce convulsive and nonconvulsive status epilepticus, continuous EEG monitoring after electroconvulsive therapy is necessary. Due to the limited clinical application of electroconvulsive therapy in the treatment of status epilepticus, no treatment plan has been agreed upon [173–176].

EEG to Guide the Treatment of Status Epilepticus

The treatment of status epilepticus requires EEG guidance because: (1) The International League against Epilepsy requires that in the treatment of epileptic status, not only does the clinical epileptic status seizure need to be terminated but also the epileptoid discharge on the electroencephalogram needs to be terminated at the same time. Many patients with convulsive status epilepticus have stopped clinical seizures after medication, but their consciousness does not recover, suggesting that convulsive status epilepticus may transform into nonconvulsive status epilepticus. It is necessary to increase the dose to fully control the occurrence of epileptic status. At this time, EEG can detect the presence of nonconvulsive status epilepticus to aid in clinical decisions on further treatment. (2) Among the diagnostic criteria for nonconvulsive status epilepticus proposed by the International League against Epilepsy in 2015, EEG revealed that epileptic discharge is a necessary criterion. (3) Many anti-status epilepticus drugs do not work immediately and may need to be monitored for a period of time before their efficacy is known. This creates uncertainty in the judgment of clinical efficacy, but EEG is very sensitive to drug treatment, and changes in EEG can be seen almost immediately after treatment; in most cases, this can reflect the efficacy of the drug and improve the treatment of patients. (4) Maintenance treatment is required for a period of time after termination of status epilepticus, but the specific time has not been defined. The basic condition for stopping maintenance therapy is that the EEG results return to normal after medication.

(5) Patients whose status epilepticus is not terminated after medication may be treated with an insufficient dose, and they may also be resistant to the drug. Dual-frequency EEG showed that 40% was the maximum tolerated dose for the patient, and it was not appropriate to increase the dose of the drug. Therefore, when treating epileptic status with recommended drugs, synchronous EEG monitoring should be performed as much as possible where proper conditions exist to improve the effect of drug therapy [95].

References

1. Trinka E, Cock H, Hesdorffer D, et al. A definition and classification of status epilepticus--Report of the ILAE Task Force on Classification of Status Epilepticus. Epilepsia. 2015;56(10):1515–23.
2. Wang X, Li S. Refractory status epilepticus. Springer Singapore; 2017.
3. Harper JR, Varakis G. Children in adult intensive therapy units. Br Med J. 1970;1(5699):810–3.
4. Fincham RW, Wiley DE, Schottelius DD. Use of phenytoin serum levels in a case of status epilepticus. Neurology. 1976;26(9):879–81.
5. Bucking PH. Electroclinical correlations during anticonvulsive therapy of status epilepticus and chronic focal epilepsies using clonazepam. Schweiz Arch Neurol Neurochir Psychiatr. 1977;121(2):187–205.
6. Pilke A, Partinen M, Kovanen J. Status epilepticus and alcohol abuse: an analysis of 82 status epilepticus admissions. Acta Neurol Scand. 1984;70(6):443–50.
7. Snodgrass SM, Tsuburaya K, Ajmone-Marsan C. Clinical significance of periodic lateralized epileptiform discharges: relationship with status epilepticus. J Clin Neurophysiol. 1989;6(2):159–72.
8. Jagoda A, Riggio S. Refractory status epilepticus in adults. Ann Emerg Med. 1993;22(8):1337–48.
9. Bosque Varela P, Machegger L, Oellerer A, et al. Imaging of status epilepticus: making the invisible visible. A prospective study on 206 patients. Epilepsy Behav. 2023;141:109130.
10. Kubota T, Tsushima T, Al-Kindi S, et al. Association between status epilepticus and cardiorespiratory comorbidity in patients with epilepsy: a population-based study. Epilepsy Behav. 2022;135:108889.
11. Lu M, Faure M, Bergamasco A, et al. Epidemiology of status epilepticus in the United States: a systematic review. Epilepsy Behav. 2020;112:107459.
12. Bergin PS, Brockington A, Jayabal J, et al. Status epilepticus in Auckland, New Zealand: incidence, etiology, and outcomes. Epilepsia. 2019;60(8):1552–64.
13. Vijiala S, Alvarez V. Epidemiology of status epilepticus in a non-urban area in Switzerland. Acta Neurol Scand. 2021;143(4):413–20.
14. Guo Y, Yu L, He B, et al. Aetiological features of elderly patients with newly diagnosed symptomatic epilepsy in Western China. Biomed Res Int. 2018;2018:4104691.
15. Donnan AM, Schneider AL, Russ-Hall S, et al. Rates of status epilepticus and sudden unexplained death in epilepsy in people with genetic developmental and epileptic encephalopathies. Neurology. 2023;100(16):e1712–e22.
16. Khor SB, Lim KS, Fong SL, et al. Cause of mortality among people with epilepsy in Malaysia: a hospital-based study. Epilepsy Res. 2022;181:106887.
17. Jin Y, Liu Y, Xu X, et al. Mortality and causes of death among people with convulsive epilepsy in northwestern China. Epilepsy Behav. 2022;127:108492.
18. Deng B, Dai Y, Wang Q, et al. The clinical analysis of new-onset status epilepticus. Epilepsia Open. 2022;7(4):771–80.

19. Zhou B, Huang Y, Wang J, et al. The aetiology of convulsive status epilepticus: a study of 258 cases in Western China. Seizure. 2014;23(9):717–21.
20. Cornwall CD, Kroigard T, Kristensen JSS, et al. Outcomes and treatment approaches for super-refractory status epilepticus: a systematic review and meta-analysis. JAMA Neurol. 2023;80(9):959–68.
21. Aminoff MJ, Simon RP. Status epilepticus. Causes, clinical features and consequences in 98 patients. Am J Med. 1980;69(5):657–66.
22. Vincent FM, Vincent T. Lorazepam in myoclonic seizures after cardiac arrest. Ann Intern Med. 1986;104(4):586.
23. Young GB, Gilbert JJ, Zochodne DW. The significance of myoclonic status epilepticus in postanoxic coma. Neurology. 1990;40(12):1843–8.
24. Walker MC, Howard RS, Smith SJ, et al. Diagnosis and treatment of status epilepticus on a neurological intensive care unit. QJM. 1996;89(12):913–20.
25. Nordt SP, Clark RF. Midazolam: a review of therapeutic uses and toxicity. J Emerg Med. 1997;15(3):357–65.
26. Dolinak D, Smith C, Graham DI. Global hypoxia per se is an unusual cause of axonal injury. Acta Neuropathol. 2000;100(5):553–60.
27. Nutma S, Ruijter BJ, Beishuizen A, et al. Myoclonus in comatose patients with electrographic status epilepticus after cardiac arrest: corresponding EEG patterns, effects of treatment and outcomes. Resuscitation. 2023;186:109745.
28. Dragancea I, Backman S, Westhall E, et al. Outcome following postanoxic status epilepticus in patients with targeted temperature management after cardiac arrest. Epilepsy Behav. 2015;49:173–7.
29. De Stefano P, Kaplan PW, Quintard H, et al. Nonconvulsive status epilepticus following cardiac arrest: overlooked, untreated and misjudged. J Neurol. 2023;270(1):130–8.
30. Limotai C, Ingsathit A, Thadanipon K, et al. How and whom to monitor for seizures in an ICU: a systematic review and meta-analysis. Crit Care Med. 2019;47(4):e366–e73.
31. Zafar A. Prevalence, electroclinical spectrum and effect on the outcome of non-convulsive status epilepticus in critically ill patients; the utility of routine electroencephalogram. Epilepsy Behav. 2023;141:109144.
32. Andal VMD, Espiritu AI, Geronimo MAG, et al. Clinical features and outcomes of nonconvulsive status epilepticus in a developing country: a 5-year retrospective study. Epilepsy Behav. 2020;113:107547.
33. Pandian JD, Cascino GD, So EL, et al. Digital video-electroencephalographic monitoring in the neurological-neurosurgical intensive care unit: clinical features and outcome. Arch Neurol. 2004;61(7):1090–4.
34. Hui AC, Cheng C, Lam A, et al. Prognosis following Postanoxic myoclonus status epilepticus. Eur Neurol. 2005;54(1):10–3.
35. Lim ML, Lim RRZ, Tien JC, et al. Lance Adams syndrome after hypoxic cardiac arrest: a case report. A A Pract. 2022;16(8):e01605.
36. Brøchner AC, Lindholm P, Jensen MJ, et al. Post-hypoxic myoclonus status following out-of-hospital cardiac arrest-does it still predict a poor outcome? A retrospective study. Healthcare (Basel, Switzerland). 2021;10(1):41.
37. Orav K, Bosque Varela P, Pruwasser T, et al. Post-hypoxic status epilepticus – a distinct subtype of status epilepticus with poor prognosis. Epileptic Disord. 2023;25(6):823–32.
38. Nath U, Warren NM, Ali H. NMDA receptor encephalitis–expanding the clinical spectrum. BMJ Case Rep. 2011;2011
39. Motta E, Gołba A, Kazibutowska Z, et al. Anti-NMDA receptor encephalitis – case report. Neurol Neurochir Pol. 2012;46(3):288–93.
40. Lopinto-Khoury C, Sperling MR. Autoimmune status epilepticus. Curr Treat Options Neurol. 2013;15(5):545–56.
41. Chanson E, Bicilli E, Lauxerois M, et al. Anti-NMDA-R encephalitis: should we consider extreme delta brush as electrical status epilepticus? Neurophysiol Clin. 2016;46(1):17–25.

42. Kachlmeier A, Adams R, Zahalka T. Anti-NMDA receptor encephalitis in a 73-year-old female with secondary progressive multiple sclerosis: a case report. Epilepsy Behav Rep. 2023;24:100618.
43. Yao L, Yue W, Xunyi W, et al. Clinical features and long-term outcomes of seizures associated with autoimmune encephalitis: a follow-up study in East China. J Clin Neurosci. 2019;68:73–9.
44. Zhang Y, Deng C, Zhu L, et al. Predisposing factors and prognosis of status epilepticus in patients with autoimmune encephalitis. Medicine (Baltim). 2020;99(13):e19601.
45. Qu XP, Vidaurre J, Peng XL, et al. Seizure characteristics, outcome, and risk of epilepsy in pediatric anti-N-methyl-d-aspartate receptor encephalitis. Pediatr Neurol. 2020;105:35–40.
46. Pandit AK, Ihtisham K, Garg A, et al. Autoimmune encephalitis: a potentially reversible cause of status epilepticus, epilepsy, and cognitive decline. Ann Indian Acad Neurol. 2013;16(4):577–84.
47. Kaaden T, Madlener M, Angstwurm K, et al. Seizure semiology in antibody-associated autoimmune encephalitis. Neurol Neuroimmunol Neuroinflammat. 2022;9(6)
48. Sheikh Z, Hirsch LJ. A practical approach to in-hospital management of new-onset refractory status epilepticus/febrile infection related epilepsy syndrome. Front Neurol. 2023;14:1150496.
49. Alemdar M, Acar T, Dalkilic S. Anti-N-methyl D-aspartate receptor encephalitis presenting with the new-onset refractory status epilepticus. North Clin Istanb. 2023;10(3):385–9.
50. Eisele A, Schwager M, Bogli SY, et al. The role of neuronal antibodies in cryptogenic new onset refractory status epilepticus. Epilepsia. 2023;64(12):e229–e36.
51. Tainski de Azevedo AL, Tedesco Tonial C, Andrades GRH, et al. New-onset refractory status epilepticus (NORSE) in paediatric patients: causes, characteristics and outcomes. BMJ Neurol Open. 2022;4(2):e000314.
52. Lee Y, Ahn SJ, Lee HS, et al. Myelin oligodendrocyte glycoprotein antibody-associated encephalitis after severe acute respiratory syndrome coronavirus 2 infection: a case report and retrospective case reviews. Encephalitis. 2023;3(2):71–7.
53. Triplett J, Vijayan S, MacDonald A, et al. Fulminant anti-GAD antibody encephalitis presenting with status epilepticus requiring aggressive immunosuppression. J Neuroimmunol. 2018;323:119–24.
54. Monnerat BZ, Velasco TR, Nakano FN, et al. Opercular myoclonic-anarthric status epilepticus due to glutamic acid decarboxylase antibody-associated encephalitis. Epileptic Disord. 2013;15(3):342–6.
55. Mitchell JW, Valdoleiros SR, Jefferson S, et al. Autoimmune encephalitis as an increasingly recognised cause of non-convulsive status epilepticus: a retrospective, multicentre evaluation of patient characteristics and electroencephalography (EEG) results. Seizure. 2020;80:153–6.
56. Cikrikcili U, Ulusoy C, Turan S, et al. Non-convulsive status epilepticus associated with glutamic acid decarboxylase antibody. Clin EEG Neurosci. 2013;44(3):232–6.
57. Juneja P, Swor D. An evidence-based approach to diagnosis and prognosis in a Young woman with new-onset super-refractory status epilepticus: a case report. Case Rep Neurol. 2022;14(1):5–11.
58. Margraf NG, Dargvainiene J, Theel E, et al. Neurofilament light (NfL) as biomarker in serum and CSF in status epilepticus. J Neurol. 2023;270(4):2128–38.
59. Chen SH, O'Dea PK, Sianati B, et al. Role of responsive neurostimulation and immunotherapy in refractory epilepsy due to autoimmune encephalitis: a case report. Front Neurol. 2022;13:1028290.
60. Koh S, Kim YS, Kim MH, et al. Encephalitis with status epilepticus and stroke as complications of non-severe COVID-19 in a young female patient: a case report. BMC Neurol. 2022;22(1):253.
61. Gugger JJ, Husari K, Probasco JC, et al. New-onset refractory status epilepticus: a retrospective cohort study. Seizure. 2020;74:41–8.
62. Pasini E, Michelucci R. The heart and seizures: friends or enemies? J Clin Med. 2023;12(18)

63. Fain AC, Daruvala S, Ayub N. Pearls & oy-sters: severe case of ictal asystole in temporal lobe epilepsy. Neurology. 2023;101(9):e978–e81.
64. Kowalik A, Bauer J, Elger CE. Asystolic seizures. Nervenarzt. 1998;69(2):151–7.
65. Rocamora R, Kurthen M, Lickfett L, et al. Cardiac asystole in epilepsy: clinical and neurophysiologic features. Epilepsia. 2003;44(2):179–85.
66. Ryvlin P, Montavont A, Kahane P. Sudden unexpected death in epilepsy: from mechanisms to prevention. Curr Opin Neurol. 2006;19(2):194–9.
67. Leung H, Kwan P, Elger CE. Finding the missing link between ictal bradyarrhythmia, ictal asystole, and sudden unexpected death in epilepsy. Epilepsy Behav. 2006;9(1):19–30.
68. Winesett P, Feliciano CA, Tatum WOt. Temporal lobe seizures triggering recurrent syncope by ictal asystole. Epilepsy Behav. 2009;14(1):258–60.
69. Zubair S, Arshad AB, Saeed B, et al. Ictal asystole–late manifestation of partial epilepsy and importance of cardiac pacemaker. Seizure. 2009;18(6):457–61.
70. Bregianni M, Lagarde S, Pizzo F, et al. Focal seizures producing loss of wakefulness without ictal asystole: does temporal lobe syncope exist? Epilepsy Res. 2022;186:107015.
71. Casciato S, Quarato PP, Mascia A, et al. Ictal asystole in drug-resistant focal epilepsy: two decades of experience from an epilepsy monitoring unit. Brain Sci. 2020;10(7):443.
72. Tenyi D, Gyimesi C, Kupo P, et al. Ictal asystole: a systematic review. Epilepsia. 2017;58(3):356–62.
73. Khalil M, Shukralla AA, Kilbride R, et al. Ictal asystole during long-term video-EEG; semiology, localization, and intervention. Epilepsy Behav Rep. 2021;15:100416.
74. Schuele SU, Bermeo AC, Alexopoulos AV, et al. Video-electrographic and clinical features in patients with ictal asystole. Neurology. 2007;69(5):434–41.
75. Negishi Y, Aoki Y, Itomi K, et al. SCN8A-related developmental and epileptic encephalopathy with ictal asystole requiring cardiac pacemaker implantation. Brain Dev. 2021;43(7):804–8.
76. Shmuely S, Surges R, Helling RM, et al. Cardiac arrhythmias in Dravet syndrome: an observational multicenter study. Ann Clin Transl Neurol. 2020;7(4):462–73.
77. Wali A, Siddiqui F. Focal cortical dysplasia with prolonged ictal asystole, a case report. Clin Neurophysiol Pract. 2021;6:10–5.
78. Kasper BS, Kraus C, Schwarz M, et al. A novel splice variant expands the LAMC3-associated cortical phenotype to frontal only polymicrogyria and adult-onset epilepsy. Am J Med Genet A. 2020;182(11):2761–4.
79. Al-Awwad AA, Katyal R, Herren CL. Ictal asystole in temporal lobe epilepsy: a possible cause of sudden unexplained death – a case report. Neurodiagn J. 2018;58(4):213–7.
80. Rossetti AO, Dworetzky BA, Madsen JR, et al. Ictal asystole with convulsive syncope mimicking secondary generalisation: a depth electrode study. J Neurol Neurosurg Psychiatry. 2005;76(6):885–7.
81. D'Souza CE, Feyissa AM. GAD65 antibody-associated autoimmune epilepsy with unique independent bitemporal-onset ictal asystole. Epileptic Disord. 2018;20(3):204–8.
82. Suski J, Ho R, Nei M. Ictal asystole in a patient with posterior reversible encephalopathy syndrome (PRES) and seizures. Epileptic Disord. 2017;19(3):374–8.
83. Legriel S, Bresson E, Deye N, et al. Cardiac arrest in patients managed for convulsive status epilepticus: characteristics, predictors, and outcome. Crit Care Med. 2018;46(8):e751–e60.
84. Leung H, Schindler K, Kwan P, et al. Asystole induced by electrical stimulation of the left cingulate gyrus. Epileptic Disord. 2007;9(1):77–81.
85. Lagarde S, Singh R, Bartolomei F, et al. Insular interictal positron emission tomography hypometabolism in patients with ictal asystole. Epilepsia. 2021;62(8):e117–e22.
86. Giovannini G, Meletti S. Ictal asystole as the first presentation of epilepsy: a case report and systematic literature review. Epilepsy Behav Case Rep. 2014;2:136–41.
87. Strzelczyk A, Bauer S, Knake S, et al. Ictal asystole in temporal lobe epilepsy before and after pacemaker implantation. Epileptic Disord. 2008;10(1):39–44.

88. Hagiwara K, Okadome T, Mukaino T, et al. Ictal asystole as a manifestation of pure insular epilepsy. Seizure. 2021;91:192–5.
89. Nguyen-Michel VH, Adam C, Dinkelacker V, et al. Characterization of seizure-induced syncopes: EEG, ECG, and clinical features. Epilepsia. 2014;55(1):146–55.
90. Kohno R, Abe H, Akamatsu N, et al. Long-term follow-up of ictal asystole in temporal lobe epilepsy: is permanent pacemaker therapy needed? J Cardiovasc Electrophysiol. 2016;27(8):930–6.
91. Bianco M, Breviario S, Fraccalini T, et al. Epilepsy and syncope – a case report and narrative review of arrhythmias connected to temporal lobe epilepsy. J Electrocardiol. 2022;73:76–8.
92. Zhang X, Cui L, Lin W. Cardiac arrest in frontal lobe epilepsy: a potential cause of sudden unexpected death in epilepsy. Neurol India. 2021;69(3):737–9.
93. Mehvari J, Fadaie F, Omidi S, et al. Cardiac arrest associated with epileptic seizures: a case report with simultaneous EEG and ECG. Epilepsy Behav Case Rep. 2014;2:145–51.
94. Etgen T, Neuberger HR. Reflex syncope-or more?: Ictal asystole! Inn Med (Heidelb). 2022;63(10):1085–91.
95. Serafini A, Gelisse P, Reana V, et al. Cardiac asystole during a cluster of right temporo-parietal seizures. Seizure. 2011;20(2):181–3.
96. Bestawros M, Darbar D, Arain A, et al. Ictal asystole and ictal syncope: insights into clinical management. Circ Arrhythm Electrophysiol. 2015;8(1):159–64.
97. van Westrhenen A, Shmuely S, Surges R, et al. Timing of syncope in ictal asystole as a guide when considering pacemaker implantation. J Cardiovasc Electrophysiol. 2021;32(11):3019–26.
98. Sowden N, Booth C, Kaye G. Syncope, epilepsy and ictal asystole: a case series and narrative review. Heart Lung Circ. 2022;31(1):25–31.
99. Benoit J, Martin F, Thomas P. Musicogenic epilepsy with ictal asystole: a video-EEG case report. Epileptic Disord. 2021;23(4):649–54.
100. Enkiri SA, Ghavami F, Anyanwu C, et al. New onset left frontal lobe seizure presenting with ictal asystole. Seizure. 2011;20(10):817–9.
101. Mbizvo GK, Derry C, Davenport R. Ictal asystole: a diagnostic and management conundrum. J R Coll Physicians Edinb. 2019;49(2):128–31.
102. Duplyakov D, Golovina G, Lyukshina N, et al. Syncope, seizure-induced bradycardia and asystole: two cases and review of clinical and pathophysiological features. Seizure. 2014;23(7):506–11.
103. Russo A, Francione S, Martinoni M, et al. Low-grade tumour over the left temporal neocortex and ictal asystole: network and surgical implications. Epileptic Disord. 2021;23(5):775–85.
104. Ballendine S, Shahab I, Perez-Careta M, et al. Resolution of ictal bradycardia and asystole following temporal lobectomy: a case report, and review of available cases using pacemakers. Epilepsy Behav Rep. 2019;12:100333.
105. Schuele SU, Bermeo AC, Locatelli E, et al. Ictal asystole: a benign condition? Epilepsia. 2008;49(1):168–71.
106. Taylor FM. Myoclonic seizure in infancy and childhood. Tex State J Med. 1952;48(9):647–9.
107. Ruijter BJ, Keijzer HM, Tjepkema-Cloostermans MC, et al. Treating rhythmic and periodic EEG patterns in comatose survivors of cardiac arrest. N Engl J Med. 2022;386(8):724–34.
108. Hirsch LJ, Claassen J, Mayer SA, et al. Stimulus-induced rhythmic, periodic, or ictal discharges (SIRPIDs): a common EEG phenomenon in the critically ill. Epilepsia. 2004;45(2):109–23.
109. Van Straten AF, Fesler JR, Hakimi R, et al. SIRPIDs: prevalence and outcome in critically ill patients. J Clin Neurophysiol. 2014;31(5):418–21.
110. Fodale V, La Monaca E. Propofol infusion syndrome: an overview of a perplexing disease. Drug Saf. 2008;31(4):293–303.
111. Paramsothy J, Gutlapalli SD, Ganipineni VDP, et al. Propofol in ICU settings: understanding and managing anti-arrhythmic, pro-arrhythmic effects, and Propofol infusion syndrome. Cureus. 2023;15:e40456.

112. Xuan G, Zhang Y, Cui J, et al. Propofol-associated serious adverse events: an analysis of the FAERS database. Biotechnol Genet Eng Rev. 2023;1–14
113. Park N, Ha TS. Successful treatment of propofol-related infusion syndrome in critically ill patient receiving low-dose propofol infusion: a case report. Acute Crit Care. 2023;38(1):144–8.
114. Barajas MB, Brunner SD, Wang A, et al. Propofol toxicity in the developing mouse heart mitochondria. Pediatr Res. 2022;92(5):1341–9.
115. Hemphill S, McMenamin L, Bellamy MC, et al. Propofol infusion syndrome: a structured literature review and analysis of published case reports. Br J Anaesth. 2019;122(4):448–59.
116. Dundee JW. New i.v. anaesthetics. Br J Anaesth. 1979;51(7):641–8.
117. Gepts E, Claeys AM, Camu F. Pharmacokinetics of propofol ('Diprivan') administered by continuous intravenous infusion in man. A preliminary report. Postgrad Med J. 1985;61(Suppl 3):51–2.
118. Raff M, Harrison GG. The screening of propofol in MHS swine. Anesth Analg. 1989;68(6):750–1.
119. NØRreslet J, Wahlgreen C. Propofol infusion for sedation of children. Crit Care Med. 1990;18(8):890–1.
120. El-Ebiary M, Torres A, Ramirez J, et al. Lipid deposition during the long-term infusion of propofol. Crit Care Med. 1995;23(11):1928–30.
121. Bray RJ. Propofol infusion syndrome in children. Paediatr Anaesth. 1998;8(6):491–9.
122. Hatch DJ. Propofol-infusion syndrome in children. Lancet. 1999;353(9159):1117–8.
123. Kelly DF. Propofol-infusion syndrome. J Neurosurg. 2001;95(6):925–6.
124. Wolf A, Weir P, Segar P, et al. Impaired fatty acid oxidation in propofol infusion syndrome. Lancet. 2001;357(9256):606–7.
125. Bray RJ. The propofol infusion syndrome in infants and children: can we predict the risk? Curr Opin Anaesthesiol. 2002;15(3):339–42.
126. Kang TM. Propofol infusion syndrome in critically ill patients. Ann Pharmacother. 2002;36(9):1453–6.
127. Ernest D, French C. Propofol infusion syndrome— report of an adult fatality. Anaesth Intensive Care. 2004;32(3):316–9.
128. Vasile B, Rasulo F, Candiani A, et al. The pathophysiology of propofol infusion syndrome: a simple name for a complex syndrome. Intensive Care Med. 2003;29(9):1417–25.
129. Roberts RJ, Barletta JF, Fong JJ, et al. Incidence of propofol-related infusion syndrome in critically ill adults: a prospective, multicenter study. Crit Care. 2009;13(5):R169.
130. Iyer VN, Hoel R, Rabinstein AA. Propofol infusion syndrome in patients with refractory status epilepticus: an 11-year clinical experience*. Crit Care Med. 2009;37(12):3024–30.
131. Li WK, Chen XJC, Altshuler D, et al. The incidence of propofol infusion syndrome in critically-ill patients. J Crit Care. 2022;71:154098.
132. Singh A, Anjankar AP. Propofol-related infusion syndrome: a clinical review. Cureus. 2022;14:e30383.
133. Romero PC, Morales RM, Donaire RL, et al. Severe lactic acidosis caused by propofol infusion: report of one case. Rev Med Chile. 2008;136(1):88–92.
134. Calvano J, Paluska MR, Armijo AJ, et al. Propofol-related infusion syndrome in a child with refractory status epilepticus: successful resuscitation with Veno-arterial extracorporeal membrane oxygenation, continuous renal replacement therapy, and therapeutic plasma exchange. Cureus. 2023;15:e47866.
135. Laquay N, Prieur S, Greff B, et al. Propofol infusion syndrome. Ann Fr Anesth Reanim. 2010;29(5):377–86.
136. Cannon ML, Glazier SS, Bauman LA. Metabolic acidosis, rhabdomyolysis, and cardiovascular collapse after prolonged propofol infusion. J Neurosurg. 2001;95(6):1053–6.
137. Hanna JP, Ramundo ML. Rhabdomyolysis and hypoxia associated with prolonged propofol infusion in children. Neurology. 1998;50(1):301–3.
138. Sabsovich I, Rehman Z, Yunen J, et al. Propofol infusion syndrome: a case of increasing morbidity with traumatic brain injury. Am J Crit Care. 2007;16(1):82–5.

139. Karasawa S, Nakada T-a, Mori N, et al. Case report: sustained mitochondrial damage in cardiomyocytes in patients with severe propofol infusion syndrome. F1000Res. 2020;9:712.
140. Mallard JM, Rieser TM, Peterson NW. Propofol infusion-like syndrome in a dog. Can Vet J. 2018;59(11):1216–22.
141. Barajas MB, Wang A, Griffiths KK, et al. Modeling propofol-induced cardiotoxicity in the isolated-perfused newborn mouse heart. Physiol Rep. 2022;10(15):e15402.
142. Subirà González A, Fernández Morales M, Sánchez Royo E, et al. Propofol infusion syndrome; are high doses always required? Revista Española de Anestesiología y Reanimación (English Edition). 2020;67(3):163–6.
143. Eriksen J, Povey HM. A case of suspected non-neurosurgical adult fatal propofol infusion syndrome. Acta Anaesthesiol Scand. 2006;50(1):117–9.
144. Lopez N, Correa A, Ammann R, et al. Propofol infusion syndrome in a refractory epileptic status case. Rev Chil Pediatr. 2018;89(3):384–90.
145. Shimada M, Sakamoto M. Propofol infusion syndrome treated successfully by early diagnosis. Kyobu Geka. 2020;73(13):1061–4.
146. Guitton C, Gabillet L, Latour P, et al. Propofol infusion syndrome during refractory status epilepticus in a young adult: successful ECMO resuscitation. Neurocrit Care. 2011;15(1):139–45.
147. Da-Silva SS, Wong R, Coquillon P, et al. Partial-exchange blood transfusion: an effective method for preventing mortality in a child with Propofol infusion syndrome. Pediatrics. 2010;125(6):e1493–e9.
148. Levin PD, Levin V, Weissman C, et al. Therapeutic plasma exchange as treatment for propofol infusion syndrome. J Clin Apher. 2015;30(5):311–3.
149. Sun J, Zhang B, Geng Q, et al. Dexmedetomidine alleviates Propofol infusion syndrome-induced myocardial injury through inhibiting Ferroptosis associated with accumulation of reactive oxygen species. Ann Clin Lab Sci. 2024;54(1):86–91.
150. Kilicaslan B, Akinci SB, Saricaoglu F, et al. Effects of coenzyme Q10 in a propofol infusion syndrome model of rabbits. Asian Biomed. 2023;17(4):173–84.
151. Shangguan Y, Liao H, Wang X. Clonazepam in the treatment of status epilepticus. Expert Rev Neurother. 2015;15(7):733–40.
152. Zhou X, Fang L, Tong X, et al. Clinical efficacy of clonazepam in the treatment of status epilepticus. Pak J Pharm Sci. 2022;35(3(Special)):891–5.
153. Rundfeldt C, Loscher W. The pharmacology of imepitoin: the first partial benzodiazepine receptor agonist developed for the treatment of epilepsy. CNS Drugs. 2014;28(1):29–43.
154. Kravljanac R, Djuric M, Jankovic B, et al. Etiology, clinical course and response to the treatment of status epilepticus in children: a 16-year single-center experience based on 602 episodes of status epilepticus. Eur J Paediatr Neurol. 2015;19(5):584–90.
155. Kunst S, Rojo M, Schmidbauer ML, et al. Phenobarbital in super-refractory status epilepticus (PIRATE): a retrospective, multicenter analysis. Epilepsia. 2023;64(6):1482–92.
156. Zheng F, Du C, Wang X. Levetiracetam for the treatment of status epilepticus. Expert Rev Neurother. 2015;15(10):1113–21.
157. Wang M, Jiang L, Tang X. Levetiracetam is associated with decrease in subclinical epileptiform discharges and improved cognitive functions in pediatric patients with autism spectrum disorder. Neuropsychiatr Dis Treat. 2017;13:2321–6.
158. Yasiry Z, Shorvon SD. The relative effectiveness of five antiepileptic drugs in treatment of benzodiazepine-resistant convulsive status epilepticus: a meta-analysis of published studies. Seizure. 2014;23(3):167–74.
159. Rossetti AO, Lowenstein DH. Management of refractory status epilepticus in adults: still more questions than answers. Lancet Neurol. 2011;10(10):922–30.
160. Riviello JJ Jr, Claassen J, LaRoche SM, et al. Treatment of status epilepticus: an international survey of experts. Neurocrit Care. 2013;18(2):193–200.
161. Fang Y, Wang X. Ketamine for the treatment of refractory status epilepticus. Seizure. 2015;30:14–20.

162. Orinx C, Legros B, Gaspard N. Recent antiseizure medications in the intensive care unit. Minerva Anestesiol. 2017;83(8):878–87.
163. Gaspard N, Foreman B, Judd LM, et al. Intravenous ketamine for the treatment of refractory status epilepticus: a retrospective multicenter study. Epilepsia. 2013;54(8):1498–503.
164. Rosati A, Ilvento L, L'Erario M, et al. Efficacy of ketamine in refractory convulsive status epilepticus in children: a protocol for a sequential design, multicentre, randomised, controlled, open-label, non-profit trial (KETASER01). BMJ Open. 2016;6(6):e011565.
165. Borris DJ, Bertram EH, Kapur J. Ketamine controls prolonged status epilepticus. Epilepsy Res. 2000;42(2–3):117–22.
166. Synowiec AS, Singh DS, Yenugadhati V, et al. Ketamine use in the treatment of refractory status epilepticus. Epilepsy Res. 2013;105(1–2):183–8.
167. Wasterlain CG, Naylor DE, Liu H, et al. Trafficking of NMDA receptors during status epilepticus: therapeutic implications. Epilepsia. 2013;54 Suppl 6(0 6):78–80.
168. Niquet J, Baldwin R, Norman K, et al. Midazolam-ketamine dual therapy stops cholinergic status epilepticus and reduces Morris water maze deficits. Epilepsia. 2016;57(9):1406–15.
169. Guilliams K, Rosen M, Buttram S, et al. Hypothermia for pediatric refractory status epilepticus. Epilepsia. 2013;54(9):1586–94.
170. Lin JJ, Lin KL, Hsia SH, et al. Therapeutic hypothermia for febrile infection-related epilepsy syndrome in two patients. Pediatr Neurol. 2012;47(6):448–50.
171. Cereda C, Berger MM, Rossetti AO. Bowel ischemia: a rare complication of thiopental treatment for status epilepticus. Neurocrit Care. 2009;10(3):355–8.
172. Legriel S, Lemiale V, Schenck M, et al. Hypothermia for neuroprotection in convulsive status epilepticus. N Engl J Med. 2016;375(25):2457–67.
173. Ferlisi M, Shorvon S. The outcome of therapies in refractory and super-refractory convulsive status epilepticus and recommendations for therapy. Brain. 2012;135(Pt 8):2314–28.
174. Gazdag G, Dragasek J, Takacs R, et al. Use of electroconvulsive therapy in central-eastern European countries: an overview. Psychiatr Danub. 2017;29(2):136–40.
175. Antosik-Wojcinska AZ, Dominiak M, Mierzejewski P, et al. Changes in the practice of electroconvulsive therapy in Poland: a Nationwide survey comparing data between 2005 and 2020. Neuropsychiatr Dis Treat. 2021;17:605–12.
176. Yang X, Wang X. Potential mechanisms and clinical applications of mild hypothermia and electroconvulsive therapy on refractory status epilepticus. Expert Rev Neurother. 2015;15(2):135–44.
177. Liu T, Wang Z, Dong M, et al. MicroRNA-26a inhibits cell proliferation and invasion by targeting FAM98A in breast cancer. Oncol Lett. 2021;21(5):367.

Chapter 7
Diagnosis and Treatment of Epilepsy Comorbidities

Yanbing Han, Yixue Gu, Yin Yan, Guohui Jiang, and Xin Tian

7.1 Effect of Sleep Apnea on Epilepsy

Epilepsy is closely related to sleep, and the two can affect each other [1]. Most seizures and sudden unexpected deaths in patients with epilepsy occur during sleep [2, 3]. In turn, seizures directly disrupt sleep and induce fragmented sleep at night, daytime somnolence, fatigue, cognitive impairment, and abnormal behavior [4–6]. Sleep deprivation can induce seizures, and both can occur at the same time, becoming the most common epilepsy comorbidity. Of comorbidities, sleep apnea has the most direct impact on epilepsy. As one of the most common sleep disorders in patients with epilepsy, obstructive sleep apnea (OSA) can increase the frequency of seizures and alleviate seizures after treatment [7, 8]. Therefore, understanding the

Y. Han
Department of Neurology, First Affiliated Hospital of Kunming Medical University, Kunming, China

Y. Gu · X. Tian
Department of Neurology, The First Affiliated Hospital of Chongqing Medical University, Chongqing, China

Y. Yan (✉)
Epilepsy rehabilitation Center, Beibei Hospital of Chongqing Medical University, Chongqing, China

G. Jiang
Department of Neurology, Affiliated Hospital of North Sichuan Medical College, Nanchong, Sichuan, China

X. Wang, L. Zhou (eds.), *Pharmacological Treatment of Epileptic Seizures*, https://doi.org/10.1007/978-981-96-8520-2_7

influence of OSA on epilepsy is particularly important for the diagnosis and treatment of epilepsy.

7.1.1 *Epidemiology of Sleep Apnea in Epilepsy Patients*

The average prevalence of OSA is 5% in females and 14% in males [9], and this proportion increases in all types of epilepsy patients. Currently, compared to those with OSA, there are few data on the prevalence of CSA in patients with epilepsy [10–12]. Al-Abri et al. [10] confirmed OSA through questionnaires, interviews, screening, and polysomnography (PSG) monitoring of 100 adult epilepsy patients who attended the Sultan Qaboos University Hospital Neurology Clinic and found that only 9% of them had OSA. The prevalence of OSA in epilepsy patients with SA symptoms was greater when PSG was used. Specifically, Pornsriniyom et al. [11] investigated 132 adult patients with epilepsy referred to the Cleveland Clinic for PSG and identified 76 patients (57.6%) with OSA. The incidence of OSA in adult patients with epilepsy is far greater than that in juveniles. Moreover, Gogou et al. [13] described 40 children with idiopathic epilepsy and 27 healthy children who underwent overnight polysomnography, and the prevalence of OSA was significantly greater in the epilepsy group (35%) than in the healthy group (7.4%). In addition, Shaheen et al. [14] included a total of 26 age- and sex-matched Egyptian children with epilepsy and 12 healthy individuals who underwent PSG in a study; eleven patients (42.3%) were found to have OSA, but none of the healthy children developed OSA. In 2017, a meta-analysis involving a total of 26 studies, including epilepsy patients aged 3–76 years from 8 countries in Europe and Asia, who all completed PSG, was performed. The results showed that the prevalence of OSA ranged from 7.7% to 75.7%, with a high level of heterogeneity [15]. Further subgroup analysis indicated that males were more susceptible to OSA than females were (44.8% vs. 25.5%), and adults were more vulnerable to OSA than children were (40.1% vs. 26.3%). However, the prevalence of OSA was not found to be significantly different for different seizure types, patients with refractory epilepsy, or patients receiving different numbers of antiseizure medications (ASMs) [15]. Furthermore, a prospective study in 84 children with epilepsy by Jain et al. [16] demonstrated that there was no significant correlation between the incidence of OSA and seizure type. However, Scharf et al. [17] reported that patients with generalized epilepsy have a greater risk of OSA than those with focal epilepsy. Nevertheless, McCarter et al. [18] reported that the incidence of focal seizures was greater in patients with OSA. From this perspective, these studies contradict each other. However, further studies are needed to confirm these findings and to clarify the relationship between epilepsy or seizure type and OSA [15, 18, 19].

At some points, mild OSA appears to be more common in epilepsy patients than in healthy individuals. After reviewing the clinical features of 86 patients with epilepsy comorbid with OSA, Cheng [20] established that 38 patients (44.2%) had mild OSA, 25 patients (29.1%) had moderate OSA, and 23 patients (26.7%) had severe OSA, indicating that mild OSA was the most common condition. Manni et al. [21] prospectively enrolled 283 adult epilepsy patients for OSA screening and reported that the incidence of OSA was mild in 66.6%, moderate in 22.2%, and severe in 11.1% of patients. In addition, a meta-analysis conducted by Lin et al. [15] in 2017 reported that the prevalence of mild OSA was significantly greater than that of moderate or severe OSA in adult patients with epilepsy. This is especially true in patients with refractory epilepsy [19].

7.1.2 The Impact of Sleep Apnea on Seizures

7.1.2.1 Sleep Apnea as an Underlying Etiology of Epilepsy

Several studies have shown that SA can induce seizures, and seizures can be stopped or reduced after treatment with SA, suggesting that SA may be a potential cause or risk factor for epilepsy [22, 23]. Miliauskas et al. [24] described a 54-year-old male with nocturnal seizures, daytime somnolence, and morning headaches whose symptoms were not relieved but were aggravated after treatment with valproate acid and clonazepam. Through nocturnal PSG monitoring, there were ten CSA events all night, two of which were accompanied by severe decreases in blood oxygen saturation and generalized tonic-clonic seizures (GTCSs). The first SA lasted for 180 s until the onset of epileptic tonic–clonic seizures. The second SA was detected 20 min later and lasted for 200 s; the blood oxygen saturation decreased to 65%, which was also terminated by the GTCS. After continuous positive airway pressure (CPAP) treatment, the seizures disappeared completely in this patient. One-year follow-up after stopping ASM revealed no seizures, and the original daytime drowsiness and headache were relieved. Hollinger et al. [25] investigated 557 patients with OSA and reported that 29 patients had seizures, 21 of whom had seizures or status epilepticus that appeared for the first time, consistent with the onset of OSA symptoms. Among the 12 epilepsy patients treated with Continuous positive airway pressure (CPAP), 4 had a significant decrease in seizure frequency. Among them, one patient was completely seizure-free after being treated with CPAP alone without using any ASM.

7.1.2.2 Sleep Apnea Aggravates Seizures

SA can aggravate or induce nocturnal seizures. In a large-sample retrospective case study, SA occurred in 78.9% of epilepsy patients only during nocturnal sleep, and the incidence of nocturnal seizures decreased significantly after the improvement of SA [26]. Furthermore, the severity of epilepsy seems to be related to OSA. According to a previous report, the frequency of seizures in children with OSA was much greater than that in children without OSA [14]. Similarly, Jain et al. [16] performed a prospective study on 84 children from the USA and reported that the prevalence of OSA in children with refractory epilepsy whose seizure frequency was >1 seizure/month was markedly greater than that in those whose seizure frequency was 0–1 seizure/month. Moreover, a study on elderly patients [7] revealed that individuals with refractory epilepsy had a greater apnea-hypopnea index (AHI) than did those without refractory epilepsy, even when age, neck circumference, number of ASMs used, and frequency of nocturnal seizures were similar.

7.1.2.3 Sleep Apnea Increases Subclinical Epileptiform Discharges

Nguyen-Michel et al. [27] described a 43-year-old female who experienced refractory left temporal lobe epilepsy after trauma, with daytime partial and secondary generalized seizures at night. MRI of the brain revealed no specific signs. PSG displayed severe OSA syndrome, in which the AHI was 75/h and the lowest oxygen saturation was 72%. Seven-day vEEG monitoring revealed that symmetrical diffuse high-amplitude spike waves of 1.5–2.5 Hz appeared simultaneously when OSA occurred. These epileptiform discharges began to appear 10 s after the onset of OSA and terminated approximately 2.5 s before or at the end of SA. After CPAP treatment, the wave disappeared, but after treatment stopped, epileptiform discharges immediately appeared. Although this is only a case report, it is highly suspected that OSA can increase epileptiform discharges on EEG.

In addition, Miano et al. [23] validated these results in children. PSG was performed in 298 children with sleep-disordered breathing, and epileptiform discharges were recorded in 16.1% of the children with OSA. Obviously, these discharges were mostly in the occipital lobe in the preschooler group. With the maturity of the nervous system, the discharge area gradually transferred to the frontal lobe, which had the greatest impact on the decrease in oxygen saturation. However, due to a lack of normal controls and the inclusion of children with sleep breathing disorders, the results of this study have yet to be verified.

7.1.3 *Effect of Seizures on Sleep Apnea*

Currently, most studies have focused on the fact that OSA can induce or aggravate seizures, but there are few studies on the effects of seizures on OSA. Ismayilova et al. [28] compared the sleep problems of 208 adult epilepsy patients with those of 212 healthy controls and found that patients with a long duration of seizures and frequent use of more than one ASM drug were more likely to develop SA. However, the assessment of sleep disorders in this study was mainly based on scales, which may have led to bias due to a lack of PSG data.

Vagus nerve stimulation (VNS) is a minimally invasive treatment for refractory epilepsy. Although the side effects are usually small, there are occasional reports of SA complications [29, 30]. Pérez-Carbonell et al. [31] reported that 3 patients with refractory epilepsy developed sleep breathing disorders after VNS treatment, of whom 2 had SA and 1 had wheezing. Kim et al. [32] performed VNS treatment on 24 drug-resistant epilepsy patients, among whom 5 patients had new mild OSA and 4 patients had worse OSA. Undoubtedly, these reports indicate that SA may occur after VNS treatment. In addition, Malow et al. [33] directly revealed the relationship between the two. In 4 patients with epilepsy, apnea and hypopnea were more frequent during VNS activation than during nonactivation. Decreasing stimulation frequency, but not reducing stimulation intensity, pulse width or time, can improve VNS-related apnea and hypopnea.

7.1.4 The Effect of Sleep Apnea on Sudden Unexpected Death in Epilepsy (SUDEP)

At present, the etiology and mechanism of SUDEP remain unclear [34]. Since SUDEP mostly occurs during nocturnal sleep [2, 3], some scholars have proposed that SA may induce SUDEP [34]. So [35] described a patient who developed respiratory depression after seizures under electroencephalogram (ECG) monitoring, followed by cardiac arrest. However, there was no evidence of airway obstruction or pulmonary edema, suggesting that central respiratory depression may be a potential risk factor for SUDEP. The findings of CSA- and hypopnea-induced death in a sheep model of epilepsy further supported the relationship between SA and SUDEP [36]. After summarizing the cases of SUDEP, Jallon [37] proposed that CSA, arrhythmia, and irreversible neurogenic pulmonary edema may lead to sudden death in epilepsy patients.

The revised SUDEP-7 list (rSUDEP-7) is widely used to assess the risk of SUDEP. Chen [20] reported that severe OSA was significantly correlated with an rSUDEP-7 score ≥ 5, suggesting that severe OSA was associated with an increased risk of SUDEP. As a treatable disease, OSA may be a modifiable risk factor for SUDEP. To further verify the reliability and accuracy of the rSUDEP-7 scale in assessing the risk of sudden death in OSA patients with epilepsy, Phabphal et al. [38] monitored 95 epilepsy patients over 15 years old by PSG and found 10 patients with moderate OSA and 7 patients with severe OSA. Although the rSUDEP-7 scale was used to evaluate the OSA and AHI scores, the results showed that there was no correlation between OSA, the AHI score, or the total rSUDEP-7 score or an rSUDEP-7 score >5. Doubtlessly, the pathophysiology behind SUDEP appears to be more complex than initially assumed. Therefore, further studies on SUDEP are needed to clarify the underlying mechanisms and susceptibility factors involved.

7.1.5 Diagnosis

The incidence and prevalence of CSA in epilepsy patients are relatively low, and CSA mainly occurs after seizures; therefore, its treatment is mainly based on the treatment of epilepsy [39]. Therefore, this review primarily focuses on the diagnosis and treatment of OSA in epilepsy patients. When epilepsy patients have daytime drowsiness and snoring, they should be screened immediately for OSA. PSG is helpful in the diagnosis of SA in epilepsy patients, and the combination of video PSG and long-term video-EEG monitoring (pVEEG-M) can improve and accelerate the detection of SA and severity in epilepsy patients [40].

7.1.5.1 Daytime Sleepiness in Epilepsy Patients Cannot Be Simply Attributed to Epilepsy, and the Side Effects of OSA and ASMs Must Be Taken into Account

Clinically, somnolence and cognitive dysfunction caused by OSA in epilepsy patients are often ignored. Manni et al. [21] described the clinical characteristics of 283 epilepsy patients and revealed that 23.1% of epilepsy patients with OSA experienced daytime sleepiness, which was much greater than that of epilepsy patients without OSA (9.0%), and treatment with CPAP could reduce daytime sleepiness. These findings suggest that daytime drowsiness may be caused by OSA in these epilepsy patients. Similarly, Malow et al. [41] examined the clinical characteristics of 158 epilepsy patients and 68 neurological patients without epilepsy and revealed that daytime sleepiness was more common and severe in epilepsy patients than in patients without epilepsy. Consequently, the authors attributed these results to the existence of SA rather than to the use of ASMs in these epilepsy patients. Therefore, when epilepsy patients exhibit daytime sleepiness, we should consider the possibility of OSA and pay attention to the possibility that OSA may cause daytime sleepiness in epilepsy patients.

In addition, some ASMs can also affect the sleep structures of epilepsy patients. For example, phenobarbital causes shortened sleep latency (SL), decreased sleep efficiency (SE), reduced awakening time, increased N1 and N2 phases of Non-Rapid Eye Movement Sleep (NREM) sleep, an unchanged N3 phase, decreased REM sleep, and increased daytime sleepiness, compared to controls. Carbamazepine results in decreased or unchanged SL and SE; decreased or increased awakening time, decreased or unchanged NREM sleep N1 phase, increased or unchanged N3 phase, unchanged N2 phase, and has no effect on REM phase or daytime sleepiness. Phenytoin can lead to a decrease in SL and SE, a decrease or no change in awakening time, a decrease or increase in N1 and N3 phases of NREM sleep, a decrease in N2 phase, a decrease in REM phase, and an increase in daytime somnolence. Valproate sodium decreased or did not change awakening time; increased or did not change REM or daytime somnolence; and had no effect on SL, SE, or the N1, N2, or N3 stages of NREM sleep. Gabapentin decreases the SL, awakening time, and N1 phase of NREM sleep and increases the N3 phase of REM, daytime somnolence, SE, and NREM sleep but has no effect on the N2 phase of NREM sleep. Lamotrigine can reduce or result in no changes in the N3 phase of NREM sleep and increase or cause no changes in REM sleep and has no effect on SL, SE, awakening time, the N1 phase of NREM sleep, the N2 phase, or daytime sleepiness [42, 43]. Levetiracetam (LEV) reduces awakening time, NREM sleep phase N3, and REM sleep; increases the SE and NREM sleep phase N2; and increases or does not change daytime somnolence but has no effect on SL or NREM sleep phase N1[44]. However, perampanel (PER), pregabalin, and tiagabine can increase the N3 phase of NREM sleep [45]. Therefore, we should also pay more attention to the drugs taken by epilepsy patients and/or understand the effects of the abovementioned ASMs on sleep to better choose appropriate drugs for OSA patients with epilepsy in the clinic.

7.1.5.2 Apnea May Be the Only Manifestation of Epilepsy, and the Coexistence of Epilepsy and Sleep Apnea Will Inevitably Increase the Difficulty of Diagnosis

Apnea may be the only manifestation of seizures without any symptoms of posture or movement. Lee et al. [46] described a 19-year-old male who only experienced apnea without motor or postural seizures. The EEGs recorded during the apnea period showed repeated sharp waves or rhythmic θ activity in the left or right temporal lobe. In addition, Nesbitt et al. [47] described a 52-year-old female who complained of apnea. From the age of 11, she repeatedly experienced excessive daytime sleepiness, loud snoring during sleep, and often woke up from sleep, accompanied by asphyxia and dyspnea. EEG revealed that this patient frequently woke up from the N2 phase of NREM sleep with transient irregular θ wave activity in the left temporal lobe. The patient was finally diagnosed with insular epilepsy. After treatment with LEV, she had no more seizures, and her daytime drowsiness and sleep quality were greatly improved. Therefore, in the clinic, the possibility of epilepsy should be considered when patients with apnea present.

In addition, when treating patients with epilepsy, we should also pay attention to the history of sleep disorders, which may provide help in diagnosis. Nishimura et al. [48] described a 12-year-old boy who presented with daily complex partial seizures and monthly generalized seizures. His follow-up medical history revealed that he often snored during sleep from an early age, PSG monitoring revealed severe OSA, and vEEG synchronous PSG revealed two episodes of paroxysmal apnea during sleep without any motor activity. EEG showed rhythmic θ wave activity in the middle temporal lobe, which appeared a few seconds before the onset of apnea and disappeared shortly after CSA stopped. Finally, temporal lobe epilepsy was diagnosed. After the prescription of ASMs and surgical treatment, his seizures were well controlled, the paroxysmal discharges disappeared, and the AHI decreased significantly. However, Schwartz et al. [49] described a 30-year-old female with refractory epilepsy and Lenox-Gastaut syndrome who had taken a variety of ASMs and fitted deep brain stimulators, but the frequency of seizures still increased. When looking for the cause, it was noted that she had obvious OSA and CSA and that the duration of apnea was related to the outbreak of epileptiform activity, which improved after treatment with CPAP. In addition to temporal lobe epilepsy and insular epilepsy, nocturnal frontal lobe epilepsy may only present as symptoms of OSA but not motor seizures. Obviously, the coexistence of epilepsy and SA brings challenges to diagnosis.

7.1.6 Treatment

CPAP is the most effective non-drug method for improving OSA and reducing seizures.

7.1.6.1 Continuous Positive Airway Pressure (CPAP)

CPAP treatment can reduce the frequency of seizures and improve the prognosis of OSA patients with epilepsy [45, 50, 51]. Vendrame et al. [52] described 41 epilepsy patients with complicated OSA from the USA who were followed for at least 6 months. Twenty-eight patients who received CPAP therapy had better seizure control, and the seizure frequency decreased from 1.8 times/month to once/month, while 13 patients who did not receive CPAP treatment did not have controlled seizures (2.1 times/month at baseline and 1.8 times/month at follow-up). Subsequently, Li et al. [53] treated 85 patients with drug-resistant epilepsy with CPAP and 112 patients with nondrug-resistant epilepsy and showed that CPAP could effectively improve seizures and the prognosis of patients with drug-resistant epilepsy. To further observe the efficacy of CPAP in the treatment of OSA patients with epilepsy, Malow et al. [54] conducted a randomized double-blind study. Among 35 epilepsy patients with OSA, 22 received CPAP therapy, and 13 received pseudoCPAP therapy. Consequently, compared with that of the controls, the AHI of the CPAP treatment group decreased significantly. In conclusion, these studies strongly suggest that CPAP is the most effective nondrug treatment for OSA patients with epilepsy.

7.1.6.2 Surgery

Adenotonsillar hypertrophy is a common cause of OSA in children and adolescents; therefore, adenotonsillectomy (AT) can be used as a first-line treatment for these individuals [55, 56]. Segal et al. [55] studied a total of 27 children (average age of 5 years) with epilepsy complicated with OSA who received AT treatment. Three months after surgery, 10 children had no seizures, 3 children had a number of seizures that was reduced by more than 50%, 6 children had a reduced seizure frequency, and only 2 children had no significant change in seizure frequency. Therefore, the authors suggest that AT is helpful for the control of seizures, especially in children who are heavier and younger at the time of surgery. In addition to AT, other surgeries are also used in epileptic children with OSA. Koh et al. [57] studied nine children with neurodevelopmental disorders associated with epilepsy and sleep apnea and four children who underwent surgery; tonsillectomy was performed in two patients, adenoidectomy in one patient, and tracheostomy in one patient. The frequency of seizures decreased within 12 months after surgery. However, since fewer children were included, large-scale prospective studies are needed to examine the effectiveness of these treatments. However, if postoperative

OSA persists or if children are unwilling to undergo AT or other operations, CPAP therapy is recommended, and automatic CPAP titration in the family environment is increasingly accepted by children [58].

For adult patients, those who are not willing to receive CPAP can choose surgical treatment. The main surgical methods include uvulopalatopharyngoplasty (UPPP), maxillary and mandibular propulsion (MMA), transoral tongue suspension (TOTS) and lateral pharyngoplasty (LP). Among these modalities, UPPP surgery involves removing the tissue in the posterior part of the pharynx and larynx and enlarging the plane and space of the tongue root in the posterior palatal area. MMA therapy expands the upper respiratory tract by physically expanding the facial skeletal framework. However, the key steps of TOTS include a translabial approach, drilling two holes in the mandible, using a suture piercer to pass the polypropylene through the hole to the root of the tongue, pulling the polypropylene back through the ring, and fastening the polypropylene to the mandible [59, 60]. Although these procedures can improve OSA, there is still a lack of evidence supporting their application in epilepsy patients with OSA.

7.1.6.3 Mechanical Therapy

A mandibular advancement device is a customizable dental mouthpiece that can move the lower jaw forward when wearing it to maintain the opening of the airway. It has a good effect on mild–moderate OSA, but the effect on severe OSA is not completely known [8, 61]. Machado et al. [62] involved 262 OSA patients in a trial in which a mandibular advancement device to treat SA was used for 4 months. Of the 83 patients surveyed at the end of the treatment, 53 (62.6%) were cured (AHI < 5). These findings suggest that this device is beneficial for patients with mild–moderate OSA. Moreover, the American College of Physicians also recommends that mandibular advancement devices can be used as an alternative to CPAP therapy for patients diagnosed with OSA who prefer to use mandibular advancement devices or for adverse reactions related to CPAP therapy [63]. Recent research on the indications for mandibular advancement devices has focused mainly on OSA patients, but there is not enough evidence for its application in epilepsy patients with OSA.

7.1.6.4 Drug Therapy

Those who cannot tolerate the above treatments or who prefer drug treatment can also choose drug treatment. Although most ASMs can affect sleep structure, there are a few ASMs that do not have adverse effects on sleep structure; for example, topiramate, zonisamide, and acetazolamide can inhibit carbonic anhydrase activity, thus significantly improving SA [64–66]. An extended-release formulation of phentermine/topiramate has been approved by the Food and Drug Administration (FDA) for the long-term treatment of obesity [67]. These ASMs, which combine anticonvulsant, sedative, and weight loss effects, are recommended for the treatment of obese patients with epilepsy [39].

Modafinil, approved by the FDA for the treatment of OSA patients with daytime sleepiness, is also recommended by the American Academy of Sleep Medicine as a standard drug for the treatment of daytime sleepiness in SA patients [68]. Although maprotiline can improve the AHI in patients with mild OSA, it is not recommended as the initial medication for OSA but can be used as a second-line drug [69]. However, most of these drugs are used for the treatment of OSA, and there is a lack of research on drug therapy for epilepsy patients with OSA. Fortunately, adenosine kinase and orexin receptor antagonists are expected to be new potential drug targets for the treatment of epilepsy patients with OSA [70].

7.1.6.5 Weight Loss

Obesity is not only a risk factor for OSA in the general population and for epilepsy but is also the most controllable factor in the treatment of OSA. Ruangkana et al. [71] reported the clinical characteristics and prevalence of OSA in 113 epilepsy patients and reported that the prevalence of OSA was 68% in epilepsy patients with a BMI >25, while that in patients with a normal BMI was 32%, suggesting that being overweight may increase the risk of OSA especially in epilepsy patients but also in the general population. Therefore, the body weights of epilepsy patients should be considered. The American College of Physicians recommends that all overweight and obese patients diagnosed with OSA be encouraged to lose weight [63]. In addition, appropriate physical exercise and/or ASM drugs that can reduce patient weight, such as topiramate, may be effective.

7.1.6.6 Other Treatments

Epilepsy patients with OSA can use wedge pillows to avoid sleeping on their backs and reduce the occurrence of OSA [72]. For many years, a ketogenic diet has been effective in the treatment of epilepsy, and recent studies have shown that a ketogenic diet may benefit epilepsy patients with comorbid OSA [73].

In summary, epilepsy with comorbid SA is very common in the clinic, but it is often ignored by doctors, who often only pay attention to only a single disease. In fact, seizures and OSA interact and promote one another, seriously affecting the patient quality of life [74]. When epilepsy patients have abnormal daytime drowsiness and snoring, PSG monitoring should be performed immediately. Moreover, for treatable risk factors, such as obesity and OSA, early intervention may prevent the occurrence of SUDEP. In conclusion, understanding and improving the level of diagnosis and treatment of OSA in epilepsy patients will help to improve seizure control, outcomes, and prognoses of patients with epilepsy and improve their happiness and well-being.

7.2 Epileptic Peri-Ictal Psychosis

Epidemiological investigations have shown that there may be a two-way relationship between psychosis and epilepsy. The risk of psychosis in patients with epilepsy is 6–12 times greater than that in the general population, and the risk of epilepsy in patients with psychosis is more than 6 times greater than that in controls [75]. The coexistence of the two diseases leads to a significant increase in incidence of each and in mortality, which has a great impact on the patient's family and society [76] and has become the most important problem in the management of chronic epilepsy. The underlying pathophysiological mechanism of periepileptic psychosis is considered to be closely related to epilepsy itself, but it is not recorded in the DSM-IV or ICD-10 or other widely used diagnostic manuals of psychosis, nor is it clearly classified into the realm of neurology or psychiatry. It is in a "fuzzy" zone between the two disciplines. Exploring the relationship between epilepsy and psychosis can help medical personnel correctly handle this special medical phenomenon [77–80].

7.2.1 Classification of Epileptic Peri-Ictal Psychosis

The classification of periepileptic psychosis was originally derived from the mental symptoms of epileptic patients summarized by Turner and others [81]. They proposed that the symptoms could be divided into four categories according to the severity of psychosis and its impact on the social function of patients: the first category was absence of mental disorder; the second category was the mental symptoms of most epileptic patients, including mental weakness, mainly memory impairment; and the third category was impairment of social and work ability in addition to memory impairment. The fourth category was the most serious; patients have epileptic insanity, which seriously affects their social and work abilities. However, the current view advocates that, according to the relationship between psychosis and epileptic seizures, periepileptic psychosis can be divided into post-epileptic psychosis, interictal psychosis, alternating psychosis (forced normalization), and psychosis after epilepsy surgery. The occurrence of mental symptoms after epileptic seizures is called postictal psychosis. The occurrence of mental symptoms in the interval between recurrent seizures is called interictal psychosis. The occurrence of mental symptoms when active seizures are controlled and the EEG is also significantly improved is called forced normalization [82].

7.2.2 Historical Evolution of Epileptic Peri-Ictal Psychosis

Since the nineteenth century, the relationship between epilepsy and psychosis has attracted increasing attention. There has been a heated discussion on whether there is a special correlation between mental symptoms and epilepsy. In 1854, Fallet [83] first proposed that there was a correlation between epilepsy and psychosis. Karagulla et al. [84] reported that the psychiatric manifestations of patients with temporal lobe epilepsy (TLE) are similar to those of patients with paranoid schizophrenia, and this epilepsy-related psychopathological state can last for several years. They suggest that this is a chronic paranoid psychosis associated with temporal lobe epilepsy. Subsequently, Glaser [85] proposed that patients with temporal lobe epilepsy are prone to epileptic psychosis and suggested that brain excitement may be one of the causes of psychosis. Since then, a close correlation between TLE and epileptic psychosis has been confirmed [86].

7.2.3 Diagnosis and Treatment of Different Types of Epileptic Peri-Ictal Psychosis

7.2.3.1 Postepileptic Psychosis

Mental symptoms occur within 7 days after seizures, and this is called postepileptic psychosis [87].

Historical Evolution

In 1986, Swamy and others [88] summarized the clinical characteristics and main manifestations of 150 patients with epileptic psychosis and proposed for the first time the concept of postepileptic psychosis. On this basis, SJ Logsdail and others [89] described the phenotypes of 14 postepileptic psychosis patients collected in 1988, summarized the rules of clinical evolution, and proposed diagnostic criteria. In 1993, Mazanda R and others [90] reported that after 298 patients with drug-resistant epilepsy underwent temporal lobectomy, 4 patients (1.3%) developed post-seizure psychosis. In 1994, K Kanemoto and others [86] compared the differences between acute interictal epileptic psychosis and postepileptic psychosis, summarized the clinical characteristics of 30 patients with postepileptic psychosis, and compared them with those of 33 patients with acute interictal psychosis and 25 patients with chronic psychosis. All patients with postepileptic psychosis had complex partial seizures, and the EEG revealed obvious temporal lobe lesions. Their mental symptoms were mainly exaggerated delusions and religious delusions, which are completely different from the mental state of schizophrenia patients. In 2002, Naoto Adachi and others [76] studied 282 patients with epileptic psychosis to evaluate the correlation between postepileptic psychosis and interictal psychosis, analyzed the characteristics of postepileptic psychosis and interictal psychosis, and compared them with those of 658 patients without psychosis. They speculated that epilepsy-related psychosis was very complex and should not be defined as a single and simple disease; rather, it should be defined as a complex disease with multiple possible subcategories. This change has pushed research on postepileptic psychosis to a new height.

Epidemiological Survey

Eva Hilger and others [91] investigated 1434 patients with epilepsy based on EEG monitoring and found that 53 patients had postseizure psychosis, suggesting that the prevalence of postseizure psychosis in patients with epilepsy was approximately 3.7%. For patients with temporal lobe epilepsy, Mercè Falip [92] reported that the prevalence of postseizure psychosis was approximately 9%. E Hilger et al. [93] investigated 684 patients with temporal lobe epilepsy and reported that 48 patients had a history of postepileptic psychosis for a prevalence rate of 7%.

In addition, for the proportion of postseizure psychosis among all epileptic psychoses, Naoto Adachi and others [76] investigated 282 epileptic patients with psychosis and found that 36 of them had post-seizure psychosis, suggesting that post-seizure psychosis accounted for approximately 12.9% of all epileptic psychoses. Mercè Falip [92] reported that postseizure psychosis accounted for approximately 25% of all epileptic psychoses.

Possible Pathogenesis

The mechanism of postepileptic psychosis is still unclear. Shingo Yasumoto and others [94] conducted single photon emission computed tomography (SPECT) examinations on patients with postepileptic psychosis and found that during the presence of postepileptic psychosis symptoms, there was excessive perfusion in the right temporal lobe and left basal ganglia. Similarly, Tomohiro Oshima and others [95] analyzed the SPECT results of brain regions in 19 patients with postseizure psychosis during the attack activation period and found that in 88% of patients, right temporal lobe perfusion was relatively increased (right temporal perfusion increased or left temporal perfusion decreased). Regardless of whether pathological lesions were suspected on the right or left side during the nonpsychiatric state, the SPECT results showed that the right side was dominant during the postseizure psychosis period. It has been suggested that the hyperperfusion of different brain regions after epilepsy may be related to the development of psychosis after epilepsy. Dubois et al. [96] used quantitative magnetic resonance imaging (MRI) to study changes in cortical structure in patients with postseizure psychosis. They found that compared with those in epilepsy patients without psychiatric manifestations and epilepsy patients with interictal mental disorders, the right anterior cingulate cortex in patients with postseizure psychosis was thicker, and the right angular gyrus and left middle temporal cortex were thinner. They speculated that this might be a marker of postseizure psychosis and that the damage to functional structures in different brain regions was the basis for the development of postseizure psychosis, which provides an argument for the theory of structural anomalies.

Clinical Features

The main feature of postepileptic psychosis is that after a series of epileptic seizures, there is an obvious waking interval, followed by a sudden outbreak of mental and behavioral abnormalities, which generally lasts for several days [97]. Although this special type of syndrome can be well-identified, it needs special attention because it is not specifically described in the standard diagnostic manual of psychiatry and is relatively ignored in the literature related to epilepsy.

Age of Onset

Logsdail et al. [89] described the age characteristics of 14 patients with psychosis after epilepsy and reported that the average age of epilepsy was 16.7 years, and the average age of psychosis after epilepsy was 32.2 years. Among the 282 patients with mental disorders described by Naoto Adachi and others [76], 36 were in line with the characteristics of postepileptic psychosis. The average age at which patients experienced the onset of epileptic seizures was 18.9 years, and the average age at which patients experienced postepileptic psychosis was 34.8 years.

Course of Disease

Fourteen cases of postepileptic psychosis described by S J Logsdail et al. [89] occurred 3–33 years after the seizure, with an average of 15.5 years. Naoto Adachi [76] reported that post-seizure psychosis occurred on average 18.9 years after the onset of epilepsy in 36 patients.

Waking Period after Seizures

Devinsky and others [98] reported that there was a clear interval between the last epileptic seizure and a psychotic seizure in 20 patients with postepileptic psychosis, with a range of 2.3–72 h (an average of 25 h). A study by B de Toffol et al. [99] suggested that the interval of wakefulness could be 2–120 h, but that it was most common within 72 h and considered to be the most obvious feature of postepileptic neuropathy.

Duration

Naoto Adachi et al. [100] followed-up with 58 patients with postepileptic psychosis for an average of 12.8 years and observed 151 seizures and reported that the average duration of psychosis after the first seizure was 10.5 days, with an average duration of 9.2 days in these 58 patients. Approximately 95% of the seizures achieved self-remission within 1 month. Devinsky et al. [98] summarized the duration of psychiatric symptoms in 20 patients with postepileptic psychosis and reported that the duration of psychiatric symptoms ranged from 16–432 h (average 83 h). de Toffol and others [101] reported that the duration of psychosis after epilepsy ranged from 15 hours to 2 months.

Main Clinical Manifestations

The clinical manifestations of postepileptic psychosis are complex and variable and mainly include paranoia delusions and clear-minded hallucinations. Strange behavior, thinking disorders, insanity, and impulsive behavior are also common, carrying the risk of personal injury and self-injury [77–80, 89, 90].

1. *Paranoia*: It often occurs suddenly and mostly manifests as acute polymorphic paranoia, and it easily changes from one theme to another. However, in the case of recurrence, the situation within a patient tends to be the same. Whether it is consistent with hallucinations or not, manic arousal-to-depression is accompanied by paranoia. Among the 14 patients described by Logsdail and others 18, one patient had primary delusions and thinking disorders, and six patients had

paranoia delusions. Among the 9 patients described by Savard G and others [102], 7 showed paranoia delusions, accompanied by obvious delusions of victimization. The paranoia attack lasted for an average of 1 week, 81% disappeared within 14 days, and 97% disappeared within 1 month after the attack. The delusions of 10–15% of the patients were of the chronic progressive type. The patient has a clear mind, a normal orientation, and a normal reaction to the outside world [82]. K Kanemoto and others [103] summarized the manifestations of mental symptoms in 30 patients with postseizure psychosis. They found that relatively frequent exaggerated delusions and religious delusions were the characteristics of postseizure psychosis, but patients with postseizure psychosis rarely showed schizophrenia-like psychotic characteristics, such as perceptual delusions.

2. *Hallucinations*: These hallucinations include auditory and visual hallucinations, and tend to mainly be auditory hallucinations, but often carry other symptoms; isolated hallucinations rarely occur [103].
3. *Aggressive Behavior*: Kanemoto and others [103] described 13 targeted violent attacks in a study of 30 patients with postseizure psychosis, and such attacks were often caused by small provocations and broke out suddenly, leading to self-injury or injury to others; the suicide rate was far greater than that of the general population. E Hilger et al. [93] reported that 22.9% of the 48 patients with post-epileptic psychosis experienced aggressive behavior at onset, and some patients experienced fear at onset.
4. *Others*: In addition to schizophrenia-like symptoms, Sakakibara and others 33 described patients who also experienced manic-like symptoms after an attack, such as a high mood and excitement.

Relationships with Seizure Type

Postepileptic psychosis is more common in temporal lobe epilepsy, which manifests as complex partial seizures or complex partial seizures secondary to generalized tonic–clonic seizures, and a small part of it manifests as primary generalized seizures. K Kanemoto et al. [102] studied 30 patients with postseizure psychosis and reported that all patients had complex partial seizures or EEG manifestations with temporal epileptogenic foci. Among the 36 patients studied by Naoto Adachi and others [76, 98] had complex partial seizures.

1. *Temporal Lobe Epilepsy*: The nine patients with paroxysmal psychosis described by Savard [102] all had conditions that originated from the temporal lobe and were accompanied by abnormally frequent complex partial seizures, sometimes secondary to generalized seizures. Using video EEG, E. Hilger and others [93] studied 684 patients with temporal lobe epilepsy and found that 48 patients had psychiatric symptoms after seizures.
2. *Primary Generalized Epilepsy*: Postepileptic psychosis is more common in temporal lobe epilepsy patients, but there are also reports of patients with primary generalized epilepsy. Eisuke Sakakibara and others [104] reported that a patient with idiopathic generalized epilepsy had their first generalized tonic clonus attack at the age of 56, and psychiatric symptoms appeared the day after the attack.

Diagnosis

Logsdail and others [89] first proposed the following diagnostic criteria for postepileptic psychosis in 1988: (1) paroxysmal mental disorder occurring within 1 week after a sudden seizure of epilepsy; (2) duration of mental disorder ranging from 15 h to 2 months; (3) disturbance of consciousness characterized by acute delirium; and (4) no history of chronic antipsychotic treatment, drug withdrawal, drug use or alcohol abuse. Later, B de Toffol [101] added the diagnostic criteria for postepileptic psychosis, which included previous and added delusions, hallucinations, strange behaviors, thinking disorders or emotional abnormalities in the case of clear consciousness; (4) mental disorders caused by antiepileptic drug toxicity, nonconvulsive status epilepticus, recent head injury, alcohol or drug poisoning or withdrawal were excluded; and (5) a clear time relationship between psychiatric symptoms and seizures, most of which have a 2–120 h (most commonly 72 h) awake period after the last seizure.

Treatment

Postattack psychosis is a self-limiting disease in most cases, and most patients recover to their pre-illness state within weeks, regardless of the intervention. Therefore, in most cases, it is not necessary to address this issue, but the serious deterioration of mental illness requires intervention [90].

The treatment of postepileptic psychosis can be categorized into the management of acute symptoms and the prevention of recurrence. Mildly ill patients can be given mild sedation in a supportive environment using benzodiazepines such as lorazepam, clonazepam, and midazolam. Patients with obvious delusions and hallucinations can also be given antipsychotics, such as risperidone, in addition to benzodiazepines, and critically ill patients can be given intramuscular injections of droperidol. If circumstances permit, people should try to avoid taking antipsychotics because antipsychotics may cause seizures again, and psychosis after seizures is closely related to seizures, leading to the deterioration of psychosis [77–80, 90].

Postseizure psychosis is a syndrome of short duration. Epilepsy is the cause, and psychotic syndrome is the result. The complete control of epilepsy through appropriate drug or surgical treatment can fundamentally prevent the recurrence of psychotic symptoms [76]. Therefore, the best way to prevent recurrence is to adjust the use of reasonable antiseizure medication, circumvent epileptic seizures, and pay special attention to preventing the use of drugs with psychiatric symptoms and side effects. In the past, it has also been reported that the preventive use of antipsychotics has achieved good results. Kanner AM [105] used atypical antipsychotics to prevent postseizure psychosis in a patient, and subsequent seizures were successfully prevented. Although the patient had a series of seizures, he did not suffer from psychosis.

Prognosis

Patients with epilepsy usually have a good prognosis, and most patients' mental symptoms disappear by themselves. Adachi et al. [100] reported that mental symptoms disappeared within 5 days in 48% of patients, within 7 days in 62%, within

14 days in 81%, and within 1 month in 97% of patients. However, there are still some patients with recurrent attacks, and a few patients can progress to interictal psychosis.

7.2.3.2 Interictal Psychosis

In contrast to postseizure psychosis, interictal psychosis (IP), which is defined as a mental disorder occurring 7 days after the onset of epilepsy, is the most common type of epileptic psychosis [106], and no epileptic seizures occur when psychosis occurs [87]. IP can be acute or chronic. If the course of disease continues or repeats for more than 3 months, it is called chronic IP, and if it does not reach 3 months, it is called acute IP [86].

Historical Evolution

In 1982, V Ramani [107] reported for the first time that 10 patients with epilepsy had interictal psychosis during epilepsy treatment in the hospital. Through video EEG and serum anticonvulsant drug monitoring, nine patients were found to have interictal psychosis that could not be distinguished from acute schizophrenia. It was thought that the occurrence of such psychosis was unexplained. In 1987, Lewis SW [108] and others described a patient with Capgras syndrome, speculating that it was a manifestation of interictal psychosis. Magnetic resonance imaging revealed bilateral subcortical lesions in the occipitotemporal and frontal regions. In 1991, R Caplan et al. [109] described the occurrence of interictal psychosis in children with epilepsy. In 2006, Oshima T and others [110] summarized the types of interictal psychosis. Subsequently, Adachi N and others [100] discussed the duration of interictal psychosis. In 2009, Falip and others [92] first noted its relationship with refractory epilepsy. In 2022, Pinto Gouveia C and others [111] described their clinical practice of using long-acting paliperidone injection to treat interictal psychosis, which greatly enriched the research on interictal psychosis.

Epidemiological Survey

Research by Tadokoro and others [112] showed that the annual incidence of interictal psychosis was approximately 0.42%. Among all patients with epilepsy, the prevalence of interictal psychosis is approximately 4.7–9.25% [87, 112–114], which is approximately 2–3 times greater than that of the general population [115].

Possible Pathogenesis

Interictal psychosis is very similar to primary schizophrenia [116], but its pathophysiological mechanism is not clear. Currently, research is mainly focusing on the following hypotheses.

White Matter Damage

The occurrence of interictal mental disorders may be related to extensive and severe white matter damage in patients. Sone et al. [117] reported that these patients had white matter damage, which mainly involved anterior thalamic radiation (ATR), the fronto-occipital fasciculus (IFOF), and the inferior longitudinal fasciculus (ILF).

These structures are related to emotion and memory, so mental disorders in patients with interictal mental disorders may be related to damage to these structures.

Hippocampal Volume Reduction

The correlation between interictal psychosis and temporal lobe epilepsy, especially medial temporal lobe epilepsy, has been confirmed [87]. Allebone et al. [118] reported that in patients with interictal psychosis and postseizure psychosis, the total volume of the left hippocampus decreased, the volume of the left hippocampus decreased moderately (13.3%), and the volume of the left and right cauda equina decreased significantly (41.5% and 36.4%, respectively).

Metabolic Disorders

Changes in metabolites in the brains of patients with epilepsy may be related to interictal psychosis. Maier et al. [119] reported that the N-acetylaspartate (NAA) concentration in the anterior hippocampi of patients with temporal lobe epilepsy combined with interictal psychosis was significantly lower than that in patients without TLE psychosis, especially in the left anterior hippocampus. The volume of this region in patients with TLE combined with psychosis was reduced, suggesting that this region may play a very important role in the etiology of psychosis.

Clinical Manifestations

Age

In the studies by Tadokoro and others [112], the age of onset in patients with epilepsy IP was 35.7 ± 13.6 years. Toone and others [120] reported that the onset age of IP patients was mostly between 30 and 40 years.

Course of Disease

Kanemoto and others [103] reported that chronic psychosis occurred approximately 14.2 ± 10.6 years after the first occurrence of epilepsy, and acute interictal psychosis occurred approximately 15.1 ± 11.6 years after the first occurrence of epilepsy.

Aura of Attack

This type of attack differs from a psychological aura, such as paroxysmal fear or a sense of déja vu, which typically occurs in individuals with mental illness after an attack. Most patients with interictal psychosis have autonomic nervous system symptoms such as an aura. Kanemoto and others [103] reported that autonomic nerve aura in patients with interictal psychosis was significantly greater than that in patients with postseizure psychosis. Further research revealed that 21% of patients with interictal psychosis and 36% of patients with chronic psychosis had autonomic nervous system aura, which was significantly greater than that in patients with postseizure psychosis (13%).

Clinical Manifestations

Different from other types of epilepsy related psychosis, the clinical manifestations of interictal psychosis are very similar to those of primary schizophrenia

Table 7.1 Main positive, negative, and general mental symptoms on the PANSS scale [106, 123]

Symptom classification	Main manifestations
Positive symptoms	Delusional hallucinations: taste, smell, touch, vision, etc.; auditory hallucinations are rare
Negative symptoms	Emotional delay, thinking disorder
General psychopathological symptoms	Tension, impulse control disorder, volitional disorder, slow action appearance and behavior

[103], and it is often misdiagnosed as schizophrenia [121]. The current research trend is to recognize the clinical symptoms of interictal psychosis according to the positive and negative symptoms of schizophrenia and use the scores of the Positive and Negative Symptoms Scale (PANSS) to evaluate the disease or conduct related research [122]. The main positive symptoms, negative symptoms, and general psychopathological symptoms of interictal psychosis are shown in Table 7.1.

Diagnosis

The definition of interictal psychosis has been controversial. Due to the confusion of the definition and the disunity of the diagnostic criteria, the grouping of patients and some conclusions have not been completely unified. The currently trending view is that (1) there is epilepsy that meets the diagnostic criteria for epilepsy and seizures established by the International Anti-Epilepsy Alliance [124]. (2) Psychosis occurred 7 days after the last epileptic seizure, and there was no epileptic seizure at the time of psychosis (at least in the early stage of psychosis). A duration of psychosis less than 3 months is called acute interictal psychosis, and a duration of ≥3 months is called interictal chronic psychosis [86, 125]. (3) Patients whose mental disorders were caused by other causes (such as encephalitis, alcohol, metabolic disorders, etc.) were excluded.

This condition needs to be differentiated from schizophrenia. Because interictal psychosis is very similar to schizophrenia, it is easily confused or misdiagnosed [126], so it is a challenge for clinicians to distinguish between interictal psychosis and schizophrenia. Maguire et al. [106] summarized the main points for distinguishing between interictal psychosis and schizophrenia: (1) Age of onset: the age of onset of schizophrenia is earlier than that of interictal psychosis. The age of presentation of mental disorders in patients with interictal psychosis is 10–15 years after the onset of epilepsy, and most patients are 30–40 years old [89]. The age at which schizophrenia is prone to occur is approximately 20 years in adolescence [106]. (2) Etiology: Patients with interictal psychosis have seizures, while patients with schizophrenia generally have no history of epilepsy [106]. (3) Clinical manifestations: schizophrenia has at least two core symptoms lasting for more than 1 month, during which social, personal, and professional abilities decline. Its core features are positive symptoms (delusions, thinking disorders, and hallucinations) and negative symptoms (indifference and social withdrawal). Hallucinations are often third-person auditory, and patients usually lack insight into their symptoms and show a decline in personality and state before illness. The main manifestations of interictal psychosis are positive symptoms such as delusions and hallucinations. There are fewer third-person auditory hallucinations, more well-preserved personality characteristics, and fewer negative symptoms. Symptoms can last for days to months or even longer [106].

Treatment

Patients with interictal psychosis may require long-term treatment with antipsychotics [127]. However, the treatment of interictal psychosis is challenging because some antipsychotics may aggravate seizures, and some antipsychotics may also aggravate psychosis [106]. At present, there is no recognized best treatment plan or guidelines for interictal psychosis. In general, treatment for interictal psychosis is better than treatment for schizophrenia, so the prognosis is also better [128].

Patients with interictal psychosis need rapid sedation during acute seizures. If the symptoms are obvious and the patient is cooperative, patients can take oral antipsychotics, usually olanzapine 2.5–20 mg/d or risperidone 0.5–6 mg/d. For patients who are uncooperative or manic, benzodiazepines are recommended as the first choice. Although there is no evidence that benzodiazepines are the most effective, studies have found that 0.5–4 mg of lorazepam or 5–10 mg of diazepam is reasonable in the acute phase, and benzodiazepines can also be used in combination with antipsychotics (such as haloperidol)[106].

Prognosis

The response to antipsychotics in patients with interictal psychosis is better than that in patients with schizophrenia [111]. Adachi et al. [129] reported that the average duration of interictal psychotic seizures was 82.7 weeks, 11.0% of patients experienced relief within 1 month, and 34.8% of patients experienced seizures lasting for 6 months or more. Young patients usually have a longer course of disease. Patients with a family history of psychosis or early psychotic episodes tend to have a longer course of disease. Early administration of antipsychotics can significantly shorten the course of the disease. Slater and others [130] speculated that the long-term prognosis of patients with epilepsy is better than that of patients with schizophrenia. Although interictal psychosis sometimes has a chronic course, its symptoms tend to ease spontaneously, and personality deterioration is rare.

7.2.3.3 Epileptic Alternating Psychosis (Forced Normalization)

Epileptic alternating psychosis, also known as epileptic forced normalization, is characterized by abnormal mental behavior and emotional activity disorders when seizures in patients with active epilepsy are controlled and when EEG signals are significantly improved [131, 132].

Historical Evolution

Forced normalization was first proposed by Landolt and others [132] in the 1950s. They found that after the seizures of patients with active epilepsy were well controlled and their EEGs basically returned to normal, there were paroxysmal psychobehavioral abnormalities and emotional disorders. In 1965, Tellenbach [133] proposed "alternating psychosis," in which patients alternate between the period when they have seizures but exhibit normal behavior and the period when the seizures disappear but the patients exhibit abnormal behavior. His view emphasizes the importance of clinical manifestations and does not necessarily mean that the EEG is completely normal. In 1991, Wolf [134] suggested that paradoxical normalization be used to emphasize the contradiction between EEG and clinical data. The normalization of EEG and epileptic activity contradicts the deterioration of mental symptoms. Although we still use the concept of forced normalization, he found that although epilepsy is still active under the cortex, the simultaneous activity of the inhibitory system will guide discharge along an uncertain path, thus inducing psychosis. In 1999, Krishnamoorthy and others [135] proposed diagnostic criteria for forced normalization, including a clear diagnosis of epilepsy and the presence of acute or subacute behavioral disorders, a reduction in epileptic activity on EEG, or the complete cessation of clinical seizures that lasts for at least 1 week. Although later generations have a clearer understanding of this disease, little is known about the clinical characteristics of forced normalization. In 2022, Yan and others [131] summarized the relationship between forced normalization of epilepsy and antiseizure medication, which enriched the research in this field.

Epidemiological Survey

Yan and others [131] summarized the reports of relevant literature collected from the MEDLINE database and suggested that the prevalence of epilepsy forced normalization might be 2–7.8%.

Possible Pathogenesis

The pathogenesis of forced normalization is not clear. The first report on the pathogenesis of forced normalization of epilepsy was published by Chhenkeli SA and others [136]. These authors reported that when the EEG signal represents "forced normalization," the deep structure of the lymphatic system may exhibit epileptic bioelectrical activity, which is speculated to be caused by the separation and inhibition of the brain stem. In 1987, R. R. Shakarashvil and others [137] reported that the cerebrospinal fluid of all patients in a study of 62 patients showed enhanced free radical oxidation and inhibition of antioxidant activity and suggested that this clinical phenomenon was related to free radical metabolism disorder. In 2022, Yan and others [131] proposed that the forced normalization after epilepsy surgery may be related to the functional disorder of the limbic system after surgical resection of part of the brain tissue of patients with epilepsy, and the forced normalization after vagus nerve stimulation and the use of antiseizure medication may be related to "electric kindling" and "dopamine pharmacological kindling." However, the exact pathogenesis is still under exploration.

Clinical Features

The main clinical manifestation of forced normalization is that patients with active epilepsy have mental disorders after seizures are controlled, and epileptiform discharges on EEG signals disappear [126, 138, 139]. Yamile calle-ló Pez and others [140] analyzed 193 patients described in the literature and reported that 69.4% of

Table 7.2 Forced normalization of epilepsy caused by different antiseizure medications [131]

Drug	Age (year)	Sex	Time of appearance	Clinical manifestations
Levetiracetam	9–56	Female	1–45 days	Mental disorders, Split personality
Ethylsuccinamide	11–49	No difference	1–3 weeks	Visual hallucinations, mania, mental disorders
Valproic acid	11	No difference	1 week	Mental disorders
Lamotrigine	10–43	More female	Uncertain	Paranoia and hallucinations
Lacosamide	42–44	Female	Unknown	Psychobehavioral abnormalities
Topiramate	33–42	Female	Several days	Auditory and visual hallucinations, irritability
Zonisamide	5–33	No difference	2 weeks	Communication difficulties, stereotyped psychosis
Aminohexanoic acid	Unknown	No difference	2 weeks	Mental disorders
Phenytoin sodium	11–26	Female	3 days to 2 weeks	Mental disorders

#Only one case was reported

them had mental disorders, 27.9% had emotional disorders, and another 10% had personality separation. Yan [131] studied 118 epileptic patients with forced normalization, including 75 (66.4%) with mental disorders, 29 (25.6%) with emotional disorders, and 9 (8%) with personality separation. The rates of forced normalization of epilepsy caused by different antiseizure medications are shown in Table 7.2.

Treatment

First, we evaluated whether the current antiepileptic drug treatment is reasonable, and then, we selected the appropriate antipsychotics. It is suspected that this condition is caused by antiseizure medication, and it needs to be reduced or stopped. Patients with severe mental symptoms need additional antipsychotic treatment, of which haloperidol and risperidone are two commonly used drugs [140]. In a study by Yamile calle-ló Pez and others [140], 73% of patients with forced normalization were treated with antipsychotics. The most commonly used drug was haloperidol (35.4%), followed by risperidone (18.7%) and quetiapine (6.2%). In addition, in 47% of the patients who were treated with suspected antiseizure medication, antiepileptic treatment was stopped completely, in 25% of the patients, antiepileptic treatment was gradually reduced, and in 28% of the patients, antiepileptic treatment was not changed. Notably, all patients receiving levetiracetam were required to stop taking the drug.

Prognosis

Different factors affect the prognoses of patients who undergo forced normalization. The forced normalization induced by antiseizure medication completely disappeared in most patients (87%) after withdrawal, while only 29% and 55% of patients who underwent epilepsy surgery and vagus nerve stimulation, respectively, were completely relieved despite antipsychotic treatment [140].

7.3 Treatment of Epilepsy with Comorbid Anxiety and Depression

Epilepsy is a common neurological disease with a prevalence rate of 7.2% that affects approximately 70 million patients worldwide [141]. Approximately 20% of patients with primary generalized epilepsy and 60% of patients with focal epilepsy are resistant to a variety of antiseizure medications and develop refractory epilepsy, among which temporal lobe epilepsy (TLE) with the hippocampus and amygdala as the focus is the most common [142]. Long-term drug use and adverse drug reactions in patients with epilepsy also cause great physical and psychological effects. In addition, the bizarre behavior of epileptic seizures is often difficult to understand. Social prejudice often causes many patients to experience shame, social discrimination, lifestyle restrictions, and other factors, making it difficult for patients to integrate into society and resulting in a sense of hopelessness; thus, the incidence of depression in epileptic patients is much greater than that in the general population.

Although experts have paid increasing attention to improving the diagnosis and treatment of depressive disorder in patients with epilepsy, there is still a lack of effective biomarkers and exact therapeutic targets because the mechanism of comorbid depression in epilepsy is not clear. In addition, there is a bidirectional relationship between epilepsy and depression. Antiseizure medication can cause anxiety or depression, and antidepressant treatment may induce epilepsy, which leads to clinicians being puzzled about the diagnosis and treatment of epilepsy and comorbid depression. Therefore, the diagnosis and treatment of comorbid epilepsy and depression have become an urgent clinical problem. The occurrence of epilepsy places a heavy burden on social development and the families of patients, and the physical and mental health of patients with epilepsy complicated by depression is far greater than that of patients with seizures alone, seriously affecting patients' quality of life. To date, the comorbidity of epilepsy and depression has become an important disease that endangers human physical and mental health. Therefore, to comprehensively improve the quality of life of patients with epilepsy and depression has become a global public health issue.

7.3.1 Historical Evolution

In the late 1980s and early 1990s, many clinical studies revealed associations between epilepsy and depression. In 1981, W. Matthews [143] described the risk of suicide in patients with epilepsy, emphasizing the necessity for doctors to be alert to the possible suicidal tendency of patients. In 1987, through the study of suicide, Barraclough [144] reported that the risk of suicide in individuals with temporal lobe epilepsy was greater than that in the general population. Subsequently, researchers began to explore the frequency and impact of depression and other mood disorders in patients with epilepsy and found that this comorbidity was much more common than previously anticipated. Although the evidence to guide the treatment of depression in patients with epilepsy is limited, relevant studies have suggested that depressive episodes have important impacts on the prognoses of patients with epilepsy, including quality of life and suicide risk. In 2019, a study by Kumar N et al. [145] supported a correlation between depressive episodes and increasing the frequency of seizures and reducing the quality of life. In the same year, Gilliam, FG [146] reported that suicide risk was associated with persistent depression but not with epilepsy or sertraline use in an effectiveness study evaluating the effects of sertraline and CBT [147] on depression, quality of life, seizures, and adverse treatment effects. Screening for early depression has gradually received increasing attention. In 2019, Shen, Y et al. [148] proposed a new method for the treatment of epilepsy and its complications. Treatment with epoxide hydrolase inhibitor (TPPU) after SE alleviated spontaneous recurrent seizures (SRSs) and epilepsy-related depressive behavior in a lithium/pilocarpine-induced rat model. In 2020, S. Murawiec et al. [149] proposed that increasing the dosage of pregabalin in patients with focal epilepsy can reduce the seizure frequency of patients with focal epilepsy and improve the symptoms of anxiety, depression, and insomnia. In 2022, Gilliam et al. [146] described the impact of moderate to severe depression management on prognosis, proposed the use of depression screening scales and questionnaires (QOLIE-89, AEP, Beck Depression Inventory, etc.) routinely used in epilepsy patients, which need to be improved, and emphasized that the wide application of artificial intelligence provides better examination methods for prognosis. In 2023, the expert consensus on the management of depression in adults with epilepsy indicated the need to develop protocols to guide health professionals in the best way to manage psychiatric comorbidities in patients with epilepsy. The guidelines state that the detection and treatment of major depression is a key factor in improving epilepsy outcomes and preventing suicide risk and emphasize the role of psychiatrists in managing patients with major depression and suicidal awareness [150].

7.3.2 Epidemiological Investigation

Epidemiologic studies have shown that people with epilepsy (PWE) have a significantly increased risk of cognitive, behavioral, and psychosocial disorders. The incidence of depression in PWE patients with good clinical seizure control is 10–20%, while the incidence of depression in patients with poor seizure control is 6–60% [151–153].

In 2003, Andres M Kanner [151] reported that depression was the most common comorbidity in patients with epilepsy. Its lifetime prevalence has been estimated to range from 6% to 30% in population-based studies and even as high as 50% in patients followed at tertiary centers. Patients with a history of depression have a 4- to 6-fold increased risk of seizures. A study from Canada showed that the incidence of depressive disorders in patients with epilepsy was 17.4%, while the incidence of depressive disorders in the general population was only 10.7%[154]. According to data from the 2009 Canadian Community Health Survey (cycle 1.1, $n = 130{,}888$), the prevalence of depression in PWE was 13.0%, compared with 7.2% in the general population [152]. In China, 16.5–43.3% of epilepsy patients in different regions were found to have depression according to different depression scales [155, 156]. The investigators also reported that the prevalence of depressive symptoms in PWE was 50.8%, and the prevalence of moderate depressive symptoms was 19.8%, which is consistent with the results reported in previous studies.

With the development of the times, the situation of patients with epilepsy suffering from depression is also changing. In 2012, Andres M Kanner [153] reintegrated the data and reported that the lifetime prevalence of depressive symptoms in epilepsy patients was as high as 30–35%. In addition, in 2015, Bosak et al. [157] studied 289 outpatients with epilepsy aged 18–80 years. The International Classification of Diseases-10 (ICD-10) was used to diagnose the subtypes of depression, and it was found that 13.1% of the patients had organic mood disorders, 9.3% had depressive episodes, and 9.3% had depressive episodes. A total of 3.8% were dysthymic.

The rate of progression to epilepsy is 3–7 times greater in depressed patients than in the general population, and antidepressant treatment may promote seizures. Studies have shown that depression-prone rats have significantly increased susceptibility to epilepsy, which also exacerbates the severity of seizures. This negatively affects patient quality of life, treatment effectiveness, and relapse rate, especially for those with major depression [158].

In 2022, in a cross-sectional study, Mekonnen Tsehay [159] analyzed epilepsy-related depression in three hospitals in the Amhara region of Ethiopia and reported that approximately 15% of caregivers of children and adolescents with epilepsy suffer from depression and that more than 10% suffer from anxiety. This study suggested that healthcare providers need to pay more attention to the mental health of all caregivers of children and adolescents with epilepsy.

The suicide rate of PWE is 5–6 times greater than that of the general population, and depression is considered to be the main factor leading to suicidal ideation or suicide attempts in people with epilepsy. Some studies suggest that the risk of suicide in people with epilepsy is 10 times greater than that in the general population. Therefore, early identification of depressive disorders and timely intervention are very important to improve the quality of life and reduce the suicide rate of patients with epilepsy.

7.3.3 Etiology of Epilepsy-Related Depression

The causes of depression in patients with epilepsy are complex and involve many factors, such as physiology, psychology, society, economy, and age. These factors act together in epilepsy and cause the occurrence of anxiety.

7.3.3.1 Epileptic Depression

Epileptic depression refers to depressive symptoms related to epilepsy in patients with epilepsy, which may be caused by a variety of factors, including seizures, side effects of antiseizure medication, reduced quality of life, and social impairment. In 2007, Siri Naess et al. [160] enrolled 597 epilepsy patients aged 16–87 years and distributed questionnaires on the Hopkins Symptom Checklist and the Self-positioning Struggle Scale. The questionnaire included information on seizure frequency, drug side effects, comorbidities, surgery, and demographic variables such as age, sex, marital status, occupational status, education, and place of residence. The results showed that seizure frequency had a significant effect on both scales and was significantly positively correlated with depression, which was supported by the findings of Kalinin V. V [161] and Seth A Mensah et al. [162].

Age at onset has a complex effect on the occurrence of depression. Sang-Ahm Lee et al. [163] proposed that the Hospital Anxiety and Depression Scale (HADS-D) score at 12 months after the first attack should be established according to the age of onset. Patients with earlier seizure onset are more likely to develop depression than are those with later seizure onset. Velissaris et al. [164] identified two trajectories of depression and three of anxiety in the 12 months following a new epilepsy diagnosis and found that these trajectories were not or were only weakly associated with sociodemographic and medical factors overall.

The occurrence of depression comorbidity in epilepsy may also be related to the type of seizure. Patients with partial seizures are generally more likely to develop depression than are those with generalized seizures [151, 165]. The reason for this is that depression may have a common anatomical basis with certain seizure types, such as temporal and frontal lobe epilepsy. Using high-resolution MRI images, it was found that the hippocampal volume was reduced in patients with epilepsy and depression [166]. However, hippocampal atrophy is more obvious in PWE with depression than in those without depression [167].

Epilepsy can be divided into drug-resistant epilepsy (DRE) and nondrug-resistant epilepsy (NDRE) according to whether the seizures can be controlled by common antiseizure medication. A meta-analysis of epidemiological studies has shown that the incidence of depression in individuals with drug-refractory epilepsy (DRE) is approximately 30% [168]. There is a difference in the severity of depression between these two types of epilepsy. In 2021, Magdalena Guała-Iwaniuk [169] conducted a study in Poland involving 193 patients with epilepsy, in which they were divided into a drug resistance group (DRE Group $n = 87$) and a nondrug resistance group (NDRE Group $n = 106$). The Beck Depression Inventory (BDI) and the Statistical-Trait Anxiety Inventory (STAT-Trait Anxiety Inventory) were used for patient assessment. The results showed that patients with DRE reported more severe depressive symptoms than did those with NDRE.

In 2014, Peng et al. [165] investigated 116 patients with epilepsy and reported that patients with moderate depressive symptoms had a longer course of epilepsy and that the course was positively correlated with depression scale scores. In 2014,

Zis et al. [170] showed that in a study of 94 patients with epilepsy, one additional episode per month increased the risk of depression in people with epilepsy by 1.38 times.

7.3.3.2 Iatrogenic Depression

Depression Induced by Antiseizure Medication

Antiseizure medication are the main means to treat epilepsy, but they may also cause some side effects, including emotional and behavioral problems, such as depression, anxiety, mood lability, and abnormal behavior. Different drugs may have different effects. It is now well-established that depression may be an adverse event after treatment with antiseizure medication (ASMs)[171]. ASM-associated depression was initially associated with long-term use of barbiturates, but over time, many different compounds, notably topiramate (TPM), vigabatrin (VGB), and levetiracetam (LEV), have been found to cause adverse psychiatric reactions (e.g., depression) during treatment [172].

Depression Caused by Different Antiseizure Medications
The occurrence of drug-induced depression may be related to the quantity and drug responsiveness in addition to the type of drug used, but the relationship between drug dosage and depression is still controversial. In 2013, Peng et al. [165] showed that taking two or more ASMs was more common in epilepsy patients with moderate depression and that the number of medications used was positively correlated with depression scale scores, suggesting that multiple ASM treatment may aggravate depression.

Vigabatrin (VGB)
VGB is an antiepileptic drug that is mainly used to control partial and generalized seizures. In 1994, R A Grunewald [173] studied patients with partial seizures treated with VGB, 9.1% of whom (two out of 22) suffered severe depression within 4 weeks of taking vigabatrin and withdrew from the study. In 1996, Thomas et al. [174] conducted a retrospective investigation of 136 patients with behavioral problems and reported that the incidence of depression as a side effect of VGB treatment was associated with a previous history of depression.

Levetiracetam (LEV)
LEV is recognized as a first-line ASM that has shown good effects in the control of seizures, but it also causes certain mental and behavioral side effects. In 2003, Mula et al. [175] studied 517 patients with epilepsy treated with LEV and reported that the incidence of depression was 2.5%, of which 0.7% had suicidal ideation. In 2012, Delanty [176] studied the occurrence of adverse psychiatric events, such as anxiety, insomnia, and depression, caused by LEV in the adjuvant treatment of 214 children, adolescents, and adults with primary generalized epilepsy. Among them, 16 patients (7.4%) had depressive symptoms. In 2014, some scholars described a case of

murder committed by a patient with epilepsy, which the authors thought might be related to the patient's decreased impulse and emotion regulation after he stopped treatment with carbamazepine and switched to levetiracetam. Such impulsive behavior can be avoided by early identification and treatment, emphasizing that when levetiracetam is used in epilepsy patients, its effects on mood should be closely tracked.

Mula [175] reported that the history of febrile seizures or status epilepticus and psychiatric history were significantly different between two groups of patients, those with and without psychiatric side effects of LEV treatment, and that the history of febrile seizures or status epilepticus was more accurate than the history of psychiatric side effects in predicting the occurrence of psychiatric adverse events. The author suggested that the former two factors may increase the biological susceptibility to psychosis.

In 2020, a report by Vajda [177] described depression caused by antiseizure medication in 2039 pregnant women with epilepsy and revealed that although antiseizure medication can effectively treat seizures, carbamazepine, and topiramate may cause teratogenicity; LEV carries low teratogenicity but may cause depression during pregnancy.

However, there are also opposing views. In 2022, Zhu [178] studied anxiety and depression scores on neuropsychological scales in patients before and after LEV monotherapy. Although the self-rating depression scale score decreased after treatment, the difference was not statistically significant.

Eslicarbazepine (ESL)

Psychobehavioral side effects (PBSEs) are the main causes of discontinuation of antiseizure medication. It has been suggested that eslicarbazepine (ESL) functions similarly to the active metabolite carbamazepine (CBZ). The experiments of Jalihal [179] showed that ESL performed well in terms of tolerance and did not produce significant effects in patients who developed psychobehavioral side effects from LEV, so there was no need to discontinue use of the drug. These findings suggest that ESL may be a treatment option for patients who experience psychobehavioral side effects with LEV and other ASMs.

Topiramate (TPM)

Topiramate is a drug used for the treatment of epilepsy. However, studies on whether this drug causes depression are inconsistent. Some studies have suggested that topiramate may increase the risk of depression in patients, while others have suggested that topiramate has little or no effect on depression or even has antidepressant effects. K Phabphal et al. [180] reported that depression was induced in patients treated with topiramate for migraine prevention.

In 2008, Mula et al. [181] conducted a retrospective study that included 423 patients with epilepsy. The results showed a 3.5-fold increase in treatment-related adverse events in consecutive patients receiving topiramate who had a history of depression. In 2013, Peng [165] collected clinical data from 2010 to 2012 and evaluated 116 PWE patients using the Hamilton Depression Scale (HAMD), National Hospital Epilepsy Severity Scale (NHS 3), and Pittsburgh Sleep Quality Index

(PSQI). It was found that TPM use may be a risk factor for depressive symptoms in PWE.

Depression is associated with hippocampal sclerosis and increased drug titration speed. Febrile seizures and a history of depression are contraindications. In the treatment of TLE with hippocampal sclerosis, topiramate is more likely to cause depression in patients. In 2003, Mula et al. [182] compared 70 patients with hippocampal sclerosis and 128 patients with cryptogenic TLE and reported that at the same starting dose and titration speed, TLE patients with hippocampal sclerosis are more likely to suffer from depression, and depression is one of its predictors.

However, there are opposing views. In 2021, Aydin S [183] also showed that TPM had antidepressant effects in animal experiments, which was consistent with the results of Molina-Hernandez [184]. In addition, Mowla [185] demonstrated in a double-blind placebo-controlled study that topiramate enhanced the efficacy of antidepressants for treating major depression.

Diazepam

Diazepam is a drug used to treat epilepsy and anxiety disorders. Its main effect is to increase the levels of serotonin and norepinephrine neurotransmitters. Although it has achieved good results in treatment, some patients may develop depressive symptoms. This adverse effect may be related to its anticholinergic effect, parasympathetic effect, and ability to interact with other drugs. A study on the relationship between diazepam dosage, plasma level, age and central nervous system depression showed that the dose and plasma level of diazepam were negatively correlated with age; in particular, elderly individuals were more sensitive to the inhibitory effect of this drug than young individuals were, thus indirectly indicating that diazepam may cause depression in some patients [186].

Others

Phenytoin sodium is a traditional antiepileptic drug. A number of studies have shown that patients using phenytoin sodium are more likely to have depressive symptoms than patients taking other drugs, which may be related to its effect on the neurotransmitter glutamate.

Carbamazepine is a widely used antiepileptic drug that is often used to treat partial epilepsy and generalized seizures. However, studies have shown that patients using carbamazepine may experience depressive symptoms. A multicenter cross-sectional study revealed that the use of two or more antiseizure medications and perceived stigma were significantly associated with depression and anxiety [187].

Postepileptic Surgery Depression

In 2011, M. Wrench et al. [188] showed that approximately one-third of patients with epilepsy after surgery had postoperative depression, 8% of whom had new-onset depression after surgery, and 25% of whom experienced recurrent depression. Most patients with depression (70%) were diagnosed within the first 3 months after surgery, and 65% of patients experienced depressive symptoms lasting at least

6 months during the follow-up period. Major depression often occurs soon after surgery and is usually persistent.

Postoperative depression associated with temporal lobe epilepsy is more common than that associated with other types of surgery, possibly because the temporal lobe region of patients with temporal lobe epilepsy is related to emotion, and surgery may have an impact on the function of this region. M. Wrench [188] showed that patients who underwent medial temporal lobectomy were more likely to have primary major depression than those who underwent nonmedial temporal lobectomy. However, in Jacoby's study [189], no relationship was found between seizure variables and preoperative depression, including seizure frequency and the location of seizure foci. This study does not support the notion that patients with limbic seizures are particularly vulnerable to depression. Moreover, A.M. Swinkels [190] used the DSM-IV criteria to assess major depression and found no difference between temporal lobe epilepsy and extratemporal epilepsy.

In 2022, D. Hue [191] conducted a systematic review of the current literature on depression after epilepsy surgery and included 18 high-quality studies. These studies reported conflicting results, suggesting that the effects of TLE surgery on depression and suicide are unclear. Although most studies have not reported an increase in the prevalence or severity of depression after surgery, the sample size was small, and there were numerous confounding factors. In addition, these studies did not include comparison groups for incident depression and suicide rates. Thus, the risk of persistent or worsening depressive symptoms, incident depression, and suicide may still increase after TLE surgery. Patients should be informed of these potential risks before undergoing TLE surgery and undergo a preoperative psychological assessment.

7.3.4 Related Factors

In 2020, Yang et al. [192] conducted 51 cross-sectional studies with sample sizes ranging from 36 to 1763 patients. The factors related to the increased risk of depression in patients were analyzed, and the following factors were found to be related to the increased risk of depression: (1) Age: This was consistent with the research viewpoints of Thomson et al. [152]: "Although increasing age is associated with a decreased risk of depression in stroke and multiple sclerosis, increasing age is associated with an increased risk of depression in epilepsy [193]." (2) Sex: Female sex is an important factor affecting the comorbidity of epilepsy and depression. It is also an established predictor of depression in the general population and patients with chronic diseases [194]. (3) Education: Various studies have shown that a low education level is associated with an increased risk of depression, while a higher education level is a protective factor [195, 196]. (4) Economic conditions: epileptic patients without stable jobs were more likely to suffer from depression than those with jobs. Studies have shown that low-income patients may be more susceptible to depression in rural or low-income areas. Due to insufficient medical resources and a lack of income, it is more difficult for them to obtain effective support for their mental health [197]. However, there is no clear evidence that a high economic level reduces the risk of depression in people with epilepsy. (5) Compliance with antiseizure medication: Patients with poor compliance are more likely to have depression [198].

In addition, self-esteem reflects an individual's overall subjective emotional evaluation of his or her own worth and is considered to be an important factor affecting mental health. The association between self-esteem and depression has been explained by two dominant models. The vulnerability model points to low self-esteem as a risk factor for the development of depression. The Scar model proposes that low self-esteem is a consequence of, rather than a cause of, depression, as the experience of depression may leave permanent damage to an individual's self-concept [199].

7.3.5 *Pathogenesis*

Depression is one of the most common psychiatric comorbidities in patients with epilepsy and is associated with frequent seizures. At present, the mechanism of comorbid depression in epilepsy is still poorly studied, and most of the mechanisms are not fully understood. It is also unclear whether there is an overall effect of comorbidities, whether depression changes independently of epilepsy, or whether there is an interaction effect between different types of epilepsy and depression. The known mechanisms associated with comorbidities may be related to the 5-HT/dopaminergic/glutamatergic/endocannabinoid system, cortisol levels, neuroinflammatory responses, neuro-pathology, genetic and anatomical factors.

7.3.5.1 Neurobiochemical Factors

In recent years, researchers have explored the universality of possible roles of the endocannabinoid system (ECS) in depression and epilepsy. The ECS includes two key components, AEA and 2-AG, and two types of cannabinoid receptors, CB1 and CB2, which can affect other neurotransmitters, such as DA, 5-HT, GABA, and glutamate [200]. Antidepressants increase the effect of AEA by increasing the expression level of the CB1 receptor and preventing its degradation. Here, the common properties of ECS receptors and degradation enzymes may be involved in depression and epilepsy comorbidity through different mechanisms: increased AEA activity is associated with antidepressant effects, but the correlations of different brain regions and different models to comorbid depression and epilepsy need to be considered. An increase in CB1 expression is speculated to have an antidepressant effect and therefore is presumed to have an effect on comorbid depression. CB2 and MAGL should be used with caution in patients with depression and epilepsy. 2-AG seems to be involved in the comorbidity of depression and epilepsy, but more studies are needed to support its safety and efficacy. Relatively little research has been conducted on MAGL, a 2-AG-degrading enzyme.

Serotonin reuptake inhibitors (SSRIs) have a good effect on epilepsy and depression comorbidity. Serotonin is involved in the regulation of complex neural networks such as those involved in depression and epilepsy susceptibility. Animal and human studies have shown that SSRIs can improve mood, control seizures, and reduce generalized tonic–clonic seizures in the remission of depression, suggesting that serotonin may have a certain relationship with the comorbidity mechanism of epilepsy and depression through the 5-HT energy system [146]. Similarly, Samia Elkommos [201] reported that serotonin dysfunction is due to a different mechanism, with reduced synaptic availability in epileptic depression patients compared to patients without epilepsy with reduced 5-HT receptor density. 5-HT is synthesized from the essential amino acid L-a tryptophan. Andrade R. [202] reviewed the understanding of serotonin in the regulation of nerve excitability. Different 5-HT receptors act in multiple ways through complex mechanisms, with specific effects on seizure susceptibility and mood [172]. It has been mentioned in studies of the progression of comorbid depression in epilepsy that the neurobiochemistry and anatomy of depression in epilepsy include decreased serotonin levels.

Previous studies have shown the effect of glutamate on epilepsy, and studies on the comorbidity of epilepsy and depression suggest that glutamate has a potential pathogenic role between the two, but the specific regulatory mechanism is not clear [203].

Neuroinflammatory factors are also thought to be involved in this association, and enhanced hippocampal interleukin-1β (IL-1β) signaling may be a mechanistic factor in TLE and clinical depression [158].

7.3.5.2 Brain Structural and Functional Changes

In 2021, Samia Elkommo et al. [201] performed a systematic review comparing differences in specific groups of structural and functional brain regions in adult patients with epileptic depression. They found that depression in TLE patients seems to be associated with different patterns of brain changes, and the pattern changes in the hippocampus and subcortical structures seem to be different from those in depression outside of epilepsy, which may support the phenomenological concept of depression in epilepsy. "All studies of patients with epilepsy and depression consistently use hippocampal volume reduction as a marker, but it is not clear whether the hippocampal structures involved are more epileptiform or more severely depressed in terms of atrophy." Another difference between MDD and epileptic depression is the changes in cortical and subcortical structures, with adult major depressive episodes characterized mainly by cortical abnormalities and no changes in subcortical structures except the hippocampus. In contrast, there are numerous subcortical structural changes in patients with epileptic depression. This indicates that there may be different phenomena occurring in depression and depression in epilepsy patients and suggests the role of temporal lobe structures in mood disorders in epilepsy patients. In TLE patients, the comorbidity of epilepsy and depression commonly observed in adults may be directly associated with hyperexcitation of bilateral temporal lobe circuits. Depression and anxiety in patients with epilepsy reflect dysfunction of a widely distributed limbic network, which may be the cause or result of epilepsy. Moreover, refractory epilepsy, seizures, and some anticonvulsant drugs can disrupt central emotional adaptive function and increase the risk of epilepsy. Vaishnav Krishnan [204] noted that more attention should be given to neural circuits and molecular axes.

7.3.5.3 HPA Axis

Studies have shown that pilocarpine-induced status epilepticus in rats accompanied by chronic epilepsy can lead to depressive disorders, which may stem from dysregulation of the hypothalamic–pituitary–adrenal cortex (HPA) axis and/or decreased serotonin transportation in the hippocampus [205]. Pineda et al. [206] reported that presynaptic and postsynaptic serotonin 1A (5-HT1A) receptors may be involved in epileptiform depression. HPA axis activity and presynaptic 5-HT1A receptor function were both increased in the rats with major depression compared with the rats with initial and moderate depression, and were assessed by forced swimming to test for major depressive behavior. However, pharmacological activation of the postsynaptic 5-HT1A receptor improves the depressive phenotype in epileptic animals. Thus, in chronic epileptic conditions, the hyperactive HPA axis activates the presynaptic 5-HT1A receptor, thereby altering the regulation of serotonin release in favor of autoinhibition. Downregulation of the expression of the postsynaptic 5-HT1A receptor may further exacerbate the severity of epileptiform depression.

Neuroinflammation may also be involved in the regulation of HPA axis function and epilepsy, and depression comorbidities [207]. Studies have shown that increased expression of interleukin-1β in the hippocampus of temporal lobe epilepsy and depression models may be related to depressive behavior. Mazarati et al. [208] suggested that increased expression of IL-1β may lead to dysfunction of the hypothalamic–pituitary–adrenal cortex (HPA) axis, which can disturb the secretion of serotonin in the hippocampus and lead to depressive symptoms. In addition, this study confirmed that drug inhibition of the hippocampal interleukin-1 receptor has an antidepressant effect on TLE rats and depressed animal models after pilocarpine-induced status epilepticus (SE). Two weeks of bilateral intrahippocampal infusion of a human recombinant interleukin-1 receptor antagonist alleviated all depressive symptoms in young rats, suggesting that hippocampal interleukin-1β signaling is associated with epileptiform depression.

Conversely, the hormonal imbalance caused by the destruction of the HPA axis by seizures and interictal epileptiform discharges may contribute to the high incidence of depression in patients with epilepsy [67]. Pineda E [209] explored the comorbidity mechanism involved in epilepsy and depression in the search for safer and effective treatment methods other than ASMs and suggested that neuroinflammation, tryptophan metabolism changes, HPA axis disorders and neuron changes were the main pathways involved in the coexistence of epilepsy and depression. Druzhkova et al. [210] reported that depression is related to HPA axis-related hormones and other hormones. There is a similar mechanism of action in patients with epilepsy and in patients with major depression, and it is speculated that this mechanism is related to comorbidities.

7.3.5.4 Others

Previous studies have shown that plasma and hippocampal BDNF levels are often correlated [211]. Low levels of serum BDNF indicate a shorter latency to status epilepticus, more frequent spontaneous seizures, a greater desperation index and greater anhedonia [212]. BNDF has long been considered to be associated with depressive behaviors. Epilepsy may promote the development of depression through exposure to chronic stress [158]. In 2021, Gulyaeva [213] mentioned epilepsy as a stress-related disorder. At present, there are few studies on the effect of genetics on the comorbidity of epilepsy and depression. Heiman's study [214] investigated the association between patients and their families with depression under the influence of known epilepsy genes, and the study elucidated the relationship between leucine-rich glioma inactivation gene (LGI1) mutations and auditory function in partial epilepsy.

7.3.6 Diagnosis of Comorbid Depression in Epilepsy

Because epilepsy and depression have great similarities in terms of their impacts on quality of life, diagnosis and treatment are difficult. It is necessary to rely on medical history and symptom assessment, psychological assessment, neurophysiological assessment and other methods to aid in diagnosis. Some auxiliary examinations, such as sleep assessment, cognitive assessment, social function assessment and imaging examination, are helpful for the diagnosis of comorbid epilepsy and depression.

7.3.6.1 Imaging

The imaging diagnosis of epilepsy comorbid with depression usually relies on brain imaging techniques, such as magnetic resonance imaging (MRI) and positron emission tomography (PET). MRI can detect brain structural abnormalities such as hippocampal atrophy and temporal lobe epilepsy. PET can show metabolic rate, blood flow, and neurotransmitter levels in brain regions. These imaging techniques help physicians determine whether there is a pathophysiological basis for epilepsy or depression and guide the development of the best treatment plan.

A 2005 study revealed that depressed individuals with right hippocampal sclerosis (RHS) may tend to have a reduced left hippocampus volume, although this could not be confirmed statistically due to the small amount of data. However, the results of this study suggest that depression may affect left hippocampal volume in patients with right hippocampal sclerosis, indicating that the neuroimaging characteristics of epilepsy patients with chronic depression are worthy of further study [215].

A 2008 imaging study used positron emission tomography (PET) and a selective antagonist radio to study brain and brainstem serotonergic receptor density in patients with major depression and temporal lobe epilepsy (TLE). The results confirmed that depressive symptoms in TLE patients were associated with alterations in central serotonergic pathways, especially in the raphe nucleus, insula, cingulate gyrus, and epileptogenic hippocampus. These changes may reflect reduced extracellular serotonin concentrations in depressed patients, with receptor expression upregulation less likely.

According to a 2021 neuroimaging study, most neuroimaging studies on epileptic depression have focused on structural abnormalities in TLE patients, and these studies have shown extensive subcortical abnormalities.

7.3.6.2 Related Scales

The comorbidity of epilepsy and depression is a common clinical phenomenon that needs to be comprehensively evaluated by a variety of methods, among which the detection scale is a commonly used tool.

Hamilton Depression Scale (HAMD)

The HAMD is a standardized tool used to assess the severity of depressive symptoms. It includes 17 items, and the scores of each item vary from 0 to 2 according to severity. The HAMD is widely used to assess the severity of depressive symptoms and treatment response [216].

Positive and Negative Emotion Regulation Scale (PANAS)

The PANAS is a widely used instrument to assess positive and negative emotion regulation. The PANAS consists of 20 items, 10 of which assess positive emotion regulation and 10 of which assess negative emotion regulation. A study in 2014 aimed to explore the relationship between depression and anxiety symptoms and the condition of patients with epilepsy; the study used the PANAS scale to evaluate the emotional state of patients and revealed that depression and anxiety symptoms were related to interictal epileptic discharges [217].

Mini-Mental State Examination (MMSE)

The MMSE is a tool used to assess the cognitive function of patients. There are 30 items covering orientation, attention, memory, calculation ability, language ability, and so on. In 2014, Lunn, J et al. [218] used the MMSE to explore the relationship between cognitive function and depressive symptoms in patients with epilepsy. The results showed that MMSE scores were negatively correlated with depressive symptoms; that is, patients with lower MMSE scores were more likely to exhibit depressive symptoms. It can be concluded that the MMSE is an important tool that can be used to assess depressive symptoms in patients with epilepsy.

In addition, there are several other scales used for the diagnosis and evaluation of depression comorbidity in patients with epilepsy, such as the Self-rating Depression Scale (ZDRS), the Self-rating Depression Scale (BDI), and Self-rating Depression and Anxiety Scale (HADS). These scales can help physicians assess the severity and type of depressive symptoms in patients and monitor patient treatment response and improvement in quality of life over the course of treatment.

7.3.7 Treatment of Depression in Epilepsy

7.3.7.1 Reduction or Withdrawal of Antiseizure Medication

In most cases, depressive symptoms caused by antiseizure medication are mild, and the drugs do not necessarily need to be discontinued. However, it is necessary to reduce the dosage of or withdraw the drug if it seriously affects the quality of life of the patient. In 2001, Post R. M. [219] described three patients with bipolar disorder whose depressive symptoms were significantly aggravated after using topiramate. These patients had depressive symptoms or worsening symptoms within 1 week after treatment or titration to 50 mg/day, and depressive symptoms were significantly relieved within 1–2 weeks after discontinuation of the drug. The authors argue that although topiramate has been shown to be effective in stabilizing mood, physicians should be aware of its possible adverse effects on depressive symptoms when topiramate is prescribed. In 1993, Ring et al. [220] described 10 patients with major depression associated with vigabatrin treatment who met the DSM IIIR criteria for major depression and found that such depression usually occurred early in treatment, at or shortly after dose increases. Depressive symptoms occurred within 4–8 weeks of vigabatrin (VGB) treatment or within 6 weeks of VGB dose escalation. With the continuation of VGB treatment-related depression, 7 patients discontinued VGB, and 3 patients reduced the VGB dose, but none of them received antidepressant treatment. The prognosis of the patients was good, and the depression disappeared 2–8 weeks after drug withdrawal, suggesting that the depressive symptoms could be rapidly relieved or dissipated by dose reduction. The dose of VGB in patients with depression is 1.5–4 g/day, and depression can also occur when the frequency of seizures decreases [220].

7.3.7.2 Antidepressant Drug Treatment

Mild patients with comorbid epilepsy and depression can self-regulate to relieve symptoms, but most of them also need treatment, and drug treatment is the main method. Many studies have shown that selective serotonin reuptake inhibitors (SSRIs) and SNRIs show good therapeutic efficacy and safety in patients with comorbid depression and epilepsy. Compared with other psychotropic drugs, SSRIs do not increase the frequency or severity of seizures and affect the prognosis and suicide risk to a certain extent. Patients with epilepsy usually experience a certain degree of improvement in seizures after the relief of depressive symptoms [221]. In 2019, Gilliam [146] conducted a 16-week study of sertraline and cognitive–behavioral therapy (CBT) treatment on 140 outpatients with epilepsy and major depression and reported that the difference in the remission time of depressive symptoms between the two groups was 2.8 days, and the lower limit of the efficacy of both groups was greater than the upper limit of 33.7% in the placebo control group. Depression improved in more than half of the subjects, confirming the effectiveness of antidepressant treatment in improving depressive symptoms. The control of depression helps to improve the quality of life of epilepsy patients.

Drug Selection

In 2021, the ILAE issued recommendations for the treatment of depression in adults with epilepsy. For patients with mild depression, psychoeducation or treatment is considered an alternative to antidepressants. If drug therapy is needed, SSRIs are the drugs of choice (grade B). For moderate-to-severe depressive episodes, serotonin reuptake inhibitors are also the drug of choice (grade B). Switching to venlafaxine appears to be reasonable in patients who are partially or nonresponsive to first-line therapy (grade C) [222].

Antidepressant treatment should be maintained for at least 6 months after the resolution of the first depressive episode, but extended to 9 months for those with a history of previous depression and longer until the resolution of symptoms in patients with major depression or residual symptoms. If monotherapy fails, the addition of lithium to ongoing antidepressant therapy is recommended. Intensive lithium therapy should be continued for 2–4 weeks to assess patient response. The recommended target lithium serum concentration is 0.6–0.8 mmol/L. If a response occurs, lithium supplementation should be continued for at least 12 months. If lithium is considered an intensive therapy after monotherapy failure in the epilepsy population, it should be used with caution, given its tolerability.

Some antiseizure medications, such as lamotrigine, carbamazepine, and valproic acid, are considered to act as mood stabilizers. According to the American Epilepsy Foundation expert consensus statement, lamotrigine can be used to improve mild depressive symptoms and prevent depressive episodes.

Interactions Between Antidepressants and Antiseizure Medication

Antidepressants are usually classified as old or classic drugs, such as tricyclic antidepressants (TCAs) and monoamine oxidase inhibitors (MAOIs), and newer antidepressants, such as SSRIs, serotonin and norepinephrine reuptake inhibitors (SNRIs), and others with different mechanisms of action. A number of studies have explored the interactions between antidepressants and antiepileptic seizures and interdrug pharmacokinetics.

Among the first-generation antiseizure medication, carbamazepine (CBZ), phenytoin sodium (PHT), and barbiturates (PBs) are strong inducers of a variety of drug metabolism enzymes, including CYP (CYP 1A2, 2A6, 2B6, 2C9, 2C19, 3A4) and UGT (1A1, 2B7, 2B15). Valproate (VPA) has traditionally been considered a broad-spectrum enzyme inhibitor of CYP (2C9, 2C19, and 3A4) and UGT (1A4 and 2B7) [223]. Since all these enzymes contribute to the metabolism of most antidepressants, it is possible that these ASMs have pharmacokinetic interactions with antidepressants.

The metabolism of TCAs is quite complex and involves multiple enzymatic pathways. A study by Mula et al. [156] showed that the interaction between TCAs and first-generation ASMs was not clinically relevant. There are two reasons for this: (1) nortriptyline and desipramine are demethylating metabolites of amitriptyline and imipramine, respectively, and (2) TCA has a broad therapeutic window.

First-generation antiseizure medication (i.e., CBZ, PHT, and PB) reduce the plasma levels of most SSRIs by at least 25% [223]. However, whether this is clinically relevant depends on individual patient differences.

All enzyme-induced ASMs appear to reduce blood levels of SSRI antidepressants by approximately one-quarter. However, there is no evidence that these changes are clinically relevant and do not require dose adjustments in routine clinical practice [224]. In contrast, fluoxetine, fluvoxamine, and sertraline are CYP2C9 inhibitors that affect the level of phenytoin sodium metabolism and, to a lesser extent, increase the level of VPA [223, 224]. Enzymatic seizure drugs, such as carbamazepine, can reduce bupropion blood levels by 90%. Unlike carbamazepine, VPA does not affect bupropion metabolism in depressed patients [225].

Seizures Caused by Antidepressants

Antidepressants may trigger seizures. Bloechliger et al. [226] conducted a retrospective follow-up study, and the risk for first seizure and its association with antidepressant exposure were estimated for patients with depression who used selective serotonin reuptake inhibitors (SSRIs), serotonin-norepinephrine reuptake inhibitors (SNRIs), tricyclic antidepressants (TCAs), “other antidepressants,” no antidepressant use or previous antidepressant use. The use of SSRIs or SNRIs was found to be associated with a twofold increased risk of first seizures compared with no use, which is consistent with the results of the study by Kamal [227].

There is no known mechanism to explain why antidepressants induce seizures. Montgomery [228] suggested that the proconvulsant effects of antidepressants may be attributed to their local anesthetic, antimuscolinic, or antihistamine properties. Although many studies have reported that older antidepressants, such as MAOIs and TCAs, are frequently associated with seizure risk and may also induce seizures in non-epileptic patients [229, 230], newer antidepressants, such as SSRIs and SNRIs, show better tolerance in most patients [231, 232].

7.3.7.3 Nonpharmacological Treatment

Currently, new ideas and technologies are being developed. Neuromodulation and stimulation provide more options for the treatment of comorbid epilepsy and depression. Low-field magnetic stimulation, transcranial pulsed electromagnetic field, transcranial direct current stimulation, epidural cortical stimulation, trigeminal nerve stimulation, transcutaneous vagus nerve stimulation, transcranial focused ultrasound, near-infrared transcranial radiation, and closed-loop stimulation have been used in clinical practice, and the application of these new interventions is gradually expanding [233].

Transcranial Magnetic Stimulation

Transcranial magnetic stimulation (rTMS), a nonpharmacological treatment for epilepsy, is often used as an adjunctive treatment for epilepsy. It has the advantages of noninvasiveness, strong adaptability, minimal discomfort, and a small stimulation range, especially for pregnant patients; however, other treatments are not effective, and patients cannot tolerate surgery, which is an ideal choice.

As one of the treatment methods for depression, rTMS can help to improve the pessimistic moods of patients and has a potential role in the treatment of patients with comorbid epilepsy and depression. In 2022, Gouveia [234] described transcranial direct current stimulation (tDCS) as a neuromodulation modality to modulate circuit dysfunction and relieve mood problems. Repetitive transcranial magnetic stimulation (rTMS) is a safe, noninvasive neuromodulatory therapy for the treatment of major depressive disorder (MDD). This therapy has been approved by the FDA [235].

Vagus Nerve Stimulation (VNS)

This method has good efficacy and safety in the treatment of epileptic depression and has a positive effect on cognitive improvement. Although it has a certain effect on refractory epilepsy, it has a poor effect on reducing the severity and duration of seizures, and at the same time, it is slightly less effective in improving depressive symptoms [236].

VNS may be an option for depressed patients with insufficient response to drug treatment, but it is mainly used for the treatment of epilepsy, and there is a lack of relevant evidence to support the clinical treatment of depression. However, some reports have shown that VNS may cause serious adverse reactions, such as cardiac arrest. In a long-term follow-up study of a patient with refractory nonconvulsive SE treated with VNS, the patient was found to have cardiac arrest [237]. One patient developed dysphonia, mild cough, and bradycardia [238].

Electroconvulsive Therapy (ECT)

Indications for first-line ECT include major depression with psychotic features, major depression with psychomotor delay, "true" treatment-resistant major depression, and refusal to eat or other special conditions requiring rapid relief of depressive symptoms, such as severe suicidal tendencies or drug contraindications (e.g., pregnancy). ECT as a first-line treatment is also indicated for patients who have had a positive response to it in the past and for patients for whom ECT is preferred for specific reasons.

Other Nerve Stimulation

Due to the continuous improvement and expansion of new technologies, neuromodulation and nerve stimulation provide more options for the treatment of epilepsy and depression comorbidity. The application prospects of low-field magnetic stimulation, transcranial pulsed electromagnetic field, transcranial direct current stimulation, epidural cortical stimulation, near-infrared transcranial radiation and closed-loop stimulation are gradually expanding [233].

7.3.7.4 Other Drugs

Some medicinal plants, such as *Achyranthes bidentata*, *Amaranth*, *European berberis*, *liquorice*, *pink flower*, *pomegranate,* and *South African nightshade*, have antidepressant and antiepileptic effects [239]. Compared with SSRIs, Hypericum (St. John's wort) therapy has been shown to be effective and safe in patients with mild to moderate depression, but its therapeutic effect on epilepsy is not clear and lacks clinical support [240]. Diterpene phytol, β-motylene, CBD, and berberine are considered potential antiseizure medications that are safer and more effective. However, whether they have antidepressant effects is not clear [241]. Preclinical and clinical data on the treatment of epilepsy and its associated complications associated with plant components have provided the basis for the discovery and development of novel antiseizure medication in the medicinal plant class. However, its efficacy and safety still need to be further verified.

7.4 Suicidal Behavior in Epileptic Patients

Since the United States FDA added warnings about the potential for suicide associated with almost every antiepileptic drug in 2008, the issue of suicide among epilepsy patients has regained widespread international attention. A substantial body of research has been published on the epidemiology, triggering factors, clinical manifestations, relationship with antiseizure medication, and diagnostic and preventive methods surrounding suicide in epilepsy patients, contributing to scientific progress in the field. This ongoing effort continues to summarize and elucidate the relevant factors associated with suicide in epilepsy patients, aiming to improve the prognosis of epilepsy treatment [242–244].

7.4.1 Suicide in Epilepsy

Despite ongoing debates, numerous studies support the notion that individuals with epilepsy have a higher suicide rate. Jakob Christensen and colleagues [245] conducted a study analyzing 21,169 suicide cases and 423,128 control cases from the Danish Death Registry, revealing a threefold higher suicide rate among epilepsy patients than among controls. Haijiao Wang and colleagues [243] analyzed 1,178,401 epilepsy patients from 2786 studies and compared them with 6,900,657 control individuals, finding elevated rates of suicidal ideation, suicide attempts, and completed suicides in epilepsy patients. They emphasized the importance for clinicians to be aware of suicide risk in epilepsy patients and to identify and prevent it at an early stage. Jose F Tellez-Zenteno [246] interviewed 36,984 participants using logistic regression to assess the mental health of epilepsy patients and concluded that epilepsy is associated with a greater prevalence of suicidal ideation, emphasizing the importance of understanding the psychological aspects of epilepsy for the comprehensive management of this patient population. Although suicide in epilepsy patients is a complex phenomenon, the majority of physicians agree that the suicide rate is higher among epilepsy patients, making screening for suicide risk appropriate [247].

7.4.2 Epidemiological Investigations

Haijiao Wang and colleagues [243] reported that the rates of suicidal ideation, suicide attempts, and completed suicides among epilepsy patients were 19.73%, 5.96%, and 0.24%, respectively. In particular, patients with temporal lobe epilepsy and drug-resistant epilepsy were more prone to suicide. Nicholas Abraham and colleagues [248] conducted a meta-analysis on suicide among epilepsy patients involving 821,594 patients in seven case–control studies and reported that the prevalence rates of suicidal ideation and suicide attempts were 23.2% (95% CI: 0.176–0.301) and 7.4% (95% CI: 0.031–0.169), respectively, with a suicide completion rate of 0.5% (95% CI: 0.002–0.016). Qian Li [249] and colleagues identified 41 out of 355 patients (11.5%) with a moderate to high risk of suicide. Daniel Friedman and colleagues [244] analyzed 770 epilepsy patients with depression and found that 155 participants (20.1%) acknowledged suicidal thoughts and behaviors. Andres M Kanner [250] described a lifetime prevalence of 25% for suicidal ideation (SI) among epilepsy patients.

7.4.3 Pathological Factors in Epilepsy Patients

Recent research indicates that three main factors are associated with suicide in individuals with epilepsy.

7.4.3.1 Antiseizure Medication (ASMs)

The U.S. FDA conducted a meta-analysis of 199 studies involving 11 antiseizure medications and revealed that among patients taking ASMs, four reported suicides, while no suicide was reported in the control group. This suggests that patients taking ASMs may face a greater risk of suicide than those taking a placebo [251]. Dreier and colleagues [252] analyzed 1759 epilepsy patients who completed suicide and reported a significant association between the use of antiseizure medication and increased suicide risk. This association could not be explained by previous suicidal tendencies or a family history of mental illness, suggesting that the use of antiseizure medication may be a significant contributing factor to the increased suicide rate among epilepsy patients.

7.4.3.2 Epileptic Psychosis

Epileptic psychosis can be categorized into postictal psychosis, interictal psychosis, forced normalization, and preictal psychosis. Interictal psychosis refers to mental abnormalities occurring within 7 days after an epileptic seizure, while postictal psychosis occurs 7 days after a seizure. Both types are significantly related to the severity of epilepsy, presenting clinical features similar to those of schizophrenia; thus, they are also known as epileptic schizophrenia. Reports indicate that postictal psychosis, interictal psychosis, and forced normalization can all contribute to suicide in epilepsy patients [251, 253]. Hesdorffer and colleagues [254] conducted a study involving 14,059 patients who experienced seizures and 56,184 control patients to understand the reasons for suicide in epilepsy patients. They found that the proportion of patients who attempted suicide for the first time was 2.9 times greater in those who experienced seizures later than in the control group (95% CI, 2.5 to 3.4 times). The risk of repeated suicide attempts on the day of a diagnosed seizure was 1.8 times greater than that in the control group, suggesting a connection between suicide or repeated suicide attempts and epilepsy before seizures occur. This indicates a potential shared biological mechanism between the two, although the exact nature of this mechanism remains unclear.

7.4.3.3 Comorbidities in Epilepsy

The co-occurrence of mental abnormalities in epilepsy patients is common Dheeraj Rai [255] interviewed 7403 adults in the UK and reported that one-third of epilepsy patients met the criteria for anxiety or depression according to international classifications, whereas only one-sixth of nonepileptic individuals had anxiety or depression. Social phobia, specific phobia, generalized anxiety disorder, and depression were all associated with suicidal tendencies.

Depression

Suicide is a core manifestation of depression, and individuals with epilepsy are more likely to have comorbid depression. Tedrus et al. [256] analyzed 271 epilepsy patients and reported that 50.6% were females, with an average age of 46.6 (± 15.8) years. Fifty patients (19.3%) were at risk of suicide, and multivariate logistic regression revealed that depression was the most significant variable inducing suicidal tendencies in epilepsy patients. Manny Bagary [257] reported that comorbid depression during the first 6 months after epilepsy surgery was a specific risk factor for suicide in epilepsy patients.

Psychosis

There is a clear inherent connection between epileptic seizures and psychosis, which often co-occur and become the most common comorbidity in epilepsy patients. Andres M Kanner [250] reported that while epilepsy patients without coexisting mental disorders had a suicide risk 2–3 times greater than that of the general population, the risk increased by 12–32 times when various mental disorders were present. Emotional and mental disorders are common risk factors for suicide in epilepsy patients. Dale C Hesdorffer [258] compared 3773 epilepsy patients aged 10–60 years with 14,025 control individuals and reported an association between epilepsy and an increase in suicide risk with or without a psychiatric diagnosis before or after epilepsy diagnosis. These relationships suggest the existence of potential shared pathophysiological mechanisms that lower the threshold for epileptic seizures and increase the risk of mental disorders and suicide.

Other Mental Abnormalities

Anxiety is also common in epilepsy patients. GMAS Tedrus [259] studied 98 outpatient epilepsy patients, with an average age of 48.1 ± 15.9 years and a history of epilepsy of 26.4 ± 16.4 years. Of these patients, 33 were at risk of suicide. According to the univariate analysis, younger age and an earlier age of onset of epilepsy were significantly associated with suicide risk. Logistic regression analysis revealed that anxiety and poor family satisfaction were the most relevant factors for the highest suicide risk. Based on a population study, Andres M Kanner [250] reported similar findings, supporting the notion that comorbidities in patients with epilepsy are crucial contributors to suicide.

7.4.4 Clinical Characteristics of Suicide in Epilepsy Patients

7.4.4.1 Age and Sex

Research by Nicholas Abraham [248] revealed that suicide attempts and completed suicides in epilepsy patients are associated with age and sex. Younger epilepsy patients may be more prone to suicide due to interpersonal relationships, while male patients may use more lethal methods in suicide attempts. The authors suggest that to improve the suicide success rate in the epilepsy population, special attention should be given to suicide in young male patients.

7.4.4.2 Timing of Occurrence

Jakob Christensen and colleagues [245] conducted a study involving 21,169 suicide cases and 423,128 control cases and revealed that the highest suicide risk among epilepsy patients occurs in the first 6 months after diagnosis (5.35, 3.43–8.33; $p < 0.0001$). Additionally, those with a history of mental illness have a greater risk during this period. The authors emphasize the vulnerability of newly diagnosed epilepsy patients during this time and the need for special attention.

7.4.4.3 Risk Factors

ASM Dosage

Wen and colleagues [260] conducted a prospective cohort study of 163 epilepsy patients and found that suicidal ideation occurs only when the dosage of antiseizure medication increases, indicating a potential association between high-dose antiepileptic drug use and suicide in epilepsy patients. Aksha M Memon [261] analyzed

443 relevant articles on PubMed and reported a positive correlation between suicidal behavior in epilepsy patients and high-dose pregabalin use.

Cultural Influence

Susanna S O'Kula [262] studied 277 Spanish-speaking and 213 non-Spanish-speaking epilepsy patients and discovered that Spanish-speaking patients had less severe depressive symptoms, but the incidence of suicidal ideation was similar. Foreign birth was unrelated to the incidence of suicidal ideation.

Intractable Epilepsy

Dale C Hesdorffer [263] and colleagues used three tools to assess lifetime and recent suicidal ideation and behavior rates in patients with intractable focal epilepsy. Among the 208 patients, 1.6–3.9% had recent suicidal ideation, 1.0–4.7% had recent suicide attempts, and the lifetime suicidal ideation rate was 12.1–14.1%. Among those with recent suicide attempts, 31.1% required referral to medical professionals, and 3.9% needed emergency referral. The rates of lifetime suicidal behavior were 21.1% in the E-CSSRS and 15.5% in the C-SSRS (including aborted suicide attempts, interrupted suicide attempts, suicide attempts, preparatory acts or behavior, and nonsuicidal self-injury), which were significantly greater than those in the general population, highlighting intractable focal epilepsy as a significant factor in patient suicide.

Temporal Lobe Epilepsy

Rene Andrade-Machado [264] assessed the suicide risk of 82 epilepsy patients and found that all 33 patients at risk of suicide had temporal lobe epilepsy, indicating a greater likelihood of suicide in patients with temporal lobe epilepsy.

7.4.4.4 Clinical Manifestations of Suicide in Epilepsy Patients

Suicide in epilepsy patients can manifest as completed suicide, suicidal ideation, suicide attempts, suicidal behavior, and suicidal depression [265]. Laura Redden [266] reported that among 1327 patients taking sodium valproate, 11 experienced suicidal events, including 2 suicide attempts and 9 with suicidal ideation. Cases described by Nicholas Abraham [248] suggested that suicide in epilepsy patients mainly presents as suicidal ideation and suicide attempts, with only 0.5% resulting in completed suicide.

7.4.4.5 Suicide Induced by Different Antiseizure Medication

Lacosamide

Aksha M Memon [261] analyzed 443 articles on PubMed and found three studies suggesting an association between lacosamide treatment for epilepsy and suicidal behavior. Despite some methodological limitations, the authors believe there is an association and call for larger prospective, randomized studies to provide conclusive evidence.

Gabapentin

Kristine S Ziemba [267] conducted a structured literature search to find evidence of a single antiepileptic drug causing suicide in epilepsy patients. One cohort study using carbamazepine as a reference revealed an increased suicide risk in patients taking gabapentin (relative risk, 13.92; 95% confidence interval, 1.82–106.38). Compared with topiramate, gabapentin, oxcarbazepine, and other drugs were found to increase suicide risk in epilepsy patients. The authors suggest that although there is limited evidence of antiseizure medication causing an increased tendency for suicide in epilepsy patients, attention should be given to the potential for gabapentin use to lead to increased suicide attempts and risk.

Other Drugs

Regarding other drugs, Pavel Klein [268] studied 4000 individuals receiving treatment with antiseizure medication and 1996 individuals receiving a placebo to investigate antiepileptic drug-induced suicide in epilepsy patients. The study revealed that eslicarbazepine acetate, perampanel, brivaracetam, and cannabidiol use did not increase the likelihood of suicide in patients. The authors concluded that there is no evidence that these four antiseizure medications increase the likelihood of suicide in epilepsy patients. To further clarify the complex relationship between antiseizure medication and suicide, Emily E Leppien and colleagues [265] used the U.S. Food and Drug Administration Adverse Event Reporting System (FAERS) to compare the impact of new antiseizure medication with that of traditional antiseizure medication on suicide rates. They analyzed a total of 6309 suicide cases, with suicide case rates involving lacosamide at 2.8%, perampanel at 10.2%, clobazam at 2.8%, brivaracetam at 4.9%, and cannabidiol at 8.0%. Compared to those for older antiseizure medications, the suicide rates were lower for the four newer antiseizure medications (lacosamide, clobazam, brivaracetam, and cannabidiol), while perampanel use significantly increased the risk.

7.4.5 Diagnosis of Suicide in Epilepsy

The diagnosis of suicide in epilepsy patients relies on self-reports from patients and information provided by caregivers. Currently, suicide assessments are primarily conducted using suicide rating scales. Commonly used tools in clinical settings include the Mini International Neuropsychiatric Interview (MINI), the Columbia-Suicide Severity Rating Scale (C-SSRS), and the Interactive Voice Response System CSSRS (E-CSSRS)[263]. Dale C Hesdorffer [263] utilized these three tools to assess lifetime and recent suicidal ideation and behavior rates in patients with intractable epilepsy. Through the validation of data from 208 patients, the authors found that these screening tools are reliable for suicide screening in epilepsy patients, with a minimal likelihood of false negatives. Additionally, they observed that the E-CSSRS slightly outperformed the C-SSRS in predicting suicidal behavior, suggesting that the E-CSSRS might be the preferred choice. Hyo Jae Kim [269] validated the assessment of suicide tendencies in epilepsy patients by screening 213 patients using the Neurological Disorders Depression Inventory for Epilepsy (NDDIE) and the Patient Health Questionnaire 9 (PHQ-9). They found that the fourth item of the NDDIE and the ninth item of the PHQ-9 demonstrated value in screening for suicidal tendencies, providing rapid identification of suicidal tendencies in epilepsy patients.

Despite the prevalence of suicide in epilepsy patients, there is still a significant issue regarding the awareness and attention given by clinicians. A survey conducted by Bassel F Shneker [270] involving 175 physicians, most of whom were epilepsy specialists practicing in academic environments, revealed that 62% of them did not use any scale to screen for depression in epilepsy patients. Although 98% of the physicians warned patients about potential side effects when initiating treatment with antiseizure medication, only 44% specifically warned about suicidal thoughts or behavior. More than half of the physicians did not know whether their patients had attempted or completed suicide.

Clinical practitioners should conduct suicide assessments, especially for patients with relevant risk factors such as a family history of psychiatric illness, a history of psychiatric illness, or significant anxiety and depression. It is crucial to identify any suicidal tendencies early, particularly when initiating treatment with antiseizure medication or transitioning from one antiepileptic drug to another. Patients should be advised to report any changes in mood and suicidal thoughts to their treating physicians.

7.4.6 Treatment of Suicide in Epilepsy

The management of suicide in epilepsy patients should adhere to the following basic principles:

7.4.6.1 Control Seizures

Suicide in epilepsy is often associated with seizures. Controlling seizures not only improves the quality of life for epilepsy patients but also eliminates the risk factors contributing to suicide. It is particularly important for patients with refractory epilepsy to seek effective treatment methods to control seizures.

7.4.6.2 Continue the Use of ASMs

While the U.S. FDA emphasizes that ASMs may increase the risk of suicide in epilepsy patients, the relationship between use of these drugs and the incidence of suicide is not entirely clear, but the incidence is not high. An expert consensus on clinical medication was developed by the International League Against Epilepsy Neurobiology Committee to guide the treatment of epilepsy patients with suicidal tendencies. According to this consensus, experts emphasize that despite the FDA warning to healthcare professionals about the potential risk of increased suicidal ideation and behavior with ASMs, subsequent retrospective cohort and case–control studies have yielded conflicting results. Therefore, although some (but not all) ASMs may be associated with psychiatric abnormalities leading to suicidal thoughts and behavior, the actual suicide risk has not been determined. The risk of stopping ASMs or refusing to initiate them is significantly more severe and may result in serious harm, including patient death. If a patient needs to discontinue the use of antiseizure medication, it is essential to establish a clear association between epilepsy-related suicide and the current use of ASMs. Epilepsy-related suicide is multifactorial, and several variables influence its risk. Clinicians should investigate the presence of such risk factors and use appropriate screening tools. If necessary, patients should be referred for psychiatric evaluation. Even if a patient is at risk of suicide, ASM treatment should not be discontinued [271]. Additionally, antiseizure medication may affect abnormal emotional activity through multiple mechanisms. Referral for psychiatric evaluation should be considered if the patient's suicidal thoughts are attributable to the ASM in use.

7.4.6.3 Target Appropriate Treatment for the Risk Factors of Epilepsy-Related Suicide

When there is significant anxiety and depression, anti-anxiety and antidepressant treatments may be warranted. In the presence of psychosis, selecting appropriate antipsychotic medications is necessary. Psychosis following seizures usually does not lead to suicide and generally does not require treatment. However, for patients with interictal psychosis and forced normalization, treatment with risperidone and fluphenazine, respectively, can be considered to prevent epilepsy-related suicide. The use of antiseizure medication that can induce suicide should be avoided.

7.4.6.4 Strengthen Care

Enhanced care is crucial for patients with suicidal tendencies and suicidal ideation, especially those with a history of suicide attempts. This helps prevent patients with suicidal tendencies from progressing to completed suicide [272].

References

1. Joyal KG, Kreitlow BL, Buchanan GF. The role of sleep state and time of day in modulating breathing in epilepsy: implications for sudden unexpected death in epilepsy. Front Neural Circuits. 2022;16:983211.
2. Bonilla-Jaime H, Zeleke H, Rojas A, Espinosa-Garcia C. Sleep disruption worsens seizures: neuroinflammation as a potential mechanistic link. Int J Mol Sci. 2021;22(22):12531.
3. Grigg-Damberger M, Foldvary-Schaefer N. Bidirectional relationships of sleep and epilepsy in adults with epilepsy. Epilepsy Behav. 2021;116:107735.
4. Nayak CS, Sinha S, Nagappa M, Thennarasu K, Taly AB. Effect of carbamazepine on the sleep microstructure of temporal lobe epilepsy patients: a cyclic alternating pattern-based study. Sleep Med. 2016;27-28:80–5.
5. Macêdo P, Oliveira PS, Foldvary-Schaefer N, Gomes MDM. Insomnia in people with epilepsy: a review of insomnia prevalence, risk factors and associations with epilepsy-related factors. Epilepsy Res. 2017;135:158–67.
6. Garg D, Charlesworth L, Shukla G. Sleep and temporal lobe epilepsy – associations, mechanisms and treatment implications. Front Hum Neurosci. 2022;16:849899.
7. Chihorek AM, Abou-Khalil B, Malow BA. Obstructive sleep apnea is associated with seizure occurrence in older adults with epilepsy. Neurology. 2007;69(19):1823–7.
8. Malow BA, Weatherwax KJ, Chervin RD, Hoban TF, Marzec ML, Martin C, et al. Identification and treatment of obstructive sleep apnea in adults and children with epilepsy: a prospective pilot study. Sleep Med. 2003;4(6):509–15.
9. Patel SR. Obstructive Sleep Apnea. Ann Intern Med. 2019;171(11):Itc81–itc96.
10. Al-Abri M, Al-Asmi A, Al-Shukairi A, Al-Qanoobi A, Ramachandiran N, Jacob P, et al. Frequency of obstructive sleep apnea syndrome among patients with epilepsy attending a tertiary neurology clinic. Oman Med J. 2015;30(1):31–5.
11. Pornsriniyom D, Kim H, Bena J, Andrews ND, Moul D, Foldvary-Schaefer N. Effect of positive airway pressure therapy on seizure control in patients with epilepsy and obstructive sleep apnea. Epilepsy Behav. 2014;37:270–5.
12. Phabphal K, Sripradit M, Alan FG, Wongsritrang K, Chongsuvivatwong T, Suwanlaong K, et al. Identifying obstructive sleep apnea in patients with epilepsy: a cross-sectional multicenter study. Seizure. 2022;100:87–94.
13. Gogou M, Haidopoulou K, Eboriadou M, Pavlidou E, Hatzistylianou M, Pavlou E. Sleep respiratory parameters in children with idiopathic epilepsy: a cross-sectional study. Epilepsy Res. 2016;126:10–5.
14. Shaheen HA, Abd El-Kader AA, El Gohary AM, El-Fayoumy NM, Afifi LM. Obstructive sleep apnea in epilepsy: a preliminary Egyptian study. Sleep Breath. 2012;16(3):765–71.
15. Lin Z, Si Q, Xiaoyi Z. Obstructive sleep apnoea in patients with epilepsy: a meta-analysis. Sleep Breath. 2017;21(2):263–70.
16. Jain SV, Simakajornboon S, Shapiro SM, Morton LD, Leszczyszyn DJ, Simakajornboon N. Obstructive sleep apnea in children with epilepsy: prospective pilot trial. Acta Neurol Scand. 2012;125(1):e3–6.
17. Scharf MT, Greenberg P, Wong S, Mani R. Obstructive sleep apnea risk in patients with focal versus generalized epilepsy. Epilepsy Behav. 2020;111:107190.

18. McCarter AR, Timm PC, Shepard PW, Sandness DJ, Luu T, McCarter SJ, et al. Obstructive sleep apnea in refractory epilepsy: a pilot study investigating frequency, clinical features, and association with risk of sudden unexpected death in epilepsy. Epilepsia. 2018;59(10):1973–81.
19. Malow BA, Levy K, Maturen K, Bowes R. Obstructive sleep apnea is common in medically refractory epilepsy patients. Neurology. 2000;55(7):1002–7.
20. Cheng JY. Risk of sudden unexpected death in people with epilepsy and obstructive sleep apnea. Epilepsy Res. 2021;176:106729.
21. Manni R, Terzaghi M, Arbasino C, Sartori I, Galimberti CA, Tartara A. Obstructive sleep apnea in a clinical series of adult epilepsy patients: frequency and features of the comorbidity. Epilepsia. 2003;44(6):836–40.
22. Stanbouly D, Radley B, Steinberg B, Ascherman JA. What are the risk factors for epilepsy among patients with Craniosynostosis? J Oral Maxillofac Surg. 2022;80(7):1191–7.
23. Miano S, Tabarrini A, Vitelli O, Mazzotta A, Del Pozzo M, Rabasco J, et al. The cooccurrence of interictal discharges and seizures in pediatric sleep-disordered breathing. Epilepsy Behav. 2013;29(3):508–12.
24. Miliauskas S, Liesiene V, Zemaitis M, Sakalauskas R. Late-onset nocturnal intractable seizure during sleep: what is the origin? Medicina (Kaunas). 2010;46(2):120–4.
25. Hollinger P, Khatami R, Gugger M, Hess CW, Bassetti CL. Epilepsy and obstructive sleep apnea. Eur Neurol. 2006;55(2):74–9.
26. Sonka K, Juklícková M, Pretl M, Dostálová S, Horínek D, Nevsímalová S. Seizures in sleep apnea patients: occurrence and time distribution. Sb Lek. 2000;101(3):229–32.
27. Nguyen-Michel VH, Pallanca O, Navarro V, Dupont S, Baulac M, Adam C. How are epileptic events linked to obstructive sleep apneas in epilepsy? Seizure. 2015;24:121–3.
28. Ismayilova V, Demir AU, Tezer FI. Subjective sleep disturbance in epilepsy patients at an outpatient clinic: a questionnaire-based study on prevalence. Epilepsy Res. 2015;115:119–25.
29. Broderick L, Tuohy G, Solymos O, Lakhani S, Staunton B, Ennis P, et al. Management of vagus nerve stimulation therapy in the peri-operative period: guidelines from the Association of Anaesthetists: guidelines from the Association of Anaesthetists. Anaesthesia. 2023;78(6):747–57.
30. Chan JHM, DelRosso LM, Ruth C, Wrede JE. A surface electrode adjacent to vagal nerve stimulator lead can aid in characterizing vagal nerve stimulator-mediated pediatric sleep-disordered breathing: a case series of 7 patients. J Clin Sleep Med. 2022;18(8):1973–81.
31. Pérez-Carbonell L, Higgins S, Koutroumanidis M, Leschziner G. Sleep-disordered breathing as a consequence of Vagus nerve stimulation. Rev Neurol. 2020;70(5):179–82.
32. Kim JS, Lee DE, Bae H, Song JY, Yang KI, Hong SB. Effects of Vagus nerve stimulation on sleep-disordered breathing, daytime sleepiness, and sleep quality in patients with drug-resistant epilepsy. J Clin Neurol. 2022;18(3):315–22.
33. Malow BA, Edwards J, Marzec M, Sagher O, Fromes G. Effects of Vagus nerve stimulation on respiration during sleep: a pilot study. Neurology. 2000;55(10):1450–4.
34. Sun X, Lv Y, Lin J. The mechanism of sudden unexpected death in epilepsy: a mini review. Front Neurol. 2023;14:1137182.
35. So EL. What is known about the mechanisms underlying SUDEP? Epilepsia. 2008;49(Suppl 9):93–8.
36. Johnston SC, Horn JK, Valente J, Simon RP. The role of hypoventilation in a sheep model of epileptic sudden death. Ann Neurol. 1995;37(4):531–7.
37. Jallon P. Sudden death of epileptic patients. Presse Med. 1999;28(11):605–11.
38. Phabphal K, Koonalintip P, Sithinamsuwan P, Wongsritrang K, Amornpojnimman T, Ekpitakdamrong N, et al. Obstructive sleep apnea and sudden unexpected death in epilepsy in unselected patients with epilepsy: are they associated? Sleep Breath. 2021;25(4):1919–24.
39. Liu F, Wang X. Diagnosis and treatment of epilepsy and sleep apnea comorbidity. Expert Rev Neurother. 2017;17(5):475–85.

40. Bergmann M, Brandauer E, Stefani A, Heidbreder A, Unterberger I, Högl B. The additional diagnostic benefits of performing both video-polysomnography and prolonged video-EEG-monitoring: when and why. Clin Neurophysiol Pract. 2022;7:98–102.
41. Malow BA, Bowes RJ, Lin X. Predictors of sleepiness in epilepsy patients. Sleep. 1997;20(12):1105–10.
42. Foldvary-Schaefer N. Sleep complaints and epilepsy: the role of seizures, antiepileptic drugs and sleep disorders. J Clin Neurophysiol. 2002;19(6):514–21.
43. Kanner AM, Bicchi MM. Antiseizure medications for adults with epilepsy: a review. JAMA. 2022;327(13):1269–81.
44. Chaneva O. Effects of levetiracetam on sleep architecture and daytime sleepiness. Folia Med (Plovdiv). 2021;63(5):631–6.
45. Jo H, Choi S, Kim D, Joo E. Effects of obstructive sleep apnea on epilepsy, and continuous positive airway pressure as a treatment option. J Clin Med. 2022;11(7):2063.
46. Lee HW, Hong SB, Tae WS, Seo DW, Kim SE. Partial seizures manifesting as apnea only in an adult. Epilepsia. 1999;40(12):1828–31.
47. Nesbitt AD, Kosky CA, Leschziner GD. Insular seizures causing sleep-related breathlessness. Lancet. 2013;382(9906):1756.
48. Nishimura Y, Saito Y, Kondo N, Matsuda E, Fujiyama M, Morizane R, et al. Ictal central apnea and bradycardia in temporal lobe epilepsy complicated by obstructive sleep apnea syndrome. Epilepsy Behav Case Rep. 2015;4:41–4.
49. Schwartz K, Lastra AC, Balabanov AJ. Obstructive and central sleep apnoea in a patient with medically intractable epilepsy. BMJ Case Rep. 2022;15(9):e245564.
50. Barone DA, Segal AZ. Obstructive sleep apnea and positive airway pressure usage in populations with neurological disease. Sleep Med Clin. 2022;17(4):619–27.
51. Sethi NK. The relationship between epilepsy, obstructive sleep apnea, and treatment outcome. Sleep Med Clin. 2022;17(4):639–45.
52. Vendrame M, Auerbach S, Loddenkemper T, Kothare S, Montouris G. Effect of continuous positive airway pressure treatment on seizure control in patients with obstructive sleep apnea and epilepsy. Epilepsia. 2011;52(11):e168–71.
53. Li P, Ghadersohi S, Jafari B, Teter B, Sazgar M. Characteristics of refractory vs. medically controlled epilepsy patients with obstructive sleep apnea and their response to CPAP treatment. Seizure. 2012;21(9):717–21.
54. Malow BA, Foldvary-Schaefer N, Vaughn BV, Selwa LM, Chervin RD, Weatherwax KJ, et al. Treating obstructive sleep apnea in adults with epilepsy: a randomized pilot trial. Neurology. 2008;71(8):572–7.
55. Kevat A, Bernard A, Harris MA, Heussler H, Black R, Cheng A, et al. Impact of adenotonsillectomy on growth trajectories in preschool children with mild-moderate obstructive sleep apnea. J Clin Sleep Med. 2023;19(1):55–62.
56. Segal E, Vendrame M, Gregas M, Loddenkemper T, Kothare SV. Effect of treatment of obstructive sleep apnea on seizure outcomes in children with epilepsy. Pediatr Neurol. 2012;46(6):359–62.
57. Koh S, Ward SL, Lin M, Chen LS. Sleep apnea treatment improves seizure control in children with neurodevelopmental disorders. Pediatr Neurol. 2000;22(1):36–9.
58. Oyegbile-Chidi T. Continuous positive airway pressure use for obstructive sleep apnea in pediatric patients. Sleep Med Clin. 2022;17(4):629–38.
59. Hsin LJ, Lee YC, Lin WN, Lu YA, Lee LA, Tsai MS, et al. Transoral tongue suspension for obstructive sleep apnea-a preliminary study. J Clin Med. 2022;11(17):4960.
60. Maniaci A, Di Luca M, Lechien JR, Iannella G, Grillo C, Grillo CM, et al. Lateral pharyngoplasty vs. traditional uvulopalatopharyngoplasty for patients with OSA: systematic review and meta-analysis. Sleep Breath. 2022;26(4):1539–50.
61. Fenton JE, Fitzgerald C, Dillon PJ, O'Shea D. Never say never: circumventing a contraindication to control apnoea-induced epileptic events with a mandibular advancement device. J Laryngol Otol. 2018;132(11):1036–8.

62. Machado MA, Juliano L, Taga M, de Carvalho LB, do Prado LB, do Prado GF. Titratable mandibular repositioner appliances for obstructive sleep apnea syndrome: are they an option? Sleep Breath. 2007;11(4):225–31.
63. Qaseem A, Holty JE, Owens DK, Dallas P, Starkey M, Shekelle P. Management of obstructive sleep apnea in adults: a clinical practice guideline from the American College of Physicians. Ann Intern Med. 2013;159(7):471–83.
64. Westwood AJ, Vendrame M, Montouris G, Auerbach SH. Pearls & Oy-sters: treatment of central sleep apnea with topiramate. Neurology. 2012;78(16):e97–9.
65. Shukralla AA, Dolan E, Delanty N. Acetazolamide: Old drug, new evidence? Epilepsia Open. 2022;7(3):378–92.
66. Scherping SC 3rd, Quigg M, Davis EM. Acetazolamide as an adjunct to positive airway pressure therapy in the treatment of combined central and obstructive sleep apnea. Ann Am Thorac Soc. 2023;20(1):131–5.
67. Winslow DH, Bowden CH, DiDonato KP, McCullough PA. A randomized, double-blind, placebo-controlled study of an oral, extended-release formulation of phentermine/topiramate for the treatment of obstructive sleep apnea in obese adults. Sleep. 2012;35(11):1529–39.
68. Javaheri S, Javaheri S. Update on persistent excessive daytime sleepiness in OSA. Chest. 2020;158(2):776–86.
69. Gaisl T, Haile SR, Thiel S, Osswald M, Kohler M. Efficacy of pharmacotherapy for OSA in adults: a systematic review and network meta-analysis. Sleep Med Rev. 2019;46:74–86.
70. Roliz AH, Kothare S. The interaction between sleep and epilepsy. Curr Neurol Neurosci Rep. 2022;22(9):551–63.
71. Ruangkana P, Chinvarun Y, Udommongkol C, Chairungsaris P, Nidhinandana S, Suwantamee J, et al. Excessive daytime sleepiness and obstructive sleep apnea in Thai epileptic patients. J Med Assoc Thail. 2014;97(Suppl 2):S175–80.
72. Hoff S, Collop N. Home sleep apnea testing for the diagnosis of obstructive sleep apnea. JAMA. 2023;329(2):169–70.
73. Barrea L, Pugliese G, Frias-Toral E, Napolitano B, Laudisio D, Aprano S, et al. Is there a relationship between the ketogenic diet and sleep disorders? Int J Food Sci Nutr. 2022;73(3):285–95.
74. Nobili L, Frauscher B, Eriksson S, Gibbs SA, Halasz P, Lambert I, et al. Sleep and epilepsy: a snapshot of knowledge and future research lines. J Sleep Res. 2022;31(4):e13622.
75. Chang YT, Chen PC, Tsai IJ, Sung FC, Chin ZN, Kuo HT, et al. Bidirectional relation between schizophrenia and epilepsy: a population-based retrospective cohort study. Epilepsia. 2011;52(11):2036–42.
76. Adachi N, Matsuura M, Hara T, Oana Y, Okubo Y, Kato M, et al. Psychoses and epilepsy: are interictal and postictal psychoses distinct clinical entities? Epilepsia. 2002;43(12):1574–82.
77. Fahed M, Ramanathan S. Psychoses of epilepsy in pregnancy: a case report. Clin Psychopharmacol Neurosci. 2021;19(2):388–90.
78. Mishra BR, Biswas T, Nath S, Jha M, Mishra S, Mohapatra D. Electroconvulsive therapy with ketamine as induction agent in refractory epilepsy with atypical postictal psychosis: a case report. J ECT. 2021;37(1):e5–6.
79. Ngo VTH, Camacho H, Singh J. You are the one who was beating me: a case report of a patient with postictal psychosis secondary to bilateral temporal lobe epilepsy. Cureus. 2019;11(11):e6069.
80. Park AK, Jesudasen SJ, Olson KR. Risperidone for successful treatment of postictal psychosis refractory to olanzapine. Proceedings (Bayl Univ Med Cent). 2021;34(2):318–20.
81. Turner WA. The mental condition in epilepsy in relation to prognosis. Med Chir Trans. 1904;87:349–72.
82. Nadkarni S, Arnedo V, Devinsky O. Psychosis in epilepsy patients. Epilepsia. 2007;48(Suppl 9):17–9.
83. Weingarten MD, Lockwood AH, Hwo SY, Kirschner MW. A protein factor essential for microtubule assembly. Proc Natl Acad Sci USA. 1975;72(5):1858–62.

84. Karagulla S, Robertson EE. Phychical phenomena in temporal lobe epilepsy and the psychoses. Br Med J. 1955;1(4916):748–52.
85. Glaser GH. The problem of psychosis in psychomotor temporal lobe epileptics. Epilepsia. 1964;5:271–8.
86. Kanemoto K, Kawasaki J, Kawai I. Postictal psychosis: a comparison with acute interictal and chronic psychoses. Epilepsia. 1996;37(6):551–6.
87. Kanemoto K, Tsuji T, Kawasaki J. Reexamination of interictal psychoses based on DSM IV psychosis classification and international epilepsy classification. Epilepsia. 2001;42(1):98–103.
88. Swamy HS, Mallikarjunaiah M, Bhatti RS, Kaliaperumal VG. A study of epileptic psychoses – 150 cases. Indian J Psychiatry. 1986;28(3):231–6.
89. Logsdail SJ, Toone BK. Post-ictal psychoses. A clinical and phenomenological description. Br J Psychiatry. 1988;152:246–52.
90. Manchanda R, Miller H, McLachlan RS. Post-ictal psychosis after right temporal lobectomy. J Neurol Neurosurg Psychiatry. 1993;56(3):277–9.
91. Hilger E, Zimprich F, Pataraia E, Aull-Watschinger S, Jung R, Baumgartner C, et al. Psychoses in epilepsy: a comparison of postictal and interictal psychoses. Epilepsy Behav. 2016;60:58–62.
92. Falip M, Carreño M, Donaire A, Maestro I, Pintor L, Bargalló N, et al. Postictal psychosis: a retrospective study in patients with refractory temporal lobe epilepsy. Seizure. 2009;18(2):145–9.
93. Hilger E, Zimprich F, Jung R, Pataraia E, Baumgartner C, Bonelli S. Postictal psychosis in temporal lobe epilepsy: a case-control study. Eur J Neurol. 2013;20(6):955–61.
94. Yasumoto S, Motooka H, Ito Y, Uchimura N. A change in electrographic activity and blood flow during interictal and postictal psychotic states in a patient with epilepsy. Epilepsy Behav Case Rep. 2015;4:13–9.
95. Oshima T, Motooka H, Kanemoto K. SPECT findings during postictal psychoses: predominance of relative increase of perfusion in right temporal lobe. Epilepsia. 2011;52(6):1192–4.
96. DuBois JM, Devinsky O, Carlson C, Kuzniecky R, Quinn BT, Alper K, et al. Abnormalities of cortical thickness in postictal psychosis. Epilepsy Behav. 2011;21(2):132–6.
97. Trimble M, Kanner A, Schmitz B. Postictal psychosis. Epilepsy Behav. 2010;19(2):159–61.
98. Devinsky O, Abramson H, Alper K, FitzGerald LS, Perrine K, Calderon J, et al. Postictal psychosis: a case control series of 20 patients and 150 controls. Epilepsy Res. 1995;20(3):247–53.
99. de Toffol B. Postictal psychosis. Rev Neurol (Paris). 2009;165(10):769–73.
100. Adachi N, Ito M, Kanemoto K, Akanuma N, Okazaki M, Ishida S, et al. Duration of postictal psychotic episodes. Epilepsia. 2007;48(8):1531–7.
101. de Toffol B, Kanemoto K. Postictal psychoses: clinical and neurobiological findings. Encéphale. 2016;42(5):443–7.
102. Savard G, Andermann F, Olivier A, Rémillard GM. Postictal psychosis after partial complex seizures: a multiple case study. Epilepsia. 1991;32(2):225–31.
103. Kanemoto K, Kawasaki J, Kawai I. Postictal psychoses: in comparison with acute interictal psychoses. Jpn J Psychiatry Neurol. 1994;48(2):209–11.
104. Sakakibara E, Nishida T, Sugishita K, Jinde S, Inoue Y, Kasai K. Acute psychosis during the postictal period in a patient with idiopathic generalized epilepsy: postictal psychosis or aggravation of schizophrenia? A case report and review of the literature. Epilepsy Behav. 2012;24(3):373–6.
105. Kanner AM, Stagno S, Kotagal P, Morris HH. Postictal psychiatric events during prolonged video-electroencephalographic monitoring studies. Arch Neurol. 1996;53(3):258–63.
106. Maguire M, Singh J, Marson A. Epilepsy and psychosis: a practical approach. Pract Neurol. 2018;18(2):106–14.
107. Ramani V, Gumnit RJ. Intensive monitoring of interictal psychosis in epilepsy. Ann Neurol. 1982;11(6):613–22.
108. Lewis SW. Brain imaging in a case of Capgras' syndrome. Br J Psychiatry. 1987;150:117–21.

109. Caplan R, Shields WD, Mori L, Yudovin S. Middle childhood onset of interictal psychosis. J Am Acad Child Adolesc Psychiatry. 1991;30(6):893–6.
110. Oshima T, Tadokoro Y, Kanemoto K. A prospective study of postictal psychoses with emphasis on the periictal type. Epilepsia. 2006;47(12):2131–4.
111. Pinto-Gouveia C, Ventura F, Carneiro M, Mota D, Renca S, Pissarra C. Long-acting paliperidone injection as a treatment option for interictal psychosis of epilepsy: a case report. Psychiatry Clin Neurosci. 2022;76(7):347–8.
112. Tadokoro Y, Oshima T, Kanemoto K. Interictal psychoses in comparison with schizophrenia–a prospective study. Epilepsia. 2007;48(12):2345–51.
113. Mendez MF, Grau R, Doss RC, Taylor JL. Schizophrenia in epilepsy: seizure and psychosis variables. Neurology. 1993;43(6):1073–7.
114. Onuma T, Adachi N, Ishida S, Katou M, Uesugi S. Prevalence and annual incidence of psychosis in patients with epilepsy. Psychiatry Clin Neurosci. 1995;49(3):S267–8.
115. Clancy MJ, Clarke MC, Connor DJ, Cannon M, Cotter DR. The prevalence of psychosis in epilepsy; a systematic review and meta-analysis. BMC Psychiatry. 2014;14:75.
116. Perez MM, Trimble MR. Epileptic psychosis–diagnostic comparison with process schizophrenia. Br J Psychiatry. 1980;137:245–9.
117. Sone D, Sato N, Shigemoto Y, Kimura Y, Maikusa N, Ota M, et al. Disrupted white matter integrity and structural brain networks in temporal lobe epilepsy with and without Interictal psychosis. Front Neurol. 2020;11:556569.
118. Allebone J, Kanaan R, Maller J, O'Brien T, Mullen SA, Cook M, et al. Bilateral volume reduction in posterior hippocampus in psychosis of epilepsy. J Neurol Neurosurg Psychiatry. 2019;90(6):688–94.
119. Maier M, Mellers J, Toone B, Trimble M, Ron MA. Schizophrenia, temporal lobe epilepsy and psychosis: an in vivo magnetic resonance spectroscopy and imaging study of the hippocampus/amygdala complex. Psychol Med. 2000;30(3):571–81.
120. Hamed SA, Attiah FA. Psychosis in adults with epilepsy and its relationship to demographic, clinical and treatment variables. Neurol Res. 2019;41(11):959–66.
121. Matsuura M, Adachi N, Oana Y, Okubo Y, Kato M, Nakano T, et al. A polydiagnostic and dimensional comparison of epileptic psychoses and schizophrenia spectrum disorders. Schizophr Res. 2004;69(2–3):189–201.
122. Upton K, Meyers M, Thorsell AG, Karlberg T, Holechek J, Lease R, et al. Design and synthesis of potent inhibitors of the mono(ADP-ribosyl)transferase, PARP14. Bioorg Med Chem Lett. 2017;27(13):2907–11.
123. Slater E, Beard AW. The schizophrenia-like psychoses of epilepsy, V: Discussion and conclusions. 1963. J Neuropsychiatry Clin Neurosci. 1995;7(3):372–8; discussion 1–2.
124. Scheffer IE, Berkovic S, Capovilla G, Connolly MB, French J, Guilhoto L, et al. ILAE classification of the epilepsies: position paper of the ILAE Commission for Classification and Terminology. Epilepsia. 2017;58(4):512–21.
125. de Toffol B, Adachi N, Kanemoto K, El-Hage W, Hingray C. Interictal psychosis of epilepsy. Encéphale. 2020;46(6):482–92.
126. Swartz CM. Misdiagnosis of schizophrenia for a patient with epilepsy. Psychiatr Serv. 2001;52(1):109.
127. Gaitatzis A, Trimble MR, Sander JW. The psychiatric comorbidity of epilepsy. Acta Neurol Scand. 2004;110(4):207–20.
128. Kanner AM. Recognition of the various expressions of anxiety, psychosis, and aggression in epilepsy. Epilepsia. 2004;45(Suppl 2):22–7.
129. Adachi N, Akanuma N, Ito M, Okazaki M, Kato M, Onuma T. Interictal psychotic episodes in epilepsy: duration and associated clinical factors. Epilepsia. 2012;53(6):1088–94.
130. Slater E, Beard AW, Glithero E. The schizophrenialike psychoses of epilepsy. Br J Psychiatry. 1963;109:95–150.
131. Yan Y, Wu JH, Peng XY, Wang XF. Effects of antiseizure medications on alternative psychosis and strategies for their application. World J Psychiatry. 2022;12(4):580–7.

132. Hanemaaijer R, Ginzburg I. Involvement of mature tau isoforms in the stabilization of neurites in PC12 cells. J Neurosci Res. 1991;30(1):163–71.
133. Tellenbach H. Epilepsy as a convulsive disorder and as a psychosis. On alternative psychoses of paranoid nature in "Forced normalization" (Landolt) of the electroencephalogram of epileptics. Nervenarzt. 1965;36:190–202.
134. Wolf P. Acute behavioral symptomatology at disappearance of epileptiform EEG abnormality. Paradoxical or "forced" normalization. Adv Neurol. 1991;55:127–42.
135. Krishnamoorthy ES, Trimble MR. Forced normalization: clinical and therapeutic relevance. Epilepsia. 1999;40(Suppl 10):S57–64.
136. Chkhenkeli SA, Geladze T. "Forced normalization" of the EEG and some mechanisms of psychopathological manifestations in epileptics. Neurosci Behav Physiol. 1982;12(2):113–7.
137. Shakarashvili RR. Clinico-electrographic correlates of free radical pathology in epileptic patients. Zh Nevropatol Psikhiatr Im S S Korsakova. 1987;87(6):825–8.
138. Agrawal N, Mula M. Treatment of psychoses in patients with epilepsy: an update. Ther Adv Psychopharmacol. 2019;9:2045125319862968.
139. Carazo Barrios L, Martín GG, Godoy JR, Acebal MR, Muñoz MIC. Forced normalization: case series from a Spanish epilepsy unit. Seizure. 2020;81:132–7.
140. Calle-López Y, Ladino LD, Benjumea-Cuartas V, Castrillón-Velilla DM, Téllez-Zenteno JF, Wolf P. Forced normalization: a systematic review. Epilepsia. 2019;60(8):1610–8.
141. Amudhan S, Gururaj G, Satishchandra P. Epilepsy in India I: epidemiology and public health. Ann Indian Acad Neurol. 2015;18(3):263–77.
142. Sankar R, Mazarati A. Neurobiology of depression as a comorbidity of epilepsy. Epilepsia. 2010;51(s5):81.
143. Matthews WS, Barabas G. Suicide and epilepsy: a review of the literature. Psychosomatics. 1981;22(6):515–24.
144. Barraclough BM. The suicide rate of epilepsy. Acta Psychiatr Scand. 1987;76(4):339–45.
145. Kumar N, Lhatoo R, Liu H, Colon-Zimmermann K, Tatsuoka C, Chen P, et al. Depressive symptom severity in individuals with epilepsy and recent health complications. J Nerv Ment Dis. 2019;207(4):284–90.
146. Gilliam FG, Black KJ, Carter J, Freedland KE, Sheline YI, Tsai WY, et al. A trial of sertraline or cognitive behavior therapy for depression in epilepsy. Ann Neurol. 2019;86(4):552–60.
147. Hudson JL, McLellan LF, Eapen V, Rapee RM, Wuthrich V, Lyneham HJ. Combining CBT and sertraline does not enhance outcomes for anxious youth: a double-blind randomised controlled trial. Psychol Med. 2023;53(5):1741–9.
148. Shen Y, Peng W, Chen Q, Hammock BD, Liu J, Li D, et al. Anti-inflammatory treatment with a soluble epoxide hydrolase inhibitor attenuates seizures and epilepsy-associated depression in the LiCl-pilocarpine post-status epilepticus rat model. Brain Behav Immun. 2019;81:535–44.
149. Murawiec S, Chudek J, Nieves W, Almgren-Rachtan A, Jedrzejczak J. Increasing the dosage of pregabalin in patients with focal epilepsy decreases the frequency of seizures and ameliorates symptoms of anxiety, depression and insomnia. Eur Rev Med Pharmacol Sci. 2020;24(24):13015–24.
150. Villanueva V, Artal J, Cabeza-Alvarez CI, Campos D, Castillo A, Flórez G, et al. Proposed recommendations for the Management of Depression in adults with epilepsy: an expert consensus. Neurol Ther. 2023;12(2):479–503.
151. Kanner AM. Depression in epilepsy: prevalence, clinical semiology, pathogenic mechanisms, and treatment. Biol Psychiatry. 2003;54(3):388–98.
152. Fuller-Thomson E, Brennenstuhl S. The association between depression and epilepsy in a nationally representative sample. Epilepsia. 2009;50(5):1051–8.
153. Kanner AM, Schachter SC, Barry JJ, Hesdorffer DC, Mula M, Trimble M, et al. Depression and epilepsy: epidemiologic and neurobiologic perspectives that may explain their high comorbid occurrence. Epilepsy Behav. 2012;24(2):156–68.
154. Devinsky O, Barr WB, Vickrey BG, Berg AT, Bazil CW, Pacia SV, et al. Changes in depression and anxiety after resective surgery for epilepsy. Neurology. 2005;65(11):1744–9.

155. Guo Y, Chen ZM, Zhang YX, Ge YB, Shen CH, Ding Y, et al. Reliability and validity of the Chinese version of the neurological disorders depression inventory for epilepsy (C-NDDI-E). Epilepsy Behav. 2015;45:225–8.
156. Chen J, Zhang Y, Hong Z, Sander JW, Zhou D. Marital adjustment for patients with epilepsy in China. Epilepsy Behav. 2013;28(1):99–103.
157. Bosak M, Dudek D, Siwek M, Szczudlik A. Subtypes of interictal depressive disorders according to ICD-10 in patients with epilepsy. Neurol Neurochir Pol. 2015;49(2):90–4.
158. Błaszczyk B, Czuczwar SJ. Epilepsy coexisting with depression. Pharmacol Rep. 2016;68(5):1084–92.
159. Tsehay M, Necho M, Belete A, Srahbzu M. Depression and anxiety and their associated factors among caregivers of children and adolescents with epilepsy in three selected hospitals in Amhara region, Ethiopia: a cross-sectional study. PLoS One. 2022;17(7):e0271885.
160. Naess S, Eriksen J, Tambs K. Psychological well-being of people with epilepsy in Norway. Epilepsy Behav. 2007;11(3):310–5.
161. Kalinin VV, Zemlyanaya AA, Krylov OE, Zheleznova EV. Handedness, alexithymia, and focus laterality as risk factors for psychiatric comorbidity in patients with epilepsy. Epilepsy Behav. 2010;17(3):389–94.
162. Mensah SA, Beavis JM, Thapar AK, Kerr M. The presence and clinical implications of depression in a community population of adults with epilepsy. Epilepsy Behav. 2006;8(1):213–9.
163. Lee SA, Jeon JY, No SK, Park H, Kim OJ, Kwon JH, et al. Factors contributing to anxiety and depressive symptoms in adults with new-onset epilepsy. Epilepsy Behav. 2018;88:325–31.
164. Velissaris SL, Saling MM, Newton MR, Berkovic SF, Wilson SJ. Psychological trajectories in the year after a newly diagnosed seizure. Epilepsia. 2012;53(10):1774–81.
165. Peng WF, Ding J, Li X, Mao LY, Wang X. Clinical risk factors for depressive symptoms in patients with epilepsy. Acta Neurol Scand. 2014;129(5):343–9.
166. Seidenberg M, Kelly KG, Parrish J, Geary E, Dow C, Rutecki P, et al. Ipsilateral and contralateral MRI volumetric abnormalities in chronic unilateral temporal lobe epilepsy and their clinical correlates. Epilepsia. 2005;46(3):420–30.
167. Shamim S, Hasler G, Liew C, Sato S, Theodore WH. Temporal lobe epilepsy, depression, and hippocampal volume. Epilepsia. 2009;50(5):1067–71.
168. Kalilani L, Sun X, Pelgrims B, Noack-Rink M, Villanueva V. The epidemiology of drug-resistant epilepsy: a systematic review and meta-analysis. Epilepsia. 2018;59(12):2179–93.
169. Gugała-Iwaniuk M, Sławińska K, Bochyńska A, Konopko M, Rola R, Ryglewicz D, et al. The prevalence of depressive and anxiety symptoms in Polish epilepsy patients – the context of pharmaco-resistance. Epilepsy Behav. 2021;114(Pt A):107522.
170. Zis P, Yfanti P, Siatouni A, Tavernarakis A, Gatzonis S. Determinants of depression among patients with epilepsy in Athens. Greece Epilepsy Behav. 2014;33:106–9.
171. Hwang S, An H, Shin DW, Lee HW. Retention rates and successful treatment with Antiseizure medications in newly-diagnosed epilepsy patients. Yonsei Med J. 2024;65(2):89–97.
172. Mula M. Developments in depression in epilepsy: screening, diagnosis, and treatment. Expert Rev Neurother. 2019;19(3):269–76.
173. Grünewald RA, Thompson PJ, Corcoran R, Corden Z, Jackson GD, Duncan JS. Effects of vigabatrin on partial seizures and cognitive function. J Neurol Neurosurg Psychiatry. 1994;57(9):1057–63.
174. Thomas L, Trimble M, Schmitz B, Ring H. Vigabatrin and behaviour disorders: a retrospective survey. Epilepsy Res. 1996;25(1):21–7.
175. Mula M, Trimble MR, Yuen A, Liu RS, Sander JW. Psychiatric adverse events during levetiracetam therapy. Neurology. 2003;61(5):704–6.
176. Delanty N, Jones J, Tonner F. Adjunctive levetiracetam in children, adolescents, and adults with primary generalized seizures: open-label, noncomparative, multicenter, long-term follow-up study. Epilepsia. 2012;53(1):111–9.

177. Vajda FJE, O'Brien TJ, Graham JE, Hitchcock AA, Mitchell J, Horgan D, et al. Antiepileptic drugs and depression during pregnancy in women with epilepsy. Acta Neurol Scand. 2020;142(4):350–5.
178. Zhu H, Deng X, Feng L, Lian Y, Han X, Guo Z, et al. Efficacy comparison of oxcarbazepine and levetiracetam monotherapy among patients with newly diagnosed focal epilepsy in China: a multicenter, open-label, randomized study. CNS Neurosci Ther. 2022;28(7):1072–80.
179. Jalihal V, Shankar R, Henley W, Parrett M, Tittensor P, McLean BN, et al. Eslicarbazepine acetate as a replacement for levetiracetam in people with epilepsy developing behavioral adverse events. Epilepsy Behav. 2018;80:365–9.
180. Phabphal K, Udomratn P. Topiramate-induced depression in cases using topiramate for migraine prophylaxis. Cephalalgia. 2010;30(6):747–9.
181. Mula M, Hesdorffer DC, Trimble M, Sander JW. The role of titration schedule of topiramate for the development of depression in patients with epilepsy. Epilepsia. 2009;50(5):1072–6.
182. Mula M, Trimble MR, Sander JW. The role of hippocampal sclerosis in topiramate-related depression and cognitive deficits in people with epilepsy. Epilepsia. 2003;44(12):1573–7.
183. Aydin S, Yazici ZG, Kilic C, Ercelen Ozozturk B, Kilic FS. An overview of the behavioral, neurobiological and morphological effects of topiramate in rats exposed to chronic unpredictable mild stress. Eur J Pharmacol. 2021;912:174578.
184. Molina-Hernández M, Téllez-Alcántara NP, Olivera-López JI, Jaramillo MT. The antidepressant-like effects of topiramate alone or combined with 17β-estradiol in ovariectomized Wistar rats submitted to the forced swimming test. Psychopharmacology. 2014;231(17):3343–50.
185. Mowla A, Kardeh E. Topiramate augmentation in patients with resistant major depressive disorder: a double-blind placebo-controlled clinical trial. Prog Neuro-Psychopharmacol Biol Psychiatry. 2011;35(4):970–3.
186. Reidenberg MM, Levy M, Warner H, Coutinho CB, Schwartz MA, Yu G, et al. Relationship between diazepam dose, plasma level, age, and central nervous system depression. Clin Pharmacol Ther. 1978;23(4):371–4.
187. Zeller AM, Lear A, Post E, McNulty S, Bentley B. A National Survey on the relationship of youth sport specialization behaviors to self-reported anxiety and depression in youth softball players. Sports Health. 2024;16(2):184–94.
188. Wrench JM, Rayner G, Wilson SJ. Profiling the evolution of depression after epilepsy surgery. Epilepsia. 2011;52(5):900–8.
189. Jacoby A, Baker GA, Steen N, Potts P, Chadwick DW. The clinical course of epilepsy and its psychosocial correlates: findings from a U.K. Community study. Epilepsia. 1996;37(2):148–61.
190. Swinkels WA, van Emde BW, Kuyk J, van Dyck R, Spinhoven P. Interictal depression, anxiety, personality traits, and psychological dissociation in patients with temporal lobe epilepsy (TLE) and extra-TLE. Epilepsia. 2006;47(12):2092–103.
191. Hue CD, Couper RG, Antaya TC, Herrera M, Parra J, Burneo JG. Depression and suicide after temporal lobe epilepsy surgery: a systematic review. Epilepsy Behav. 2022;134:108853.
192. Yang Y, Yang M, Shi Q, Wang T, Jiang M. Risk factors for depression in patients with epilepsy: a meta-analysis. Epilepsy Behav. 2020;106:107030.
193. Viguera AC, Fan Y, Thompson NR, Lapin B, Chaitoff A, Griffith SD, et al. Prevalence and predictors of depression among patients with epilepsy, stroke, and multiple sclerosis using the Cleveland Clinic Knowledge Program Within the Neurological Institute. Psychosomatics. 2018;59(4):369–78.
194. Lacey CJ, Salzberg MR, D'Souza WJ. Risk factors for depression in community-treated epilepsy: systematic review. Epilepsy Behav. 2015;43:1–7.
195. Stefanello S, Marín-Léon L, Fernandes PT, Li LM, Botega NJ. Depression and anxiety in a community sample with epilepsy in Brazil. Arq Neuropsiquiatr. 2011;69(2b):342–8.

196. Tegegne MT, Mossie TB, Awoke AA, Assaye AM, Gebrie BT, Eshetu DA. Depression and anxiety disorder among epileptic people at Amanuel Specialized Mental Hospital, Addis Ababa. Ethiopia BMC Psychiatry. 2015;15:210.
197. Wang HJ, Tan G, Deng Y, He J, He YJ, Zhou D, et al. Prevalence and risk factors of depression and anxiety among patients with convulsive epilepsy in rural West China. Acta Neurol Scand. 2018;138(6):541–7.
198. Faught RE, Weiner JR, Guérin A, Cunnington MC, Duh MS. Impact of nonadherence to antiepileptic drugs on health care utilization and costs: findings from the RANSOM study. Epilepsia. 2009;50(3):501–9.
199. Shahar G, Davidson L. Depressive symptoms erode self-esteem in severe mental illness: a three-wave, cross-lagged study. J Consult Clin Psychol. 2003;71(5):890–900.
200. Epps SA. Commonalities for comorbidity: overlapping features of the endocannabinoid system in depression and epilepsy. Front Psych. 2022;13:1041460.
201. Elkommos S, Mula M. A systematic review of neuroimaging studies of depression in adults with epilepsy. Epilepsy Behav. 2021;115:107695.
202. Andrade R. Serotonergic regulation of neuronal excitability in the prefrontal cortex. Neuropharmacology. 2011;61(3):382–6.
203. Machado-Vieira R, Salvadore G, Ibrahim LA, Diaz-Granados N, Zarate CA Jr. Targeting glutamatergic signaling for the development of novel therapeutics for mood disorders. Curr Pharm Des. 2009;15(14):1595–611.
204. Krishnan V. Depression and anxiety in the epilepsies: from bench to bedside. Curr Neurol Neurosci Rep. 2020;20(9):41.
205. Singh T, Goel RK. Epilepsy associated depression: An update on current scenario, suggested mechanisms, and opportunities. Neurochem Res. 2021;46(6):1305–21.
206. Pineda EA, Hensler JG, Sankar R, Shin D, Burke TF, Mazarati AM. Plasticity of presynaptic and postsynaptic serotonin 1A receptors in an animal model of epilepsy-associated depression. Neuropsychopharmacology. 2011;36(6):1305–16.
207. Alhashimi R, Thoota S, Ashok T, Palyam V, Azam AT, Odeyinka O, et al. Comorbidity of epilepsy and depression: associated pathophysiology and management. Cureus. 2022;14(1):e21527.
208. Mazarati AM, Pineda E, Shin D, Tio D, Taylor AN, Sankar R. Comorbidity between epilepsy and depression: role of hippocampal interleukin-1beta. Neurobiol Dis. 2010;37(2):461–7.
209. Pineda E, Shin D, Sankar R, Mazarati AM. Comorbidity between epilepsy and depression: experimental evidence for the involvement of serotonergic, glucocorticoid, and neuroinflammatory mechanisms. Epilepsia. 2010;51 Suppl 3(Suppl 3):110–4.
210. Druzhkova TA, Yakovlev AA, Rider FK, Zinchuk MS, Guekht AB, Gulyaeva NV. Elevated serum cortisol levels in patients with focal epilepsy, depression, and comorbid epilepsy and depression. Int J Mol Sci. 2022;23(18):10414.
211. Klein AB, Williamson R, Santini MA, Clemmensen C, Ettrup A, Rios M, et al. Blood BDNF concentrations reflect brain-tissue BDNF levels across species. Int J Neuropsychopharmacol. 2011;14(3):347–53.
212. Becker C, Bouvier E, Ghestem A, Siyoucef S, Claverie D, Camus F, et al. Predicting and treating stress-induced vulnerability to epilepsy and depression. Ann Neurol. 2015;78(1):128–36.
213. Gulyaeva NV. Stress-associated molecular and cellular hippocampal mechanisms common for epilepsy and comorbid depressive disorders. Biochemistry (Mosc). 2021;86(6):641–56.
214. Heiman GA, Kamberakis K, Gill R, Kalachikov S, Pedley TA, Hauser WA, et al. Evaluation of depression risk in LGI1 mutation carriers. Epilepsia. 2010;51(9):1685–90.
215. Baxendale SA, Thompson PJ, Duncan JS. Epilepsy & depression: the effects of comorbidity on hippocampal volume–a pilot study. Seizure. 2005;14(6):435–8.
216. Fu CW, Tan AW, Sheng F, Luan RS, Zhan SY, Chen WQ, et al. The prevalence of anxiety symptoms and depressive symptoms in patients with somatic disorders in urban China: a multi-center cross-sectional study. Int J Psychiatry Med. 2007;37(2):185–99.

217. Salpekar JA, Mishra G. Key issues in addressing the comorbidity of attention deficit hyperactivity disorder and pediatric epilepsy. Epilepsy Behav. 2014;37:310–5.
218. Lunn J, Lewis C, Sherlock C. Impaired performance on advanced theory of mind tasks in children with epilepsy is related to poor communication and increased attention problems. Epilepsy Behav. 2015;43:109–16.
219. Post RM, Altshuler LL, Frye MA, Suppes T, Rush AJ, Keck PE Jr, et al. Rate of switch in bipolar patients prospectively treated with second-generation antidepressants as augmentation to mood stabilizers. Bipolar Disord. 2001;3(5):259–65.
220. Ring HA, Crellin R, Kirker S, Reynolds EH. Vigabatrin and depression. J Neurol Neurosurg Psychiatry. 1993;56(8):925–8.
221. Gilliam FG, Hecimovic H, Gentry MS. Serotonergic therapy in epilepsy. Curr Opin Neurol. 2021;34(2):206–12.
222. Słupska A, Słupski J. Are the self-administered questionnaires appropriate to uncover undiagnosed depression among people with epilepsy? Epilepsy Res. 2022;180:106868.
223. Italiano D, Spina E, de Leon J. Pharmacokinetic and pharmacodynamic interactions between antiepileptics and antidepressants. Expert Opin Drug Metab Toxicol. 2014;10(11):1457–89.
224. Mula M. The pharmacological management of psychiatric comorbidities in patients with epilepsy. Pharmacol Res. 2016;107:147–53.
225. Ketter TA, Jenkins JB, Schroeder DH, Pazzaglia PJ, Marangell LB, George MS, et al. Carbamazepine but not valproate induces bupropion metabolism. J Clin Psychopharmacol. 1995;15(5):327–33.
226. Bloechliger M, Ceschi A, Rüegg S, Kupferschmidt H, Kraehenbuehl S, Jick SS, et al. Risk of seizures associated with antidepressant use in patients with depressive disorder: follow-up study with a nested case-control analysis using the clinical practice research datalink. Drug Saf. 2016;39(4):307–21.
227. Kamal SM. Combination of valproate and paroxetine in mice exposed to picrotoxin. Int J Nanomedicine. 2012;7:2583–9.
228. Montgomery SA. Antidepressants and seizures: emphasis on newer agents and clinical implications. Int J Clin Pract. 2005;59(12):1435–40.
229. Igelström KM. Preclinical antiepileptic actions of selective serotonin reuptake inhibitors–implications for clinical trial design. Epilepsia. 2012;53(4):596–605.
230. Kwon OY, Park SP. Depression and anxiety in people with epilepsy. J Clin Neurol. 2014;10(3):175–88.
231. Hashimoto Y, Kotake K, Watanabe N, Fujiwara T, Sakamoto S. Lamotrigine in the maintenance treatment of bipolar disorder. Cochrane Database Syst Rev. 2021;9(9):Cd013575.
232. Barry JJ, Ettinger AB, Friel P, Gilliam FG, Harden CL, Hermann B, et al. Consensus statement: the evaluation and treatment of people with epilepsy and affective disorders. Epilepsy Behav. 2008;13(Suppl 1):S1–S29.
233. Vlaicu A, Bustuchina VM. New neuromodulation techniques for treatment resistant depression. Int J Psychiatry Clin Pract. 2020;24(2):106–15.
234. Gouveia FV, Germann J, Oliveira CC, Castro MC, Antunes GF, Gomes GCV, et al. Transcranial direct current stimulation reduces anxiety, depression and plasmatic corticosterone in a rat model of atypical generalized epilepsy. Neuroscience. 2022;480:32–41.
235. McClintock SM, Reti IM, Carpenter LL, McDonald WM, Dubin M, Taylor SF, et al. Consensus recommendations for the clinical application of repetitive transcranial magnetic stimulation (rTMS) in the treatment of depression. J Clin Psychiatry. 2018;79(1):35.
236. Möbius H, Welkoborsky HJ. Vagus nerve stimulation for conservative therapy-refractive epilepsy and depression. Laryngorhinootologie. 2022;101(S 01):S114–S43.
237. De Herdt V, Waterschoot L, Vonck K, Dermaut B, Verhelst H, Van Coster R, et al. Vagus nerve stimulation for refractory status epilepticus. Eur J Paediatr Neurol. 2009;13(3):286–9.
238. Sierra-Marcos A, Maestro I, Rodríguez-Osorio X, Miró J, Donaire A, Aparicio J, et al. Successful outcome of episodes of status epilepticus after vagus nerve stimulation: a multicenter study. Eur J Neurol. 2012;19(9):1219–23.

239. Goel RK, Gawande D, Lagunin A, Randhawa P, Mishra A, Poroikov V. Revealing medicinal plants that are useful for the Comprehensive Management of Epilepsy and Associated Comorbidities through in Silico Mining of Their Phytochemical Diversity. Planta Med. 2015;81(6):495–506.
240. Miller AL. St. John's Wort (Hypericum perforatum): clinical effects on depression and other conditions. Altern Med Rev. 1998;3(1):18–26.
241. Kaur J, Famta P, Famta M, Mehta M, Satija S, Sharma N, et al. Potential anti-epileptic phytoconstituents: an updated review. J Ethnopharmacol. 2021;268:113565.
242. Shamabadi A, Ahmadzade A, Pirahesh K, Hasanzadeh A, Asadigandomani H. Suicidality risk after using cannabis and cannabinoids: an umbrella review. Dialogues Clin Neurosci. 2023;25(1):50–63.
243. Wang H, Zhang Y, Tan G, Chen D, Fu Y, Liu L. Suicidality and epilepsy: a systematic review and meta-analysis. Front Psych. 2023;14:1097516.
244. Friedman D, Spruill TM, Liu H, Tatsuoka C, Stoll S, Jobst BC, et al. Depressive symptoms and suicidality among individuals with epilepsy enrolled in self-management studies: results from the US Centers for Disease Control and Prevention Managing Epilepsy Well (MEW) Network. Epilepsy Behav. 2018;87:235–40.
245. Christensen J, Vestergaard M, Mortensen PB, Sidenius P, Agerbo E. Epilepsy and risk of suicide: a population-based case-control study. Lancet Neurol. 2007;6(8):693–8.
246. Tellez-Zenteno JF, Patten SB, Jetté N, Williams J, Wiebe S. Psychiatric comorbidity in epilepsy: a population-based analysis. Epilepsia. 2007;48(12):2336–44.
247. Mula M, Sander JW. Suicide and epilepsy: do antiepileptic drugs increase the risk? Expert Opin Drug Saf. 2015;14(4):553–8.
248. Abraham N, Buvanaswari P, Rathakrishnan R, Tran BX, Thu GV, Nguyen LH, et al. A meta-analysis of the rates of suicide ideation, attempts and deaths in people with epilepsy. Int J Environ Res Public Health. 2019;16(8):1451.
249. Li Q, Zhu LN, Wang HJ, Lin X, Xu D, Chen D, et al. Validation of the neurological disorders depression inventory for epilepsy (NDDIE) as a rapid suicidality screening tool in Chinese people with epilepsy. Epilepsy Behav. 2019;94:216–21.
250. Kanner AM. Suicidality in patients with epilepsy: why should neurologists care? Front Integr Neurosci. 2022;16:898547.
251. Bell GS, Mula M, Sander JW. Suicidality in people taking antiepileptic drugs: what is the evidence? CNS Drugs. 2009;23(4):281–92.
252. Dreier JW, Pedersen CB, Gasse C, Christensen J. Antiepileptic drugs and suicide: role of prior suicidal behavior and parental psychiatric disorder. Ann Neurol. 2019;86(6):951–61.
253. Bell GS, Sander JW. Suicide and epilepsy. Curr Opin Neurol. 2009;22(2):174–8.
254. Hesdorffer DC, Ishihara L, Webb DJ, Mynepalli L, Galwey NW, Hauser WA. Occurrence and recurrence of attempted suicide among people with epilepsy. JAMA Psychiatry. 2016;73(1):80–6.
255. Rai D, Kerr MP, McManus S, Jordanova V, Lewis G, Brugha TS. Epilepsy and psychiatric comorbidity: a nationally representative population-based study. Epilepsia. 2012;53(6):1095–103.
256. Tedrus G, Souza DCM. I would be better off dead: investigating suicidal ideation in people with epilepsy. Arq Neuropsiquiatr. 2022;80(7):718–24.
257. Bagary M. Epilepsy, antiepileptic drugs and suicidality. Curr Opin Neurol. 2011;24(2):177–82.
258. Hesdorffer DC, Ishihara L, Mynepalli L, Webb DJ, Weil J, Hauser WA. Epilepsy, suicidality, and psychiatric disorders: a bidirectional association. Ann Neurol. 2012;72(2):184–91.
259. Tedrus G, Souza DCM, Crepaldi CR, Petrarca YM. Suicide risk in epilepsy: clinical variables, psychiatric disorders, and social support. Rev Neurol (Paris). 2023;179(3):183–7.
260. Wen X, Meador KJ, Loring DW, Eisenschenk S, Segal R, Hartzema AG. Is antiepileptic drug use related to depression and suicidal ideation among patients with epilepsy? Epilepsy Behav. 2010;19(3):494–500.

261. Memon AM, Katwala J, Douille C, Kelley C, Monga V. Exploring the complex relationship between antiepileptic drugs and suicidality: a systematic literature review. Innov Clin Neurosci. 2023;20(7–9):47–51.
262. O'Kula SS, Briggs FBS, Brownrigg B, Sarna K, Rosales O, Shegog R, et al. Depression and suicidality among Hispanics with epilepsy: findings from the Managing Epilepsy Well (MEW) Network integrated database. Epilepsy Behav. 2021;125:108388.
263. Hesdorffer DC, French JA, Posner K, DiVentura B, Pollard JR, Sperling MR, et al. Suicidal ideation and behavior screening in intractable focal epilepsy eligible for drug trials. Epilepsia. 2013;54(5):879–87.
264. Andrade-Machado R, Ochoa-Urrea M, Garcia-Espinosa A, Benjumea-Cuartas V, Santos-Santos A. Suicidal risk, affective dysphoric disorders, and quality-of-life perception in patients with focal refractory epilepsy. Epilepsy Behav. 2015;45:254–60.
265. Leppien EE, Doughty BJ, Hurd KL, Strong KN, Piper BJ, McCall KL. Newer Antiseizure medications and suicidality: analysis of the Food and Drug Administration Adverse Event Reporting System (FAERS) Database. Clin Drug Investig. 2023;43(6):393–9.
266. Redden L, Pritchett Y, Robieson W, Kovacs X, Garofalo M, Tracy K, et al. Suicidality and divalproex sodium: analysis of controlled studies in multiple indications. Ann General Psychiatry. 2011;10(1):1.
267. Ziemba KS, O'Carroll CB, Drazkowski JF, Wingerchuk DM, Hoffman-Snyder C, Wellik KE, et al. Do antiepileptic drugs increase the risk of suicidality in adult patients with epilepsy?: a critically appraised topic. Neurologist. 2010;16(5):325–8.
268. Klein P, Devinsky O, French J, Harden C, Krauss GL, McCarter R, et al. Suicidality risk of newer Antiseizure medications: a meta-analysis. JAMA Neurol. 2021;78(9):1118–27.
269. Kim HJ, Jeon JY, Kim HW, Lee SA. Validation of items on the NDDIE and PHQ-9 associated with suicidal ideation during suicidality screening in patients with epilepsy. Seizure. 2022;99:99–104.
270. Shneker BF, Cios JS, Elliott JO. Suicidality, depression screening, and antiepileptic drugs: reaction to the FDA alert. Neurology. 2009;72(11):987–91.
271. Mula M, Kanner AM, Schmitz B, Schachter S. Antiepileptic drugs and suicidality: an expert consensus statement from the task force on therapeutic strategies of the ILAE commission on Neuropsychobiology. Epilepsia. 2013;54(1):199–203.
272. Jones JE, Hermann BP, Barry JJ, Gilliam FG, Kanner AM, Meador KJ. Rates and risk factors for suicide, suicidal ideation, and suicide attempts in chronic epilepsy. Epilepsy Behav. 2003;4(Suppl 3):S31–8.

Chapter 8
Side Effects of Anti-seizure Medication

Liming Zhang, Wen-Hung Chung, Xin Xu, Zucai Xu, Songyan Liu, Ling Li, Fei Xiao, Zan Wang, Zhen Hong, Ying Wang, and Huapin Huang

L. Zhang
Department of Neurology, The First Affiliated Hospital of Harbin Medical University, Harbin, Heilongjiang, China

W-H. Chung
Department of Dermatology, Xiamen Chang Gung Hospital, Xiamen, China

X. Xu · F. Xiao (✉)
Department of Neurology, The First Affiliated Hospital of Chongqing Medical University, Chongqing, China

Z. Xu
Department of Neurology, Affiliated Hospital of Zunyi Medical University, Zunyi, Guizhou, China

S. Liu
Department of Neurology, China-Japan Union Hospital, Jilin University, Changchun, Jilin, China

L. Li
Department of Neurology, Qilu Hospital (Qingdao), Cheeloo College of Medicine, Shandong University, Qingdao, China

Z. Wang
Department of Neurology, The First Affiliated Hospital of Chongqing Medical University, Chongqing, China

Z. Hong (✉)
Department of Neurology, West China Hospital, Sichuan University, Chengdu, China

Y. Wang
Department of Neurology, The First Affiliated Hospital of DaLian Medical University, DaLian, China

H. Huang
Department of Neurology, Fujian Medical University Union Hospital, Fuzhou, China

X. Wang, L. Zhou (eds.), *Pharmacological Treatment of Epileptic Seizures*,
https://doi.org/10.1007/978-981-96-8520-2_8

Anti-seizure medication (ASM) can effectively control epileptic seizures but can also convey side effects, which are pharmacological effects that coexist with the targeted effects of ASMs. There is no drug that does not carry a possibility of side effects. However, some side effects are acceptable, while others can cause fatal harm to patients and are not acceptable. Therefore, based on the degree of damage to the patient, some side effects of ASMs can be divided into fatal side effects, such as fatal epidermolysis, hypersensitivity syndrome, cardiac arrest, and sudden death. Some ASMs do not cause death but have serious effects on the patient and their offspring, such as birth malformation, mental abnormalities, metabolic encephalopathy, and malignant hyperthermia syndrome. Some side effects, such as weight gain, nausea, and hair growth, are acceptable. Clinicians should be highly concerned about fatal side effects and should do their best to avoid them.

8.1 Effects of ASMs on Cardiac Function

For many years, studies on the adverse effects of ASMs in humans have focused mainly on skin allergic reactions, liver function damage, or leukopenia, and little attention has been given to the effects of ASMs on the heart. In recent years, people have gradually recognized the adverse effects ASMs can have on the cardiovascular system while also controlling epileptic seizures. Rupak Desai et al. [1] surveyed 1,424,320 patients with epilepsy and reported that 277,230 patients (23.9%) had arrhythmias, of which 9.7% had atrial fibrillation, 7.3% had no clear cause, 1.4% had cardiac arrest, 1.2% had bundle branch block (BBB), and 1% had ventricular tachycardia. In addition, Altun Y et al. [2] conducted a study on 63 patients taking ASMs and reported that the Tp-e interval and the Tp-e/QT and Tp-e/QTc ratios were greater in the patient group than in the control group ($p < 0.05$), and the QTmax ratio was lower. It has been suggested that ASMs have significant effects on cardiac function, and more intense follow-up of patients using ASMs is needed. Clinical practice has shown that many ASMs have adverse effects on cardiac function, including long-term consequences, such as an increased risk of atherosclerosis and subsequent cardiovascular diseases due to their effects on lipids and the proinflammatory environment and a potentially fatal risk of arrhythmia due to their effects on ion channels [3].

Kloster [4] and Opeskin [5] described patients with epilepsy who died suddenly and found that the patients had pathological changes in their myocardium, such as coronary arteriole wall fibrosis, myocardial atrophy, myocardial fibrosis, leukocyte infiltration and atrial conduction abnormalities, suggesting that these problems deserve attention.

8.1.1 Historical Evolution

In 1950, Harris AS et al. [6] reported that phenytoin sodium (an ASM) had a significant effect on ectopic ventricular tachycardia. In 1965, Centa A et al. [7] first noted that ASMs could cause cardiac development disorders and heart malformations. Subsequently, Pfammatter [8] reported that two brothers who had been receiving ASM treatment for a long time had recurrent syncope attacks, which were ultimately confirmed to be long QT syndrome caused by ASMs. In 1994, Steinhoff et al. [9] noted chest pain and electrocardiogram changes in a patient taking lamotrigine, suggesting that lamotrigine may have cardiotoxic side effects. T Tomson et al. [10] retrospectively analyzed clinical evidence regarding arrhythmia and changes in heart rate variability caused by a variety of ASMs and reported that phenytoin use was mainly associated with bradyarrhythmias, some of which were fatal. Carbamazepine inhibits the conduction system of the heart, and this side effect occurs mainly in elderly or other susceptible patients; thus, this drug has attracted widespread attention. Subsequently, Kenneback et al. [11] reported that sudden discontinuation of antiseizure drugs caused heart rhythm disturbances that may be associated with sudden death in patients with epilepsy. These studies have enriched the evidence in this field and have brought attention to the effects of drugs on heart function; moreover, some people have proposed the idea of an epileptic heart phenotype [12].

8.1.2 Epidemiology

Christensen [13] studied 91,949 people who took lamotrigine. Among the patients with no history of heart disease ($n = 86{,}769$), 194 (0.23%) had cardiac conduction disorders. Among those with heart disease ($n = 5180$), 1150 (22.2%) died, suggesting that lamotrigine may have an effect on heart function. Elinor Lee-Lane et al. [14] conducted a study on 10,241 patients receiving anti-seizure drugs and found that the patients had an increased risk of major cardiovascular events compared to the control group (hazard ratio = 1.58, $p < 0.001$). Since then, it has been observed that patients with epilepsy have a significantly greater mortality rate due to circulatory disorders and a significantly increased overall risk of cardiovascular events and that epilepsy is more common in patients with cardiovascular diseases (CVD) comorbidities and may be a predictor of death in patients with acute myocardial infarction.

8.1.3 Effects of ASMs on Cardiac Function

8.1.3.1 Ventricular Late Potentials (VLPs)

VLPs are high-frequency and low-amplitude fragmented waves that occur in the late stage of ventricular electrical activity and represent delayed electrical excitation conduction and depolarization in the myocardial ischemic area. The emergence of VLPs, reflecting an instability of myocardial electrical activity, is an important mechanism for the occurrence of reentry ventricular arrhythmias and a predictive signal of sudden death in patients with ventricular arrhythmias [15]. Rejdak et al. [16] studied the electrocardiograms of 45 epileptic patients and 19 healthy controls and found that 23 epileptic patients had VLPs, while only 2 healthy volunteers had VLPs, suggesting that epileptic patients were more prone to VLPs than healthy individuals were. Rejdak et al. [16] subsequently divided the 45 patients with epilepsy into a VLP group and a no-VLP group for analysis and reported that patients with VLPs had a longer disease course and that a large proportion of them had refractory epilepsy. Rejdak et al. [16] suggested that this characteristic of cardiac electrical activity in epilepsy patients may be the basis for susceptibility to arrhythmia after the use of ASMs. However, there have been no clear reports on whether there is a direct relationship between VLP- and ASM-induced arrhythmia.

8.1.3.2 Impact on Cardiovascular Metabolism

Some ASMs have an impact on cardiovascular metabolism and can induce metabolic changes, especially atherosclerotic changes that are directly related to heart function. Carbamazepine, phenytoin sodium, phenobarbital, valproic acid, oxcarbazepine, and eslicarbazepine can significantly increase the total cholesterol, triglyceride, low-density lipoprotein, apolipoprotein, and valproic acid levels and reduce high-density lipoprotein (HDL) levels. Enzyme-induced ASMs (carbamazepine, phenytoin, phenobarbital, and primidone) have a strong lipid-raising effect, while oxcarbazepine and eslicarbazepine do not have the same lipid-raising effect [17–19]. In addition, HDL-C levels were significantly reduced in patients treated with topiramate [20]. In 2020, a population-wide study of a large database was reported, which revealed a significantly greater incidence of hyperlipidemia in older patients treated with enzyme-induced ASMs than in those treated with non-enzyme-induced ASMs, consistent with the metabolic effects of enzyme-induced ASMs described above [21].

Inflammation is a recognized cause of CVD. Carbamazepine, oxcarbazepine, phenytoin, valproic acid, topiramate, and levetiracetam are proinflammatory drugs. Carbamazepine, phenytoin, and valproic acid increase levels of inflammatory biomarkers (such as C-reactive protein), and valproic acid increases homocysteine levels. The new generation of ASMs (LEV, OXC, and TPM) are associated with a mild increase in homocysteine levels, while folic acid levels do not change significantly

[18]. However, replacing CBZ or PHT with a member of the new generation of ASMs (LEV or LTG) results in reduced homocysteine levels [22].

Serum uric acid level is also a risk factor for proinflammatory and pro-oxidative conditions and increases cardiovascular risk [23]. VPA can increase uric acid, and CBZ and PHT can reduce uric acid [17].

Weight gain is also a risk factor for CVD, and several ASMs are associated with weight gain. Specifically, carbamazepine, valproic acid, pregabalin, gabapentin, oxcarbazepine, eslicarbazepine, and vigabatrin can increase weight; the effect of valproic acid on weight gain is particularly obvious. VPA is also associated with nonalcoholic fatty liver disease, metabolic syndrome, and increased thickness of epicardial adipose tissue, which is a marker of subclinical atherosclerosis [20, 24]. Increased carotid intima-media thickness measured by ultrasound is also considered a surrogate marker of atherosclerosis in epilepsy patients, and this marker has been evaluated in several clinical studies. Meta-analyses of such studies have shown significantly greater carotid wall thickness in ASM users, particularly CBZ and VPA users [25].

ASMs also have anti-inflammatory and cardiovascular protective effects. For example, VPA and LTG reduce the expression of nuclear DNA-binding proteins and proteolytic enzymes (matrix metalloproteinase-9) that induce inflammation and vascular disease [26], resulting in vascular protection and antiseizure effects [27]. In experimental models of myocarditis, myocardial infarction, and cardiomyopathy, cannabidiol has been shown to lower blood pressure, be an anti-inflammatory and antioxidant (reducing free radicals) and antiapoptotic agent, and play a protective role in the heart [28]. In obese animal models, cannabidiol reduces triglyceride levels and increases HDL-C concentrations [29].

Elevated blood lipid levels, increased inflammatory marker levels, elevated uric acid levels, and weight gain are the main causes of arteriosclerosis. All of these adverse metabolic factors ultimately lead to atherosclerosis, which is a direct cause of myocardial infarction, and atherosclerosis itself can lead to arrhythmias.

Tetiana Litovchenko et al. [30] summarized the cardiovascular effects of antiepileptic drugs, which manifested as autonomic nervous balance disorder, increased sympathetic nervous tension, and decreased parasympathetic nerve activity; they proposed that the occurrence of acute vascular events may increase the frequency of seizures and paroxysmic electroencephalogram phenomena. Levetiracetam has a more favorable effect on cardiac autonomic balance than carbamazepine and valproic acid.

8.1.3.3 Impact on Cardiac Structure

Cardiac structure abnormalities are also among the causes of cardiac function abnormalities induced by ASMs. In recent years, to explore the treatment of Dravet syndrome, treatment methods including the administration of stiripentol (STP) combined with clobazam and fenfluramine (FFA) have been used. To date, there have been no reports of cardiac dysplasia. FFA was initially used for weight loss, and it was later found to cause valvular disease and was discontinued. Since the initiation of its use in the treatment of Dravet syndrome, there have been increasing reports of heart valve disease caused by FFA. In addition, primary pulmonary hypertension, mitral stenosis, thickening, and even mural thrombosis are all present during long-term FFA administration. FFA has dose-dependent side effects on cardiac structure. It has been reported that long-term administration of 60 mg of FFA has adverse effects on cardiac structure, while low-dose administration has not been reported to cause negative cardiac structural changes [31]. An excessive dose can induce heart valve disease. The issue of FFA dose control has caught people's attention.

8.1.3.4 The Toxic Effects of ASMs on the Heart

Arrhythmia in patients with epilepsy is particularly prominent in heart disease patients. Arrhythmias are caused by changes in the electrical characteristics of heart tissue, leading to atrial and ventricular excitation and conduction disorders. These disorders can cause the heart rate to decrease or increase and can be regular or irregular, possibly interfering with the coordinated contraction of the atrium and ventricle. Typical clinical manifestations include palpitations and syncope signs and symptoms. Arrhythmias may also manifest indirectly through embolic events (such as stroke due to Atrial fibrillation). ECG recording is the key to diagnosing arrhythmias. A study of clinical data from approximately 1.5 million hospitalized epilepsy patients revealed that approximately 24% of patients had arrhythmias during hospitalization [31].

ASMs can also affect coronary arteries, resulting in insufficient blood flow and impaired oxygen supply, which can lead to reversible or irreversible myocardial ischemia. In the context of preexisting coronary artery disease, seizures associated with sustained systemic muscle activity and severe cardiopulmonary dysfunction can further increase the risk of myocardial ischemia.

Compared with the general population, people with epilepsy have a two- to three-fold increased risk of premature death, a considerable proportion of which (15%) is due to sudden cardiac death or acute myocardial infarction [32]. In adults with epilepsy, the overall incidence of SUDEP is approximately 1:1000/year, and the risk is greater in people with epilepsy who have frequent convulsive attacks that are associated with heart disease.

ASMs improve the control of seizures, thereby reducing the burden of negative effects of seizures on the heart. Regarding SUDEP, one meta-analysis reported that the use of an effective dose of ASM reduced the incidence of definitive or probable SUDEP by more than seven-fold compared to placebo use in patients with hard-to-control seizures [33]. In a case–control study, a specific combination of multiple treatments and ASM was associated with a reduced risk of SUDEP, while failure to adhere to ASM therapy was associated with an increased risk of SUDEP [34].

ASMs also have toxic effects on the cardiovascular system. Previous studies have suggested that ASM use may be an independent risk factor for sudden cardiac death even in the absence of epilepsy, especially in patients taking sodium channel blockers (SCBs). According to a study of acute coronary events confirmed at autopsy, patients treated with ASMs had a greater rate of sudden cardiac death (SCD) than did controls, and the use of ASMs was associated with a small increase in myocardial infarction [35].

8.1.4 Possible Mechanisms Through Which Drug-Related Seizures Affect Heart Function

8.1.4.1 Effects on the Tail Currents of Cardiomyocytes

In 2003, Danielsson et al. [36] confirmed that ASMs could cause arrhythmia based on tail current data. The QT interval represents the time it takes for a cardiac cycle to depolarize the ventricles. A rapid delay in the rectifier potassium ion current (IKr) can induce QT interval prolongation, which may lead to fatal arrhythmias, such as tip torsion and ventricular tachycardia. Tail currents, on the other hand, are thought to be closely related to the hERG. Danielsson et al. [36] used a cell patch clamp and reported that carbamazepine could block 20% of the tail current of cardiomyocytes at concentrations of 250 μmol/L and 500 μmol/L. Moreover, they also found that gabapentin could block 40% of the tail current at a concentration of 100 mmol/L. At 54 mmol/L, the tail current was inhibited by 20%, while at 1000 μmol/L and 87 μmol/L, the tail current was inhibited by 35% and 20%, respectively. Therefore, carbamazepine, gabapentin, and topiramate potentially block IKr, increasing the risk of causing arrhythmia. Moreover, the data suggest that the greater the concentrations of gabapentin and topiramate administered are, the more obvious the blocking effect, and the greater the risk of arrhythmia. Phenytoin, phenobarbital, and lamotrigine may have similar effects. In 2007, Danielsson et al. [37] confirmed in their experiments on embryonic mice that multidrug combination therapy with anti-seizure drugs blocking ion channels was more likely to block IKr than single-drug therapy was, significantly prolonging the repolarization time of cardiomyocytes and leading to difficulty in controlling arrhythmias.

8.1.4.2 Effects on Ion Channels

ASM use can influence the activity of ion channels to play a role in preventing seizures. Some ASMs primarily act on excitatory volt-gated sodium channels (VGSCs), which play an important role in brain neuron excitability and epilepsy mechanisms. Because the excitation and contraction of cardiomyocytes are caused by the transmembrane flow of ions, there is overlap in some subtypes of ion channels expressed in the heart and brain. ASMs may affect cardiac ion channels. Excessive intake of Na+ channel blockers (SCBs) alone or in combination with other SCBs in the context of preexisting underlying heart disease can lead to arrhythmia. The literature has shown that SCB drugs such as CBZ, PHT, OXC, eslicarbazepine (ESL), lamotrigine (LTG), and lacosamide (LCM) can specifically affect the voltage-gated sodium current; the PR interval can be extended to varying degrees; and the cardiac QT interval is also a key ASM target. Changes in the QT interval reflect the time required for the ventricles to depolarize and repolarize, and lengthening or shortening of the QT interval can cause fatal damage to the heart, leading to cardiac syncope or sudden death. When patients are given SCBs to combat seizures, the risk of sudden cardiac death increases [38]. OXC, PHT, ESL, LCM, and LTG mainly affect the PR interval, resulting in a prolonged PR interval. Brivaracetam, cannabidiol, clobazam, perampanel, and vigabatrin can shorten the PR interval. Cenobamate, rufinamide, and primidone can shorten the QT interval. Fenfluramine has a mild adverse effect of increasing the QT interval. Zonisamide (ZNS) can induce heart rate changes, Atrial fibrillation, and syncope. Carbamazepine, phenytoin, fenfluramine, phenobarbital, and lamotrigine can change the QT interval [3]. Potassium channels determine the formation of action potentials and are involved in mediating the heart electrical signal transmission. Therefore, altering the voltage-dependent gating of potassium channels with drugs can also cause changes in cardiac conduction function, including the period between the PR and phase change in the QT. In vitro studies have also shown that lamotrigine, phenytoin sodium, and phenobarbital affect the heart's fast delayed IKr [36, 39], which may lead to a prolonged QT interval and promote ventricular flutter or ventricular fibrillation [38].

Calcium channels are also expressed in both the brain and the heart, with varying preferential expression patterns depending on the channel type. CBZ, LTG, and phenytoin not only are classical SCBs but also inhibit calcium channels, while LEV appears to mediate antiseizure effects by binding to presynaptic synaptic vesicle protein 2A. It can also act on calcium channels [40].

ASM use affects cardiac electrophysiology only in specific populations with underlying genetic or acquired changes [41]. For example, SCBs affect patients with inherited long QT syndrome (LQTS) differently depending on the mutated gene, and patients with LQTS2 (in which the affected gene encodes a potassium channel carrying a rapid inward recirculating current (IK)) are twice as likely to have a serious cardiac event (cardiac arrest and ventricular arrhythmia) than are those who do not take such drugs. Patients with LQTS1 (in which the α subunit of the affected gene encoding the KvLQT1 potassium channel is altered) had an 80% lower incidence of these cardiac events when taking SCBs [42]. Thus, depending on the specific genetic mutations in a patient with LQTS, SCBs can have arrhythmogenic or protective effects. In addition, drug-induced Brugada syndrome, a typical electrocardiogram (ECG) pattern that can lead to ventricular tachycardia, ventricular fibrillation, and sudden death, is an example of the specific cardiotoxic effects of ASMs (primarily SCBs). Brugada syndrome is a congenital heart disease that is not associated with any structural heart disease and is associated with mutations in the gene encoding heart sodium channels (SCN5A). It was recently observed that similar Brugada ECG patterns may be caused by multiple SCB treatments or high doses of intravenous PHT [43, 44].

8.1.4.3 Excitatory Changes in the Autonomic Nerves

ASMs can indirectly cause cardiac dysfunction and arrhythmias by regulating the central autonomic nervous system and by directly binding to heart tissue.

In 2001, Druschky et al. [45] at the University of Erlangen-Nuremberg, Germany, quantitatively analyzed the innervation of cardiac sympathetic postganglionic fibers via metaiodobenzylguanidine single-photon computed tomography (MIBG-SPECT). The time-domain and frequency-domain parameters of heart rate variability (HRV) were used to analyze the function of autonomic nervous regulation.

The study included 22 patients with temporal lobe epilepsy (11 treated with carbamazepine and 11 not taking carbamazepine) and 16 healthy individuals. The results showed that the MIBG uptake rate decreased significantly in temporal lobe epilepsy patients compared to healthy individuals, but there was no significant difference between the carbamazepine and carbamazepine subgroups. The results of the time domain parameter analysis suggest that both temporal lobe epilepsy and carbamazepine may affect the regulatory function of the autonomic nervous system and that abnormal regulatory function may be the basis of arrhythmia. In 2012, Lotufo et al. [46] reviewed and analyzed 30 articles on HRV in epilepsy patients before July 2011. Epilepsy patients had a lower high-frequency power spectrum (HF) than did the control group. In patients treated with ASMs, a higher low-frequency (LF) power spectrum is present, suggesting that increased excitability of the sympathetic nervous system is a risk factor for CVD and even a predictor of morbidity and mortality. A reduced HRV is also a potential biomarker of sudden cardiac death. Leosuthamas et al. [47] analyzed patients hospitalized in an epilepsy care unit from January 2013 to December 2021 and selected two 5-min electrocardiograms from each patient's waking and sleeping periods for HRV analysis. The results showed that carbamazepine, levetiracetam, lamotrigine, and clonazepam were significantly correlated with changes in sleep HRV parameters. Only CBZ had a negative effect on the HRV, which was represented by a decrease in the standard deviation of the RR interval (SDNN). Even after adjusting for other ASMs and beta-blockers used simultaneously, there was a near-significant trend ($p = 0.052$). The combined use of levetiracetam and clonazepam, adjusted for significant clinical features and other ASMs, had the opposite effect on increasing HRV. The authors suggest that CBZ has a negative effect on HRV and should be used with caution in patients known to be at risk for sudden death. In addition, HRV assessments should be performed before starting the use of CBZ and reconducted after long-term use. Changes in autonomic excitability in epileptic patients and patients treated with ASMs constitute the pathological basis of arrhythmia induced by ASMs.

Interestingly, reports of ASM-induced HRV changes remain somewhat controversial, and according to a meta-analysis that included six original studies, ASMs had no significant effect on HRV [47].

8.1.5 Clinical Manifestations

The effects of antiseizure drugs on cardiac function are mainly manifested by effects on cardiac structure, myocardial metabolism, and vascular function, and the most obvious manifestation is the effect on heart rhythm. Ruchi Yadav et al. [48] studied the effect of lacosamide on cardiac function and reported that lacosamide can significantly affect cardiac function; among these effects, ventricular tachycardia was the most common (29.4%). This was followed by new atrial fibrillation (17.6%), complete heart block (17.6%), Mobitz type 1 atrioventricular block (11.8%), sinus arrest (11.8%), pulseless electrical activity (5.9%), and QRS group broadening (5.9%). It is suggested that the effects of ASMs on patients are multifaceted.

8.1.6 Adverse Effects of Different ASMs on Cardiac Function

8.1.6.1 Carbamazepine (CBZ)

Carbamazepine is one of the most common ASMs that causes arrhythmia. Wang [49] studied 2699 epileptic patients out of a population of 329,432 people and reported that, compared with nonepileptic patients, epileptic patients had an increased risk of arrhythmia, and these associations were not affected by genetic predisposition. In particular, patients taking carbamazepine have a greater risk of arrhythmia. The need for regular monitoring and management of heart rhythm in patients with epilepsy should be emphasized to reduce the risk of cardiovascular complications.

Historical Evolution

Carbamazepine is currently the most highly studied ASM agent that causes arrhythmia. In 1975, Levy et al. [50] proposed that carbamazepine overdose could lead to arrhythmia. In 1987, Jacome [51] reported the syncope and death of a patient with epilepsy after carbamazepine was used, which was thought to be related to the abnormal cardiac function of the patient caused by the drug. In 1995, Checchini et al. [52], an Italian scholar, reported a case of persistent sinus tachycardia in a patient whose blood concentration of carbamazepine was within the therapeutic range. Since then, the results of many studies have indicated that CBZ can cause or aggravate sinus node dysfunction or atrioventricular block. A survey that was conducted at the Cardiff Epilepsy Center in New Zealand revealed that among 14 epilepsy patients who died suddenly of unknown cause, 11 patients were taking CBZ at the time of death; these patients accounted for 79% of the total study population, and the cause of death was related to arrhythmia caused by a prolonged QT interval [53].

Epidemiological Investigation

Although carbamazepine has been widely reported to cause cardiac dysfunction, there are few epidemiological data. To explore the effects of carbamazepine on sinus node function and atrioventricular conduction, S Matteoli et al. [54] conducted 24-h ECG monitoring on 10 patients with epilepsy without heart disease and found that 7 patients had ectopic supraventricular pulsation. Konrad Rejdak et al. [16] studied 45 patients with epilepsy taking carbamazepine and reported that 22 patients had abnormal VLPs.

Clinical Features

The main mechanism of action of carbamazepine is to inhibit voltage-gated sodium ion channels and activate potassium ion channels. As an inhibitor of sodium ion channels, carbamazepine has similar effects on nerves and the heart and can reduce the speed of automatic depolarization of cardiac pacemaker cells in stage 4, thus inhibiting the automaticity of ventricular pacemaker cells and exacerbating bradycardia caused by complete atrioventricular block [55]. Therefore, the effects of carbamazepine on cardiac function are mainly focused on heart rhythm.

Effects of Carbamazepine on Heart Rhythm

In 1990, A Donnet et al. [56] reported that carbamazepine can cause complete atrioventricular blockage. In 1997, C D Johnson et al. [57] noted that carbamazepine can cause sinus node dysfunction in patients, which brought attention to the cardiac side effects of carbamazepine. Later, E Spina et al. [58] conducted 24-h electrocardiogram imaging on 25 patients taking carbamazepine and found that 6 patients had abnormal electrocardiogram results, suggesting that attention should be given to the impact of carbamazepine use on cardiac function; this may be one of the main side effects of carbamazepine. Boesen, E [59] reported that three patients had carbamazepine-induced intermittent complete atrioventricular block, sinus block with borderline rhythm, and Stokes–Adams attack caused by intermittent cardiac arrest. It has been suggested that carbamazepine affects the heart rhythm of patients mainly through complete atrioventricular block, sinus node dysfunction, and intermittent cardiac arrest.

Susceptible Population and Related Factors

Japanese scholars have studied cases of arrhythmia caused by carbamazepine, as reported in the literature, and have summarized two different causes of arrhythmia caused by CBZ: sinus tachycardia caused by overdose, which mainly occurs in young people. Additionally, heart blockage caused by a therapeutic dose or low dose is more common in elderly women and often occurs after long-term drug treatment. The incidence is related to blood concentration and can quickly recover after drug withdrawal [55]. In 1995, Kenneback et al. [11] also demonstrated mild prolongation of the PR interval in healthy volunteers taking CBZ. In addition, it has been reported that bradycardia induced by therapeutic doses of CBZ can also occur in younger patients (24-year-old women) [60]; therefore, there is no uniform conclusion on the effect of age on the cardiac conduction system effects of carbamazepine.

Experimental Studies

Several scholars have studied the effects of carbamazepine on atrial, atrioventricular junction, and ventricular conduction in normal dogs and found that carbamazepine prolongs the duration of atrioventricular conduction and slows the duration of stage 4 depolarization of autonomic nerve fibers; therefore, carbamazepine may cause bradycardia in individuals with a normal cardiac conduction system structure [61].

Treatment

In most cases, the effect of carbamazepine on cardiac function is mild, and patients generally do not need to stop taking the drug; however, it is necessary to stop taking the drug when complete atrioventricular block and sinus node dysfunction frequently occur. Carbamazepine was discontinued in two of the three patients included in the study by Boesen, E et al. [59]. E Benassi et al. [62] reported that two patients had cardiac conduction disorders induced by carbamazepine. After stopping carbamazepine treatment, the abnormal heart rhythms of both patients disappeared; after resuming treatment, the abnormal heart rhythm of one patient reappeared.

Prevention

Since carbamazepine affects the conduction function of the heart as its main side effect, it is recommended that electrocardiography be performed before carbamazepine is used and that the conduction function of the heart be comprehensively evaluated. Heart function should be regularly monitored during administration, and patients with abnormal cardiac conduction function (such as sick sinus syndrome) should avoid this drug because of the increased risk of arrhythmia and even death. Moreover, other drugs with similar mechanisms of action, such as tricyclic antidepressants and antiarrhythmic drugs, should be avoided.

8.1.6.2 Lamotrigine (LTG)

LTG can inhibit sodium channels to stabilize the neuronal membrane and prevent the release of excitatory neurotransmitters. The results of an in vitro study have also indicated that LTG significantly inhibits the fast delayed rectifier potassium ion current (IKr) [39], thus demonstrating potential arrhythmogenic properties.

Historical Evolution

Lamotrigine was introduced in the 1990s. In 1994, Steinhoff BJ et al. [9] noted that LTG might affect the heart rhythms of patients. In 1997, Peano C et al. [63] reported that a patient treated with lamotrigine and venlafaxine developed ventricular arrhythmia. In 2000, Pricone MG et al. [64] reported for the first time that an overdose of lamotrigine can cause significant ECG changes, emphasizing the safety of lamotrigine use. In 2003, Walczak T [65] first proposed that LTG might be related to the sudden and unexplained death of epilepsy patients, which has attracted widespread attention. In 2005, Danielsson BR et al. [39] described the effect of lamotrigine on the myocardial hERG current. In 2021, the ILAE Task Force issued a safety warning about the impact of lamotrigine on heart function [66], bringing wider attention to the effects of lamotrigine on heart rhythms in epilepsy patients.

Epidemiology

Although lamotrigine has been used clinically for more than 30 years, there have been no epidemiological reports of lamotrigine causing cardiac dysfunction. Biehl A [67] reviewed the data of 233 patients taking lamotrigine, 96 of whom underwent electrocardiography during medication, and found that 7 (7.3%) patients had lamotrigine-related arrhythmias. Christensen [13] studied 91,949 epileptic patients taking lamotrigine; 194 (0.23%) out of 86,769 patients with no history of heart disease developed arrhythmias, suggesting that lamotrigine-induced cardiac conduction disorders were less common.

Animal Experiments

ASMs usually play an antiepileptic role by affecting ion channels, and most of these ion channels are simultaneously distributed in the brain and the heart; therefore, antiepileptic drugs may affect cardiomyocytes in addition to playing an antiepileptic role, causing cardiac dysfunction. Hulbert J et al. [68] studied the effects of lamotrigine on cardiomyocytes in animals and reported that increasing the lamotrigine concentration reversibly inhibited the electromechanical coupling of cardiomyocytes. Therefore, the author suggested that lamotrigine could reversibly damage the excitation and contraction of the heart. Similarly, Simon P Hagley [69] experimented on dogs and reported that after administering large amounts of lamotrigine to the dogs, an electrocardiogram showed sinus tachycardia with a prolonged QT interval.

Clinical Manifestations

Arrhythmia

Restrepo JA [70] analyzed the data of 1606 elderly epileptic patients who consumed lamotrigine and reported that lamotrigine increased QRS waves by 3.5 ± 13.1 milliseconds on average, while another six patients had Brugada syndrome and one had QTc prolongation in their medical records. Moore et al. [71] studied 57 epileptic patients taking LTG and reported that 2 patients had prolonged QRS (114–116 ms) and 4 had prolonged QT intervals (463–586 ms). Saetre et al. [72] reported that in a group of elderly epileptic patients taking a small dose of LTG (110 mg/day, blood concentration 2.6 μg/mL), the PQ interval increased by an average of 8.8 ms. Genevieve Davis [73] described a case of bradycardia in an adolescent patient who began taking lamotrigine to enhance the effects of antidepressants, and the heart rate gradually returned to normal with gradual reduction and withdrawal of the drug. These findings suggest that lamotrigine may affect heart function in patients with arrhythmia.

Death

In recent years, the ILAE working group has raised concerns about the adverse effects of lamotrigine on the heart and has warned against its use. The drug's sodium channel blocking (SCB) effect may increase the risk of arrhythmia and related sudden cardiac death; lamotrigine was thus classified as a Class IB arrhythmogenic drug. It is speculated that LTG can slow ventricular conduction, widen the QRS wave group, and cause obvious arrhythmogenic effects, including sudden death in patients with structural heart disease or myocardial ischemia; however, this approach has not been widely accepted. Christensen et al. [13] conducted a 2-year follow-up of 91,949 patients aged ≥15 years on initial lamotrigine treatment, 94 (0.23%) of whom developed cardiac conduction disorders. The authors compared the risks during current and past LTG treatment with those during the study period. Lamotrigine use was not associated with the risk of cardiac conduction disorders in people without prior heart disease or with mortality in people with prior heart disease. A systematic review reported by Restrepo et al. [70] included the published literature on Web of Science and PubMed from the inception of the database through August 2021 for patients who had recorded ECG changes, laboratory abnormalities, or sudden cardiac death while taking lamotrigine. A total of 8 randomized controlled trials, 9 nonrandomized observational studies, and 24 case reports were included, for a total of more than 3054 participants, more than 1606 of whom were treated with LTG. The final conclusion was that the evidence is insufficient to support the FDA's warning about the cardiac risks of lamotrigine and that therapeutic doses of lamotrigine may be associated with moderate, nonhazardous QRS widening.

Excessive Reactions

Wang W et al. [74] studied the relationship between the blood concentrations of LTG and the death rate of 7286 patients who consumed LTG and reported that the mortality rate of patients older than 65 years was closely related to the blood concentration of LTG. When patients died due to cardiovascular factors, the blood concentration of LTG was within the toxic range. Lamotrigine can cause death in patients through its effects on the cardiovascular system. Wang W [74] reported that a 48-year-old epileptic patient developed pulseless wide-QRS tachycardia and junctional tachycardia after taking excessive LTG (blood concentration 74.7 μg/mL, 3–14 μg/mL required for treatment). In the same year, Kicka et al. [75] studied a large number of LTG poisoning cases and observed many cardiac dysfunctions, such as ventricular arrhythmia, atrioventricular block, cardiogenic shock, and ventricular fibrillation, suggesting malignant arrhythmia or death, which is a common overdose reaction to lamotrigine. Alyahya B, F, et al. [76] analyzed 48 patients in whom lamotrigine overdose occurred in eight databases; the potentially life-threatening complications included seizures (55%), a glaucoma score ≤ 8 (20%), hypotension (12%), wide-complex tachycardia (WCT), and cardiac arrest (6%). The authors noted that severe toxicity, central nervous system depression, and seizures may occur when serum concentrations in humans are greater than 25 mg/L.

Sudden Death of Unknown Cause

Sudden death of unknown cause is a special phenomenon in patients with epilepsy. Patients often die suddenly and in an unexplained manner at night or after a seizure, and autopsies cannot find anything that could have contributed to the patient's death. In 2012, there were four deaths from SUDEP among women with idiopathic epilepsy receiving LTG monotherapy. In a case–control study, the incidence of SUDEP was significantly greater in female epilepsy patients treated with LTG [77]. Decreased heart rate variability (HRV) is a potential biomarker of sudden cardiac death. Leosuthamas D et al. [47] demonstrated that there was a statistically significant difference between patients taking lamotrigine and controls regarding HRV parameters during sleep. SUDEP, Brugada syndrome, or refractory ventricular fibrillation have also been reported in patients treated with LTG. Interestingly, genetic analysis of two of these patients revealed new mutations in the genes encoding sodium channel subunits (SCN5A and SCN9A) in heart tissue [78, 79], while genetic testing for SNC5A mutations in the other patient was negative [80].

Bunschoten et al. [81] analyzed 26 studies with 24,962 participants, 2326 of whom used lamotrigine. Twelve studies showed no significant risk of SUDEP in

LTG users. One study reported sudden cardiac death, and three studies with unclear definitions of sudden death did not find an increased risk of death in LTG users compared to controls.

Treatment

Although the role of lamotrigine in causing arrhythmias is controversial, caution should be taken in the use of lamotrigine in high-risk populations with cardiac conduction disorders (such as degree II or III atrioventricular block), ventricular arrhythmias, and other cardiac diseases (such as myocardial ischemia, heart failure, structural heart disease, and sodium channel diseases such as Brugada syndrome). In addition, concurrent use of other SCBs may increase the risk of arrhythmia, and these SCBs should not be combined with each other. Once arrhythmia occurs, reduction or withdrawal is necessary.

When sodium channel inhibition occurs in lamotrigine excess, alkalization of urine and intravenous use of fat emulsions may be beneficial for saving patient lives. Chavez P [82] described an adult patient with a prolonged QRS wave group on ECG after excessive administration of lamotrigine. Treatment with sodium bicarbonate failed, and intravenous fat emulsion was instead used; ECG abnormalities disappeared immediately. It has been suggested that in the case of lamotrigine overdose, intraventricular conduction through the heart may be delayed, resulting in prolonged QRS and QTc waves, and intravenous use of fat emulsion can successfully treat the cardiotoxicity of lamotrigine.

Overall, there is no evidence that lamotrigine use has a greater risk of induced arrhythmia than other SCBs, so lamotrigine can still be used in healthy individuals with no change in ventricular conduction (QRS time limit) or in patients with epilepsy without heart disease.

8.1.6.3 Lacosamide (LCM)

LCM is a new type of antiepileptic drug. In 2008, the US FDA approved LCM for the adjunctive treatment of partial seizures with or without secondary generalized seizures. The mechanism of action is to enhance the slow deactivation of voltage-gated sodium channels. Experimental and clinical trials have shown that LCM acts on neurons and the heart and may increase the risk of arrhythmia.

Historical Evolution

Although there have been reports of arrhythmias caused by lacosamide in the early clinical stage, the effect of lacosamide on patient cardiac function was first observed by Degiorgio CM et al. [83], who reported that an epileptic patient developed atrial flutter/atrial fibrillation after taking a large dose of lacosamide (600 mg/day).

Subsequently, Nizam A [84] noted that second-degree atrioventricular block may occur in patients using LCM. They reported a case of second-degree atrioventricular block in a patient with epilepsy while taking lacosamide. The atrioventricular block caused hypotension and bradycardia, which aggravated the seizures, and the patient was completely normal after withdrawal of the drug. In 2012, Kaufman KR et al. [85] reported that atrial fibrillation can occur when patients are taking small doses of LCM, emphasizing the need to monitor patients' heart function when using LCM. In 2021, when Kim HK et al. [86] used LCM to treat status epilepticus, patients also exhibited significant cardiac dysfunction. Subsequently, Sumbul O et al. [87] replicated the effects of LCM on cardiac function through animal experiments, and the effects of LCM on cardiac function have received widespread attention.

Epidemiology

Kim HK [88] conducted a survey of 85 patients using LCM and reported that 28 (32.9%) had cardiac function impairment. Yadav R [48] described 38 patients taking LCM, 2 of whom developed arrhythmias. Bamgbose O [89] studied the use of LCM in 38 neonates, 2 of whom (5%) developed arrhythmias. Davidson KE et al. [90] compared the effects of different medication methods on cardiac function in 166 patients and reported that 2.3% and 2.6% of patients treated with intravenous drip and push injection, respectively, had bradycardia, 8% and 10.3%, respectively, had hypotension, and one patient in each group had a prolonged PR interval. Overall, the incidence of LCM-induced cardiac function injury was 2.3–32.9%.

Clinical Manifestations

The manifestations of cardiac dysfunction caused by LCM vary. Kim HK et al. [86] conducted a study on 38 patients with heart dysfunction treated with lacosamide and found that 19 patients presented with first-degree atrioventricular block, 7 patients presented with hypotension, 2 patients had atrial fibrillation and bradycardia, and 1 patient presented with atrial flutter. After intravenous LCM loading, the mean PR interval increased from 169.3 to 184.5 ms, and the mean heart rate increased from 91.7 to 86.9, suggesting that the manifestations of cardiac dysfunction caused by LCM varied.

Bradycardia

Fong SL [91] studied 686 infants and 28 newborns taking LCM and reported that one of them presented with bradycardia. Among the 38 patients with abnormal heart function reported by Kim HK [86], 2 had bradycardia.

Sinus Arrest and Death

Shibata M et al. [92] described a patient with sinus node dysfunction and atrioventricular block after receiving lacosamide treatment who subsequently died due to septic shock. Bainbridge J [92] treated diabetes mellitus with 600 mg/d LCM, and one patient died of cardiac arrest. Huberman MA [93] also reported a case of cardiac arrest after lacosamide use. Among the patients described by Yadav R [48], 11.8% had sinus arrest.

Wide QRS Tachycardia

Takai C [88] reported a case of wide-QRS tachycardia in a patient poisoned by lacosamide, which was successfully treated by veno-arterial extracorporeal membrane oxygenation. Ng PC [94] reported a case of suspected single LCM overdose with prolonged QRS. Wide QRS tachycardia was observed in 5.9% of the patients in the study by Yadav R [48].

Refractory Ventricular Tachycardia

Marcellino C [95] described a 60-year-old female patient who developed a state of status epilepticus after taking an overdose of LCM, accompanied by refractory ventricular tachycardia. The patient gradually recovered through cutaneous stellate ganglion block combined with extracorporeal membrane oxygenation. The authors suggest that attention should be given to the damage caused to cardiac function by high-dose LCM. Eleftheriou G [84] reported a case of multiple episodes of life-threatening ventricular fibrillation requiring cardioversion after first taking lacosamide as an adjuvant treatment for epilepsy. DeGiorgio AC [96] reported a case of severe ventricular tachycardia in a 49-year-old man with intractable frontal lobe epilepsy after the addition of 400 mg LCM to his treatment; this tachycardia persisted during hospitalization and did not progress until LCM was discontinued, suggesting a link between the arrhythmia and LCM.

Atrioventricular Block

Among the cases reported by Kim HK et al. [86], 19 patients presented with first-degree atrioventricular block. Nizam et al. [92] reported that when combined with other ASMs that can prolong the PR interval, LCM can cause second-degree atrioventricular block and eventually lead to hypotension and bradycardia. Yan-Ting Lu [97] retrospectively analyzed the electrocardiograms and blood pressures of 38 patients in the neurological intensive care unit before and after routine intravenous injection of LCM for 30 min. The results showed that 2 patients developed cardiac side effects after LCM loading—one (3.0%) with a new first-degree atrioventricular block and the other (3.0%) with an atrial premature beat. Stamm et al. [98] reported that a healthy young man developed a second-degree atrioventricular block a few hours after intravenous lacosamide treatment, which disappeared after discontinuation. The authors suggest that routine ECG should be considered for all patients receiving LCM. Lachuer C [99] described an 88-year-old female patient who developed atrioventricular block after taking a small dose of lacosamide, and the stability of her vital signs could be maintained only by placing a pacemaker. Among the cases reported by Yadav R [48], 15.9% of the patients presented with heart block, suggesting that atrioventricular block is a common manifestation of LCM affecting the heart.

Atrial Fibrillation and Flutter

Atrial fibrillation and flutter are common manifestations of the effects of lacosamide on cardiac function. Among the cases reported by Kim HK [86], two patients developed atrial fibrillation and one patient developed atrial flutter. Degiorgio CM [83] described a patient with epilepsy who developed atrial flutter/atrial fibrillation after taking a high dose of LCM (600 mg/day). The patient had no significant risk factors for heart disease, and his symptoms were relieved after stopping LCM therapy. Kaufman KR et al. [85] noted that small doses (200 mg) of LCM can induce atrial fibrillation in patients with epilepsy; therefore, cardiac monitoring may be required during the use of LCM.

Other

Marilyn E [100] conducted a study of 32 patients and reported that after 2 h of medication, the heart rates of epilepsy patients increased, and the average extension of the PR interval was approximately 6 ms. Kim HK et al. [86] also observed that the mean PR interval increased from 169.3 to 184.5 ms, and the mean heart rate increased from 91.7 to 86.9 when LCM was delivered intravenously at the loading dose. Bamgbose O [89] reported that atrial coupling occurred in 2 neonates out of 38 children receiving LCM.

Relevant Factors

Dose

Rudd GD [101] conducted a study of 944 patients randomized to receive different doses of LCM and compared the results with those of 364 patients taking placebo; no impairment of cardiac function was found in patients taking either 200 mg/day or 400 mg/day LCM, but when the dose was increased to 600 mg/day, no impairment of cardiac function was found. The patients began to show cardiac function impairment, an increased PR interval, and reported atrioventricular block, suggesting that lacosamide had a pharmacodynamic effect during the PR interval. Kropeit D [102] revealed no impairment of heart function at 400 mg/day LCM in healthy people. However, as the dose was increased to 800 mg/day, the PR interval was only slightly extended, suggesting that the effect of lacosamide on cardiac function in patients is dose dependent.

Age

Bainbridge J et al. [15] compared responses to lacosamide and found that, compared with patients under 65 years of age, patients over 65 years of age were more likely to have cardiac function impairment during lacosamide monotherapy. The incidence of cardiac impairment was 7.7% in the older subjects and 4.0% in the younger group when LCM was administered at 600 mg/day.

8.1.6.4 Other ASMs

Levetiracetam (LEV)

LEV is a derivative of pyrrolidone. In 2011, Rojano et al. [103] first proposed that acquired long QT syndrome (ALQTS) might be related to LEV administration. ALQTS is a clinical syndrome involving changes in ventricular repolarization caused by various factors. The ECGs of ALQTS patients are characterized by prolonged QTc, requiring ≥450 ms for males and ≥460 ms for females. Rojano et al. [103] reported that an 88-year-old female epilepsy patient was treated with LEV (500 mg, i.v., and q12h) for 24 h, an electrocardiogram indicated sinus bradycardia (heart rate 55 times/copy, QTc 480 ms), and a 24 h Holter electrocardiogram indicated sinus bradycardia and transient atrial fibrillation. This change in ventricular repolarization disappeared within 48 h after the patient was switched to valproic acid treatment rather than with LEV. Many scholars believe that the mechanism of action of LEV involves the binding of synaptic vesicle protein 2A. In formal QT/QTc studies in healthy volunteers, no effect on cardiac repolarization has been observed [104] nor have changes in the QT interval been observed in patients with poststroke epilepsy [105]. Aydin et al. [106] studied the records of 30 patients diagnosed with epilepsy and treated with levetiracetam. The mean age of the patients was 10.93 ± 3.74 (4–17) years. Sixteen patients (53.33%) were boys. A total of 13 patients (43.3%) presented with focal seizures, and 17 patients (56.7%) presented with generalized seizures. A comparison of ECG parameters (PR interval, QTc, QT interval, and QRS duration) revealed that the PR interval and QTc were decreased at 6 months of treatment; however, these changes were not statistically significant. There were no significant differences in ECG parameters associated with sex or epilepsy type before treatment or at 6 months ($p > 0.05$). The authors concluded that LEV had no effect on ECG parameters. Nonclinical evaluation combined with the comprehensive in vitro proarrhythmia assay (CIPA) has indicated that there is no QT prolongation in patients receiving LEV. The risk of arrhythmia is at least 10 times that of FTPC, which is in good agreement with clinical and postmarketing

LEV data but does not rule out the very rare case of QT prolongation in patients with potential risk factors [107].

In prospective studies of the effect of LEV on lipids, LEV was not associated with significant changes in lipid levels, except for in one study that reported elevated LDL levels [108]. Switching from enzyme-induced ASM therapy to LEV therapy significantly reduced TC, TG, LDL-C, and non-HDL-C levels in young and elderly patients [109]. In another small study in children, LEV also improved lipid status, suggesting a possible protective effect against atherosclerosis [110].

Phenobarbital (PB)

PB affects the heart's fast delayed rectified potassium ion current (IKr) and therefore may have a potential arrhythmogenic effect [36]. In 2014, Siniscalchi et al. [105] conducted a study on 49 patients who used PB for epileptic seizures after stroke and found that the QTc interval was significantly prolonged.

Rufinamide (RUF)

RUF is approved by the FDA in the United States for the adjuvant treatment of Lennox–Gastaut syndrome. A small study conducted by Schimpf et al. [110] on 19 patients with Lennox–Gastaut syndrome showed that the mean QTc interval was slightly shortened before and after oral treatment, but no serious adverse reactions, such as symptomatic arrhythmia or sudden cardiac death, were observed during a follow-up of 3.04 ± 1.09 years after treatment. However, these findings suggest that the RUF carries a potential risk of arrhythmia [111].

To date, no arrhythmic effects of RUF have been reported. In patients with congenital short QT syndrome or who are receiving other ASM treatments that may shorten the QT interval, such as CNB and PRI, it may be wise to avoid the use of RUF. ECG should be regularly repeated during use to avoid damage caused by adverse events such as arrhythmias.

Gabapentin (GBP) and Pregabalin (PGB)

Both drugs block L-type calcium channels. Previous case reports and observational studies have suggested that GBP may be associated with an increased risk of atrial fibrillation. However, all the evidence is based on patients older than 65 years with comorbidities that predispose to arrhythmia. Park et al. [112] described the case of an African American male in his 20s who presented to a chronic pain clinic with lumbar radiculitis and developed atrial fibrillation 4 days after starting GBP. It is suggested that GBP can induce new atrial fibrillation in young people.

Recently, there have also been reports on the protective effect of GBP on the myocardium. Wu et al. [113] reported that GBP was administered to rats before myocardial ischemia–reperfusion (I/R), and the results showed that gabapentin preconditioning successfully alleviated myocardial ischemia–reperfusion injury, including reducing the myocardial infarction size and cell apoptosis. The myocardial protective effect of GBP may be related to the activation of PI3K/Akt in the myocardium and the upregulation of GABAARδ in the spinal cord. Therefore, GBP may have a protective effect on the myocardium during routine clinical treatment.

In one in vitro study, the QT interval was significantly prolonged after a single dose of PGB in rabbits, while GBP had no inhibitory effect on the interaction between the cardiac rapid currents [114]. Patients in a population-based cohort study who were treated with PGB or GBP for unknown reasons were at a higher risk of starting treatment with medications specifically designed to treat atrial fibrillation [115]. An 80-year-old woman was reported to have a prolonged QT interval and syncope episodes during treatment with PGB [116].

Cannabidiol (CBD)

CBD is a nonpsychoactive cannabinoid whose mechanism of action has not been fully determined. Although in vitro experimental studies with purified CBD have shown that the drug can inhibit a variety of cardiac ion channels [117, 118], formal QT/QTc studies in healthy volunteers showed no effect on cardiac electrophysiology after treatment with oral mucosal sprays containing THC and CBD at both therapeutic and ultratherapeutic doses [119]. Wang et al. [120] used perfluorooctane sulfonate (PFOS) to study the effect of CBD on cardiomyocytes. PFOS is a fluorinated organic compound that can be widely detected in the environment and in organisms, can cross biological barriers, and cause cardiotoxicity. Mice were fed PFOS (5 mg/kg) and/or CBD (10 mg/kg). In vitro, H9C2 cells were treated with PFOS (200 μM) and/or CBD (10 μM). The results showed that CBD could alleviate PFOS-induced mitochondrial dynamic imbalance and energy metabolism disorders in cardiomyocytes by improving antioxidant capacity, suggesting that CBD may have a novel protective effect on PFOS-induced cardiomyocytes.

Valproic Acid (VPA)

In 2022, Yildiz et al. [121] studied the effects of high and low doses of VPA on the hearts of nonepileptic female rats, and the results showed that the intensity of caspase-3 staining increased in a dose-dependent manner, while the intensity of connexin-43 and troponin-T staining decreased significantly. The administration of high doses of VPA led to an increase in MDA levels in cardiac tissue, and these results support that VPA treatment increases cardiac risk markers. In a Danish cohort study, VPA treatment was shown to be associated with a greater risk of heart failure and death from heart failure in elderly patients with epilepsy with heart failure than was lamotrigine or levetiracetam treatment [122].

Despite the potential role of VPA in weight gain, the effect of VPA treatment on lipid levels is unclear. Guo et al. [123] conducted a meta-analysis of pediatric epilepsy patients, including a case–control study on the effects of VPA treatment on lipid profiles, and the results showed that VPA treatment was associated with a significant decrease in total cholesterol and low-density lipoprotein levels, as well as high-density lipoprotein and triglyceride levels, with no significant effects observed. Muller et al. [124] studied the negative effects of ASMs on lipid levels; specifically, participants who used valproic acid had lower HDL levels ($p = 0.002$) and greater triglyceride levels ($p = 0.002$) than participants who did not use VPA.

George et al. [125] compared the prevalence of insulin resistance (IR) in children treated with valproate sodium (VPA) and phenytoin sodium (PS) monotherapy for >1 year. A total of 150 children aged 6–18 years were divided into Group A (VPA), Group B (PS), and Group C (healthy control group age- and sex-matched with Group A), with 50 patients in each group. Regardless of age, sex, adolescence, and nutritional status, the prevalence of IR and nonalcoholic fatty liver disease in children in the VPA group was significantly greater than that in the PS and healthy control groups (12% and 34%, respectively). Central obesity, acanthosis, hypertension, and dyslipidemia were significantly correlated with IR, but multivariate analysis showed no independent correlation. VPA treatment predisposes children to metabolic complications, so close monitoring facilitates early detection and timely intervention.

Cenobamate (CNB)

CNB mainly acts on voltage-gated sodium currents and GABAA receptors [126]. In 2022, Darpo et al. [127] conducted a phase I clinical study on the effect of CNB on the QT interval in which they tested the effect of CNB on the normal QT interval (QTc) in healthy adults ($n = 108$) at both therapeutic and supratherapeutic doses (maximum recommended dose 400 mg/day). The results suggest that CNB has no clinically relevant prolonging effect on ECG parameters (e.g., PR or QRS), and the HR in patients is similar to that of the placebo controls. CNB was associated with a slight dose-related reduction in QTc, but the extent of change was not clinically relevant (no reduction ≤340 ms). The authors concluded that CNB had no clinically relevant effect on HR or ECG parameters, nor did it have a QTc prolongation effect at therapeutic or supratherapeutic doses. In another formal QT study, at a supratherapeutic dose of 500 mg of CNB, the drug shortened the QT interval in up to 66% of subjects [3].

In combination with the above studies, use of this drug is not recommended in patients with familial short QT syndrome, and this drug should be used with caution in combination with other drugs that shorten the QT interval, such as primidone or rufinamide.

8.1.7 Treatment

The effect of most ASMs on heart function is mild and needs to only be monitored if there is no obvious dysfunction; if one cannot stop or reduce the use of antiseizure drugs, a small number of patients with severe impacts on heart function need to reduce or stop use of the drug (specifically, see the treatment of heart function with different antiseizure drugs).

8.1.8 Prevention

The application of some ASMs has adverse effects on the heart, which directly leads to the risk of fatal arrhythmia; long-term administration of these agents, due to associated elevated blood lipids, promotes inflammation and can cause atherosclerosis. It appears that to avoid adverse cardiac effects of ASMs, the following considerations should be taken: Enzyme-induced ASMs should be avoided in patients at cardiovascular risk as these drugs may aggravate cardiovascular risk factors, including weight gain associated with specific ASMs. For patients with new episodes of syncope or brief loss of consciousness, a 12-lead electrocardiogram (or Holter recording) is recommended for identifying ASM-induced arrhythmias. In patients with epilepsy who are older than 60 years or have heart disease, an electrocardiogram (ECG) should be performed before the use of ASM agents, such as SCBs. If antiepileptic therapy involving SCBs is to be adjusted, 12-lead electrocardiography (before adjustment and 2 weeks after adjustment) is recommended to rule out atrioventricular block or sinus node dysfunction. It is especially recommended for patients taking other cardioactive medications, such as antihypertensive or antiarrhythmic drugs, or for those taking high doses or combinations of SCBs. The use of two or more SCBs should be avoided in combination therapy with ASMs.

8.2 Drug-Induced Liver Injury Induced by ASMs in Patients with Epilepsy

Liver injury is the most common adverse effect of ASM and can range from mild injury to fatal damage. It can occur independently or as part of drug hypersensitivity syndrome, making it one of the most common side effects in patients with epilepsy. The mechanisms underlying drug-induced liver injury (DILI) caused by ASMs are diverse and involve immune-mediated responses, direct cell toxicity, or specific reactions. This warrants attention.

8.2.1 Epidemiology

Harshad Devarbhavi et al. [128] studied patients with DILI caused by ASMs in a large single-center database from 1998 to 2021. Among 1067 patients using ASMs, they found that DILI was caused by 18 different ASMs, including carbamazepine (n = 36), phenytoin (n = 71), phenobarbital (n = 8), and sodium valproate (n = 14), with 13 fatalities (85%). They concluded that DILI is primarily caused by first-generation ASMs, while DILI caused by newer generation drugs makes up less than 10% of cases. Brad K Kamitaki et al. [129] reported that many earlier and newer generation ASMs, including valproate, phenytoin, carbamazepine, phenobarbital, lamotrigine, levetiracetam, oxcarbazepine, and diazepam, are associated with DILI. However, zonisamide, perampanel, stiripentol, lacosamide, clobazam, pregabalin, felbamate, topiramate, gabapentin, ethosuximide, brivaracetam, and pexidartinib rarely cause liver injury. In 2011, Harshad Devarbhavi et al. [130] conducted a study on children who developed DILI between 1997 and 2004 (retrospective) and between 2005 and 2010 (prospective). Among 450 patients with DILI, 39 were children (8.7%). ASM use, including that of phenytoin (n = 10) and carbamazepine (n = 6), were among the common causes. The overall mortality rate was high (30.7%). Naga Chalasani et al. [131] reported a significant decrease in the incidence of ASM-related liver injury (from 8.5% in 2004–2007 to 2.6% in 2015–2020; $p = 0.01$). ASMs other than phenytoin are commonly used to treat nonseizure disorders. Compared to those of non-ASM patients, those of ASM-related liver injury were younger (mean age 38.5 years vs. 50.1 years, $p < 0.001$), more likely to be African American (27% vs. 12%, $p = 0.008$), and more often associated with skin hypersensitivity reactions. To date, there have been no reports in the literature of vigabatrin, tiagabine, or rufinamide causing DILI.

A retrospective cohort analysis of 661 patients with drug-induced acute liver failure from 1987 to 2006 in the United Network for Organ Sharing (UNOS) database was performed. These cases accounted for 12% of acute liver failure transplants during this period [132]. However, due to underreporting or misdiagnosis, the incidence of DILI may have been higher than expected [133].

8.2.2 Clinical Manifestations of ASM-Induced Liver Injury

8.2.2.1 Age and Sex

Harshad Devarbhavi et al. [128] conducted a study on patients with DILI caused by ASM use in a large single-center DILI registry and found that, compared to patients with DILI caused by other drugs, patients with DILI caused by ASMs were younger (31 years vs. 41 years; $p = 0.31$) and more likely to be female (52% vs. 46%; $p = 0.19$); additionally, the incidence of jaundice was lower (41% vs. 59%, $p = 0.001$), and the Model for End-Stage Liver Disease (MELD) score was lower

(14.5 vs. 16.5; $p = 0.02$). Additionally, topiramate-induced hyperammonemia was also associated with age and sex, with a greater proportion of drug-induced liver injury events observed in male patients aged 75 years or older. Sanja Petrović [134] reported that newer generation ASMs can also cause DILI in older adults.

8.2.2.2 Severity

Lamotrigine, levetiracetam, oxcarbazepine, topiramate, and zonisamide have each led to one or more cases of DILI. An analysis of 1947 hepatotoxicity events from safety reports (ICSRs) revealed that 56.97% occurred in females, 67.05% were severe, and 3.36% died, indicating that liver injury caused by ASMs can be severe [134]. Similarly, Brad K Kamitaki et al. [129] studied 2175 cases of DILI attributed to ASMs, with 97.2% classified as severe reactions, including death, hospitalization, disability, and other life-threatening outcomes.

8.2.2.3 Fatal Liver Function Injury

DILI induced by ASMs is one of the most important causes of drug-induced death in patients and is the third most common type of drug used by adults with DILI [135]. Koenig et al. [136] conducted a questionnaire survey among German doctors from 1994 to 2003 and described a total of 9 patients with fatal liver injury. Zimmerman et al. [137] studied the pathological specimens of 23 patients with fatal hepatotoxicity caused by valproic acid in the United States and reported that 80% of the patients had microvesicular steatosis, most of which were accompanied by central necrosis or cirrhosis. Dreifuss et al. [138] reported that among children under 2 years of age who received treatment with multiple ASMs, patients with developmental delays, neurological diseases and congenital developmental abnormalities had the highest risk of liver disease-related death. The overall mortality rate is 1 in 10,000; most cases occur within 90 days after treatment. These results indicate that fatal liver injury is a manifestation of liver injury caused by ASMs.

8.2.2.4 Hypersensitivity Syndrome

Reactive metabolite syndrome (RMS), also known as hypersensitivity syndrome (HRMS), is a common manifestation of liver function injury caused by ASMs and is characterized by fever, rash, eosinophilia, and organ damage [128]. DILI induced by ASMs is often observed in patients with hypersensitive rash syndrome, including drug-induced hypersensitivity syndrome (DIHS), Stevens–Johnson syndrome (SJS), and toxic epidermal necrolysis (TEN) [128]. ASMs that can cause hypersensitivity syndrome include phenytoin (PHT), carbamazepine (CBZ), phenobarbital (PB), and lamotrigine (LTG) [139, 140]. The incidence of RMS is approximately 10–100/100,000, with symptoms usually occurring 1–8 weeks after initiation of

ASM treatment. Approximately 50% of ASMs patients have abnormal liver function, especially abnormal liver enzyme levels, but this may also manifest as severe hepatitis [141]. Approximately 9% of patients taking phenobarbital develop liver damage caused by reactive metabolic syndrome [142]. The drugs that can induce RMS include phenytoin (PHT), carbamazepine (CBZ), and phenobarbital (PB), and the onset of RMS often occurs early in the course of treatment, with a greater risk among individuals who have a first-degree relative with RMS [140].

8.2.2.5 Others

Valproic acid (VPA) administration is a common cause of hepatotoxicity, and 10–15% of patients using valproic acid experience transient elevation of liver enzyme levels; 1 in 10,000 of these patients may develop fatal injury. Long-term use of phenytoin (PHT) can also lead to mild elevation of liver enzyme levels; the total incidence is 10–25%, but severe liver injury is rare [142]. Severe liver toxicity caused by carbamazepine is specific, and risk factors include young age and longer duration of treatment [139]. Among these patients, 61% may experience asymptomatic elevation of liver enzyme levels, but this increase is usually transient [143]. The incidence of liver enzyme level elevation in patients taking lamotrigine is less than 1%, and severe hepatotoxicity is even rarer [144].

8.2.3 Drug-Induced Liver Injury Caused by Different ASM Agents

8.2.3.1 Valproic Acid (VPA)

Valproic acid is widely used for the treatment of partial and generalized seizures, migraines, cluster headaches, and bipolar affective disorders [145]. A study conducted by Enrique S Meseguer et al. [146] involving 60 patients revealed that 15 patients experienced liver dysfunction, suggesting that liver injury is still the biggest obstacle to the use of valproic acid and that it is also a commonly used drug that causes liver damage.

Historical Evolution of VPA-Induced Liver Injury

The antiseizure properties of VPA were first described in 1962, and it was approved by the U.S. Food and Drug Administration (FDA) for clinical use as an ASM in 1978. In 1979, Donat JF [147] first described fatal VPA-induced hepatitis, and subsequently, Suchy et al. [148] described VPA-related acute liver failure. In 1980, Jacobi G [149] described lethal hepatotoxicity caused by sodium valproate administration in children, which has led to widespread attention being given to

VPA-induced hepatotoxicity. In 1984, Palm R et al. [150] noted that VPA hepatotoxicity can be induced by phenytoin poisoning, causing severe liver impairment in patients and becoming the first recognized symptom of phenytoin poisoning. In 1986, Nomura F et al. [151] confirmed the hepatotoxicity and possible underlying mechanisms of VPA through animal experiments, thereby advancing the understanding of its hepatotoxicity. Subhash [152] reported that VPA can cause hepatic encephalopathy. Recently, Wong YJ et al. [153] conducted a systematic analysis of the phenomenon of elevated blood ammonia levels caused by VPA, emphasizing its relationship with liver dysfunction. Atef MM [154] also noted a potential protective effect of liraglutide against valproic acid-induced hepatotoxicity, thus enriching the research on valproic acid hepatotoxicity.

Epidemiology of VPA-Induced Liver Injury

Liu et al. [155] analyzed reports of pediatric hepatic adverse events from the U.S. Food and Drug Administration Adverse Event Reporting System. They identified a total of 14,143 cases in children, 511 of which were attributed to VPA. Cano-Paniagua et al. [156] studied 286 patients with elevated liver enzyme levels after taking VPA; among these patients, 18 had DILI (6%), indicating that VPA was one of the drugs responsible for liver damage in these patients. Schmid et al. [157] evaluated all cases of severe adverse liver reactions caused by VPA reported to the German Federal Institute for Drugs between 1993 and 2009. They identified 132 patients with severe VPA-related liver failure. Approximately, one-third (34.8%) of the adverse events occurred during monotherapy with VPA, while the majority occurred during combination therapy with VPA, with 34 cases (25.8%) indicating a significant impact of VPA on the occurrence of nonfatal and fatal liver failure. Cotariu et al. [158] reported that approximately 10–15% of patients using VPA experienced transient elevation of liver enzyme levels, and 44% of patients had hyperbilirubinemia. Elevations in alkaline phosphatase (ALP) and gamma-glutamyl transferase (GGT) levels were less common.

The Main Clinical Manifestations of VPA Hepatotoxicity

The hepatotoxicity of VPA is rare and idiosyncratic, which typically occurs within the first 3 months of drug use.

Susceptibility factors

Dreifuss et al. [138] reported that the highest risk of developing hepatotoxicity occurred in patients who were taking ASMs and had congenital metabolic deficiencies and psychomotor delays. In patients with nonfatal disease, early recognition of VPA-related hepatotoxicity, discontinuation of the drug, and intravenous carnitine supplementation may aid in recovery. Schmid et al. [157] summarized cases of VPA hepatotoxicity that were reported to the German Federal Institute for Drugs and

Medical Devices between 1993 and 2009. They reported a greater incidence of hepatotoxicity in patients receiving treatment with multiple antiseizure medications (ASMs) and concurrent treatment with benzodiazepines or antipsychotic drugs. However, multidrug use did not increase mortality rates.

Fatal Liver Injury
Donat et al. [147] were the first researchers to notice fatal liver injury associated with VPA, and they found that patients taking VPA developed fatal hepatitis. Miguil et al. [159] described the case of a 19-year-old male with absence seizures who had been treated with VPA for 2 months. Several weeks later, he developed jaundice and hepatic encephalopathy, which led to death. Pourahmad et al. [160] also identified VPA as the third most commonly used heterophylly that causes liver injury and death. Stewart et al. [161] reported that VPA can cause fatal liver dysfunction and that its development is related to genetic factors. Using lipidomic analyses, Xu et al. [162] analyzed the mechanisms of VPA-induced hepatotoxicity, suggesting that this effect might be related to the disruption of lipid metabolism.

Liver injury in patients with drug hypersensitivity syndrome
Although some drug hypersensitivity syndromes caused by valproic acid are acceptable when because of the importance of antiepileptic drug therapy, the most severe adverse effects of VPA should be considered. Robert G Bota et al. [163] described a 25-year-old female patient who developed drug hypersensitivity syndrome while using VPA, leading to liver injury after renal and cardiac dysfunction. Yau-Li Huan et al. [164] studied liver biopsy specimens from a patient with hypersensitivity syndrome caused by sodium valproate and reported that the patient had obvious toxic hepatitis and microvesicular steatosis.

Valproic acid (VPA)-induced hyperammonemia and hepatic encephalopathy
Clinically, determining the significance of VPA-induced hyperammonemia is challenging because it can cause varying degrees of damage or no symptoms. In a prospective study, the prevalence of hyperammonemia (defined as an ammonium level exceeding twice the normal upper limit) was reported to range from 70% to 100%. However, the results of this study did not establish a relationship between elevated blood ammonia levels and clinical symptoms [165]. Yiu-Ching Jennifer Wong et al. [166] analyzed 204 published reports and reported that the incidence of asymptomatic elevation of blood ammonia levels was much greater than that of symptomatic elevation. They also observed a gradual normalization of blood ammonia levels with the discontinuation of VPA, suggesting that VPA-induced hyperammonemia may not have significant clinical implications. However, Hidetada Yamada et al. [167] reported that a patient developed consciousness disorder and subsequent cerebral edema and status epilepticus as their blood ammonia levels increased after 3 days of treatment with VPA. They emphasized the importance of monitoring blood ammonia levels when using VPA, even in patients receiving monotherapy with VPA. Amit Chopra [168] summarized the characteristics of VPA-induced hyperammonemia encephalopathy and identified factors such as interactions with other drugs, intellectual disability, carnitine deficiency, and urea cycle disorders as

risk factors. The duration and dosage of VPA treatment, as well as the serum VPA and ammonia levels, do not appear to be related to the occurrence or severity of hyperammonemia encephalopathy. Although hyperammonemia encephalopathy is rare clinically, patients may experience psychiatric symptoms, usually at the beginning of VPA treatment or several months into treatment. Hyperammonemia encephalopathy usually improves with the discontinuation of VPA [169, 170]. For epilepsy patients with liver dysfunction, as long as the elevation in ammonium levels is less than twice the normal upper limit, antiseizure therapy can be continued.

The Mechanism of VPA-Induced Liver Injury

VPA is an ASM agent that can cause specific liver damage and is primarily metabolized by the liver. The metabolite 2-propyl-4-pentenoic acid has been associated with VPA-induced hepatotoxicity [171]. The main mechanisms by which VPA induces liver injury are as follows

1. Release of the 2-propyl-4-pentenoic acid metabolite: Due to the potential cytotoxic effects of VPA and its major metabolite 2-propyl-4-pentenoic acid (4-ene VPA), close monitoring of plasma VPA concentrations is necessary during clinical use to circumvent severe side effects [172].
2. Reduction in glutathione (GSH) storage and antioxidant levels, leading to oxidative stress: Amjad S. Aljarboa [173] reported significantly decreased levels of hepatic glutathione (GSH) and superoxide dismutase (SOD) activity in VPA-treated patients. These results suggest that indole-3-acetic acid may be a promising protective agent against VPA-induced hepatotoxicity.
3. Inhibition of fatty acid β-oxidation, induction of mitochondrial DNA depletion and hypermethylation, reduced proton leakage, oxidative phosphorylation impairment, and decreased ATP synthesis: Targeted metabolomic analysis of acylcarnitines (ACs) in pediatric serum revealed decreased expression of genes involved in fatty acid β-oxidation (carnitine palmitoyltransferase (CPT) 1, CPT2, and long-chain acyl-CoA dehydrogenase (LCAD)) due to VPA-induced liver dysfunction, indicating that fatty acid β-oxidation (FAO) is disrupted. The upregulation of gene expression after fenofibrate treatment suggests an improvement in FAO, indicating that the disruption of fatty acid β-oxidation induced by VPA may contribute to liver injury and that reversing fatty acid metabolism has a significant protective effect against VPA-induced hepatotoxicity [174].
4. Inhibition of carnitine palmitoyltransferase I enhances the activation of peroxisome proliferator-activated receptor-gamma and acyl-CoA synthetase 1 and induces long-chain fatty acid uptake and triglyceride synthesis, leading to steatosis. Studies have shown that VPA treatment depletes carnitine, coenzyme A, and antioxidant enzymes, further impairing liver function [171].

Treatment for VPA-Induced Hepatotoxicity

Treatment for VPA-related hepatotoxicity usually involves discontinuation of VPA. Since carnitine is an essential amino acid in fatty acid metabolism, it has been hypothesized that the cause of VPA hepatotoxicity and hyperammonemia may be carnitine deficiency. This hypothesis suggests that carnitine can be used as a treatment for drug-induced liver injury caused by VPA. It has also been reported that carnitine can improve the blood ammonia clearance rate in some patients with encephalopathy [175, 176].

8.2.3.2 Phenytoin (PHT)

Phenytoin sodium (PHT) was the first ASM to be evaluated through preclinical studies rather than through clinical observation, and it is also the first nonsedative ASM. PHT is one of the ASMs used for the treatment of generalized tonic–clonic seizures [177].

Historical Evolution of PHT-Induced Liver Injury

Phenytoin (PHT) was first synthesized in 1908 and was subsequently used as an ASM until 1938. In 1984, Pineda JA et al. [178] described a case of active hepatitis in an epileptic patient receiving PHT therapy and proposed that PHT could cause liver dysfunction. In 1999, N R Temkin et al. [179] conducted a randomized, double-blinded trial and reported that patients with epilepsy treated with phenytoin experienced severe adverse events, including coagulation abnormalities and liver damage, but the difference compared with patients not taking phenytoin was not significant. This supports the notion that liver injury is a common adverse reaction associated with phenytoin.

Epidemiology of PHT-Induced Liver Injury

PHT-induced severe liver injury is rare. Kamitaki et al. [129] analyzed adverse events of ASM-induced liver injury reported in the FDA Adverse Event Reporting System (FAERS) from 2018 to 2020. Among a total of 3200 patients who underwent PHT therapy, 126 (3.9%) experienced DILI. Russo M et al. [132] evaluated 137 patients with drug-induced acute liver failure in the United Network for Organ Sharing (UNOS) liver transplantation database from 1990 to 2002 and described 10 patients with acute liver failure caused by PHT, accounting for 7.3% of all patients. Chronic mild liver enzyme-level elevations are relatively common in long-term PHT treatment, occurring in 10–25% of patients. H W Aiges et al. [142] evaluated liver function in 63 epilepsy patients who had been receiving PHT treatment for 12 months. They found that 56 patients (88.9%) had elevated serum alanine aminotransferase levels. Among the 11 patients who initially had elevated aspartate aminotransferase and alanine aminotransferase levels, 6 had persistent abnormal transaminase levels for more than 20 weeks. These six patients continued to take the same dose of PHT, and their transaminase levels normalized within 8–14 months. These data indicate that most patients who experience elevated liver enzyme levels after PHT treatment will gradually recover due to adaptation. Increased gamma-glutamyl transferase (GGT) content is observed in 50–90% of patients receiving PHT treatment, while alkaline phosphatase (ALP) level elevation is less common. The most common pattern of liver damage associated with PHT is cholestatic or mixed. The clinical incidence of liver toxicity is estimated to be 1 in 10,000–150,000 cases [180]. Naga Chalasani et al. [131] reviewed the clinical data of patients with epilepsy treated with phenytoin prior to 2020 and reported that among 16 HT-related DILI patients, 3 (19%) died or needed liver transplantation.

Mechanism of PHT-Induced Liver Injury

Ninety-five percent of PHT is metabolized by the liver, and 5% is excreted by the kidneys [181]. PHT is metabolized to aromatic oxide by cytochrome P450, which is mainly converted by epoxide hydrolase. A decrease in the level of epoxide hydrolase leads to an increase in the level of aromatic oxides. Aromatic oxides are reactive electrophilic compounds that can bind proteins and lead to cell death, mutation, tumor formation, as well as liver damage [182, 183]. Eita Sasaki et al. [184] reported that PHT can reduce the liver glutathione (GSH) content, and that depletion of GSH exacerbates liver injury induced by PHT in mice. They also found that aromatic oxide intermediates, which can be converted into mercaptan complexes, are involved in the liver damage induced by PHT.

Clinical Features of PHT-Induced Liver Injury

PHT-induced liver injury is typically observed within the first 6 weeks of treatment and does not show a sex difference. In addition to symptoms associated with ASM hypersensitivity syndrome, the most common symptoms include nausea and fatigue.

Susceptibility factors
Nicoletti et al. [185] reported that HLA-B53:01 is a susceptibility factor for phenytoin-induced DILI in African Americans. Among 21 patients with ASM-related DILI, there was a significant association between HLA-B53:01 and aromatic ASM-related liver injury (ASM-DILI). The strongest association was found between phenytoin-induced DILI and HLA-B53:01. They also discovered that out of 9 patients with phenytoin-induced DILI, 8 carried the HLA-B53:01 allele.

Reversible liver dysfunction
Most hepatotoxicity is acute in onset and rapidly reverses after discontinuation of the drug. Yüksel Altuntaş et al. [186] described the case of a 47-year-old woman

who developed toxic cholestatic hepatitis induced by phenytoin. After 25 days of phenytoin treatment, she presented with exfoliative dermatitis, elevated liver enzymes, a cholestatic pattern, and increased eosinophil numbers. After discontinuation of phenytoin treatment, her liver function test results returned to normal within 3 weeks.

Chronic Persistent Liver Dysfunction
There have been reports of irreversible chronic liver damage caused by PHT-induced liver injury. A.K. Roy et al. [187] described an asymptomatic 52-year-old woman who had been receiving sodium phenytoin treatment for 11 years and was found to have elevated serum transaminase levels. Tests for hepatitis A, B, and C were negative. Liver biopsy revealed chronic persistent hepatitis. The authors attributed phenytoin-related chronic liver enzyme abnormalities to enzyme induction. Patients who have experienced RMS may experience recurrent hepatotoxicity if PHT is used again. Fatal cases have been described among patients with symptomatic hepatotoxicity, with mortality ranging from 10% to 40%. Liver biopsies in patients with fatal hepatotoxicity demonstrate liver necrosis and/or hepatocellular damage [142].

Treatment for PHT-Induced Liver Injury

For persistent or severe liver injury, discontinuation of PHT is necessary. When hepatotoxicity does not improve after drug discontinuation, treatment with activated charcoal and the molecular adsorbent recirculating system (MARS) has been successful [61]. A MARS is a blood purification system that filters albumin. The concentration of albumin inside the filter is significantly greater than the plasma concentration. When a patient undergoes MARS therapy, PHT preferentially binds to the albumin within the filter, after which the charcoal column removes the PHT from the blood [188]. Moreover, high-flux cellulose membranes used in blood dialysis can lower the levels of uremic toxins and free PHT [189].

8.2.3.3 Carbamazepine (CBZ)

Carbamazepine (CBZ) is widely used to treat partial seizures, partial secondary generalized seizures, and generalized tonic–clonic seizures [190]. CBZ is also one of the ASMs most likely to cause clinical liver injury.

Historical Evolution of CBZ-Induced Liver Injury

In 1964, CBZ was first approved by the FDA for the treatment of trigeminal neuralgia and became widely used as an ASM in 1974. In 1981, M Levy [191] first described three cases of granulomatous hepatitis caused by carbamazepine (CBZ). Each patient developed hepatitis within 1 month of taking CBZ, and their symptoms rapidly disappeared after discontinuing CBZ. Histologically, all patients had granulomatous hepatitis. In 1998, F.E. Berkowitz [192] described a case of acute liver failure in a 10-year-old boy 4 days after carbamazepine treatment, enriching the research on CBZ-induced liver injury.

Epidemiology of CBZ-Induced Liver Injury

Askmark et al. [193] analyzed 713 adverse reactions to CBZ reported by the Swedish Adverse Drug Reactions Advisory Committee between 1965 and 1987. They found that adverse liver reactions accounted for approximately 10% of all adverse events related to CBZ. Kamitaki et al. [129] analyzed adverse DILI events caused by ASM reported in the FDA Adverse Event Reporting System (FAERS) from 2018 to 2020. Among the 4737 patients treated with CBZ, 225 (4.7%) experienced DILI. Naga Chalasani et al. [194] conducted a retrospective analysis of the etiology, clinical features, and outcomes of DILI among self-identified African Americans and non-Hispanic white individuals between September 2004 and February 2016. The authors found that the use of the causative drugs varied by race, with a higher incidence of phenytoin-induced DILI in African Americans (5% vs. 1%). African Americans often experienced more severe disease than white individuals did, with a significantly greater frequency of severe skin reactions (2.1% vs. 0.36%). The rate of liver transplantation or liver-related death within 6 months (10.2% vs. 5.8%) and the rate of chronic DILI were also greater in African Americans (24% vs. 16%).

Mechanism of CBZ-Induced Liver Injury

CBZ is primarily metabolized by hepatic cytochrome P450 enzymes through epoxidation, hydroxylation, and, to a lesser extent, coupling [195]. The resulting metabolites can cause hepatotoxicity through direct damage or immune-related mechanisms. The most important metabolite of CBZ is 10,11-epoxide, which possesses pharmacological activity and is associated with hepatotoxicity [196]. Other metabolites, such as 3-OH CBZ, play a significant role in CBZ-induced liver toxicity by causing mitochondrial dysfunction through the generation of reactive oxygen species, inhibition of glutathione expression, and alteration of oxidative stress markers [197].

Clinical Features of CBZ-Induced Liver Injury

Sixty-one percent of patients with CBZ-induced liver injury present with asymptomatic liver enzyme elevation, which is usually transient and reversible after discontinuation. Severe carbamazepine hepatotoxicity usually manifests as acute granulomatous hepatitis and can be self-limiting after withdrawal. The most common laboratory test abnormality was elevated GGT levels, and liver function impairment was usually observed within 2 months of CBZ treatment, for a median onset time of 5 weeks. Severe hepatotoxicity can have multiple [198] pathological manifestations. The prognosis can be improved by early identification of CBZ-induced hepatotoxicity and drug withdrawal. The overall mortality rate is estimated to be 17% [139].

Vanishing Bile Duct Syndrome

Vanishing bile duct syndrome is a rare manifestation of CBZ-induced liver toxicity. Forbes GM [199] described the case of a 59-year-old male who developed vanishing bile duct syndrome after 2 months of carbamazepine treatment for glossopharyngeal neuralgia. This syndrome is characterized by elevated levels of gamma-glutamyl transferase (GGT) or alkaline phosphatase (ALP), along with loss of small bile ducts, jaundice, and liver dysfunction. Due to its rarity, little is known about the risk factors for vanishing bile duct syndrome. Reported cases include patients receiving long-term CBZ therapy as well as those who have recently started CBZ treatment [200].

Liver Injury in Hypersensitivity Syndrome Patients

Approximately 30% of CBZ-induced liver injuries exhibit hypersensitivity. In a study of 570 patients with drug-induced liver injury, E Björnsson et al. reported that a favorable prognosis of CBZ-induced hepatotoxicity was associated with increased eosinophil numbers, whereas liver necrosis was related to poor outcomes.

CBZ-Induced Granulomatous Hepatitis

Liver injury caused by CBZ can present as jaundice and cholangitis, with histological findings of noncaseating granulomatous hepatitis that resolves upon discontinuation of the drug. M Levy et al. [191] described three cases of CBZ-induced granulomatous hepatitis. Each patient took carbamazepine for less than 1 month and subsequently developed fever with biliary tract infection. The symptoms disappeared quickly after carbamazepine was discontinued. Histologically, all patients had granulomatous hepatitis.

Pathological Characteristics of CBZ-Induced Liver Injury

The pathological manifestations of liver injury include cholestasis or hepatocellular damage, and more severe cases show greater hepatocellular injury and evidence of liver necrosis on biopsy [139]. The currently identified pathological manifestations of CBZ hepatotoxicity include bile duct loss, liver necrosis, granulomatous hepatitis, and immune-mediated hepatitis.

8.2.3.4 Lamotrigine (LTG)

Lamotrigine (LTG) is a type of phenyltriazine drug and is a broad-spectrum ASM used for the treatment of simple partial seizures, complex partial seizures, secondary generalized tonic–clonic seizures, and primary generalized tonic–clonic seizures [201]. It has also shown efficacy in treating partial seizures, absence seizures, and atonic seizures in children [202]. Lamotrigine works by blocking voltage-gated sodium channels, thereby inhibiting the release of excitatory neurotransmitters (including glutamate and aspartate) associated with seizure activity [202].

Historical Evolution of LTG-Induced Liver Injury

In 1992, LTG was approved for use as an ASM [203]. In 1998, A Gómez Caturla [204] described a case of acute hepatitis caused by LTG. In 2009, Georges Ouellet et al. [144] reported that a 40-year-old female patient developed fulminant hepatitis after 2 weeks of LTG use, which improved after the discontinuation of lamotrigine and supportive therapy, suggesting that LTG can cause fulminant hepatitis independent of the dose, titration, or combination of drugs. In 2002, Kerith Overstreet [205] described the case of a patient receiving lamotrigine treatment who experienced fatal progressive hepatotoxicity. Liver dysfunction and failure occurred after the patient developed a rash and fever. Initially, liver biopsy showed approximately 50% hepatocellular necrosis, but 3 weeks later, postmortem examination revealed extensive liver necrosis with marked bile duct proliferation. Subsequently, LTG-induced liver injury has received significant attention.

Epidemiology of LTG-Induced Liver Injury

The incidence of elevated transaminase levels in LTG patients is low, and severe hepatotoxicity is rare. When it does occur, it is typically idiosyncratic and presents as hepatocellular damage. Sanja Petrović [134] reported 1947 liver toxicity events out of 1399 safety reports (ICSR), 166 of which were attributed to lamotrigine. Both cholestasis and hepatocellular necrosis accounted for 16% of the cases of LTG-induced hepatotoxicity. Kamitaki et al. [129] analyzed liver injuries caused by lamotrigine reported in the FDA Adverse Event Reporting System (FAERS) from 2018 to 2020. Among the 9308 patients treated with lamotrigine, 317 (3.4%) experienced DILI. There have also been reports of acute liver failure [144], which usually occurs in patients taking multiple medications, including other ASMs and non-ASM drugs.

Mechanism of LTG-Induced Liver Injury

Lamotrigine is metabolized primarily by the liver, is metabolized to aromatic oxides in a manner similar to CBZ and PHT, and causes liver toxicity via RMS. The most common side effect of these drugs is a skin reaction, which occurs in approximately 10% of patients and is usually accompanied by fever and eosinophilia [206].

Characteristics of LTG-Induced Liver Injury

Liver function impairment in patients with drug hypersensitivity syndrome
Drug hypersensitivity syndrome caused by LTG has long been recognized, and the most serious adverse effect of LTG is often accompanied by liver function impairment. Liver damage usually occurs within 1 month of LTG initiation and is associated with rapid drug titration, status epilepticus, and younger age. A 21-year-old female epileptic patient was reported to have developed skin lesions, pruritus, cholestatic hepatitis, and systemic symptoms—fever, lymphadenopathy, extensive exfoliating erythema papulosis, and jaundice—after 30 days of treatment with lamotrigine. Hematological examination revealed peripheral eosinophilia. Fulminant liver failure was diagnosed, and orthotopic liver transplantation was performed. Histology of the transplanted liver showed hepatic necrosis, and the residual portal space and lobules showed mixed inflammatory infiltration of lymphocytes and eosinophils. These findings indicate an association between lamotrigine and acute liver failure and between drug rash and eosinophilia and systemic symptoms syndrome (DRESS) [207]. Oren K Fix [208] described the case of a 20-year-old female epilepsy patient who developed elevated liver enzyme levels and histological evidence of eosinophilic hepatitis after 6 weeks of lamotrigine use. Discontinuation of lamotrigine and treatment with corticosteroids resulted in a significant improvement in liver enzyme levels within a few weeks.

Acute liver failure in LTG-Induced liver injury
Acute liver failure is associated with rash, diffuse intravascular coagulation, rhabdomyolysis, and high temperature. In most cases, liver toxicity resolves after discontinuation, but fatal liver necrosis has been reported. Georges Ouellet et al. [144] described the case of a female patient diagnosed with bipolar disorder who developed anticonvulsant hypersensitivity syndrome (AHS) with fulminant hepatitis after taking lamotrigine for 2 weeks. The patient improved after stopping lamotrigine treatment and receiving supportive treatment.

8.2.3.5 Phenobarbital (PB)

PB was first discovered to have antiepileptic properties in 1912. It was subsequently used as an ASM to treat local and secondary generalized tonic–clonic seizures and status epilepticus effectively [209]. PB can enhance the effect of GABA, thereby increasing the seizure threshold [210].

Historical Evolution of PB-Induced Liver Injury

In 1912, phenobarbital (PB) was introduced as an ASM. In 1964, P B HERDSON et al. [211] reported for the first time that PB could cause changes in the fine structures of the rat liver. In 1976, M Weisburst et al. [212] described a case of hepatitis in an 18-year-old female who was taking PB. The patient recovered clinically after discontinuing the medication and receiving methylprednisolone and diphenhydramine treatment for 2 weeks. This case study brought widespread attention to the hepatotoxicity caused by phenobarbital. In 1992, Sawaishi Y et al. [213] reported that phenobarbital treatment led to impaired liver function, and liver biopsy revealed moderate parenchymal damage with subacute cellular infiltration. This study further contributed to our understanding of phenobarbital-induced hepatotoxicity [207].

Epidemiology of PB-Induced Liver Injury

Kamitaki et al. [129] analyzed the adverse liver injury events caused by LTG reported in the FDA Adverse Event Reporting System (FAERS) from 2018 to 2020. A total of 1250 patients who used PB were reported, 59 of whom (4.7%) had DILI. Approximately 9% of phenobarbital patients develop liver damage caused by metabolic syndrome, accompanied by fever, rash, eosinophilia, and lymph node enlargement [142]. A prospective study showed that elevated aminotransferase levels caused by long-term PB treatment were observed in less than 1% of patients [214].

Characteristics of PB-Induced Liver Injury

Elevated Aminotransferase Activity Caused by Phenobarbital

Hepatic injury caused by PB is not commonly observed and is usually mild. Discontinuation of the medication can alleviate symptoms in most patients, and long-term PB treatment-induced elevations in alkaline phosphatase (ALP) or gamma-glutamyl transferase (GGT) levels are typically asymptomatic and clinically insignificant [142]. H.W. Aiges et al. [142] assessed liver function in 63 epilepsy patients who had been receiving PB treatment for more than 12 months. Elevated serum gamma-glutamyl transferase activity was found in 56 patients. Among the 11 individuals with elevated transaminase levels, 6 had persistently abnormal transaminase levels for more than 20 weeks. Optical microscopy revealed uniform hepatocyte swelling without cell necrosis, inflammation, fibrosis, or disruption of liver structure. These 6 patients continued on the same dose of PB, and their transaminase activity returned to normal within 8–14 months.

Hepatic Impairment in Hypersensitivity Syndrome Induced by PB

Hepatic impairment is a common and often severe manifestation of PB-induced hypersensitivity syndrome, and it tends to occur suddenly. G Mockli [215] described a case of massive liver necrosis in a 2-year-old child who developed an allergic reaction to phenobarbital. Despite discontinuing phenobarbital, the child experienced fulminant liver failure and died. Liver dysfunction is one of the manifestations of phenobarbital-related drug hypersensitivity syndrome. Y. Sawaishi et al. [213] described the case of a 5-year-old girl who developed liver dysfunction and severe exfoliative dermatitis after 3 weeks of phenobarbital treatment. Gradual improvement in liver function was observed after phenobarbital treatment was discontinued. During the recovery phase, mild renal impairment initially worsened due to hemolysis following blood transfusion. Liver biopsy showed moderate parenchymal damage with subacute cellular infiltration, while kidney biopsy revealed interstitial nephritis, ruling out acute tubular necrosis caused by hemolysis. A continuous lymphocyte transformation test and skin patch test demonstrated positive results for phenobarbital.

8.2.3.6 Levetiracetam (LEV)

Levetiracetam (LEV) is a broad-spectrum, second-generation ASM that has quickly become one of the most commonly prescribed medications for epilepsy patients due to its good tolerability and ability to be rapidly titrated. There is limited literature regarding severe liver injury associated with LEV treatment, likely because LEV is primarily eliminated through renal excretion and undergoes minimal hepatic metabolism.

Historical Evolution of LEV-Induced Liver Injury

In 2004, J Gavilan [216] first described DILI in epilepsy patients taking LEV. In 2010, several scholars reported that LEV-induced drug hypersensitivity syndrome led to acute liver failure [217]. In 2021, Andreas Rogalewski et al. [218] described a case of severe drug-induced liver injury caused by levetiracetam, increasing awareness of LEV-associated hepatotoxicity. These studies have contributed to a growing understanding of LEV-induced liver injury.

Epidemiology of LEV-Induced Liver Injury

Kamitaki et al. [129] conducted an analysis of adverse events reported in the FDA Adverse Event Reporting System (FAERS) from 2018 to 2020 regarding liver injury associated with LEV. The study included a total of 14,682 patients treated with LEV, among whom 380 (2.59%) reported drug-induced liver injury.

Mechanism of LEV-Induced Liver Injury

Levetiracetam (LEV) does not bind to plasma proteins and is not metabolized in the liver; therefore, it does not undergo specific hepatic pharmacokinetics [190]. Additionally, LEV metabolism is unrelated to the hepatic cytochrome P450 system and does not inhibit or induce liver enzymes. The exact mechanism of liver injury associated with LEV remains unclear, but LEV-related injury is speculated to be a hypersensitivity reaction. Some researchers believe that this type of liver injury represents a specific drug-induced liver injury (DILI) with different histological patterns involving hepatocellular, cholestatic, and mixed features [218].

Characteristics of LEV-Induced Liver Injury

Liver Enzyme-Level Elevation due to LEV
LEV-induced liver injury is a rare adverse reaction that can range from asymptomatic transaminase level elevation to fulminant liver failure [218]. Andreas Rogalewski [218] described the case of a young woman who developed DILI 2 months into LEV treatment. Researchers collected literature on LEV-induced liver injury from 1999 to April 2021. They identified 21 patients (13 males and 8 females) with liver injury, with an average age of 31 years (range: 0.13–76). The average duration of liver injury was 19 days (range: 3–120), 5 patients had asymptomatic liver enzyme level elevation (23.8%), and 16 patients had fever, gastrointestinal symptoms, and rash (76.2%). The median alanine aminotransferase (ALT) and aspartate aminotransferase (AST) levels were 773 IU/L (range: 60–4800) and 667.5 IU/L (range: 53–10,387), respectively. Liver biopsies revealed hepatocellular necrosis. After LEV was discontinued, liver function normalized within a median time of 9 days (range: 2–270 days).

Fulminant Liver Failure due to LEV
Researchers analyzed the VigiBase database and found that among elderly patients with epilepsy who experienced drug-induced liver injury caused by newer ASMs, the most common fatal events of levetiracetam-induced drug-induced liver injury were acute liver failure and fulminant hepatitis [134]. Sun et al. [219] conducted an analysis of a series of LEV-induced liver injury cases, considering factors such as indications for LEV, preexisting liver diseases, concomitant medications, LEV dosage, and duration during drug-induced liver injury (DILI). They found that DILI can occur within days to up to 5 months after beginning LEV treatment, and in the worst cases, liver transplantation may be required or the injury may result in death. During the course of the disease, it may be helpful to monitor the serum transaminase concentration. LEV treatment withdrawal is the first choice for treatment. In addition, for severe cases, treatment with immunosuppressants such as cortisone may be considered.

8.2.3.7 Others

Nonamphetamines

Nonamphetamines are dicarbamate derivatives that were approved by the FDA for use as ASMs in 1993. They can be used to treat both partial and generalized seizures, and common side effects include nausea, dizziness, drowsiness, and fatigue [220]. Although the incidence of hepatotoxicity caused by nonamphetamines is low, it is typically severe and often occurs within the first 6 months of treatment [221]. M.G. O'Neil et al. [222] described 36 cases of hepatotoxicity related to nonamphetamine treatment collected by the U.S. Food and Drug Administration. Five of the patients died. They described a patient with generalized tonic–clonic seizures who developed acute liver failure and died within 40 days of nonamphetamine treatment. However, the mechanism of toxicity induced by nonamphetamines is still unclear.

Gabapentin

Gabapentin is an antiseizure drug that is also used to treat neuropathic pain [223]. Kamitaki et al. [129] analyzed reports of liver injury caused by gabapentin in the FDA Adverse Event Reporting System (FAERS) from 2018 to 2020. Among a total of 18,903 patients treated with gabapentin, 191 (1%) reported drug-induced liver injury. Contreras-Mota et al. [224] described a case of acute liver injury in a 56-year-old male patient with a history of chronic kidney disease undergoing hemodialysis. The patient was diagnosed with lumbar spinal stenosis and developed acute liver injury after receiving gabapentin treatment. The liver injury resolved after the medication was discontinued, but the underlying mechanism remains unclear. Therefore, this drug has been reported to cause liver toxicity and should be used with caution.

8.2.4 Prognosis of Patients with ASM-Induced Liver Function Injury (ASM-DILI)

ASM can cause liver damage, and although most patients have mild symptoms, there have been cases of acute liver failure (ALF) and death. Ayse L Mindikoglu et al. [135] conducted a retrospective cohort study using the United Network for Organ Sharing (UNOS) liver transplantation database from 1987 to 2006; the study included 661 patients diagnosed with DILI. The results showed that the 1-year survival rate of patients with acute liver failure caused by ASMs was 52%, and the survival rate of children with liver injury caused by ASMs was even lower. Among the 22 patients under 18 years of age who developed ALF due to ASM use, 73% died within 1 year. The authors concluded that the risk of death in children due to ASM-induced ALF is much greater than that due to other drugs, with a 1-year survival rate of only 27% for patients under 18 years old; the survival rate is 75% for patients older than 18 years old, indicating a more than fourfold increase in the risk of death for children.

Patients who undergo liver transplantation for ASM-induced DILI also have a higher rate of retransplantation than non-ASM patients (approximately 4–9% vs. 24%) [135]. Ezhilarasan D [99] suggested that monitoring medication use and regular measurements of serum transaminase levels, blood ammonia concentrations, and lipid parameters during ASM use may help improve drug safety or prevent the progression of DILI.

8.2.5 Summary

Treatment of epilepsy can sometimes lead to severe liver injury. However, over the past 20 years, several new drugs have been approved for treating ASMs that have a lower incidence of toxicity and milder liver toxicity than older generation ASMs. Based on our experience, the incidence of ASM-related liver injury has significantly decreased in the past 20 years, possibly due to a decrease in the use of older generation ASMs. Several unique characteristics of liver injury related to ASMs, including hypersensitivity syndrome and fatal liver function impairment, exist, the outcome of which depends on the type of ASM involved.

8.3 Endocrine Effects of ASMs in Patients

Unlike the effects on other systems of the human body, the effects of ASMs on a patient's endocrine system are insidious and not easily detectable, but they can seriously affect a patient's quality of life and require monitoring.

8.3.1 ASM-Related Dysfunction

Antiseizure medications (ASMs) have a significant effect on sexual function in patients with epilepsy. Sexual dysfunctions (SDs) are characterized by disturbances in sexual desire and by psychophysiological changes associated with the sexual response cycle. Since the 1960s, self-reporting techniques for assessing sexual function have been developed to both diagnose and rate the severity of SD. The diagnosis of SD related to ASMs should be based on the causal relationship between the ASMs and SD.

8.3.1.1 ASM-Related Dysfunction

As early as 1954, the relationship between SD and epilepsy was first described in patients with epilepsy by Gastaut [225]. As this field has attracted increased attention, ASMs have been found to be important factors causing SD. In 1980, Beran et al. [226] reported that among 19 epilepsy patients treated with sodium valproate, one had improved libido. In 1985, a multicenter, 1-year, randomized controlled trial by Mattson et al. [227] reported that traditional ASMs were associated with a high incidence of impotence or decreased libido, as indicated by the use of carbamazepine (13%), phenobarbital (16%), phenytoin (11%), and primidone (22%). New

ASMs have fewer adverse effects than traditional ASMs, but their effects on sexual function have also been recently described. In 1999, Clark et al. [228] reported that gabapentin (900 mg/day) treatment induced orgasmic dysfunction in a man with neuropathic pain. Subsequently, several ASMs used for patients with epilepsy, including oxcarbazepine, pregabalin, topiramate, lamotrigine, and levetiracetam, were reported to cause changes in sexual function. The main clinical manifestations of SD are as follows.

Hyposexuality

Hyposexuality is a relatively common problem for patients with epilepsy taking ASMs. In two multicenter, randomized controlled trials by Mattson et al. [227, 229], patients receiving treatment with traditional ASMs had a high incidence of impotence or decreased libido during the 1-year follow-up (valproate 10%, carbamazepine 7–13%, phenobarbital 16%, phenytoin 11%, and primidone 22%). In a cross-sectional study, 40 of 63 (63.5%) men with epilepsy taking carbamazepine had sexual intercourse less than three times a week, whereas only 9 of 55 (16.4%) healthy controls had such a low frequency. Grant et al. [230] described two female epileptic patients. One patient who took 1800 mg/day gabapentin complained of decreased libido and anorgasmia, and her symptoms were resolved after the withdrawal of gabapentin. The other patient complained of anorgasmia when her gabapentin dose reached 1800 mg/day. Her sexual function recovered after her 300 mg evening dose was moved to bedtime.

Hypersexuality

According to an investigation of outpatients with epilepsy, 4 of 21 (19%) patients receiving valproate monotherapy, 3 of 40 (8%) patients receiving carbamazepine monotherapy, and 1 of 29 (3%) patients receiving oxcarbazepine monotherapy exhibited enhanced sexual function. Grabowska-Grzyb et al. [231] described two hypersexuality patients treated with LTG. One patient was a 55-year-old man with temporal lobe epilepsy who had not had sexual intercourse for 7 years. When the LTG dose was increased to 100 mg/day, the patient had obsessive thoughts about sexual activity and experienced several daily erections. He could not accept this enhanced sexual activity, and discontinuation of lamotrigine returned him to his original state. The other patient was a 50-year-old man with frontal lobe epilepsy. He had sexual intercourse approximately once every 6 months, and the infrequency was attributed to his age. When he received 100 mg/day lamotrigine, he experienced several erections each day. He accepted this increased sexual activity and had sexual intercourse 2–3 times a day.

Erectile Dysfunction (ED)

ED may be a common problem in epileptic patients treated with traditional ASMs. In an observational study by Kuba et al. [232], sexual function was prospectively analyzed among 40 men with intractable epilepsy, 31 of whom were treated with traditional ASMs, using the International Inventory of Erectile Function Questionnaire. Six (15%) patients developed ED, six (15%) patients developed orgasmic dysfunction, 16 (40%) patients developed a loss of sexual desire, 22 (55%) patients became dissatisfied with sexual intercourse, and 20 (50%) patients became dissatisfied with their sexual life. Case reports revealed that new ASM agents, such as levetiracetam, topiramate, pregabalin, gabapentin, and zonisamide, may also cause ED.

Ejaculation Disorders

Few case reports on ejaculation disorders have been published. Leris et al. [233] described a 61-year-old man with trigeminal neuralgia who experienced ejaculatory failure and anorgasmia shortly after taking carbamazepine. After discontinuation of carbamazepine, his sexual function returned to normal. However, when he took carbamazepine again, he immediately experienced ejaculatory failure. Elia et al. [234] described a 59-year-old man with epilepsy. He had taken valproate and phenytoin for 15 years, but he complained of orgasmic anejaculation in the preceding 6 months. Spermatozoa were found in his postorgasmic urine, confirming the diagnosis of retrograde ejaculation. The authors hypothesized that this symptom resulted from ASM use, which may cause bladder sphincter inhibition and receptor alterations.

8.3.2 *Effects of ASMs on Thyroid and Parathyroid Function*

8.3.2.1 ASMs Associated with Thyroid Dysfunction

Thyroid hormones are essential for development, neural differentiation, and metabolic regulation in mammals, and thyroid dysfunction may impede growth and development in children and adversely affect endocrine function in adults [235]. Certain ASMs, such as carbamazepine (CBZ), phenobarbital (PHB), phenytoin (PHT), valproate (VPA), and oxcarbazepine (OXC), are known to interfere with normal thyroid function. ASMs may accelerate thyroid hormone metabolism by affecting the hepatic microsomal enzyme system and interfering with the competitive binding of thyroid hormone to thyrotropin-binding globulin [235, 236].

8.3.2.2 Traditional ASMs

Liver Enzyme-Induced Antiseizure Medications (EIASMs)

It is now generally accepted that EIASMs such as phenobarbital (PHE) and carbamazepine (CBZ) can affect the production, release, transport, metabolism, and secretion of thyroid hormones through a variety of mechanisms, and the most-researched mechanism is the hepatic microsomal enzyme system, which is an induction of the hepatic P450 enzyme system, leading to a decrease in T [236], increased human uridine diphosphate glucuronosyltransferase (UGT) function, increased thyroid hormone metabolism, and decreased levels of T4 and FT4 [235].

Tanaka et al. [237] found in a long-term follow-up of 287 children with epilepsy that after 3 years of carbamazepine use and 6 years of phenobarbital use, triiodothyroid acid (T3) and thyroxine (T4) levels decreased in the children. Verrotti et al. [238] reported that serum T4 and FT4 levels returned to normal after CBZ was discontinued for 6 months. Lossuis et al. [239] reported a significant increase in the serum FT4 concentration in epileptic patients after 4 months of CBZ discontinuation. In other words, the effect of EIASM treatment on thyroid hormones is reversible. A 2014 study [236] showed that changes in thyroxine levels induced by carbamazepine administration returned to normal after discontinuation of the drug. This study revealed that the serum FT4 concentration in children treated with phenobarbital significantly decreased at months 1 and 6, but this reduction did not persist until month 12, whereas the serum TSH level increased progressively over the 12-month treatment period and gradually returned to normal after the discontinuation of phenobarbital; thus, the effects of phenobarbital on thyroid function appear to be reversible. In other words, the effects of EIASM treatment on thyroid hormones are reversible [235].

Enzyme Inhibitor: Sodium Valproate (VPA)

Another effect of ASMs on thyroid hormones may be due to interference with the competitive binding of thyroid hormones to thyrotropin-binding globulin. The peripheral conversion of T4 to active T4 is also increased, resulting in a decrease in FT4. A reduced serum T4-binding globulin concentration, protein-binding site displacement, and decreased T4 5′-deiodination enzyme activity are possible explanations for the effects of VPA on thyroid hormones [235]. According to Olcay Güngör, and others [240], 15.2% of patients had subclinical hypothyroidism after the 12th month of VPA treatment. Attilakos et al. [241] suggested that serum TSH levels returned to normal in children 3 months after VPA withdrawal; hence, the effect of VPA on thyroid function is also reversible.

8.3.2.3 New ASMs

Studies in adult patients with epilepsy have shown that carbamazepine-induced reductions in the serum thyroid hormone level return to normal when oxcarbazepine therapy is used to replace carbamazepine [242]. Another prospective study of children with epilepsy treated with oxcarbazepine showed a significant decrease in FT4 levels and a significant increase in TSH levels after 8 and 18 months of treatment [243]. After OXC treatment is stopped, the FT4 concentration decreases and returns to normal; OXC, therefore, has fewer and safer effects on thyroid function than carbamazepine [244].

The results of a study conducted by Nishiyama et al. [107] suggest that LEV monotherapy does not affect thyroid function. It has also been suggested that the use of LEV may lead to subclinical hypothyroidism [245]. A study by Attilakos et al. [246] in children with new-onset epilepsy treated with LEV monotherapy showed a significant reduction in triglyceride levels at 6 and 12 months of LEV therapy. The triglyceride/LDL cholesterol ratio was significantly lower at 6 and 12 months of LEV treatment, while the LDL cholesterol/HDL cholesterol ratio was significantly lower at 12 months of LEV treatment ($p = 0.025$). There were no significant changes in the other parameters. It was concluded that long-term LEV monotherapy does not cause adverse changes in thyroid hormones or lipid levels in children with epilepsy. Whether LEV can be considered a safer alternative to prevent cardiovascular complications caused by ASMs in adult life is unknown. The safety of levetiracetam should be monitored dynamically to further determine the safety of the drug.

Among the new antiseizure medications, the antiseizure medication least harmful to thyroid hormone function is lamotrigine [245].

8.3.2.4 ASMs Associated with Parathyroid Dysfunction

Secondary parathyroid dysfunction caused by ASMs mainly manifests as hyperparathyroidism. It has been found that phenobarbital, phenytoin sodium, carbamazepine, and even some of the newer ASM agents, such as gabapentin, topiramate, and lamotrigine, may stimulate the upregulation of hepatic cytochrome enzyme P450 activity and inhibit mitochondrial vitamin D3 25-hydroxylase activity, resulting in lower 25-hydroxyvitamin D (25-OHD) levels, decreased small intestinal calcium absorption, lower blood calcium levels, and secondary compensatory serum parathyroid hormone levels. Misra et al. [247] prospectively compared 25-hydroxyvitamin D, parathyroid hormone, calcium, phosphorus, and alkaline phosphatase levels in children at the start of and 6 months into carbamazepine treatment and correlated them with carbamazepine levels. The mean parathyroid hormone concentration increased from 34.24 ± 21.38 pg/mL S.D. to 45.01 ± 24.46 pg/mL S.D. ($p = 0.001$). Changes in vitamin D concentrations were negatively correlated with changes in parathyroid hormone levels ($r = -0.404$, $p = 0.022$). The serum alkaline phosphatase concentration increased from 283.50 ± 100.10 IU/L S.D. to 364.25 ± 126.98 IU/L S.D. ($p < 0.001$). Changes in vitamin D and parathyroid hormone levels were not significantly correlated with carbamazepine levels. Carbamazepine treatment is thought to reduce vitamin D levels; therefore, monitoring of vitamin D levels and supplementation may help prevent alterations in bone metabolism.

8.3.3 ASM-Related Bone Density Changes

Patients with epilepsy are prone to fractures, with an increased risk of fracture 2–6 times that of healthy people [248], and a large number of patients with epilepsy have skeletal abnormalities (ranging from 4% to 70% according to different studies) [249]. ASMs can increase the catabolism of 25-hydroxyvitamin D by inducing increased catabolism of the hepatic P-450 enzyme system, which can lead to relative hypocalcemia, increased levels of parathyroid hormone (PTH), and a subsequent decrease in bone mineral density (BMD) [250, 251], which may ultimately result in a range of bone-related side effects, including but not limited to, rickets, reduced BMD, altered bone conversion, and increased fracture risk [252–255]. However, some studies have shown that the use of nonenzymatically induced ASMs can also significantly reduce BMD [256]. Other environmental and epidemiological parameters, including age, sex, diet, and mobility, may also influence mineral metabolism.

8.3.3.1 Liver Enzyme-Induced ASMs (EIASMs)

Enzyme-induced ASMs have a more significant negative impact on bone mass and osteoporosis than non-enzyme-induced ASMs. A variety of ASMs are commonly used as hepatic cytochrome P450 (CYP450) inducers, such as phenytoin, phenobarbital, and carbamazepine. Oxcarbazepine, a 10-keto structural derivative of carbamazepine, is a weak inducer of CYP2B and CYP3A4 activity [257]. These drugs cause a number of endocrine disturbances, such as increased vitamin D metabolism, decreased vitamin D levels, decreased calcium absorption, and subsequent hypocalcemia. These changes lead to the activation of bone resorption secondary to osteoclast bone resorption, which results in bone loss and impaired mineralization and ultimately decreases BMD and 25-OH-vitamin D levels in patients. In addition, several ASM agents (carbamazepine, phenytoin, and phenobarbital) also have direct effects on osteoblast activity, including osteoclast inhibition and osteoclast activation, which leads to further negative effects on bone metabolism.

In addition to CYP450 dysregulation related to vitamin D deficiency and bone loss, a study by Wilson et al. [258] showed that sodium phenytoin administration reduces the electrophoretic mobility of the collagen I protein produced by osteoblast-like cells, which is ultimately involved in bone loss. Petty et al. [259], conversely, found that Na+ currents in mouse osteoblasts were blocked by carbamazepine and phenytoin, which in turn affected osteoclast function and bone strength. A retrospective study revealed lower serum calcium and phosphorus levels and greater alkaline phosphatase activity in epilepsy patients taking phenytoin sodium than in healthy individuals [260]. However, another study found no decrease in BMD in patients treated with phenytoin sodium monotherapy [261]. Phenytoin may have direct, toxic effects on bone cells [262]. Carbamazepine may act on bone metabolism through induction of hepatic enzyme activity [263], and it may alter vitamin D metabolism and reduce vitamin D levels [264].

8.3.3.2 Nonenzymatic-Induced ASMs

Sodium valproate is a CYP450 inhibitor, and there are various hypotheses regarding the mechanism by which it affects BMD and bone metabolism, including by directly affecting growth plate chondrocyte proliferation, activating osteoclasts leading to bone loss, activating constitutive androstane receptors and pregnane X receptors to interfere with bone metabolism, and activating apoptosis [265, 266]. A study conducted in 2005 showed that the serum osteocalcin concentration in children treated with sodium valproate was significantly lower than that in the control group, suggesting that sodium valproate administration can significantly affect bone formation [267]. In addition, in patients receiving long-term oral treatment with sodium valproate, there are occasional complications of Fanconi syndrome, a proximal tubular dysfunction characterized by proteinuria, glycosuria, phosphaturia, hyperaminoaciduria, hypokalemia, hypophosphatemia, and type II renal tubular acidosis [268]. In contrast, in patients with concomitant Fanconi syndrome, approximately 98% had hypophosphataemia, and 25.9% had pathological fractures [269].

8.3.3.3 Other ASMs

Several reports have suggested that topiramate [270] and lamotrigine [253] may cause femoral and lumbar spine injuries. Although a number of single studies have suggested the presence of effects of levetiracetam, topiramate, and lamotrigine on BMD and bone metabolism, a meta-analysis [271] concluded that these drugs had no statistically significant effect on these indicators. Another study in which phenytoin sodium treatment was replaced with levetiracetam treatment demonstrated significant increases in BMD in the lumbar spine and left femur and a rebound in 25-(OH)-vitamin D levels in patients who either replaced or discontinued phenytoin sodium treatment. In contrast, patients who continued phenytoin treatment had significantly decreased BMD and low 25-(OH)-vitamin D levels at both sites [272].

8.3.4 *Hyponatremia Induced by Antiseizure Medications in Patients with Epilepsy*

Treatment with antiseizure medications (ASMs) is associated with adverse effects of varying degrees of severity. Certain reactions, such as cardiac arrhythmias or hypersensitivity syndrome, are clearly unacceptable and potentially life-threatening. These subtle adverse events are easily missed but may escalate to serious or even fatal consequences if they are not identified and managed in a timely fashion. Hyponatremia stands out as a prime example of such a potentially overlooked adverse effect.

Clinically, hyponatremia typically presents with neurological and muscular system disturbances. The condition arises from reduced serum sodium concentrations, leading to lower extracellular fluid osmolality and subsequent cellular swelling. In the brain, this swelling can manifest as headache, nausea, vomiting, fatigue, restlessness, disorientation, and decreased reflexes. Severe acute hyponatremia can result in cerebral herniation, potentially accompanied by convulsions, coma, permanent brain damage, apnea, or even death. The involvement of gastrointestinal smooth muscle can also contribute to symptoms such as nausea and vomiting. In general, females tend to have greater susceptibility to drug-induced hyponatremia than males do.

8.3.4.1 Hyponatremia Induced by Different ASMs

1. Carbamazepine (CBZ): CBZ is among the ASMs most frequently identified as a cause of hyponatremia in the epileptic population. As early as 1966, Braunhofer et al. [273] reported the anti-diuretic properties of CBZ and suggested that this could lead to adverse effects on sodium balance.

   Kalff et al. [274] conducted a larger study involving 573 epilepsy patients treated with CBZ across two centers and reported that 28 participants (4.8%) presented serum sodium concentrations below 135 mmol/L. Kuz et al. [275] identified the initial 3 months following the commencement of CBZ therapy as the period presenting the greatest risk for developing hyponatremia in individuals with epilepsy. Individuals aged 2080 years appear most susceptible to developing hyponatremia induced by CBZ. It has been hypothesized that lower sodium intake contributes to the increased susceptibility observed in older patients. The dose of CBZ is linked to the risk of hyponatremia, as indicated by numerous studies; specifically, a higher dosage corresponds to an increased risk. Furthermore, pretreatment serum sodium levels (baseline levels) influence the likelihood of hyponatremia developing. Specifically, low baseline sodium levels can increase the risk of persistent hyponatremia to as high as 64.7%, whereas the risk decreases to 7% when baseline levels are within the normal range. Therefore, the use of CBZ as an initial therapy might be inappropriate for patients who already have low baseline sodium values.

2. Oxcarbazepine (OXC): Dong et al. [276] examined serum sodium in 97 OXC-treated epilepsy patients and reported hyponatremia (<134 mmol/L) in 29.9% and severe hyponatremia (<129 mmol/L) in 12.4%. According to Asconapé et al. [277], hyponatremia typically emerges during the initial 3 months post-OXC initiation, coinciding with the stabilization period of plasma OXC concentrations. Likewise, Schmidt et al. [278] observed that reduced serum sodium levels often occur within the first 2 months of treatment among epilepsy patients receiving OXC. Conversely, findings from a retrospective study by Kim et al. [279] involving 1009 epilepsy patients on OXC suggested a potentially longer latency for hyponatremia onset than previously assumed; their data revealed that nearly 59.4% developed symptomatic hyponatremia within 2 years of starting OXC. This same study also identified age as an independent risk factor for developing severe hyponatremia associated with this medication.

   Patients who take OXC alongside other ASMs face a heightened risk of hyponatremia than do those who use OXC alone. Lin et al. [280] demonstrated that OXC-induced hyponatremia risk escalates with concurrent ASM use, as evidenced by hyponatremia rates of 16% (4/25) with OXC monotherapy, 25% (6/24) with dual ASM therapy, and 80% (4/5) with quadruple ASM therapy. Specific combinations, such as OXC with VPA, have been shown by Kim et al. [279] to independently increase risk, whereas combinations with topiramate or LEV did not have the same effect in their study. Conversely, Dong et al. [276] found a significant association only between the OXC-LEV combination and the occurrence of hyponatremia. Furthermore, Kim et al. [279] reported that concurrent use of OXC and diuretics is an independent risk factor for severe and symptomatic hyponatremia, while combinations with ACE inhibitors, calcium channel blockers, or aspirin might also increase the risk of severe/symptomatic events.
3. Eslicarbazepine (ESL): ESL is a third-generation ASM that structurally resembles CBZ and OXC, and epilepsy patients receiving ESL may experience hyponatremia. Sperling et al. [281] reported that 5.1% of ESL-treated patients experienced a decrease in sodium concentration greater than 10 mmol/L, with 1.5% developing severe hyponatremia (<125 mmol/L). In Hufnagel A et al.'s [282] 1-year open-label study evaluating ESL as adjunctive therapy in 325 adults with epilepsy, decreased blood sodium was reported as an adverse event in only 4 patients (1.2%), with mean sodium levels remaining stable throughout the study period. ESL-induced hyponatremia appears to be dose dependent, as shown in Sperling MR et al.'s [283] randomized historical-control study examining adults with seizures on ESL monotherapy. Their data revealed serum sodium reductions ≥10 mmol/L from baseline in 11.7% of patients taking 1600 mg ESL compared with 20.3% taking 1200 mg ESL, whereas severe hyponatremia (sodium ≤125 mmol/L) occurred in 3.9% and 4.7% of these groups, respectively.
4. Others: A report from VigiBase, the WHO/Uppsala Monitoring Centre's adverse drug reaction database, documented by Beers et al. [284], described severe hyponatremia induced by VPA in four elderly individuals with epilepsy. A distinct association between VPA and hyponatremia was confirmed via the reporting odds ratio (ROR) methodology (ROR: 1.83, 95% CI 1.61–2.08). Lamotrigine

(LTG), recognized as a broad-spectrum ASM, is utilized for managing simple and complex partial seizures as well as secondary and primary generalized tonic–clonic seizures. Three case reports documenting hyponatremia induced by LTG in epilepsy patients exist within adverse drug reaction databases [9, 66]. A study published in Lancet in 2000 involved two children diagnosed with cranial diabetes insipidus; these children, treated with LTG for seizures, subsequently showed reduced requirements for desmopressin. Levetiracetam (LEV), a newer ASM, is indicated for treating partial seizures in adults and children over the age of four. Two case reports concerning LEV-induced hyponatremia have been published. In one instance, an individual with seizures had previously developed hyponatremia attributed to CBZ prior to starting LEV therapy. Notably, this individual's serum sodium concentration increased within 2 days following LEV discontinuation, an effect potentially linked to LEV's swift peak effect (approx. 1 h postadministration) and brief elimination half-life (6–8 h). Among 3100 epilepsy patients taking gabapentin (GBP), Wilton et al. [285] identified two individuals who experienced hyponatremia. Hyponatremia persisted in one patient who continued taking the medication; conversely, the second patient ceased GBP treatment and experienced sodium level recovery, which suggested that GBP was the likely etiology for the occurrence of hyponatremia.

8.3.4.2 Proposed Mechanisms for ASM-Associated Hyponatremia

The precise mechanisms responsible for hyponatremia induced by ASMs remain incompletely understood. The syndrome of inappropriate antidiuretic hormone secretion (SIADH) may be a significant factor in the development of ASM-associated hyponatremia. Kloster et al. [286] specifically suggested that SIADH triggered by OXC is the likely mechanism responsible for hyponatremia caused by this drug. The antidiuretic effects of CBZ and OXC might be attributable to the activation of the vasopressin 2 receptor (V2R)/aquaporin 2 (AQP2) pathway, as suggested by Berghuis et al. [287, 288]. In brief, this pathway involves the interaction of vasopressin with V2Rs on the basolateral membrane, which subsequently activates adenylyl cyclase via the Gs protein, leading to cAMP production from ATP; cAMP-dependent protein kinase A then phosphorylates AQP2 within intracellular vesicles, promoting its translocation to the apical membrane to increase water permeability. It is thought that CBZ/OXC might stimulate renal water reabsorption through direct action on the V2R-Gs protein complex and by promoting AQP2 expression. SIADH has also been implicated in the pathogenesis of hyponatremia associated with VPA. Observations in patients experiencing VPA-induced hyponatremia include elevated ADH levels, reduced plasma osmolality, and increased urinary sodium and osmolality. Beers et al. [284] proposed that inadequate renal compensation might underlie the development of SIADH in certain patients treated with VPA. Furthermore, LTG is thought to influence voltage-sensitive sodium channels, thereby diminishing calcium conductance, which could lead to SIADH and hyponatremia.

Aldosterone may also contribute to the mechanism of hyponatremia induced by OXC. A study by Isojarvi et al. [288] examined ten epilepsy patients who transitioned from CBZ to OXC; six maintained stable serum sodium despite increased aldosterone levels, while the remaining four exhibited low serum sodium without a corresponding change in aldosterone. This pattern suggests that the elevated aldosterone observed is probably a compensatory reaction of the renin–angiotensin–aldosterone system, aimed at preventing further sodium depletion rather than rectifying existing low sodium levels.

8.3.4.3 Managing Hyponatremia Associated with ASM Therapy

Prior to initiating ASM therapy, assessing a patient's serum sodium level is crucial for identifying any preexisting low baseline levels. Regular monitoring of serum sodium during the initial 3 months following the start of ASM treatment, particularly for OXC or CBZ, is recommended, as advised by Asconapé et al. [277]. Within this initial 3-month period, the frequency of monitoring should be guided by specific clinical circumstances. The serum sodium concentration should be measured during the second week after initiating ASM therapy. If the sodium level remains at or above 130 mmol/L without any identified risk factors, subsequent monitoring can be performed on the basis of the clinician's judgment, and routine long-term checks are generally unnecessary. If sodium levels fall between 125 and 130 mmol/L in the presence of risk factors, testing should occur every 3–4 weeks, or as deemed appropriate by the physician, to monitor for potential deterioration. For asymptomatic patients with sodium levels less than 125 mmol/L, management involves initiating fluid restriction, reducing the medication dosage, and performing weekly sodium checks until levels rise above 125 mmol/L. Should sodium levels persist below 125 mmol/L despite fluid restriction and dose adjustment, discontinuation of the medication is warranted. If sodium levels stay below 125 mmol/L concurrently with the emergence of symptoms such as lethargy, diffuse disease, or vomiting, it becomes necessary to consider a diagnosis of water intoxication. Dose adjustments based on sodium level fluctuations are appropriate only when seizures are fully managed. For patients with inadequately controlled seizures, subtherapeutic drug levels, and serum sodium concentrations ranging from 125 to 135 mmol/L, increasing the medication dosage until seizure control is achieved is the recommended course. Weekly sodium monitoring should continue alongside the application of fluid restriction. Consideration should be given to withdrawing the drug if the serum sodium level persistently decreases or falls below 125 mmol/L following the initiation of ASM therapy. Additionally, regarding pharmacological options for correcting hyponatremia, demeclocycline has been shown to be effective in improving hyponatremia induced by CBZ and LEV and is employed for treating severe SIADH-related hyponatremia. Lithium also demonstrates effectiveness in managing hyponatremia associated with CBZ.

Hyponatremia occurs frequently in epilepsy patients undergoing treatment with OXC and CBZ, whereas its occurrence with other ASM therapies is considerably less common or not well established. This particular adverse effect might be overlooked in clinical practice because of its frequent presentation with nonspecific and subtle manifestations. Nevertheless, awareness among clinicians is vital regarding risk factors such as advanced age, substantial ASM dosages, low baseline sodium, polytherapy, and female sex in epilepsy patients receiving ASM treatment. Striving for both the clinical effectiveness of ASMs and the minimization of associated adverse effects should be the central objectives when managing individuals with epilepsy.

8.4 Psychiatric Behavioral Abnormalities Induced by New ASMs

Epilepsy is a chronic neurological disorder characterized by recurrent seizures. Epidemiological studies indicate a prevalence of 7%, with approximately 50 million individuals affected globally. Despite the availability of various treatments for epilepsy, medication remains the primary therapeutic approach. Over the past two decades, more than 16 new ASMs have been developed, introduced into clinical practice, and demonstrated favorable treatment outcomes. However, issues arising from their use have been identified. One notable concern is the occurrence of psychiatric behavioral abnormalities after drug administration, which often leads to treatment failure [289, 290]. Insufficient awareness and delayed intervention regarding these issues not only increase patient suffering but also may result in severe adverse consequences. Therefore, it is imperative for clinicians, when selecting medications and monitoring treatments, to be familiar with and vigilant about the serious adverse reactions associated with these new drugs, as this knowledge could lead to the development of appropriate preventive measures.

8.4.1 Epidemiological Findings

Weintraub D et al. [291] studied 1394 epilepsy patients taking one or more new ASM agents. They observed that gabapentin, lamotrigine, levetiracetam, perampanel, nonamphetamines, oxcarbazepine, tiagabine, topiramate, and zonisamide could induce psychiatric behavioral abnormalities, the incidence of which ranged from 0.6% to 8.8%. In another study by Stephen et al. [292] involving 1058 epilepsy patients receiving topiramate (n = 170), levetiracetam (n = 170), pregabalin (n = 135), zonisamide (n = 203), lacosamide (n = 160), eslicarbazepine acetate (n = 52), retigabine (n = 64), or perampanel (n = 54) treatment, a survey on drug side effects revealed that 12.1% of patients with generalized hereditary epilepsy and 20.1% of patients with focal seizures experienced statistically significant psychiatric abnormalities. Among these patients, 1.9–16.7% of patients discontinued medication due to drug-induced psychiatric abnormalities.

8.4.2 *Susceptibility Factors*

Not all epilepsy patients taking anti-seizure medications experience psychiatric symptoms. The most prominent feature distinguishing patients with psychiatric symptoms from those without is a biological susceptibility to psychotropic adverse reactions. This susceptibility is multifactorial and involves different mechanisms and triggering factors that collectively contribute to the occurrence of such side effects.

8.4.2.1 History of Psychiatric Illness and Family History of Mental Disorders

Patients with epilepsy and a history of psychiatric illness are more prone to experiencing psychiatric abnormalities following medication. Akanuma et al. [289] analyzed 105 occurrences of psychiatric abnormalities in 89 patients taking anti-seizure medications and found a significant correlation between a history of psychiatric illness and psychiatric abnormalities postmedication. Multiple regression analysis revealed that a past psychiatric history was closely associated with the manifestation of psychiatric symptoms after treatment with anti-seizure medications. Studies by Stephen et al. [292] and Ogunsakin et al. [293] further support these findings, emphasizing the need for special attention given to epilepsy patients with a history of psychiatric illness when monitoring and identifying psychotropic adverse reactions related to antiseizure medications. Additionally, Mula et al. [294] and Weintraub et al. [295] highlighted that a history of psychiatric illness is a crucial predictive indicator for the development of medication-related psychiatric disorders in epilepsy patients, underscoring the importance of vigilant monitoring in clinical settings.

8.4.2.2 Medication Dosage and Rapid Titration

The occurrence of psychiatric symptoms in epilepsy patients after taking ASMs is associated with medication dosage. Trimble et al. [296] conducted a retrospective study on 89 patients experiencing psychiatric symptoms while being treated with carbamazepine, valproic acid, or topiramate and revealed that the incidence of carbamazepine-related psychiatric symptoms increased with increasing dosage. Moreover, research on perampanel has shown a greater incidence of psychiatric behavioral abnormalities (aggressive behavior, suicidal thoughts, irritability, etc.) during the first 6 weeks of rapid titration and with higher perampanel doses, with the frequency of aggressive behavior correlating with daily doses [295, 297]. While limited data exist for zonisamide (ZNS), studies suggest that approximately 10% of patients receiving high doses of ZNS may experience mood disorders [298]. In most cases, using a single anti-seizure medication and gradual titration can reduce the occurrence of psychiatric disorders.

8.4.2.3 Seizure Type

In a study by Stephen et al. [292] involving 1058 epilepsy patients, 12.1% of those with generalized hereditary seizures experienced psychiatric abnormalities, while 20.1% of patients with focal seizures exhibited psychiatric symptoms. This finding suggests that patients with focal seizures are more prone to psychiatric abnormalities when taking anti-seizure medications.

8.4.2.4 Other Factors

Patients with refractory epilepsy, secondary generalized seizures, or no seizures may experience psychiatric behavioral abnormalities when taking anti-seizure medications. This association may be related to the pathological damage of the disease itself and the involvement of neural networks, which increase susceptibility to medication-induced psychiatric side effects. However, confirmation is needed [291]. Akanuma et al. [289] also reported a correlation between postmedication psychiatric symptoms and epilepsy-related variables (a longer duration of epilepsy and a greater frequency of seizures). Additionally, research on the safety of anti-seizure medications suggests that female patients are more susceptible to medication-related psychiatric behavioral abnormalities, although the underlying mechanism remains unclear [292].

8.4.3 New ASMs Causing Psychiatric Abnormalities

In clinical practice, the introduction of primidone is commonly used as a point of distinction between new and old ASMs. ASMs initiated for use after the introduction of primidone are referred to as new ASMs. Table 8.1 provides a list of new ASMs associated with psychiatric behavioral side effects.

Research indicates that novel ASMs can lead to psychiatric behavioral abnormalities. Commonly implicated drugs include levetiracetam, topiramate, gabapentin, lamotrigine, zonisamide, and perampanel. In particular, perampanel (PER) is associated with psychiatric symptoms such as aggression, hostility, emotional or behavioral anomalies, and homicidal thoughts and threats [299]. Zonisamide is linked to a higher incidence of depressive mood [300].

Table 8.1 ASMs Inducing Psychiatric Symptoms

Author	Journal	Publication time	Medication	Manifestation
Andres M, et al	Curr Pain Headache Rep	2011;15(3):164–9	VPA, GBP, TPM	Suicide, behavioral abnormalities
Baibing Chen, et al.	Epilepsy Behav	2017:76:24–31.	LEV, ZNS, VPA, LB, GBP, LTG, OXC	Depressive mood, psychosis, anxiety, suicidal thoughts, irritability, aggression, anger
Lea Julia Mertens et al.	Epilepsy Behav	2018:83:175–180	Several medications	Emotional instability, depression, aggression/irritability, psychosis, suicidal risk
Linda J Stephen, et al.	Epilepsy Behav	2017;71A:73–78	TPM, LEV, ZNS, LSD, PBL, RGB, PPA, RGB, BVT	Somatic symptoms
Brivaracetam et, al	Epilepsy Behav	2020;103:106864		Aggressive behavior, mental disorders, anger, aggression, excitement, hallucinations, panic attacks, anxiety
W H Theodore et al.	Epilepsia	1995;36(11):1105–10.	FBA	Suicide, behavioral abnormalities

Note: *LEV* levetiracetam, *ZNS* zonisamide, *LTG* lamotrigine, *GBP* gabapentin, *OXC* oxcarbazepine, *VPA* valproic acid, *LB* lacosamide, *TPM* topiramate, *PBL* pregabalin, *LSD* lacosamide, *EZA* eslicarbazepine acetate, *RGB* rufinamide, *PPA* pirlindole, *BVT* brivaracetam, *FBA* felbamate

8.4.4 Psychiatric Abnormalities Induced by ASMs

ASMs can lead to various psychiatric symptoms, as illustrated in Table 8.1. These symptoms manifest in various ways, encompassing general psychiatric manifestations such as emotional instability (anxiety, anger, tension), behavioral abnormalities (personality changes, hyperactivity, impulsivity, aggressive behavior, self-harm), and irritability (easily angered, excited, furious, even engaging in disputes). In severe cases, individuals may also experience depression, paranoia delusions, suicidal tendencies, changes in personality, cognitive impairments, and other manifestations (Table 8.1). Lim HW and colleagues [301] employed the BDI, SCL-90-R, and SSI-Beck scoring systems to assess the impact of antiepileptic drug use on the mental well-being of 257 epileptic patients. Their findings indicated that patients exhibited symptoms such as obsessive-compulsive disorder, depression, hostility, paranoia, and cognitive impairments. In a study by Kennedy GM [302] investigating psychiatric behavioral abnormalities induced by GBP, patients exhibited manifestations including depression, anxiety/excitability/neuroticism, behavioral abnormalities/personality changes/aggressive behavior, cognitive impairments/thought disorders, and memory impairments. Machado RA et al. [303] conducted a prospective cohort study involving 131 epilepsy patients over a 5-year follow-up period. The results suggest a potential risk of suicide with the use of lamotrigine and a 33.3% incidence of depressive episodes in patients treated with topiramate (TPM). Ketter TA and colleagues [304], in their research on patients taking lamotrigine, observed aggressive behavior, agitation, restlessness, confusion, and hallucinations. These psychiatric abnormalities can generally be categorized into five types.

8.4.4.1 Neurotic Symptoms

Manifesting as emotional instability, the core symptoms include anxiety, anger, and tension. Berkovic SF [305] observed 164 patients with refractory generalized epilepsy treated with levetiracetam for 6–12 months and found that one patient exhibited abnormal angry emotions. Frey LC [306] conducted a retrospective chart review and reported that in patients treated with lamotrigine monotherapy, six individuals experienced significant psychiatric symptoms including anxiety and emotional instability.

8.4.4.2 Behavioral Abnormalities

These abnormalities are characterized by personality changes, hyperactivity, impulsivity, aggressive behavior, and even self-harm. Goldberg-Stern H [307] analyzed 78 patients with refractory epilepsy (0.5–39 years old) and reported that 26.9% of patients exhibited behavioral abnormalities, including irritability, and impulsivity. Anhut H [308] conducted a multicenter, double-blind, randomized, placebo-controlled study to evaluate the effectiveness and safety of adding gabapentin (GBP) to the treatment regimens of 272 patients with refractory partial epilepsy. Among these patients, 7.2% experienced euphoria. Molokwu OA [309] described two cases: one, a 29-year-old male with posttraumatic epilepsy, experienced explosive anger and violent behavior after sodium valproate and phenobarbital were replaced with levetiracetam. The symptoms disappeared after discontinuation. The second patient, a 23-year-old female with refractory epilepsy, experienced anger, excitement, and multiple suicide attempts after the addition of levetiracetam. Kawai [310] used standardized scoring scales to study aggressive behavior induced by ASMs in 266 epilepsy patients. The results showed that the levetiracetam group had significantly greater scores than did the carbamazepine (CBZ) group ($p = 0.001$) and lacosamide group ($p = 0.029$), especially for physical aggression, verbal aggression, and hostility.

8.4.4.3 Irritability

This abnormality is characterized by extreme anger, excitability, fury, and persistent disputes. Matsuo M [311], in a retrospective evaluation of levetiracetam efficacy, included 76 epilepsy patients who were followed for at least 18 months, and found two patients with noticeable irritability.

8.4.4.4 Cognitive Impairments

These impairments can manifest as perceptual, thinking, or memory disorders, along with difficulty finding words, lack of concentration, and language problems. Adelman J [312] conducted a randomized double-blind placebo-controlled trial evaluating the safety and tolerability of topiramate (TPM) in 1580 epilepsy patients and reported that TPM-related cognitive impairment was common, reaching 9%, mainly including sensory and memory impairments. In a prospective study of 170 patients with refractory epilepsy, Stephen LJ [313] observed sensory and language impairments in 8% of patients taking TPM. In a systematic review of new ASMs, Marson AG [314] included 3091 patients with refractory epilepsy and found that patients treated with TPM experienced cognitive impairments. In two independent open-label, double-blinded studies on the addition of GBP to treatment regimens of pediatric patients with partial epilepsy and generalized tonic–clonic epilepsy, Reife RA [315] also described delayed thinking, lack of concentration, and sensory impairments.

8.4.4.5 Psychosis-Like Symptoms

These symptoms manifest as depression, schizophrenia, delusions, or suicidal tendencies. Vande Griend JP [316] described a 73-year-old patient with complex partial seizures and a history of renal insufficiency who was treated with levetiracetam (500 mg BID) for 5 months, which resulted in poor mood, weight loss, and fatigue. After the patient was diagnosed with depression, her symptoms almost disappeared after discontinuation of LEV. Another patient, a 92-year-old woman with focal epilepsy and chronic kidney disease, was treated with 500 mg/day levetiracetam for 5 weeks, which led to depressive symptoms such as a lack of pleasure, twitching, and decreased appetite. Emotion and cognition improved within 8 days of discontinuation. Brandt C [306] described a 52-year-old female with hippocampal sclerosis and poorly controlled epilepsy who was switched from oxcarbazepine and levetiracetam (4000 mg) to levetiracetam and lamotrigine treatment. After the dose of lamotrigine was increased, the patient exhibited psychotic symptoms and delusions (fearing threats from the police and debts from lawyers). Despite the addition of clonazepam (3 mg/day) and aripiprazole (2 mg) on the fourth day, these symptoms persisted for 7 days. Patorno E [317] conducted a cohort study of 297,620 epilepsy patients to compare the risk of suicide, violent death, and suicide attempts between patients taking GBP, lamotrigine, and TPM. The results revealed 801 suicide attempts, 26 suicides, and 41 violent deaths within a 2-month follow-up, suggesting an increased risk of suicide when ASMs such as GBP and lamotrigine were used.

8.4.5 Different Characteristics of Psychiatric Behavioral Abnormalities Induced by Novel ASMs

8.4.5.1 Gabapentin (GBP)

GBP is a derivative of gamma-aminobutyric acid (GABA), and its pharmacological action is primarily associated with sedation. Although there is literature suggesting that GBP improves mood, reduces depression and anxiety, treats social phobia, and decreases suicide risk in epilepsy patients, there have been reports of psychiatric behavioral abnormalities induced by GBP [314, 318]. A study of 240 epilepsy patients treated with GBP revealed that 10 patients (4%) discontinued treatment due to adverse events, including one case of neurotic symptoms, one case of depression, and one case of memory impairment [319].

Susceptibility Factors

Age and Intellectual Impairment: Adverse psychiatric reactions to GBP are age-related and more common among pediatric patients than older patients. Patients with a history of cognitive impairment are also prone to psychiatric behavioral abnormalities [318, 320]. For example, a 10-year-old female with refractory complex partial seizures and a history of right temporal lobe lesions and intellectual disability developed uncontrolled behavioral problems, including mood swings, food throwing, screaming, indiscriminate urinating, and aggressive behavior after 3 months of GBP treatment. The behavior significantly improved after a 2-week withdrawal [318]. Tallian KB [320] described another case involving a 6-year-old girl with complex partial seizures, learning disabilities, and attention deficit hyperactivity disorder (ADHD) who exhibited severe disruptive behavior after 6 months of GBP treatment. Behavior improved after the GBP dose was reduced [320].

Drug Dosage: Dose selection is crucial. An increase in GBP dose to 900 mg/d led to mild manic behavior, which transiently improved upon GBP dose reduction and disappeared after complete discontinuation [318]. It has been suggested that aggression may occur when the GBP dose is between 1000 and 1200 mg/day.

Clinical Features

Onset Time: Psychiatric behavioral abnormalities induced by GBP often occur early in the course of treatment [321]. For instance, a 37-year-old female developed excitement, an elevated mood, and aggressive behavior after 5 days of GBP monotherapy. Symptoms completely disappeared after discontinuation [321]. In another case, a 7-year-old male with refractory complex partial seizures and intellectual impairment developed severe behavioral disturbances, including overactivity, aggression, and making strange animal-like sounds, after 2 weeks of GBP monotherapy. Behavioral improvement was observed 1 week after discontinuation [318].

Neurotic Symptoms: GBP has been associated with neurotic symptoms. In a study of 32 children with refractory focal epilepsy and intellectual disability or ADHD, 7 patients exhibited noticeable neurotic symptoms [322]. Another study of 2074 epilepsy patients treated with GBP revealed that 2.4% of patients experienced neurotic symptoms.

Behavioral Abnormalities: A 10-year-old female with refractory complex partial seizures and a history of learning disabilities developed severe behavioral disturbances, including unprovoked explosive anger and aggressive behavior, after 2 weeks of GBP monotherapy. Symptoms significantly improved after a 5-week withdrawal [318]. In another case, an adult with intellectual disabilities and refractory epilepsy exhibited mild manic behavior after use of GBP [323]. A randomized, double-blind, placebo-controlled trial involving 43 patients with generalized tonic–clonic seizures revealed that one patient exhibited clear mania after GBP was added to the treatment regimen [324].

Cognitive Impairment: In a multicenter, double-blind, randomized, placebo-controlled study of 272 patients with refractory partial epilepsy, one patient exhibited significant cognitive impairment after GBP was added to the treatment regimen [325].

Severity: A 16-year-old male with intellectual disabilities and tonic–clonic seizures developed appetite and sleep disturbances, aggression, and behavioral disturbances after 5 days of GBP treatment. Symptoms improved after GBP was discontinued [326].

Management

Early reduction, discontinuation, or switching of medications are recommended. In most cases, symptoms self-resolve or disappear after dose reduction, discontinuation, or switching to an alternative medication [320, 326]. For instance, seven children with epilepsy and comorbid attention-deficit/hyperactivity disorder (ADHD) exhibited behavioral problems, irritability, hyperactivity, defiance, and aggressive behavior during GBP combination therapy. Improvement was observed after dose reduction or discontinuation [327].

8.4.5.2 Lamotrigine

Lamotrigine is a voltage-gated sodium channel blocker. It can inhibit seizures induced by pentetrazol and electrical stimulation, shorten the discharge time after excitation in the focus, cortex, and hippocampus, and combat partial and generalized seizures. Research suggests that lamotrigine may be used to treat bipolar disorder. Psychiatric behavioral abnormalities induced by lamotrigine are relatively rare and mainly manifest as depression, delusions, hallucinations, and other schizophrenia-like symptoms [302].

Susceptibility Factors

Risk factors for lamotrigine-induced adverse psychiatric reactions mainly include a history of psychiatric disorders, hemispheric lesions, and rapid titration (increasing the dose by more than 25 mg per week) [306, 328].

Age: Lamotrigine also has mood-stabilizing properties in addition to its antiepileptic effects. Elderly epilepsy patients often have concomitant depressive symptoms. Therefore, caution is needed when using lamotrigine in elderly epilepsy patients, especially those with a history of psychiatric disorders or cerebral hemispheric lesions. For example, a 53-year-old patient with symptomatic epilepsy, left hippocampal sclerosis, and a long history of antiepileptic drug use developed sleep disturbances, incoherent speech, and paranoid delusions after switching from carbamazepine and clonazepam to lamotrigine treatment. Symptoms attributed to lamotrigine were unresponsive to treatment with flupentixol and clonazepam, but they disappeared within 7 days of lamotrigine discontinuation [329]. Another patient, a 52-year-old female with hippocampal sclerosis and focal epilepsy, developed psychotic symptoms and aggression with lamotrigine augmentation [329].

Drug Dosage: In clinical use, lamotrigine should be initiated with a cautious initial dose, and the weekly dose should not exceed 25 mg [303]. For instance, a 27-year-old male patient with complex partial seizures developed restlessness after his lamotrigine dose was increased to 250 mg/day. The symptoms disappeared after the lamotrigine dose was reduced [328]. Another patient, a 44-year-old patient with symptomatic epilepsy, developed severe anxiety and paranoid delusions after the dose of lamotrigine was increased to 375 mg/day. Treatment with flupentixol (10 mg) and reducing the lamotrigine dose to 200 mg resulted in symptom resolution within 4 days [329].

Clinical Presentations

Onset Time: Psychiatric behavioral abnormalities induced by lamotrigine occur relatively late. For example, a 29-year-old female patient developed severe behavioral abnormalities, including irritability, frequent crying, screaming, tantrums, restlessness, and hyperactivity 1 month after lamotrigine was added to 1500 mg/day primidone. The abnormal behavior persisted for 9 months and disappeared 3 weeks after lamotrigine discontinuation [328]. Another patient, a 43-year-old patient with epilepsy who, after receiving treatment with various ASMs for an extended period, developed restlessness, irritability, and hyperactivity within 3 months of lamotrigine therapy. The abnormal behaviors persisted for 6 months, and the symptoms disappeared after lamotrigine discontinuation [328].

Neurotic Symptoms: A 27-year-old male patient developed neurotic symptoms during treatment with lamotrigine combined with phenytoin. Another patient, a 29-year-old female patient, frequently developed screaming and anger during treatment with lamotrigine combined with primidone therapy [328].

Behavioral Abnormalities: In a study of 3071 epilepsy patients receiving lamotrigine adjunctive therapy, 5 patients discontinued treatment due to severe aggressive behavior, including shouting, damaging objects, and threatening others [330].

Schizophrenia-like Symptoms: In a randomized, double-blind trial using the Hostility-Aggression Scale to evaluate the effects of lamotrigine adjunctive therapy in adults with partial epilepsy, 3% of patients experienced depressive episodes [331]. Another study of 3071 epilepsy patients receiving lamotrigine adjunctive therapy revealed 12 cases of severe depression [332]. In a case report, a 35-year-old male patient developed visual hallucinations (seeing people, graves, candles, etc.) and illusions after his lamotrigine dose was increased to 200 mg. Symptoms improved after lamotrigine discontinuation [312].

Management

Currently, it is believed that psychiatric behavioral abnormalities induced by lamotrigine can be eliminated by reducing the dose or discontinuing the drug [333, 334]. For instance, a 53-year-old patient with focal epilepsy and lesions started treatment with lamotrigine at a low dose, which was gradually increased to 250 mg; the patient developed paranoia. Reducing the dose of lamotrigine to 100 mg and adding flupentixol (4 mg) and diazepam (10 mg) resulted in symptom resolution within a few days [329]. Another patient, a 49-year-old male with idiopathic generalized epilepsy, developed visual hallucinations and anxiety with lamotrigine, and his symptoms rapidly improved after lamotrigine discontinuation for 3 months [329].

8.4.5.3 Topiramate (TPM)

Topiramate is a novel antiepileptic drug that substitutes a sulfamate group for monosaccharides. Recent research indicates that psychiatric behavioral abnormalities induced by TPM are mainly characterized by depression and cognitive impairment. The mechanism may be related to the increase in brain GABA levels and activity, as well as the inhibition of glutamate activity [303]. Clinical trials have shown that 17% of patients receiving TPM treatment experience depression [335].

Susceptibility Factors

The main risk factors for TPM-induced depression are a history of psychiatric disorders, hippocampal sclerosis, and cognitive impairment, which are significantly correlated with the daily dose. The higher the daily dose is, the more pronounced the cognitive impairment [336, 337].

Age: Since TPM mainly leads to adverse central nervous system reactions, especially affecting attention and memory, caution is advised when administering it to school-age children. Patients with a history of psychiatric disorders and hippocampal sclerosis are at a greater risk of developing depression.

Drug Dosage: Studies have shown that patients with hippocampal sclerosis are more prone to depression when they are treated with similar starting doses and titration rates as patients without hippocampal sclerosis. Patients with a history of febrile seizures and depression are at a higher risk of developing depression with rapid titration of TPM [336, 338]. Cognitive impairment is also significantly correlated with the daily dose of TPM. Higher daily doses result in more apparent cognitive dysfunction [339]. A study of 423 epilepsy patients treated with TPM revealed that the risk of depression was fivefold greater in patients who underwent rapid titration than in those who did not [338].

Clinical Presentations

Onset Time: Cognitive impairment induced by TPM often appears within 2–3 weeks after treatment initiation and continues or worsens with increasing drug doses [340, 341]. For example, a study involving healthy volunteers showed that symptoms such as drowsiness, psychomotor slowing, speech disorders, attention deficits, and memory difficulties appeared 2–3 weeks after the target dose of TPM was reached [340].

Neurotic Symptoms: In a randomized, double-blind, placebo-controlled study of TPM in 113 epilepsy patients, 8 patients experienced neurotic symptoms [342]. Another study of 47 patients with refractory partial epilepsy receiving TPM 400 mg/day found that 6 patients experienced neurotic symptoms [343].

Cognitive Impairment: Studies on the impact of TPM on patient mental behavior have shown that 13 patients experienced thought disorders and that 20 patients experienced sensory disturbances in a study involving 181 patients with refractory partial epilepsy [344]. Another double-blind, placebo-controlled trial involving 124 adults with partial-onset seizures revealed that 36 patients experienced thought disorders during TPM treatment [345].

Depression: An observational study of 44,300 epilepsy patients suggested that the use of high-potency drugs (including TPM) increased the risk of depression and self-harm or suicidal behavior threefold compared to those not using ASMs in the previous year [346].

Severity: In a randomized, double-blind, placebo-controlled trial evaluating TPM safety, 8% of patients withdrew from the study due to cognitive impairment

[312]. In a clinical trial involving 181 patients with refractory partial epilepsy, 9% of patients experienced mild or moderate central nervous system symptoms but none withdrew from the study [337].

Management

Psychiatric behavioral abnormalities induced by TPM appear early, and reducing or discontinuing the drug can eliminate these symptoms [347, 348]. A study of 431 epilepsy patients using TPM revealed that the main psychiatric event induced by TPM was depressive episodes. For such patients with depression, early reduction or discontinuation of the drug is recommended, as these patients generally have a good prognosis. After reducing or discontinuing the drug, 87% of patients fully recovered, and only a small percentage required hospitalization or additional drug therapy [336].

8.4.5.4 Levetiracetam

Levetiracetam is a pyrrolidone derivative with a chemical structure unrelated to those of existing ASMs. It is a highly effective novel antiepileptic drug. Reports suggest that levetiracetam has a role in improving patient cognitive functions, but there have also been reports of psychiatric side effects. Cramer JA and colleagues [349] conducted an efficacy and safety evaluation of levetiracetam treatment in 2871 adult epilepsy patients. They found that 0.7% of patients experienced anxiety, 1.4% exhibited hostility, 1.5% had mood instability, 1.7% reported depression, and 2% experienced tension. Tekgül H and others [350] conducted a retrospective study on 351 epilepsy patients (6 months to 18 years old) receiving levetiracetam treatment; the results revealed irritability (67%), hyperactivity (8%), behavioral disorders (5%), neuroticism (5%), and suicide attempts (2%) during the 12-month treatment period. Feng XF and colleagues [351] reported significant psychiatric behavioral abnormalities in children and adolescents with epilepsy who were treated with levetiracetam. The most common adverse reactions were irritability (38.7%) and learning disorders (16%), with 13.3% of the participants experiencing behavioral abnormalities.

Susceptibility Factors

Psychiatric side effects are most commonly associated with levetiracetam, and major risk factors include drug titration speed, genetic variations, a history of psychiatric illness, intellectual disabilities, autism, or attention deficit hyperactivity disorder [352, 353].

Genetic Variations: Helmstaedter C and others [352] analyzed 290 epilepsy patients treated with levetiracetam and found an association between psychiatric abnormalities and genetic variations. Patients with psychiatric abnormalities had reduced dopamine activity-related gene expression. Subsequent analysis of the rs1800497 polymorphism in 100 epilepsy patients suggested a correlation between genetic variations in dopamine activity and levetiracetam-induced psychiatric abnormalities. Although further verification is needed to show causality, pharmacogenomic approaches to behavioral side effects may become useful tools in the future.

Drug Dosage: Studies have shown that rapid titration can lead to psychiatric behavioral abnormalities. Vaisleib II and colleagues [354] conducted a retrospective chart review study of 3219 epilepsy patients and reported that rapid administration of levetiracetam (1–14 days) was tolerable, but the incidence of adverse events ranged from 12% to 22%. Nakken KO [353] reported a case of a 4-year-old boy with Lennox-Gastaut syndrome who was initially unresponsive to levetiracetam treatment. After titration to 33 mg/kg, aggressive behavior occurred 30 min later, leading to hospitalization. Discontinuation of levetiracetam for 48 h resolved the aggressive behavior. Another patient involved a girl with focal epilepsy who had 15 seizures per day. Levetiracetam titration from 10 to 30 mg/kg reduced the seizure frequency to 5–7 times per day, but at 40 mg/kg, the frequency increased to 20 times per day. The dose was reduced to 15 mg/kg or less, and the number of seizures was maintained at a frequency of 5–7 times per day.

Sex and Age: Bilo L and colleagues [355] treated 200 epilepsy patients with levetiracetam, with a follow-up period of at least 6 months. Forty-six patients (23%) withdrew from the study due to adverse reactions, and females (30.6%) experienced higher rates of adverse reactions than males (13.2%). Verrotti A and others [356] conducted a meta-analysis involving 2832 patients, 26 of whom experienced tension and irritability. No correlation was found with age, sex, or dose assessment variables.

Others: Numerous studies have suggested that individuals with a history of febrile seizures or status epilepticus, psychiatric and behavioral issues, intellectual disabilities, autism, or attention deficit hyperactivity disorder have a greater risk of developing psychiatric behavioral abnormalities after taking levetiracetam [294]. Brodtkorb E and colleagues [357] conducted an open study on 184 refractory epilepsy patients with a mean follow-up period of 8.1 months. After levetiracetam treatment, the rate of side effects in patients with and without learning disabilities was 23% and 10%, respectively, suggesting that patients with learning disabilities have more frequent and greater risk of behavioral problems. Youroukos S [358] reported the case of a 12-year-old epileptic girl with a history of cognitive or behavioral disorders. She received sodium valproate and levetiracetam as add-on therapy. Ten days later, despite seizure control, she developed hallucinations, anxiety, and self-harm. Discontinuation of levetiracetam for 1 week resolved the psychiatric behavioral abnormalities. Kossoff EH [359] described the case of a 13-year-old patient with complex partial seizures in the left temporal lobe and a history of learning disabilities. Levetiracetam monotherapy led to hallucinations, screaming, and depression after approximately 3 months. Symptoms disappeared after discontinuation. Another patient, a 5-year-old girl, had a mild cognitive delay. After receiving levetiracetam treatment at a dose of 25 mg/kg/day BID and a ketogenic diet, she developed visual hallucinations and restlessness 2 weeks later. Oral diazepam (DZP) treatment improved restlessness, but the hallucinations persisted. Symptoms resolved without recurrence within 24 h after discontinuation. The third patient was a 16-year-old patient with complex partial seizures, a tumor in the right temporal parietal area, and an IQ of 76. She became extremely agitated and attempted to run away 2 days after receiving levetiracetam treatment at a dose of 500 mg BID (15 mg/kg/day). Local law enforcement revealed her engaging in suicidal and homicidal behavior with persecutory delusions. Symptoms improved 1 day after discontinuation, and she apologized 3 days later. Subsequent 6-month psychological testing occasionally revealed paranoia but no hallucinations.

Clinical Manifestations

Levetiracetam, among the new generation of ASMs, is most commonly associated with psychiatric behavioral abnormalities and manifests in various forms.

Onset: Psychiatric behavioral abnormalities after medication typically appear within 2–3 weeks of drug initiation and may intensify or persist with continued use. Tamarelle C [358] described the case of a 5-year-old boy with partial seizures who had no psychiatric or behavioral abnormalities before medication. After he had been taking levetiracetam for 3 weeks, he developed irritability, a loss of interest in enjoyable activities, and aggressive behavior at school. Symptoms lasted for 4 weeks, and improvement was observed after discontinuation. Youroukos S [359] reported a case in which a 12-year-old girl with idiopathic epilepsy developed hallucinations, anxiety, and self-harm 10 days after levetiracetam at a dose of 60 mg/kg was added to her treatment regimen. Complete resolution of psychiatric behavioral abnormalities occurred after the discontinuation of levetiracetam for 1 week.

Neuroticism: Briggs DE and others [360] studied 1030 patients with partial seizures in a multicenter, double-blinded clinical trial of levetiracetam efficacy and safety. They found that 1.8% exhibited neuroticism. Glauser TA and colleagues [361] treated 24 children with refractory partial seizures with levetiracetam, 5 of whom reported neuroticism. Delanty N and others [362] conducted a multicenter, randomized, double-blind, placebo-controlled study of levetiracetam add-on therapy for epilepsy and reported that 3.7% of patients experienced tension and 3.2% had anxiety.

Behavioral Abnormalities: Opp J and others [363] conducted a multicenter study on levetiracetam add-on therapy in 285 pediatric epilepsy patients. They found that 15.4% of children exhibited behavioral abnormalities and that 10.5% engaged in aggressive behavior. Lagae L and colleagues [364] conducted a prospective trial on 67 pediatric epilepsy patients to assess the efficacy and safety of levetiracetam add-on therapy, revealing that 5% of patients experienced aggressive behavior. De la Loge C and others [365] conducted a randomized, double-blind, placebo-controlled study on refractory pediatric epilepsy using the Child Behavior Checklist (CBCL) and Pediatric Health Questionnaire (CHQ-PF50) to assess behavior and mental function before and after levetiracetam monotherapy. The results showed that children treated with levetiracetam were more likely to exhibit aggressive behavior than were those treated with a placebo. Gao ZJ and others [366] conducted an open study on 32 pediatric epilepsy patients (8 months to 12 years old) receiving levetiracetam monotherapy, with a target dose of 20–40 mg/kg/day and a follow-up of more than 3 months. They found that 19.4% of patients experienced emotional and behavioral changes.

Irritability: Briggs DE and others [360] conducted a multicenter, double-blind controlled study on the efficacy and safety of levetiracetam treatment involving 1030 patients with partial seizures. They found that 3.8% of patients experienced irritability. Pina-Garza JE and others [362] conducted a multicenter, double-blind, randomized study on levetiracetam monotherapy and combination therapy for partial epilepsy in children aged 1 month to 4 years. The authors found that the most common adverse event was irritability (11.7%).

Psychosis-like Symptoms: Briggs DE and others [360] conducted a multicenter, double-blinded controlled study on the efficacy and safety of levetiracetam treatment involving 1030 patients with partial seizures. They found that 0.7% of patients experienced psychosis-like symptoms, and 0.5% had suicidal tendencies. Kumar N [367] described a 52-year-old patient with acute seizures who developed severe behavioral abnormalities, including emotional excitement, irritability, hostility, and personality disintegration, after receiving levetiracetam treatment at a dose of 500 mg/day for 3 days. Psychiatric assessment revealed characteristic depression, emotional and thought abnormalities, suspicion, and withdrawal states with visual hallucinations. Shorvon SD and others [368] conducted a multicenter, double-blinded, randomized, placebo-controlled trial to assess the efficacy and tolerability of levetiracetam in 324 patients with refractory partial-onset seizures. Patients received levetiracetam add-on therapy at doses of 1000 mg/day and 2000 mg/day BID. The results showed that 5.7% of patients developed depression.

Severity: Nakken KO and others [353] analyzed 44 children with epilepsy treated with levetiracetam and found that 1 child experienced severe aggressive behavior and that 1 had psychiatric symptoms of forced normalization, requiring discontinuation. Kossoff EH and others [369] reported the case of a 17-year-old girl with temporal lobe epilepsy, mild cognitive impairment, and depression. After levetiracetam was added to her treatment regimen at a dose of 33 mg/kg/day for 2 weeks, she developed headache, somnolence, and auditory hallucinations. Symptoms disappeared after discontinuation. A month later, a low dose of 500 mg BID was administered, and psychiatric symptoms recurred. Kuba R and others [370] retrospectively analyzed 218 adult epilepsy patients treated with levetiracetam, with a follow-up period of 36 months. Four patients experienced mood instability, 3 had depression, and 4 had aggressive behavior, leading to study withdrawal.

Management

Currently, it is believed that levetiracetam-induced psychiatric behavioral abnormalities develop early and that reducing the dose or discontinuing the medication can eliminate these effects [371]. Major P and others [372] conducted a retrospective chart summary and questionnaire survey of 90 patients aged 3–19 years receiving levetiracetam and vitamin B6 (pyridoxine) treatment, with a follow-up of 6 months. The results showed a significant improvement in behavior in 41% of patients, suggesting that vitamin B6 supplementation may improve the behavioral problems caused by levetiracetam. However, there is no scientific basis to support this supposition, and the interaction mechanism between levetiracetam and vitamin B6 requires further evaluation, including the dose and timing of combination therapy.

8.4.5.5 Perampanel

Perampanel is the first AMPA receptor antagonist and a novel antiepileptic drug. A study by Rugg-Gunn [297] compared patients taking perampanel with those receiving a placebo and revealed that patients taking perampanel were more prone to psychiatric abnormalities, with 9.1% of patients needing to discontinue perampanel, while only 4.8% of patients in the placebo group discontinued perampanel use, suggesting that psychiatric behavioral abnormalities may be an important side effect of perampanel. Although perampanel may cause psychiatric abnormalities in patients with epilepsy, effective control of seizures with perampanel may lead to improvements in preexisting psychiatric and behavioral abnormalities [292].

Epidemiology

Hasegawa N [292] conducted a retrospective study of 135 patients taking perampanel and reported that 32 patients (23.7%) developed psychiatric behavioral abnormalities, including irritability, aggression, and anxiety, after starting perampanel treatment. Lossius [373] studied 175 patients taking perampanel and reported that 34% of patients developed psychiatric behavioral abnormalities, suggesting that the incidence of psychiatric behavioral abnormalities in patients taking perampanel may range from 23.7% to 34%.

Susceptibility Factors

History of Psychiatric Disorders: Patients with a history of psychiatric disorders are more likely to develop psychiatric behavioral abnormalities after taking new ASMs. Kanner [374] compared the rate of psychiatric abnormalities after taking perampanel in 352 patients (16.1%) with a history of psychiatric disorders and 1835 patients (83.9%) without a history of psychiatric disorders. The results showed that patients with a positive history of psychiatric disorders had a greater rate of psychiatric abnormalities after perampanel administration. In patients without a history of psychiatric disorders, the incidence of psychiatric abnormalities while taking perampanel at doses of 2–4 mg/day was not greater than that in the placebo group. Among patients with a history of psychiatric disorders, those taking perampanel at doses of 8–12 mg had a greater incidence of psychiatric abnormalities.

Drug Dose: Ettinger [291] studied patients taking different doses of perampanel and reported that 17.2% of patients taking 8 mg/day of perampanel developed psychiatric behavioral abnormalities, while 22.4% of patients taking 12 mg/day of perampanel developed psychiatric behavioral abnormalities. The incidences of hostile/aggressive psychiatric abnormalities in the 8 mg and 12 mg perampanel groups were 2.8% and 6.3%, respectively. The authors suggest that these side effects be monitored during the dose titration period and at higher doses. Kanner [374] also reported that patients taking perampanel at doses above 4 mg/day were more likely to develop psychiatric behavioral abnormalities.

Intellectual Disabilities: Yamamoto [375] followed 895 Japanese epilepsy patients taking perampanel and reported that patients with intellectual disabilities were more likely to develop psychiatric behavioral abnormalities related to drug concentration. The authors suggested that caution should be exercised in titrating perampanel in patients with intellectual disabilities, and drug concentration monitoring is necessary.

Others: Hasegawa N [292] described 32 patients who developed psychiatric and behavioral abnormalities after taking perampanel and reported significant correlations with structural abnormalities, concomitant use of nitrazepam, and the presence of restlessness and depression.

Clinical Manifestations

Psychiatric behavioral abnormalities induced by perampanel mainly manifest as behavioral changes, irritability, aggression, agitation, anxiety, and mood changes [376]. Liu P [377] observed adverse events related to perampanel in 17 randomized controlled trials (RCTs) involving 5711 subjects and reported that 11 adverse events (aggression, ataxia, balance disorders, dizziness, falls, fatigue, irritability, rash, somnolence, vertigo, and weight gain) were significantly associated with perampanel. Among these adverse events, aggression, ataxia, and irritability were the most pronounced. Steinhoff [378] conducted an epidemiological survey of four major behavioral abnormalities caused by perampanel and reported that the incidence of irritability was 5.6%, that of anger was 3.3%, and that of aggression was 2.5%. The average discontinuation rate due to irritability was 0.8%, and the discontinuation rate due to aggression was 2%.

Aggression: This includes physical aggression, verbal aggression, anger, hostility, etc., and is the most common psychiatric adverse reaction to ASMs. Perampanel and levetiracetam are the ASMs most likely to cause aggressive behavior. Kawa

[379] evaluated aggression using a standardized assessment scale in 144 patients taking levetiracetam or perampanel and reported that patients taking perampanel exhibited significantly more overt aggressive behavior, while those taking levetiracetam exhibited more covert aggressive behavior.

Agitation: Hasegawa et al. [292] assessed the differences in agitation side effects between patients receiving levetiracetam and those receiving perampanel treatment, and the results showed that both levetiracetam and perampanel could cause agitation in different patient groups. Patients with temporal lobe epileptiform discharges were more sensitive to levetiracetam and more likely to experience agitation, while those without temporal lobe discharges were more sensitive to perampanel, possibly due to differences in the regulation of AMPA receptors between the hippocampus and neocortex.

Irritability: Hasegawa [380] studied 98 patients taking levetiracetam and perampanel; 7 patients in the levetiracetam group and 17 patients in the perampanel group experienced irritability. Logistic multivariate regression analysis revealed a significant correlation between temporal lobe focal discharge and levetiracetam-induced irritability. As the dose was increased, the incidence of perampanel-induced irritability decreased. Nontemporal lobe focal discharges were associated with perampanel-induced irritability, and higher doses of perampanel were more likely to cause irritability.

Restlessness: Hasegawa N [380] studied 32 patients who developed psychiatric and behavioral abnormalities after taking perampanel and found a significant correlation of perampanel with restlessness.

Related Factors

The incidence of psychiatric and behavioral abnormalities is significantly reduced when perampanel is used in combination with carbamazepine. It is believed that combination therapy comprising perampanel and carbamazepine may be associated with favorable outcomes for patients with epilepsy, as indicated by psychiatric and behavioral symptoms [292].

Treatment

The psychiatric side effects of perampanel, often characterized by aggression, may require dose reduction or discontinuation. Out of 32 patients with psychiatric and behavioral abnormalities studied by Hasegawa N [292], 5 patients were able to tolerate adverse events by reducing the perampanel dose, while 14 patients with ongoing psychiatric symptoms experienced a transient exacerbation of psychiatric symptoms when continuing the medication. Please note that the information provided here is based on the sources available up to my last knowledge update in January 2022, and there may be further developments or new research

8.4.6 Diagnosis

In addition to clinical descriptions, various scales are used as primary diagnostic criteria for identifying psychiatric behavioral abnormalities induced by ASMs. Commonly used assessment tools can be found in Table 8.2.

Commonly used scales for assessing the personalities of epilepsy patients include the Minnesota Multiphasic Personality Inventory (MMPI), the Washington Psychosocial Seizure Inventory (wPSi), and the Eysenck Personality Questionnaire

Table 8.2 Assessment tools for identifying antiepileptic drug-related psychiatric behavioral abnormalities

Scale Name	Brief Characteristics	References
CBCL	First used in the United States in 1970, widely used among similar child scales. Comprehensive content, good reliability, and excellent predictive validity for determining children with social and behavioral problems. Suitable for children aged 4–16.	[9]
SCL-90-R	Developed in 1975, it is currently the most widely used outpatient scale for mental disorders and psychological diseases. Assists in understanding one's mental health across ten aspects. Applicable to individuals aged 16 and older.	[10, 12]
NDDI-E	In 2006, scholars in the United States, led by Gilliam, formulated a rapid and accurate epilepsy depression scale. This self-assessment scale consists of six questions and can quickly identify depressive disorders in epilepsy patients. It is currently routinely used in epilepsy clinics in the United States.	[13]
MMSE	Developed in 1975, it is one of the most influential tools for screening cognitive impairment. The scale includes seven aspects: time orientation, place orientation, immediate memory, attention and calculation, delayed memory, language, and visuospatial ability.	[10]
QOL IE-31	Shortened to QOLIE-31 in 1998, it covers the most important quality of life issues in the daily lives of epilepsy patients, with a total of 31 items divided into seven aspects: seizure worry, overall quality of life, emotional health, energy/fatigue, cognitive function, medication side effects, and work-driving-social restrictions. It can be used in clinical trials to assess patient responses after changing treatment plans.	[10, 11, 14, 15]
BDI-II	Developed in 1961, it is one of the most widely used self-assessment scales for depressive symptoms. The scale can be used to assess the severity of depressive symptoms in psychiatric patients and in the general population.	[12, 13]
DSM-IV	Officially published in May 1994, it is the American diagnostic standard for mental disorders, serving as a tool to assess mental status. The depression scale is one portion of it.	[15, 16]
SSI-Beck	Developed in 1979, it is a questionnaire used to quantify and assess suicidal ideation.	[12]
BAI	Developed in 1985, it is a self-assessment scale with 21 items, mainly assessing the degree to which the subject is bothered by various anxiety symptoms. Suitable for adults with anxiety symptoms.	[12]

(EPQ). Classic depression scales such as the Hamilton Rating Scale for Depression (HRSD) are recognized for their simplicity, clear standards, and ease of use (although they may not effectively distinguish anxiety). The Beck Depression Inventory (BDI) is the most commonly used self-assessment scale for depression. Other psychiatric examination scales commonly used for epilepsy patients include the Halstead-Reitan Neuropsychological Battery (H-R), Symptom Checklist-90 (SCL-90), and Hospital Anxiety and Depression Scale, which provide a more comprehensive and objective diagnostic approach for evaluating psychiatric symptoms induced by ASMs.

Mertens [290] utilized the BDI, the expanded Neurological Disorders Depression Inventory-Epilepsy (NDDI-E), and the Fragebogen (FPZ) scale to assess the emotions, personality, and behavior of 494 epilepsy patients. The assessment revealed the presence of emotional instability, aggression/irritability, psychosis, suicidal tendencies, somatization, and other psychiatric symptoms. The authors speculate that these tools can help identify damage caused by ASMs.

Currently, there is a lack of unified diagnostic classification criteria and treatment consensus for psychiatric symptoms induced by ASMs. The occurrence of psychiatric symptoms in epilepsy patients is associated with many factors, and epileptic seizures can also trigger abnormal behaviors. Therefore, when diagnosing and treating epilepsy patients with psychiatric symptoms, clinicians should first try to identify the causes of these symptoms. It is crucial to determine whether the symptoms are due to primary psychiatric disorders, psychiatric symptoms induced by ASMs, or other factors. This determination is essential for subsequent treatment choices. Misdiagnosing psychiatric symptoms induced by ASMs as primary psychiatric disorders or due to other causes may lead to serious consequences. As long as treatment with pathogenic ASMs continues, the induced psychiatric symptoms are likely to persist. Moreover, while enduring the adverse reactions caused by ASMs, patients may also face the potential risk of exacerbating epilepsy through additional treatment with antipsychotic medications. Therefore, clinicians need to first identify the cause of psychiatric symptoms to help distinguish between psychiatric symptoms induced by ASMs and other forms of epileptic mental disorders.

8.4.7 Treatment

If the onset of a patient's psychiatric symptoms strongly correlates with the use of ASMs, suspicion should be raised regarding the possibility of drug-induced effects. Generally, psychiatric symptoms induced by ASMs improve after use of the causative agents is discontinued. Therefore, when there is a high suspicion that a patient's psychiatric symptoms are triggered by ASMs, it is essential to promptly adjust the treatment plan, modify the dosage of the causative ASMs, and discontinue them if necessary; in subsequent antiepileptic drug treatments, drugs with similar or identical mechanisms of action should be avoided.

Although most psychiatric symptoms induced by ASMs are mild, transient, and reversible, severe symptoms often do not resolve spontaneously. Treatment for these patients involves more than just reducing the dose or discontinuing the causative ASMs; individualized measures such as the judicious use of antipsychotic medications are needed to control psychiatric symptoms. Examples include benzodiazepines, clozapine, levetiracetam, olanzapine, flupenthixol, and selective serotonin reuptake inhibitors (SSRIs) [381, 382].

Every clinician adjusting medication regimens for epilepsy patients, especially when adding or adjusting drugs such as levetiracetam, PER, or TPM, should be vigilant in identifying patients at high risk for psychiatric symptoms. This approach is particularly crucial for individuals with a history of psychiatric disorders or familial susceptibility, as it enables informed communication of the potential occurrence of psychiatric adverse reactions. Additionally, efforts should be made to titrate medications gradually to prevent the onset of psychiatric symptoms due to rapid titration, which could worsen seizures. Regular follow-up for epilepsy patients is also crucial to circumvent overlooking early, mild, or reversible psychiatric symptoms and preventing their progression into chronic psychiatric disorders such as schizophrenia, depression, anxiety disorders, or manic-depressive illnesses.

New generation ASMs are associated with psychiatric behavioral abnormalities that can significantly impact patient quality of life and even pose a threat to life. This should be given high priority, necessitating a thorough understanding of their clinical manifestations and risk factors. Various preventive measures should be implemented to guard against the occurrence of adverse psychiatric reactions. When selecting medications, a personalized treatment approach should be adopted, taking into account the specific circumstances of each patient to mitigate risks. After initiating medication, timely identification is crucial for early detection and intervention, thereby circumventing risks to the patient's life.

8.5 Effects of ASMs on Cognitive Function in Patients with Epilepsy

Patients with epilepsy often report cognitive impairment, especially memory impairment, and neuropsychological tests can also determine that patients with epilepsy have cognitive impairment. However, there are many sources of cognitive impairment in patients with epilepsy, seizures, and epileptic encephalopathy, and comorbidities in patients with epilepsy can cause cognitive impairment; ASMs are only one of the reasons for this. Wang L et al. [383] analyzed the cognitive dysfunction of 257 patients with epilepsy and reported that education level, frequency of seizures, and type of ASM used were related to the cognitive dysfunction of epilepsy patients. In many cases, the roles of these factors are unclear. However, the use of ASMs is very important, and rational use of ASMs is expected to improve the cognitive function of patients.

8.5.1 Historical Evolution

Phenobarbital (PB) is an older generation ASM. Although it has long been recognized that PB has a clear effect on cognitive function in patients, the first report describing the effects of PB on cognitive function in patients was published in 1991. Bigarella MM et al. [384] measured the cognitive function of 20 patients with focal seizure epilepsy who took PB and found that PB had a significant effect on the cognitive function of patients. In 2003, Salinsky MC et al. [385] used quantitative EEG to study the effects of ASMs on the cognitive function of patients. The study included 20 patients who started treatment with ASMs, 12 patients who stopped ASM use, 33 patients who received stable ASM treatment, and 73 healthy controls, and revealed that ASMs had a significant effect on patient cognition. The authors speculate that although EEG is not a direct measure of cognitive function, it can still reflect the side effects of the drug. In 2013, Kim SM et al. [386] noted that oxcarbazepine had a significant impact on the cognitive function of patients and suggested that cognitive side effects should be considered when selecting such drugs. Videman M et al. [387] noted that the cognitive function of offspring whose mothers consumed valproic acid, oxcarbazepine, and carbamazepine before birth was significantly affected. Recently, Salinsky M [388] described the effect of pregabalin on cognitive function. In 2016, Callisto SP et al. [389] systematically summarized the effects of the new ASM topiramate (TPM) on the cognition of epilepsy patients, which enriched the related research.

8.5.2 Epidemiology

Due to the limitations of detection methods and the complexity of clinical manifestations, there are no epidemiological data on the effects of ASMs on cognitive dysfunction in patients with epilepsy. Lauren Feldman et al. [390] investigated 670 patients taking ASMs and reported that 270 (40%) had cognitive dysfunction. Marco Mula et al. [391] analyzed the characteristics of cognitive impairment caused by TPM and reported that 10% of patients taking TPM had cognitive impairment.

8.5.3 Clinical Manifestations and Drug Characteristics

8.5.3.1 Clinical Manifestations

Human cognition is a very complex mental function involving attention, intelligence, language skills, nonverbal memory, executive function, and psychomotor speed. Sung-Pa Park et al. [392] reported that the effects of ASMs on cognitive function were mainly reflected in attention, alertness, and psychomotor speed. R

Trimble [393] highlighted memory deficits, attention problems, psychomotor slowness, and reading and writing difficulties as the main manifestations of cognitive impairment in epilepsy patients.

8.5.3.2 ASMs

Not all medications cause cognitive impairment in people with epilepsy. Adam Strzelczyk et al. [394] conducted a study on frequently used ASMs in clinical practice and found that TPM and ZNS were associated with language disorders and cognitive delay/memory problems. Frank M C Besag [395] reported that PB, TPM, and phenytoin had negative effects on cognition, especially because TPM caused more obvious word-finding difficulties and other language defects. R Kalviainen et al. [396] reported that PB, phenytoin, carbamazepine, and valproic acid had significant damaging effects on cognitive function. Newer ASMs, with the exception of ZNS and TPM, caused fewer adverse cognitive effects than older drugs.

Traditional ASMs

Compared with new ASMs, almost all traditional ASMs can cause cognitive dysfunction in patients. Voorhies et al. [397] conducted a study on the influence of traditional ASMs on cognitive function and reported that valproic acid and carbamazepine had different degrees of influence on patient cognitive function. The effects of PB on cognitive function are often dose dependent. Frank M C Besag et al. [395] also reported that PB and phenytoin had negative impacts on cognition. M R Trimble [398] reported that phenytoin caused the most severe cognitive deficits. PB and sodium valproate can cause moderate cognitive impairment. Carbamazepine appears to be relatively free of this toxicity. The authors suggest that further research is needed on the relationship between anticonvulsant type and cognitive function. Teiichi Onuma et al. [399] also emphasized the need to pay attention to the effects of traditional ASMs on cognitive function. Most classical ASM agents (PB, PHT, CBZ, and VPA), especially PB, have adverse effects on cognition.

1. Carbamazepine (CBZ)

   The evidence for the effect of CBZ on cognitive ability comes mainly from comparative studies with other ASMs. Children treated with CBZ were compared with those taking levetiracetam, and the cognitive function test results did not significantly differ from baseline; moreover, there were no significant differences between the two drugs [384]. Similarly, the Wechsler Intelligence Scale for Children (WISC) scores of the CBZ group did not differ from baseline, and there were no significant differences between groups in total IQ, verbal IQ, or operational IQ. In children with BECTS, moderate doses of CBZ caused a decrease in visual motor coordination, sustained attention, and instant word recall tests [400, 401]. Among patients taking CBZ and eslicarbazepine (ESL), executive ability and selective attention in the CBZ group were worse than those in the ESL group [402]. It is thought that CBZ may have an effect on memory, coordination, and attention, as well as vocabulary, arithmetic, and comprehension, compared to some other ASMs.

2. Phenytoin sodium (PHT)

   PHT inhibits high-frequency neuronal firing by preferentially binding deactivated sodium ion channels [403]. However, because the therapeutic dose and toxic dose are very close, the toxic side effects are severe, there are many adverse reactions, and the clinical application of PHT has been significantly reduced. Although PHT has been on the market for a long time, research on the effects of PHT on cognitive function has been limited. After receiving 360 mg of PHT, healthy volunteers showed decreases in scores on the number cancellation, word expression, visual response, story recall, and other cognitive tests [404], suggesting that PHT may affect cognitive function. Moreover, the cognitive impairment caused by the drug continues to persist after withdrawal [405].

3. Valproic acid (VPA)

   VPA is a broad-spectrum ASM. The evidence for the effects of VPA on cognition comes mainly from comparisons with other ASMs. A comparison of VPA, CBZ, and PB revealed no difference in visual motor function scores according to the WSC-R or Bender-Gestalt tests [401]. In the focused attention test and the number symbol test, the scores of the VPA group were significantly worse than those of the CBZ group [400]. In studies of patients treated with VPA or CBZ for up to 6 years, the VPA group performed well on tests of immediate word recall, selectivity, and focused attention, while reaction times were slower on single-attention tests. Compared with that in the ESL and LTG groups [406], the incidence of attention disorders in the VPA group was significantly greater. Compared with those of the OXC, LEV, LTG, and TPM groups, the assessment of the executive function system in the VPA group was decreased, the working memory of the VPA group was weaker than that of the LTG group, the numerical breadth test score was lower than that of the OXC or LTG group, and the classification fluency score was lower than that of the OXC group [407]. In summary, VPA is generally not associated with severe cognitive impairment; however, compared with CBZ, LEV, LTG, and OXC, VPA may have an impact on memory, attention, and executive function.

4. Phenobarbital

   Phenobarbital is the oldest ASM agent in widespread use, especially in developing countries [408]. In children with febrile convulsions treated with PB, memory impairment is associated with high PB blood concentrations, and a longer duration of treatment reduces comprehension levels [407]. After 2 years of treatment, the mean IQ of the PB group was significantly lower than that of the placebo group [409], and even after 6 months of tapering and discontinuation, the mean IQ of the PB group remained lower than that of the placebo group. The reading scores of children treated with PB for a long period of time were also decreased significantly, and the average IQ was still lower than that of the placebo group after 2 years of drug withdrawal [384]. Bigarella et al. [384] studied 20 patients with focal epilepsy aged 17–52 years who took PB and found that patients who took PB had more pronounced cognitive deficits than patients taking other drugs. However, further research is needed to determine the factors associated with cognitive dysfunction in patients with epilepsy. According to studies comparing PB with other ASMs, children treated with PB may have greater cognitive deficits. Compared with those in the VPA group, the children in the PB group had lower scores on cognitive tests, especially memory tests [410]. PB is generally believed to be associated with a range of cognitive impairments, particularly with respect to memory function, and is generally associated with worse cognitive conditions than the control group. The defects persisted even after the drug was stopped.

5. Others

   Primidone is considered to be a precursor drug for PB and is rapidly converted into PB in the body. Its cognitive effects can be inferred from the cognitive research regarding PB. Clonazepam is a benzodiazepine, and when it was first introduced, it was considered an improvement over barbiturates. The most common cognition-related adverse effects of clonazepam were drowsiness, behavior, and personality changes (inattentive, disruptive, and aggressive behaviors) [411]. Withdrawal may result in acute anxiety, insomnia, confusion, and other symptoms [412].

Novel ASMs

Lars Brunbech et al. [413] compared the effects of the new ASMs oxcarbazepine, vigabatrin, lamotrigine, zonisamide, gabapentin, tiagabine, topiramate, and levetiracetam on patient cognitive function. The results showed that, compared with "old" ASMs (such as phenytoin, PB, valproic acid and carbamazepine), the effect of new ASMs on cognitive function may be less pronounced, suggesting that the effect of new ASMs on the cognitive function of epilepsy patients is slight. However, the authors also argue that this aspect has not been systematically studied and that methodological issues in neuropsychological testing obscure the results and require different analyses for different drugs.

1. Lacosamide

   Christoph Helmstaedter et al. [414] studied the effects of lacosamide on cognition in patients with epilepsy through the use of EpiTrack, verbal memory, and subjective ratings of self-perceived side effects (cognition, emotion) and compared the findings with those of patients taking TPM and lamotrigine (LTG). The results showed that the three drugs had significant effects on the cognitive impairment of epilepsy patients. Among the patients using TPM, 53% had cognitive impairment, while that of patients taking LCM was 14% and that of patients taking LTG was 27%, suggesting that LCM use leads to less cognitive impairment than TPM and that LTG and LCM are relatively safe drugs.

Kuan-Ying Li [415] obtained a total of 251 records, including two meta-analyses, one randomized controlled trial, and 14 observational studies after screening. Most studies are in agreement that LCM carries a low risk of cognitive impairment and is significantly superior to carbamazepine, TPM, and perampanel. Despite its low incidence, depression remains the most commonly associated mental change. The authors suggest that the effects of LCM on cognitive and emotional states are limited. DMIJf et al. [416] conducted a study on 33 patients taking LCM and reported that LCM treatment had no significant impact on the speed of information response and no significant negative impact on other cognitive functions.

2. Perampanel (PER)

   Meschede C [417] studied 94 patients taking ASMs, 57 of whom were taking PER and 37 of whom were taking LCM. Cognitive ability was assessed with the EpiTrack screening for executive function and the VLMT short-form assessment of verbal memory, with a median follow-up interval of 36 weeks. The results revealed no negative effects on cognition from long-term use of PER or increased self-reports of irritability or aggression.

3. Brivaracetam (BRV)

   Levetiracetam is a precursor of brivaracetam. To understand whether BRV has an effect on patient cognition, Alexander Witt et al. [418] analyzed 43 patients with epilepsy. The results showed that taking BRV not only significantly positively affected cognitive function, but there was also no change in mood or aggression scores. Kuan-Ying Li et al. [419] searched relevant literature in three major databases and revealed that BRV was not found to have an impact on human or animal cognitive. Patients who are intolerant to levetiracetam and have side effects related to levetiracetam may benefit from a change in BRV.

4. Topiramate (TPM)

   Edgar Kockelmann [420] conducted a study on 42 patients taking TPM and used patients taking LTG as a control. The results showed that patients taking TPM scored poorly on speech fluency, memory span, and working memory, indicating that patients had cognitive impairment in performing specific functions, the severity of which was dose dependent. When the dose is too high, cognitive function impairment becomes more obvious. Michael E Smith et al. [421] studied the effects of TPM on EEG and evoked potential changes related to cognitive function in 29 healthy people. The results showed that both EEG and evoked potential changes were damaged after participants consumed TPM, suggesting that TPM has a significant effect on cognitive function. Frank M C Besag [395] also reported that TPM had a negative impact on cognition, especially in individuals who had obvious word-finding difficulties and other language deficits. Sung-Pa Park et al. [392] noted that, regardless of which ASM it was compared with, the damage caused by TPM to patient cognitive function was very obvious. Marco Mula et al. [391] analyzed the characteristics of cognitive impairment caused by TPM and reported that 10% of patients taking TPM had cognitive impairment. Most of the adverse cognitive events caused by this drug occur early in treatment (i.e., within 6 weeks), are dose-dependent and are generally mild to moderate.

5. Lamotrigine (LTG)

   To understand the effects of LTG on the cognition of healthy people, Meador [422] conducted a study in which TPM was used as a control. The results showed that LTG performance was significantly improved across 33 (80%) variables in 47 controls. Therefore, compared with TPM, LTG has little effect on adverse cognition and behavior.

6. Pregabalin (PGB)

   Salinsky M [388] conducted a double-blinded parallel study of 32 healthy volunteers taking PGB, and 30 subjects completed the experiment (94%). Three of the six target cognitive measures showed significant differences between the PGB and placebo groups, suggesting that PGB has negative effects on patient cognition and that these effects are one of the factors to consider when choosing a drug.

7. Felbamate (FBM)

   FBM was originally approved as an adjunct for focal and general seizures associated with Lennox–Gastaut syndrome (LGS) [423]. However, due to its serious adverse reactions, such as aplastic anemia and hepatotoxicity, its use is significantly limited [423]. Few studies have evaluated cognitive function related to FBM. In a study of children with LGS receiving FBM treatment, it was found that the social interaction, intelligence assessment, attention, initiative performance, and memory improved [424]. However, after stopping FBM treatment, these cognitive functions showed a trend toward degeneration, so the improvement in cognitive function may be related to the reduction in seizures. When evaluating the effectiveness and safety of FBM, emotional and behavioral disorders were found in a small number of cases [425]. There are too few data on the effects of FBM on cognition to draw firm conclusions at this time.

8. Vigabatrin (VGB)

   VGB is a GABA structural analog that acts by irreversibly inhibiting GABA aminotransferase and causing elevated levels of GABA. It is currently approved for the monotherapy treatment of infantile spasms in children from 1 month to 2 years of age and as an adjunct treatment for refractory focal seizures in adults and children aged 10 years and older. Due to the high incidence of adverse effects related to visual field defects, the clinical application of this drug is limited. After taking VGB, there was an increase in adverse psychobehavioral events in patients with focal epilepsy, which were associated with depression and mild mental disorders [426]. According to the digital cancellation test cognitive assessment, VGB dose was associated with a decrease in scores, but VBG had little effect on various other cognitive tests in the study [426, 427]. It is currently thought that the cognitive improvements observed with VGB use in the treatment of infantile spasms are more likely to be the result of reduced seizures. In patients with focal seizures, VGB may be associated with depression and mental disorders.

9. Zonisamide (ZNS)

   ZNS is a carbonic anhydrase inhibitor. Its antiseizure mechanism is mainly related to inhibiting repeated discharges of voltage-gated sodium channels and reducing voltage-sensitive T-type calcium currents [428].

   ZNS may be associated with negative cognition and mood. In general, adverse effects on executive function are reversed when the drug is discontinued. However, in a ZNS long-term follow-up study, deficits in cognition (memory and attention), mood (anxiety and depression), and language persisted even 1 year after treatment, mainly in delayed word recall, connection tests, and verbal fluency. This effect mainly occurred in the high-dose group but also in a small number of low-dose patients. A study of children with epilepsy also revealed that, in the low-dose group (3–4 mg/kg/day), the picture arrangement test scores improved significantly from baseline. In the high-dose group, the word test scores deteriorated significantly, but there was no difference in the percentage of seizure-free patients between the dose groups. In follow-up studies, it was found that the ZNS group had no significant deterioration in school performance based on the Child Behavior Checklist (CBCL) or controlled oral word association test (COWAT) [429].

   In general, studies on the cognitive effects of ZNS are rare. In addition to the impairment of specific language abilities found at higher doses, the effects on cognitive abilities are small.

10. Retigabine (RTG)

    RTG can selectively activate voltage-gated potassium channels (KCNQ2 and KCNQ3) and is mainly used to treat refractory focal seizures in adults [430]. However, due to reports of adverse reactions to retinal and skin pigmentation, the use of the drug was limited, and it was voluntarily withdrawn from the market in the U.S. in 2017. In earlier studies, there was no significant difference between the RTG group and the placebo group in terms of cognitive assessment results, such as the Wisitory Assessment Scale (WISA) memory test, Stroop test, digital cancellation test, and oral fluency test [431, 432].

11. Rufinamide (RUF)

    RUF is a triazole derivative approved in 2008 for the additive treatment of LGS-associated seizures. The mechanism of action of RUF may be related to the prolonged deactivation of voltage-gated sodium channels, which maintains the stability of the neural membrane [433].

    Among children with LGS, CBCL scores (including behavioral and emotional problems, attention, and sleep) in the RUF treatment group did not change significantly from baseline [434]. In patients aged 7–58 years with LGS assessed using the Leiter-R, VABS, and CBCL, there was also no significant change in cognitive scores at baseline or treatment endpoints [435]. Even at different doses (200–1600 mg/day), there was no significant deterioration in cognitive function in the RUF dose group [436]. Therefore, RUF does not seem to be associated with negative cognitive effects, but the sample sizes of the studies were small, and additional evidence is needed.

12. Eslicarbazepine (ESL)

    ESL is a voltage-gated sodium channel blocker for the treatment of focal seizures in patients 4 years of age and older [437]. In studies of adjunctive therapy for ESL, there was no significant difference from baseline scores on the Cognitive Drug Study (CDR) system for attention, continuity of attention, quality of working memory, or memory speed, but ESL had a significant negative effect on episodic memory that worsened over time [438]. However, in the assessment of healthy volunteers, ESL and oxcarbazepine are considered to have similar cognitive characteristics and do not cause clinically relevant cognitive impairment. Compared to oxcarbazepine, ESL has a lower incidence of adverse events [439].
13. Cannabidiol (CBD)

    CBD is indicated for the treatment of patients older than 2 years of age with Dravet syndrome, LGS, or refractory epilepsy. A number of studies on the treatment of refractory epilepsy with CBD have shown no differences in adaptive behavior or cognitive function between the CBD treatment group and the placebo group [440]. Although the samples in these studies were small, no negative effects on cognitive outcomes were reported.
14. Fenfluramine (FFA)

    FFA is used to treat Dravet syndrome in patients older than 2 years. The antiseizure mechanism of FFA may be related to its stimulating effect on the release of serotonin. Evidence from short-term placebo-controlled trials [441, 442] suggests that there is no deterioration in cognitive function in Dravet syndrome patients treated with FFA and that there is some degree of improvement in some cognitive subdomains. However, cognitive improvements may be associated with seizure control.
15. Everolimus (EVO)

    EVO acts as a mammalian target of rapamycin (mTOR) inhibitor and is primarily used to treat seizures associated with tuberous sclerosis complex (TSC) [443]. In TSC children, as assessed by the WISC, the CBCL, the Dutch Children's Communication Checklist, and the Short Sensor Profile, EVO was found to have no significant effect on cognitive outcomes [444]. The overall conclusion was that EVO treatment did not cause additional cognitive impairment or developmental defects in children with TSC. The effects of EVO on cognitive and developmental outcomes in patients with TSC may be difficult to determine due to the cognitive and developmental impairments associated with this condition, but early successful treatment of seizures may help mitigate developmental deficits.
16. Gabapentin (GBP)

    GBP is an analog of gamma-aminobutyric acid (GABA), whose antiseizure effect is mediated by the inhibition of voltage-gated calcium channels [445]. GBP is often used clinically as an adjunct to other ASMs. GBP can lead to behavioral disorders [318] and can worsen existing behavioral problems in children, especially attention deficit hyperactivity disorder (ADHD) [327]. The worsening of behavioral disorders may have adverse effects on cognition. However, other researchers hold the opposite view, and according to the Rutter scale assessment, GBP does not cause behavior deterioration [446]. Therefore, further studies on the effects of GBP on cognition are needed.

17. Clobazam (CLB)

    CLB is widely used to treat developmental and epileptic encephalopathy, including Dravet syndrome, due to its well-tolerated, safe, and broad-spectrum anti-seizure activity. In children previously treated with CLB, there was no significant decline in cognitive ability [408], but attention should be given to the tolerance of CLB treatment [447]. There are relatively few drug studies on CLB, and it is generally believed that CLB has little impact on cognitive function and that the sedative effects of higher doses of CBL are correspondingly increased. For example, in Dravet syndrome, in combination with other ASMs (VPA or CBD), timely dose adjustment is required to reduce drowsiness [448].

18. Oxcarbazepine (OXC)

    OXC is a carbamazepine analog whose antiseizure effect is mediated by voltage-sensitive sodium channel blockade. In OXC versus CBZ and/or VPA studies, the duration of a computer search task was similar between groups [449, 450]. In a comparative study of OXC and PHT, OXC was slightly superior to PHT only in the energy assessment portion of the Brief Profile of Mood States (BPOMS) [404], suggesting that OXC may not be associated with patient cognitive impairment. Improvements in some cognitive areas may be the result of improved seizure control rather than a direct effect of medication.

In summary, patients using different ASMs have different cognitive characteristics, and the drug dose, blood concentration, drug titration speed, drug combination and drug treatment duration affect patient cognitive function. Clinicians should pay attention to changes in the cognitive functions of patients to balance the relationship between adverse reactions and drugs.

8.5.3.3 Prenatal Injury

Mari Videman [387] studied 56 children born to mothers who had taken ASMs before birth. In comparison with 62 children who did not receive ASMs before birth, the children of mothers taking CBZ, OXC, or VPA had significant cognitive impairment after birth, while those taking LEV or LTG had no effect on cognitive function. This finding suggests that prenatal exposure to ASMs may impair speech and that this effect may occur as early as infancy.

8.5.3.4 Developmental and Epileptic Encephalopathy (DEE)

DEE is one of the most common clinical epileptic syndromes. These patients often have significant cognitive impairments, and frequent seizures often require the use of ASMs. Adam Strzelczyk et al. [394] investigated the selection of drugs for patients with DEE. VPA, CLB, TPM, CBD, FFA, LEV, BRV, TPM, ZNS, PER, stiripentol, LTG, RUF, VGB, LCM, and EVO were studied. LEV, ZNS, and PER may have some effect on the emotional activity of patients but not on obvious cognitive function damage. TPM and ZNS were associated with language impairment and cognitive retardation/memory problems. The remaining ASMs do not appear to have harmful effects.

8.5.3.5 Relevant Factors

1. The extent of cognitive dysfunction that occurs after taking ASMs is often related to the number of drugs taken. Robert J Quon et al. [451] analyzed 224 patients from three datasets and reported that patients receiving multiple drugs had worse subjective cognitive impairment than did those taking only one ASM agent. Lei Wang [383] studied the cognitive dysfunction of 257 patients with epilepsy and also found that there were significant differences in the impact on cognitive function between the single-drug group and the group taking more than two ASMs. Pranvera Hoxhaj [452] analyzed 25 papers on cognitive impairment in epilepsy in PubMed and the Cochrane Library and reported that the cognitive impairment of patients may be related to the use of multiple ASMs.
2. Dose and blood concentration: The effect of ASMs on the cognitive function of patients is related not only to the type and quantity of drugs used but also to the doses of drugs taken. The combination of drugs and the use of large doses of ASM are more likely to cause cognitive impairment [453].

8.5.4 Diagnosis

Neuropsychological testing has been the primary method for objectively examining cognitive dysfunction associated with ASM use [454]. The ABNAS, the Depression Health Questionnaire (PHQ-9), the Generalized Anxiety Disorder 7-Item (GAD-7) scale, the Epilepsy Quality of Life (QOLIE-10), and the EuroQOL five-dimensional questionnaire (EQ-5D) are all commonly used scales for neuropsychological measurement. The Oldenkamp Baker Neuropsychological Assessment Form (ABNAS) is a patient-reported scale that has been validated to measure the adverse cognitive effects of ASMs. Lauren Feldman [390] studied the cognitive impairment of 670 patients with epilepsy and reported that the variables most closely related to subjective cognitive impairment were the PHQ-9 score, the number of ASMs taken, and the frequency of seizures. Identifying these three predictors provides a clear framework for understanding and addressing subjective cognitive complaints in adults with epilepsy.

8.5.5 Treatment

1. Optimizing the use of ASMs

   Adverse cognitive events associated with ASM use can be avoided by slow dosing, the use of the lowest effective dose, and the avoidance of multiple treatments [392]. Marco Mula et al. [391] also noted that the cognitive impairment caused by TPM could be significantly reduced by using monotherapy, individualized dosing, and titration schemes. Early detection and treatment of cognitive impairment can help minimize its impact on patients' quality of life [452]. Teiichi Onuma [399] proposed that, from a therapeutic perspective, simplifying the use of ASMs, avoiding multiple medications, and avoiding overdoses are important in almost all cases.
2. Reducing or stopping the medications

   At present, studies have not shown that ASMs cause cognitive impairment severe enough to require reduction or withdrawal of medication. However, when necessary, reduction and withdrawal are still the main methods used to reduce injury.

8.6 Anti-Seizure Medications and SUDEP

8.6.1 Definition and Classification

Sudden unexpected death in epilepsy (SUDEP) is not a specific disease but rather a cause of death in patients with epilepsy. In 1997, Nashef first proposed a definition of SUDEP: sudden, unexpected, witnessed or unwitnessed, nontraumatic, and nondrowning death in patients with epilepsy, with or without evidence for a seizure and excluding documented status epilepticus, in which postmortem examination does not reveal a toxicological or anatomic cause for death [455]. Nashef's definition of SUDEP is based on rigorous autopsy results and is suitable for studying its pathogenesis. In the same year, to meet the needs of epidemiological investigation and research, Annergers classified SUDEP into four types: defined (autopsy required), probable (no autopsy, no clear cause of death), possible (cannot be excluded but lacks sufficient evidence to indicate SUDEP), and unlikely (with other clear causes of death) [456]. In 2012, Nashef et al. revised the previous definition of precise diagnosis, clarifying the use of "unexpected" instead of "unexplained" in the terminology. SUDEP should occur within 1 h after onset, and status epilepticus is defined as having an onset time $\geq$30 min or no recovery period between them. Three new classifications were also added: definite SUDEP plus, near-SUDEP, or near-SUDEP plus and unclassified (Table 8.3).

Table 8.3 Research classification for sudden unexpected death in epilepsy [457]

Classification	Definition
Definite sudden unexpected death in epilepsy (SUDEP)	Sudden, unexpected, witnessed or unwitnessed, nontraumatic, and nondrowning death that occurs in benign circumstances in an individual with epilepsy; with or without evidence for a seizure; and excludes documented status epilepticus, in which postmortem examination does not reveal a cause of death
Definite SUDEP plus	A death satisfying the criteria for definite SUDEP; if a concomitant condition other than epilepsy is identified before or after death; if the death might have been due to the combined effect of both conditions; and if autopsy or direct observations or recording of the terminal event did not prove the concomitant condition to be the cause of death
Probable SUDEP or probable SUDEP plus	Same definition as definite SUDEP or SUDEP plus but without autopsy
Possible SUDEP	A competing cause of death is present
Near-SUDEP or near-SUDEP plus	A patient with epilepsy who survives resuscitation for more than an hour after cardiorespiratory arrest and has no structural cause identified after investigation
Not SUDEP	A clear alternative cause of death is identified
Unclassified	Incomplete information available; impossible to classify

8.6.2 Historical Evolution

In 1975, Terrence CF. [458] first reported the presence of unexplained SUDEP. They reported the autopsy results of 36 cases of SUDEP, no anatomical or chemical evidence was found to explain this phenomenon. Eight years later, they performed an autopsy on eight epilepsy patients who died suddenly of unknown causes, noting evidence of neuronal pulmonary edema, and they concluded that the patient was generally considered to have died instantly, but the presence of neurogenic pulmonary edema may provide an opportunity for them to be cured [459]. In 1985, Lund A [460] noted that ASMs may play an important role in the death of these patients. In 1986, Dasheiff RM et al. [461] suggested that patients tended to have fatal arrhythmias before death. They [462] reported the characteristics of seven cases of unexplained SUDEP patients who were to be treated with surgery. In 1993, m E Drake et al. [463] reported the absence of heart disease in SUDEP cases, suggesting that arrhythmias may not be the only pathological mechanism. In 1997, Shorvon S [464]. Li et al. summarized for the first time the risk factors for SUDEP, deepening the understanding of the death of this patient.

8.6.3 Epidemiology

In a 2017 American Academy of Neurology meta-analysis on the incidence of SUDEP that included 12 studies, the overall incidence of SUDEP was 0.58 cases per 1000 person-years, the incidence of SUDEP in children was 0.22 cases per 1000 person-years, the incidence of SUDEP in adults was 1.2 cases per 1000 person-years, and the risk of SUDEP in adults was higher than that in children [465]. Previous studies have shown that SUDEP is the most important cause of death in young patients with epilepsy [466]. Therefore, it is very important to identify and intervene early in the risk factors for SUDEP.

8.6.4 Possible Mechanisms of SUDEP

8.6.4.1 Respiratory Dysfunction

Respiratory depression and apnea occur during and after a seizure, which contributes to the development of SUDEP. Central apnea after seizures is closely associated with SUDEP. A study reviewing cardiorespiratory arrest occurring in multiple epilepsy monitoring units between January 2008 and December 2009 reported video-EEG and ECG data for 10 SUDEP patients who developed rapid breathing (18–50 breaths/min) after generalized tonic–clonic seizure (GTCS), died immediately after sudden cardiorespiratory arrest within 3 min of onset, or developed transient cardiorespiratory arrest, followed by recovery of this cardiorespiratory dysfunction; additionally, cardiorespiratory arrest recurred within 11 min after the end of the attack, during which apnea tended to precede cardiac arrest [467]. Another study yielded similar results and concluded that central apnea following seizure can occur both in focal and generalized epilepsy, representing a phenomenon that may serve as a biomarker of SUDEP [468]. The mechanism of central apnea following seizures is currently unknown. Previous studies have shown that central apnea is associated with the limbic system, including the amygdala, hippocampus, parahippocampal gyrus, etc. [469]. A study using intracranial electrodes to record seizures in patients with intractable epilepsy while performing high-resolution head MRI and monitoring respiration revealed that central apnea and oxygen desaturation developed when seizures spread to the amygdala, and direct electrical stimulation of the amygdala also showed similar respiratory manifestations, suggesting that there may be a functional link between the amygdala and brainstem respiratory structures, resulting in the development of SUDEP [470].

8.6.4.2 Cardiac Dysfunction

Altered cardiac function and respiratory depression during seizures are associated with oxygen desaturation. Myers et al. reported that QT prolongation on an electrocardiogram reading was associated with the proportion and duration of oxygen desaturation during seizures, suggesting that abnormal repolarization of the heart during seizures is associated with respiratory depression [471]. In addition, inherited ion channel disorders and arrhythmias resulting from ASMs are possible mechanisms of SUDEP. Researchers have identified multiple genetic mutations, including mutations in the KCNAl, SCN1A, SCN8A, HCN2, PRR72, KCNQ1, KCNH2, SCN5A, and RYR2 genes, in patients who died suddenly from epilepsy [472]. Mutations in KCNQ1 (Kv7.1), KCNH2 (Kv11.1), and SCN5A (Nav1.5) are the most frequent mutations in known genes related to congenital long QT syndrome (LQTS) [473]. Patients with LQTS are susceptible to ventricular tachycardia and torsade de pointes and are at risk of sudden death. SCN1A encodes the α1 subunit of a sodium channel and is the most common genetic mutation found in patients with Dravet's syndrome (DS) [474]. SCN1A is expressed in both the brain and heart, and its mutations can cause fatal bradycardia and inhibit heart rate variability [475–477]. Although the cardiac mechanism of SUDEP has been investigated, it remains unknown whether respiratory dysfunction is involved in SUDEP of DS patients. In addition, lamotrigine may inhibit the delayed rectifier potassium current, which is associated with an increased risk of QT interval prolongation, cardiac arrhythmias, and sudden death [39]. Phenytoin and carbamazepine act as sodium ion channel blockers that slow cardiac conduction [10]. Carbamazepine also reduces heart rate variability, which is associated with SUDEP risk [478].

8.6.4.3 Sympathetic Denervation

Sympathetic activation occurs and continues during and after GTCS seizures. Elevated cerebrospinal fluid and serum norepinephrine and epinephrine concentrations have been reported to persist for more than 30 min following GTCS attacks [479]. Parasympathetic activity also gradually increases after attacks, and together with sympathetic activity, it promotes the development of SUDEP [480]. Heart rate variability (HRV) is a widely used objective method to assess cardiac autonomic activity and is considered a biomarker for predicting SUDEP. Sivathamboo et al. compared 5-min HRV during sleep and wakefulness in 31 SUDEP patients and 56 controls and found that short-term low-frequency power decreased and high-frequency power increased in the SUDEP group compared with the control group, indicating relative parasympathetic activation in SUDEP [481]. Cardiopulmonary dysfunction in SUDEP patients in epilepsy monitoring units, as well as the findings on HRV in this study, suggest that tachyarrhythmia caused by increased sympathetic activity is not the main mechanism of SUDEP, and increased parasympathetic activity causes bradyarrhythmia, which may be the mechanism of most SUDEPs.

8.6.4.4 Postictal Generalized EEG Suppression (PGES)

PGES is common after GTCS, and PGES was observed in all SUDEP patients in the epilepsy monitoring unit study [467]. Alexandre et al. also described a significantly increased risk of PGES when GTCS occurred during sleep and without early oxygen administration [482]. An extended PGES (>50 s) may have the greatest predictive value for SUDEP [483]. Tao et al. reported that nearly all patients were inactive or unresponsive to speech and stimuli during PGES, and this unresponsiveness may affect brainstem protective reflexes and prevent arousal and postural changes [484]. PGES is associated with respiratory dysfunction, arousal disorders, and autonomic dysregulation [484–486]. More studies are needed to confirm the role of PGES in the pathophysiology of SUDEP.

8.6.4.5 Postictal Arousal Deficits

Impaired consciousness and arousal: Abnormal cortical discharges can spread to the midbrain and medulla oblongata and affect specific nuclei in the ascending arousal system (AAS). This system is composed of discrete neurotransmitter-specific nuclei, including the raphe nuclei [487], the locus coeruleus [488], the ventral tegmental area [489], the pedunculopontine and laterodorsal tegmental nuclei [490], and the parabrachial complex [491], which may alter the levels of consciousness in people with epilepsy. Blumenfeld proposed the network inhibition hypothesis, which states that consciousness is maintained through interactions between cortical and subcortical structures [492]. Once aberrant discharges start in the cortex, they travel along known anatomical connections to subcortical structures and activate GABAergic interneurons that inhibit the AAS. Following AAS inhibition, cortical activity is suppressed, resulting in loss of consciousness. Single photon emission computed tomography imaging showed that cerebral blood flow increased from temporal lobe structures and decreased in the midbrains and brainstems of patients with complex partial seizures of the temporal lobe [493]. Recordings of cholinergic neurons in the pedunculopontine tegmental nuclei demonstrated that acetylcholine-responsive neurons in the AAS are inhibited during limbic seizures [35]. Loss of consciousness due to AAS inhibition leaves a patient with epilepsy at greater risk for SUDEP, as protective reflexes are suppressed during the postictal coma.

8.6.4.6 Other Molecular Mechanisms

Brainstem neurotransmitters, including adenosine, 5-hydroxytryptamine (5-HT), norepinephrine, acetylcholine, and glutamate, play important roles in the development of SUDEP [480]. Adenosine and 5-HT have opposite effects on respiration; adenosine induces apnea, whereas 5-HT is associated with recovery from apnea. In a recent study, Faingold et al. proposed a hypothesis regarding the roles of adenosine and 5-HT in SUDEP. GTCS leads to the release of neuroactive adenosine substances. Adenosine induces respiratory depression by acting on neurons in the rostroventral nucleus of the medulla oblongata, which in turn reduces central drive to the lungs, resulting in apnea. Moreover, apnea leads to an increase in pCO2, which activates pontine raphe neurons and increases the release of 5-HT, which triggers the automatic recovery mechanism of respiration by activating periaqueductal gray neurons. If these mechanisms are insufficient to overcome apnea, SUDEP can occur [494].

8.6.5 Epilepsy and SUDEP

Currently known risk factors for SUDEP include GTCS frequency, nocturnal seizures, early age of onset, and long duration of epilepsy [495].

One study showed that GTCS frequency was the main risk factor for SUDEP, even after Hesdorffer et al. fully adjusted the confounding factors of GTCS frequency. The results showed that GTCS frequency increased the risk of SUDEP. The risk in patients who developed GTCS 1–2 times per year increased 2.94-fold compared with that in patients who did not have GTCSs, while the risk of SUDEP in patients who developed GTCS more than 50 times per year increased 14.51-fold compared with that in patients who did not have GTCSs [496]. Moreover, studies conducted in Sweden, the United States, and the United Kingdom revealed that the risk of SUDEP in patients who had experienced one or more GTCS episodes was 7.1-fold greater than that in epileptic patients without GTCS, and the more frequent the GTCS was, the greater the risk of SUDEP was [497].

Clark et al. analyzed autopsy findings in 123 SUDEP patients in Australia and reported that approximately 70% of these patients died at night [498]. Lamberts et al. studied 154 SUDEP patients and 616 controls and reported that the SUDEP group was more likely to experience epileptic seizures at night than was the nonsurviving group; nocturnal seizures tended to increase the risk of SUDEP, with a 3.9-fold greater incidence of SUDEP than in the control group, suggesting that nocturnal seizures may be an independent risk factor for SUDEP [499]. In addition, SUDEP patients are often found in the prone position at night, and Liebenthal et al. described 253 SUDEP patients whose body position at the time of death. A total of 73.3% of these patients reportedly died in the prone position; random-effects model analysis revealed a significant relationship between nocturnal prone position and SUDEP compared with the nonprone position [500]. Nilsson et al. found a relative risk of 7.72-fold for SUDEP with onset between 0 and 15 years of age compared to epilepsy with onset after 45 years of age [470]. In a prospective case–control study, the risk of SUDEP was 13.9 times greater in patients with a disease duration ≥30 years than in those with a disease duration <15 years [500].

8.6.6 ASMs and SUDEP

In recent years, the relationship between ASMs and SUDEP, including the effective doses and appropriate choices of ASMs, the number of ASMs taken by a patient, and ASM regimen compliance, has been intensively studied.

Effective doses and appropriate choices of ASM therapy reduce the risk of SUDEP. In a large case–control study in 2005, Langan et al. reviewed the case data of 154 autopsied patients and reported that SUDEP occurred 21.7 times more frequently in patients who did not receive any ASMs than in patients who received 1–2 ASMs [501]. In a 2011 meta-analysis that included 112 randomized double-blinded controlled studies, data on 33 deaths, including 20 deemed SUDEP deaths, were extracted from the 112 eligible randomized trials. Eighteen deaths were classified as definite or probable SUDEP, and two were classified as possible SUDEP. Definite or probable SUDEP, all SUDEP, and all causes of death were significantly less frequent in the efficacious ASM group than in the placebo group, with odds ratios of 0.17 (95% CI 0.05–0.57), 0.17 (0.05–0.57), and 0.37 (0.17–0.81), respectively. The rates of definite or probable SUDEP per 1000 person-years were 0.9 (95% CI 0.2–2.7) in patients who received efficacious ASM doses and 6.9 (3.8–11.6) in those allocated to the placebo group [33]. There appears to be broad agreement that if a significant difference is detected between the proportion of SUDEP victims taking a certain ASM and the proportion taking the same drug among controls, then when evaluating whether there is a causal relationship, the numbers should be corrected for the frequency of GTCSs [497, 502, 503]. Importantly, however, it has not been acknowledged that in correcting for seizure frequency, the influence of ASM efficacy, which has been demonstrated to be crucial in the prevention of SUDEP, is simultaneously eliminated [33]. A relationship could be regarded as causal, in the sense that an increased occurrence of SUDEP may be caused by an unfavorable choice of ASM that provides inferior protection against GTCSs. Although treatment of refractory epilepsy with ASMs sometimes fails to provide good seizure control and may even lead to side effects, effective doses of ASMs and appropriate choices of ASM therapy reduce the occurrence of SUDEP.

Noncompliance to ASM therapy has also been proposed as a precipitating factor for SUDEP. Noncompliance to ASM therapy tends to induce seizures, especially poorly controlled GTCS seizures, thereby increasing the incidence of SUDEP. In 1999, Opeskin et al. compared postmortem ASM levels in 44 patients who died of SUDEP and 44 patients who died of other causes, suggesting noncompliance if ASMs were undetectable or if ASMs did not reach therapeutic levels. The study revealed no significant differences in undetectable ASMs, those not reaching therapeutic levels, or those reaching therapeutic levels between the SUDEP group and the control group, indicating that compliance with ASM treatment was not reduced in the SUDEP group [504]. Drugs are redistributed in the body after death in humans, so the reliability of detecting ASM levels in autopsied blood needs to be confirmed. Human hair grows at a rate of 1 cm per month, and the drugs taken can penetrate the hair and remain relatively stable; therefore, changes in postmortem hair ASM concentrations are considered to reflect changes in patient antemortem ASM intake. Williams et al. described greater changes in hair ASM concentrations in SUDEP patients than in patients with common epilepsy, suggesting that compliance with antemortem ASM medication was reduced in the SUDEP group [505]. Nilsson et al. found a significantly greater incidence of SUDEP with frequent changes in ASM dose than with stable-dose therapy in a retrospective study (RR = 6.08) [506]. Shankar et al. combined findings regarding changes in hair ASMs and self-reports in patients to define SUDEP, and the results were consistent with those of previous studies [507]. After multivariate adjustment, Faught et al. assessed adherence to treatment with ASMs by drug occupancy and found that noncompliance tripled mortality rates in patients with epilepsy [508]. In general, noncompliance with ASM therapy increases the risk of SUDEP, but there is no uniform definition or assessment criteria for adherence to medication usage, which may be responsible for the different results across studies. Improper treatment or poor compliance with ASM therapy leads to poor control of seizures, especially GTCSs, and promotes the development of SUDEP through various mechanisms, including cardiopulmonary dysfunction, autonomic dysfunction, arousal deficits, PGES, and brainstem dysfunction [480].

Combined treatment with multiple ASMs does not increase the risk of SUDEP. In a 1995 Canadian cohort study, the incidence of SUDEP increased with the number of ASMs taken, with men who used ≥3 ASMs having the highest incidence of SUDEP. Poisson regression analysis showed that the incidence of SUDEP increased 1.7-fold with each increase in the maximum dose of ASMs [509]. In a case–control study published in Lancet in 1999, the risk of SUDEP increased with the number of ASMs used, and the incidence of SUDEP was 9.89-fold greater in epileptic patients treated with three ASMs simultaneously than in those treated with monotherapy [507]. Similar results were described in two subsequent studies [501, 510]. A recent Swedish study including 255 epileptic patients who died of SUDEP and 1148 controls showed that polypharmacy with ASMs, particularly the use of three or more ASMs, was associated with a reduced risk of SUDEP (OR = 0.31), and combinations including lamotrigine (OR = 0.55, 95% CI: 0.31–0.97), valproic acid (OR = 0.53, 95% CI: 0.29–0.98), and levetiracetam (OR = 0.49, 95% CI: 0.27–0.90) reduced the risk. No specific ASMs were associated with increased risk. Regarding monotherapy, levetiracetam users had the lowest risk of SUDEP (OR = 0.10, 95% CI: 0.02–0.61) [34], although this difference was limited. Therefore, the number of ASMs taken has little to do with the high risk of SUDEP, which may only reflect the severity of seizures [497].

There is insufficient evidence to support an association between particular ASMs and the risk of SUDEP. In 1998, Timmings et al. reported that 85% of SUDEP victims who were on ASM therapy at the time of death were treated with CBZ, while only 38% were treated with CBZ [53]. In this cohort, as many as 10 of the 14 SUDEP victims had idiopathic generalized epilepsy (IGE) [511], and 11/14 were taking CBZ, which, when used to treat IGE, may cause aggravation of seizures [512]. In a 2001 study, serum CBZ concentrations were greater in SUDEP patients than in controls, particularly in patients receiving polypharmacy or frequent dose changes [513]. This may be because patients with severe epilepsy tend to be treated with higher doses of drugs; CBZ cannot be identified as an independent risk factor for SUDEP. A large study that included 216 SUDEP patients concluded after correcting for the frequency of GTCSs that neither the use of CBZ nor that of any other ASM could increase the risk of SUDEP [497]. Lamotrigine is another common sodium channel blocker. On October 9, 2020, the US FDA issued a safety warning regarding lamotrigine: taking lamotrigine increases the risk of arrhythmias. The avoidance of lamotrigine is recommended for patients with structural heart disease or cardiac conduction abnormalities. This warning is based on the findings of in vitro studies regarding lamotrigine that have shown that therapeutic doses of lamotrigine lead to class IB antiarrhythmic effects, which widen QRS waves and may induce new arrhythmias and sudden death. However, it is important to note that the FDA did not have sufficient clinical evidence to issue this warning. To address this issue, Bunschoten et al. conducted a rapid systematic review of studies related to lamotrigine and sudden death/electrocardiographic abnormalities in 2022, which included a total of 26 studies and assessed the quality of the included studies using the American Academy of Neurology's Risk of Bias Assessment Tool. Most of the included studies had a high risk of bias, so there was insufficient evidence to support or refute that lamotrigine was associated with sudden death/electrocardiographic changes [81]. In a UK study of pregnant patients with epilepsy, 11 of 14 epilepsy-related deaths were considered to have resulted from SUDEP, and 9 of these patients were taking lamotrigine, which seems to suggest that lamotrigine is associated with SUDEP. However, recent observations from the European and International Antiepileptic Drug and Pregnancy Registry suggest that women taking lamotrigine have decreased plasma concentrations during pregnancy and that epilepsy during pregnancy is difficult to effectively control, which may provide a reasonable explanation for the association between lamotrigine and SUDEP [514]. Appropriate dosage increases should be made during pregnancy to maintain plasma concentrations of lamotrigine, to prevent seizures as much as possible, and to reduce the risk of potential adverse events such as SUDEP. Dono et al. evaluated the effects of perampanel (PER) administration on cardiac autonomic control in patients affected by drug-resistant temporal lobe epilepsy (TLE) and found that at baseline, no differences were detected between the PER group and the non-PER group according to time-domain and frequency-domain HRV parameters. At follow-up, in the PER group, a multiplicative effect for the interaction between treatment and time was observed for MeanRR, LnRMSSD, LnHF, HF, and HF%, with increased values, supporting the notion that PER increases vagal tone in DRTLE. This activity may exert a cardioprotective effect by reducing the risk of developing cardiac arrhythmias, and future studies will need to test the protective effects of PER on SUDEP [515].

Congenital long QT syndrome (cLQTS) is a group of arrhythmia syndromes caused by mutations in genes encoding myocardial cell membrane ion channel proteins, resulting in ion channel dysfunction. Clinically, it is characterized by a prolonged QT interval, QT variability, multiform ventricular tachycardia, torsade de pointe ventricular tachycardia, episodic syncope, and sudden cardiac death, and it is the main cause of paroxysmal syncope and sudden death in children and young people [516, 517]. Increasing amounts of evidence suggest that heart and neuronal channel diseases overlap. Many cardiac ion channel genes that cause cLQTS are also expressed in the brain [518]. Animal studies [519, 520], clinical studies [512, 521], and randomized reports [81, 514, 515, 517] suggest that heart channel disease may also be associated with epilepsy. In randomized reports of SUDEP in patients with generalized epilepsy accompanied by high fever convulsive syndrome (GEFS+) and DS, the genetic predisposition to fatal arrhythmias has been discussed, as the gene product of SCN1A (NaV1.1) is expressed in the hearts of mammals. Although nonchannel or noncardiac mechanisms may be involved in the association between ASMs and SUDEP, the key question is whether drugs with the potential to prolong QT intervals increase the risk of fatal epilepsy-related arrhythmias in genetically susceptible individuals. Several ASMs are associated with abnormalities in the cardiac conduction system and rhythmicity, mainly in predisposed individuals [72, 522]. CBZ and intravenous PHT can give rise to sinus bradycardia, sinus arrest, and atrioventricular block [523], whereas lacosamide has shown a tendency to induce atrioventricular block [524]. In addition, the QT interval can be increased by retigabine and CBZ, and primidone can shorten it [521, 525]. PHT, phenobarbital (PB), and LTG have been shown to inhibit IKr [39, 496], and a possible role in SUDEP has been suggested. However, among epidemiological studies focusing on a possible relationship between ASMs and SUDEP, only CBZ and LTG have been implicated [77].

In addition, the use of ASMs can reduce the number of red blood cells, and the resulting insufficient oxygen supply can lead to cardiopulmonary and metabolic conditions during seizures [514, 526]. Evidence from patients taking CBZ to control seizures suggests that ASM use may also alter plasma fatty acid profiles since fatty acids contribute to membrane properties, and disruption of this profile may affect neural and cardiac excitability [527]. However, the clinical relevance of ASMs to the development of SUDEP remains unclear and requires further investigation.

There is a growing body of evidence that ASMs are not associated with an increased risk of SUDEP at the population level. Nevertheless, there is evidence that carbamazepine and lamotrigine may be associated with QT prolongation and arrhythmias, and that carbamazepine can affect the cardiac conduction system and reduce HRV in susceptible patients. Whether these effects of lamotrigine and carbamazepine lead to an increased risk of SUDEP remains to be evaluated. The effects of these ASMs may be limited to genetically susceptible individuals and may be too rare to be identified in epidemiological studies or clinical trials. The latest evidence from a meta-analysis of randomized, placebo-controlled clinical trials of effective dose-assisted ASMs strongly supports the protective effect of combination therapy with ASMs against multiple drugs. Meta-analyses have shown that seizure control can prevent SUDEP, and combined ASM therapy has a protective effect on SUDEP occurrence in patients with refractory epilepsy. This information provides guidance to doctors and highlights the need to control seizures to prevent SUDEP.

8.7 The Impact of ASMs on Pregnancy

Globally, approximately 12.5 million women of childbearing age suffer from epilepsy. The prevalence of women with epilepsy (WWE) of childbearing age in the United States is between 1.1 and 1.5 million, with approximately 24,000 WWE giving birth each year [528]. Given the high prevalence of epilepsy in women, ASMs are commonly taken before and during pregnancy. Changes in physiology and metabolic parameters during pregnancy can lead to fluctuations in ASM blood concentrations, increasing variability in patient responses to these medications. Subtherapeutic concentrations of ASMs in mothers may increase seizure frequency, as well as the risk of miscarriage and preterm birth. Conversely, exposure to ASMs can affect WWE in multiple ways. It is worth exploring whether ASMs could impact fertility and contraceptive efficacy in women of childbearing age, potentially leading to failed pregnancies or contraception; furthermore, exposure to ASMs can lead to various potential fetal abnormalities, including abnormal neurodevelopment. For the WWE population, the key to ASM therapy is maintaining seizure control while minimizing the potential adverse impacts of ASMs before and after pregnancy, including during planned conception, contraception, pregnancy, and breastfeeding. Since epilepsy is a chronic condition that often requires lifelong treatment, considerations for potential pregnancies should begin at the time of diagnosis to determine the most appropriate, and especially the safest, treatment using ASMs. The safest therapeutic approach should also be selected according to the woman's needs, concerns, and desires. Comprehensive preconception counseling should cover the control of seizures and the risks associated with medication therapy for both the individual and the fetus.

This chapter focuses on the adverse effects of ASMs on WWE, with specific attention given to the impacts of prepregnancy administration of ASMs on conception, contraception, reproductive ability in WWE, fetal exposure during pregnancy, and the effects of ASMs on breastfeeding.

8.7.1 Impact of ASM on Contraception in WWE

Contraception failure, defined as unintended pregnancy during treatment, can have a significant effect on emotional health and overall wellness. Hormonal contraceptives, particularly oral formulations, are widely used globally for family planning. The real-world effectiveness of these drugs is determined by factors such as obesity, smoking status, adherence to therapy, and potential drug interactions.

Interactions between ASMs and hormonal contraceptives have significant implications for WWE. Liver enzyme-inducing ASMs accelerate the metabolism of estrogens and progestins, leading to contraception failure, as observed with phenytoin, carbamazepine, phenobarbital, and topiramate [529, 530]. Moreover, the use of oral contraceptives may reduce the concentrations of ASMs like lamotrigine, thereby increasing the risk of epileptic seizures [530]. Greater awareness of these interactions may assist in optimizing epilepsy treatment for women.

The hepatic metabolism of estrogen and progestin is most pronounced when ASMs that induce cytochrome P450 enzymes, such as phenytoin, phenobarbital, and carbamazepine, are used. ASMs that induce uridine diphosphoglucuronosyltransferase (UGT) enzymes, such as lamotrigine and oxcarbazepine, to a lesser extent influence estrogen and progestin metabolism [529–531]. Topiramate is an exception among UGT enzyme inducers; its impact on estrogen and progesterone levels is minimal at doses less than 200 mg/day but increases significantly at doses greater than 200 mg/day [532]. Recent real-world research has also confirmed that low-dose (≤200 mg/day) topiramate probably does not affect oral contraceptive effectiveness [533].

Table 8.4 categorizes ASMs into those capable of reducing the effectiveness of oral contraceptive pills (OCPs) via enzyme-inducing effects and those without this action [3]. For WWE taking ASMs that can affect OCP levels, it is preferable to avoid OCPs, if possible, and to use barrier methods (i.e., condoms, diaphragms, or sponges) or intrauterine devices (IUDs). These latter contraceptive devices include traditional IUDs, the Copper T, and the modern levonorgestrel-releasing IUD [530].

Approximately half of WWE reported their pregnancies as unplanned [534]. Recent research from the Epilepsy Birth Control Registry (EBCR) indicates that nearly 60% of WWE are at risk of unintended pregnancy [535]. Most women (approximately 65%) taking enzyme-inducing ASMs are unaware of the interaction with hormonal contraceptives, increasing the risk of unintended pregnancy [536]. This finding underscores the importance of advising on contraception and preconception. Contraceptive counseling should be a crucial aspect of care for WWE.

Table 8.4 List of ASMs that do and do not affect hormonal contraception through hepatic enzyme induction

ASMs That Decrease the Effectiveness of Hormonal Contraceptives	ASMs That Do Not Change the Effectiveness of Hormonal Contraceptives
Carbamazepine (Tegretol, Tegretol XR, Carbatrol, Equetri)	Acetazolamide (Diamox)
Phenobarbital	Clonazepam (Klonopin)
Phenytoin (Dilantin)	Diazepam (Valium)
Primidone (Mysoline)	Valproic Acid (Depakote, Depakene)
Clobazam (Onfi)	Ethosuximide (Zarontin)
Felbamate (Felbatol)	Gabapentin (Neurotin, Graslise, Horizant)
Eslicarbazepine (Aptiom)	Lacosamide (Vimpat)
Lamotrigine (Lamictal)[a]	Levetiracetam (Keppra)
Oxcarbazepine (Trileptal)	Lorazepam (Ativan)
Preampanel[b]	Pregabalin (Lyrica)
Rufinamide (Banzel)	Tigabine (Gabitril)
Topiramate (Topamax)[c]	Vigabatrin (Sabril)
	Zonisamide (Zonegran)

Adapted from Reddy [530]

[a]Lamictal is a weak inducer at doses of 300 mg daily or more

[b]Perampanel is a weak inducer at doses of 12 mg or higher

[c]Topiramate induces hormonal contraceptives at doses of 200 mg daily or higher

8.7.2 Impact of ASM on the Fertility and Reproductive Capability (Fecundity) of WWE

A survey from the UK indicated that 33% of WWE respondents chose not to have children due to epilepsy [532]. For women with a desire to conceive, whether they can conceive and have live births like their peers of the same age is a matter of concern.

Recent research on whether the fertility and fecundity of women with epilepsy are impaired has produced conflicting results. Most studies suggest that the fertility rate of WWE ranges from 37% to 88% of that observed in other groups. For instance, data from a group of patients collected in Rochester from 1935 to 1974 showed that fertility rates declined to 80% of the expected values in affected males and 85% in affected females [537]. Additionally, a retrospective survey of reproductive histories of nearly 1000 WWE was conducted via the EBCR to assess infertility (nonpregnancy within a year) and impaired fecundity (percentage of infertility or failure to achieve live birth) [538]. They reported an infertility rate of 9.2% and an impaired fecundity rate of 20.7% among WWE, which are higher than the approximate 6.5% and 12.7%, respectively, reported in the general population [538]. The EBCR study also revealed a trend toward impaired fecundity among individuals receiving multi-therapy ASMs, with live-birth/pregnancy rates being greater in those receiving lamotrigine therapy than in those receiving valproate therapy [538]. Contrasting with these results, a retrospective cohort study from Iceland revealed no overall difference in birth rates between WWE and age-matched controls or between patients with barring epilepsy combined with cerebral palsy or intellectual disability [539].

Fertility rates are influenced by multiple factors, including social factors, frequency of intercourse, and biological factors. Even if previous studies reported lower birth rates in WWE, it is challenging to distinguish between biological and social contributions. Pennell and colleagues designed the first prospective study on this topic [540]. A unique feature of the WEPOD cohort is that all women planned their pregnancies in advance, which differs from pregnancy registries or population studies. An advantage of this study is its use of digital diaries to record medication use, seizures, sexual activity, and menstrual bleeding. Together with the measurement of progesterone levels to confirm ovulation, these findings enabled the investigation of potential previously unexplored fertility factors [540]. This study revealed that WWE seeking to conceive without known infertility or related diseases had similar likelihoods, times to conception, and live birth rates as did their peers without epilepsy [540].

By comparing the infertility risk associated with ASMs, several studies have indicated that multiple-drug and single-drug treatment plans have similar successful pregnancy rates for WWE [541]. However, a prospective cohort study from India reported that the use of three or more AEDs and phenobarbital was associated with increased infertility risk [542]. Studies from the International Registry of ASMs and Pregnancy report that polytherapy with ASMs increases miscarriage risk, and part of the research (including the WEPOD cohort) might not have detected this difference because fewer women received polytherapy.

Research indicates a greater incidence of anovulatory cycles and sexual dysfunction in WWE than in women without epilepsy. Enzyme-inducing ASMs (including valproate/sodium valproate) have been shown to influence female hormones and cause high rates of menstrual disorders. For instance, Isojarvi JI reported that VPA could cause menstrual disorders in up to 45% of WWE (menstrual disorders were defined as amenorrhea, oligomenorrhea, a long cycle, or irregular menses for at least 6 months) [543]. Women taking sodium valproate for epilepsy often experience menstrual irregularities and hyperandrogenism. Valproate therapy is associated with polycystic ovary syndrome (PCOS), which is even more common when used before the age of 20 [543]. Some ASMs (such as PHT, PB, VPA, CBZ, etc.) may interfere with the hypothalamic-pituitary-gonadal axis, leading to imbalances in estrogen and progesterone secretion. All these side effects could be potential factors affecting the fertility and fecundity of WWE (for details, please see the part "8.3 Endocrine Effects of ASMs in patients").

8.7.3 *Impact on Fetal Outcomes of ASM Exposure During Pregnancy*

8.7.3.1 ASM-Related Teratogenic Risk-Established Pregnancy Registry

This registry provides observations on potential teratogenicity due to the use of ASMs. The first 12 weeks of pregnancy are the key period for embryonic organ development. Major congenital malformations (MCMs) that threaten life or require surgical intervention, such as cardiac malformation, neural tube defects, urogenital malformation, skeletal malformation, and cleft palate, often occur during this period [544]. Overall, when embryos are exposed to ASMs in utero, the probability of MCMs occurring is approximately 4–9%, which is 2–3 times greater than that in the general population (approximately 1–2%) [545].

Studies have shown that the teratogenic risk of ASMs is related to the type of medication and dosage of treatment and whether it involves multidrug treatment. These findings can help rational selection of these medications. A study of the UK Epilepsy and Pregnancy Register showed that pregnant WWE exposed to ASMs during pregnancy had an overall incidence rate of fetal MCMs of only 4.2%, which was slightly greater than that of pregnant WWE who were not exposed to ASMs (3.5%). However, the rate significantly increased in the multidrug treatment groups, especially when valproic acid was included [545]. A prospective study by the EURAP compared the incidence of MCMs with the use of eight types of ASMs. The most common compound was valproic acid (10.3%), followed by phenobarbital (6.5%), and phenytoin (6.4%), with carbamazepine (5.5%) and topiramate (3.9%) in the middle [546]. Oxcarbazepine (3.0%), lamotrigine (2.9%), and levetiracetam (2.8%) had relatively high safety levels, with the incidence of MCMs corresponding to pregnant WWE who were not taking ASMs [546]. The data related to topiramate and phenytoin should be interpreted cautiously because, in that study, the sample sizes exposed to these two drugs were smaller [546]. The North American Registry of Pregnancy in Epilepsy also showed that ASMs such as sodium valproate and phenobarbital have a greater risk of major deformities than newer ASMs such as lamotrigine and levetiracetam [547]. Compared to a reference population, topiramate is associated with an increased risk of cleft lips [547]. Additionally, dose-dependent studies in the EURAP series of registered studies suggest a dose-dependent risk of ASM teratogenicity [548]. When the LTG dose is <300 mg/day, the teratogenic risk is the lowest (2.0%), and this dose was therefore used as an internal reference for the study. When the VPA dose is >1500 mg/day, the teratogenic risk is particularly high, with an incidence rate exceeding 25%. In comparison, all the doses of VPA used in the study, PB and the highest dose of CBZ (>1000 mg/day) significantly increased the risk of congenital malformations. The teratogenic risk when the VPA dose is <700 mg/day is equivalent to that when the dose is CBZ <1000 mg/day, PB <150 mg/day, or LTG >300 mg/day, reaching approximately 6.3%. Therefore, it is equally important to adjust drug doses and select drug types when managing epilepsy in pregnant women. In addition, the study revealed that those with a family history of congenital malformations are more than four times more likely to have malformations in their offspring.

As our understanding of the pregnancy safety of ASMs has improved, there has been a shift in prescription practices for ASMs by medical professionals. Reports on ASM prescription practices are available worldwide. In the UK, France, Italy, and Nordic countries such as Denmark, Finland, Iceland, Norway, and Sweden, lamotrigine is the most commonly used ASM for pregnant women with epilepsy [549, 550]. Several studies have reported trends in ASM use during pregnancy in the United States. A NEAD study showed that between 1999 and 2004, carbamazepine, sodium valproate, phenytoin, and lamotrigine were the most commonly prescribed single therapies. In contrast, the newer Maternal Outcomes and Neurodevelopmental Effects of Anti-Epileptic Drugs (MONEAD) study showed that between 2012 and 2016, lamotrigine and levetiracetam were the most common monotherapies, and their combined use was the most common multiple-drug therapy [551]. The increasing trend of lamotrigine and levetiracetam use has also been reflected in research from North America and Italy [547, 552].

In the past decade, following the introduction of new third-generation ASMs to the market, the use of ASMs associated with increased MCM risks has further declined. Compared to traditional ASMs, newer ASMs are generally regarded as having more favorable pharmacokinetics, but they are not without risk, as they may undergo significant pharmacokinetic changes when an individual becomes pregnant. The inclusion population of pregnancy registry studies on the teratogenic risk of newer ASMs is still small, and the level of evidence is relatively low [553]. In recent years, as doctors' prescriptions of ASMs have gradually switched to newer ASMs, the incidence of MCMs in fetuses born to mothers receiving single-drug treatment has significantly declined. These findings suggest that newer ASM agents may be effective at ensuring pregnancy safety [553]. However, due to the unknown changes in pharmacokinetics during pregnancy and the lack of evidence related to medication safety during pregnancy, choosing these drugs still presents a challenge.

8.7.3.2 Impact of ASM on Psychomotor Development in Infants Postbirth

The long-term effects of in utero ASM exposure on fetal brain development are also worth noting. Recent research results have suggested that VPA exposure during pregnancy in women with epilepsy is related to decreased IQ, decreased learning ability, and autism spectrum disorders [554, 555]. No evidence suggests that other ASM agents have adverse effects on psychomotor development after birth in infants. Meta-analyses have confirmed that the effect of ASMs on the IQ of children who have been exposed to ASMs in utero depends on the dosage [556]. There was no significant difference in the impact on IQ among the four drugs, including lamotrigine, carbamazepine, phenytoin, and sodium valproate, in the low-dose group. In the high-dose group, the impact of VPA was significant.

8.7.3.3 Low Folic Acid Levels and Teratogenic Risks

While the probability of birth defects in children born to women with epilepsy (WWE) is greater than that in those born to healthy individuals, more than 90% of children can be completely normal through careful selection of medications, dosages, and proper interventions. A low level of folic acid is associated with neural tube defects, miscarriages, and intrauterine fetal growth restriction; thus, daily supplementation with small doses of folic acid plays a significant role in preventing fetal neural tube defects [544]. The results from the NEAD study [557] showed that the consumption of folic acid by women suffering from epilepsy is also beneficial to the psychomotor development of the fetus postbirth. It is generally suggested that WWE who are taking ASMs require more folic acid supplementation than does the general population, especially when they are concurrently using ASM, which counteract folic acid, such as valproic acid, phenobarbital, phenytoin, and carbamazepine [558].

8.7.3.4 Obstetric and Perinatal Outcomes

The MONEAD study [559] involved the prospective examination of a cohort of 351 pregnant WWE for severe adverse events. Generally, maternal use of ASMs does not seem to correlate with early adverse outcomes in newborns. There were no differences in head circumference, gestational age at birth, 5-min Apgar score, or birth weight between neonates born to WWE and those born to control individuals. However, specific monotherapies seem to influence fetal growth. On average, among infants born to epileptic mothers receiving monotherapy with topiramate, the largest decrease in birth weight *Z* scores was observed [559].

There have also been studies indicating that ASM may have an effect on gestational age in newborns. In a multinational, prospective, observational study carried out in the U.S. and the U.K. [560], the effect of single antiepileptic medication on gestational age was examined. "Small for gestational age" was defined as a birth weight lower than the 10th percentile for that specific gestational age. The results showed that the risk of a newborn being small for gestational age was greater for mothers who consumed valproic acid (VPA) during pregnancy than for those who consumed phenytoin (PHT) or lamotrigine (LTG) and was greater for those who consumed carbamazepine (CBZ) than for those who consumed PHT and LTG. The presence of microcephaly suggests poor neurodevelopment during the embryonic and fetal stages. Among newborns and 12-month-old infants, those exposed to CBZ and VPA during the embryonic stage had a greater incidence of microcephaly.

8.7.4 Breastfeeding

Breastfeeding has many benefits, including promoting an intimate relationship between the mother and baby, reducing the risk of the mother developing conditions such as breast cancer and ovarian cancer, decreasing the likelihood of diabetes, infections, and sudden infant death syndrome, and positively influencing infant neurocognitive development. WWE who are on long-term oral antiepileptic medications often express greater concerns about the safety of breastfeeding for their babies. Studies indicate that the rate of commencement of breastfeeding among WWE is 30% lower than that among other pregnant women [561].

By measuring the levels of antiepileptic medications in breast milk and the sera of breastfeeding infants, it is currently suggested that almost all ASMs can make their way into breast milk. For instance, a recent study by Birnbaum and colleagues assessing the serum antiepileptic drug levels in 138 breastfeeding infants, while also testing the corresponding concentrations in postpartum mothers exposed to ASMs, revealed that infant serum drug concentrations were much lower than maternal serum levels and were usually below the lower limit of the serum concentration reference range [561]. The infant serum ASM concentrations are generally lower, ranging from 0.3% to 44.2% of maternal concentrations.

Despite the fact that ASMs can be secreted into breast milk, breastfeeding by women exposed to ASMs is largely safe. Women with epilepsy should be encouraged to breastfeed their children, whether or not they are on antiepileptic medication [562]. The relative infant dose (RID) is a significant parameter for evaluating the risk of drug excretion in breast milk, with an RID of less than 10% considered safe. The RID of most ASMs is less than 10%, but those of phenobarbital and topiramate exceed 10, at 24% and 24.5%, respectively [561, 563]. Moreover, maternal use of ASMs while continuing to breastfeed does not impede mental or motor development in their children, either immediately or later in life [564]. However, during the breastfeeding period, it is important to closely monitor the newborn for any adverse reactions related to ASMs (including somnolence, difficulty breastfeeding, hyperirritability, and crying); if present, breastfeeding should be temporarily ceased.

Surveys have shown that about half of pregnant WWE receive counseling about breastfeeding from a neurologist, and those who do so are more likely to breastfeed their babies. In fact, counseling about breastfeeding can increase the likelihood of continuing breastfeeding after 6 weeks. As such, counseling on breastfeeding is crucial for WWE.

8.8 Rhabdomyolysis Caused by ASMS

Rhabdomyolysis (RM) is a clinical syndrome that results in muscle cell degradation products and contents being released into the systemic circulation, resulting in a series of symptoms, such as electrolyte imbalance, acid–base disorder, coagulation abnormality, and renal dysfunction [565–567]. The clinical manifestations are acute myasthenia, myalgia, and muscle swelling, with creatine kinase (CK) levels elevated to >1000 U/L. Mild RM is defined as CK levels that are more than 5 times the upper limit of normal. Myoglobinuria and acute kidney injury (AKI) suggest that severe RM [568–571] may occur in patients using ASMs, leading to asymptomatic elevated serum CK levels and more serious complications, such as arrhythmia, electrolyte disturbance, acute renal failure, hypovolemic shock, and diffuse intravascular coagulation (DIC) [572].

8.8.1 Epidemiology

Rhabdomyolysis was first described in Germany in 1881 [573] but was not described in detail until World War II by Bywaters and Beall et al. [574]. Because the diagnostic criteria for rhabdomyolysis syndrome do not have a unified consensus, clinical data and clinical statistics are relatively rare. Some patients with mild rhabdomyolysis syndrome may not be clearly diagnosed, and prospective studies of its incidence are lacking, with approximately 26,000 patients diagnosed with rhabdomyolysis syndrome in the U.S. each year [568]. A study by Chamberlain et al. [575] revealed that out of 1500 pediatric patients who came for counseling, 4 were diagnosed with rhabdomyolysis syndrome.

8.8.2 Etiology

The etiology of rhabdomyolysis syndrome can be roughly divided into physical and nonphysical factors. Physical factors include trauma and tissue crushing injury, excessive exercise, muscle ischemia, and temperature changes. Nonphysical factors include the use of medicine and drugs, infections, electrolyte disorders, endocrine diseases, autoimmune diseases, and genetic defects [572]. Use of ASMs is among the most common causes of rhabdomyolysis.

8.8.3 Clinical Manifestations

The clinical manifestations of rhabdomyolysis vary from a single asymptomatic increase in the serum creatine kinase concentration to severe electrolyte disturbance, arrhythmia, acute renal failure, DIC, etc. [576], which is closely related to the extent of muscle injury.

8.8.3.1 Main Clinical Manifestations

Early manifestations of rhabdomyolysis syndrome are difficult to diagnose and have a missed diagnosis rate of 50%. Rhabdomyolysis may be characterized by many nonspecific symptoms, such as myalgia, swelling, weakness, fever, nausea, vomiting, confusion, delirium, and anuria [577]. However, rhabdomyolysis is typically characterized by acute or subacute onset myalgia, transient myasthenia, and chromaturia, which is known as the triad of rhabdomyolysis. Muscle weakness can occur anywhere in the body, but the most common area is near the lower extremities. Chromaturia refers to the presence of large amounts of myosin (>1.5–3.0 mg/L) in the urine [567]; however, the probability of triad co-occurrence is less than 10% [578].

8.8.3.2 Major Complications

Acute Renal Failure

The most serious complication of rhabdomyolysis is acute renal failure, which is caused by tubular necrosis due to myosin accumulation, the incidence of which is 14–46% [579], and the incidence of acute renal failure in children with rhabdomyolysis syndrome is 42–50% [580]. Studies have shown that when the serum creatine kinase concentration is 5000–15,000 IU/L, the incidence of acute renal failure is 35%, and when the serum creatine kinase concentration is greater than >15,000 IU/L, the incidence is 70% [581].

Liver Failure

In 25% of patients, liver failure occurs as a result of liver inflammation caused by the release of proteases from liver cells [582].

Inflammatory Response and Multiple Organ Dysfunction Syndrome (MODS)

After rhabdomyolysis, a large number of inflammatory mediators and cytokines are released that promote endothelial damage, resulting in inflammation. Sepsis tends to occur when vascular intima or skin damage and coagulation dysfunction promote the occurrence of MODS, and multiple-organ failure often causes death [578].

Others

Other complications include compartment syndrome, hypercalcemia (late stage), hypocalcemia, hyperphosphatemia, hyperkalemia, and disseminated intravascular coagulation (DIC). Severe hyperkalemia can lead to arrhythmia, resulting in cardiac arrest, and a large amount of phosphate release can lead to hypocalcemia, which can also cause arrhythmia [583].

8.8.3.3 Imaging Examination

B-ultrasonography or magnetic resonance imaging of locally swollen tissue can reveal muscle necrosis, determine the extent of muscle injury and liquefaction, and constitute a noninvasive method for diagnosing muscle necrosis.

8.8.4 Rhabdomyolysis Caused by Different ASM Agents

8.8.4.1 Levetiracetam

Levetiracetam is an acetylpyrrolidine compound that has recently been used in the clinic. In December 1999, the FDA officially approved this adjunctive treatment for partial seizures in adults older than 16 years, and in June 2005, the indication was expanded to children older than 4 years [584]. Hisanao Akiyama et al. [585] described a 29-year-old female patient with a history of epilepsy who had been taking 1000 mg/day valproic acid and 20 mg/day oxazepam orally. The patient was treated for recurrent epilepsy, and levetiracetam (1000 mg/day) and valproic acid (800 mg/day) were added to her treatment regimen on the third day after admission. On the fourth day, the patient began to experience back muscle pain and weakness in both lower limbs, and the symptoms gradually worsened. Laboratory tests revealed CK values greater than 2410 IU/L. Levetiracetam treatment was stopped immediately, her symptoms improved rapidly, and her serum CK level returned to normal. Isaacson JE et al. [586] described a case of rhabdomyolysis caused by levetiracetam. The patient was a 19-year-old male with a history of epilepsy who presented with two convulsions. A significant increase in creatine phosphokinase (CPK) was observed after treatment with levetiracetam, and CK levels quickly returned to normal after withdrawal of levetiracetam. A similar case involving a 13-year-old girl was described by Incecik F et al. [587]. Moinuddin et al. [588] reviewed previous case reports of 13 patients with LEV-induced rhabdomyolysis and found that most of the patients were young adults or adolescents aged between 19 and 30 years, and only one patient was over 60 years old. The peak serum CK concentrations varied widely, ranging from 1368 IU/L to 49,539 IU/L, and these differences may have been related to differences in muscle mass. Elevated CK levels were observed within 12–36 h of LEV initiation, indicating a need for close observation during the initial treatment phase. In most cases, it takes 3–5 days from LEV initiation to achieve peak CK levels, and CK levels gradually recover after discontinuation. Clinical symptoms (back pain and muscle pain) were present in 5 of the 13 patients. The exact mechanism by which LEV causes rhabdomyolysis is unclear, but the current hypothesis is that LEV interacts with the SV2A protein in the motor nerve endings of slow-twitch muscle fibers, resulting in enhanced cholinergic neurotransmission and increased muscle stress and leading to rhabdomyolysis [588].

8.8.4.2 Phenytoin Sodium

Phenytoin sodium has been used for antiepileptic treatment since 1938, and its main side effects include nystagmus, gingival hyperplasia, hypersensitivity, hematopoietic dysfunction, etc. [589] The first case of PHT-induced rhabdomyolysis was described in 1986 [590] in a 22-year-old male with epilepsy who was diagnosed with PHT-induced rhabdomyolysis after 3 months of PHT (300 mg/day) therapy for myalgia, fever, and rash, elevated serum creatine kinase (CK) levels (242,000 IU/L), and brown urine. After admission, PHT was discontinued, and 30 mg of intravenous infusion of methylprednisolone was given for 3 days, followed by 100 mg of prednisone orally once a day. Hormone therapy was gradually discontinued on the 7th day after admission, and the patient's condition gradually improved. Santos-Calle et al. [591] described a 46-year-old patient with sudden generalized tonic–clonic seizures. After intravenous infusion of 1250 mg PHT and intravenous infusion of 150 mg Q8h, the CK level increased significantly (54,000 IU/L) 5 days later, and the CK level finally decreased and gradually returned to normal after drug withdrawal. Clinical symptoms disappeared, supporting the diagnosis of PHT-induced rhabdomyolysis. Korman et al. [592] described a similar case of PHT-induced rhabdomyolysis with renal and liver failure. Similarly, PHT (1000 mg/day) treatment in a 33-year-old male epilepsy patient resulted in elevated serum CK levels (2370 UI/L), which returned to normal 6 days after withdrawal [593]. Intravenous PHT was administered to a 37-year-old male with status epileptic disorder for 7 consecutive days, resulting in increased serum CK levels (3825 IU/L), and CK levels returned to normal after withdrawal [594], supporting the report that phenytoin sodium can cause rhabdomyolysis.

8.8.4.3 Sodium Valproate

Sodium valproate began to be used clinically in 1963 because of its high permeability to the blood–brain barrier and low incidence of toxic side effects, it is often used in children. Its side effects include intestinal reactions, pancreatitis, liver injury, headache, nystagmus, ataxia, dizziness, etc. [595].

In 1990, Roodhooft et al. [596] first described a child with progressive disturbance of consciousness, anuria, and rhabdomyolysis due to overdose of VPA, followed by renal failure. In 1997, Pinkston [593] described a patient with drowsiness, headache, and no urine for 24 h when the dosage of sodium valproate was increased to 500 mg BID. The CK level in the patient's urine was 1242 IU/L, suggesting that rhabdomyolysis was related to VPA toxicity. Patients with carnitine fatty acyltransferase type II (CPAII) deficiency are prone to rhabdomyolysis after treatment with valproic acid. Patients with CPAII defects have intermittent myoglobinuria and even rhabdomyolysis. The diagnosis is supported by acute rhabdomyolysis and renal failure after valproic acid administration. The authors speculate that patients with CPAII type defects (typical 113 serine-to-leucine mutations) should be particularly cautious in the administration of valproic acid [597] and that carnitine should be added to valproic acid treatment of high-risk patients with rhabdomyolysis [598]. In addition to adults, rhabdomyolysis due to valproic acid has also occurred in newborns [599]. Valproic acid may also be associated with rhabdomyolysis in the treatment of bipolar disorder or the prevention of migraine. Creatine kinase levels should be closely monitored for early treatment of rhabdomyolysis.

8.8.4.4 Gabapentin

Gabapentin was approved by the FDA in 1994 for the treatment of partial seizures [592], and it has common adverse effects, including vertigo, drowsiness, fatigue, and ataxia. Rhabdomyolysis syndrome is a rare complication of gabapentin [572]. Bilgir et al. [600] described rhabdomyolysis in a 63-year-old woman with diabetes after taking gabapentin. Patients started treatment at a dose of 900 mg/day, and after 3 weeks, they developed pain and weakness in the lower limbs, a decreased urine volume, and changes in urine color. Laboratory tests revealed increased CK levels, positive urine myoglobin, myogenic injury on electromyography, and rhabdomyolysis synthesis by muscle biopsy. Falconi et al. [601] reported that after 3 days of gabapentin administration in a 65-year-old diabetic male patient, laboratory examination confirmed an increase in the muscle necrosis index. Immediate discontinuation of the drug and peritoneal dialysis treatment was applied, and both clinical and biochemical indicators improved. Tuccori Mario et al. [600] described a similar case of severe birth myopathy in a diabetic female treated with gabapentin (450 mg/day), which recovered completely after 10 days of discontinuation. Similarly, a 31-year-old female patient had elevated serum CK levels (44,360 UI/L) after

3 weeks of gabapentin treatment (3000 mg/day). Recent reports of gabapentin-induced rhabdomyolysis and the need for renal replacement therapy at both normal and excessive doses suggest that muscular toxicity during gabapentin therapy is not dependent on dosage or time.

8.8.4.5 Lamotrigine

Lamotrigine was developed and synthesized in the UK in 1978 and began to be marketed in 1990. It is used for the treatment of partial seizures and general tonic–clonic seizures [602], and adverse reactions, including headache, fatigue, nausea, dizziness, lethargy, and insomnia, have been reported. It can even cause severe skin erythema and multiple organ failure [572]. In 1994, Schaub JE et al. [603] reported that a patient taking 1000 mg/day carbamazepine and 2 mg/day clonazepam had poor epileptic control and was switched to lamotrigine. When the initial dose of 25 mg/day was increased to 100 mg/d within 2 weeks, skin lesions, maculopapules, hyperthermia, lethargy, ataxia and other symptoms appeared. Laboratory tests revealed a CK value of 7770 IU/L, a myoglobin level of 3600 g/L, and a creatinine level of 234 μmol/L, suggesting lamotrigine hypersensitivity syndrome combined with rhabdomyolysis syndrome. Chattergoon et al. [604] described two cases of multiple-organ dysfunction and DIC 9 days after the addition of LTG. Michael et al. [605] described a patient with depression who overdosed on lamotrigine in an attempt to commit suicide. Her blood CK level at admission was 616 IU/L, which increased to 6517 IU/L 1 day after admission, and her creatinine level was 1.1 mg/dL (normal value 0.3–1.3 mg/dL), indicating moderate rhabdomyolysis syndrome. After treatment, her creatine phosphokinase level decreased, and her symptoms were relieved, suggesting the possibility of drug-induced rhabdomyolysis. Later, Kicka M [75] reported other related events. Kicka M [75] also described a case of a suicide attempt in a patient taking lamotrigine, leading to deep coma, respiratory depression, epileptic status, hyperkalemia, and rhabdomyolysis.

8.8.4.6 Propofol

Propofol was approved by the FDA in 1989 and has been increasingly used to treat status epilepticus [606]. Propofol perfusion-related syndrome (PRIS) may occur during the use of propofol and is characterized by symptoms and signs related to metabolic acidosis, hyperkalemia, heart failure, and rhabdomyolysis that cannot be explained by other reasons based on long-term massive infusion of propofol. In 1992, Parke [607] reported that a pediatric patient developed PRIS after receiving 7.5–10 mg/kg/h propofol for 66–115 h. To study the incidence, risk factors, and biomarkers of PRIS caused by propofol, Diaz JH et al. [608] conducted a 1-year retrospective study and showed that the incidence of PRIS was 4.1%, the mortality rate was 33%, and the duration of propofol infusion was positively and linearly correlated with the blood triglyceride level. In 1998, Hanna JP [609] et al. reported a case of rhabdomyolysis, progressive hypoxia, and metabolic acidosis in a child and an adolescent treated with propofol for refractory status epilepticus. One patient, a 17-year-old male, was given 80 mg of propofol (167 pg/kg/min for the first hour), after which the dose was increased from 147 mg/kg/min to 292 mg/kg/min. After 44 h of use, propofol was discontinued due to severe hypoxia, brown urine, and a creatine kinase level of 83,000 UL. The total dose of propofol given was 19,275 mg (482 mg/kg). The patient died 84 h after treatment, and an autopsy indicated rhabdomyolysis. The other patient was a 7-year-old male who received a propofol dose starting at 33.3 mg/kg/min, which was subsequently increased to 449 mg/kg/min. Brown urine appeared 38 h after propofol administration, and his creatine kinase level was elevated to 49,992 UL. Propofol treatment was discontinued after 63 h, at which time the total dose was 35,330 mg (1275 mg/kg), and the autopsy indicated rhabdomyolysis. Some experts believe that for children with serious diseases, the use of propofol should be limited to 67 μg/kg/min [610]. Zarovnaya [611] described a case in which adult epileptic patients also developed PRIS after receiving large amounts of propofol. When PRIS occurs, propofol treatment should be stopped immediately, and cardiopulmonary support should be provided. Hemodialysis and plasma exchange may be helpful.

8.8.4.7 Pregabalin

Pregabalin is a novel calcium channel regulator that is mainly used to treat peripheral neuralgia [612]. In 2004, it was approved in the United States and the European Union as an adjunctive treatment for focal epilepsy in adults and has since been approved in the United States for focal seizures in children older than 4 years of age [612]. Several reports from phase III clinical trials before it was marketed as an ASM suggested that pregabalin could cause CPK level elevation [613].

Gunathilake et al. [614] described a 66-year-old female patient with an ankle fracture who was treated with 75 mg pregabalin twice a day and subsequently developed severe muscle pain. During the physical examination, the patient had weakness in the proximal upper and lower extremities and decreased muscle tone. Urine tests were positive for myosin, increased creatine kinase, acute renal failure, and neutrophilia. The diagnosis of rhabdomyolysis syndrome can be based on clinical signs, biochemical results, and reactions after withdrawal. Diuretics are added to cope with renal failure, and humoral therapy is actively administered. Kidney function returned to normal at 48 h, creatine kinase levels returned to normal after 7–8 days, and muscle strength improved.

8.8.5 Diagnosis

Early detection, diagnosis, and treatment of rhabdomyolysis are key to preventing death.

8.8.5.1 Clinical Manifestations

A high awareness of the possibility of ASMs causing rhabdomyolysis is the most important condition for early diagnosis and treatment because less than 10% of patients experience the RM triad. Clinicians need to be alert to the presence of other nonspecific symptoms. Detailed neuromuscular examination of limbs, blood pressure, sensory disturbance, muscle strength, and volume abnormalities are important diagnostic clues.

8.8.5.2 Laboratory Diagnosis

An important basis for laboratory diagnosis is the serum creatine kinase concentration. Although there is no consensus on diagnostic criteria, it is generally considered that a level more than 5 times the highest normal value indicates RMS [577]. The level of CK can predict the incidence of acute renal failure, and when the CK value is greater than 5000 IU/L, kidney damage is likely to occur [615].

Urine test strips can be used to determine whether the patient is positive for myoglobinuria. Myoglobinuria is an important basis for diagnosing RM, but negative myoglobinuria does not exclude RM [616]. Since the half-life of myoglobin is shorter than that of serum creatine kinase, myoglobin concentrations return to normal after 6–8 h of muscle injury, so myoglobin levels are not sensitive to CK values.

A large amount of creatine released by muscle destruction is converted into creatinine in the blood, so the increase in creatinine in rhabdomyolysis patients is often greater than the increase in urea nitrogen, and the BUN/creatinine ratio is reduced; this helps to distinguish the renal failure from that of other causes [617].

8.8.6 Differential Diagnosis

8.8.6.1 Myositis

Symptoms of myositis may persist for more than a week, with elevated CK values persisting until treatment begins. In patients with rhabdomyolysis, CK levels automatically return to normal after a few days or a week. A muscle biopsy can help diagnose this disease.

8.8.6.2 Rhabdomyolysis due to Epilepsy or Status Epilepticus

The increase in CK levels in patients with postseizure rhabdomyolysis syndrome usually peaks at 24–48 h, whereas the CK level in ASM-induced rhabdomyolysis syndrome tends to peak at approximately 7 days.

8.8.7 Therapy

Identifying the cause of RM and timely treatment are the keys to treatment. If RM is caused by ASMs, their use should be stopped immediately. Routine treatments include intravenous fluids, alkalizing urine, correcting metabolic disorders, and kidney replacement therapy.

8.8.7.1 Fluid Therapy

Early rehydration with isotonic saline or balanced crystals can help protect the kidneys by increasing the glomerular filtration rate and urine output. The infusion must start within 6 h of muscle injury, the infusion speed should be maintained at 1.5 L/h, and the urine volume should be maintained at 200–300 mL/h. Intravenous fluids should be continued until CK levels drop below 1000 IU/L. Close monitoring is also needed to prevent large amounts of fluid from entering the body, which can lead to congestive heart failure and pulmonary edema, especially in elderly individuals or those with cardiopulmonary conditions.

8.8.7.2 Fixing Electrolyte Imbalance

The administration of carbonate can correct acidosis and hyperkalemia, and hemodialysis should be performed when fatal hyperkalemia and metabolic acidosis occur [578].

8.8.7.3 Alkaline Urine

Alkaline urine can accelerate myoglobin clearance and prevent renal tubule blockage, and urine and plasma pH should be maintained at >6.5 and >7.5, respectively [618].

8.8.7.4 Corticosteroids

Corticosteroid toxicity is low. Short-term, high-dose corticosteroids may be an effective treatment option for recurrent rhabdomyolysis that does not respond well to rehydration therapy [619].

8.8.7.5 Kidney Replacement Therapy

Approximately 8–65% of patients with RM require kidney replacement therapy. Early continuous renal replacement therapy (CRRT) can significantly improve the prognosis in patients with RM and AKI. However, for RM without AKI, there is insufficient evidence to show that early blood purification therapy is more effective than conventional drug therapy in preventing AKI.

8.8.8 Prognosis

The prognosis of rhabdomyolysis syndrome depends mainly on the complications and its underlying cause, and if it is managed promptly and properly, the prognosis is better. When the disease progresses to acute renal failure, the prognosis is poor, and the mortality rate of rhabdomyolysis syndrome is 8–10% [620], 42% of patients with acute renal failure, and 8% of patients without acute renal failure [621]. The mortality rate of rhabdomyolysis syndrome in children is 7–10%.

8.8.9 Prevention

ASMs can induce rhabdomyolysis, although the incidence of this disease is low, and can still lead to fatal consequences if they are not detected early. Factors contributing to the increase in ADR caused by ASMs include older age, female sex, comorbidities, combined drug use, etc. [565] In addition, large doses and prolonged ASM use may lead to an increased risk of muscular toxicity. For safe use of ASMs, it is recommended that the dose of ASMs be titrated gradually in clinical practice and that serum CK levels and kidney function be regularly monitored so that prompt diagnosis and treatment can be provided if side effects occur. Recently, there has been increasing evidence that genetic polymorphisms related to pharmacokinetics (such as drug receptors, transporters, and metabolic enzymes) and pharmacodynamics (such as muscle enzymes) contribute to an increased risk of myopathy. In particular, there is ample evidence of an association between certain human leukocyte antigen (HLA) alleles and an increased risk of specific adverse drug reactions. In patients with epilepsy with HLA-B genetic markers, treatment with carbamazepine, phenytoin, lamotrigine, and oxcarbazepine is associated with an increased risk of Stevens–Johnson syndrome. The rarity of ASM-induced myotoxicity in the existing literature may reaffirm the importance of genetic factors in ASM-induced adverse events. In the future, genetic polymorphisms in patients with ASM-induced rhabdomyolysis could help explain the occurrence of this adverse event and help clinicians adjust the type and dose of ASM administered to improve treatment outcomes in these patients.

References

1. Desai R, Rupareliya C, Patel U, et al. Burden of arrhythmias in epilepsy patients: a nationwide inpatient analysis of 1.4 million hospitalizations in the United States. Cureus. 2017;9(8):e1550.
2. Altun Y, Yasar E. Effects of valproate, carbamazepine and levetiracetam on Tp-e interval, Tp-e/QT and Tp-e/QTc ratio. Ideggyogy Sz. 2020;73(3–4):121–7.
3. Zaccara G, Lattanzi S, Brigo F. Cardiac adverse effects of antiseizure medications. Expert Opin Drug Saf. 2022;21(5):641–52.
4. Kloster R, Engelskjøn T. Sudden unexpected death in epilepsy (SUDEP): a clinical perspective and a search for risk factors. J Neurol Neurosurg Psychiatry. 1999;67(4):439–44.
5. Opeskin K, Thomas A, Berkovic SF. Does cardiac conduction pathology contribute to sudden unexpected death in epilepsy? Epilepsy Res. 2000;40(1):17–24.
6. Harris AS, Kokernot RH. Effects of diphenylhydantoin sodium (dilantin sodium) and phenobarbital sodium upon ectopic ventricular tachycardia in acute myocardial infarction. Am J Phys. 1950;163(3):505–16.
7. Centa A, Rasore-Quartino A. The "digito-cardiac" malformative syndrome (Holt-Oram): genetic forms and phenocopy. Probable teratogenic action of antiepileptic drugs. Pathologica. 1965;57(853):227–32.
8. Pfammatter JP, Gertsch M, Weber JW, et al. Stress-induced polymorphous ventricular tachyarrhythmias in two brothers: unusual pattern of inheritance in the long QT syndrome. Clin Cardiol. 1993;16(6):517–20.
9. Steinhoff BJ, Stodieck SR, Tiecks FP, et al. Cardiac side effects and ECG changes with lamotrigine? A clinical study. Schweiz Arch Neurol Psychiatr (1985). 1994;145(3):8–12.
10. Tomson T, Kennebäck G. Arrhythmia, heart rate variability, and antiepileptic drugs. Epilepsia. 1997;38(11 Suppl):S48–51.
11. Kennebäck G, Ericson M, Tomson T, et al. Changes in arrhythmia profile and heart rate variability during abrupt withdrawal of antiepileptic drugs. Implications for sudden death. Seizure. 1997;6(5):369–75.
12. Verrier RL, Pang TD, Nearing BD, et al. The Epileptic Heart: concept and clinical evidence. Epilepsy Behav. 2020;105:106946.
13. Christensen J, Trabjerg BB, Dreier JW. Cardiac morbidity and mortality associated with the use of lamotrigine. Epilepsia. 2022;63(9):2371–80.
14. Lee-Lane E, Torabi F, Lacey A, et al. Epilepsy, antiepileptic drugs, and the risk of major cardiovascular events. Epilepsia. 2021;62(7):1604–16.
15. Avitia RL, Reyna MA, Bravo-Zanoguera ME, et al. QRS complex duration enhancement as ventricular late potential indicator by signal-averaged ECG using time-amplitude alignments. Biomed Tech (Berl). 2013;58(2):179–86.
16. Rejdak K, Rubaj A, Głowniak A, et al. Analysis of ventricular late potentials in signal-averaged ECG of people with epilepsy. Epilepsia. 2011;52(11):2118–24.
17. Ertek S, Cicero AF. Hyperthyroidism and cardiovascular complications: a narrative review on the basis of pathophysiology. Arch Med Sci. 2013;9(5):944–52.
18. Sarecka-Hujar B, Szołtysek-Bołdys I, Kopyta I, et al. Concentrations of the selected biomarkers of endothelial dysfunction in response to antiepileptic drugs: a literature review. Clin Appl Thromb Hemost. 2019;25:1076029619859429.
19. Vyas MV, Davidson BA, Escalaya L, et al. Antiepileptic drug use for treatment of epilepsy and dyslipidemia: systematic review. Epilepsy Res. 2015;113:44–67.
20. Carmona-Vazquez CR, Ruiz-Garcia M, Pena-Landin DM, et al. The prevalence of obesity and metabolic syndrome in paediatric patients with epilepsy treated in monotherapy with valproic acid. Rev Neurol. 2015;61(5):193–201.
21. Mintzer S, Yi M, Hegarty S, et al. Hyperlipidemia in patients newly treated with anticonvulsants: a population study. Epilepsia. 2020;61(2):259–66.

22. Mintzer S, Skidmore CT, Abidin CJ, et al. Effects of antiepileptic drugs on lipids, homocysteine, and C-reactive protein. Ann Neurol. 2009;65(4):448–56.
23. Yang Y, Zhang X, Jin Z, et al. Association of serum uric acid with mortality and cardiovascular outcomes in patients with hypertension: a meta-analysis. J Thromb Thrombolysis. 2021;52(4):1084–93.
24. Karatoprak E, Tosun O. Effects of valproic acid and levetiracetam monotherapy on carotid intima-media and epicardial adipose tissue thickness in non-obese children with epilepsy. Brain Dev. 2020;42(2):165–70.
25. Lai Q, Shen C, Zheng Y, et al. Effects of antiepileptic drugs on the carotid artery intima-media thickness in epileptic patients. J Clin Neurol. 2017;13(4):371–9.
26. Wahid A, Chen W, Wang X, et al. High-mobility group box 1 serves as an inflammation driver of cardiovascular disease. Biomed Pharmacother. 2021;139:111555.
27. Tao S, Sun J, Hao F, et al. Effects of sodium valproate combined with lamotrigine on quality of life and serum inflammatory factors in patients with poststroke secondary epilepsy. J Stroke Cerebrovasc Dis. 2020;29(5):104644.
28. Kicman A, Toczek M. The effects of cannabidiol, a non-intoxicating compound of cannabis, on the cardiovascular system in health and disease. Int J Mol Sci. 2020;21(18):6740.
29. Shayesteh MRH, Haghi-Aminjan H, Mousavi MJ, et al. The protective mechanism of cannabidiol in cardiac injury: a systematic review of non-clinical studies. Curr Pharm Des. 2019;25(22):2499–507.
30. Litovchenko T, Grymailo V, Tondiy O, et al. The peculiarities of the heart rate variability and electroencephalogram changes in patients with epilepsy and cardiovascular pathology. Wiad Lek. 2019;72(2):165–8.
31. Frampton JE. Fenfluramine: a review in Dravet and Lennox-Gastaut syndromes. Drugs. 2023;83(10):923–34.
32. Surges R, Shmuely S, Dietze C, et al. Identifying patients with epilepsy at high risk of cardiac death: signs, risk factors and initial management of high risk of cardiac death. Epileptic Disord. 2021;23(1):17–39.
33. Ryvlin P, Cucherat M, Rheims S. Risk of sudden unexpected death in epilepsy in patients given adjunctive antiepileptic treatment for refractory seizures: a meta-analysis of placebo-controlled randomised trials. Lancet Neurol. 2011;10(11):961–8.
34. Sveinsson O, Andersson T, Mattsson P, et al. Pharmacologic treatment and SUDEP risk: a nationwide, population-based, case-control study. Neurology. 2020;95(18):e2509–e18.
35. Hookana E, Ansakorpi H, Kortelainen ML, et al. Antiepileptic medications and the risk for sudden cardiac death caused by an acute coronary event: a prospective case-control study. Ann Med. 2016;48(1–2):111–7.
36. Danielsson BR, Lansdell K, Patmore L, et al. Phenytoin and phenobarbital inhibit human HERG potassium channels. Epilepsy Res. 2003;55(1–2):147–57.
37. Danielsson C, Azarbayjani F, Sköld AC, et al. Polytherapy with hERG-blocking antiepileptic drugs: increased risk for embryonic cardiac arrhythmia and teratogenicity. Birth Defects Res A Clin Mol Teratol. 2007;79(8):595–603.
38. Redfern WS, Carlsson L, Davis AS, et al. Relationships between preclinical cardiac electrophysiology, clinical QT interval prolongation and torsade de pointes for a broad range of drugs: evidence for a provisional safety margin in drug development. Cardiovasc Res. 2003;58(1):32–45.
39. Danielsson BR, Lansdell K, Patmore L, et al. Effects of the antiepileptic drugs lamotrigine, topiramate and gabapentin on hERG potassium currents. Epilepsy Res. 2005;63(1):17–25.
40. Surges R, Volynski KE, Walker MC. Is levetiracetam different from other antiepileptic drugs? Levetiracetam and its cellular mechanism of action in epilepsy revisited. Ther Adv Neurol Disord. 2008;1(1):13–24.
41. Zaccara G, Lattanzi S. Comorbidity between epilepsy and cardiac arrhythmias: implication for treatment. Epilepsy Behav. 2019;97:304–12.

42. Auerbach DS, Biton Y, Polonsky B, et al. Risk of cardiac events in Long QT syndrome patients when taking antiseizure medications. Transl Res. 2018;191:81–92.e7.
43. Brugada J, Brugada P, Brugada R. The syndrome of right bundle branch block, ST segment elevation in V1 to V3 and sudden death. Cardiovasc Drugs Ther. 2002;16(1):25–7.
44. Al Aloul B, Adabag AS, Houghland MA, et al. Brugada pattern electrocardiogram associated with supratherapeutic phenytoin levels and the risk of sudden death. Pacing Clin Electrophysiol. 2007;30(5):713–5.
45. Druschky A, Hilz MJ, Hopp P, et al. Interictal cardiac autonomic dysfunction in temporal lobe epilepsy demonstrated by [(123)I]metaiodobenzylguanidine-SPECT. Brain. 2001;124(Pt 12):2372–82.
46. Lotufo PA, Valiengo L, Benseñor IM, et al. A systematic review and meta-analysis of heart rate variability in epilepsy and antiepileptic drugs. Epilepsia. 2012;53(2):272–82.
47. Leosuthamas D, Limotai C, Unwanatham N, et al. Is anti-seizure medication the culprit of SUDEP? Neurol Sci. 2023;44(10):3659–68.
48. Yadav R, Schrem E, Yadav V, et al. Lacosamide-related arrhythmias: a systematic analysis and review of the literature. Cureus. 2021;13(12):e20736.
49. Wang J, Huang P, Yu Q, et al. Epilepsy and long-term risk of arrhythmias. Eur Heart J. 2023;44(35):3374–82.
50. Levy RH, Pitlick WH, Troupin AS, et al. Pharmacokinetics of carbamazepine in normal man. Clin Pharmacol Ther. 1975;17(6):657–68.
51. Jacome DE. Syncope and sudden death attributed to carbamazepine. J Neurol Neurosurg Psychiatry. 1987;50(9):1245.
52. Checchini M, Magni M, Scaglione M, et al. Cardiac effects of carbamazepine therapy. Minerva Cardioangiol. 1995;43(9):379–81.
53. Timmings PL. Sudden unexpected death in epilepsy: is carbamazepine implicated? Seizure. 1998;7(4):289–91.
54. Matteoli S, Trappolini M, Curione M, et al. Effects of carbamazepine on heart conduction in young patients: a serial study using ambulatory ECG. G Ital Cardiol. 1994;24(4):391–7.
55. Ide A, Kamijo Y. Intermittent complete atrioventricular block after long term low-dose carbamazepine therapy with a serum concentration less than the therapeutic level. Intern Med. 2007;46(9):627–9.
56. Donnet A, Milandre L, Habib G, et al. Complete atrioventricular block induced by carbamazepine. Ann Med Interne (Paris). 1990;141(5):489–90.
57. Johnson CD, Rivera H, Jiménez JE. Carbamazepine-induced sinus node dysfunction. P R Health Sci J. 1997;16(1):45–9.
58. Spina E, Kenneback G, Bergfeldt L, et al. Prevalence of cardiac conduction disturbances during carbamazepine treatment: preliminary data. Funct Neurol. 1987;2(4):563–7.
59. Boesen F, Andersen EB, Jensen EK, et al. Cardiac conduction disturbances during carbamazepine therapy. Acta Neurol Scand. 1983;68(1):49–52.
60. Kaul S, Meena AK, Murthy JM. Carbamazepine induced bradycardia. Neurol India. 2000;48(4):403–4.
61. Hewetson KA, Ritch AE, Watson RD. Sick sinus syndrome aggravated by carbamazepine therapy for epilepsy. Postgrad Med J. 1986;62(728):497–8.
62. Benassi E, Bo GP, Cocito L, et al. Carbamazepine and cardiac conduction disturbances. Ann Neurol. 1987;22(2):280–1.
63. Peano C, Leikin JB, Hanashiro PK. Seizures, ventricular tachycardia, and rhabdomyolysis as a result of ingestion of venlafaxine and lamotrigine. Ann Emerg Med. 1997;30(5):704–8.
64. Pricone MG, King CV, Drummer OH, et al. Postmortem investigation of lamotrigine concentrations. J Forensic Sci. 2000;45(1):11–5.
65. Walczak T. Do antiepileptic drugs play a role in sudden unexpected death in epilepsy? Drug Saf. 2003;26(10):673–83.

66. French JA, Perucca E, Sander JW, et al. FDA safety warning on the cardiac effects of lamotrigine: an advisory from the Ad Hoc ILAE/AES Task Force. Epilepsy Curr. 2021;21(3):1535759721996344.
67. Biehl A, Taube M, Kotloski RJ, et al. Lamotrigine use and potential for adverse cardiac effects: a retrospective evaluation in a Veteran population. Epilepsy Behav. 2023;149:109496.
68. Hulbert J, Elger CE, Meyer R, et al. Antiepileptic drugs impair shortening of isolated cardiomyocytes. Front Neurol. 2017;8:133.
69. Hagley SP, Epstein SE, Stern JA, et al. Lamotrigine toxicosis treated with intravenous lipid emulsion therapy in a dog. J Am Anim Hosp Assoc. 2020;56(4):226–30.
70. Restrepo JA, MacLean R, Celano CM, et al. The assessment of cardiac risk in patients taking lamotrigine; a systematic review. Gen Hosp Psychiatry. 2022;78:14–27.
71. Moore PW, Donovan JW, Burkhart KK, et al. A case series of patients with lamotrigine toxicity at one center from 2003 to 2012. Clin Toxicol (Phila). 2013;51(7):545–9.
72. Saetre E, Abdelnoor M, Amlie JP, et al. Cardiac function and antiepileptic drug treatment in the elderly: a comparison between lamotrigine and sustained-release carbamazepine. Epilepsia. 2009;50(8):1841–9.
73. Davis G, Ward K, Mohiuddin S. Sinus bradycardia in an adolescent taking lamotrigine. Case Rep Psychiatry. 2022;2022:3353684.
74. Wang W, Battini V, Carnovale C, et al. A novel approach for pharmacological substantiation of safety signals using plasma concentrations of medication and administrative/healthcare databases: a case study using Danish registries for an FDA warning on lamotrigine. Pharmacol Res. 2023;193:106811.
75. Kicka M, Kłopotowski T, Picheta S, et al. Massive lamotrigine poisoning—case report. Przegl Lek. 2011;68(8):543–5.
76. Alyahya B, Friesen M, Nauche B, et al. Acute lamotrigine overdose: a systematic review of published adult and pediatric cases. Clin Toxicol (Phila). 2018;56(2):81–9.
77. Aurlien D, Larsen JP, Gjerstad L, et al. Increased risk of sudden unexpected death in epilepsy in females using lamotrigine: a nested, case-control study. Epilepsia. 2012;53(2):258–66.
78. Aurlien D, Leren TP, Taubøll E, et al. New SCN5A mutation in a SUDEP victim with idiopathic epilepsy. Seizure. 2009;18(2):158–60.
79. Banfi P, Coll M, Oliva A, et al. Lamotrigine induced Brugada-pattern in a patient with genetic epilepsy associated with a novel variant in SCN9A. Gene. 2020;754:144847.
80. Sotero FD, Silva CS, Cunha N, et al. Lamotrigine-induced Brugada syndrome: a rare adverse event. Seizure. 2022;94:7–9.
81. Bunschoten JW, Husein N, Devinsky O, et al. Sudden death and cardiac arrythmia with lamotrigine: a rapid systematic review. Neurology. 2022;98(17):e1748–e60.
82. Chavez P, Casso Dominguez A, Herzog E. Evolving electrocardiographic changes in lamotrigine overdose: a case report and literature review. Cardiovasc Toxicol. 2015;15(4):394–8.
83. Degiorgio CM. Atrial flutter/atrial fibrillation associated with lacosamide for partial seizures. Epilepsy Behav. 2010;18(3):322–4.
84. Eleftheriou G, Butera R, Gallo M, et al. Lacosamide-induced recurrent ventricular fibrillation: a case report. Int J Clin Pharmacol Ther. 2020;58(12):736–9.
85. Kaufman KR, Velez AE, Wong S, et al. Low-dose lacosamide-induced atrial fibrillation: case analysis with literature review. Epilepsy Behav Case Rep. 2013;1:22–5.
86. Kim HK, Lee H, Bae EK, et al. Cardiac effects of rapid intravenous loading of lacosamide in patients with epilepsy. Epilepsy Res. 2021;176:106710.
87. Sumbul O, Aygun H. Electrocorticographic and electrocardiographic evaluation of lacosamide in a penicillin-induced status epilepticus model. Epilepsy Res. 2022;180:106866.
88. Ng PC, Schimmel J, Wang GS. Lacosamide overdose: a case of QRS prolongation and seizure. J Emerg Med. 2019;56(6):652–6.
89. Bamgbose O, Boyle F, Kean AC, et al. Tolerability and safety of lacosamide in neonatal population. J Child Neurol. 2023;38(3–4):137–41.

90. Davidson KE, Newell J, Alsherbini K, et al. Safety and efficiency of intravenous push lacosamide administration. Neurocrit Care. 2018;29(3):491–5.
91. Fong SL, Utidjian L, Kaur M, et al. Safety of intravenous lacosamide in hospitalized children and neonates. Epilepsia. 2023;64(9):2297–309.
92. Shibata M, Hoshino R, Shimizu C, et al. Lacosamide-induced sinus node dysfunction followed by severe agranulocytosis. BMC Neurol. 2021;21(1):217.
93. Huberman MA, Mallar C, Kalika PM. Neonatal cardiac arrest following lacosamide treatment: a case report. Pediatr Neurol. 2023;149:184–6.
94. Takai C, Misumi K, Kaito D, et al. Lacosamide intoxication-induced wide QRS tachycardia successfully treated with veno-arterial extracorporeal membrane oxygenation. Intern Med. 2023;62(8):1185–9.
95. Marcellino C, Ransom CC, Wijdicks EF. Refractory ventricular tachycardia and seizures with lacosamide overdose. Cureus. 2022;14(9):e29547.
96. DeGiorgio AC, Desso TE, Lee L, et al. Ventricular tachycardia associated with lacosamide co-medication in drug-resistant epilepsy. Epilepsy Behav Case Rep. 2013;1:26–8.
97. Lu YT, Lin CH, Ho CJ, et al. Evaluation of cardiovascular concerns of intravenous lacosamide therapy in epilepsy patients. Front Neurol. 2022;13:891368.
98. Stamm B, Sheikh A, Schuele S, et al. Lacosamide-associated second-degree atrioventricular block in a healthy, young athlete. Epilepsy Behav Rep. 2020;14:100372.
99. Lachuer C, Corny J, Bézie Y, et al. Complete atrioventricular block in an elderly patient treated with low-dose lacosamide. Cardiovasc Toxicol. 2018;18(6):579–82.
100. Luk ME, Tatum WO, Patel AV, et al. The safety of lacosamide for treatment of seizures and seizure prophylaxis in adult hospitalized patients. Neurohospitalist. 2012;2(3):77–81.
101. Rudd GD, Haverkamp W, Mason JW, et al. Lacosamide cardiac safety: clinical trials in patients with partial-onset seizures. Acta Neurol Scand. 2015;132(5):355–63.
102. Kropeit D, Johnson M, Cawello W, et al. Lacosamide cardiac safety: a thorough QT/QTc trial in healthy volunteers. Acta Neurol Scand. 2015;132(5):346–54.
103. Rojano Martín B, Maroto Rubio M, Bilbao Ornazabal N, et al. Elderly patient with acquired long QT syndrome secondary to Levetiracetam. Neurologia. 2011;26(2):123–5.
104. Rosillon D, Astruc B, Hulhoven R, et al. Effect of brivaracetam on cardiac repolarisation—a thorough QT study. Curr Med Res Opin. 2008;24(8):2327–37.
105. Aydin H, Korkut O. Effect of levetiracetam therapy on electrocardiographic parameters. Arch Pediatr. 2023;30(3):149–52.
106. Delaunois A, Mathy FX, Cornet M, et al. Testing the nonclinical Comprehensive In Vitro Proarrhythmia Assay (CiPA) paradigm with an established anti-seizure medication: levetiracetam case study. Pharmacol Res Perspect. 2023;11(1):e01059.
107. Nishiyama M, Takami Y, Ishida Y, et al. Lipid and thyroid hormone levels in children with epilepsy treated with levetiracetam or carbamazepine: a prospective observational study. Epilepsy Behav. 2019;90:15–9.
108. Okada S, Nishina M, Koizumi K, et al. Impact of enzyme-inducing anti-epilepsy drugs on lipid levels in elderly patients with epilepsy. Epilepsy Res. 2020;166:106428.
109. Siniscalchi A, Scaglione F, Sanzaro E, et al. Effects of phenobarbital and levetiracetam on PR and QTc intervals in patients with post-stroke seizure. Clin Drug Investig. 2014;34(12):879–86.
110. Schimpf R, Veltmann C, Papavassiliu T, et al. Drug-induced QT-interval shortening following antiepileptic treatment with oral rufinamide. Heart Rhythm. 2012;9(5):776–81.
111. Shah RR. Drug-induced QT interval shortening: potential harbinger of proarrhythmia and regulatory perspectives. Br J Pharmacol. 2010;159(1):58–69.
112. Park SH, Hunter K, Berry H, et al. Atrial fibrillation induced by gabapentin: a case report. J Med Case Rep. 2023;17(1):236.
113. Wu B, Cao Y, Meng M, et al. Gabapentin alleviates myocardial ischemia-reperfusion injury by increasing the protein expression of GABA(A)Rδ. Eur J Pharmacol. 2023;944:175585.

114. Mintzer S, Dimova S, Zhang Y, et al. Effects of lacosamide and carbamazepine on lipids in a randomized trial. Epilepsia. 2020;61(12):2696–704.
115. Ortiz de Landaluce L, Carbonell P, Asensio C, et al. Gabapentin and pregabalin and risk of atrial fibrillation in the elderly: a population-based cohort study in an electronic prescription database. Drug Saf. 2018;41(12):1325–31.
116. Adar A, Cakan F, Önalan O. Pregbalin induced recurrent syncopal attacks with prolong QT interval. Ann Noninvasive Electrocardiol. 2018;23(4):e12489.
117. Le Marois M, Ballet V, Sanson C, et al. Cannabidiol inhibits multiple cardiac ion channels and shortens ventricular action potential duration in vitro. Eur J Pharmacol. 2020;886:173542.
118. Orvos P, Pászti B, Topal L, et al. The electrophysiological effect of cannabidiol on hERG current and in Guinea-pig and rabbit cardiac preparations. Sci Rep. 2020;10(1):16079.
119. Sellers EM, Schoedel K, Bartlett C, et al. A multiple-dose, randomized, double-blind, placebo-controlled, parallel-group QT/QTc study to evaluate the electrophysiologic effects of THC/CBD spray. Clin Pharmacol Drug Dev. 2013;2(3):285–94.
120. Wang X, Xu T, Luo D, et al. Cannabidiol alleviates perfluorooctanesulfonic acid-induced cardiomyocyte apoptosis by maintaining mitochondrial dynamic balance and energy metabolic homeostasis. J Agric Food Chem. 2023;71(14):5450–62.
121. Yıldız A, Vardı N, Parlakpınar H, et al. Effects of low- and high-dose valproic acid and lamotrigine on the heart in female rats. Cardiovasc Toxicol. 2022;22(4):326–40.
122. Liang D, Gardella E, Kragholm K, et al. The relationship between valproate and lamotrigine/levetiracetam use and prognosis in patients with epilepsy and heart failure: a Danish register-based study. J Card Fail. 2022;28(4):630–8.
123. Guo HL, Dong N, Chen F, et al. Effect of long-term valproic acid therapy on lipid profiles in paediatric patients with epilepsy: a meta-analysis. Epileptic Disord. 2022;24(5):822–30.
124. Muller AL, Diaz-Arias L, Cervenka MC, et al. The effect of anti-seizure medications on lipid values in adults with epilepsy. Epilepsy Behav. 2023;144:109260.
125. George LJ, Singh P, Aneja S, et al. Insulin resistance in children on sodium valproate – a hospital based cross-sectional study in Indian children. Trop Dr. 2023;53(1):91–6.
126. Roberti R, De Caro C, Iannone LF, et al. Pharmacology of cenobamate: mechanism of action, pharmacokinetics, drug-drug interactions and tolerability. CNS Drugs. 2021;35(6):609–18.
127. Darpo B, Sager PT, Xue H, et al. A phase 1 clinical study evaluating the effects of cenobamate on the QT interval. Clin Pharmacol Drug Dev. 2022;11(4):523–34.
128. Devarbhavi H, Sridhar A, Kurien SS, et al. Clinical and liver biochemistry phenotypes, and outcome in 133 patients with anti-seizure drug-induced liver injury. Dig Dis Sci. 2023;68(5):2099–106.
129. Kamitaki BK, Minacapelli CD, Zhang P, et al. Drug-induced liver injury associated with antiseizure medications from the FDA adverse event reporting system (FAERS). Epilepsy Behav. 2021;117:107832.
130. Devarbhavi H, Karanth D, Prasanna KS, et al. Drug-induced liver injury with hypersensitivity features has a better outcome: a single-center experience of 39 children and adolescents. Hepatology. 2011;54(4):1344–50.
131. Chalasani N, Bonkovsky HL, Stine JG, et al. Clinical characteristics of antiepileptic-induced liver injury in patients from the DILIN prospective study. J Hepatol. 2022;76(4):832–40.
132. Russo MW, Galanko JA, Shrestha R, et al. Liver transplantation for acute liver failure from drug induced liver injury in the United States. Liver Transpl. 2004;10(8):1018–23.
133. Larrey D. Epidemiology and individual susceptibility to adverse drug reactions affecting the liver. Semin Liver Dis. 2002;22(2):145–55.
134. Petrović S, Kovačević M, Vezmar Kovačević S, et al. Drug-induced liver injury associated with the use of newer antiseizure medications in the elderly: an analysis of data from VigiBase. Expert Opin Drug Metab Toxicol. 2023;19(3):175–83.
135. Mindikoglu AL, Magder LS, Regev A. Outcome of liver transplantation for drug-induced acute liver failure in the United States: analysis of the United Network for Organ Sharing database. Liver Transpl. 2009;15(7):719–29.

136. Dreifuss FE, Santilli N, Langer DH, et al. Valproic acid hepatic fatalities: a retrospective review. Neurology. 1987;37(3):379–85.
137. Zimmerman HJ, Ishak KG. Valproate-induced hepatic injury: analyses of 23 fatal cases. Hepatology. 1982;2(5):591–7.
138. Koenig SA, Buesing D, Longin E, et al. Valproic acid-induced hepatopathy: nine new fatalities in Germany from 1994 to 2003. Epilepsia. 2006;47(12):2027–31.
139. Björnsson E, Kalaitzakis E, Olsson R. The impact of eosinophilia and hepatic necrosis on prognosis in patients with drug-induced liver injury. Aliment Pharmacol Ther. 2007;25(12):1411–21.
140. Vittorio CC, Muglia JJ. Anticonvulsant hypersensitivity syndrome. Arch Intern Med. 1995;155(21):2285–90.
141. Knowles SR, Uetrecht J, Shear NH. Idiosyncratic drug reactions: the reactive metabolite syndromes. Lancet. 2000;356(9241):1587–91.
142. Aiges HW, Daum F, Olson M, et al. The effects of phenobarbital and diphenylhydantoin on liver function and morphology. J Pediatr. 1980;97(1):22–6.
143. Strolin Benedetti M, Ruty B, Baltes E. Induction of endogenous pathways by antiepileptics and clinical implications. Fundam Clin Pharmacol. 2005;19(5):511–29.
144. Ouellet G, Tremblay L, Marleau D. Fulminant hepatitis induced by lamotrigine. South Med J. 2009;102(1):82–4.
145. Nalivaeva NN, Belyaev ND, Turner AJ. Sodium valproate: an old drug with new roles. Trends Pharmacol Sci. 2009;30(10):509–14.
146. Meseguer ES, Elizalde MU, Borobia AM, et al. Valproic acid-induced liver injury: a case-control study from a prospective pharmacovigilance program in a tertiary hospital. J Clin Med. 2021;10(6):1153.
147. Donat JF, Bocchini JA Jr, Gonzalez E, et al. Valproic acid and fatal hepatitis. Neurology. 1979;29(2):273–4.
148. Suchy FJ, Balistreri WF, Buchino JJ, et al. Acute hepatic failure associated with the use of sodium valproate. N Engl J Med. 1979;300(17):962–6.
149. Jacobi G, Thorbeck R, Ritz A, et al. Fatal hepatotoxicity in child on phenobarbitone and sodium valproate. Lancet. 1980;1(8170):712–3.
150. Palm R, Silseth C, Alván G. Phenytoin intoxication as the first symptom of fatal liver damage induced by sodium valproate. Br J Clin Pharmacol. 1984;17(5):597–9.
151. Nomura F, Hatano H, Ohnishi K, et al. Effects of anticonvulsant agents on halothane-induced liver injury in human subjects and experimental animals. Hepatology. 1986;6(5):952–6.
152. Subhash HS, Heddle RJ, Schultz DW, et al. Hepatic encephalopathy precipitated by sodium valproate therapy. Med J Aust. 2008;188(9):549.
153. Wong YJ, Fan J, Wan A, et al. Valproic acid-associated hyperammonemia: a systematic review. J Clin Psychopharmacol. 2023;43(3):283–94.
154. Atef MM, Abou Hashish NA, Hafez YM, et al. The potential protective effect of liraglutide on valproic acid induced liver injury in rats: targeting HMGB1/RAGE axis and RIPK3/MLKL mediated necroptosis. Cell Biochem Funct. 2023;41(8):1209–19.
155. Liu Y, Li H, Huang L, et al. Liver injury in children: signal analysis of suspected drugs based on the food and drug administration adverse event reporting system. BMC Pediatr. 2023;23(1):492.
156. Cano-Paniagua A, Amariles P, Angulo N, et al. Epidemiology of drug-induced liver injury in a University Hospital from Colombia: updated RUCAM being used for prospective causality assessment. Ann Hepatol. 2019;18(3):501–7.
157. Schmid MM, Freudenmann RW, Keller F, et al. Non-fatal and fatal liver failure associated with valproic acid. Pharmacopsychiatry. 2013;46(2):63–8.
158. Cotariu D, Zaidman JL. Valproic acid and the liver. Clin Chem. 1988;34(5):890–7.
159. Miguil M, Chlihi A, Mjahed K, et al. Fatal hepatic necrosis during treatment with sodium valproate. Cah Anesthesiol. 1995;43(3):325–6.

160. Pourahmad J, Eskandari MR, Kaghazi A, et al. A new approach on valproic acid induced hepatotoxicity: involvement of lysosomal membrane leakiness and cellular proteolysis. Toxicol In Vitro. 2012;26(4):545–51.
161. Stewart JD, Horvath R, Baruffini E, et al. Polymerase γ gene POLG determines the risk of sodium valproate-induced liver toxicity. Hepatology. 2010;52(5):1791–6.
162. Xu S, Chen Y, Ma Y, et al. Lipidomic profiling reveals disruption of lipid metabolism in valproic acid-induced hepatotoxicity. Front Pharmacol. 2019;10:819.
163. Bota RG, Ligasan AP, Najdowski TG, et al. Acute hypersensitivity syndrome caused by valproic acid: a review of the literature and a case report. Perm J. 2011;15(2):80–4.
164. Huang YL, Hong HS, Wang ZW, et al. Fatal sodium valproate-induced hypersensitivity syndrome with lichenoid dermatitis and fulminant hepatitis. J Am Acad Dermatol. 2003;49(2):316–9.
165. Chicharro AV, de Marinis AJ, Kanner AM. The measurement of ammonia blood levels in patients taking valproic acid: looking for problems where they do not exist? Epilepsy Behav. 2007;11(3):361–6.
166. Wong YJ, Mihic T, Wan A, et al. Valproic acid-associated hyperammonemia: a systematic review-reply to comments by Dr Aney. J Clin Psychopharmacol. 2024;44(1):73–4.
167. Yamada H, Shishido T, Mukai T, et al. Valproic acid-induced hyperammonemic encephalopathy in a patient receiving valproic acid monotherapy. Rinsho Shinkeigaku. 2019;59(5):258–63.
168. Chopra A, Kolla BP, Mansukhani MP, et al. Valproate-induced hyperammonemic encephalopathy: an update on risk factors, clinical correlates and management. Gen Hosp Psychiatry. 2012;34(3):290–8.
169. Dealberto MJ. Valproate-induced hyperammonaemic encephalopathy: review of 14 cases in the psychiatric setting. Int Clin Psychopharmacol. 2007;22(6):330–7.
170. Wadzinski J, Franks R, Roane D, et al. Valproate-associated hyperammonemic encephalopathy. J Am Board Fam Med. 2007;20(5):499–502.
171. Stahl SM. Anticonvulsants as mood stabilizers and adjuncts to antipsychotics: valproate, lamotrigine, carbamazepine, and oxcarbazepine and actions at voltage-gated sodium channels. J Clin Psychiatry. 2004;65(6):738–9.
172. Wu CY, Lu CY. Derivatization oriented strategy for enhanced detection of valproic acid and its metabolites in human plasma and detection of valproic acid induced reactive oxygen species associated protein modifications by mass spectrometry. J Chromatogr A. 2014;1374:14–22.
173. Aljarboa AS, Alhusaini AM, Sarawi WS, et al. The implication of LPS/TLR4 and FXR receptors in hepatoprotective efficacy of indole-3-acetic acid and chenodeoxycholic acid. Life Sci. 2023;334:122182.
174. Ma Y, Wang M, Guo S, et al. The serum acylcarnitines profile in epileptic children treated with valproic acid and the protective roles of peroxisome proliferator-activated receptor a activation in valproic acid-induced liver injury. Front Pharmacol. 2022;13:1048728.
175. Schiavo A, Maldonado C, Vázquez M, et al. Quantitative systems pharmacology model to characterize valproic acid-induced hyperammonemia and the effect of L-carnitine supplementation. Eur J Pharm Sci. 2023;183:106399.
176. Lheureux PE, Hantson P. Carnitine in the treatment of valproic acid-induced toxicity. Clin Toxicol (Phila). 2009;47(2):101–11.
177. Walker M. Status epilepticus: an evidence based guide. BMJ. 2005;331(7518):673–7.
178. Riera Velasco JR, Rodrigo Sáez LR, Pérez Alvarez R, et al. Chronic active hepatitis caused by diphenylhydantoin. Med Clin. 1986;87(5):214.
179. Temkin NR, Dikmen SS, Anderson GD, et al. Valproate therapy for prevention of posttraumatic seizures: a randomized trial. J Neurosurg. 1999;91(4):593–600.
180. Sano J, Kawada H, Yamaguchi N, et al. Effects of phenytoin on serum gamma-glutamyl transpeptidase activity. Epilepsia. 1981;22(3):331–8.
181. Bajpai M, Roskos LK, Shen DD, et al. Roles of cytochrome P4502C9 and cytochrome P4502C19 in the stereoselective metabolism of phenytoin to its major metabolite. Drug Metab Dispos. 1996;24(12):1401–3.

182. Dwivedi R, Gogtay N, Kharkar V, et al. In-vitro lymphocyte toxicity to a phenytoin metabolite in phenytoin induced cutaneous adverse drug eruptions. Indian J Dermatol Venereol Leprol. 2004;70(4):217–20.
183. Spielberg SP, Gordon GB, Blake DA, et al. Predisposition to phenytoin hepatotoxicity assessed in vitro. N Engl J Med. 1981;305(13):722–7.
184. Sasaki E, Iwamura A, Tsuneyama K, et al. Role of cytochrome P450-mediated metabolism and identification of novel thiol-conjugated metabolites in mice with phenytoin-induced liver injury. Toxicol Lett. 2015;232(1):79–88.
185. Nicoletti P, Dellinger A, Li YJ, et al. HLA-B*53:01 is a significant risk factor of liver injury due to phenytoin and other antiepileptic drugs in African Americans. Am J Gastroenterol. 2024;119(1):200–2.
186. Altuntaş Y, Oztürk B, Erdem L, et al. Phenytoin-induced toxic cholestatic hepatitis in a patient with skin lesions: case report. South Med J. 2003;96(2):201–3.
187. Roy AK, Mahoney HC, Levine RA. Phenytoin-induced chronic hepatitis. Dig Dis Sci. 1993;38(4):740–3.
188. Sen S, Ratnaraj N, Davies NA, et al. Treatment of phenytoin toxicity by the molecular adsorbents recirculating system (MARS). Epilepsia. 2003;44(2):265–7.
189. Frenchie D, Bastani B. Significant removal of phenytoin during high flux dialysis with cellulose triacetate dialyzer. Nephrol Dial Transplant. 1998;13(3):817–8.
190. Bialer M. Chemical properties of antiepileptic drugs (AEDs). Adv Drug Deliv Rev. 2012;64(10):887–95.
191. Levy M, Goodman MW, Van Dyne BJ, et al. Granulomatous hepatitis secondary to carbamazepine. Ann Intern Med. 1981;95(1):64–5.
192. Berkowitz FE, Henderson SL, Fajman N, et al. Acute liver failure caused by isoniazid in a child receiving carbamazepine. Int J Tuberc Lung Dis. 1998;2(7):603–6.
193. Askmark H, Wiholm BE. Epidemiology of adverse reactions to carbamazepine as seen in a spontaneous reporting system. Acta Neurol Scand. 1990;81(2):131–40.
194. Chalasani N, Reddy KRK, Fontana RJ, et al. Idiosyncratic drug induced liver injury in African-Americans is associated with greater morbidity and mortality compared to caucasians. Am J Gastroenterol. 2017;112(9):1382–8.
195. Bernus I, Dickinson RG, Hooper WD, et al. Dose-dependent metabolism of carbamazepine in humans. Epilepsy Res. 1996;24(3):163–72.
196. Park BK, Kitteringham NR, Powell H, et al. Advances in molecular toxicology-towards understanding idiosyncratic drug toxicity. Toxicology. 2000;153(1–3):39–60.
197. Lu W, Uetrecht JP. Peroxidase-mediated bioactivation of hydroxylated metabolites of carbamazepine and phenytoin. Drug Metab Dispos. 2008;36(8):1624–36.
198. Mitchell MC, Boitnott JK, Arregui A, et al. Granulomatous hepatitis associated with carbamazepine therapy. Am J Med. 1981;71(4):733–5.
199. Forbes GM, Jeffrey GP, Shilkin KB, et al. Carbamazepine hepatotoxicity: another cause of the vanishing bile duct syndrome. Gastroenterology. 1992;102(4 Pt 1):1385–8.
200. Ramos AM, Gayotto LC, Clemente CM, et al. Reversible vanishing bile duct syndrome induced by carbamazepine. Eur J Gastroenterol Hepatol. 2002;14(9):1019–22.
201. Brodie MJ. Lamotrigine versus other antiepileptic drugs: a star rating system is born. Epilepsia. 1994;35(Suppl 5):S41–6.
202. Culy CR, Goa KL. Lamotrigine. A review of its use in childhood epilepsy. Paediatr Drugs. 2000;2(4):299–330.
203. Timmings PL, Richens A. Lamotrigine in primary generalised epilepsy. Lancet. 1992;339(8804):1300–1.
204. Gómez Caturla A, Arteta Jiménez M, Fernández Planelles C, et al. Acute hepatitis associated with lamotrigine administration. Med Clin. 1998;111(17):675–6.
205. Overstreet K, Costanza C, Behling C, et al. Fatal progressive hepatic necrosis associated with lamotrigine treatment: a case report and literature review. Dig Dis Sci. 2002;47(9):1921–5.

206. Maggs JL, Naisbitt DJ, Tettey JN, et al. Metabolism of lamotrigine to a reactive arene oxide intermediate. Chem Res Toxicol. 2000;13(11):1075–81.
207. Amante MF, Filippini AV, Cejas N, et al. Dress syndrome and fulminant hepatic failure induced by lamotrigine. Ann Hepatol. 2009;8(1):75–7.
208. Fix OK, Peters MG, Davern TJ. Eosinophilic hepatitis caused by lamotrigine. Clin Gastroenterol Hepatol. 2006;4(4):xxvi.
209. Jain P, Aneja S, Cunningham J, et al. Treatment of benzodiazepine-resistant status epilepticus: systematic review and network meta-analyses. Seizure. 2022;102:74–82.
210. Kim JJ, Gharpure A, Teng J, et al. Shared structural mechanisms of general anaesthetics and benzodiazepines. Nature. 2020;585(7824):303–8.
211. Herdson PB, Garvin PJ, Jennings RB. Fine structural changes in rat liver induced by phenobarbital. Lab Invest. 1964;13:1032–7.
212. Weisburst M, Self T, Peace R, et al. Jaundice and rash associated with the use of phenobarbital and hydrochlorothiazide. South Med J. 1976;69(1):126–7.
213. Sawaishi Y, Komatsu K, Takeda O, et al. A case of tubulo-interstitial nephritis with exfoliative dermatitis and hepatitis due to phenobarbital hypersensitivity. Eur J Pediatr. 1992;151(1):69–72.
214. Gaskill CL, Miller LM, Mattoon JS, et al. Liver histopathology and liver and serum alanine aminotransferase and alkaline phosphatase activities in epileptic dogs receiving phenobarbital. Vet Pathol. 2005;42(2):147–60.
215. Mockli G, Crowley M, Stern R, et al. Massive hepatic necrosis in a child after administration of phenobarbital. Am J Gastroenterol. 1989;84(7):820–2.
216. Gavilán JC, Bermúdez F, Romero M, et al. Levetiracetam hepatitis. Med Clin. 2004;122(1):38.
217. Lens S, Crespo G, Carrión JA, et al. Severe acute hepatitis in the DRESS syndrome: report of two cases. Ann Hepatol. 2010;9(2):198–201.
218. Rogalewski A, Zuhorn F, Wilkens L, et al. Severe drug-induced liver injury caused by levetiracetam – a case report and review of the literature. Epilepsy Behav Rep. 2021;16:100464.
219. Sun W, He Y, Li Z, et al. Analysis of the clinical characteristics of the liver injury induced by levetiracetam. J Pharm Pharmacol. 2022;74(3):409–14.
220. Vidaurre J, Gedela S, Yarosz S. Antiepileptic drugs and liver disease. Pediatr Neurol. 2017;77:23–36.
221. Dieckhaus CM, Thompson CD, Roller SG, et al. Mechanisms of idiosyncratic drug reactions: the case of felbamate. Chem Biol Interact. 2002;142(1–2):99–117.
222. O'Neil MG, Perdun CS, Wilson MB, et al. Felbamate-associated fatal acute hepatic necrosis. Neurology. 1996;46(5):1457–9.
223. Takahashi H, Shimoyama N. A prospective open-label trial of gabapentin as an adjuvant analgesic with opioids for Japanese patients with neuropathic cancer pain. Int J Clin Oncol. 2010;15(1):46–51.
224. Contreras-Mota M, Rosales-Cortés V. Hepatotoxicity probably associated with gabapentin. Rev Med Inst Mex Seguro Soc. 2021;59(2):157–62.
225. Gastaut H, Collomb H. Sexual behavior in psychomotor epileptics. Ann Med Psychol (Paris). 1954;112(2 5):657–96.
226. Beran RG, Read T, Reid M, et al. Individualized patient assessment in the treatment of epilepsy with sodium valproate. Epilepsia. 1980;21(4):379–86.
227. Mattson RH, Cramer JA, Collins JF, et al. Comparison of carbamazepine, phenobarbital, phenytoin, and primidone in partial and secondarily generalized tonic-clonic seizures. N Engl J Med. 1985;313(3):145–51.
228. Clark JD, Elliott J. Gabapentin-induced anorgasmia. Neurology. 1999;53(9):2209.
229. Mattson RH, Cramer JA, Collins JF. A comparison of valproate with carbamazepine for the treatment of complex partial seizures and secondarily generalized tonic-clonic seizures in adults. The Department of Veterans Affairs Epilepsy Cooperative Study No. 264 Group. N Engl J Med. 1992;327(11):765–71.

230. Grant AC, Oh H. Gabapentin-induced anorgasmia in women. Am J Psychiatry. 2002;159(7):1247.
231. Grabowska-Grzyb A, Nagańska E, Wolańczyk T. Hypersexuality in two patients with epilepsy treated with lamotrigine. Epilepsy Behav. 2006;8(3):663–5.
232. Kuba R, Pohanka M, Zákopcan J, et al. Sexual dysfunctions and blood hormonal profile in men with focal epilepsy. Epilepsia. 2006;47(12):2135–40.
233. Leris AC, Stephens J, Hines JE, et al. Carbamazepine-related ejaculatory failure. Br J Urol. 1997;79(3):485.
234. Elia J, Imbrogno N, Delfino M, et al. Retrograde ejaculation and abnormal hormonal profile in a subject under treatment with valproate and phenytoin. Arch Ital Urol Androl. 2010;82(4):193–4.
235. Yılmaz U, Yılmaz TS, Akıncı G, et al. The effect of antiepileptic drugs on thyroid function in children. Seizure. 2014;23(1):29–35.
236. Vestergaard P. Effects of antiepileptic drugs on bone health and growth potential in children with epilepsy. Paediatr Drugs. 2015;17(2):141–50.
237. Tanaka K, Kodama S, Yokoyama S, et al. Thyroid function in children with long-term anticonvulsant treatment. Pediatr Neurosci. 1987;13(2):90–4.
238. Verrotti A, Laus M, Scardapane A, et al. Thyroid hormones in children with epilepsy during long-term administration of carbamazepine and valproate. Eur J Endocrinol. 2009;160(1):81–6.
239. Lossius MI, Taubøll E, Mowinckel P, et al. Reversible effects of antiepileptic drugs on thyroid hormones in men and women with epilepsy: a prospective randomized double-blind withdrawal study. Epilepsy Behav. 2009;16(1):64–8.
240. Güngör O, Özkaya AK, Temiz F. The effect of antiepileptic drugs on thyroid hormonal function: valproic acid and phenobarbital. Acta Neurol Belg. 2020;120(3):615–9.
241. Attilakos A, Katsarou E, Prassouli A, et al. Thyroid function in children with epilepsy treated with sodium valproate monotherapy: a prospective study. Clin Neuropharmacol. 2009;32(1):32–4.
242. Adhimoolam M, Arulmozhi R. Effect of antiepileptic drug therapy on thyroid hormones among adult epileptic patients: an analytical cross-sectional study. J Res Pharm Pract. 2016;5(3):171–4.
243. Garoufi A, Koemtzidou E, Katsarou E, et al. Lipid profile and thyroid hormone concentrations in children with epilepsy treated with oxcarbazepine monotherapy: a prospective long-term study. Eur J Neurol. 2014;21(1):118–23.
244. Hamed SA. The effect of antiepileptic drugs on thyroid hormonal function: causes and implications. Expert Rev Clin Pharmacol. 2015;8(6):741–50.
245. Han Y, Yang J, Zhong R, et al. Side effects of long-term oral anti-seizure drugs on thyroid hormones in patients with epilepsy: a systematic review and network meta-analysis. Neurol Sci. 2022;43(9):5217–27.
246. Attilakos A, Dinopoulos A, Tsirouda M, et al. Effect of levetiracetam monotherapy on lipid profiles and thyroid hormones in children with epilepsy: a prospective study. Epilepsy Res. 2019;155:106162.
247. Misra A, Aggarwal A, Singh O, et al. Effect of carbamazepine therapy on vitamin D and parathormone in epileptic children. Pediatr Neurol. 2010;43(5):320–4.
248. Jetté N, Lix LM, Metge CJ, et al. Association of antiepileptic drugs with nontraumatic fractures: a population-based analysis. Arch Neurol. 2011;68(1):107–12.
249. Souverein PC, Webb DJ, Petri H, et al. Incidence of fractures among epilepsy patients: a population-based retrospective cohort study in the General Practice Research Database. Epilepsia. 2005;46(2):304–10.
250. Farhat G, Yamout B, Mikati MA, et al. Effect of antiepileptic drugs on bone density in ambulatory patients. Neurology. 2002;58(9):1348–53.

251. Menon B, Harinarayan CV. The effect of anti epileptic drug therapy on serum 25-hydroxyvitamin D and parameters of calcium and bone metabolism—a longitudinal study. Seizure. 2010;19(3):153–8.
252. Linde J, Molholm Hansen J, Siersbaek-Nielsen K, et al. Bone density in patients receiving long-term anticonvulsant therapy. Acta Neurol Scand. 1971;47(5):650–1.
253. Guo CY, Ronen GM, Atkinson SA. Long-term valproate and lamotrigine treatment may be a marker for reduced growth and bone mass in children with epilepsy. Epilepsia. 2001;42(9):1141–7.
254. Verrotti A, Greco R, Latini G, et al. Increased bone turnover in prepubertal, pubertal, and postpubertal patients receiving carbamazepine. Epilepsia. 2002;43(12):1488–92.
255. Coppola G, Fortunato D, Auricchio G, et al. Bone mineral density in children, adolescents, and young adults with epilepsy. Epilepsia. 2009;50(9):2140–6.
256. Nettekoven S, Ströhle A, Trunz B, et al. Effects of antiepileptic drug therapy on vitamin D status and biochemical markers of bone turnover in children with epilepsy. Eur J Pediatr. 2008;167(12):1369–77.
257. Tamber MS, Mountz JM. Advances in the diagnosis and treatment of epilepsy. Semin Nucl Med. 2012;42(6):371–86.
258. Wilson EL, Garton M, Fuller HR. Anti-epileptic drugs and bone loss: phenytoin reduces pro-collagen I and alters the electrophoretic mobility of osteonectin in cultured bone cells. Epilepsy Res. 2016;122:97–101.
259. Petty SJ, Milligan CJ, Todaro M, et al. The antiepileptic medications carbamazepine and phenytoin inhibit native sodium currents in murine osteoblasts. Epilepsia. 2016;57(9):1398–405.
260. Lifshitz F, Maclaren NK. Vitamin D-dependent rickets in institutionalized, mentally retarded children receiving long-term anticonvulsant therapy. I. A survey of 288 patients. J Pediatr. 1973;83(4):612–20.
261. Phabphal K, Geater A, Limapichart K, et al. The association between BsmI polymorphism and bone mineral density in young patients with epilepsy who are taking phenytoin. Epilepsia. 2013;54(2):249–55.
262. Takahashi A, Onodera K, Shinoda H, et al. Phenytoin and its metabolite, 5-(4-hydroxyphenyl)-5-phenylhydantoin, show bone resorption in cultured neonatal mouse calvaria. Jpn J Pharmacol. 2000;82(1):82–4.
263. Tjellesen L, Nilas L, Christiansen C. Does carbamazepine cause disturbances in calcium metabolism in epileptic patients? Acta Neurol Scand. 1983;68(1):13–9.
264. Mintzer S, Boppana P, Toguri J, et al. Vitamin D levels and bone turnover in epilepsy patients taking carbamazepine or oxcarbazepine. Epilepsia. 2006;47(3):510–5.
265. Gunes A, Bilir E, Zengil H, et al. Inhibitory effect of valproic acid on cytochrome P450 2C9 activity in epilepsy patients. Basic Clin Pharmacol Toxicol. 2007;100(6):383–6.
266. Cerveny L, Svecova L, Anzenbacherova E, et al. Valproic acid induces CYP3A4 and MDR1 gene expression by activation of constitutive androstane receptor and pregnane X receptor pathways. Drug Metab Dispos. 2007;35(7):1032–41.
267. Song XQ, Wang ZP, Bao KR, et al. Effect of carbamazepine and valproate on bone metabolism in children with epilepsy. Zhonghua Er Ke Za Zhi. 2005;43(10):728–32.
268. Foreman JW. Fanconi Syndrome. Pediatr Clin N Am. 2019;66(1):159–67.
269. Wang C, Zhou Y, Song L, et al. Valproic-induced Fanconi syndrome: clinical features, risk factors, diagnosis and management. Front Med (Lausanne). 2022;9:945244.
270. Heo K, Rhee Y, Lee HW, et al. The effect of topiramate monotherapy on bone mineral density and markers of bone and mineral metabolism in premenopausal women with epilepsy. Epilepsia. 2011;52(10):1884–9.
271. Zhuo L, Zhang Y. Effects of new antiseizure medication on bone metabolism and bone mineral density in children: a meta-analysis. Front Pediatr. 2022;10:1015691.
272. Gordon CM, Baim S, Bianchi ML, et al. Special report on the 2007 Pediatric Position Development Conference of the International Society for Clinical Densitometry. South Med J. 2008;101(7):740–3.

273. Braunhofer J, Zicha L. Does Tegretal offer new possibilities of therapy in several neurologic and endocrine diseases? A clinical electroencephalographic and thin-layer chromatographic study. Med Welt. 1966;36:1875–80.
274. Kalff R, Houtkooper MA, Meyer JW, et al. Carbamazepine and serum sodium levels. Epilepsia. 1984;25(3):390–7.
275. Kuz GM, Manssourian A. Carbamazepine-induced hyponatremia: assessment of risk factors. Ann Pharmacother. 2005;39(11):1943–6.
276. Dong X, Leppik IE, White J, et al. Hyponatremia from oxcarbazepine and carbamazepine. Neurology. 2005;65(12):1976–8.
277. Asconapé JJ. Some common issues in the use of antiepileptic drugs. Semin Neurol. 2002;22(1):27–39.
278. Schmidt D, Arroyo S, Baulac M, et al. Recommendations on the clinical use of oxcarbazepine in the treatment of epilepsy: a consensus view. Acta Neurol Scand. 2001;104(3):167–70.
279. Kim YS, Kim DW, Jung KH, et al. Frequency of and risk factors for oxcarbazepine-induced severe and symptomatic hyponatremia. Seizure. 2014;23(3):208–12.
280. Lin CH, Lu CH, Wang FJ, et al. Risk factors of oxcarbazepine-induced hyponatremia in patients with epilepsy. Clin Neuropharmacol. 2010;33(6):293–6.
281. Sperling MR, Abou-Khalil B, Harvey J, et al. Eslicarbazepine acetate as adjunctive therapy in patients with uncontrolled partial-onset seizures: results of a phase III, double-blind, randomized, placebo-controlled trial. Epilepsia. 2015;56(2):244–53.
282. Hufnagel A, Ben-Menachem E, Gabbai AA, et al. Long-term safety and efficacy of eslicarbazepine acetate as adjunctive therapy in the treatment of partial-onset seizures in adults with epilepsy: results of a 1-year open-label extension study. Epilepsy Res. 2013;103(2–3):262–9.
283. Sperling MR, Harvey J, Grinnell T, et al. Efficacy and safety of conversion to monotherapy with eslicarbazepine acetate in adults with uncontrolled partial-onset seizures: a randomized historical-control phase III study based in North America. Epilepsia. 2015;56(4):546–55.
284. Beers E, van Puijenbroek EP, Bartelink IH, et al. Syndrome of inappropriate antidiuretic hormone secretion (SIADH) or hyponatraemia associated with valproic acid: four case reports from the Netherlands and a case/non-case analysis of vigibase. Drug Saf. 2010;33(1):47–55.
285. Wilton LV, Shakir S. A postmarketing surveillance study of gabapentin as add-on therapy for 3,100 patients in England. Epilepsia. 2002;43(9):983–92.
286. Kloster R, Børresen HC, Hoff-Olsen P. Sudden death in two patients with epilepsy and the syndrome of inappropriate antidiuretic hormone secretion (SIADH). Seizure. 1998;7(5):419–20.
287. Berghuis B, de Haan GJ, van den Broek MP, et al. Epidemiology, pathophysiology and putative genetic basis of carbamazepine- and oxcarbazepine-induced hyponatremia. Eur J Neurol. 2016;23(9):1393–9.
288. Isojärvi JI, Huuskonen UE, Pakarinen AJ, et al. The regulation of serum sodium after replacing carbamazepine with oxcarbazepine. Epilepsia. 2001;42(6):741–5.
289. Akanuma N, Adachi N, Fenwick P, et al. Individual vulnerabilities to psychosis after antiepileptic drug administration. BMJ Neurol Open. 2020;2(2):e000036.
290. Adachi N, Onuma T, Kato M, et al. Psychoses after an antiepileptic drug administration: frequency, timing, and duration. Epilepsy Behav. 2023;140:109087.
291. Chen B, Choi H, Hirsch LJ, et al. Psychiatric and behavioral side effects of antiepileptic drugs in adults with epilepsy. Epilepsy Behav. 2017;76:24–31.
292. Stephen LJ, Wishart A, Brodie MJ. Psychiatric side effects and antiepileptic drugs: observations from prospective audits. Epilepsy Behav. 2017;71(Pt A):73–8.
293. Ogunsakin O, Tumenta T, Louis-Jean S, et al. Levetiracetam induced behavioral abnormalities in a patient with seizure disorder: a diagnostic challenge. Case Rep Psychiatry. 2020;2020:8883802.
294. Mula M, Trimble MR, Sander JW. Are psychiatric adverse events of antiepileptic drugs a unique entity? A study on topiramate and levetiracetam. Epilepsia. 2007;48(12):2322–6.

295. Ettinger AB, LoPresti A, Yang H, et al. Psychiatric and behavioral adverse events in randomized clinical studies of the noncompetitive AMPA receptor antagonist perampanel. Epilepsia. 2015;56(8):1252–63.
296. Trimble MR, Rüsch N, Betts T, et al. Psychiatric symptoms after therapy with new antiepileptic drugs: psychopathological and seizure related variables. Seizure. 2000;9(4):249–54.
297. Rugg-Gunn F. Adverse effects and safety profile of perampanel: a review of pooled data. Epilepsia. 2014;55(Suppl 1):13–5.
298. Mula M, Sander JW. Negative effects of antiepileptic drugs on mood in patients with epilepsy. Drug Saf. 2007;30(7):555–67.
299. Dussaule C, Bouilleret V. Psychiatric effects of antiepileptic drugs in adults. Geriatr Psychol Neuropsychiatr Vieil. 2018;16(2):181–8.
300. Bagary M. Epilepsy, antiepileptic drugs and suicidality. Curr Opin Neurol. 2011;24(2):177–82.
301. Lim HW, Song HS, Hwang YH, et al. Predictors of suicidal ideation in people with epilepsy living in Korea. J Clin Neurol. 2010;6(2):81–8.
302. Kennedy GM, Lhatoo SD. CNS adverse events associated with antiepileptic drugs. CNS Drugs. 2008;22(9):739–60.
303. Machado RA, Espinosa AG, Melendrez D, et al. Suicidal risk and suicide attempts in people treated with antiepileptic drugs for epilepsy. Seizure. 2011;20(4):280–4.
304. Ketter TA, Post RM, Theodore WH. Positive and negative psychiatric effects of antiepileptic drugs in patients with seizure disorders. Neurology. 1999;53(5 Suppl 2):S53–67.
305. Berkovic SF, Knowlton RC, Leroy RF, et al. Placebo-controlled study of levetiracetam in idiopathic generalized epilepsy. Neurology. 2007;69(18):1751–60.
306. Frey LC, Strom LA, Shrestha A, et al. End-of-dose emergent psychopathology in ambulatory patients with epilepsy on stable-dose lamotrigine monotherapy: a case series of six patients. Epilepsy Behav. 2009;15(4):521–3.
307. Goldberg-Stern H, Feldman L, Eidlitz-Markus T, et al. Levetiracetam in children, adolescents and young adults with intractable epilepsy: efficacy, tolerability and effect on electroencephalogram—a pilot study. Eur J Paediatr Neurol. 2013;17(3):248–53.
308. Anhut H, Ashman P, Feuerstein TJ, et al. Gabapentin (Neurontin) as add-on therapy in patients with partial seizures: a double-blind, placebo-controlled study. The International Gabapentin Study Group. Epilepsia. 1994;35(4):795–801.
309. Molokwu OA, Ezeala-Adikaibe BA, Onwuekwe IO. Levetiracetam-induced rage and suicidality: two case reports and review of literature. Epilepsy Behav Case Rep. 2015;4:79–81.
310. Kawai M, Goji H, Kanemoto K. Aggression as psychiatric side effect of newer AEDs in patients with epilepsy: cross-sectional study based on Buss-Perry Aggression Questionnaire. Epilepsy Behav. 2021;115:107546.
311. Matsuo M, Fuji A, Matsuzaka T, et al. Effectiveness and safety of long-term levetiracetam treatment in patients with refractory epilepsy. No To Hattatsu. 2015;47(4):272–8.
312. Adelman J, Freitag FG, Lainez M, et al. Analysis of safety and tolerability data obtained from over 1,500 patients receiving topiramate for migraine prevention in controlled trials. Pain Med. 2008;9(2):175–85.
313. Stephen LJ, Sills GJ, Brodie MJ. Topiramate in refractory epilepsy: a prospective observational study. Epilepsia. 2000;41(8):977–80.
314. Marson AG, Kadir ZA, Hutton JL, et al. The new antiepileptic drugs: a systematic review of their efficacy and tolerability. Epilepsia. 1997;38(8):859–80.
315. Reife RA, Pledger GW. Topiramate as adjunctive therapy in refractory partial epilepsy: pooled analysis of data from five double-blind, placebo-controlled trials. Epilepsia. 1997;38(Suppl 1):S31–3.
316. Vande Griend JP, Linnebur SA, Bainbridge JL. Probable levetiracetam-associated depression in the elderly: two case reports. Am J Geriatr Pharmacother. 2009;7(5):281–4.
317. Patorno E, Bohn RL, Wahl PM, et al. Anticonvulsant medications and the risk of suicide, attempted suicide, or violent death. JAMA. 2010;303(14):1401–9.

318. Wolf SM, Shinnar S, Kang H, et al. Gabapentin toxicity in children manifesting as behavioral changes. Epilepsia. 1995;36(12):1203–5.
319. The long-term safety and efficacy of gabapentin (Neurontin) as add-on therapy in drug-resistant partial epilepsy. The US Gabapentin Study Group. Epilepsy Res. 1994;18(1):67–73.
320. Tallian KB, Nahata MC, Lo W, et al. Gabapentin associated with aggressive behavior in pediatric patients with seizures. Epilepsia. 1996;37(5):501–2.
321. Trinka E, Niedermüller U, Thaler C, et al. Gabapentin-induced mood changes with hypomanic features in adults. Seizure. 2000;9(7):505–8.
322. Khurana DS, Riviello J, Helmers S, et al. Efficacy of gabapentin therapy in children with refractory partial seizures. J Pediatr. 1996;128(6):829–33.
323. Short C, Cooke L. Hypomania induced by gabapentin. Br J Psychiatry J Ment Sci. 1995;166(5):679–80.
324. Sivenius J, Kälviäinen R, Ylinen A, et al. Double-blind study of gabapentin in the treatment of partial seizures. Epilepsia. 1991;32(4):539–42.
325. Crawford P, Ghadiali E, Lane R, et al. Gabapentin as an antiepileptic drug in man. J Neurol Neurosurg Psychiatry. 1987;50(6):682–6.
326. Childers MK, Holland D. Psychomotor agitation following gabapentin use in brain injury. Brain Inj. 1997;11(7):537–40.
327. Lee DO, Steingard RJ, Cesena M, et al. Behavioral side effects of gabapentin in children. Epilepsia. 1996;37(1):87–90.
328. Ettinger AB, Weisbrot DM, Saracco J, et al. Positive and negative psychotropic effects of lamotrigine in patients with epilepsy and mental retardation. Epilepsia. 1998;39(8):874–7.
329. Brandt C, Fueratsch N, Boehme V, et al. Development of psychosis in patients with epilepsy treated with lamotrigine: report of six cases and review of the literature. Epilepsy Behav. 2007;11(1):133–9.
330. Beran RG, Gibson RJ. Aggressive behaviour in intellectually challenged patients with epilepsy treated with lamotrigine. Epilepsia. 1998;39(3):280–2.
331. Labiner DM, Ettinger AB, Fakhoury TA, et al. Effects of lamotrigine compared with levetiracetam on anger, hostility, and total mood in patients with partial epilepsy. Epilepsia. 2009;50(3):434–42.
332. Messenheimer J, Mullens EL, Giorgi L, et al. Safety review of adult clinical trial experience with lamotrigine. Drug Saf. 1998;18(4):281–96.
333. Meador KJ, Loring DW, Ray PG, et al. Differential cognitive and behavioral effects of carbamazepine and lamotrigine. Neurology. 2001;56(9):1177–82.
334. Viteri C, Codina M, Cobaleda S, et al. Quality of life and treatment satisfaction in Spanish epilepsy patients on monotherapy with lamotrigine or valproic acid. Seizure. 2010;19(7):432–8.
335. Arroyo S, Dodson WE, Privitera MD, et al. Randomized dose-controlled study of topiramate as first-line therapy in epilepsy. Acta Neurol Scand. 2005;112(4):214–22.
336. Mula M, Trimble MR, Lhatoo SD, et al. Topiramate and psychiatric adverse events in patients with epilepsy. Epilepsia. 2003;44(5):659–63.
337. Privitera M, Fincham R, Penry J, et al. Topiramate placebo-controlled dose-ranging trial in refractory partial epilepsy using 600-, 800-, and 1,000-mg daily dosages. Topiramate YE Study Group. Neurology. 1996;46(6):1678–83.
338. Mula M, Hesdorffer DC, Trimble M, et al. The role of titration schedule of topiramate for the development of depression in patients with epilepsy. Epilepsia. 2009;50(5):1072–6.
339. Fröscher W, Schier KR, Hoffmann M, et al. Topiramate: a prospective study on the relationship between concentration, dosage and adverse events in epileptic patients on combination therapy. Epileptic Disord. 2005;7(3):237–48.
340. Martin R, Kuzniecky R, Ho S, et al. Cognitive effects of topiramate, gabapentin, and lamotrigine in healthy young adults. Neurology. 1999;52(2):321–7.
341. Fritz N, Glogau S, Hoffmann J, et al. Efficacy and cognitive side effects of tiagabine and topiramate in patients with epilepsy. Epilepsy Behav. 2005;6(3):373–81.

342. Cramer JA, Fisher R, Ben-Menachem E, et al. New antiepileptic drugs: comparison of key clinical trials. Epilepsia. 1999;40(5):590–600.
343. Sharief M, Viteri C, Ben-Menachem E, et al. Double-blind, placebo-controlled study of topiramate in patients with refractory partial epilepsy. Epilepsy Res. 1996;25(3):217–24.
344. Faught E, Wilder BJ, Ramsay RE, et al. Topiramate placebo-controlled dose-ranging trial in refractory partial epilepsy using 200-, 400-, and 600-mg daily dosages. Topiramate YD Study Group. Neurology. 1996;46(6):1684–90.
345. Shorvon SD. Safety of topiramate: adverse events and relationships to dosing. Epilepsia. 1996;37(Suppl 2):S18–s22.
346. Andersohn F, Schade R, Willich SN, et al. Use of antiepileptic drugs in epilepsy and the risk of self-harm or suicidal behavior. Neurology. 2010;75(4):335–40.
347. Guberman A, Neto W, Gassmann-Mayer C. Low-dose topiramate in adults with treatment-resistant partial-onset seizures. Acta Neurol Scand. 2002;106(4):183–9.
348. Zhang L, Huang J, Zhuang JH, et al. Topiramate as an adjunctive treatment for refractory partial epilepsy in the elderly. J Int Med Res. 2011;39(2):408–15.
349. Cramer JA, De Rue K, Devinsky O, et al. A systematic review of the behavioral effects of levetiracetam in adults with epilepsy, cognitive disorders, or an anxiety disorder during clinical trials. Epilepsy Behav. 2003;4(2):124–32.
350. Tekgül H, Gencpinar P, Çavuşoğlu D, et al. The efficacy, tolerability and safety of levetiracetam therapy in a pediatric population. Seizure. 2016;36:16–21.
351. Feng XF, Chen YX, Liu L, et al. Retention rates of levetiraceram in Chinese children and adolescents with epilepsy. Eur J Paediatr Neurol. 2015;19(2):143–8.
352. Helmstaedter C, Mihov Y, Toliat MR, et al. Genetic variation in dopaminergic activity is associated with the risk for psychiatric side effects of levetiracetam. Epilepsia. 2013;54(1):36–44.
353. Nakken KO, Eriksson AS, Lossius R, et al. A paradoxical effect of levetiracetam may be seen in both children and adults with refractory epilepsy. Seizure. 2003;12(1):42–6.
354. Vaisleib II, Neft RA. Rapid dosage titration of levetiracetam in children. Pharmacotherapy. 2008;28(3):393–6.
355. Bilo L, de Leva MF, Meo R. Levetiracetam in clinical practice: efficacy and tolerability in epilepsy. Can J Neurol Sci. 2010;37(3):376–82.
356. Verrotti A, Prezioso G, Di Sabatino F, et al. The adverse event profile of levetiracetam: a meta-analysis on children and adults. Seizure. 2015;31:49–55.
357. Brodtkorb E, Klees TM, Nakken KO, et al. Levetiracetam in adult patients with and without learning disability: focus on behavioral adverse effects. Epilepsy Behav. 2004;5(2):231–5.
358. Tamarelle C, Pandit F, Mazarati A, et al. Levetiracetam-induced depression in a 5-year-old child with partial epilepsy. Seizure. 2009;18(3):235–6.
359. Youroukos S, Lazopoulou D, Michelakou D, et al. Acute psychosis associated with levetiracetam. Epileptic Disord. 2003;5(2):117–9.
360. Briggs DE, French JA. Levetiracetam safety profiles and tolerability in epilepsy patients. Expert Opin Drug Saf. 2004;3(5):415–24.
361. Glauser TA, Pellock JM, Bebin EM, et al. Efficacy and safety of levetiracetam in children with partial seizures: an open-label trial. Epilepsia. 2002;43(5):518–24.
362. Delanty N, Jones J, Tonner F. Adjunctive levetiracetam in children, adolescents, and adults with primary generalized seizures: open-label, noncomparative, multicenter, long-term follow-up study. Epilepsia. 2012;53(1):111–9.
363. Opp J, Tuxhorn I, May T, et al. Levetiracetam in children with refractory epilepsy: a multicenter open label study in Germany. Seizure. 2005;14(7):476–84.
364. Lagae L, Buyse G, Ceulemans B. Clinical experience with levetiracetam in childhood epilepsy: an add-on and mono-therapy trial. Seizure. 2005;14(1):66–71.
365. de la Loge C, Hunter SJ, Schiemann J, et al. Assessment of behavioral and emotional functioning using standardized instruments in children and adolescents with partial-onset seizures treated with adjunctive levetiracetam in a randomized, placebo-controlled trial. Epilepsy Behav. 2010;18(3):291–8.

366. Gao ZJ, Jiang YW. Follow-up study on levetiracetam monotherapy in children with epilepsy. Zhongguo Dang Dai Er Ke Za Zhi. 2008;10(6):711–4.
367. Kumar N, Swaroop HS, Chakraborty A, et al. Levetiracetam induced acute reversible psychosis in a patient with uncontrolled seizures. Indian J Pharmacol. 2014;46(5):560–1.
368. Shorvon SD, Löwenthal A, Janz D, et al. Multicenter double-blind, randomized, placebo-controlled trial of levetiracetam as add-on therapy in patients with refractory partial seizures. European Levetiracetam Study Group. Epilepsia. 2000;41(9):1179–86.
369. Kossoff EH, Bergey GK, Freeman JM, et al. Levetiracetam psychosis in children with epilepsy. Epilepsia. 2001;42(12):1611–3.
370. Kuba R, Novotná I, Brázdil M, et al. Long-term levetiracetam treatment in patients with epilepsy: 3-year follow up. Acta Neurol Scand. 2010;121(2):83–8.
371. Farooq MU, Bhatt A, Majid A, et al. Levetiracetam for managing neurologic and psychiatric disorders. Am J Health Syst Pharm. 2009;66(6):541–61.
372. Major P, Greenberg E, Khan A, et al. Pyridoxine supplementation for the treatment of levetiracetam-induced behavior side effects in children: preliminary results. Epilepsy Behav. 2008;13(3):557–9.
373. Lossius IMB, Svendsen T, Sødal HF, et al. Effect and tolerability of perampanel in patients with drug-resistant epilepsy. Epilepsy Behav. 2021;119:107965.
374. Kanner AM, Patten A, Ettinger AB, et al. Does a psychiatric history play a role in the development of psychiatric adverse events to perampanel… and to placebo? Epilepsy Behav. 2021;125:108380.
375. Yamamoto Y, Shiratani Y, Asai S, et al. Risk factors for psychiatric adverse effects associated with perampanel therapy. Epilepsy Behav. 2021;124:108356.
376. Fan PF, Zhuo C, Huang M. Efficacy and safety of perampanel for epilepsy: a systematic review and meta-analysis of real-world studies. Eur Rev Med Pharmacol Sci. 2023;27(13):6027–39.
377. Liu P, Zhu Z, Wu H. The safety of perampanel in different disorders and doses: a meta-analysis. Seizure. 2023;106:22–8.
378. Steinhoff BJ, Klein P, Klitgaard H, et al. Behavioral adverse events with brivaracetam, levetiracetam, perampanel, and topiramate: a systematic review. Epilepsy Behav. 2021;118:107939.
379. Kawai M, Goji H, Kanemoto K. Differences in aggression as psychiatric side effect of levetiracetam and perampanel in patients with epilepsy. Epilepsy Behav. 2022;126:108493.
380. Hasegawa N, Tohyama J. Differences in levetiracetam and perampanel treatment-related irritability in patients with epilepsy. Epilepsy Behav. 2021;116:107644.
381. Langosch JM, Trimble MR. Epilepsy, psychosis and clozapine. Hum Psychopharmacol. 2002;17(2):115–9.
382. Nickl-Jockschat T, Paulzen M, Schneider F, et al. Drug interaction can lead to undetectable serum concentrations of quetiapine in the presence of carbamazepine. Clin Neuropharmacol. 2009;32(1):55.
383. Wang L, Chen S, Liu C, et al. Factors for cognitive impairment in adult epileptic patients. Brain Behav. 2020;10(1):e01475.
384. Bigarella MM, Mäder MJ, Doro MP, et al. Cognitive functions of epileptic patients on monotherapy with phenobarbitone and healthy controls. Arq Neuropsiquiatr. 1991;49(2):136–41.
385. Salinsky MC, Oken BS, Storzbach D, et al. Assessment of CNS effects of antiepileptic drugs by using quantitative EEG measures. Epilepsia. 2003;44(8):1042–50.
386. Kim SM, Song JY, Lee C, et al. Effect of oxcarbazepine on background EEG activity and cognition in epilepsy. J Epilepsy Res. 2013;3(1):7–15.
387. Videman M, Stjerna S, Roivainen R, et al. Evidence for spared attention to faces in 7-month-old infants after prenatal exposure to antiepileptic drugs. Epilepsy Behav. 2016;64(Pt A):62–8.
388. Salinsky M, Storzbach D, Munoz S. Cognitive effects of pregabalin in healthy volunteers: a double-blind, placebo-controlled trial. Neurology. 2010;74(9):755–61.

389. Callisto SP, Illamola SM, Birnbaum AK, et al. Severity of topiramate-related working memory impairment is modulated by plasma concentration and working memory capacity. J Clin Pharmacol. 2020;60(9):1166–76.
390. Feldman L, Lapin B, Busch RM, et al. Evaluating subjective cognitive impairment in the adult epilepsy clinic: effects of depression, number of antiepileptic medications, and seizure frequency. Epilepsy Behav. 2018;81:18–24.
391. Mula M. Topiramate and cognitive impairment: evidence and clinical implications. Ther Adv Drug Saf. 2012;3(6):279–89.
392. Park SP, Kwon SH. Cognitive effects of antiepileptic drugs. J Clin Neurol. 2008;4(3):99–106.
393. Trimble R. Cognitive effects of antiepileptic drugs. Rev Neurol. 1987;143(5):420–8.
394. Strzelczyk A, Schubert-Bast S. Psychobehavioural and cognitive adverse events of anti-seizure medications for the treatment of developmental and epileptic encephalopathies. CNS Drugs. 2022;36(10):1079–111.
395. Besag FMC, Vasey MJ. Neurocognitive effects of antiseizure medications in children and adolescents with epilepsy. Paediatr Drugs. 2021;23(3):253–86.
396. Kälviäinen R, Äikiä M, Riekkinen PJ Sr. Cognitive adverse effects of antiepileptic drugs: incidence, mechanisms and therapeutic implications. CNS Drugs. 1996;5(5):358–68.
397. Voorhies TM. Cognitive and behavioral effects of antiepileptic drugs. Semin Neurol. 1988;8(1):35–41.
398. Trimble MR. Anticonvulsant drugs and cognitive function: a review of the literature. Epilepsia. 1987;28(Suppl 3):S37–45.
399. Onuma T. Cognitive dysfunction and antiepileptic drugs. Brain Nerve. 2011;63(4):379–83.
400. Stores G, Williams PL, Styles E, et al. Psychological effects of sodium valproate and carbamazepine in epilepsy. Arch Dis Child. 1992;67(11):1330–7.
401. Chen YJ, Kang WM, So WC. Comparison of antiepileptic drugs on cognitive function in newly diagnosed epileptic children: a psychometric and neurophysiological study. Epilepsia. 1996;37(1):81–6.
402. Meador KJ, Seliger J, Boyd A, et al. Comparative neuropsychological effects of carbamazepine and eslicarbazepine acetate. Epilepsy Behav. 2019;94:151–7.
403. Yaari Y, Selzer ME, Pincus JH. Phenytoin: mechanisms of its anticonvulsant action. Ann Neurol. 1986;20(2):171–84.
404. Salinsky MC, Spencer DC, Oken BS, et al. Effects of oxcarbazepine and phenytoin on the EEG and cognition in healthy volunteers. Epilepsy Behav. 2004;5(6):894–902.
405. Williams J, Bates S, Griebel ML, et al. Does short-term antiepileptic drug treatment in children result in cognitive or behavioral changes? Epilepsia. 1998;39(10):1064–9.
406. Glauser TA, Cnaan A, Shinnar S, et al. Ethosuximide, valproic acid, and lamotrigine in childhood absence epilepsy. N Engl J Med. 2010;362(9):790–9.
407. Camfield CS, Chaplin S, Doyle AB, et al. Side effects of phenobarbital in toddlers; behavioral and cognitive aspects. J Pediatr. 1979;95(3):361–5.
408. Bawden HN, Camfield CS, Camfield PR, et al. The cognitive and behavioural effects of clobazam and standard monotherapy are comparable. Canadian Study Group for Childhood Epilepsy. Epilepsy Res. 1999;33(2–3):133–43.
409. Farwell JR, Lee YJ, Hirtz DG, et al. Phenobarbital for febrile seizures—effects on intelligence and on seizure recurrence. N Engl J Med. 1990;322(6):364–9.
410. Vining EP, Mellitis ED, Dorsen MM, et al. Psychologic and behavioral effects of antiepileptic drugs in children: a double-blind comparison between phenobarbital and valproic acid. Pediatrics. 1987;80(2):165–74.
411. Dokkedal-Silva V, Berro LF, Galduróz JCF, et al. Clonazepam: indications, side effects, and potential for nonmedical use. Harv Rev Psychiatry. 2019;27(5):279–89.
412. Rosebush PI, Mazurek MF. Catatonia after benzodiazepine withdrawal. J Clin Psychopharmacol. 1996;16(4):315–9.
413. Brunbech L, Sabers A. Effect of antiepileptic drugs on cognitive function in individuals with epilepsy: a comparative review of newer versus older agents. Drugs. 2002;62(4):593–604.

414. Helmstaedter C, Witt JA. The longer-term cognitive effects of adjunctive antiepileptic treatment with lacosamide in comparison with lamotrigine and topiramate in a naturalistic outpatient setting. Epilepsy Behav. 2013;26(2):182–7.
415. Li KY, Huang LC, Chang YP, et al. The effects of lacosamide on cognitive function and psychiatric profiles in patients with epilepsy. Epilepsy Behav. 2020;113:107580.
416. IJff DM, van Veenendaal TM, Majoie HJ, et al. Cognitive effects of lacosamide as adjunctive therapy in refractory epilepsy. Acta Neurol Scand. 2015;131(6):347–54.
417. Meschede C, Witt JA, Rademacher M, et al. Evaluating the longer-term cognitive effects of adjunctive perampanel compared to lacosamide in a naturalistic outpatient setting. Seizure. 2018;58:141–6.
418. Witt JA, Elger CE, Helmstaedter C. Short-term and longer-term effects of brivaracetam on cognition and behavior in a naturalistic clinical setting-preliminary data. Seizure. 2018;62:49–54.
419. Li KY, Hsu CY, Yang YH. A review of cognitive and behavioral outcomes of Brivaracetam. Kaohsiung J Med Sci. 2023;39(2):104–14.
420. Kockelmann E, Elger CE, Helmstaedter C. Cognitive profile of topiramate as compared with lamotrigine in epilepsy patients on antiepileptic drug polytherapy: relationships to blood serum levels and comedication. Epilepsy Behav. 2004;5(5):716–21.
421. Smith ME, Gevins A, McEvoy LK, et al. Distinct cognitive neurophysiologic profiles for lamotrigine and topiramate. Epilepsia. 2006;47(4):695–703.
422. Meador KJ, Loring DW, Vahle VJ, et al. Cognitive and behavioral effects of lamotrigine and topiramate in healthy volunteers. Neurology. 2005;64(12):2108–14.
423. Pellock JM. Felbamate. Epilepsia. 1999;40(Suppl 5):S57–62.
424. Gay PE, Mecham GF, Coskey JS, et al. Behavioral effects of felbamate in childhood epileptic encephalopathy (Lennox-Gastaut syndrome). Psychol Rep. 1995;77(3 Pt 2):1208–10.
425. Shah YD, Singh K, Friedman D, et al. Evaluating the safety and efficacy of felbamate in the context of a black box warning: a single center experience. Epilepsy Behav. 2016;56:50–3.
426. Bresnahan R, Gianatsi M, Maguire MJ, et al. Vigabatrin add-on therapy for drug-resistant focal epilepsy. Cochrane Database Syst Rev. 2020;7(7):Cd007302.
427. Dodrill CB, Arnett JL, Sommerville KW, et al. Effects of differing dosages of vigabatrin (Sabril) on cognitive abilities and quality of life in epilepsy. Epilepsia. 1995;36(2):164–73.
428. Leppik IE. Zonisamide: chemistry, mechanism of action, and pharmacokinetics. Seizure. 2004;13 Suppl 1:S5–9; discussion S10.
429. Guerrini R, Rosati A, Bradshaw K, et al. Adjunctive zonisamide therapy in the long-term treatment of children with partial epilepsy: results of an open-label extension study of a phase III, randomized, double-blind, placebo-controlled trial. Epilepsia. 2014;55(4):568–78.
430. Porter RJ, Dhir A, Macdonald RL, et al. Mechanisms of action of antiseizure drugs. Handb Clin Neurol. 2012;108:663–81.
431. Kälviäinen R, Aikiä M, Mervaala E, et al. Long-term cognitive and EEG effects of tiagabine in drug-resistant partial epilepsy. Epilepsy Res. 1996;25(3):291–7.
432. Dodrill CB, Arnett JL, Sommerville KW, et al. Cognitive and quality of life effects of differing dosages of tiagabine in epilepsy. Neurology. 1997;48(4):1025–31.
433. Hakimian S, Cheng-Hakimian A, Anderson GD, et al. Rufinamide: a new anti-epileptic medication. Expert Opin Pharmacother. 2007;8(12):1931–40.
434. Arzimanoglou A, Ferreira J, Satlin A, et al. Evaluation of long-term safety, tolerability, and behavioral outcomes with adjunctive rufinamide in pediatric patients (≥1 to <4 years old) with Lennox-Gastaut syndrome: final results from randomized study 303. Eur J Paediatr Neurol. 2019;23(1):126–35.
435. Operto FF, Verrotti A, Marrelli A, et al. Cognitive, adaptive, and behavioral effects of adjunctive rufinamide in Lennox-Gastaut syndrome: a prospective observational clinical study. Epilepsy Behav. 2020;112:107445.
436. Aldenkamp AP, Alpherts WC. The effect of the new antiepileptic drug rufinamide on cognitive functions. Epilepsia. 2006;47(7):1153–9.

437. Moavero R, Santarone ME, Galasso C, et al. Cognitive and behavioral effects of new antiepileptic drugs in pediatric epilepsy. Brain Dev. 2017;39(6):464–9.
438. Jóźwiak S, Veggiotti P, Moreira J, et al. Effects of adjunctive eslicarbazepine acetate on neurocognitive functioning in children with refractory focal-onset seizures. Epilepsy Behav. 2018;81:1–11.
439. Milovan D, Almeida L, Romach MK, et al. Effect of eslicarbazepine acetate and oxcarbazepine on cognition and psychomotor function in healthy volunteers. Epilepsy Behav. 2010;18(4):366–73.
440. Miller I, Scheffer IE, Gunning B, et al. Dose-ranging effect of adjunctive oral cannabidiol vs placebo on convulsive seizure frequency in Dravet syndrome: a randomized clinical trial. JAMA Neurol. 2020;77(5):613–21.
441. Lagae L, Sullivan J, Knupp K, et al. Fenfluramine hydrochloride for the treatment of seizures in Dravet syndrome: a randomised, double-blind, placebo-controlled trial. Lancet. 2019;394(10216):2243–54.
442. Nabbout R, Mistry A, Zuberi S, et al. Fenfluramine for treatment-resistant seizures in patients with Dravet syndrome receiving stiripentol-inclusive regimens: a randomized clinical trial. JAMA Neurol. 2020;77(3):300–8.
443. Wiegand G, May TW, Ostertag P, et al. Everolimus in tuberous sclerosis patients with intractable epilepsy: a treatment option? Eur J Paediatr Neurol. 2013;17(6):631–8.
444. Overwater IE, Rietman AB, Mous SE, et al. A randomized controlled trial with everolimus for IQ and autism in tuberous sclerosis complex. Neurology. 2019;93(2):e200–e9.
445. Taylor CP. Mechanisms of action of gabapentin. Rev Neurol. 1997;153(Suppl 1):S39–45.
446. Morris GL. Gabapentin. Epilepsia. 1999;40(Suppl 5):S63–70.
447. Bateson AN. Basic pharmacologic mechanisms involved in benzodiazepine tolerance and withdrawal. Curr Pharm Des. 2002;8(1):5–21.
448. Strzelczyk A, Schubert-Bast S. A practical guide to the treatment of Dravet syndrome with anti-seizure medication. CNS Drugs. 2022;36(3):217–37.
449. Donati F, Gobbi G, Campistol J, et al. The cognitive effects of oxcarbazepine versus carbamazepine or valproate in newly diagnosed children with partial seizures. Seizure. 2007;16(8):670–9.
450. Donati F, Gobbi G, Campistol J, et al. Effects of oxcarbazepine on cognitive function in children and adolescents with partial seizures. Neurology. 2006;67(4):679–82.
451. Quon RJ, Mazanec MT, Schmidt SS, et al. Antiepileptic drug effects on subjective and objective cognition. Epilepsy Behav. 2020;104(Pt A):106906.
452. Hoxhaj P, Habiya SK, Sayabugari R, et al. Investigating the impact of epilepsy on cognitive function: a narrative review. Cureus. 2023;15(6):e41223.
453. American Academy of Pediatrics. Behavioral and cognitive effects of anticonvulsant therapy. Committee on Drugs. Pediatrics. 1985;76(4):644–7.
454. Valton L, Mascott CR. What is the role of neuropsychological testing in the investigation and management of pharmacologically intractable partial epilepsy? Rev Neurol. 2004;160 Spec No 1:5S154–63.
455. Nashef L. Sudden unexpected death in epilepsy: terminology and definitions. Epilepsia. 1997;38(11 Suppl):S6–8.
456. Annegers JF. United States perspective on definitions and classifications. Epilepsia. 1997;38(11 Suppl):S9–12.
457. Nashef L, So EL, Ryvlin P, et al. Unifying the definitions of sudden unexpected death in epilepsy. Epilepsia. 2012;53(2):227–33.
458. Terrence CF Jr, Wisotzkey HM, Perper JA. Unexpected, unexplained death in epileptic patients. Neurology. 1975;25(6):594–8.
459. Terrence CF, Rao GR, Perper JA. Neurogenic pulmonary edema in unexpected, unexplained death of epileptic patients. Ann Neurol. 1981;9(5):458–64.
460. Lund A, Gormsen H. The role of antiepileptics in sudden death in epilepsy. Acta Neurol Scand. 1985;72(4):444–6.

461. Dasheiff RMDL. Sudden unexpected death of epileptic patient due to cardiac arrhythmia after seizure. J Arch Neurol. 1986;43(2):194–6.
462. Dasheiff RM. Sudden unexpected death in epilepsy: a series from an epilepsy surgery program and speculation on the relationship to sudden cardiac death. J Clin Neurophysiol. 1991;8(2):216–22.
463. Drake ME, Reider CR, Kay A. Electrocardiography in epilepsy patients without cardiac symptoms. Seizure. 1993;2(1):63–5.
464. Shorvon S. Risk factors for sudden unexpected death in epilepsy. Epilepsia. 1997;38(11 Suppl):S20–2.
465. Harden C, Tomson T, Gloss D, et al. Practice guideline summary: sudden unexpected death in epilepsy incidence rates and risk factors: report of the Guideline Development, Dissemination, and Implementation Subcommittee of the American Academy of Neurology and the American Epilepsy Society. Epilepsy Curr. 2017;17(3):180–7.
466. Karlovich E, Devinsky O, Brandsoy M, et al. SUDEP among young adults in the San Diego County Medical Examiner Office. Epilepsia. 2020;61(3):e17–22.
467. Ryvlin P, Nashef L, Lhatoo SD, et al. Incidence and mechanisms of cardiorespiratory arrests in epilepsy monitoring units (MORTEMUS): a retrospective study. Lancet Neurol. 2013;12(10):966–77.
468. Vilella L, Lacuey N, Hampson JP, et al. Postconvulsive central apnea as a biomarker for sudden unexpected death in epilepsy (SUDEP). Neurology. 2019;92(3):e171–e82.
469. Lacuey N, Hampson JP, Harper RM, et al. Limbic and paralimbic structures driving ictal central apnea. Neurology. 2019;92(7):e655–e69.
470. Dlouhy BJ, Gehlbach BK, Kreple CJ, et al. Breathing inhibited when seizures spread to the amygdala and upon amygdala stimulation. J Neurosci Off J Soc Neurosci. 2015;35(28):10281–9.
471. Seyal M, Pascual F, Lee CY, et al. Seizure-related cardiac repolarization abnormalities are associated with ictal hypoxemia. Epilepsia. 2011;52(11):2105–11.
472. Klassen TL, Bomben VC, Patel A, et al. High-resolution molecular genomic autopsy reveals complex sudden unexpected death in epilepsy risk profile. Epilepsia. 2014;55(2):e6–12.
473. Massey CA, Sowers LP, Dlouhy BJ, et al. Mechanisms of sudden unexpected death in epilepsy: the pathway to prevention. Nat Rev Neurol. 2014;10(5):271–82.
474. Claes L, Del-Favero J, Ceulemans B, et al. De novo mutations in the sodium-channel gene SCN1A cause severe myoclonic epilepsy of infancy. Am J Hum Genet. 2001;68(6):1327–32.
475. Maier SK, Westenbroek RE, Yamanushi TT, et al. An unexpected requirement for brain-type sodium channels for control of heart rate in the mouse sinoatrial node. Proc Natl Acad Sci USA. 2003;100(6):3507–12.
476. Kalume F. Sudden unexpected death in Dravet syndrome: respiratory and other physiological dysfunctions. Respir Physiol Neurobiol. 2013;189(2):324–8.
477. Delogu AB, Spinelli A, Battaglia D, et al. Electrical and autonomic cardiac function in patients with Dravet syndrome. Epilepsia. 2011;52(Suppl 2):55–8.
478. Persson H, Ericson M, Tomson T. Carbamazepine affects autonomic cardiac control in patients with newly diagnosed epilepsy. Epilepsy Res. 2003;57(1):69–75.
479. Simon RP. Heart and lung in the postictal state. Epilepsy Behav. 2010;19(2):167–71.
480. Devinsky O, Hesdorffer DC, Thurman DJ, et al. Sudden unexpected death in epilepsy: epidemiology, mechanisms, and prevention. Lancet Neurol. 2016;15(10):1075–88.
481. Sivathamboo S, Friedman D, Laze J, et al. Association of short-term heart rate variability and sudden unexpected death in epilepsy. Neurology. 2021;97(24):e2357–e67.
482. Alexandre V, Mercedes B, Valton L, et al. Risk factors of postictal generalized EEG suppression in generalized convulsive seizures. Neurology. 2015;85(18):1598–603.
483. Shorvon S, Tomson T. Sudden unexpected death in epilepsy. Lancet. 2011;378(9808):2028–38.
484. Tao JX, Yung I, Lee A, et al. Tonic phase of a generalized convulsive seizure is an independent predictor of postictal generalized EEG suppression. Epilepsia. 2013;54(5):858–65.

485. Kuo J, Zhao W, Li CS, et al. Postictal immobility and generalized EEG suppression are associated with the severity of respiratory dysfunction. Epilepsia. 2016;57(3):412–7.
486. Sarkis RA, Thome-Souza S, Poh MZ, et al. Autonomic changes following generalized tonic clonic seizures: an analysis of adult and pediatric patients with epilepsy. Epilepsy Res. 2015;115:113–8.
487. Azmitia EC, Gannon PJ. The primate serotonergic system: a review of human and animal studies and a report on Macaca fascicularis. Adv Neurol. 1986;43:407–68.
488. Aston-Jones G, Cohen JD. An integrative theory of locus coeruleus-norepinephrine function: adaptive gain and optimal performance. Annu Rev Neurosci. 2005;28:403–50.
489. Bromberg-Martin ES, Matsumoto M, Hikosaka O. Dopamine in motivational control: rewarding, aversive, and alerting. Neuron. 2010;68(5):815–34.
490. Jones BE. Activity, modulation and role of basal forebrain cholinergic neurons innervating the cerebral cortex. Prog Brain Res. 2004;145:157–69.
491. Fuller PM, Sherman D, Pedersen NP, et al. Reassessment of the structural basis of the ascending arousal system. J Comp Neurol. 2011;519(5):933–56.
492. Blumenfeld H. Impaired consciousness in epilepsy. Lancet Neurol. 2012;11(9):814–26.
493. Blumenfeld H, McNally KA, Vanderhill SD, et al. Positive and negative network correlations in temporal lobe epilepsy. Cereb Cortex. 2004;14(8):892–902.
494. Faingold CL, Feng HJ. A unified hypothesis of SUDEP: seizure-induced respiratory depression induced by adenosine may lead to SUDEP but can be prevented by autoresuscitation and other restorative respiratory response mechanisms mediated by the action of serotonin on the periaqueductal gray. Epilepsia. 2023;64(4):779–96.
495. Tomson T, Surges R, Delamont R, et al. Who to target in sudden unexpected death in epilepsy prevention and how? Risk factors, biomarkers, and intervention study designs. Epilepsia. 2016;57(Suppl 1):4–16.
496. Hesdorffer DC, Tomson T, Benn E, et al. Combined analysis of risk factors for SUDEP. Epilepsia. 2011;52(6):1150–9.
497. Hesdorffer DC, Tomson T, Benn E, et al. Do antiepileptic drugs or generalized tonic-clonic seizure frequency increase SUDEP risk? A combined analysis. Epilepsia. 2012;53(2):249–52.
498. Clark D, Riney K. A population-based post mortem study of sudden unexpected death in epilepsy. J Clin Neurosci. 2016;23:58–62.
499. Lamberts RJ, Thijs RD, Laffan A, et al. Sudden unexpected death in epilepsy: people with nocturnal seizures may be at highest risk. Epilepsia. 2012;53(2):253–7.
500. Liebenthal JA, Wu S, Rose S, et al. Association of prone position with sudden unexpected death in epilepsy. Neurology. 2015;84(7):703–9.
501. Langan Y, Nashef L, Sander JW. Case-control study of SUDEP. Neurology. 2005;64(7):1131–3.
502. Tomson T, Hirsch LJ, Friedman D, et al. Sudden unexpected death in epilepsy in lamotrigine randomized-controlled trials. Epilepsia. 2013;54(1):135–40.
503. Pack AM. SUDEP: what are the risk factors? Do seizures or antiepileptic drugs contribute to an increased risk? Epilepsy Curr. 2012;12(4):131–2.
504. Opeskin K, Burke MP, Cordner SM, et al. Comparison of antiepileptic drug levels in sudden unexpected deaths in epilepsy with deaths from other causes. Epilepsia. 1999;40(12):1795–8.
505. Williams J, Lawthom C, Dunstan FD, et al. Variability of antiepileptic medication taking behaviour in sudden unexplained death in epilepsy: hair analysis at autopsy. J Neurol Neurosurg Psychiatry. 2006;77(4):481–4.
506. Nilsson L, Farahmand BY, Persson PG, et al. Risk factors for sudden unexpected death in epilepsy: a case-control study. Lancet. 1999;353(9156):888–93.
507. Shankar R, Walker M, McLean B, et al. Steps to prevent SUDEP: the validity of risk factors in the SUDEP and seizure safety checklist: a case control study. J Neurol. 2016;263(9):1840–6.
508. Faught E, Duh MS, Weiner JR, et al. Nonadherence to antiepileptic drugs and increased mortality: findings from the RANSOM Study. Neurology. 2008;71(20):1572–8.

509. Tennis P, Cole TB, Annegers JF, et al. Cohort study of incidence of sudden unexplained death in persons with seizure disorder treated with antiepileptic drugs in Saskatchewan, Canada. Epilepsia. 1995;36(1):29–36.
510. Walczak TS, Leppik IE, D'Amelio M, et al. Incidence and risk factors in sudden unexpected death in epilepsy: a prospective cohort study. Neurology. 2001;56(4):519–25.
511. Timmings PL. Sudden unexpected death in epilepsy: a local audit. Seizure. 1993;2(4):287–90.
512. Thomas P, Valton L, Genton P. Absence and myoclonic status epilepticus precipitated by antiepileptic drugs in idiopathic generalized epilepsy. Brain J Neurol. 2006;129(Pt 5):1281–92.
513. Nilsson L, Bergman U, Diwan V, et al. Antiepileptic drug therapy and its management in sudden unexpected death in epilepsy: a case-control study. Epilepsia. 2001;42(5):667–73.
514. Hauser E, Seidl R, Freilinger M, et al. Hematologic manifestations and impaired liver synthetic function during valproate monotherapy. Brain Dev. 1996;18(2):105–9.
515. Dono F, Evangelista G, Consoli S, et al. Perampanel enhances the cardiovagal tone and heart rate variability (HRV) in patients with drug-resistant temporal lobe epilepsy. Seizure. 2022;99:16–23.
516. Da Costa A, Chalvidan T, Belounas A, et al. Predictive factors of ventricular fibrillation triggered by pause-dependent torsades de pointes associated with acquired long QT interval: role of QT dispersion and left ventricular function. J Cardiovasc Electrophysiol. 2000;11(9):990–7.
517. Refsgaard L, Holst AG, Sadjadieh G, et al. High prevalence of genetic variants previously associated with LQT syndrome in new exome data. Eur J Hum Genet. 2012;20(8):905–8.
518. Nashef L, Hindocha N, Makoff A. Risk factors in sudden death in epilepsy (SUDEP): the quest for mechanisms. Epilepsia. 2007;48(5):859–71.
519. Jawad S, Mercer A, Jamil N, et al. Haematological values of epileptic patients entering drug trials. Int J Clin Pharmacol Res. 1988;8(5):363–6.
520. Edey S, Moran N, Nashef L. SUDEP and epilepsy-related mortality in pregnancy. Epilepsia. 2014;55(7):e72–4.
521. Yuen AW, Sander JW, Flugel D, et al. Erythrocyte and plasma fatty acid profiles in patients with epilepsy: does carbamazepine affect omega-3 fatty acid concentrations? Epilepsy Behav. 2008;12(2):317–23.
522. Kennebäck G, Bergfeldt L, Vallin H, et al. Electrophysiologic effects and clinical hazards of carbamazepine treatment for neurologic disorders in patients with abnormalities of the cardiac conduction system. Am Heart J. 1991;121(5):1421–9.
523. Kasarskis EJ, Kuo CS, Berger R, et al. Carbamazepine-induced cardiac dysfunction. Characterization of two distinct clinical syndromes. Arch Intern Med. 1992;152(1):186–91.
524. Ben-Menachem E, Biton V, Jatuzis D, et al. Efficacy and safety of oral lacosamide as adjunctive therapy in adults with partial-onset seizures. Epilepsia. 2007;48(7):1308–17.
525. DeSilvey DL, Moss AJ. Primidone in the treatment of the long QT syndrome: QT shortening and ventricular arrhythmia suppression. Ann Intern Med. 1980;93(1):53–4.
526. Lehnart SE, Mongillo M, Bellinger A, et al. Leaky Ca2+ release channel/ryanodine receptor 2 causes seizures and sudden cardiac death in mice. J Clin Invest. 2008;118(6):2230–45.
527. MacCormick JM, Crawford JR, Chung SK, et al. Symptoms and signs associated with syncope in young people with primary cardiac arrhythmias. Heart Lung Circ. 2011;20(9):593–8.
528. King A, Gerard EE. Contraception, fecundity, and pregnancy in women with epilepsy: an update on recent literature. Curr Opin Neurol. 2022;35(2):161–8.
529. Anderson GD. Pharmacogenetics and enzyme induction/inhibition properties of antiepileptic drugs. Neurology. 2004;63(10 Suppl 4):S3–8.
530. Reddy DS. Clinical pharmacokinetic interactions between antiepileptic drugs and hormonal contraceptives. Expert Rev Clin Pharmacol. 2010;3(2):183–92. https://doi.org/10.1586/ecp.10.3.
531. Parekh K, Kravets HD, Spiegel R. Special considerations in the management of women with epilepsy in reproductive years. J Pers Med. 2022;12(1):88.

532. Doose DR, Wang SS, Padmanabhan M, et al. Effect of topiramate or carbamazepine on the pharmacokinetics of an oral contraceptive containing norethindrone and ethinyl estradiol in healthy obese and nonobese female subjects. Epilepsia. 2003;44(4):540–9.
533. Sarayani A, Winterstein A, Cristofoletti R, et al. Real-world effect of a potential drug-drug interaction between topiramate and oral contraceptives on unintended pregnancy outcomes. Contraception. 2023;120:109953.
534. Davis AR, Pack AM, Kritzer J, et al. Reproductive history, sexual behavior and use of contraception in women with epilepsy. Contraception. 2008;77(6):405–9.
535. Herzog AG, Mandle HB, MacEachern DB. Prevalence of highly effective contraception use by women with epilepsy. Neurology. 2019;92(24):e2815–e21.
536. Pack AM, Davis AR, Kritzer J, et al. Antiepileptic drugs: are women aware of interactions with oral contraceptives and potential teratogenicity? Epilepsy Behav. 2009;14(4):640–4.
537. Webber MP, Hauser WA, Ottman R, et al. Fertility in persons with epilepsy: 1935–1974. Epilepsia. 1986;27(6):746–52.
538. MacEachern DB, Mandle HB, Herzog AG. Infertility, impaired fecundity, and live birth/pregnancy ratio in women with epilepsy in the USA: findings of the Epilepsy Birth Control Registry. Epilepsia. 2019;60(9):1993–8.
539. Olafsson E, Hauser WA, Gudmundsson G. Fertility in patients with epilepsy: a population-based study. Neurology. 1998;51(1):71–3.
540. Pennell PB, French JA, Harden CL, et al. Fertility and birth outcomes in women with epilepsy seeking pregnancy. JAMA Neurol. 2018;75(8):962–9.
541. Larsen MD, Jølving LR, Fedder J, et al. The efficacy of assisted reproductive treatment in women with epilepsy. Reprod Biomed Online. 2020;41(6):1015–22.
542. Unnikrishnan G, Jacob NS, Salim S, et al. Enduring language deficits in children of women with epilepsy and the potential role of intrauterine exposure to antiepileptic drugs. Epilepsia. 2020;61(11):2442–51.
543. Isojärvi JI, Laatikainen TJ, Pakarinen AJ, et al. Polycystic ovaries and hyperandrogenism in women taking valproate for epilepsy. N Engl J Med. 1993;329(19):1383–8.
544. Harden CL, Pennell PB, Koppel BS, et al. Management issues for women with epilepsy—focus on pregnancy (an evidence-based review): III. Vitamin K, folic acid, blood levels, and breast-feeding: report of the Quality Standards Subcommittee and Therapeutics and Technology Assessment Subcommittee of the American Academy of Neurology and the American Epilepsy Society. Epilepsia. 2009;50(5):1247–55.
545. Morrow J, Russell A, Guthrie E, et al. Malformation risks of antiepileptic drugs in pregnancy: a prospective study from the UK Epilepsy and Pregnancy Register. J Neurol Neurosurg Psychiatry. 2006;77(2):193–8.
546. Tomson T, Battino D, Bonizzoni E, et al. Comparative risk of major congenital malformations with eight different antiepileptic drugs: a prospective cohort study of the EURAP registry. Lancet Neurol. 2018;17(6):530–8.
547. Hernández-Díaz S, Smith CR, Shen A, et al. Comparative safety of antiepileptic drugs during pregnancy. Neurology. 2012;78(21):1692–9.
548. Tomson T, Battino D, Bonizzoni E, et al. Dose-dependent risk of malformations with antiepileptic drugs: an analysis of data from the EURAP epilepsy and pregnancy registry. Lancet Neurol. 2011;10(7):609–17.
549. Cohen JM, Cesta CE, Furu K, et al. Prevalence trends and individual patterns of antiepileptic drug use in pregnancy 2006–2016: a study in the five Nordic countries, United States, and Australia. Pharmacoepidemiol Drug Saf. 2020;29(8):913–22.
550. Hurault-Delarue C, Morris JK, Charlton R, et al. Prescription of antiepileptic medicines including valproate in pregnant women: a study in three European countries. Pharmacoepidemiol Drug Saf. 2019;28(11):1510–8.
551. Meador KJ, Pennell PB, May RC, et al. Changes in antiepileptic drug-prescribing patterns in pregnant women with epilepsy. Epilepsy Behav. 2018;84:10–4.

552. Clavenna A, Campi R, Putignano D, et al. Changes in antiepileptic drug prescriptions over a decade in childbearing women in Lombardy region, Italy. Br J Clin Pharmacol. 2022;88(3):1152–8.
553. Avachat C, Barry JM, Lyu X, et al. Management of anti-seizure medications during pregnancy: advancements in the past decade. Pharmaceutics. 2022;14(12):2733.
554. Meador KJ, Baker GA, Browning N, et al. Fetal antiepileptic drug exposure and cognitive outcomes at age 6 years (NEAD study): a prospective observational study. Lancet Neurol. 2013;12(3):244–52.
555. Adab N, Kini U, Vinten J, et al. The longer term outcome of children born to mothers with epilepsy. J Neurol Neurosurg Psychiatry. 2004;75(11):1575–83.
556. Meador KJ, Baker GA, Browning N, et al. Cognitive function at 3 years of age after fetal exposure to antiepileptic drugs. N Engl J Med. 2009;360(16):1597–605.
557. Meador KJ, Pennell PB, May RC, et al. Effects of periconceptional folate on cognition in children of women with epilepsy: NEAD study. Neurology. 2020;94(7):e729–e40.
558. Hernández-Díaz S, Werler MM, Walker AM, et al. Folic acid antagonists during pregnancy and the risk of birth defects. N Engl J Med. 2000;343(22):1608–14.
559. Van Marter LJ, Pennell PB, Brown C, et al. Neonatal outcomes in the MONEAD study of pregnant women with epilepsy. J Pediatr X. 2021;7:100073.
560. Pennell PB, Klein AM, Browning N, et al. Differential effects of antiepileptic drugs on neonatal outcomes. Epilepsy Behav. 2012;24(4):449–56.
561. Birnbaum AK, Meador KJ, Karanam A, et al. Antiepileptic drug exposure in infants of breastfeeding mothers with epilepsy. JAMA Neurol. 2020;77(4):441–50.
562. Meador KJ. Breastfeeding and antiepileptic drugs. JAMA. 2014;311(17):1797–8.
563. Anderson PO. Antiepileptic drugs during breastfeeding. Breastfeed Med. 2020;15(1):2–4.
564. Meador KJ, Baker GA, Browning N, et al. Breastfeeding in children of women taking antiepileptic drugs: cognitive outcomes at age 6 years. JAMA Pediatr. 2014;168(8):729–36.
565. Liu P, He M, Xu X, et al. Real-world safety of Lacosamide: a pharmacovigilance study based on spontaneous reports in the FDA adverse event reporting system. Seizure. 2023;110:203–11.
566. Arai Y, Okanishi T, Kanai S, et al. Identifying risk factors for adverse events of pyridoxal phosphate in infantile epileptic spasms syndrome. Epilepsy Behav. 2023;145:109348.
567. MacVicar S, Hetherington A, Strickland M. Desmond Beall – a Canadian's contribution to understanding rhabdomyolysis. Can J Surg. 2023;66(4):E409–e10.
568. Stahl K, Rastelli E, Schoser B. A systematic review on the definition of rhabdomyolysis. J Neurol. 2020;267(4):877–82.
569. Mathew DM, Chilakala A, Elfert K. Rhabdomyolysis in the setting of severe hyponatremia: a case report. Cureus. 2023;15(6):e39993.
570. Harris AS, Aratani S, Johmura Y, et al. In vivo dynamics of senescence in rhabdomyolysis-induced acute kidney injury. Biochem Biophys Res Commun. 2023;673:121–30.
571. Boparai S, Lakra R, Dhaliwal L, et al. Therapeutic plasma exchange in severe rhabdomyolysis: a case-control study. Cureus. 2023;15(5):e39748.
572. Otsuki T. Epilepsy care network. Nihon Rinsho. 2014;72(5):947–51.
573. Vanholder R, Sever MS, Erek E, et al. Rhabdomyolysis. J Am Soc Nephrol. 2000;11(8):1553–61.
574. Bywaters EG, Beall D. Crush injuries with impairment of renal function. Br Med J. 1941;1(4185):427–32.
575. Chamberlain MC. Rhabdomyolysis in children: a 3-year retrospective study. Pediatr Neurol. 1991;7(3):226–8.
576. Huerta-Alardín AL, Varon J, Marik PE. Bench-to-bedside review: rhabdomyolysis—an overview for clinicians. Crit Care. 2005;9(2):158–69.
577. Cervellin G, Comelli I, Lippi G. Rhabdomyolysis: historical background, clinical, diagnostic and therapeutic features. Clin Chem Lab Med. 2010;48(6):749–56.
578. Bosch X, Poch E, Grau JM. Rhabdomyolysis and acute kidney injury. N Engl J Med. 2009;361(1):62–72.

579. Sauret JM, Marinides G, Wang GK. Rhabdomyolysis. Am Fam Physician. 2002;65(5):907–12.
580. Watanabe T. Rhabdomyolysis and acute renal failure in children. Pediatr Nephrol. 2001;16(12):1072–5.
581. Veenstra J, Smit WM, Krediet RT, et al. Relationship between elevated creatine phosphokinase and the clinical spectrum of rhabdomyolysis. Nephrol Dial Transplant. 1994;9(6):637–41.
582. Lane R, Phillips M. Rhabdomyolysis. BMJ. 2003;327(7407):115–6.
583. Chatzizisis YS, Misirli G, Hatzitolios AI, et al. The syndrome of rhabdomyolysis: complications and treatment. Eur J Intern Med. 2008;19(8):568–74.
584. Crepeau AZ, Treiman DM. Levetiracetam: a comprehensive review. Expert Rev Neurother. 2010;10(2):159–71.
585. Akiyama H, Haga Y, Sasaki N, et al. A case of rhabdomyolysis in which levetiracetam was suspected as the cause. Epilepsy Behav Case Rep. 2014;2:152–5.
586. Isaacson JE, Choe DJ, Doherty MJ. Creatine phosphokinase elevation exacerbated by levetiracetam therapy. Epilepsy Behav Case Rep. 2014;2:189–91.
587. Incecik F, Herguner OM, Besen S, et al. Acute rhabdomyolysis associated with levetiracetam therapy in a child. Acta Neurol Belg. 2016;116(3):369–70.
588. Moinuddin IA. Suspected levetiracetam-induced rhabdomyolysis: a case report and literature review. Am J Case Rep. 2020;21:e926064.
589. Haruda F. Phenytoin hypersensitivity: 38 cases. Neurology. 1979;29(11):1480–5.
590. Engel JN, Mellul VG, Goodman DB. Phenytoin hypersensitivity: a case of severe acute rhabdomyolysis. Am J Med. 1986;81(5):928–30.
591. Santos-Calle FJ, Borrás-Blasco J, Navarro-Ruiz A, et al. Unsuspected rhabdomyolysis associated with phenytoin. Int J Clin Pharmacol Ther. 2005;43(9):436–40.
592. Korman LB, Olson MJ. Phenytoin-induced hepatitis, rhabdomyolysis, and renal dysfunction. Clin Pharm. 1989;8(7):514–5.
593. di Russo P, Perrini P, Benedetto N, et al. Phenytoin-induced rhabdomyolysis: timely recognition for safely remission. Neurol India. 2016;64(4):793–4.
594. Zwaenepoel B, Le Roy S, Decruyenaere A, et al. Letter to the editor: phenytoin-induced rhabdomyolysis. Acta Neurol Belg. 2019;119(2):293–4.
595. Kim H, Jo S, Park KW, et al. A case of phenytoin-induced rhabdomyolysis in status epilepticus. J Epilepsy Res. 2016;6(1):36–8.
596. Ponchaut S, Van Hoof F, Veitch K. Valproate and cytochrome c oxidase deficiency. Eur J Pediatr. 1995;154(1):79.
597. Wieser T. Carnitine palmitoyltransferase II deficiency. In: Adam MP, Feldman J, Mirzaa GM, et al., editors. GeneReviews(®). Seattle: University of Washington, Seattle. Copyright © 1993–2024, University of Washington, Seattle. GeneReviews is a registered trademark of the University of Washington, Seattle. All rights reserved; 1993.
598. Lheureux PE, Penaloza A, Zahir S, et al. Science review: carnitine in the treatment of valproic acid-induced toxicity – what is the evidence? Crit Care. 2005;9(5):431–40.
599. Meyer S, Martin T, Löffler G, et al. Severe rhabdomyolysis caused by valproic acid in a neonate with seizures and chromosomal abnormalities. Klin Padiatr. 2011;223(7):434–5.
600. Tuccori M, Lombardo G, Lapi F, et al. Gabapentin-induced severe myopathy. Ann Pharmacother. 2007;41(7):1301–5.
601. Falconi D, Tattoli F, Brunetti C, et al. Rhabdomyolysis from gabapentin: a case report. G Ital Nefrol. 2015;32(2):gin/32.2.37.
602. Gilman JT. Lamotrigine: an antiepileptic agent for the treatment of partial seizures. Ann Pharmacother. 1995;29(2):144–51.
603. Schaub JE, Williamson PJ, Barnes EW, et al. Multisystem adverse reaction to lamotrigine. Lancet. 1994;344(8920):481.
604. Chattergoon DS, McGuigan MA, Koren G, et al. Multiorgan dysfunction and disseminated intravascular coagulation in children receiving lamotrigine and valproic acid. Neurology. 1997;49(5):1442–4.

605. Schwartz MD, Geller RJ. Seizures and altered mental status after lamotrigine overdose. Ther Drug Monit. 2007;29(6):843–4.
606. Rossetti AO, Logroscino G, Bromfield EB. Refractory status epilepticus: effect of treatment aggressiveness on prognosis. Arch Neurol. 2005;62(11):1698–702.
607. Parke TJ, Stevens JE, Rice AS, et al. Metabolic acidosis and fatal myocardial failure after propofol infusion in children: five case reports. BMJ. 1992;305(6854):613–6.
608. Diaz JH, Prabhakar A, Urman RD, et al. Propofol infusion syndrome: a retrospective analysis at a level 1 trauma center. Crit Care Res Prac. 2014;2014:346968.
609. Hanna JP, Ramundo ML. Rhabdomyolysis and hypoxia associated with prolonged propofol infusion in children. Neurology. 1998;50(1):301–3.
610. Cornfield DN, Tegtmeyer K, Nelson MD, et al. Continuous propofol infusion in 142 critically ill children. Pediatrics. 2002;110(6):1177–81.
611. Zarovnaya EL, Jobst BC, Harris BT. Propofol-associated fatal myocardial failure and rhabdomyolysis in an adult with status epilepticus. Epilepsia. 2007;48(5):1002–6.
612. Toth C. Pregabalin: latest safety evidence and clinical implications for the management of neuropathic pain. Ther Adv Drug Saf. 2014;5(1):38–56.
613. Krasowski MD, McMillin GA. Advances in anti-epileptic drug testing. Clin Chim Acta. 2014;436:224–36.
614. Gunathilake R, Boyce LE, Knight AT. Pregabalin-associated rhabdomyolysis. Med J Aust. 2013;199(9):624–5.
615. Torres PA, Helmstetter JA, Kaye AM, et al. Rhabdomyolysis: pathogenesis, diagnosis, and treatment. Ochsner J. 2015;15(1):58–69.
616. Bagley WH, Yang H, Shah KH. Rhabdomyolysis. Intern Emerg Med. 2007;2(3):210–8.
617. Petejova N, Martinek A. Acute kidney injury due to rhabdomyolysis and renal replacement therapy: a critical review. Crit Care. 2014;18(3):224.
618. Cabral BMI, Edding SN, Portocarrero JP, et al. Rhabdomyolysis. Dis Mon. 2020;66(8):101015.
619. Antoon JW, Chakraborti C. Corticosteroids in the treatment of alcohol-induced rhabdomyolysis. Mayo Clin Proc. 2011;86(10):1005–7.
620. Gabow PA, Kaehny WD, Kelleher SP. The spectrum of rhabdomyolysis. Medicine. 1982;61(3):141–52.
621. Ward MM. Factors predictive of acute renal failure in rhabdomyolysis. Arch Intern Med. 1988;148(7):1553–7.

Chapter 9
Role of Artificial Intelligence Technology in Drug Therapy of Epilepsy

Richard Shek-kwan Chang, Zhibin Chen, Emma Foster, Terence J. O'Brien, and Patrick Kwan

9.1 Introduction

Epilepsy is a prevalent chronic neurological disorder worldwide, affecting people of all ages and ethnic backgrounds. The lifetime risk of epilepsy is approximately 760 per 100,000 individuals. More than 50 million people live with epilepsy, accounting for 13 million disability-adjusted life years (DALYs) globally [1]. The disease burden is significant at both the individual and societal levels. Recurrent seizures can lead to physical and psychosocial disabilities, while comorbidities such as learning disabilities and psychiatric disorders complicate epilepsy management [2]. Premature mortality can be attributed to status epilepticus and Sudden Unexpected Death in Epilepsy (SUDEP). Epilepsy is associated with social stigma, unemployment, and marital problems across different cultural backgrounds [3–5]. Substantial healthcare resources are allocated to epilepsy care, with an average annual cost of over US $1000 per person in high-income countries and an estimated global healthcare cost of US $119 billion per year [6].

Currently, pharmacological therapies remain the primary treatment modality for epilepsy. Antiseizure medications (ASMs) control seizures via various putative mechanisms of action [7], which include sodium channel blockers (e.g., phenytoin and carbamazepine), GABA agonists (e.g., benzodiazepines and barbiturates), calcium channel blockers (e.g., ethosuximide), as well as agents targeting molecular substrates such as synaptic vesicle protein 2A (SV2A) receptors (e.g., levetiracetam and brivaracetam), and AMPA receptors (e.g., perampanel). The number of ASMs available has significantly increased in the past two decades, with more than 20 in the market

R. S.-k. Chang · Z. Chen · E. Foster · T. J. O'Brien · P. Kwan (✉)
Department of Neuroscience, Central Clinical School, Monash University, Melbourne, VIC, Australia
e-mail: shek.chang@monash.edu; ben.chen1@monash.edu; emma.foster@monash.edu; terence.obrien@monash.edu; patrick.kwan@monash.edu

X. Wang, L. Zhou (eds.), *Pharmacological Treatment of Epileptic Seizures*,
https://doi.org/10.1007/978-981-96-8520-2_9

currently [8]. Newer ASMs generally exhibit improved adverse event profiles and fewer drug interactions. However, the effectiveness of these new ASMs in seizure control does not surpass their older counterparts. Recent studies have shown that the proportion of people with drug-resistant epilepsy (DRE) remains steady at around 30% of all people living with epilepsy, despite the expanded pharmacological options [9]. This implies the ASMs are not effective in reversing the course of the disease.

Currently, the pharmacological management of epilepsy is largely empirical. Once the diagnosis of epilepsy is confirmed, a patient is typically prescribed an ASM. The choice of drug depends on the clinician's discretion, considering factors such as epilepsy classification, patient demographics (e.g., childbearing potential), comorbidities, and potential drug interactions. The decision-making process may vary depending on the individual clinician's experience. If the initial ASM fails to control seizures, a second ASM may be added to or substitute for the first. According to the criteria of International League Against Epilepsy (ILAE), a diagnosis of DRE can be made if a patient does not achieve sustained (12 months or more) seizure freedom after adequate trials of two appropriately ASMs [10]. Currently, there are no reliable biomarkers to predict DRE at the time of epilepsy diagnosis. Patients often undergo a trial-and-error process until the right ASM may be selected, which can take months or even years to achieve the goal of seizure freedom or confirm the diagnosis of DRE [11].

On the other hand, the concept of Personalized Medicine or Precision Medicine has gained significant attention in recent years [12]. In the conventional treatment paradigm, various guidelines on the selection of ASMs are based on clinical trials conducted with stringently selected patient groups. These studies draw conclusions by using large patient cohorts to ensure sufficient statistical power and minimize confounding factors. However, this evidence-based practice has been criticized as an "one-size-fits-all" approach that neglects the specific characteristics of individuals. In contrast, Personalized Medicine aims to customize therapy on the individual level. By gathering personal profiles, including demographics, genomics, radiographic, and physiological features, the most suitable therapy can be tailored to each patient. In the field of epilepsy, Personalized Medicine promises to be an achievable goal with advances in technology [13, 14]. For example, the development of pharmacogenomic panels may allow the prediction of responsiveness and potential adverse effects of ASMs of an individual patient [15]. Neuroimaging processing can detect subtle structural substrates of epileptogenicity, thereby enhancing the success rate of surgical treatment [16]. Automated analysis of electroencephalogram (EEG) signals can be used to detect seizures and predict the prognosis of epilepsy [17]. All these techniques involve a huge amount of data that overwhelms manual analytical capacity.

9.2 Artificial Intelligence and Machine Learning

Artificial intelligence (AI) refers to the capability of a machine to imitate intelligent human thinking and learning. AI has a wide application in medicine. It has the advantage of precision, efficiency, and perpetuity. Hence, investment in AI in health care industry may save cost by reducing medical errors, streamlining workflow, and reducing manpower [18]. Novel applications emerge continuously, some notable examples are given below.

Robotics powered by AI has revolutionized the surgical field. Robotic-assisted surgery refers to specialized robotic system to assist or replace the surgeon in certain procedures to enhance precision and minimize complication risk. For example, robotic systems have improved the accuracy and efficiency of electrode implantation for stereoelectroencephalography (SEEG) for epilepsy surgery. These robotic systems even allow telesurgery, in which surgeons can operate on patients remotely [19, 20].

In the journey of management, a patient may have multiple consultations by various specialists or receive treatment from different institutes. Reconstruction of patient's natural history from electronic medical records from different sources is now possible with Natural Language Processing (NLP) [21]. NLP is a subfield of AI that focuses on how the computer could understand and generate human language.

An automatic medical image reporting system involves both computer vision and NLP. Computer vision algorithms process and analyze medical images. These algorithms employ various techniques such as image segmentation, object detection, and image classification to identify anatomical structures and abnormalities in the images. The findings of the input image are expressed as a structured and coherent textual report with the help of NLP.

The concept of applying AI in decision-making or problem-solving processes can be traced back to the mid-twentieth century. Clinical Decision Support Systems (CDSS) are software systems designed to facilitate daily clinical decisions [22]. With the incorporation of AI, the capabilities of CDSS can be enhanced. An exemplary example is the MYCIN system developed in the 1970s, which aimed to facilitate the management of bacterial infections [23]. It consisted of three major components: the knowledge base, inference engine, and user interface. The knowledge base contained facts provided by human experts, while the user interface facilitated communication between the computer software and the user. The data input into the inference engine by the user was then interpreted using a preset logic flow. The MYCIN system employed a backward chaining technique, which is a top-to-bottom approach that tracks backward to prove the truth of facts. Other examples of CDSS include an alert warning system in computerized prescription program, where a warning signal appears if a patient has a potential drug allergy or drug interaction to the prescribed medication. Over the past two decades, there have been spectacular advances in computer technology, including the emergence of high-performance processors, massive storage, the internet, and cloud computing, nurturing the next generation of AI.

Machine Learning (ML) is a branch of AI that may help to solve many practical problems. ML can be broadly divided into supervised learning and unsupervised learning [24]. In supervised learning, a human-labeled training dataset is used to train the ML algorithm [25]. The training dataset consists of labeled input features matched with corresponding categorized outputs. Examples of supervised learning models include regression, random forest (RF), support vector machine (SVM), *k*-nearest neighbor (*k*NN), and Gradient Boosting Tree (GBT) [26–28]. Supervised learning has wide-ranging applications, such as classification, NLP, and image recognition. Classification predicts categorical outputs; NLP is used for analyzing text data (e.g., automated translators) and image recognition is used for recognizing images (e.g., face recognition systems). Unsupervised learning is usually used in hidden pattern recognition and association. Examples of unsupervised learning techniques include K-Means Clustering, Principal Component Analysis (PCA), and Autoencoders. Deep learning is a more advanced type of ML. It does not require manual input in feature selection, rather the model could extract features from raw data. The algorithm structure is in the form of multilayered artificial neural network. The inputs go through artificial neuron layers in a nonlinear way and map into outputs. The deep learning model can also improve its own performance as the size of the training data grows.

To develop an ML model, several key steps are involved, including data preprocessing and feature selection, algorithm selection, model training and validation, and performance evaluation. In the data preprocessing and feature selection stage, data is collected from various sources, and any missing or irrelevant data are removed. Sometimes, features or variables in a dataset are transformed, such as conversion from a continuous scale to categorical value, for the convenience of model fitting.

Next, suitable algorithms are selected based on the specific problem to be solved. In some cases, multiple models are developed and compared to select the one with the best performance.

Once the algorithm is selected, the dataset is divided into a training set and a validation set. The training set is used to train the supervised learning model to make meaningful predictions. After training is completed, the model will then be validated to assess its performance and generalizability. Various validation techniques can be employed, such as k-fold cross-validation and leave-one-out cross-validation (LOOCV). In k-fold cross-validation, the whole dataset is divided into equal portions or folds of number k. The model is then trained on $k - 1$ folds, and one fold is left out for validation. The model is trained for k times, so that each of the k folds is used for validation [29]. In LOOCV, each observation is selected as validation set, while the rest of observations ($N - 1$) are considered as a training set. The choice of validation approach depends on the size of the dataset, and the complexity of the computation involved.

Several metrics are commonly used to assess the performance of ML models. For example, in a classification task, performance metrics usually include accuracy, precision, recall, F-score, positive predictive value (PPV), negative predictive value (NPV), and area under the receiver operating characteristic curve (AUC). The AUC varies from zero to one, where one signifies a perfect classifier and 0.5 suggests a random classifier that is not better than chance.

It is valuable to understand the relative contribution of each feature in making a prediction within an ML model. This provides insights into the relationships between features and outcomes and helps improve the model. Established methods, such as model coefficient and permutation importance, can be used to assess the relative importance of different features in a predictive model. Model coefficient reflects the weight of a feature in a linear model, with the higher coefficient value indicating greater importance. Permutation importance is a model-agnostic approach that measures the impact of shuffling the value of a feature on the model's performance. By evaluating the drop in performance after shuffling each feature, one can determine its relative importance.

ML may be applied to solve many problems in the development and clinical use of ASMs. In this chapter, we will focus on two main clinical applications: ASM response and DRE prediction.

9.3 Prediction of ASM Response

Devinsky et al. developed a RF model to predict the ASM with the highest likelihood of seizure control for individual patients utilizing claims data [30]. About 6 years of medical claims data was retrieved from a nationwide comprehensive claim database in the US. Adults with epilepsy were identified based on International Classification of Diseases, Ninth Revision (ICD-9) coding and pharmacy claim for ASMs. The researchers recruited cases with any one of the three conditions: (1) initiation of first ever ASM, (2) addition of ASM to an existing regimen, and (3) substitution of an ASM by another ASM. The date of these major changes in regimen was defined as the index date. Patient's features and the treatment outcomes were extracted from 12 months before and after the index date respectively. ASM substitution or addition of ASM to an existing regimen or complete withdrawal of the ASM was presumed to be treatment failure due to either inefficacy or intolerability.

A huge number of features, about 5000, covering demographics, comorbidities, therapeutic mechanism of ASMs, were available in each case. To avoid overfitting, a selection process with statistical criteria was implemented to filter out irrelevant features. The final training dataset included 34,990 patients, and the validation dataset comprised 8292 patients.

The trained RF model selected the ASM with the highest probability of successful outcome as output. The machine-selected ASM was compared to the ASM chosen by physicians. The RF model achieved an AUC of 0.72. The ASM selected by the model matched with the physician's choice in only 13% of the cases. In this group, the treatment outcomes were found to be better with a lower chance of altering the ASM regimen. Other secondary outcomes such as health service utilization also favored ASM selection by the ML model.

This study used a claim database as the data source for developing ML model. This kind of administrative database has certain advantages. It contains a large number of cases and is readily available. If the database has a broad coverage, the cohort obtained could minimize selection bias.

However, claim database also has its limitations. Clinical details could not be directly retrieved. Clinical conditions have to be presumed by surrogate markers. In Devinsky's study, any change in ASM was supposed to be treatment failure, but it could not distinguish whether it was due to lack of efficacy or medication intolerability. Moreover, the database could not differentiate whether the ASMs are prescribed for seizure prophylaxis or other purposes, for instance valproate could be used as a mood stabilizer and prophylaxis of migraine; gabapentin and pregabalin are commonly used to treat neuropathic pain. The diagnosis defined by coding may be subject to the pitfalls of either over-coding or under-coding. Commonly used clinical outcomes such as seizure freedom or 50% seizure reduction could not be obtained directly from the claim database.

Ouyang et al. designed a SVM model to identify biomarkers to predict the therapeutic outcomes of ASMs [31]. Quantitative EEG (QEEG) analysis of patients' background EEG was utilized as a biomarker to assess therapeutic efficacy. A total of 20 children with epilepsy, 11 of whom responded to ASMs and 9 had DRE, were enrolled. EEG recordings were obtained from each patient at different time points before and after initiation or change of ASM regimen. The EEG recordings were then analyzed by QEEG technique. Discriminative features of the EEG were selected and fed into the SVM model to classify the treatment outcomes. A tenfold cross-validation approach was adopted for internal validation. Finally, six EEG feature descriptors were found crucial in differentiating treatment effective (seizure reduction >50%) and ineffective groups. The performance metrics of the model yielded an accuracy of 83%.

This study integrated clinical and electrophysiological features to enhance the predictive capabilities of ML model. However, there are drawbacks in the study that undermine its generalizability. First, the number of patients was small. Also, the recruited patients had different seizure subtypes including both focal and generalized seizures. The EEG features of these seizure subtypes are known to have great discrepancies. On the other hand, the ASMs used by the patients could also affect the EEG tracing. In this study, the ineffective group more commonly had patients using ASM combinations, while the effective group more commonly used monotherapy. The effects of multiple ASMs or their drug interactions may cause bias in QEEG analysis when compared to single ASM. Further study with a larger and more homogeneous patient population is needed to verify the results.

Zhang et al. attempted to estimate the therapeutic outcomes of specific ASMs by using ML [32]. A SVM classifier was developed to predict seizure freedom in epilepsy patients receiving levetiracetam based on both clinical and QEEG features. The study recruited 46 patients receiving levetiracetam from a single center in China. Twenty-two patients achieved seizure freedom, while 24 did not. Eleven clinical features were selected as input, including (1) age, (2) duration of epilepsy, (3) family history of epilepsy, (4) seizure subtype (generalized, focal, or unknown onset), (5) seizure frequency in the 12 months before levetiracetam, (6) psychiatric comorbidities, (7) seizure circadian rhythm, (8) temporal lobe epilepsy, (9) time between last seizure and levetiracetam initiation before treatment, (10) interictal spikes in EEG, and (11) positive MRI findings. For the EEG features, sample entropy of alpha, beta, theta, and delta frequencies was used to describe the data [33]. Sample entropy is a measurement used in signal processing and time-series analysis to quantify the regularity or predictability of a signal. Four frequency bands of alpha, beta, theta, and delta were reconstructed and then used to calculate sample entropy for each patient in every channel.

To prevent overfitting, only strictly selective bands were extracted and incorporated into the input dataset. Consequently, four bands from four different channels were selected: beta bands from EEG lead Fp2, alpha bands from F4, theta bands from C3, and beta bands from F8. The 11 clinical and four QEEG features (sample entropy of alpha, beta, theta, and delta) of all patients formed the dataset and were then used to train and validate the SVM model. The algorithm was validated by fivefold cross-validation, hold-out validation, and jack-knife validation. Mean Impact Value (MIV) was then assessed the contribution of each individual feature to the model [34]. The results showed that the beta band from Fp2 played a crucial role in the classifier model. Clinical features of temporal lobe epilepsy, family history, circadian rhythm of seizure, MRI findings, comorbidity, time between last seizure and levetiracetam initiation before treatment, and duration of epilepsy had descending importance. As for QEEG features, beta band from Fp2 has a significant contribution. Interestingly, age, seizure type, interictal spikes, and seizure frequency before levetiracetam did not have a notable impact on the model.

The combined model of both clinical and EEG features yielded an AUC of 0.95 in the training dataset and AUC of 0.96 in the validation dataset. The researchers tried to compare the performance of SVM model with input of clinical features only, EEG features only, and combination of clinical and EEG features. The model with combined input demonstrated the best results.

The superior performance of the combined input integrating clinical and EEG inputs made clinical sense, as multiple modalities probably enhanced the accuracy of the classifier's prediction. However, the small number of recruited patients is a main drawback of the study. The specific bands of the four EEG channels showed significant difference between seizure-free and non-seizure-free groups, but the authors did not postulate the electrophysiological mechanisms behind their findings. The high AUC values in both training and validation may imply the model has high generalizability. It is worthwhile to further evaluate the model in external validation by using an independent cohort.

Yao et al. constructed ML models to predict the outcomes of ASM in new-onset epilepsy [35]. A total of 287 patients with newly diagnosed epilepsy were recruited from a single center. The cohort had at least 3 years of follow-up. Fourteen demographic and clinical features were selected as input features of the model, including: (1) sex, (2) living area, (3) occupation, (4) education level, (5) age at seizure onset, (6) risk factors of epilepsy (including brain trauma, stroke intracranial infection, perinatal hypoxia, brain tumor), (7) family history of epilepsy, (8) seizure types (focal, generalized, or unknown onset), (9) number of seizures before treatment, (10) history of febrile seizure, (11) duration of previous treatment, (12) presence of multiple seizure types (more than one seizure type including focal aware, focal impaired awareness, focal to bilateral tonic–clonic, generalized onset, and unknown onset seizures), (13) EEG findings, and (14) MRI findings.

In their treatment protocol, monotherapy of ASM was selected by the attending epileptologist. One of the seven ASMs were selected: carbamazepine, oxcarbazepine, valproate, lamotrigine, levetiracetam, topiramate, and gabapentin. Outcomes from the first ASM were classified into three groups: early remission (less than

6 months after ASM commencement), late remission (more than 6 months after ASM commencement), and no remission (ongoing seizures after 1 year of ASM treatment). In the dataset, there were 207 remission cases, in which 140 were early remission and 67 were late remission, along with 80 cases of no remission.

The researchers compared the performance of five supervised ML models: Decision Tree, RF, SVM, Extreme Gradient Boosting (XGBoost), and Logistic Regression. Two experiments were conducted. In the first experiment, all 287 patients' data was used as a training dataset, aiming to predict remission versus no remission status. In the second experiment, data from 207 patients in the remission group were used as a training dataset, aiming to predict early versus late remission. A fivefold cross-validation was carried out for internal validation.

Among the five models, XGBoost algorithm achieved the best metrics in predicting remission versus no remission, with an F1 score of 0.95 and an AUC of 0.98. The best predictor for remission versus no remission was the number of seizures before treatment. XGBoost model also performed the best in predicting early remission versus later remission, with F1 score of 0.84 and AUC of 0.92. The presence of multiple seizure types had the most significant impact in predicting early versus late remission.

This study compares different ML models instead of preselection of a single model, therefore enhancing transparency in model selection. Another notable point is that the input features cover investigational results in addition to other clinical features from medical history and demographics. Both the EEG and MRI findings are incorporated as categorical features in the dataset. The XGBoost model achieved impressively high F1 and AUC values in predicting early remission versus late remission and remission versus no remission. One of the contributing factors was the application of grid search to optimize the hyperparameter set in hyperparameter tuning. Hyperparameters are parameters that are not learned during the training process, but they are set before training and determine how the model learns and generalizes from the data. Hyperparameter optimization is the process of finding the best set of hyperparameters for a ML model. Of course, grid search also has its drawbacks such as requirement of additional computational resources and inability to deal with a large number of hyperparameters or extensive ranges of hyperparameter values.

Two related studies, conducted by Petrovski et al. and Shazadi et al., aimed to predict response to ASM in newly diagnosed epilepsy patients by exploiting pharmacogenomic markers [36, 37].

Petrovski et al. developed a multi-single-nucleotide polymorphisms (SNPs) classification model to predict the treatment outcome of the first ASM in patients with newly diagnosed epilepsy [36]. A total of 115 patients with newly diagnosed epilepsy from two hospitals in Australia were enrolled. Treatment response was assessed at the end of the follow-up period of 1 year. Drug responders were defined as seizure freedom with the first ASM, while non-responders were defined as those with recurrent seizures while on the initial ASM.

Genotyping for 4041 SNPs in 279 candidate genes was performed. These candidate genes were chosen based on their roles in pathogenesis of epilepsy or drug metabolism, as well as their high expression levels in the brain. The list of SNPs was further narrowed down, and five sophistically selected SNPs were finally included in the ML model development. The algorithm of *k*NN was employed as a classifier.

A fivefold cross-validation approach was employed for internal validation. In addition, the model was further externally validated by two independent validation cohorts. The first validation cohort comprised 63 newly diagnosed epilepsy patients from the same population, and the second cohort comprised 108 community-treated chronic epilepsy patients. The performance of multi-SNP model was further compared with models based on individual SNAPs alone in each validation cohort.

The performance metrics showed promising results. In the cross-validation, the model achieved an accuracy of 84%. In the validation using the 63 newly diagnosed epilepsy patients, the model yielded a sensitivity of 91% and specificity of 53%. For the chronically treated epilepsy validation cohort, the multi-SNP classifier model achieved a sensitivity of 81% and specificity of 50%. The multi-SNP models consistently outperformed the single-SNP models in both independent validation cohorts.

Shazadi et al. further investigated Petrovski's multi-SNP model by externally validating it with larger independent cohorts [37]. They utilized two cohorts from the UK: the Glasgow cohort, consisting of 281 new-onset epilepsy patients, and a subset of patients from the SANAD study, which included 491 patients with genetic sampling [38]. The genotyping process was the same as in Petrovski's study, focusing on the five specific SNPs. The *k*NN algorithm retained identical input features as the original model. The UK cohorts were used to validate the multi-SNP model in three ways: (1) Petrovski's training dataset served as the training dataset and each of the two UK cohorts as the test datasets; (2) retraining the *k*NN model using the SANAD cohort as both training and test datasets. A random 70:30 train-test split was adopted. The parameters of *k*NN were identical to those employed in original Petrovski's model; (3) testing the performance of Petrovski's *k*NN model using a LOOCV approach in the UK cohorts.

The results showed that the multi-SNAPs model could reasonably predict the treatment responses in carbamazepine or valproate in both Glasgow and SANAD cohorts (Glasgow: odds ratio [OR] = 3.1, 95% confidence interval [CI] = 1.4–6.6, $p = 0.018$; SANAD: OR = 2.8, 95% CI: 1.3–6.1, $p = 0.048$). However, the model could not reliably predict lamotrigine and other ASM treatment responses in both UK cohorts.

These two studies tried to predict the response to ASM by genetic approach. The hypothesis that multiple SNPs could have a better prediction than single SNP is sensible, as response to ASM is probably a trait influenced by multiple genetic variants. The possible reason of the failed external validation of the ML model on the two UK cohorts may be because of different prescription patterns between the Australian and UK cohorts. Carbamazepine and valproate were more commonly used for the new-onset epilepsy in the Australian cohorts, while lamotrigine or other ASMs were used more commonly in the UK cohorts [37]. This highlights the preference for prescription in different institutions or countries could be a source of bias in the dataset. It would be optimal to collect the developmental dataset from a diverse range of institutions and countries.

De Jong et al. combined both clinical and genetic data to develop a ML to predict the response to brivaracetam [39]. The data sources consisted of two patient cohorts from two randomized placebo-controlled clinical trials of adjunctive brivaracetam. The first cohort consisted of 235 patients, while the second cohort consisted of other 47 patients. The data from the larger cohort was used for the developmental dataset for both training and internal validation, while the smaller group severed as the retrospective validation dataset. The treatment response was defined as a >50% reduction in seizure frequency after 12 weeks. Both the clinical and genetic features were incorporated into the ML models. Whole-genome sequencing (WGS) data of the patient cohorts was available. The huge amount of genetic data from WGS was robustly narrowed down to a workable list of genetic features that related to mechanisms of epilepsy and drug action. Finally, four data modalities were employed, including (1) mutational load scores, (2) polygenic risk score, (3) SV2A structural variance (the molecular target of brivaracetam), and (4) clinical data.

As some of the input features may be associated with placebo response, the researchers further validated the models with an extra placebo dataset. A cohort of 235 patients who were assigned to placebo arm in the same clinical trial was used as the placebo dataset. However, genetic data was not available in this placebo cohort. The researchers assessed the placebo response in the model trained only on clinical data instead.

The researchers compared five different ML models, including sparse multi-block partial least squares discriminant analysis, multimodal neural network, elastic net classifier, GBT, and logistic regression-based stacking. The ML models underwent internal cross-validation and were further validated externally using the validation dataset.

Among the tested models, the GBT achieved the best performance parameters, with an AUC of 0.76 (95% CI: 0.76 ± 0.014) in the training dataset and 0.75 (95% CI: 0.75 ± 0.15) in the validation dataset. Analysis of the placebo cohort ensured that model trained on the clinical data modality was not associated with placebo effect.

The researchers demonstrated that the integration of genetic and clinical data modalities improved the model's performance (AUC of 0.76) compared to using clinical data alone (AUC of 0.71). Genetic factors included the presence of structural variants overlapping the SV2A gene and the mutational load in a gene set representing microtubule minus end binding. The only clinical factor that predicted brivaracetam responsiveness was prior levetiracetam use. Failure in levetiracetam use predicted a poor brivaracetam response.

This study has demonstrated that a meaningful model could be developed with a relatively small cohort. Such a drug response prediction model focusing on a single ASM could facilitate enrichment trials. Eligible subjects with a high probability of non-responsiveness could be screened out using a ML model before being recruited into a drug trial. This measure could effectively reduce the sample size by increasing the responder rate, making it easier to achieve statistically significant differences between the treatment and placebo groups in randomized controlled trials. It would also shorten the drug trial process and reduce the cost of drug development.

However, the short duration of follow-up (12 weeks) and small absolute difference in seizure frequency in the corresponding clinical trials make the reliability of developmental dataset questionable. On the other hand, the contribution of genetic data to the final model was surprisingly small, as reflected by the small increase from AUC 0.71 of the model with clinical features alone to AUC 0.76 of model with the combination of clinical plus genetic features [40]. The cost effectiveness of incorporating genetic data into the ML model is challenged.

Hakeem et al. have developed and validated a deep leaning model to predict the response of the first ASM for new-onset epilepsy [41]. Five cohorts from Scotland, Malaysia, Australia, and China comprised 1798 adults with newly diagnosed epilepsy were included for model development. An attention-based deep learning Transformer model was adopted in this study [42]. The model consists of an encoder and decoder, both of which have a multi-head attention mechanism. In this mechanism, each head is a separate attention layer that learns to attend to different relationships or patterns in the input data. By using multiple heads, the model can extract useful information from complex relationships and make more reliable predictions.

Sixteen clinical features were input into the model: (1) sex, (2) age group at ASM initiation, (3) history of febrile convulsion, (4) history of childhood CNS infection, (5) history of head trauma, (6) history of hypoxic brain injury, (7) history of alcohol abuse, (8) history of alcohol abuse, (9) epilepsy in first-degree relative, (10) history of cerebrovascular disease, (11) intellectual disability, (12) psychiatric disorder, (13) number of pretreatment seizure, (14) type of epilepsy, (15) EEG findings, and (16) brain imaging findings. Shapley additive explanations (SHAP) value was used to assess the relative impact of each feature to the model. The output was one of the seven ASMs (carbamazepine, lamotrigine, levetiracetam, oxcarbazepine, phenytoin, topiramate, or valproate), being considered as the best choice giving the highest chance of treatment success as defined as seizure freedom while still using the first ASM within the first year of treatment. The study had two parts. In the first part, data from pooling the five study cohorts was randomly selected for training and validation. Approach of 80:20 train-test split was adopted. In the second part, the ML model was trained by using the Glasgow cohort, which is the largest of the five cohorts. The model was then validated on each of the remaining four cohorts. The researchers compared six different ML models including transformer, multilayered perceptron (MLP), XGBoost, SVM, RF, and logistic regression in both parts of the study.

Among the six models, the transformer model attained the best performance with an AUC of 0.65 (95% CI: 0.65 ± 0.02) and a weighted balanced accuracy of 0.62 (95% CI: 0.62 ± 0.02) on the test set.

In the second part of the study, the transformer model was trained using the largest cohort and achieved AUCs in the range of 0.52–0.60 and a weighted balanced accuracy in the range of 0.51–0.62 in validation cohorts. A number of pre-treatment seizures, EEG, and neuroimaging findings had the highest SHAP values in the pooled cohort and hence contributed most to the prediction model.

This study has two remarkable features. First, the dataset in the ML model development was derived from some of the largest, best characterized adult cohorts of newly diagnosed epilepsy in the world [43, 44]. Second, a deep learning ML model instead of traditional statistical learning models was selected to predict the best ASM in new-onset epilepsy. This transfer learning technique allows their model to expand to diverse patient populations, tasks, and datasets with small sample sizes, with comparable performance as their large developmental dataset [45, 46]. The model could bring clinical implication if it could be further improved and validated.

9.4 Prediction of DRE

Silva-Alves et al. attempted to use both clinical and genetic parameters to predict drug responsiveness in patients with mesial temporal epilepsy [47]. They used RF classifier for prediction. They gathered a cohort of 237 patients with mesial temporal lobe epilepsy, in which 75 responsive to ASM and 162 were drug-resistant, from a single center in Brazil. ASM responsiveness was defined as seizure freedom for at least 12 months. DRE was regarded as a failure in reaching seizure freedom despite taking two or more ASMs either sequentially or in combination. Clinical features included gender, age of seizure onset, febrile seizures, and presence of hippocampal sclerosis on MRI. They genotyped 119 SNPs in 11 different genes. They ran the algorithm with the clinical features only, genetic features only, and a combination of both clinical and genetic features. In addition, the researchers tried different combinations of features to train the model to obtain the best results. They validated their model by LOOCV. Mean decreased accuracy (MDA) value is used to show the most relevant features contributing to the best model [48].

The results showed that the clinical plus genetic features contributed model had the best performance. The best model included the presence of hippocampal sclerosis and 56 SNPs. Finally, the model based on a combination of clinical and genetic data achieved an AUC of 0.82, compared with AUC of 0.46 for the model with clinical data only and AUC of 0.80 with genetic data only. SNP in CYP1A2 gene had the greatest MDA value and hence had the greatest contribution in the prediction model, followed by the presence of hippocampal sclerosis on MRI.

In current study, the genetic component has a dominant contribution. It is reflected in the AUC of 0.80 for genetic data only model compared with the AUC of 0.46 for clinical only model. It contrasts with the aforementioned model developed by de Jong et al., in which clinical data bears more weight. This could be explained by the homogeneity of localization of epilepsy focus, that is the temporal lobe, in this study, while in the de Jong's study the epilepsy foci were variable. It may imply that epilepsy subtype should be targeted if genetic features are to be incorporated into ML model.

An et al. aimed to predict DRE by making use of administrative data through a ML model [49]. They made use of a large claim database in the US. The researchers identified epilepsy and DRE cases indirectly. Epilepsy was defined by three criteria: (1) cases with one or more epilepsy diagnosis claim with ICD-9 or ICD-10 for epilepsy and recurrent seizures, or two claims for convulsion with appropriate ICD-9 or ICD-10 codes, (2) cases with more than one claim for an ASM, and (3) cases with the first ASM prescribed as monotherapy for at least 60 days of supply. The authors identified 292,892 epilepsy patients for inclusion in the dataset. Drug-responsive cases were defined as ordering of same ASM regimen without the need of change for at least a year. Treatment failure was defined as a different ASM and claimed no matter if it was an add-on, replacement of a current agent, or as rescue therapy. The definition of DRE in this study was different from the widely accepted consensus endorsed by the ILAE, which states failure of two appropriated chosen ASMs [10]. In this study, failure of three ASMs was considered as DRE instead. Those who just failed one or two ASMs were excluded from the analysis. The proportion of DRE in their cohort was about 13%. For each patient, an index date was defined as the date when the first ASM was claimed. The period preceding the index date, traced back to the commencement of health care plan, was defined as observation window. The period following the index date, up until the date of the last claim, was defined as evaluation window. The data extracted from the observation window was used to predict drug responsiveness of epilepsy. Three ML algorithms were compared: multivariate logistic regression (MLR), SVM, and RF. A total of 1270 features were extracted from each patient, encompassing the demographics, comorbidities, insurance policy, treatments, and encounters. Half of the extracted features were finally used in the dataset to build the model. The dataset was randomly divided into a training set (60%), validation set (20%), and test set (20%). As a reference, the researchers formulated a benchmark model, which only contained two features, namely the age at epilepsy onset and sex. Information Gain value was used to demonstrate relative contribution of features to the predictive model [50]. They used Brier scores and calibration plots to assess the reliability of the predicted probabilities output by the ML models [51, 52].

The RF was the best model in this study and achieved an AUC of 0.76 (95% CI: 0.76–0.77), outperforming the benchmark model with an AUC of 0.66 (95% CI: 0.65–0.66). Moreover, predicted probabilities for DRE were well calibrated with the observed frequencies in the data. The research group analyzed the time period from the index date to the date of initiation of the third ASM regimen, which was used as a surrogate marker of failure of the second ASM that fulfilled the ILAE's definition of DRE. The period was 1.97 years on average. In other words, the RF model could predict ILAE-defined DRE approximately 2 years before a patient failed two ASMs.

The limitation of the study based on the claim database has been discussed before. Another major drawback of this study is that the definition of DRE departs from the definition accepted globally. A proxy of failure of three, rather than two, ASM regimens was considered as DRE. The aim of this maybe to enable a greater contrast in data between DRE and non-DRE and hence enhance the model performance [53]. This may again highlight the limitations of performing clinical study by employing administrative database.

Delen et al. aimed to predict DRE by training ML algorithms on data retrieved from a nationwide electronic medical record (EMR) database [54]. The researchers identified epilepsy patients by the ICD code of epilepsy in the diagnosis record. Drug responsiveness was assessed indirectly. DRE was defined by the use of non-ASM treatments, namely epilepsy surgery or VNS, while all cases with solely ASM treatment were assumed to be non-DRE. A total of 37,024 were finally recruited in the cohort. Among them, 806 had DRE and 36,218 had non-refractory disease. The features listed in the dataset included patient's demographic features namely age, gender, race, and marital status; physician's initial diagnosis; total comorbidity count; and presence of eight common comorbidities: hypertension, depression and anxiety, hyperlipidemia, drug abuse, head and neck symptoms, esophageal disease, anemia, and diabetes mellitus. The dataset was randomly split into a 70:30 ratio for training and validation, respectively. The contribution of each feature was evaluated by excluding features one at a time when running the model repeatedly. In each iteration, the performance difference of the model between including and excluding the specific feature could be calculated, reflecting the importance of the feature. Since the cohort was grossly imbalanced with a very small fraction of DRE cases (2.2%), the researchers used additional balancing measures to avoid biases.

Three ML algorithms were compared, including the decision tree, RF and GBT. The performances of the three classifiers adopting each of the different balancing approaches were compared. The best combination attained F1-score of 0.59, accuracy of 75%, and AUC of 0.83. The analysis of relative importance of input feature showed that comorbidity count was the most important feature in the prediction of DRE, followed by drug abuse, hypertension, and hyperlipidemia.

This study defines DRE with an unusual criterion, only cases with epilepsy surgery or VNS were considered as DRE. This is a marked discrepancy with the global consensus. It is well known that epilepsy surgery is underused in DRE population. The reasons are multifactorial including under-referral, lack of expertise, and low patient acceptance. The pitfall is reflected by the very low proportion (only 2.2%) of DRE in the cohort, compared to the commonly quoted proportion of around 30%. Although complex statistical measures have been employed, trying to balance the biased figure, the limitation could not be overcome. The high AUC but a relatively low F1 may imply the skewed dataset. The findings of comorbidities including hypertension and hyperlipidemia play an important role in predicting DRE are not entirely convincing.

The studies discussed above were summarized in Table 9.1.

Table 9.1 Summary of the aim, strengths and limitations of the included studies

Author (year)	Aim of study	Highlights of study design	Number of patients recruited	Strength of the study	Limitation of the study
Prediction of ASM response					
Devinsky et al. [30] (2016)	To develop a ML model to select ASM with highest successful outcome for an individual	ML model: RF Retrospective recruitments from claims database for both training and validation Index date of ASM change (initiation of new claim, add-on or substitution) was used to train the ML to predict ASM regimen with lowest likelihood of regimen change	34,990 patients from a claim database	Very large number of recruited cases from a national wide claims database	Important clinical features such as frequency of seizure, indication of ASM, etc. could not be obtained from the claim databases
Ouyang et al. [31] (2018)	To develop a ML model to differentiate ASM effective and ineffective groups	ML model: SVM EEG recorded before and 1–3 months after ASM initiation or change for QEEG features selection and model training EEG recorded before and 6 months after ASM initiation or change for model validation	20 patients from single center	Biomarkers of EEG was employed and analyzed by QEEG technique in the ML development	Small number of patients were recruited

(continued)

Table 9.1 (continued)

Author (year)	Aim of study	Highlights of study design	Number of patients recruited	Strength of the study	Limitation of the study
Zhang et al. [32] (2018)	To develop a ML model to predict probability of seizure freedom in patients treated with LEV	ML model: SVM Retrospective recruitment of patients on LEV, employing both clinical and EEG sample entropy in various frequency band as input features	46 patients from single center	Combination of biomarkers of EEG and clinical features were employed in the ML development Comparison of clinical features only model with EEG and clinical combination model proved the better performance of the combined model	Small number of patients were recruited The reasons of why some frequency bands of certain electrodes of EEG had relatively greater contribution to the ML model outcome than the others were not explained
Yao et al. [35] (2019)	To develop a ML model to predict the outcomes ASM of patients with newly diagnosed epilepsy	ML models: decision trees, RF, SVM, logistic regression, XGBoost Retrospective recruitment of patients, employing 14 clinical features to train and validate the model	287 patients from single center	Different ML models were compared to choose the best performing one	Patients were recruited from single center, prescription preference, disease pattern may affect the model's generalizability

(continued)

Table 9.1 (continued)

Author (year)	Aim of study	Highlights of study design	Number of patients recruited	Strength of the study	Limitation of the study
Petrovski et al. [36] (2009) and Shazadi et al. [37] (2014)	To develop and externally validate a ML model to predict the outcomes ASM of patients with newly diagnosed epilepsy	ML model: *k*NN Prospectively recruited patient cohort was employed for genetic data collection. Selected SNPs were input to train the model The model was validated by Australian and then the UK cohorts	115 Australian patients in training dataset; 63 patients from same hospital population for validation; 108 community-treated patients for external validation; further external validation on two independent UK cohorts (281 from Glasgow and 491 from SANAD trial)	Genetic features were incorporated into the ML model. Multi-SNP model were compared to individual SNPs models and proved to be outperforming	The model failed to predict treatment response other than with CBZ or VPA in other independent cohorts upon external validation

(continued)

Table 9.1 (continued)

Author (year)	Aim of study	Highlights of study design	Number of patients recruited	Strength of the study	Limitation of the study
De Jong [39] (2021)	To develop a ML model to predict the response to BRV	ML models: sMBPLS-DA, multi-modal neural network, elastic net classifier, GBT, and logistic regression-based stacking Retrospective recruiting patients from two clinical trials on BRV Both clinical and highly selected genetic features were employed to develop the model Placebo dataset was used to train the model to prove the absence of placebo effects in the final results	235 patients from the treatment arm of a multicenter clinical trial as training dataset; 47 patients from the treatment arm of another multicenter clinical trial as validation dataset; 235 patients from the placebo arm of the same study of training dataset as placebo dataset	Both clinical and genetic features including those related specifically to BRV pharmacodynamics were incorporated in the ML model Relative high AUC (0.75) was achieved in external validation in independent cohort Comparison between genetics plus clinical model to the clinical only model proves that the combined model was superior	Small contribution of pharmacogenetics may indicate cost-ineffectiveness of employment of genetic data or a need of improvement of genetic input selection

(continued)

Table 9.1 (continued)

Author (year)	Aim of study	Highlights of study design	Number of patients recruited	Strength of the study	Limitation of the study
Hakeem et al. [41] (2022)	To develop a ML model to predict the outcome of first ASM for newly diagnosed epilepsy	ML models: transformer, MLP, XGBoost, SVM, RF, and Logistic Regression Sixteen clinical features as input for model development Two approaches to train and validate in order to select the best model	1798 patients from five cohorts from four countries	Large number of patients from cohorts from different countries were recruited for model development Deep learning model of transformer was employed	Moderate AUC (0.62) suggested room for further improvement
Prediction of DRE					
Silva-Alves et al. [47] (2017)	To develop a ML model to predict drug resistant mesial TLE	ML model: RF Both clinical and genetic (SNP) variables as input to develop the model	237 patients from single center	Employment of both clinical and genetics (multi-SNPs) in ML development Combination of genetics and clinical features greatly improve the model when compare with clinical only model	High sensitivity but low specificity of the model probably limit its application. It may be more suitable in screening rather than diagnosing.

(continued)

Table 9.1 (continued)

Author (year)	Aim of study	Highlights of study design	Number of patients recruited	Strength of the study	Limitation of the study
An et al. [49] (2018)	To develop a ML model to predict DRE	ML models: SVM, RF, MLR Retrospective recruitments from claims database for both training and validation Proxy indicators, such as changes in ASM claim, as surrogates for clinical features	292,892 patients from a claim database	A great number of cases from a claim database were employed	Unusual definition of DRE (those who failed three ASMs rather than two) was used
Delen et al. [54] (2020)	To develop a ML model to predict DRE	ML model: decision trees, RF, GBT Retrospective recruitments from claims database for both training and validation Proxy indicators as surrogates for clinical features	37,024 patients from a EMR database	A great number of cases from a nationwide EMR database were employed	Unusual definition of DRE (those with VNS and epilepsy surgery) was used resulting in very low proportion of DRE

ASM antiseizure medication, *AUC* area under curve, *DRE* drug resistant epilepsy, *EMR* electronic medical record, *GBT* gradient boosting tree, *kNN* *k*-nearest neighbor, *ML* machine learning, *MLP* multilayer perceptron, *MLR* multivariate logistic regression, *QEEG* quantitative EEG, *RF* random forest, *sMBPLS-DA* sparse multi-block partial least squares - discriminant analysis, *SNP* single nucleotide polymorphism, *SVM* support vector machine, *TLE* temporal lobe epilepsy, *VNS* vagus nerve stimulation, *XGBoost* extreme gradient boosting

9.5 Conclusions

The application of AI in epilepsy prognosis prediction is still in its infancy, albeit and growing number of research studies have shown encouraging results. A crucial factor in the successful development of a powerful predictive model lies in the availability of high-quality developmental datasets. An optimal cohort from which the dataset is generated should consist of reliable diagnoses, comprehensive investigations, and longitudinal follow-up history. It would be ideal if the dataset could be collected from different centers to minimize biases in prescription preferences, patient demographics, and clinical backgrounds. External validation is an essential step to ensure the generalizability of an ML model. It involves testing the model on a new dataset independent of the model development. Unfortunately, this important step is lacking in most of the existing published models. Furthermore, the inclusion of genetics, radiological, and EEG features holds great potential to enhance the performance of the ML model. Similar to therapeutic agents or medical devices, the ultimate assessment of an ML model prior to widespread clinical use is a randomized controlled trial to verify its efficacy and safety in practice.

Achieving all these goals requires close collaboration between clinicians, data scientists, and ML specialists. The synergistic efforts of such interdisciplinary teams could lead to a paradigm shift in the management of epilepsy, ultimately achieving the goal of Personalized Medicine for epilepsy.

References

1. WHO. Epilepsy: a public health imperative. Geneva: World Health Organization; 2019. Contract No.: Licence: CC BY-NC-SA 3.0 IGO
2. Keezer MR, Sisodiya SM, Sander JW. Comorbidities of epilepsy: current concepts and future perspectives. Lancet Neurol. 2016;15(1):106–15.
3. Asadi-Pooya AA, Barzegar Z. Marital status in young adult patients with seizures: epilepsy vs. functional seizures. Epilepsy Behav. 2021;121(Pt A):108066.
4. Jacoby A, Austin JK. Social stigma for adults and children with epilepsy. Epilepsia. 2007;48(Suppl 9):6–9.
5. Lim KS, Wo SW, Wong MH, Tan CT. Impact of epilepsy on employment in Malaysia. Epilepsy Behav. 2013;27(1):130–4.
6. Begley C, Wagner RG, Abraham A, Beghi E, Newton C, Kwon CS, et al. The global cost of epilepsy: a systematic review and extrapolation. Epilepsia. 2022;63(4):892–903.
7. Hakami T. Neuropharmacology of antiseizure drugs. Neuropsychopharmacol Rep. 2021;41(3):336–51.
8. Chen Z, Brodie MJ, Kwan P. What has been the impact of new drug treatments on epilepsy? Curr Opin Neurol. 2020;33(2):185–90.
9. Perucca E, Brodie MJ, Kwan P, Tomson T. 30 years of second-generation antiseizure medications: impact and future perspectives. Lancet Neurol. 2020;19(6):544–56.
10. Kwan P, Arzimanoglou A, Berg AT, Brodie MJ, Allen Hauser W, Mathern G, et al. Definition of drug resistant epilepsy: consensus proposal by the ad hoc Task Force of the ILAE Commission on Therapeutic Strategies. Epilepsia. 2010;51(6):1069–77.
11. Chen Z, Brodie MJ, Liew D, Kwan P. Treatment outcomes in patients with newly diagnosed epilepsy treated with established and new antiepileptic drugs: a 30-year longitudinal cohort study. JAMA Neurol. 2018;75(3):279–86.
12. Chen Z, Rollo B, Antonic-Baker A, Anderson A, Ma Y, O'Brien TJ, et al. New era of personalised epilepsy management. BMJ. 2020;371:m3658.
13. Nabbout R, Kuchenbuch M. Impact of predictive, preventive and precision medicine strategies in epilepsy. Nat Rev Neurol. 2020;16(12):674–88.
14. Walker LE, Mirza N, Yip VLM, Marson AG, Pirmohamed M. Personalized medicine approaches in epilepsy. J Intern Med. 2015;277(2):218–34.
15. Chung WH, Hung SI, Hong HS, Hsih MS, Yang LC, Ho HC, et al. Medical genetics: a marker for Stevens-Johnson syndrome. Nature. 2004;428(6982):486.

16. Bernasconi A, Antel SB, Collins DL, Bernasconi N, Olivier A, Dubeau F, et al. Texture analysis and morphological processing of magnetic resonance imaging assist detection of focal cortical dysplasia in extra-temporal partial epilepsy. Ann Neurol. 2001;49(6):770–5.
17. Liu G, Xiao R, Xu L, Cai J. Minireview of epilepsy detection techniques based on electroencephalogram signals. Front Syst Neurosci. 2021;15:685387.
18. Mintz Y, Brodie R. Introduction to artificial intelligence in medicine. Minim Invasive Ther Allied Technol. 2019;28(2):73–81.
19. Falagario U, Veccia A, Weprin S, Albuquerque EV, Nahas WC, Carrieri G, et al. Robotic-assisted surgery for the treatment of urologic cancers: recent advances. Expert Rev Med Devices. 2020;17(6):579–90.
20. Barba P, Stramiello J, Funk EK, Richter F, Yip MC, Orosco RK. Remote telesurgery in humans: a systematic review. Surg Endosc. 2022;36(5):2771–7.
21. Najafabadipour M, Zanin M, Rodriguez-Gonzalez A, Torrente M, Nunez Garcia B, Cruz Bermudez JL, et al. Reconstructing the patient's natural history from electronic health records. Artif Intell Med. 2020;105:101860.
22. Middleton B, Sittig DF, Wright A. Clinical decision support: a 25 year retrospective and a 25 year vision. Yearb Med Inform. 2016;Suppl 1(Suppl 1):S103–16.
23. Shortliffe EH, Davis R, Axline SG, Buchanan BG, Green CC, Cohen SN. Computer-based consultations in clinical therapeutics: explanation and rule acquisition capabilities of the MYCIN system. Comput Biomed Res. 1975;8(4):303–20.
24. Abbasi MU, Rashad A, Basalamah A, Tariq M. Detection of epilepsy seizures in neo-natal EEG using LSTM architecture. IEEE Access. 2019;7:179074–85.
25. Bzdok D, Krzywinski M, Altman N. Machine learning: supervised methods. Nat Methods. 2018;15(1):5–6.
26. Fix E, Hodges JL Jr. Discriminatory analysis – nonparametric discrimination: consistency properties. Int Stat Rev. 1989;57(3):238–47.
27. Hearst MA, Dumais ST, Osuna E, Platt J, Scholkopf B. Support vector machines. IEEE Intell Syst Appl. 1998;13(4):18–28.
28. Chen T, Guestrin C, editors. XGBoost: a scalable tree boosting system. Association for Computing Machinery; 2016.
29. Steyerberg E. Clinical prediction models: a practical approach to development, validation, and updating. 2nd ed. New York: Springer; 2019.
30. Devinsky O, Dilley C, Ozery-Flato M, Aharonov R, Goldschmidt Y, Rosen-Zvi M, et al. Changing the approach to treatment choice in epilepsy using big data. Epilepsy Behav. 2016;56:32–7.
31. Ouyang CS, Chiang CT, Yang RC, Wu RC, Wu HC, Lin LC. Quantitative EEG findings and response to treatment with antiepileptic medications in children with epilepsy. Brain Dev. 2018;40(1):26–35.
32. Zhang JH, Han X, Zhao HW, Zhao D, Wang N, Zhao T, et al. Personalized prediction model for seizure-free epilepsy with levetiracetam therapy: a retrospective data analysis using support vector machine. Br J Clin Pharmacol. 2018;84(11):2615–24.
33. Jia Y, Gu H, Luo Q. Sample entropy reveals an age-related reduction in the complexity of dynamic brain. Sci Rep. 2017;7(1):7990.
34. Jiang JL, Su X, Zhang H, Zhang XH, Yuan YJ. A novel approach to active compounds identification based on support vector regression model and mean impact value. Chem Biol Drug Des. 2013;81(5):650–7.
35. Yao L, Cai M, Chen Y, Shen C, Shi L, Guo Y. Prediction of antiepileptic drug treatment outcomes of patients with newly diagnosed epilepsy by machine learning. Epilepsy Behav. 2019;96:92–7.
36. Petrovski S, Szoeke CE, Sheffield LJ, D'Souza W, Huggins RM, O'Brien TJ. Multi-SNP pharmacogenomic classifier is superior to single-SNP models for predicting drug outcome in complex diseases. Pharmacogenet Genomics. 2009;19(2):147–52.
37. Shazadi K, Petrovski S, Roten A, Miller H, Huggins RM, Brodie MJ, et al. Validation of a multigenic model to predict seizure control in newly treated epilepsy. Epilepsy Res. 2014;108(10):1797–805.

38. Marson AG, Al-Kharusi AM, Alwaidh M, Appleton R, Baker GA, Chadwick DW, et al. The SANAD study of effectiveness of valproate, lamotrigine, or topiramate for generalised and unclassifiable epilepsy: an unblinded randomised controlled trial. Lancet. 2007;369(9566):1016–26.
39. de Jong J, Cutcutache I, Page M, Elmoufti S, Dilley C, Frohlich H, et al. Towards realizing the vision of precision medicine: AI based prediction of clinical drug response. Brain. 2021;144(6):1738–50.
40. Terman SW. Rise of the machines? Predicting brivaracetam response using machine learning. Epilepsy Curr. 2022;22(2):111–3.
41. Hakeem H, Feng W, Chen Z, Choong J, Brodie MJ, Fong SL, et al. Development and validation of a deep learning model for predicting treatment response in patients with newly diagnosed epilepsy. JAMA Neurol. 2022;79(10):986–96.
42. Ashish V, Noam S, Niki P, Jakob U, Llion J, Aidan NG, et al. Attention is all you need. arXiv:1706.03762. 2023. Available from: https://arxiv.org/abs/1706.03762.
43. Kwan P, Brodie MJ. Early identification of refractory epilepsy. N Engl J Med. 2000;342(5):314–9.
44. Lawn N, Chan J, Lee J, Dunne J. Is the first seizure epilepsy--and when? Epilepsia. 2015;56(9):1425–31.
45. Chiang S, Rao VR. Choosing the best antiseizure medication – can artificial intelligence help? JAMA Neurol. 2022;79(10):970–2.
46. Terman SW. Deep thoughts-predicting initial treatment response in newly diagnosed epilepsy. Epilepsy Curr. 2023;23(2):90–2.
47. Silva-Alves MS, Secolin R, Carvalho BS, Yasuda CL, Bilevicius E, Alvim MK, et al. A prediction algorithm for drug response in patients with mesial temporal lobe epilepsy based on clinical and genetic information. PLoS One. 2017;12(1):e0169214.
48. Hastie T, Tibshirani R, Friedman J. The elements of statistical learning: data mining, inference, and prediction. 2nd ed ed. New York: Springer; 2009.
49. An S, Malhotra K, Dilley C, Han-Burgess E, Valdez JN, Robertson J, et al. Predicting drug-resistant epilepsy – a machine learning approach based on administrative claims data. Epilepsy Behav. 2018;89:118–25.
50. Michalski R, Carbonell J, Mitchell T. Machine learning: an artificial intelligence approach. Springer Science & Business Media; 2013.
51. Brier G. Verification of forecasts expressed in terms of probability. Mon Weather Rev. 1950;78:1–3.
52. Niculescu-Mizil A, Caruana R, editors. Predicting good probabilities with supervised learning. In: The 22nd international conference on machine learning, Bonn, Germany. 2005.
53. Smolyansky ED, Hakeem H, Ge Z, Chen Z, Kwan P. Machine learning models for decision support in epilepsy management: a critical review. Epilepsy Behav. 2021;123:108273.
54. Delen D, Davazdahemami B, Eryarsoy E, Tomak L, Valluru A. Using predictive analytics to identify drug-resistant epilepsy patients. Health Informatics J. 2020;26(1):449–60.

MIX
Papier aus verantwortungsvollen Quellen
Paper from responsible sources
FSC® C105338
FSC
www.fsc.org

If you have any concerns about our products,
you can contact us on
ProductSafety@springernature.com

In case Publisher is established outside the EU,
the EU authorized representative is:
Springer Nature Customer Service Center GmbH
Europaplatz 3, 69115 Heidelberg, Germany

Printed by Libri Plureos GmbH
in Hamburg, Germany